Current Chemotherapy and Immunotherapy

Proceedings of the 12th International Congress of Chemotherapy

Volume I

DEL GOVERNO
DELLA PESTE,

E DELLE MANIERE DI GUARDARSENE,

Trattato del Signor

LODOVICO ANTONIO MURATORI

BIBLIOTECARIO DEL SERENISS. SIGN.

DVCA DI MODENA.

Diviſo in Politico, Medico, & Eccleſiaſtico.

Da conſervarſi, & averſi pronto per le occaſioni, che Dio tenga ſempre lontane;

Ed in queſta ſeconda Edizione accreſciuto dall' Autore con nuove aggiunte poſte in fine del Libro.

CONSAGRATO

A SUA SAGRA REAL MAESTA.

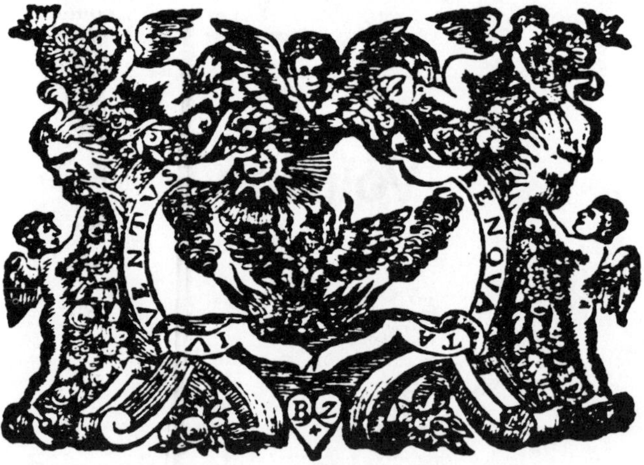

IN TORINO, MDCCXXI.

Per Pietro Giuſeppe Zappata, Stampatore dell'Illuſtriſſima Città.
Con licenza de' Superiori, e Privilegio di S. M.

Frontispiece of the treatise of L. Muratori (1721) on the management of the plague, in three parts: political, medical, and ecclesiastic management.

Current Chemotherapy and Immunotherapy

Proceedings of the 12th International Congress of Chemotherapy

Florence, Italy
19-24 July 1981

Editors:

Piero Periti

Chair of Chemotherapy
University of Florence
Istituto di Farmacologia
Florence, Italy

Giuliana Gialdroni Grassi

Chair of Chemotherapy
Istituto Carlo Forlanini
Pavia, Italy

Volume I

Published by
The American Society for Microbiology
Washington, D.C.
U.S.A.

1913 I Street, N.W.
Washington, DC 20006

Library of Congress Cataloging in Publication Data

International Congress of Chemotherapy (12th: 1981: Florence, Italy)

Current chemotherapy and immunotherapy.

Includes indexes.
1. Chemotherapy—Congresses. 2. Immunotherapy—Congresses. I. Periti, Piero. II. Gialdroni Grassi, G. (Giuliana) III. Title.
RM260.2.I57 1981 615.5'8 82-3922

ISBN 0-914826-39-5 AACR2

Printed in the United States of America

CONTENTS

VOLUME I

Section I. Antimicrobial Agents

VOLUME II

Section II. Antiviral Agents

Section III. Interferon

Section IV. Immunology

Section V. Anticancer Chemotherapy

Preface

Since the first in Geneva in 1959, the International Society of Chemotherapy has held congresses biannually, and the most recent is the 12th International Congress of Chemotherapy.

Twenty years have gone by since the first Congress in Italy was held in Naples in 1961, and we are again together in Italy for the 12th International Congress. The comparison of the chemotherapy of twenty years ago with that of today reveals the considerable development which has occurred in both the antimicrobial and antiblastic drug fields. On the occasion of the 12th International Congress of Chemotherapy many more accomplishments in these areas have come to the fore, accompanied by a new area of research and therapeutic application which concerns immunoactive drugs. The field of chemotherapy, with its wide scope and its methods of research, provides an ideal framework for the study of immunopharmacology. At the Florence meeting, the third and youngest component of chemotherapy, the immunomodulant, was affirmed.

The largest of the three areas, for historic reasons and for past successes, is naturally enough antimicrobial chemotherapy, which was the first to achieve the aim of therapeutic efficacy and is perfecting this progress with the advent of antiviral drugs. The beta-lactam antibiotics show great promise, as do the semisynthetic penicillins, the cephalosporins, and the monobactam molecules.

In the antiblastic chemotherapy field, the anthracyclines, anthracenediones, and cisplatin and their derivatives are prominent among the new antiproliferative chemical agents. Progress in development of anticancer drugs is still very slow, but there is the positive factor that research continues, aided by much greater laboratory and clinical knowledge of the individual agents of past years and improvement on their pharmacological properties with structurally analogous agents. Even for these types of drugs there is proof of an immunomodulant pro-host effect distinguishing the molecules that have had greater antiblastic success, which emphasizes the importance of such a parameter along with the direct cytoreductive attribute.

Immunomodulation and its pharmacological aspects link together the different sectors of chemotherapy, from vaccines in general to the role of subinhibitory concentrations of antimicrobial drugs, from anticancer agents to interferon and its various intraspecies matrices of humoral factors of natural immunity, from cytotoxic agents to immunomodulant chemotherapeutics.

We have cause to believe that the 12th International Congress of Chemotherapy has affirmed without question, as an integral whole, the image of modern chemotherapy, and these two volumes of the Proceedings, entitled *Current Chemotherapy and Immunotherapy,* are a valid assertion of this. The success of the Congress was demonstrated by the presence of more than 5,000 participants who evidenced the vastness of the scientific and applicative interest which continues in the development of chemotherapy, now clearly differentiated from other branches of pharmacology and playing a complex role ranging from preclinical research work and clinical pharmacology to medical therapy.

Last, but not least, the success of the 12th International Congress of Chemotherapy can be attributed also to the beauty of the city of Florence, and to the contribution of the local and regional political authorities and the police force, who helped to render the participants' stay in Florence pleasant and peaceful, in a Florence enjoying springtime weather although it was mid-July, and so helped to make the meeting of the chemotherapists unforgettable for everybody.

The Editors

Piero Periti
Florence, Italy

Giuliana Gialdroni-Grassi
Pavia, Italy

12th International Congress of Chemotherapy

19–24 July 1981 *Florence, Italy*

ORGANIZATION

Organizing Committee

Piero Periti, *President*
Giuliana Gialdroni Grassi, *Co-President*
Michelangelo Rizzo, *Financial Secretary*
Ernesto Pozzi, *Organizing Secretary*
Teresita Mazzei, *Scientific Secretary*

Scientific Committee

Enzo Bonmassar, Italy
Ryochi Fujii, Japan
Guglielmo Gargani, Italy
Felice Gavosto, Italy
Giuliana Gialdroni Grassi, Italy
Thomas H. Hall, U.S.A.
Kurt Hellmann, Great Britain
John Kosmidis, Greece
Zdenek Modr, Czechoslovakia
Luciano Rausa, Italy
Karl H. Spitzy, Austria
Carlo Zanussi, Italy

Administrative Committee

Angelo Lamanna
Teresita Mazzei
Emiliano Panconesi
Piero Periti
Michelangelo Rizzo

Executive Committee of the International Society of Chemotherapy

Helmut P. Kuemmerle, *President*
Carlo Grassi, *Past-President*
Fernando Baquero, *Vice-President*
George K. Daikos, *Vice-President*
Ryochi Fujii, *Vice-President*
Giuliana Gialdroni Grassi, *Vice-President*
Janusz Jeljaszewicz, *Vice-President*
Karl Karrer, *Vice-President*
J. David Williams, *Secretary General*
Jack W. Frankel, *Treasurer*
Georges H. Werner, *Treasurer*

Advisory Committee

Leonardo Donatelli
Harold Neu
Paolo Preziosi

The Changing Horizons of Chemotherapy

P. SENSI

Lepetit Research Laboratories, Milan, Italy

First, I want to express my gratitude to Prof. Periti and Prof. Gialdroni Grassi and to the members of the Organizing Committee for the honor to be invited to deliver the opening lecture at the 12th International Congress of Chemotherapy.

The topic I have originally selected for this lecture is so broad that considering the short available time of 20 minutes I decided to present only a very schematic outline of the successes, failures, and prospects in a field which was opened exactly 90 years ago, when Ehrlich in 1891 coined the word "chemotherapy."

In reality we should recall that, from earliest times, man has searched empirically for remedies against those diseases which are now known to be caused by invading pathogenic organisms. In the past centuries, remedies of various origins, animal, vegetable, and mineral, have achieved some reputation in spite of their now known inefficacy.

As an example, one of the most extensive treatises concerning the management of the plague, written by L. Muratori in the 18th century, reports, in the second part concerning the medical management, more than 130 different remedies mainly prepared with several herbs or herbal extracts (a typical combined therapy, according to the present terminology). But the same author, as a reflection of the inefficacy of the proposed therapies, reports in the third part many religious practices to be followed and prayers to be recited in order to hopefully stimulate divine intervention in the calamity. Among the innumerable empirical remedies developed in the past, only a very limited number of them have resisted scientific challenge (Table 1).

The rational bases of chemotherapy were given by Ehrlich, who introduced several concepts which are still valid: (i) the concept of selective toxicity, (ii) the principle of chemical action on some specific structure of the pathogen, (iii) the screening of a large number of compounds and the chemical modification of active leads, (iv) the role of appropriate animal models, and (v) the problem of development of resistance.

The initial successes of chemotherapy (Table 2) were obtained in the first three decades of this century practically only in parasitic diseases, a field which later suffered a declining interest, with some periodical exceptions. For example, the intensive programs in malaria, in connection with the problems created by World Wars I and II and the conflict in Southeast Asia, yielded a very interesting series of antimalarial drugs to be used for prophylaxis and therapy.

With the exception of the arsphenamines for the chemotherapy of syphilis, until the middle of the 1930s there was no drug for the systemic treatment of bacterial diseases. The discovery of sulfanilamide as a metabolite of Prontosil opened the way to the development of several sulfonamides and to the beginning of the antibacterial chemotherapeutic era.

The discovery of penicillin and the demonstration of its safety and therapeutic value in 1940 initiated the golden period of discoveries of antibacterial microbial metabolites. In the following 20 years (1940–1960), the initial examples of all important classes of antibiotics were found. The last example of an important family of antibiotics was the rifamycins, isolated at the end of the 1950s in our laboratories.

From 1960 to 1980 many derivatives of the primary antibiotics were obtained, either by biosynthesis or by semisynthesis.

If we compare the list of antimicrobial drugs of choice reported in *Medical Letters* in 1980 with the same list reported in 1970, we notice an increase in the number of members of certain families, without inclusion of any completely novel entity.

The number and variety of antibiotics and chemotherapeutic agents available today for the treatment of bacterial diseases have markedly reduced the fatality rates of these illnesses, in many cases to zero, as well as the duration of chronic infections. In bacterial diseases, therapeutic failures, which still occur, are only in a minority of cases due to the lack of appropriate drugs; more often they are related to several other reasons, the most important one probably being the misuse of the available antibacterial agents. A better knowledge of the biological properties of the present drugs and a continuous improvement of the diagnostic procedures should lead to more effective antibacterial chemotherapy. But at the same time there is a great deal of activity in looking for new agents

TABLE 1. *Examples of old remedies for parasitic diseases containing active substances*

Disease	Remedy	Active substance
Malaria	Cinchona barks	Quinine
Malaria	Dichroa febrifuga (Ch'ang Shan)	Febrifugine
Amebiasis	Ipecacuanha	Emetine
Roundworms	Artemisia	Santonin

that are more effective, with fewer side effects and capable of overcoming some problems created by the use of the already available drugs (resistance, allergic reactions, increasing frequency of pathogens very rare in the past, etc.). The screening for new antibiotics is going on in many laboratories in the world, using various new sophisticated techniques. The semisynthetic and biosynthetic approach to the discovery of analogs of old antibiotics continues to generate new highly effective agents, but also in many cases "me-too" drugs. Besides some new aminoglycosides and the great number of new semisynthetic penicillins and cephalosporins, the nonclassical beta-lactams represent probably the most promising novel class of compounds.

The interest in the treatment of neoplastic diseases with chemicals began in the early 1940s with the discovery of the carcinolytic effect of nitrogen mustard. The dramatic severity and the increasing incidence of neoplastic diseases have stimulated intensive research programs in order to find chemical compounds capable of inhibiting or delaying the uncontrolled proliferation of abnormal cells at doses acceptable to the normal cells. This huge effort has yielded a series of drugs of various chemical classes (alkylating agents, antimetabolites, nitrosoureas, antibiotics, and alkaloids), which, in spite of their rather low chemotherapeutic ratio, have provided increasing cure rates in several forms of human cancer. Improvements in the combined use of various chemotherapeutic agents, and also with surgery and radiation, could provide better responses and response rates. But there is no doubt that many neoplastic diseases do not respond to the available drugs and the search for more effective agents must be intensively pursued. The main problem is that there is not enough knowledge on the unique characteristics of cancer cells that can be identified as selective targets. Therefore, blind screening or chemical modification of products already known to have some effect on neoplastic cells are now the main approaches for finding new agents. In the absence of a deeper knowledge of the biochemical differences between normal and cancer cells, further studies on screening tests and animal models which can be extrapolated to the human disease represent also an important contribution to the discovery of new agents.

In the field of viral infections, where the immunological approach has led to brilliant results such as the complete eradication of some viral diseases, chemotherapy has not yet given impressive results, and much remains to be done in the development of effective antiviral drugs.

Although mass screening of thousand of compounds has detected many with antiviral activity, most of them do not possess sufficient selectivity toward specific viral functions or structures and therefore do not give good therapeutic responses in vivo. The result is that today only a minor part of the viral diseases benefit from appropriate chemotherapeutic treatments. Also in this area, progress in the knowledge of viral biology can give new ideas for the synthesis of target-oriented agents.

On the basis of the scientific literature, I have evaluated the comparative research efforts made in the last 5 years in the various fields of chemotherapy. From this survey I found that the chemotherapy of microbial diseases, where the most impressive successes have already been achieved, is still the area of research most pursued and constitutes approximately 60 to 70% of the scientific papers concerning synthesis of new compounds, in vitro and in vivo evaluation, pharmacology, and clinical trials.

Also, the research efforts made in the field of neoplastic diseases are impressive. Excluding the papers concerning the basic studies on the biology of cancer cells, the chemotherapeutic approach ranks in the order of 20 to 30% of the total chemotherapeutic papers. Viral chemotherapy represents about 5 to 10%. Despite the fact that some parasitic diseases, such as malaria, schistosomiasis, and filariasis, each affect more than 200 million people with high rates of incapacitation and death, the research efforts made to find more effective drugs, adequate for the socioeconomic conditions of the countries where these diseases are widespread, are relatively small (only 2 to 5%).

This distribution of research interest in the different fields is unfortunately determined by the probability of commercial success more than by the real medical needs of humanity. For this reason since 1976, WHO has sponsored a special program for research and training in six selected tropical diseases: malaria, schistosomiasis, filariasis, trypanosomions, leishmaniasis, and leprosy. Among other provisions, WHO plans to facilitate the clinical-pharmacological evaluation of new drugs, minimizing the delay between preclinical experimentation and clinical use.

TABLE 2. *Some milestones in chemotherapy*

Diseases	1900–10	1910–20	1920–30	1930–40	1940–50	1950–60	1960–70	1970–80
Parasitic	Methylene blue Atoxyl Trypan red		Suramin Pamaquine	Quinacrine Carbarsone	Chloroquine Chlorguanide Lucanthone	Carbamazine Primaquine Nitroimidazoles	Pyrimethamine Niridazole Levamisole	Mefloquine Oxamniquine
Bacterial	Arsphenamine			Prontosil Sulfonamides	Penicillin Nitrofurans Chloramphenicol Tetracyclines	Isoniazid Erythromycin Nystatin Lincomycin Cephalosporin C Amphotericin B Vancomycin Rifamycins	Methicillin Ampicillin Cephalothin Cephaloridine Gentamicin Nalidixic acid Co-trimoxazole Rifampin Clindamycin	Many semisynthetic penicillins and cephalosporins Nonclassical β-lactams Other aminoglycosides
Neoplastic					Nitrogen mustards Methotrexate	Mercaptopurine Chlorambucil Cyclophosphamide Melphalan Actinomycin D Vinblastine	Nitrosoureas Procarbazine L-Asparaginase Daunomycin Adriamycin	*cis*-Platinum — New entities under evaluation —
Viral						Methisazone Interferon	Idoxuridine Cytarabine	Vidarabine Ribavirin

This program, which should be followed by the commitment of the scientific community and of the industrial organizations, could reverse the declining trend in chemotherapeutic research on tropical diseases.

Parallel to the continuous development of the treatment of diseases caused by invading organisms through use of chemicals which block or kill the pathogens, the concept of chemotherapy is becoming broader and includes other approaches, some of which have already reached very interesting results. In recent years there has been an impressive development in immunopharmacology with a great proliferation of experimental studies on nonspecific immunostimulants and on compounds which have been identified as modulators of the immune response. Also, products affecting chemotaxis and chemokinesis could have significant application in the suppression of metastasis of neoplastic cells or in increasing the bactericidal activity of neutrophils against various organisms.

The preparation and use of immunochemotherapeutic complexes between drugs and specific antibodies represent a way of carrying therapeutic agents to specific tissue sites and therefore can constitute a more effective treatment than either of the component parts of the complex. The recent advent of the monoclonal hybridoma technique is opening new perspectives in this field. Studies on the significance of bacterial adhesion as a pathogenic factor are suggesting the possibility of finding compounds, interfering with this phenomenon, to be used in the treatment or prophylaxis of infectious bacterial diseases. Finally, I want to mention the research on products which increase the sensitivity of hypoxic cells to radiation and therefore improve the efficiency of this treatment.

The examples I have shown indicate that the search for fighting against invading pathogens is going on not only with the classical approaches but also in many other directions.

The International Congresses of Chemotherapy which have taken place every 2 years since 1959 have represented the best arena where the confrontation of new ideas, approaches, and experimental models has had fruitful results. All the steps in the chemotherapeutic advances during the last 20 years can be identified by looking at the proceedings of these congresses. If we consider that at the first international congress, the chemotherapy of neoplastic diseases was considered only a promise and not yet a therapeutic reality and that the semisynthetic penicillins and cephalosporins were discussed for the first times, respectively, at the second and third international congresses, we can derive how many innovative steps have been made since then.

The exciting scientific program of the next days in Florence and the participation of highly qualified scientists will give us a picture of the progress achieved in the last 2 years and an outlook on the perspectives for future successes of chemotherapy.

Section I: Antimicrobial Agents

Symposia

R-Plasmid Resistance

S. MITSUHASHI *Moderator*	*Laboratory of Drug Resistance in Bacteria* *Department of Microbiology, School of Medicine* *Gunma University, Maebashi, Japan*
K. N. TIMMIS *Moderator*	*Max Planck Institute for Molecular Genetics* *Berlin-Dahlem, West Germany*
F. H. KAYSER	*Institute of Medical Microbiology* *University of Zurich* *Zurich, Switzerland*
F. E. HAHN	*Division of Communicable Disease and Immunology* *Walter Reed Army Institute of Research* *Washington, D.C. 20012, U.S.A.*
N. DATTA	*Royal Postgraduate Medical School* *London, England*
T. YAMAMOTO S. YAMAGISHI S. MITSUHASHI	*Faculty of Pharmaceutical Sciences* *Chiba University* *Chiba, Japan* and *School of Medicine* *Gunma University* *Maebashi, Gunma, Japan*
M. INOUE A. FUSE H. KAWASHIMA S. MITSUHASHI	*Laboratory of Drug Resistance in Bacteria* *School of Medicine* *Gunma University* *Maebashi, Gunma, Japan*
B. W. HOLLOWAY C. CROWTHER M. NAYUDU N. S. WILLETTS	*Department of Genetics* *Monash University* *Clayton, Victoria, Australia* and *Department of Molecular Biology* *University of Edinburgh* *Edinburgh, Scotland*
T. TOKOTA T. YAMAMOTO R. SEKIGUCHI	*Department of Bacteriology* *School of Medicine* *Juntendo University* *Tokyo 113, Japan*
K. N. TIMMIS P. A. MANNING J. K. TIMMIS A. MOLL	*Max Planck Institute for Molecular Genetics* *Berlin-Dahlem, West Germany*

Conjugative (R) and nonconjugative (r) drug resistance plasmids and their worldwide spread have caused many problems in medicine, stock farming, and fish breeding industries. In addition, the prevalence of drug resistance plasmids and the discovery of transposons have broadened our perspective on the role that genetic exchanges play in the natural history of bacterial species. This symposium consists of four main topics: (i) pharmaceutical approaches to the problems caused by drug resistance plasmids, (ii) transposons, (iii) mobilization mechanisms of nonconjugative plasmid and conjugal transfer of bacterial chromosomes, and (iv) plasmids conferring toxicity or invasiveness of pathogenic bacteria.

Mechanisms and Genetic Basis of Resistance to Aminocyclitols in Gram-Positive Cocci

F. H. Kayser

Resistance of *Staphylococcus aureus* to the aminocyclitol antibiotics gentamicin (GM), sisomicin, amikacin, and netilmicin has not been a problem until recently in the Zurich area. From 1979 to 1980, however, an increase in the frequencies of isolation of strains resistant to GM/sisomicin (2 to 21%), tobramycin (2 to 22%), amikacin (1 to 13%), and netilmicin (1 to 9%) has been observed in strains isolated from patients at the University Hospital.

Examination of the biochemical mechanism of resistance in these strains revealed aminocyclitol-modifying enzymes long known to be due to resistant phenotypes in various bacteria. *S. aureus* strains mostly produced APH(3′) and APH(2″) simultaneously with AAC(6′); rarely, ANT(4′,4″) was produced. The latter enzyme was more frequently observed in *Staphylococcus epidermidis*. The genetic determinants of aminocyclitol resistance often were integrated into plasmids of various sizes (3 to 36 megadaltons). Strains also have been observed in which no evidence for plasmid-mediated aminocyclitol resistance was found.

Aminocyclitols are relatively inactive against enterococci, but are able to produce bactericidal synergy in combination with penicillins. Synergy is dependent upon a low level of resistance to aminocyclitols. Examination of nearly 400 enterococci in agar dilution tests revealed that 35% of isolates showed high-level resistance (MIC, 1,250 mg/liter) to kanamycin and streptomycin, but none to GM/sisomicin, tobramycin, netilmicin, or amikacin. Kanamycin-resistant *Streptococcus faecalis* strains produced APH(3′). Half of the streptomycin-resistant isolates produced AAD(6), and the other half had ribosomal resistance. APH(3′) and AAD(6) were indistinguishable from respective staphylococcal transferase enzymes. ANT(4′,4″) has not been found in our isolates, but has been observed occasionally in *S. faecalis* by other researchers. *Streptococcus faecium* strains with high-level resistance also produced APH(3′) and AAD(6). In addition, low amounts of a transferase acetylating GM/sisomicin, tobramycin, and netilmicin AAC(6′) were observed in many cultures. High-level resistance to aminocyclitols could be transferred by mixed cultivation from *S. faecalis* to appropriate receptors. Molecular weight determinations by means of measurement of DNA length showed plasmids of 38 to 50 megadaltons in size. No transfer of antibiotic resistance could be achieved with *S. faecium* isolates as donors.

Pharmacological Approaches to the R-Plasmid Problem

F. E. Hahn

Pharmacological approaches to the R-plasmid problem fall into three major categories: (i) chemotherapy of plasmids per se, aimed at their elimination from bacteria; (ii) selective inhibition of plasmid-carrying bacteria; and (iii) evasion or antagonism of the actions of plasmid gene products. The first class of such inhibitors includes substances which intercalate preferentially into supercoiled DNA. Substituted phenanthridines, acridines, anthracyclines, thioxanthenones, fluorenes, phenoxazines, and phenothiazines restored in vitro drug susceptibility to cultures of plasmid-bearing bacteria. The second class of antiplasmid inhibitors were those of the enzyme DNA gyrase. Nalidixic acid inhibited the nicking and closing of circular duplex DNA; sodium dodecyl sulfate promoted double-stranded cleavage of circular DNA and covalent attachment of the denatured gyrase; and novobiocin inhibited the DNA-dependent introduction of negative supercoils into circular DNA by the gyrase. These compounds eliminate drug resistance from plasmid-containing bacteria.

Selective inhibition of plasmid-containing bacteria has been obtained with certain phosphorus-containing antibiotics which are inhibitors of cell wall peptidoglycan polymer synthesis. Macarbomycin and especially Flavomycin inhibit preferentially the growth of plasmid-containing bacteria. It is conceivable that the attachment of plasmids to a membrane fraction renders plasmid-containing bacteria more susceptible to the action of macarbomycin or Flavomycin than bacteria which have unoccupied membranes.

Evasion or antagonism of the actions of plasmid gene products (enzymes) involves two different approaches. The first approach consists of molecular modification of antibiotics to delete those groups which are derivatized by plasmid-encoded enzymes, while maintaining antibacterial potency of the modified drugs.

The second approach is based upon the use of inhibitors of plasmid gene products in combination with antibiotics. Resistance to penicillins and cephalosporins is caused by enzymatic hydrolysis of their β-lactam rings. The β-lactamases of resistant bacteria can be plasmidic or chromosomal gene products. A methodical search for β-lactamase inhibitors in fermentation broths of *Streptomyces* spp. discovered clavulanic acid, a fused β-lactam structure, different from the β-lactam antibiotics. Clavulanic acid itself has only weak antibacterial activity but inhibits a variety of bacterial β-lactamases at low concentration and sensitizes bacteria to inhibition by β-lactam antibiotics. A semisynthetic penicillanic acid sulfone, designated CP-45,899, is a preferential inhibitor of plasmid-encoded β-lactamases and acts in vitro synergistically with penicillin. Theoretical considerations suggest that superior β-lactamase inhibitors might be obtained by systematic derivatization of penicillanic acid.

Transposons in the Spread of Resistance to Trimethoprim and GM

N. Datta

The study of R plasmids in many laboratories has contributed to our present understanding of their evolution. A diversity of plasmids exist in bacteria and can be classified by various means, including incompatibility grouping. R plasmids are ones that have acquired genes for antibiotic resistance, often carried on transposons, the specialized DNA sequences that can transpose themselves from one replicon to another.

The spread of resistance genes among bacteria and their plasmids depends upon many factors, including (i) the degree of selection imposed in the environment and (ii) the frequency of their transposition. The first transposon to be identified as such, Tn*A*, determines resistance to ampicillin and other penicillins. Intense selection has been exerted on a world scale for the spread of this character, by the use of ampicillin (ABPC) and, more recently, other broad-spectrum penicillins. Tn*A* (Tn*1* or Tn*3*) transposes at high frequency. The successful dissemination of this DNA sequence and its acquisition by *Haemophilus influenzae* and *Neisseria gonorrhoeae* is a remarkable evolutionary phenomenon.

Two transposons, Tn*7* and Tn*402*, determining trimethoprim resistance have been described. We have recently identified a third, designated Tn*735*. Trimethoprim, like ABPC, is a broad-spectrum, nontoxic, orally administered antibacterial and therefore is extensively used, with sulfamethoxazole as co-trimoxazole or alone. Tn*7*, like Tn*1*, transposes at high frequency, so it is not surprising that the incidence of trimethoprim resistance, determined by Tn*7*, is increasing. Trimethoprim resistance is still relatively uncommon among bacteria causing infection in the community (outside hospitals), but when it is found it is frequently Tn*7* determined. It is more common in bacteria causing infection in hospital. In a recent survey of strains of *Escherichia coli* causing urinary infections, 1% of those from the community and 10% of those from hospital were trimethoprim resistant. In either case, we found evidence for the presence of transposon Tn*7* in the trimethoprim-resistant strains, 2 of 3 of the community ones and 24 of 27 of the hospital ones. Tn*402* and Tn*735*, though determining the same high level of trimethoprim resistance, transpose between replicons at 1,000-fold lower frequency in laboratory experiments. This is reflected in their relative rarity in bacteria isolated from clinical material.

In hospitals, but not in the nonhospital community, there has been strong selection for GM-resistant bacteria. Much of the GM resistance found is plasmid determined and in some cases is carried on transposons. We have identified transposon Tn*732*, which determines resistance to GM and tobramycin and is mediated by an aminoglycoside-adenylylating enzyme, and Tn*733*, which gives GM resistance and is mediated by an acetyltransferase. C. E. Rubens et al. (1979) have found transposons determining resistance to multiple antibiotics including GM. No GM resistance transposon so far identified is transposable at the high frequencies seen with Tn*1* or Tn*7*. The dissemination of these genes seems, at present, to depend more upon the transmission of resistant bacteria between patients and of plasmids between bacteria than upon transposition of DNA sequences.

Transposition of Various β-Lactamase Genes Specified by R Plasmids

T. Yamamoto, S. Yamagishi, S. Mitsuhashi

A large number of antibiotic resistance genes on plasmids have been recognized to be located in a discrete DNA sequence, called a transposon. Transposons are able to translocate from one replicon to another in the absence of the bacterial *recA* gene function. Because of their ability to move freely from plasmid to plasmid, transposons can be thought to have played a large part in the rapid evolutionary spread and accumulation of drug resistance genes on plasmids.

Plasmid-mediated resistance to β-lactam antibiotics is mostly associated with the elaboration of β-lactamase. Many β-lactamases have been well characterized and roughly classified into five groups with respect to substrate specificity. Among them, the type I (or the TEM type) enzyme is by far the most widespread and is found on a wide variety of naturally occurring plasmids. The second type is the oxacillin-hydrolyzing enzyme, which can be differentiated from the others by its ability to hydrolyze oxacillin or methicillin at an appreciable rate.

Since the first recognition of a transposon, Tn*1* on plasmid RP4, many ABPC transposons (Tn*A*'s) have been reported which specify the type I enzyme. We also identified two kinds of Tn*A*, Tn*2601* and Tn*2602*, on plasmids Rms212 and Rms325, respectively, which are about 4.7

kilobase pairs and flanked by short inverted repeat sequences at both ends. The type I β-lactamase is very uniform in biochemical and immunochemical properties but is heterogeneous in absolute levels of enzyme activity. By a comparative study of the transcription of the β-lactamase gene (*bla*) specified by both Tn*A*'s, we clarified that the difference in the rate of transcription of each *bla* gene plays a key role in determining the heterogeneity of absolute levels of enzyme activity among the type I β-lactamases. Furthermore, we demonstrated that Tn*2602* was capable of transposition at 8 to 50 times higher frequency than other Tn*A*'s, e.g., Tn*2601* and Tn*3*.

Next, we found that the type II (or OXA-1) β-lactamase gene, which is one of the subgroups in oxacillin-hydrolyzing enzymes, can transpose to various plasmids in a *recA* background. We designated this transposon Tn*2603*. Tn*2603* has a molecular size of 20 kilobase pairs and is flanked by small inverted repeat sequences of about 0.2 kilobase pair. Tn*2603* encodes resistance to streptomycin, sulfonamide, and mercury in addition to the type II β-lactamase. In most cases, the type II β-lactamase gene has been recognized together with streptomycin, sulfonamide, and mercury resistance genes on naturally occurring plasmids. We have also recognized transposons indistinguishable from Tn*2603* on R455 and R656a. Therefore, it may be speculated that Tn*2603* plays a major role in the generation and distribution of R plasmids which mediate the type II β-lactamase.

Mobilization of ColE1 Derivatives by the Concomitant Presence of Nonconjugative and Conjugative Plasmids

M. Inoue, A. Fuse, H. Kawashima, S. Mitsuhashi

It has long been recognized that certain nonconjugative plasmids such as ColE1 can be mobilized to other bacteria at high frequency by F or other conjugative plasmids. However, some nonconjugative plasmids, such as pSC101, are mobilized poorly by the fertility systems. Recently, evidence has accumulated to show a strong relation between the ability of ColE1 plasmid DNA to be relaxed and its ability to be transferred by conjugation. This mobilization is governed in part by a ColE1 gene, called *mob*. Some ColE1 derivatives, pBR313 and pBR322, are *mob*; hence, these plasmids are mobilized by a conjugative plasmid at a very low frequency compared with the mobilization frequencies of ColE1 plasmids.

pMS76 is a nonconjugative, 5.54-megadalton plasmid that contains a single site susceptible to digestion by different restriction endonucleases. This plasmid, which mediates the hypersynthesis of type I β-lactamase, is present in *E. coli* K-12 cells at about 20 copies per chromosome. In addition, plasmid pMS76 can be mobilized by conjugative plasmids and it shares a number of other properties with the amplifiable ColE1 plasmid, including the ability to amplify copy number in the presence of chloramphenicol. Tn*5* derived from pSC101::Tn*5* was transposed into pMS76, and the recombinant plasmids were constructed. Then we tested incompatibility between pMS76 and other amplifiable plasmids. However, pMS76 is compatible with ColE1-derived replicons pBR322 and pCR1 and with other multicopy plasmids, RSF1030 and pACYC184.

When pMS76-1 DNA was transformed into the *E. coli* K-12 *recA* strain carrying both pBR322 and R9-5, mobilization of both pMS76-1 and pBR322 plasmids by R9-5 was tested. R9-5 is one of the chloramphenicol resistance plasmids isolated from R100-1. The mobilization frequency of pBR322 from the *recA* strain was at >10% efficiency by R9-5; i.e., over half of the recipients which received R9-5 also contained pMS76-1, but about 10% of the recipients which received R9-5 contained pBR322. A number of R9-5$^-$ pBR322$^+$ recipients could be recovered. However, the mobilization of pBR322 from *E. coli* K-12 having R9-5 was reduced by a factor of 10^6 to 10^7 compared with the presence of plasmid pMS76-1. This type of mobilization was observed by the presence of plasmid pMS76-1 F *lac tra*(ΔI). Hence, it is noteworthy that the *mob* mutant of ColE1, pBR322, is complemented in *trans* by *mob*$^+$ pMS76, a naturally occurring plasmid that is not closely related to ColE1 in incompatibility testing. This finding suggested that plasmid pMS76 produces a diffusible gene product(s) involved in its own transfer. Another mutant of pMS76, pMS76-2, cannot mobilize plasmid pBR322 with the presence of plasmid R9-5. From restriction endonuclease analysis, pMS76-2 lost the *Sma*I site from pMS76. Accordingly, the mobilization of plasmid pBR322 will be related to the *Sma*I site on plasmid pMS76. We also found nine small cryptic plasmids from *Shigella* spp. which were about 2.6 megadaltons in size. pBR322 was mobilized with these cryptic plasmids at a frequency of 10% per R9-5.

Acquisition of Genome Segments by R Plasmids

B. W. Holloway, C. Crowther, M. Nayudu, N. S. Willetts

Whereas only about 2% of *Pseudomonas aeruginosa* strains isolated from patients carry a transmissible plasmid with antibiotic resistance determinants, about 30% of such strains carry transmissible FP plasmids which can promote bacterial chromosome transfer but do not carry any antibiotic resistance determinants. FP plasmids can readily acquire transposons, and it is possible that FP plasmids may have a role in the development of R plasmids in *P. aeruginosa.* In one case, a close relationship between an R plasmid, R18-1, and an FP plasmid, FP110, has been shown.

The ability of naturally occurring R plasmids to promote bacterial chromosome transfer has been demonstrated for a wide variety of bacterial genera. The best known of such plasmids is R68.45. It has been demonstrated that R68.45 and other similar plasmids carry a duplication of a region of the plasmid chromosome located immediately counter-clockwise from the kanamycin resistance determinant region of the plasmid genome. This duplicated region has been identified by its characteristic pattern of restriction endonuclease sites. A previously unidentified insertion sequence, IS*21,* has been shown to occur in this tandemly duplicated region of the R68.45 genome. IS*21* was shown to transpose to a variety of sites in plasmid pED815, a derivative of pBR325. R68 variants have been isolated which have increased chromosome mobilizing ability for *E. coli,* but not for *P. aeruginosa.* Moreover, these variants do not have the same tandemly duplicated region of the plasmid chromosome as is found in R68.45. Instead, they contain a 1.2-kilobase DNA insert at either of two plasmid regions, one near the carbenicillin resistance determinant and the other located counter-clockwise from the *Eco*RI site.

Plasmids such as R68.45 can form plasmid primes, a hybrid plasmid containing both plasmid and bacterial DNA. These plasmids retain normal transfer functions as well as the wide bacterial host range of the IncP-1 plasmids, so they are an efficient means of constructing bacterial hybrids which possess the normal genome of the recipient together with a fragment of chromosome of the bacterium in which the plasmid prime was formed.

Enterotoxin Plasmids Harboring Drug Resistance Genes

T. Yokota, T. Yamamoto, R. Sekiguchi

Enterotoxin plasmids producing both heat-labile and heat-stable enterotoxins (LT and ST) derived from *E. coli* H10407(pJH104) and one encoding only the LT obtained from *E. coli* TD218C1(pJY20) (both strains of human origin) were labeled with drug resistance transposons by two different methods. One, an R plasmid, RP4 *amp tet kan,* was transferred to the enterotoxigenic strains, and the ABPC resistance of transconjugants was further transferred to the plasmid-free strain of *E. coli* 20SO. The subclones of the second transconjugants resistant to ABPC but not to tetracycline and kanamycin were selected, and their enterotoxigenicities were assayed. The second, an R plasmid susceptible to high temperature for replication, R402 *amp str spc,* was transferred to the enterotoxigenic strains, and the transconjugants were successively subcultured in L broth containing 100 μg of ABPC per ml at 42°C for 10 days. The ABPC resistance of transconjugants was further transferred to *E. coli* 20SO at 42°C, and the second transconjugants were confirmed to be sensitive to streptomycin and spectinomycin and to be enterotoxigenic. Retransfer of ENT-R plasmids (enterotoxin plasmids harboring drug resistance genes) thus obtained was performed with *E. coli* CSH2, *E. coli* YE100 *cya,* and *E. coli* CA7902 *cya* as the recipients.

Although the cotransfer of enterotoxigenicity and ABPC resistance in the ENT-R plasmids derived from *E. coli* TD218C1 by both labeling methods was always stable (pJY14), that of the ENT-R plasmids obtained from *E. coli* H10407 by either labeling method was found to be unstable, and the enterotoxigenicity was easily lost by conjugative transfer and transformation.

Agarose gel electrophoresis of the cleared lysates of *E. coli* 20SO bearing pJY10 or its segregants, from which either enterotoxigenicity or ABPC resistance was spontaneously eliminated (pJY12 and pJY11), revealed that the three substrains harbored only one size each of covalently closed circular DNA of about 63 kilobases in size. A DNA segment containing LT^+ and ST^+ regions, which consisted of two *Eco*RI fragments, was inserted into a cloning vehicle, ColE1-Tn*5,* by *Eco*RI digestion and subsequent ligation.

Although the LT^+ gene itself was confirmed not to be a transposon, a rather wide region of DNA containing the LT^+ gene and AT transposon was found to be flanked by repeated DNA sequences, three in a set (designated β). This novel DNA structure (β-Tn *toxS-toxL*-β-β) suggested the possibility that the LT^+ region is on a higher transposon containing an ST transposon within the structure. Unlike the unstable ENT-R plasmid derived from *E. coli* H10407, the stable ENT-R plasmids obtained from *E. coli* TD218C1 did not contain such a complicated DNA structure. In this case, the LT^+ DNA region was confirmed not to be flanked by any inverted repeat nucleotide sequences.

Involvement of Antibiotic Resistance Plasmids in Bacterial Resistance to Serum

K. N. Timmis, P. A. Manning, J. K. Timmis, A. Moll

Animal blood contains a number of nonspecific (complement, lysozyme, phagocytes, ion-binding proteins, etc.) and specific (antibodies, lymphocytes) agents that alone or in combination lyse, kill, or prevent the growth of the majority of bacteria with which they make contact. Abilities to resist, evade, or inactivate these host defenses thus constitute major virulence components of invasive bacterial pathogens that distinguish them from their noninvasive relatives. Epidemiological studies that have shown invasive gram-negative pathogens, but not non-invasive or nonpathogenic bacteria, to be generally highly resistant to serum, as well as results from experimental infections in animal models with serum-resistant and serum-susceptible bacteria, are consistent with this conclusion.

Thus far, efforts to analyze plasmid-mediated serum resistance have focused on the IncFII group R plasmids, R6-5 and R100, and IncFI group Col plasmid, ColV, I-K94. Transposon mutagenesis and gene cloning experiments have shown that the serum resistance gene of R6-5/R100 is *traT,* one of two genes for plasmid surface exclusion. The *traT* protein, *traT*p, is a 25,000-dalton polypeptide that is present in about 20,000 copies per cell in the outer membrane of *E. coli* K-12. Iodination of whole cells, using lactoperoxidase, revealed that *traT*p is highly exposed on the cell surface; this is consistent with its function of preventing compliment attack of the cell surface. The ColV-encoded serum resistance factor is also an outer membrane protein but is distinct from *traT*p.

Comparison of the binding of complement components of *E. coli* K-12 cells that do, or do not, carry the *traT* gene has revealed no difference in the binding of any complement component to serum-susceptible and serum-resistant bacteria. This indicates that *traT*p inhibits the activity of the complement membrane attack unit and not its assembly. The tendency of *traT*p to self-aggregate and the estimation of 30,000 complement binding sites per bacterium indicate that complement may only damage bacteria at specific surface sites and that *traT*p may be localized at such sites.

Significance of Low Concentrations of Antibiotics in Infections

VICTOR LORIAN *Moderator*	*The Bronx-Lebanon Hospital Center Bronx, New York 10456, U.S.A.*
LEON D. SABATH *Moderator*	*Minnesota University Minneapolis, Minnesota 55455, U.S.A.*
MICHAEL T. REYMAN	*Brookwood Medical Center Baptist Medical Center-Montclair Birmingham, Alabama 35294, U.S.A.*
ILARIO VIANO	*Institute of Pharmacology Turin, Italy*
KLAUS VOSBECK	*Pharmaceuticals Division Ciba-Geigy Ltd. Basel, Switzerland*
SAIDA BEN REDJEB	*Hôpital Charles Nicoll Tunis, Tunisia*
ALI BOUJNAH	*Faculty of Medicine Tunis, Tunisia*
CURTIS G. GEMMELL	*University of Glasgow Glasgow, U.K.*
ROBERTA FONTANA	*Institute of Microbiology Padova, Italy*
BARBARA ATKINSON	*The Bronx-Lebanon Hospital Center Bronx, New York 10456, U.S.A.*

The effects of antibiotics at low concentrations were first observed by Gardner, an associate of Flemming, in 1940. During the years some reports have been published describing the morphological changes of bacteria under the effect of low concentrations of various antibiotics. Systematic investigations about the effects of sub-MICs on bacteria started in the early 1970s with Stille in Germany, Koike in Japan, and in our laboratory in New York. During the last 5 years, an increasing number of publications have been devoted to this subject. Three symposia were dedicated to this subject: Effects of Subinhibitory Concentrations of Antibiotics on Bacteria, at the 10th International Congress of Chemotherapy (*Current Chemotherapy*, 1977, p. 72–78); Significance of Subinhibitory Concentrations of Antibiotics, Turin, 8, September (Proceedings of the Symposium on Significance of Subinhibitory Concentrations of Antibiotics, Rev. Infect. Dis. **1**:780–879); and Subminimal Doses of Antibiotics, at the XI Triennial World Congress of Pathology, 20–25 September 1981. In addition to the various reports about the ultrastructure of bacteria exposed to sub-MIC of antibiotics, the changes in their biochemical constitution and in their virulence showed the relevance of results obtained in this area. Abnormal forms of bacteria produced by sub-MICs of antibiotics were observed in specimens from patients treated with antibiotics. The minimum antibiotic concentration (MAC) and its relationship to the MIC, the MIC/MAC, has been shown to be valuable for the evaluation of new antibiotics as well as the old antibiotics. Sub-MICs were shown to be therapeutically active in experimental infections in animals, and some recent studies showed that, to reproduce the ultrastructure of bacteria as seen in infections, it is necessary to grow them on a solid-phase support rather than in a liquid medium.

This symposium brought very new data related to the chemical constitution of bacteria exposed to sub-MICs of antibiotics, new data about the fixation of drugs at low concentrations on the penicillin-binding proteins, and the effect of drugs in the production of pathogenic substances. To be virulent, bacteria have to adhere at the surface of cells. This is a relatively new area that has been developing during the last few years. Sub-MICs of antibiotics have been shown to interfere with adherence and therefore with virulence, and new data about this very new subject are presented. Filaments of gram-negative bacteria produced by many beta-lactam antibiotics are suspected, because of their size, to be more resistant to defense mechanisms. Figure 1 shows, however, how one single polymorphonuclear cell engulfs a filament at least 30 μg long. Most important, however, are clinical data related to sub-MICs of antibiotics. It is shown how sub-MICs of ampicillin in the urine, which were produced with a tiny dose of 10 mg a day, can cure urinary infections.

Treatment of Serious Gram-Negative Bacillary Infections with Sub-MICs of Aminoglycoside Antibiotics

M. T. Reymann

A prospective clinical study of 120 patients with serious gram-negative bacillary disease caused by a large variety of *Enterobacteriaceae* and *Pseudomonas* species, and who were treated with one of several dosage regimens utilizing gentamicin or tobramycin, was previously reported (Antimicrob. Agents Chemother. **16:**353–361, 1979). During the course of therapy, numerous parameters were monitored, including peak serum aminoglycoside (AMG) levels and MICs of the infecting organism(s).

A comparison made of peak AMG serum levels achieved versus the MIC for the infecting pathogen revealed that 17 to 33% of the peak serum AMG concentrations in our three dosage ranges failed to exceed the MIC of the patient's organism. Dosages used were those routinely recommended in seriously ill patients, with appropriate adjustments made for impaired renal function.

The overall mortality of patients in the study group was 37% (44 of 120). There was no significant difference in mortality between the gentamicin and tobramycin groups. A comparison was made between mortality in those patients with serum AMG levels less than 1/8 of the MIC compared with those with inhibitory levels greater than 1/8, and there was found to be no significant difference. At the time of the original study no comparison was made between patients with subinhibitory concentrations and the remainder of the study population.

A retrospective evaluation was performed on those patients whose peak AMG serum concentration to MIC ratio was <1 (subinhibitory) on more than 50% of occasions. A comparison was made with the other study patients with regard to toxicity and patient characteristics. We identified 22 patients who had >60% of their measured peak AMG serum concentrations classified as subinhibitory. A total of 101 serum levels were drawn on these patients over the course of their period of therapy with AMG ($\bar{x} = 4.6$ levels per patient). Of these serum levels, 90 of 101 (89%) were <1 × MIC; 47 of 90 (52%) were <0.50 × MIC; and 16 of 90 (18%) were <0.25 × MIC. Nine patients received gentamicin and 13 received tobramycin.

With regard to the types of infectious processes present in this subgroup, 11 of 22 had sepsis documented by positive blood cultures. Of these the genitourinary tract was believed to be the source in four. Pneumonia was present in 11 of 22 as a primary or coexisting infection, and 2 of 22 patients had serious wound infections. Patients with uncomplicated urinary tract infection were not included in the overall study group.

In addition to the AMG administered, 20 of 22 patients in this subgroup also received one or more additional antibiotics for longer than 48 h. A cephalosporin antibiotic was the most frequent second agent. The gram-negative bacillus pathogen isolated was ultimately shown to be susceptible to one or more of the additional antibiotics in only 5 of these 20 patients. In the other 15 patients who received a second antibiotic, the gram-negative pathogen was susceptible only to the AMG agent being administered.

As noted previously, overall mortality for the entire study group was 37% (44 of 120). When those patients with subinhibitory concentrations of AMG were removed from consideration, the overall mortality remained unchanged at 37% (36 of 98). Among the group of patients with subinhibitory concentrations, 36% (8 of 22) died. Of these eight patients, all had documented sepsis and three had pneumonia. Three of the eight patients who died received also other antibiotics to which their gram-negative pathogen was susceptible. Therefore, 14 patients survived of whom 12 were actually cured by subinhibitory concentrations of AMG alone. All 14 patients had a normal immunodefense system; two patients, however, received large doses of steroids. *Escherichia coli* was the pathogen in eight cases; of the other six, two were caused by *Klebsiella*, three by *Serratia*, and one by *Proteus*. All surviving patients experienced clinical and bacteriological cure.

Overall nephrotoxicity secondary to AMG therapy in our original study group was 13% (13 of 100). In 17 nondialysis patients in the subinhibitory group, there was no evidence of renal toxicity attributable to AMG therapy.

In the absence of a prospective study of seri-

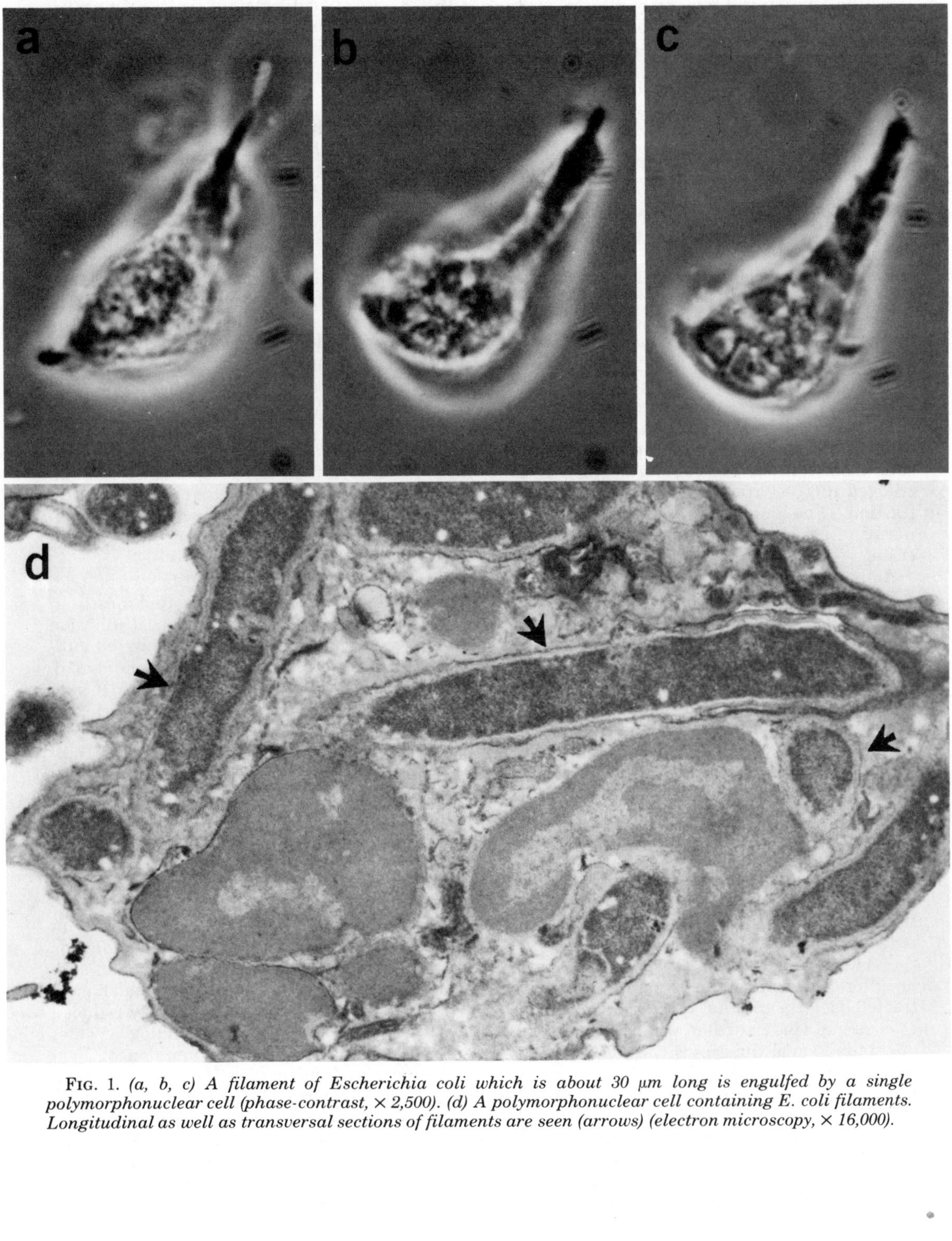

FIG. 1. *(a, b, c) A filament of Escherichia coli which is about 30 μm long is engulfed by a single polymorphonuclear cell (phase-contrast, × 2,500). (d) A polymorphonuclear cell containing E. coli filaments. Longitudinal as well as transversal sections of filaments are seen (arrows) (electron microscopy, × 16,000).*

ously ill patients, in whom subinhibitory anti- that there could well be justification for exam- biotic dosages have been used, our data suggest ining the efficacy and toxicity of AMGs, used in subinhibitory concentrations, alone or in combination with other antibiotic agents.

Effects of Sub-MIC of Antibiotics on the Biochemical Constitution of Gram-Negative Bacilli

I. Viano, M. Marchisio, M. Santiano, M. Eandi

This study reports qualitative and quantitative alterations of cytoplasm protein of some gram-negative bacilli grown in the presence of sub-MICs of ampicillin, cefoperazone, and gentamicin.

The bacteria were exposed to the antibiotics by the membrane technique, using filter membranes placed on Trypticase soy agar (BBL Microbiology Systems). After a proper period of incubation at 37°C, the organisms were displaced into saline and washed two times with saline. The bacteria were disrupted in an ultrasonic disintegrator. The cellular debris was centrifuged at 60,000 rpm to remove the membrane fraction. The supernatant was analyzed by means of gel electrophoresis and isoelectric focusing.

Ampicillin produced filaments with *E. coli* ATCC 10536 and one clinical isolate each of *Salmonella typhimurium* and *Proteus vulgaris* at concentrations of 0.75, 1, and 1.5 μg/ml, respectively. The cytoplasm of these filaments contained four proteins of high molecular weight at low electrophoretic mobility which were not present in the cytoplasm of the untreated organisms. Cefoperazone induced the formation of long filaments of *E. coli* ATCC 10536 at a concentration of 0.25 μg/ml and induced the formation of filaments of a strain of *Klebsiella pneumoniae* at a concentration of 4 μg/ml. The cytoplasm of these filaments showed a small number of acidic proteins with a low isoelectric point not present in the cytoplasm of the controls. The same strains of *K. pneumoniae* and *P. vulgaris* exposed to gentamicin at concentrations of 0.15 and 0.3 μg/ml, respectively, showed no difference between the protein content of the treated bacteria and that of the controls.

These data indicate that, while the final target of beta-lactam antibiotics is the cell wall, these antibiotics at sub-MICs can produce alterations in the protein synthesis without significantly affecting the cell wall. Gentamicin inhibits irreversibly the assemblage of ribosomes but does not affect the protein synthesis of active ribosomes. That exposure of gram-negative bacilli to sub-MICs of gentamicin did not alter qualitatively the protein content of the cells exposed is another confirmation of this mechanism.

Interference of Sub-MIC of Antibiotics with Bacterial Adhesion to Epithelial Surfaces

K. Vosbeck

Bacterial adhesion to epithelial surfaces has been recognized as an important contributing factor in the pathogenesis of a number of infectious diseases. There is good evidence that adhesive factors are of primary significance in the pathogenesis of *E. coli* diarrhea. Adhesiveness of *E. coli* strains has also been associated with their ability to cause urinary tract infections. Adhesion of streptococci to fibrin has been shown to constitute the first step in the development of endocarditis, and adhesion of streptococci to tooth surfaces is instrumental in the development of dental caries. Agents interfering with bacterial adhesion may be of prophylactic as well as of therapeutic value, be it alone or in combination with classical antibiotics.

The classical methods of microscopically counting bacteria adhering to exfoliated cells and the assays measuring binding of radiolabeled bacteria to tissue culture cells or to exfoliated cells, hemagglutination, yeast agglutination, or hydrophobicity measurements should be used to complement each other.

The effect of sub-MICs of antibiotics on bacterial adhesion has been investigated mostly in *E. coli* and streptococci. Streptococcal adhesion to eucaryotic cells appears to be mediated indirectly by the lipid moiety of lipoteichoic acid. Treatment of streptococci with sub-MICs of benzylpenicillin leads to a release of lipoteichoic acid and to a concomitant decrease of streptococcal adhesion to human buccal cells. Sub-MICs of benzylpenicillin, as well as of rifampin, have been reported to decrease the hydrophobicity of streptococci, which is thought to be an expression of their adhesiveness.

Adhesion of *E. coli* strains may be mediated by a number of different adhesions, which are commonly classified as those causing mannose-sensitive and those causing mannose-resistant hemagglutination. Mannose-sensitive adhesion, as measured by agglutination of mannan-containing yeast cells and adhesion to human buccal cells, was reported to be significantly reduced after growth in sub-MICs of aminoglycosides and tetracycline, but not chloramphenicol.

We measured the binding of radiolabeled bacteria to monolayers of the human epithelioid tissue-culture cell line, Intestine 407. The specific adhesion of one *E. coli* strain (SS142) was found to be inhibited after growth in sub-MICs of trimethoprim-sulfametrole, tetracycline, or clindamycin, but not streptomycin, chloramphenicol, or a number of beta-lactam antibiotics. Inhibition of adhesion was paralleled by a loss of bacterial piliation. In contrast, adhesion of filamentous *E. coli* obtained by growth in sub-MIC of nalidixic acid was increased. When adhesion of a larger number of different *E. coli* strains was tested after growth in sub-MICs of these antibiotics, we found that trimethoprim-sulfametrole caused the most consistent decrease of adhesion, followed by streptomycin, tetracycline, and chloramphenicol, whereas clindamycin was less effective.

Although adhesion of gram-negative bacteria appears to be mediated by species- and even strain-specific factors, it can be concluded that, at least in *E. coli*, antibiotics affecting protein synthesis are in general effective in inhibiting adhesion. The effects of beta-lactam antibiotics remain unclear due to the morphological changes they produce. The effect of protein synthesis inhibitors may be due to the selective inhibition of the synthesis of protein adhesion factors.

Treatment of Urinary Infections with 10 mg of Ampicillin per Day

S. Ben Redjeb, A. Slim, A. Horchani, S. Zmerli, A. Boujnah, V. Lorian

This study encompassed 38 patients with various urinary infections. All patients had over 10^5 *E. coli* per ml in two consecutive urinary specimens. The patients were alternatively included either in the group receiving ampicillin or in the control group. Each of the patients in the treatment group received 10 mg of ampicillin per day. The ampicillin was dissolved in water and was given with a large glass of water in the morning, after lunch, and before dinner. The control group received just the glass of water. All patients, treated as well as controls, were given a total of 2 liters of liquid per day. During the first 3 days and on day 7 from the beginning of the investigation, all patients were monitored for the number of organisms in the urine, the presence of filaments, the number of leukocytes in the urine, the concentration of ampicillin in the urine for those receiving the drug, and finally the total urine output.

Those patients who, on day 3 or earlier as well as on day 7, had a urinary colony-forming unit (CFU) count of *E. coli* below 10,000/ml and a leukocyte count lower than 10^4/ml were classified as "cured." Of the 20 patients receiving 10 mg of ampicillin per day and 2 liters of liquids, 16 were cured; of the 18 patients receiving only 2 liters of liquids, none was cured.

There were twice the number of females as males in the study, and the group receiving ampicillin had a slightly higher proportion of females. The clinical types of urinary infections in both groups were about the same. Cystitis represented about one-half. The other half consisted of complicated cystitis due to operated or nonoperated lithiasis and one tumor compressing the ureter. The MICs for isolated *E. coli* ranged between 1 and 4 μg/ml; most were 4 μg of ampicillin per ml. The concentrations of ampicillin in the urine were between 5 and 0.5 μg/ml and ranged between 1/8 of the MIC and the MIC. The majority were between 1/5 and 1/2 of the MIC of the respective *E. coli* of each patient. After 24 h, 8 of the 20 patients receiving ampicillin showed a CFU count lower than 10^5. On days 2 and 3, as well as on day 7 after the beginning of treatment, 16 treated cases showed CFU counts below 10^4. In contrast, the control patients not receiving the drug showed practically no changes in the number of organisms in the urine. Filaments 10 to 25 μm long were observed on eight occasions in the urine sediment during the first day of administration of ampicillin. The decrease in the number of *E. coli* in the urine in the ampicillin group is paralleled by the decrease in the number of leukocytes which, on day 3 of treatment as well as on day 7, showed practically normal figures. The control group showed no change in the numbers of leukocytes in the urine.

Sub-MICs of ampicillin as low as 1/8 of the MIC were shown to produce a 1-log decrease in the bacterial population exposed in vitro. This concentration was called the MAC. All urines contained ampicillin at the MAC, and it is likely that this was one reason for cure. Filaments were observed in the urine of nine patients. Filaments were shown not to adhere to the urinary endothelium, and this fact is likely to be the second reason for the therapeutic success. These results proved that sub-MICs of antibiotics at the site of infection can be therapeutic. Low dosage of antibacterial agents in the treatment of infection should, therefore, be considered as one form of therapy for bacterial urinary infections.

Expression of Virulence Factors of Bacteria Grown with Sub-MICs of Antibiotics

C. G. Gemmell

Some pathogenic bacteria produce disease by the elaboration of exotoxins. Alteration in the bacterium's ability to express these virulence factors in the presence of antibiotics is reviewed. Clindamycin, in contrast to chloramphenicol and erythromycin, impaired the ability of toxinogenic strains of *Staphylococcus aureus* to elaborate coagulase, alpha- and delta-hemolysin, heat-stable DNase, and epidermolytic toxin. Fucidin, which acts at a different locus in the ribosomal biosynthesis of proteins, inhibited only the production of certain of these toxins and enzymes. Chloramphenicol and erythromycin did not affect toxinogenesis at any sub-MIC level. It is postulated that clindamycin specifically acts on membrane-associated ribosomes by interfering with the biosynthesis and secretion of the toxins into the periplasmic space of the bacterial cell. Subsequent treatment of such antibiotic-altered cells with polymyxin, known to affect membrane permeability, caused the late release of the nuclease but not of the other toxins.

Experimental infections with *S. aureus* in mice have been used to estimate the production of various toxins intraperitoneally and subcutaneously; alpha-hemolysin and DNase can be readily detected in such infections. However, when mice are challenged with clindamycin-grown staphylococci, little or none of these toxins is produced. Thus, it appears that antibiotic therapy could alter the toxinogenicity of *S. aureus* both in vitro and in vivo without altering the growth characteristics of the organism. Similar experiments have also been conducted with *Streptococcus pyogenes* with similar results. Expression of streptolysins O and S, DNase, and hyaluronidase were altered by the presence of sub-MIC levels of clindamycin.

Sublethal concentrations of ampicillin and vancomycin have been shown to induce beta-hemolysis in certain strains of *S. aureus* and *Streptococcus pneumoniae* detectable on sheep blood agar. The identity of the toxin (hemolysin) responsible has not yet been made. Penicillinase production by *S. aureus* can either be enhanced or inhibited by growth in the presence of antibiotics.

There is conflicting experimental evidence for the effects of antibiotics on toxin production in the anaerobic clostridia. For example, clindamycin can inhibit the production of the alpha-hemolysin (phospholipase C) of *Clostridium perfringens* completely in vitro. However, with regard to the cytotoxin produced by *Clostridium difficile*, now associated with pseudomembranous (or antibiotic associated) colitis, the ability of some strains to elaborate this toxin in vitro is impaired by clindamycin, whereas in others its production is stimulated 100-fold. Enterotoxin production by *Vibrio cholerae* and *E. coli* is stimulated by growth in the presence of lincomycin. The mechanism involved is thought to be based upon an action of the antibiotic on the synthesis of a repressor protein controlling the gene responsible for enterotoxin production. Failure of the cells to elaborate sufficient amounts of this repressor results in the uncontrolled synthesis of the enterotoxin. Streptomycin was shown to impair hemolytic activity of *E. coli* at concentrations which failed to significantly affect growth rate.

Protease activity of *Pseudomonas aeruginosa* is partially responsible for lesions in lung tissue in pseudomonal pneumonia. Experiments have shown that tetracycline can inhibit enzyme production in vitro without impairing growth. Chloramphenicol and polymyxin were without effect. Lysozyme-release experiments with washed tetracycline-treated cells indicated that the protease enzyme did not accumulate intracellularly but was inhibited at the ribosomal level.

These examples serve to show that toxinogenesis by pathogenic bacteria can be directly influenced by antibiotics, and such an interaction may affect the outcome of treatment of infections in humans.

Binding of Sub-MIC of Beta-Lactam Antibiotics to Penicillin-Binding Proteins of Bacteria

R. Fontana

Beta-lactam antibiotics interfere with bacterial cell physiology and cause alterations at concentrations which do not cause complete inhibition of growth (sub-MICs).

We have analyzed the penicillin-binding protein (PBP) pattern and the peptidoglycan synthesis in cells grown in liquid medium in the presence of benzylpenicillin at sub-MICs that caused morphological alterations. One strain each of *Streptococcus faecalis* ATCC 9790, *S. aureus* A8, and *E. coli* W7 was analyzed. The first alteration caused by benzylpenicillin in *S. faecalis* was elongation. This effect could be observed during the first 2 h of incubation in the presence of 0.01 μg/ml (1/4 of the MIC). Upon further incubation, long chains of irregular-shaped cocci appeared. Electron microscopy showed that the elongated cells contained several incomplete septa, whereas the chains consisted of cells held together by abnormal septa. These findings indicated that sub-MICs blocked or retarded the completion of the septa but did not block either the septum initiation or the peripheral cell wall growth. Below the MIC, the minimum concentration causing alteration morphology, [^{14}C]benzylpenicillin did not bind to PBPs in growing cells, but at concentrations of 0.01 μg/ml (1/4 of the MIC) up to the MIC the antibiotic bound only to one of the six PBPs of *S. faecalis* (PBP 3). Concentrations lower than the MIC did not interfere with peptidoglycan synthesis.

The lowest concentration causing alterations in *S. aureus* was 0.004 μg/ml (1/8 of the MIC). After its exposure to 1/8 of the MIC for 2 h, the cells appeared larger than normal but, contrary to *S. faecalis*, they maintained their spheroidal configuration. Inside most cells, electron microscopy showed a septum which appeared thicker than normal and irregular in shape. After 14 h of incubation the majority of the cells contained many thick septa. These findings suggest that, in contrast to *S. faecalis*, septa of *S. aureus* are both initiated and completed in the presence of sub-MICs of penicillin. Concentrations equal to 1/4 of the MIC did not affect the incorporation of radioactive precursors into peptidoglycan. Penicillin bound to PBP 3 at 1/8 of the MIC and to PBP 1, 2, and 3 at 1/4 and 1/2 of the MIC.

The lowest concentration of benzylpenicillin that affected the morphology of *E. coli* was 3 μg/ml (1/8 the MIC). Furthermore, 1/4 and 1/8 of the MIC did not interfere with peptidoglycan synthesis. Radioactive benzylpenicillin bound to both PBP 4 (not 3) and 7 at 1/4 and 1/8 of the MIC and to PBP 7 alone at lower concentrations which did not affect morphology.

Since penicillin binds to PBPs at concentrations below the MIC, PBPs are targets for penicillin effects not necessarily leading to bacterial death. Such effects can be brought about by partial saturation of only one PBP in both *S. faecalis* and *S. aureus* and of two PBPs in *E. coli*. The bacterial function most sensitive to sub-MIC of penicillin was cell division without the inhibition of peptidoglycan synthesis. For practical purposes, therefore, abnormal morphology alone does not lead to the death of the cell. The morphological responses to sub-MICs observed in the three species suggest different mechanisms for the inhibition of cell divison: inhibition of septum initiation in *E. coli*, inhibition of septum completion in *S. faecalis*, and inhibition of septum lysis in *S. aureus*.

Phagocytosis and Serum Complement Activity on Bacteria Exposed to Antibiotics

B. Atkinson

The bactericidal effects of the immunodefense mechanisms of the normal host against abnormal bacteria appear to vary with the bacterial species (most are serum resistant and only one-half of the *E. coli* species are serum susceptible), antibiotic concentration, time of exposure, and the technique used.

Sub-MICs of rifampin and mecillinam have been shown to convert serum-resistant *E. coli* to a serum-susceptible state. Tetracycline and streptomycin at sub-MICs have been shown to increase bacterial susceptibility to the killing action of serum. Polymyxin B has been shown to accelerate the effect of serum on *Serratia marcescens*.

In our studies, the organisms were grown on filter membranes placed on agar containing ampicillin or mecillinam at sub-MICs before exposure to serum. Filaments or round cells (mecillinam) resulted. Serum-susceptible, moderately susceptible, and serum-resistant *E. coli* as well as *Proteus mirabilis*, *S. marcescens*, and *Klebsiella pneumoniae* were studied. Except for a highly serum-susceptible *E. coli* (K-12), which showed 100% killing of normal as well as antibiotic-exposed organisms, the filaments and round cells showed less susceptibility or equal susceptibility to the organisms grown on drug-free medium. The effect of fresh defibrinated blood on filaments and round cells gave similar results.

Various results have been reported with antibiotic-treated bacilli exposed to human polymorphonuclear cells (PMNs). A 10-min exposure to chloramphenicol (4 × MIC) was shown to render *E. coli* more susceptible to killing by PMNs. Exposure of *P. aeruginosa* to carbenicillin at sub-MICs also enhanced bacterial susceptibility of PMNs. In our studies using five strains each of serum-resistant but phagocytosis-sensitive *P. aeruginosa* and *E. coli* grown with sub-MICs of beta-lactam antibiotics on membranes, three strains showed less susceptibility to the effect of the PMN after 1 and 2 h. The remaining two strains showed equal susceptibility.

Serum produces little effect on staphylococci. Exposure to sub-MICs of nafcillin, penicillin, or vancomycin of staphylococci and streptococci grown in broth has been shown to enhance the killing of PMNs, whereas gentamicin and chloramphenicol at sub-MICs produced no effect. When *S. aureus* is grown on membranes on agar at 1/3 MIC of oxacillin and exposed to PMNs, killing is 25% less in 0.5 h and 1 h, but similar to the control at 2 and 3 h.

Streptococcus pyogenes strains which possess M protein resist phagocytosis by preventing opsonization. Preexposure of the streptococcus to sub-MICs of clindamycin resulted in a greater phagocytosis and killing due to the loss of M protein and consequent opsonization.

Legionellosis: Update on Diagnosis and Therapy

ALBERT BALOWS
Moderator

Center for Infectious Diseases
Centers for Disease Control
Atlanta, Georgia 30333, U.S.A.

WILLIAM B. BAINE
DONATO GRECO

Departments of Internal Medicine and Microbiology
University of Texas Southwestern Medical School
Dallas, Texas 75235, U.S.A.
and
Department of Infectious and Communicable Diseases
Laboratory of Epidemiology and Biostatistics
Istituto Superior di Sanita
Rome, Italy

INGEGERD M. KALLINGS

The National Bacteriological Laboratory
Stockholm, Sweden

CLYDE THORNSBERRY

Center for Infectious Diseases
Centers for Disease Control
Atlanta, Georgia 30333, U.S.A.

PIETER L. MEENHORST

University Hospital
Leiden, The Netherlands

Resume

A. Balows

Seldom has the discovery of a "new" bacterial pathogen and the disease it produces exerted such a pronounced international impact as has the group of bacteria named *Legionella* and the disease legionellosis. Since 1977, when the etiological role of what was then referred to as "Legionnaires' disease bacterium" was established, there has been a tremendous amount of interest in this unusual disease and its etiological agent. From this interest, a considerable amount of data, information, and experience have been generated on an international scale. This symposium was designed specifically to provide an update, with emphasis on the diagnosis and therapy of legionellosis, and at the same time to prevent an overview of new information on the etiological agents, host-parasite interactions, and possible mechanisms of pathogenesis.

Currently, legionellosis is defined as an acute bacterial disease caused by legionellae belonging to *Legionella pneumophila* or one of five other defined species. Two of the species have been further characterized by having antigenically distinct serogroups. Characteristically, legionellosis is a bronchopneumonia which may involve other organs or systems. The incubation period is about 2 to 10 days. A febrile illness without pneumonia or involvement of other systems and a short incubation period of 1 to 3 days has been termed "Pontiac fever" and is caused by *L. pneumophila*.

Epidemiologically, legionellosis has occurred in several outbreaks usually associated with dissemination by water or aerosols from central air conditioning systems; it has been associated with dust from recent excavations and as nosocomial disease. The latter has generally occurred in compromised patients and in some instances has created serious problems because of high morbidity and mortality. Outbreaks of a less severe form of "flulike" illness, involving only the upper respiratory tract, have also occurred. Sporadic cases as well as outbreaks have been reported from the United States, Canada, England, almost all European countries, Israel, Australia, New Zealand, and some African countries. The geographic distribution of cases appears to be linked to the effort exerted in diagnosing previously undiagnosed pneumonia. The seasonal occurrence is primarily in summer and fall and supports the concept of transmission by aerosolization of water from cooling towers and evaporative condensers and by airborne dust from construction areas. Spread by water droplets is another potential mechanism as the organisms can survive in tap water for 1 year or longer and have been found in shower heads and in potable water. Person-to-person spread has not been documented. Middle-aged males are infected more frequently than females, and cigarette smoking and excessive intake of alcohol are recognized risk factors.

The first organism shown to be an etiological agent of legionellosis was named *Legionella pneumophila*. Subsequently, this species was found to contain at least six antigenically distinct serogroups, and five additional species were found belonging to the same genus: *L. bozemanii, L. micdadei, L. dumoffii, L. gormanii,* and *L. longbeachae*. The five species will infect guinea pigs when injected intraperitoneally, and infected guinea pig tissue can be used to infect embryonated hens' eggs. Growth on agar media has been obtained by using several formulations that contain L-cysteine and ferric iron as two known growth requirements. Adding activated charcoal to the medium enhances growth and reduces the incubation time by 3 or more days; however, activated charcoal is not a growth requirement. The organisms are gram-negative, motile, pleomorphic bacilli that grow from about 25 to 60°C, with the optimum temperature at 35°C with 2.5% CO_2. Primary cultivation of legionellae on cysteine-yeast extract (CYE) agar (with activated charcoal) from clinical specimens does occur, but it may take 7 more days of growth before typical white, ground-glass-appearing colonies appear. The legionellae are catalase positive, gelatinase positive, and usually oxidase negative and are not known to metabolize carbohydrate substrates. Some species fluoresce and all species show marked in vitro susceptibility to erythromycin and rifampin. All species reveal large quantities of branched-chain fatty acids and show gas-liquid chromatography patterns that are usually pathognomonic of the species.

The diagnosis of legionellosis is largely dependent upon laboratory findings. Positive cultures of legionellae have been obtained from respiratory tract secretions, biopsy material, pleural fluid, blood, and autopsy specimens; however, adequate clinical specimens are infrequently obtainable. Consequently, the diagnosis is most often made retrospectively by using serological methods to detect a significant rise in antibody titers. Progress has been made in developing one or more antigen detection assays, but all current attempts lack either sensitivity or specificity. The indirect immunofluorescent-antibody test has been well standardized and has provided the most commonly used diagnostic tool. While paired sera are preferred to provide a basis for demonstrating a fourfold rise in titer to at least 1:128, a standing titer of 1:256 in a single convalescent serum specimen is diagnostically useful in conjunction with clinical findings and history consistent with legionellosis.

All species of *Legionella* when tested in vitro against a variety of antimicrobial agents show varying degrees of susceptibility to all agents tested except vancomycin. However, the most active drug is rifampin, followed by erythromycin. The susceptibility to beta-lactam antibiotics varies with the amount of beta-lactamase produced by the species being tested. *L. micdadei* does not produce beta-lactamase and is most susceptible to cephalosporins; this may provide a therapeutic alternative when the infective species is known.

One of the major problems that require the combined skills of the clinician and the laboratory scientist is management of patients who acquire legionellosis while hospitalized. Nosocomial disease has created an international dilemma that requires an integrated diagnostic, therapeutic, and environmental control program to reduce incidence and fatality rates. Such programs are being developed and evaluated. Total control and prevention will come only with more rapid diagnostic procedures, better understanding of the pathogenesis, effective environmental control, and the development of a vaccine for individuals at greatest risk.

Update on Epidemiology

William B. Baine, Donato Greco

A great deal was known about the epidemiology of infection with *L. pneumophila* before the nature of the etiological agent was even suspected, but we are only beginning to learn about the epidemiology of infections with the other, more recently discovered species of *Legionella*. It is premature to speculate on the extent to which the same concepts will apply to infections with other species of *Legionella*.

Legionellosis was first recognized as an epidemic phenomenon, and other acute, apparently self-limited episodes have been described. Elsewhere, legionellosis, once recognized, has appeared as an endemic problem. Legionellosis is a seasonal disease, at least in the United States and in the United Kingdom. Both outbreaks and sporadic cases have been most common in the summer and early fall.

Cases are now known to have occurred at least as early as 1947, and the first recognized outbreak dates from 1965, over a decade before the historic episode in Philadelphia.

Cases of legionellosis in children have been documented in the United States and Europe, but clinical illness resulting from *Legionella* infection is typically a disease of the middle-aged and elderly. Data from outbreaks and sporadic cases show a consistent tendency for attack rates to be higher in men than in women.

Smokers are at higher risk than nonsmokers. Legionellosis is more closely related to smoking than are clinically similar cases of pneumonia without evidence of *Legionella* infection. Some evidence for alcohol consumption as a risk factor independent of smoking has also been found. Legionellosis is particularly frequent in travelers.

Persons with renal failure, diabetes mellitus, and cancer and those receiving immunosuppressive therapy contribute disproportionately to the incidence of recognized *Legionella* infections in the community. Clusters of legionellosis cases in renal transplantation programs and oncology units have been reported from several countries. In many instances nosocomial acquisition of legionellosis in compromised hosts has been unequivocally demonstrated.

Once the disease had been described and specific diagnostic tests had been developed, indigenous or imported cases of legionellosis were soon recognized in northern and southern Europe, Australia, Israel, and Africa, as well as in North America.

On a smaller scale, outbreaks of legionellosis have repeatedly been linked to certain settings. Transmission of legionellosis in or near hotels has been a recurrent epidemiological theme. From the 1965 outbreak at St. Elizabeth's in Washington, D.C., clusters of cases have been reported in association with hospitals.

Apart from specific types of buildings, the general category of excavation and construction sites is involved in several outbreaks (including some associated with hotels or hospitals) and in many apparently sporadic cases of the disease.

Legionellosis has been repeatedly linked to exposure to heat-exchange devices known as cooling towers and evaporative condensors, and *L. pneumophila* has been isolated from water samples from these devices in several cities during outbreak investigations. It is worth pointing out that recovery of *Legionella* from cooling towers has also occurred in the absence of evidence of cases of infection.

Legionella organisms have also been recovered from other artificially warmed water, including thermal effluents from power plants in Indiana and South Carolina and from soft-water lakes in the latter state in the absence of recognized cases of infection.

L. pneumophila has joined the sparse ranks of those pulmonary pathogens for which the inanimate environment is the source of infection. Freshwater, soil, or both may also be the ultimate reservoir, as well as the proximate source, of *L. pneumophila*. Alternatively, by analogy with leptospirosis, although transmission occurs through contact with the inanimate environment, animals might serve as the reservoir of the etiological agent.

Some support for the hypothesis that the reservoir of this pathogen is freshwater lies in the observation by Tison and colleagues that the blue-green alga *Fischerella* can provide all the carbon and energy sources required for growth of *L. pneumophila*. In addition, Rowbotham has shown that *Legionella* is capable of multiplying within species of the free-living amoebae *Acanthamoeba* and *Naegleria*, which are common inhabitants of soil and freshwater. The work that has been done by Kaufmann and Patton to identify carriers of *Legionella* in wild animals has been negative.

Tobin and colleagues have isolated *L. pneumophila* from showers and other potable water sources in hospitals and hotels in England, and Cordes and colleagues have found the organism in shower heads in three hospitals in the United States. In this country, Mazzotti and Castellani-Pastoris have recovered *L. pneumophila* from a shower head in a hotel room that had been used by a man who later developed *Legionella* pulmonary infection. It has not yet been possible, however, to document an epidemiological association between showering and legionellosis.

The weight of evidence from investigations of outbreaks of legionellosis argues that the principal mode of transmission is by the airborne route, with inhalation of aerosols of contaminated water or dust.

In the Philadelphia outbreak of 1976, consumption of water from the implicated hotel was a significant risk factor. Of course, fountains and faucets, like showers, splash water and could conceivably play a role in transmission through the generation of aerosols instead of by introducing the pathogen to an enteric portal of entry. Of interest is the report that guinea pigs are refractory to infection when fed *Legionella*.

Rare anecdotes raising the possibility of patient-to-physician transmission of infection are difficult to evaluate.

One final possibility is that some legionellosis cases reported relapses of chronic infection, but it is more interesting to think about putative chronic infection with *L. pneumophila* in terms of the role it might play in various chronic inflammatory conditions.

Bacteriology of Legionellosis

A. Balows

Following the discovery of the etiological relationship between *L. pneumophila* and Legionnaires disease by McDade et al. and the subsequent isolation of *L. pneumophila* on agar media by McDade and Weaver, research on this unusual bacterium and closely related isolates was approached both retrospectively and prospectively. Retrospective literature research as well as communication with several of the authors revealed the following important historical scientific incidents.

(i) Organisms now known to belong to the genus *Legionella* were first isolated from human clinical specimens in 1943 by Tatlock, in 1947 by Jackson et al., and in 1959 by Bozeman et al. These investigators, however, were able to isolate the organism only in guinea pigs and in the yolk sac of embryonated hen's eggs. They believed their respective isolates to be rickettsialike organisms, but they were unable to demonstrate an etiological relationship between their isolates and disease in humans.

(ii) Dumoff appears to have been the first person to have isolated *L. pneumophila* by direct inoculation of clinical specimens on commercially prepared enriched chocolate agar plates. He was convinced that this organism was responsible for the patient's pneumonia and pleural effusion (the patient was also compromised with systemic lupus erythematosus), but he was unable to identify the isolate or to clearly establish its pathogenicity. The first of his isolates was ultimately received in the reference laboratories of the Bacteriology Division of the Centers for Disease Control very shortly after McDade and Weaver had successfully cultivated *L. pneumophila* from guinea pig tissue previously infected with human lung tissue from a victim of Legionnaires disease in the Philadelphia outbreak. This sheer coincidence made it possible to identify Dumoff's first isolate as resembling those associated with the Legionnaires disease in Philadelphia.

(iii) The first known environmental isolate was obtained from water samples taken in 1968 from an evaporative condenser of a central air conditioning unit as part of an investigation of a bizarre illness of unknown etiology called Pontiac fever. These water samples were stored at −70°C until 1978, when *L. pneumophila* was isolated using the methods perfected by Orrison et al. and Feeley et al.

These are important historic landmarks in the bacteriological research on legionellosis because they provide much of the insight needed to better understand the organisms, their habitats, growth requirements, and possible modes of transmission in causing disease in humans. Considerable interest in legionellae has developed throughout the world as both the organisms and the disease are being recognized with increasing frequency in a growing number of countries. All of the species isolated from individuals with recognized illness have also been isolated from man's environment and, when carefully investigated, most cases are associated with water- or airborne transmission. The evidence is now rather convincing that legionellosis is not a new disease but only newly recognized and that the legionellae are long-time inhabitants of freshwater and possibly soil.

Currently one genus, *Legionella*, is recognized in the family *Legionellaceae*, and six species within the genus have been identified: *L. pneumophila* (with six serogroups), *L. bozemanii*, *L. micdadei*, *L. dumoffii*, *L. gormanii*, and *L. longbeachae* (with two serogroups). Other possible new species within the genus *Legionella* are currently being studied, and the possibility exists that new genera of the family will also be described. All species are essentially similar morphologically. The cells are bacillary to filamentous and are gram negative. Filamentous forms of up to 20 to 30 μm are common when grown on agar media and occasionally in yolk sacs; bacillary forms of about 2 to 3 μm in length are seen in infected tissue. The width varies between 0.4 and 0.6 μm. Bizarre shapes are seen when the organisms are grown in semisynthetic broth media.

Several medium formulations have been described that can be used successfully to isolate or cultivate legionellae. The three agar media that appear to be used most frequently are CYE or buffered CYE, Mueller-Hinton agar supplemented with 1% powdered hemoglobin and 1% IsoVitaleX, and clear medium (F-G agar) that uses Mueller-Hinton agar supplemented with an iron salt and L-cysteine. Other adaptations, including selective antibotics or selenium salts to stimulate growth, have been used with varying degrees of success. Two essential growth requirements are iron and L-cysteine. Hemoglobin, soluble ferric pyrophosphate, or ferric nitrate has been used to provide the iron, and L-glutathione may be substituted for L-cysteine. Growth in the laboratory occurs best at 35 ± 1°C, but survival (and growth?) in a freshwater environment has occurred at temperatures as low as 6°C and as high as 63°C (thermally polluted ponds). The pH range for growth on laboratory media is 6.9 ± 1. Carbohydrate utilization has not been observed, and the carbon source is most likely obtained from one or more essential amino acids. After suitable incubation, very small colonies, best observed with a hand lens, are seen after 3 days; after 5 to 7 days the colonies vary in size from 3 to 4 mm in diameter. The colony appearance is not remarkable unless viewed with oblique light at a 10° angle, when a ground-glass appearance is seen. When grown on a clear agar medium such as F-G agar, *L. pneumophila, L. bozemanii*, and *L. dumoffii* will produce a browning of the agar around the areas of heavy growth. On CYE agar, colonies of *L. bozemanii* and *L. dumoffii* give a blue-white fluorescence under long-wave UV light; *L. pneumophila, L. micdadei*, and *L. longbeachae* give a dull yellow fluorescence. All six species are catalase and gelatinase positive; there are species variations with the oxidase test and the ability to produce beta-lactamase. All species are negative for urease production and nitrate reduction; only *L. pneumophila* will hydrolyze hippurate. None of the six species will grow on commonly used blood agar formulations.

Although it should not present a major problem to most laboratories to isolate and presumptively identify those legionellae that have been described, genus and species identification can best be done by using species (and serogroup, where applicable)-specific direct immunofluorescent-antibody conjugates. The use of direct immunofluorescent-antibody species- and serogroup-specific conjugates is usually definitive, but rarely occurring cross-reactions with nonlegionellae have been observed. Another very useful method for genus, and in most cases species, identification of the legionellae is the determination of cellular fatty acids by gas-liquid chromatography. Moss has clearly demonstrated that characteristic long-chain cellular fatty acid profiles exist for each of the six species, although in some instances (*L. pneumophila* versus *L. longbeachae*) it is the relative amounts of the major acids that vary in *L. longbeachae* but are fairly constant in *L. pneumophila*.

Finally, efforts to identify one or more mechanisms of virulence in legionellae have so far not been productive. An endotoxin-like substance has been demonstrated, and production of hemolysin and lymphocytotoxin have been reported. Plasmids have been detected in some but not all species, but no virulence or invasive factors are known to be coded on the plasmids. Wong et al. have demonstrated that legionellae cells maintained in yolk sac will readily penetrate or be engulfed by phagosomes of human embryonic lung monolayer cell culture, and in 2 to 3 days the monolayer is virtually destroyed by the rapidly multiplying legionellae. Agar-maintained cultures (supplemented Mueller-Hinton) seemingly have lost this capability and require a longer incubation on the pulmonary fibroblast cells. After a lag phase of about 10 days, the fibroblast cell line invasion and the destruction by rejuvenated *Legionella* is again a matter of 2 to 3 days.

Our knowledge of the bacteriology of this "new" group of bacteria is in its infancy; as such, it provides an excellent opportunity as well as a stimulating challenge for scientists to use their ingenuity and innovative thinking to further unravel the biology of the legionellae.

Serological Diagnosis of Legionellosis

I. M. Kallings

The majority of reported cases of legionellosis have been diagnosed by serology ever since McDade and co-workers developed the indirect immunofluorescence method for detection of antibodies during their work to solve the Philadelphia outbreak in 1976. Additional methods to detect antibodies against *Legionella* have been described since then, e.g., microagglutination, microhemagglutination, and a micro-enzyme-linked immunosorbent assay (micro-ELISA). Agglutination methods are less sensitive than immunofluorescence and have not found very much use. The micro-ELISA test that has been described was based on a soluble antigen, which was not very well defined. There are works in progress to purify and characterize antigens that can be used in ELISA.

The indirect immunofluorescence assay, which is still the most commonly used method for serodiagnosis of legionellosis, is very reproducible (98%), specific (99%), and sensitive (ca. 99%). It is essential that the anti-human immunoglobulin conjugate used contain all immunoglobulin classes, e.g., IgG, IgM, and IgA. Strains of different serogroups can be mixed to provide a polyvalent antigen suitable for screening procedures.

The criteria for serological diagnosis of legionellosis have been suggested by the Centers for Disease Control (Atlanta, Ga.) to be a ≥4-fold rise in antibody to at least 1/128 for a serologically confirmed diagnosis and to ≥1/256 in a single serum sample for a presumptive diagnosis.

There have been several reports on seroreactivity against *L. pneumophila* and other microorganisms, e.g., *Mycoplasma pneumoniae, Chlamydia psittaci, Bacteroides fragilis, Pseudomonas pseudomallei*, and *Pseudomonas fluorescens*. Some of these cross-reactions can be eliminated by the use of a heat-killed or yolk sac-grown antigen instead of the Formalin-killed antigen that was first described. It can also be eliminated by treating sera with an immunosorbent prepared from *Escherichia coli* O13:K92:H4.

Antibody formation in legionellosis has been said to occur late during the course of the disease. In an outbreak in Västerås, Sweden, with 68 confirmed cases, antibodies at a level of ≥1/

128 were detected on day 7 or earlier in 15 of 47 patients who had their first serum sample drawn within the first week after onset of illness. The geometric mean titer (GMT) exceeded 1/256 on day 11. None of 56 patients from whom paired sera were available showed a titer rise later than 3 weeks after onset of illness (Fig. 1).

After 6 months there was a significant decrease in antibody titer measured with a polyvalent immunoglobulin (IgG), and after 1 year the GMT was close to 1/64 (Fig. 2a). IgM titers measured in 44 patients were similar, except the decline appeared by the third month. The GMT for IgM was 1/20 after 1 year. The deviation was large, however; thus, a titer of 1/1,024 IgM was seen in one patient after 12 months (Fig. 2b). These persisting high titers, although rare, underline the necessity to be careful in the interpretation of antibody levels in single serum samples.

Direct fluorescent-antibody staining used to detect *Legionella* organisms provides a rapid diagnosis. It has a specificity of 100% when compared with culture and 88% when compared with antibody detection. This test can be performed on sputum, transtracheal aspirates, bronchial washings, and tissues. The tissues can be examined also if they have been formalinized or kept frozen.

Radioimmunoassay and ELISA have been adopted to detect soluble *Legionella* antigen in urine. Radioimmunoassay is the more sensitive of the two and it is also a method that gives an early diagnosis.

Clinical and Therapeutic Aspects in Legionellosis

P. L. Meenhorst

Legionellosis is defined as an acute disease caused by all defined *Legionella* species. Pneumonia is the major clinical manifestation of an infection caused by legionellae, and so far all but one of the identified species have been isolated from lungs of patients suffering from pneumonia.

***L. pneumophila* infections: (i) Legionnaires disease.** Infection with *L. pneumophila* may give rise to a pneumonic form of illness

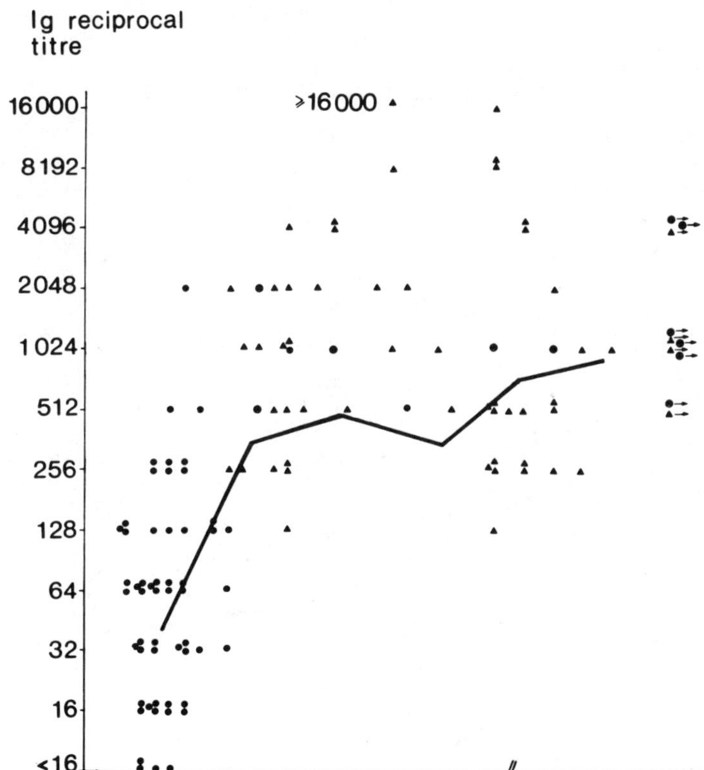

FIG. 1. *GMTs of Legionella antibodies in patients during an outbreak in Västerås, Sweden.*

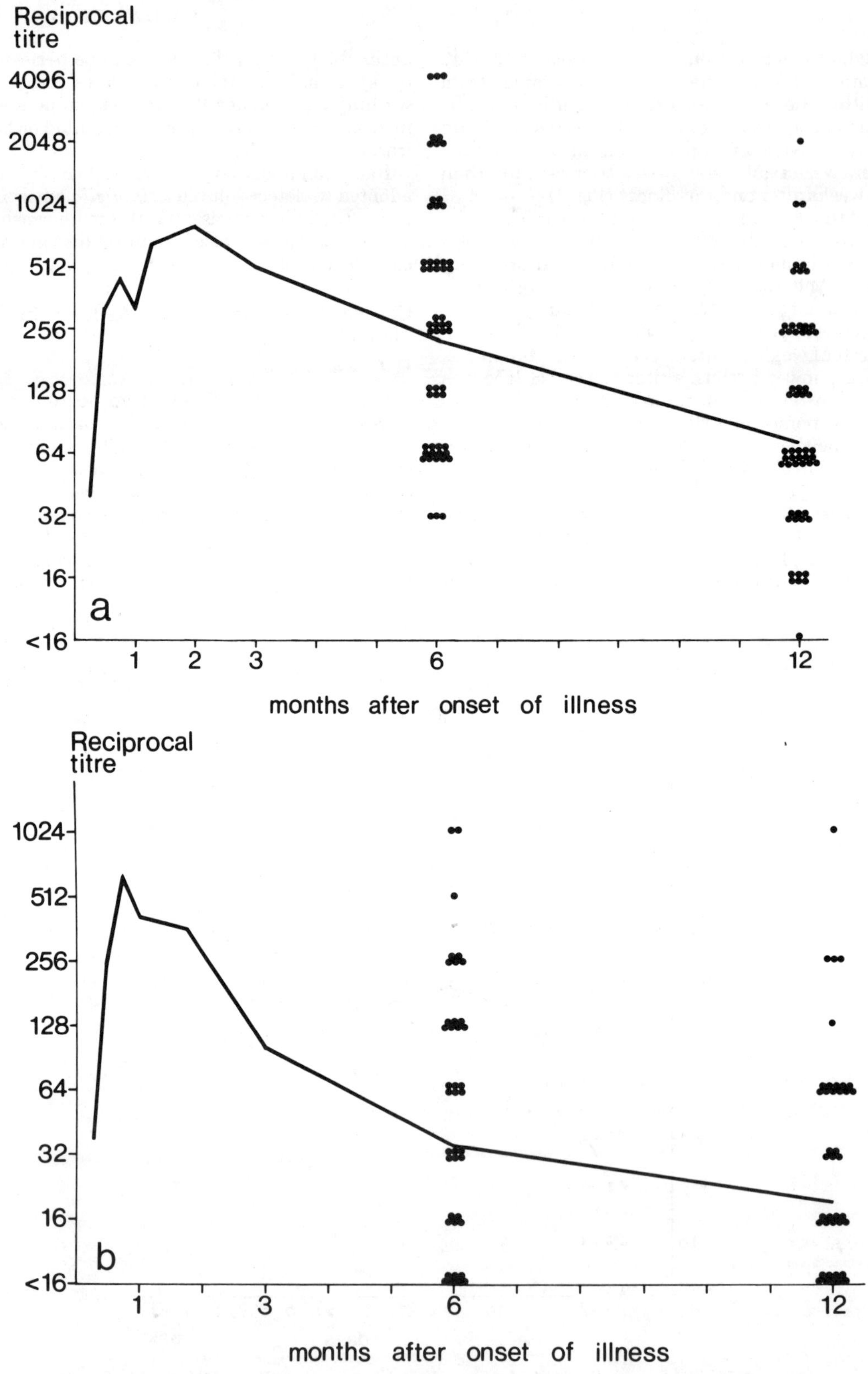

FIG. 2. *GMTs of antibodies against L. pneumophila serogroup 1 by indirect immunofluorescence: (a) polyvalent conjugant; (b) IgM conjugate.*

called Legionnaires disease and a febrile, nonpneumonic form of illness called Pontiac fever. Cases of Legionnaires disease without pneumonia have been identified; therefore, the disease caused by *L. pneumophila*, as well as by the other *Legionella* species, in which pneumonia is a prominent feature, might more appropriately be called *Legionella* pneumonia.

In the typical case, initial symptoms of *Legionella* pneumonia caused by *L. pneumophila* include malaise, anorexia, myalgia, gastrointestinal complaints, and headache, followed within 48 h by a high fever and often preceded by recurrent rigors. During the progression of the disease many organ systems may be involved. Neurological disorders, hepatic dysfunction, cardiac involvement, hematological and immunological disorders, renal failure, and shock are seen. In uncomplicated *Legionella* pneumonia spontaneous resolution of the infection may start on day 8 to 10 of the illness.

(ii) Pontiac fever. In Pontiac fever the major symptoms are myalgia, headache, and fever. The sickness is self-limiting, lasting from 2 to 7 days.

Other *Legionella* species infections. Only a limited number of patients suffering from an infection with the other *Legionella* species have been described. Meanwhile, it seems that the clinical picture caused by these bacteria is not essentially distinct from that of Legionnaires disease. *L. micdadei* has been incriminated as the cause of a febrile, self-limiting nonpneumonic form of illness lasting 3 to 5 days. The major symptoms and signs are fever, a maculopapular eruption limited to the legs, and splenomegaly.

Immunology. It has been shown that *L. pneumophila* behaves as a facultative intracellular microorganism. Thus, it is conceivable that cellular immunity plays a major role in overcoming the infection and the ultimate clearance of *L. pneumophila*. This may be true for the other *Legionella* species as well. Therefore, patients with a defect in cellular immunity due to either underlying disease or the type of antibiotic therapy used may have difficulties in overcoming an infection with legionellae when no effective therapy is given.

Therapy. (i) Pontiac fever and Fort Bragg fever. It is not clear whether specific therapy is indicated for the nonpneumonic forms of *Legionella* infections or whether it will be effective.

(ii) *Legionella* pneumonia. In vitro, legionellae are susceptible to many antimicrobial agents. In vitro, erythromycin and rifampin are the most active drugs against all *Legionella* species, whereas those drugs prevented death of guinea pigs infected intraperitoneally with a lethal dose of *L. pneumophila*.

Rectrospectively collected data on the Philadelphia outbreak of Legionnaires disease showed the lowest case/fatality ratio in patients treated with either oxytetracycline or erythromycin. However, this benefit was not statistically significant.

On the foregoing data, erythromycin has been advocated as the drug of choice in cases of *Legionella* pneumonia and has been used most extensively. However, recovery from *Legionella* pneumonia has been related to therapy with many antimicrobial agents. No controlled clinical trials of antimicrobial agents in *Legionella* pneumonia have been performed. A major disadvantage in studying the effect of various antimicrobial agents on the clinical course of community-acquired cases of *Legionella* pneumonia is the delay between onset of symptoms and treatment in hospital. It may well be that, in view of the natural course of the disease, clinical improvement has been often unjustifiedly ascribed to the antimicrobial agents given.

However, particularly in nosocomial cases of *Legionella* pneumonia, in which the majority of patients are immunosuppressed, a striking beneficial influence of erythromycin therapy on the clinical course and on the case/fatality ratio has been shown by Kirby et al. and by others.

On the other hand, culture-proven treatment failures of erythromycin therapy have been documented. We have experienced a failure of combined therapy with intravenous (i.v.) erythromycin and i.v. rifampin in a previously healthy patient with *Legionella* pneumonia. Combined therapy was given for 6 days and i.v. erythromycin alone was given for another 7 days. *L. pneumophila* was isolated from the sputum before treatment and from the lungs at autopsy. The isolates were highly susceptible in vitro to erythromycin and rifampin.

In contrast to rifampin, not much is known about the capacity of most antimicrobial agents which show in vitro activity against legionellae to penetrate phagocytic cells and their intracellular activity. Even when bactericidal concentrations of antimicrobial agents for legionellae may be attained in the lungs, it is conceivable that eradication of legionellae can only be obtained when host defense mechanisms contribute to the clearance of legionellae. On the one hand, in two patients with impaired cellular immunity due to end-stage Hodgkin's disease, we observed that prolonged treatment (>3 weeks) with erythromycin failed to eradicate *L. pneumophila*, and, on the other hand, we observed successful treatment with erythromycin in combination with tobramycin or cefamandole in four severely granulocytopenic (granulocytes, $<500/mm^3$) patients due to acute leukemia, with *Legionella* pneumonia caused by *L. pneumophila*. Another patient was treated from the onset with erythromycin (four daily doses of 500 mg i.v.) alone for 7 days and was maintained on oral therapy (in view of a persistent granulocytopenia) for another 52 days. The patient died of causes unrelated to *Legionella* pneumonia. At autopsy, 59 days after the onset of the *Legionella* pneumonia, *L. pneumophila* could not be demonstrated in the lungs by direct fluorescent antibody or by culture.

In view of our experience and that of others, the addition of rifampin to erythromycin early in the disease in immunosuppressed patients, particularly those with impaired cellular immunity, and in critically ill patients is beneficial. These antibiotics should be given parenterally: erythromycin, four daily doses of 1 g i.v., and rifampin, two daily doses of 600 mg i.v. Treatment should be continued for at least 3 weeks, because a shorter therapy may result in a relapse in some cases. Oral treatment can be started when clinical improvement has been achieved with parenteral therapy. In a more benign case of *Legionella* pneumonia, oral therapy with erythromycin, four daily doses of 500 mg to 1 g, may be considered.

The role of the tetracyclines in the treatment of *Legionella* pneumonia remains unclear. Clinical improvement has been ascribed to oxytetracycline and doxycycline.

In Vitro Susceptibility of *Legionella* Species to Antimicrobial Agents

Clyde Thornsberry, Linda Kirven McDougal

Legionnaires disease, first described in 1977, is generally an atypical pneumonia with acute febrile illness. Patients generally failed to respond to treatment with the beta-lactam compounds often used in the therapy of pneumonias. The infection was shown to be caused by a bacterium that had not been previously described and which was subsequently named *L. pneumophila.* Since the isolation and classification of *L. pneumophila* as the etiological agent of Legionnaires disease, four additional new species of bacteria, phenotypically similar to *L. pneumophila,* have also been implicated as causative agents of human pneumonia. These newly recognized bacterial species are *L. micdadei, L. bozemanii, L. dumoffii,* and *L. longbeachae.* A fifth new bacterial species with similar phenotypic characteristics, *L. gormanii,* was isolated from the environment and has been serologically, although not culturally, implicated in human pneumonia.

Erythromycin was demonstrated to be efficacious for therapy of Legionnaires disease, and the prognosis was improved with prompt and adequate therapy. In vitro susceptibility data also showed that these organisms were susceptible to erythromycin, with MICs of 0.12 μg/ml. Therefore, erythromycin was recommended as the drug of choice for therapy of these infections. Successful therapy has been achieved with other drugs, e.g., doxycycline, but experience with these drugs is limited. Commonly used beta-lactam antibiotics, particularly cephalosporins, have not been efficacious in treating Legionnaires disease. This lack of effectiveness is due, in part, to the production of a beta-lactamase by most species of *Legionella* and also, in part, to the intracellular nature of this pathogen. The necessity of obtaining intracellular levels of drug may also contribute to the less than optimal results with drugs such as aminoglycosides, which have low MICs.

The purpose of this paper is to review the in vitro antimicrobial susceptibility of earlier isolates of *L. pneumophila* and to report the susceptibility data for recent isolates of *L. pneumophila* and newly recognized *Legionella* species. Isolates were obtained from various geographic areas in the United States and include both clinical and environmental strains. The six recognized *Legionella* species and the representative strains that were tested are as follows: *L. pneumophila*, 6 serogroups; *L. bozemanii* WIGA, MI 15, and Arizona 1; *L. gormanii* LS 13; *L. dumoffii* Tex K-L and NY 23; *L. micdadei* Tatlock, PPA, California 1, and Virginia 1; and *L. longbeachae* LB 4, LA 24, Atlanta 0963, Concord 051, and Tucker 377.

We first reported the in vitro susceptibility of *L. pneumophila* tested on Mueller-Hinton agar supplemented with 1% hemoglobin and 1% IsoVitaleX, the first artificial medium on which the bacterium was grown. Subsequently, we reported susceptibility tests performed by microdilution with Feeley-Gorman iron broth. These media were not entirely satisfactory, in that high inocula were required to produce growth, multiple passages of strains were necessary after isolation on media which did not optimally support their growth, and some *L. pneumophila* strains grew inconsistently on these media. In addition, isolates of the newer species, *L. micdadei,* could not be grown on Mueller-Hinton agar supplemented as above or Feeley-Gorman agar. The best artificial medium developed to date for isolating *Legionella* is CYE agar. CYE medium is not an ideal susceptibility testing medium because of apparent inactivation of some antimicrobials, but it is the only medium currently available which readily supports the primary growth of all recognized species of *Legionella.* Susceptibility tests were done by the agar dilution method with a Steers replicator.

TABLE 1. *Geometric mean MICs (micrograms per milliliter) for six Legionella species*

Drug	*L. pneumophila*	*L. bozemanii*	*L. dumoffii*	*L. micdadei*	*L. gormanii*	*L. longbeachae*
Cephalothin	16.0	4.0	24.0	1.0	8.0	32.0
Cefoperazone	12.0	≤0.12	8.0	≤0.12	1.0	2.0
Cefotaxime	1.0	0.25	4.0	≤0.12	0.25	1.0
Moxalactam	6.0	0.5	1.0	≤0.12	≤0.12	0.75
Penicillin	4.0	1.0	8.0	≤0.12	8.0	6.0
Cefoxitin	0.38	0.38	0.5	0.12	0.5	
Erythromycin	0.12	0.5	0.18	0.75	0.12	0.5
Rifampin	0.03	0.03	0.06	0.03	0.03	0.18
Sulfamethoxazole-trimethoprim	9.5/0.5	1.2/0.06	≤0.6/0.03	9.5/0.5	1.2/0.06	1.2/0.06
Gentamicin	0.75	1.0	0.5	0.5	0.5	1.0
Chloramphenicol	1.0	2.0	2.0	3.0	2.0	

The inoculum was 24-h growth from CYE agar suspended in sterile distilled water and diluted to contain approximately 3×10^8 colony-forming units/ml (McFarland no. 1).

The susceptibility results for six species of *Legionella*, tested against 11 different antimicrobial agents, are shown in Table 1. The most active drug for all species was rifampin, although *L. longbeachae* was less susceptible than the other species. All species were susceptible to erythromycin, but *L. pneumophila* was more susceptible to erythromycin than the other species.

Although all species appear susceptible to the sulfamethoxazole-trimethoprim combination, there was a distinct division between species, due primarily to the activity of trimethoprim. In a separate study to determine whether identification of *Legionella* to the species level would be aided by disk diffusion tests, we observed large zones of inhibition when 5-μg trimethoprim disks were used to test isolates of *L. bozemanii, L. dumoffii, L. gormanii*, and *L. longbeachae*. With isolates of *L. pneumophila* and *L. micdadei*, we observed virtually no zone with the trimethoprim disks.

The susceptibility of *Legionella* species to chloramphenicol varied slightly. Most isolates of *L. pneumophila* had chloramphenicol MICs 1 to 2 dilutions lower than the other species, whose MICs fell in a moderately susceptible range.

All isolates were tested for beta-lactamase production by a chromogenic cephalosporin method. *L. micdadei* was the only recognized species that was beta-lactamase negative. All other species produced varying amounts of beta-lactamase, although, depending on the age of the culture, isolates of *L. bozemanii* varied from a very weak positive reaction to a strong positive. The susceptibility of *Legionella* species to enzyme-susceptible beta-lactam antibiotics varied significantly with the amount of beta-lactamase produced. Cefoxitin was the most active cephalosporin against all species of *Legionella*, including the new third-generation cephalosporins. Several therapeutic failures, however, have been observed with cefoxitin in treating Legionnaires disease.

TABLE 2. *Effect of CYE agar on antimicrobial activity*

Drug	Effect[a] of:				
	pH	Yeast extract	Charcoal	Ferric pyrophosphate	Cysteine
Penicillins	–	>	–	–	–
Erythromycin	<	–	–	–	–
Tetracyclines	>	>	<	≪	–
Aminoglycosides	–	≪	–	–	–
Rifampin	–	–	<	–	–
Sulfamethoxazole-trimethoprim	–	<	–	–	–

[a] –, No effect; <, decreased; >, increased; ≪, greatly decreased.

The MICs of erythromycin, rifampin, gentamicin, and sulfamethoxazole-trimethoprim for the control strains were higher than those reported with conventional media. This was particularly true for tetracycline, doxycycline, and minocycline, and those results are not included in Table 1. The in vitro results, however, showed that doxycycline and minocycline were relatively more active than tetracycline.

To determine the inhibitory effects of specific components, or combination of components, in CYE agar, each ingredient was tested by agar diffusion, separately and in different combinations, against 18 antimicrobial agents with three standard control strains. The results (Table 2) indicate that the yeast extract in CYE agar inhibited the aminoglycosides and sulfamethoxazole-trimethoprim. The charcoal and ferric pyrophosphate were inhibitory for the tetracyclines. The lower pH of CYE medium (6.9) appeared to suppress the activity of erythromycin, whereas the charcoal reduced the activity of rifampin.

In conclusion, all species of *Legionella*, with the exception of *L. micdadei*, produced a beta-lactamase when tested by a chromogenic cephalosporin test but not by the starch-iodine or acidometric techniques. CYE agar provided growth requirements for *Legionella* that gave adequate and consistent growth for susceptibility testing. A valid comparison, thus, could be made of susceptibility profiles among the different species of *Legionella*. Finally, all *Legionella* species were susceptible in vitro to rifampin and erythromycin, the recommended drugs of choice for therapy of Legionnaires disease.

Chemotherapy of Infectious Diarrheal Diseases

K. GYR *Moderator*	*The University Hospital (Kantonsspital Basel)* *CH-4031 Basel, Switzerland*
A. VON GRAEVENITZ	*University of Zurich* *CH-8028 Zurich, Switzerland*
T. H. FLEWETT	*Regional Virus Laboratory* *East Birmingham Hospital* *Birmingham B9 5ST, U.K.*
D. A. SACK	*Baltimore City Hospitals* *Johns Hopkins University* *Baltimore, Maryland 21224, U.S.A.* and *International Centre for Diarrhoeal Disease Research* *Dacca, Bangladesh*
J.-P. BUTZLER	*St. Pierre University Hospital* *B-1000 Brussels, Belgium*
M. H. RICHMOND	*University of Bristol Medical School* *Bristol BS8 1TD, U.K.*
R. FEKETY	*The University of Michigan Medical Center* *Ann Arbor, Michigan 48109, U.S.A.*

Diarrhea: a Global Problem

K. Gyr

Infectious diarrhea is one of the principal causes of illness in the world, children and old people being particularly at risk. Acute viral gastroenteritis is extremely common in industrialized nations, and among illnesses affecting United States families it is second only to the common cold. Diarrheal infections may befall up to 50% of tourists from the United States and Northern Europe travelling to risk areas. Diarrhea is a much more dramatic problem for the Third World. A major study by the World Health Organization covering seven countries in Africa, the Middle East, Asia, and South America showed that, in children aged 0 to 6 years, the monthly rate of diarrhea was as high as 40%. Field investigations in Guatemala, India, and Indonesia revealed that up to the age of 3 years every child suffered from one or two bouts of diarrhea yearly and that these were fatal in 1 to 4% of cases. Taking these data as a basis, it was calculated that, from a population of almost 500,000 children under 5 years of age in Asia, Africa, and Latin America, the morbidity would be about 460,000 cases of diarrhea in 1975. With a fatality of 1 to 4%, this would signify 5,000 to 18,000 deaths due to diarrhea.

The importance of infectious diarrhea has long been misjudged, and it is not until very recently that the World Health Organization launched a worldwide diarrheal disease control program which, besides diagnostic, pathophysiological, and immunological aspects, mainly concentrates on oral rehydration therapy.

Bacterial Diarrheas—Etiological Stratification and Diagnosis

A. von Graevenitz

Excluding viral and parasitological diarrheas, one must nowadays distinguish between members of about 12 bacterial genera causing diarrhea. Individual species include: *Bacillus cereus, Clostridium perfringens, C. difficile, Staphylococcus aureus, Aeromonas* spp., *Plesiomonas shigelloides, Vibrio cholerae* (O-1 and non-agglutinable species), *V. parahaemolyticus, Vibrio* F (EF-6), *Campylobacter fetus* subsp. *jejuni, Escherichia coli* (enterotoxic, enteroinvasive, "enteropathogenic"), *Salmonella* spp., *Shigella* spp., and *Yersinia enterocolitica*. Certain agents have geographical preferences. The mechanisms by which these bacteria cause diarrhea include invasion, production of enterotoxin, and cytotoxicity. Infecting doses are usually larger for the enterotoxin-forming agents, whereas incubation periods are shorter if preformed toxin is ingested.

Culture of stool for *Salmonella* and *Shigella*

only is unsatisfactory today. The diagnostic laboratory needs some epidemiological and nosological information on the patient if it is to proceed correctly in identifying diarrheal agents. Transport media are necessary. The laboratory has to advise the physician whether stool *and* food (the latter possibly quantitatively) should be cultured and has to inform him of the limitations of routine procedures (e.g., in the diagnosis of toxin-forming *E. coli*). For epidemiological purposes, typing may be indicated. Finally, almost each genus listed requires different primary and enrichment media.

A detailed list of epidemiological facts and suggestions for identification of the causative agents were presented.

Viral Diarrhea: Etiology and Prevention

T. H. Flewett

Most acute infectious diarrhea in infancy and childhood appears to be caused by viruses, of which the rotaviruses are by far the most important. The proportion of cases of acute infectious diarrhea caused by rotaviruses varies at different times of the year and in different centers. In England, from 40 to 65% of cases of winter diarrhea in young children have been found to be caused by rotaviruses in different studies. In tropical countries the epidemiology is quite variable. Comparatively few studies have been made of the epidemiology in varying climatic conditions and many more are required.

Other viruses causing acute infection with diarrhea are adenoviruses, coronaviruses, astroviruses, viruses of the Norwalk group, and caliciviruses. In temperate countries the adenoviruses seem to be the next most important after rotaviruses, but in tropical countries coronaviruses may turn out to be much more important than we know at present.

Pathogenesis. All of the diarrhea viruses cause diarrhea by infecting, damaging, and ultimately destroying enterocytes lining the small intestine. An early consequence of virus infection is a change in the membrane permeability of infected cells, and as these cells control the flux of sodium, chloride, glucose, and other electrolytes between the lumen of the bowel and the bloodstream, it can easily be understood how the infection of these cells may precipitate an attack of diarrhea.

Serotypes. At least three, and probably four and perhaps more, serotypes of rotavirus exist. We do not know yet to what extent infection by a serotype would confer subsequent immunity against infection by other serotypes or even against a subsequent infection by the same serotype.

Prevention. It is a general rule that viruses which infect the enterocytes of the human small intestine are extremely reluctant to grow in monolayer tissue cultures. However, this problem has recently been overcome for the rotaviruses. One serotype has been adapted to tissue culture after 11 serial passages through gnotobiotic piglets. More recently, it has been found possible to make recombinants by using an uncultivable human rotavirus and a calf rotavirus which has been adapted to tissue culture, having the antigenic property of the human virus and the growth capacity of the calf virus. The first trials of candidate vaccine viruses in human volunteers have just taken place, but it will be some time before we get to the stage of field trials of live attenuated oral vaccines in children. But there is no guarantee that such vaccines will confer good protection. However, if a live oral virus vaccine does not work, there are other approaches. Techniques now exist for splicing a piece of genetic material from a virus into a bacterial cell, and the bacterial cell will then make the protein specified by that particular piece of nucleic acid. It might be possible to clone in bacterial cells the piece of rotavirus genome which specifies the immunizing protein; if this were put into a strain of *E. coli* which had the capacity for colonizing the small intestine, it might perhaps be immunogenic for rotaviruses.

Pathophysiology of Enterotoxin-Induced Diarrhea and Therapeutic Approaches

D. A. Sack

The pathophysiology of the diarrhea caused by the enterotoxigenic bacterium *V. cholerae* and enterotoxigenic *E. coli* is perhaps better understood than any other of the infectious diarrhea pathogens. Enterotoxigenic diarrhea therefore serves as a model diarrheal disease. Many aspects of bacterial colonization, bacterial genetics, and pathophysiology are understood at a basic level, and this knowledge allows for the development of new therapies aimed at interrupting a particular stage of the disease. The important stages in the development of enterotoxigenic diarrhea include: (i) colonization of the small intestine and association of the bacteria with the mucosa; (ii) release of toxin from the bacteria and its attachment to specific ganglioside receptors on the intestinal cells; (iii) stimulation of cellular enzymes, resulting in an elevation of cyclic nucleotides; (iv) after a lag period, hypersecretion of isotonic small intestinal fluid with subsequent hypovolemia and dehydration; (v) development of an intestinal immune response which clears the organism and neutralizes the toxin. This immune response leads to recovery and protection from subsequent exposure.

Intervention in the pathogenesis of the disease process can occur at several of these stages, and this intervention is the basis for therapy. The first goal of current therapy is rehydration to prevent the complications of dehydration. Rehydration can usually utilize an oral rehydration solution, although some patients who are so dehydrated as to be in shock will require intravenous rehydration. Antibiotics which are active in the intestine, and to which the organism is susceptible, kill the bacteria and stop the production of enterotoxin and thereby shorten the disease. The usual antibiotic is tetracycline; however, other antibiotics may be indicated in certain situations. Antibiotics are not a substitute for rehydration.

Newer therapies which offer promise for control of enterotoxigenic diarrhea in the future include: (i) toxin and colonization factor receptor blockade; (ii) toxin neutralization; (iii) antisecretory agents; and (iv) oral vaccines. Since cholera toxin binds to a specific receptor, GM_1 ganglioside, it may be possible to saturate these binding sites with the binding subunit of cholera toxin (B subunit). B subunit is not physiologically active, but it can competitively inhibit holotoxin from binding to the mucosa. This receptor blockade would have the further advantage of immunizing the intestine, since the B subunit is antigenically similar to the holotoxin and will stimulate a local antitoxic immune response when given orally. The B subunit could be either a nonliving antigen or in the form of a genetically engineered live vaccine strain which produces the antigen in vivo. A similar approach might be used to block the colonization factor receptor with purified colonization factor; however, colonization factor receptor blockade is at present more speculative. Theoretically, the toxin-receptor relationship could also be used to neutralize the toxin before its attachment to the mucosa. Several materials, including nonspecific absorbents, antitoxin, or GM_1 ganglioside, will neutralize toxin. To date, however, clinical studies with these materials have not demonstrated a clinically significant benefit, and this failure is likely due to the close association of the bacteria to the mucosa. There is little chance to neutralize the toxin before it attaches.

The crucial role of the elevation of cyclic nucleotides in enterotoxigenic diarrhea should allow for the development of pharmacological agents which will reverse these biochemical changes and thereby act as antisecretory agents. Several such agents have been found in animal experiments, but to date only chlorpromazine has been tested successfully in humans. Although effective in decreasing purging, this drug has limitations and should be used only in certain situations such as severe cholera. An effective vaccine against enterotoxigenic diarrhea would be especially desirable. Likely a successful vaccine will be an oral vaccine which will combine certain antigens or the virulent bacteria in such a way as to stimulate a local antibody response. Candidate vaccines include both killed antigens and live mutant bacteria.

Diarrhea of a Nonenterotoxic Nature: Clinical and Chemotherapeutic Implications

J.-P. Butzler

There are three cogent reasons to administer antimicrobial agents to patients with gastroenteritis: to abbreviate the clinical course, to shorten the period of excretion of the causative organisms, and to reduce the contact spread of infection within households. The choice of an effective antimicrobial agent is complicated by the emergence of multiresistant bacteria. Therefore, a stool culture should be obtained and antibiotic susceptibility of the enteropathogen should be determined to insure optimal therapy. Antimicrobial agents should not be used routinely for gastroenteritis of unknown etiology.

Salmonella. A distinction must be made between the five clinical syndromes: gastroenteritis, carrier state, bacteremia, enteric fever, and localized suppuration (septic joints, osteomyelitis). In cases of mild gastroenteritis and nontyphoid carriers, antimicrobials are contraindicated, as they may prolong duration of excretion and lead to increase incidence of resistant strains. In patients with nontyphoid *Salmonella* bacteremia, ampicillin or co-trimoxazole should be administered. In enteric fever, ampicillin and amoxicillin are the drugs of choice. They have the disadvantage of being much more expensive than chloramphenicol. At this time the main value of co-trimoxazole is in the treatment of chloramphenicol-resistant strains.

Campylobacter jejuni. Usually the disease starts with fever coupled with a general feeling of weakness, headache, and confusion. This prodromal state lasts for up to 2 days and is followed by nausea and abdominal cramps. These are rapidly followed by diarrhea, which may be profuse, watery, or slimy and foul-smelling. In 50% of cases there is fresh blood in the stools. The clinical features vary from those of a brief insignificant gastroenteritis to an enterocolitis with abdominal pain and bloody diarrhea. In general, *Campylobacter* enteritis has a very good prognosis, and the isolation of *Campylobacter* from the stools does not necessarily require chemotherapy. Indeed, by the time a bacteriological diagnosis is made, it is common to find that the patient is already recovering. *Campylobacter* enteritis can be treated successfully by diet; however, if the abdominal pain is severe or there is the possibility of complications, it is preferable to administer an antimicrobial agent. Erythromycin stearate (500 mg twice a day) for adults or erythromycin ethylsuccinate (40 mg/kg per day) for children are treatment regimens that have been successful. It is preferable to carry out susceptibility tests because cases of erythromycin resistance have been described.

Yersinia enterocolitica. Enterocolitis is the most frequent manifestation, and it occurs especially in the 0- to 5-year age group. The diarrhea may have different appearances: it may be watery, slimy, or, more seldom, bloody. Diarrhea may be the only symptom, but it may also be found in association with fever and abdominal pain. The enterocolitis is usually benign and spontaneous recovery occurs within a short time. There is little information at present to indicate that antibiotics shorten the course of gastroenteritis. However, various authors have had good results with the following antibiotics: tetracyclines, chloramphenicol, and co-trimoxazole. Furazolidone has a good in vitro activity but does not seem to have a good in vivo activity. When treatment is judged to be necessary, we prefer to give co-trimoxazole.

Shigella. Shigellosis appears to be a two-organ disease: a proximal bowel secretory diarrhea and an acute bacterial colitis resulting in dysentery. Sequence of involvement of these organs is paralleled by changes in clinical symptomatology from watery diarrhea to dysentery syndrome, including abdominal cramps, tenesmus, and blood in stools. There are three arguments to consider the use of an antimicrobial: reduction in duration of symptoms; shortening of the period of postinfection carriage; and reduction of the spread of infection within a household. Because of the high incidence of antibiotic resistance, the susceptibility pattern of the strain should be determined before initiating antibiotic treatment. The drug of choice is ampicillin; however, resistance, especially in *S. sonnei*, may limit its utility. In children it is given in a dosage of 100 mg/kg per day for 5 days. In adults the dosage is 2 g/day for 5 days. When isolates are ampicillin resistant, co-trimoxazole is the drug of choice (trimethoprim, 10 mg, and sulfamethoxazole, 50 mg/kg per day) in divided doses for 5 days. In adults a single oral dose of 2.5 g of tetracycline may be an alternative and perhaps the most practical therapy.

Antibiotic-Resistant *Enterobacteriaceae* in Non-Hospital Surroundings

M. H. Richmond

Three main areas are of interest when one considers the incidence of antibiotic-resistant members of the *Enterobacteriaceae* outside hospitals: (i) the human population outside hospital, including people who are well and those who are ill; (ii) the animal and poultry population, most of it having a strong connection with humans via the food chain; and (iii) the environment, where contamination by organisms of human, animal, and poultry origin may be widespread. Of these, the first and last are often in close connection with the human population in hospitals. As far as the first is concerned, humans move in and out of hospitals, whereas with the third, organisms arising in hospitals are steadily and continuously dispatched into the sewage sytem. Whether they thereby cease to be a matter for concern depends greatly on the extent to which the systems achieve adequate containment of the organisms. Many studies over the years have shown that the incidence of antibiotic-resistant members of the *Enterobacteriaceae* in at least some of these areas is high. The human population outside hospitals commonly carries a significant number of resistant enteric bacteria in its collective alimentary tract, and the values found on direct examination of individuals fit reasonably well with the incidence of resistant bacteria in the sewage system. In general, although the proportion of enteric bacteria resistant to antibiotics is much higher in hospitals than outside, in terms of absolute numbers there are many more resistant organisms of this group outside hospitals. Indeed, some estimates put the distribution of resistant bacteria at 95% in favor of the external environment, including humans living outside hospitals.

The one place where resistant members of the *Enterobacteriaceae* are really prevalent outside hospitals is in a limited range of domestic animals and poultry which are being raised by intensive rearing procedures. This is largely because the use of antibiotics for various nontherapeutic uses forms an important part of such procedures—with a consequent powerful selective effect for resistant organisms. Currently, in the United Kingdom, upwards of 50% of *E. coli* isolates made from animals under intensive rearing conditions are resistant to more than one antibiotic, whereas analogous measurements on bacteria isolated from animals and poultry raised by conventional means commonly show an incidence of resistance of less than 5%.

This large reservoir of resistant organisms in farm animals and poultry has often been identified as a serious source of human infection, and legislation has been introduced in many countries to try to limit the human morbidity alleged to arise from animal and poultry sources. In practice, it seems that this source of human disease may well have been overestimated. Certainly zoonotic infections do occur, and on occasion they are serious—even life-threatening. But it is very doubtful that more than a very small proportion of human infections involving members of the *Enterobacteriaceae* have their origin outside humans. Nor is there much need to seek a source of antibiotic use outside humans to account for the incidence of antibiotic resistance in human strains. In the United Kingdom, for example, the use of tetracycline for human therapy seems adequate to account for the incidence of tetracycline resistance among members of the *Enterobacteriaceae* isolated from the human population. It follows from this line of argument that success in reducing the incidence of resistance in bacteria of human relevance is more likely to follow a limitation on the human rather than the veterinary use of antibiotics.

Antibiotic-Induced Diarrhea: Diagnosis and Treatment

R. Fekety

Studies in humans and hamsters have shown that *Clostridium difficile* is the most important cause of antibiotic-associated colitis. One or more toxins produced by the organism are responsible for the disease. When either they or the organism are detected in stools of patients with antibiotic-associated diarrhea, there is a high probability of colitis. Proctosigmoidoscopy is the quickest as well as the most accurate way to establish the diagnosis. The responsible organisms are always very susceptible to vancomycin, which is highly effective in treatment of the disease. Vancomycin is also remarkably free of systemic side effects, since it is not significantly absorbed when given orally. We have treated 30 patients with antibiotic-associated colitis with vancomycin, in a total daily oral dose of either 500 or 2,000 mg. The efficacy of these two regimens is comparable. Intravenous vancomycin is less reliably effective. Alternatively, therapy can be given with oral metronidazole, bacitracin, or cholestyramine. The latter appears to act by binding the toxin. None of these alternatives is superior to vancomycin. Tetracycline or erythromycin may be useful in mild cases, but many isolates of *C. difficile* are resistant to them. About 10% of patients treated with any regimen will relapse. They respond well to retreatment with the same regimen; resistant organisms are not the reason for relapses following vancomycin. Persistence of the organism, possibly in spore form, or reacquisition of the organism may be the mechanism of recurrences. Naturally acquired immunity to the toxin and disease is uncommon, if it occurs at all. Most diarrhea associated with antibiotic use is benign, unassociated with colitis, not treatable with vancomycin, and self-limited when the precipitating antibiotics are discontinued.

Sexually Transmitted Diseases I: Nongonococcal Urethritis

J. D. ORIEL *Moderator*	*Department of Genito-Urinary Medicine University College Hospital, London, U.K.*
G. L. RIDGWAY *Moderator*	*Department of Medical Microbiology University College Hospital, London, U.K.*
P.-A. MÅRDH	*Department of Medical Microbiology University of Lund Lund, Sweden*
K. K. HOLMES	*Department of Medicine University of Washington Seattle, Washington 98114, U.S.A.*
L. WESTRÖM	*Department of Obstetrics and Gynaecology University of Lund Lund, Sweden*
M. O. BEEM	*Department of Pediatrics University of Chicago Chicago, Illinois 60637, U.S.A.*
W. M. McCORMACK	*Diagnostic Laboratories Department of Public Health Jamaica Plain, Massachusetts 02130, U.S.A.*
J. SCHACHTER	*Hooper Foundation University of California San Francisco, California 94143, U.S.A.*
W. R. FAIR	*Department of Surgery Washington University St. Louis, Missouri 63110, U.S.A.*

Etiology of NGU

Per-Anders Mårdh

Nongonococcal urethritis (NGU), earlier called nonspecific urethritis by some, appears to be increasing, judging by information from the few countries where an official register of cases of NGU is kept. One of the controversies surrounding this condition stems from differences of opinion as to which criteria are used to confirm the diagnosis and to differentiate NGU from posterior urethritis, which is one manifestation of nonbacterial prostatitis.

Chlamydia trachomatis seems to be one of the most important etiological agents of NGU. This organism occurs in roughly one-fourth of all cases of gonorrhea, one-half of all cases of NGU, and three-fourths of all cases of postgonococcal urethritis. The latter condition is NGU occurring after the treatment of gonorrhea with beta-lactam antibiotics. The etiology in approximately one-half of all cases of NGU remains unknown.

Ureaplasma urealyticum is claimed by certain workers to be the cause of a large proportion of cases of NGU, whereas others are still far from convinced. In a small proportion of NGU cases, herpesvirus (which can be difficult to diagnose when the lesion is located in the anterior urethra), *Trichomonas vaginalis*, and *Staphylococcus saprophyticus* seem to be etiologically involved.

The use of unsuitable sampling, transportation, or isolation techniques and the low sensitivity of established diagnostic methods may lead to failure to diagnose urethritis due to *Neisseria gonorrhoeae* and other specific microorganisms.

Chlamydial Infection in Men

King K. Holmes

The seroepidemiology of chlamydial antibodies in homosexual and heterosexual men indicates that the overall presence of antibody is similar in both groups. The urethral isolation rate of *C. trachomatis* is much higher in the heterosexual group despite a similar prevalence of antibody, which suggests that infection of other sites (e.g., the anorectum) is of greater importance in homosexuals. The presence of *C. trachomatis* in the absence of urethral discharge and dysuria shows that symptomless chlamydial infection of the genital tract can occur in men as well as in women.

The etiology of acute epididymitis is now better understood. In men under the age of 35 years the most likely causative organism is *C. trachomatis*, whereas in older men coliform bacilluria is more likely to be associated with the condition. In one group of men with epididymitis who were studied, *N. gonorrhoeae* was not recovered from any men in either category.

The association of *C. trachomatis* with "nonspecific" proctitis in homosexual men has been studied. Two forms of clinical proctitis are defined: one is associated with LGV (lymphogranuloma venereum) serotypes, and the other is associated with "genital" chlamydial serotypes. The former is associated with granuloma formation, and symptomatically and histologically may closely resemble Crohn's disease or other inflammatory bowel disorder. The latter may be symptomless or associated with a mucoid, mucopurulent or blood-stained discharge. Serology of single serum samples is unhelpful for the diagnosis of infection by non-LGV serotypes, but a late fourfold rise in titer may aid diagnosis. The presence of other bowel pathogens, in particular, *Campylobacter* spp. and *Entamoeba histolytica*, should not be overlooked in this group.

The use of tetracyclines to treat chlamydial epididymitis and proctitis is usually successful.

Chlamydial Infection in Women

Lars Weström

In a defined population of about 14,000 women 15 to 34 years of age registered in Lund, Sweden, the annual incidences per 1,000 women of genital chlamydial and gonococcal infections during 1977 to 1980 were 47.9 and 10.1, respectively. In sexually active women regarded as being at risk of sexually transmitted diseases, the annual incidences of both infections decreased with increasing age of the women.

Asymptomatic chlamydial infection was more common than asymptomatic gonococcal infection and was proportionally more common in the older women.

During the 4 years of the study, a decrease was observed in the annual incidences of both chlamydial and gonococcal infections, especially in the teenage group of women.

The risk of acute salpingitis in women with genital chlamydial infection was the same (11.2%) as that for women with gonorrhea (10.7%). The risk of acute salpingitis in women with genital chlamydial infection decreased with increasing age; in the teenage group it was 19%, but in the age group 30 to 34 years it was 7%.

Chlamydial Infection in Infants

M. O. Beem

Surveys of pregnant women for *C. trachomatis* infection have found prevalence values ranging from 2% to as high as 21%. Among a relatively small number of the infants of infected women identified in these studies who were closely followed for evidence of chlamydial infection after birth, observed transmission rates have ranged from 21 to 70%. Infants with *C. trachomatis* infection yield organisms from three sampling sites: conjunctivae, nasopharynx, and rectum. Either the conjunctivae or the respiratory tract or both may serve as the portal of entry of natally acquired infection. Since conjunctival infection always extends to involve the respiratory tract, the latter site is the one most consistently culture positive in infected infants. Gastrointestinal tract shedding of *C. trachomatis* is uncommon during the first 3 weeks of life, but subsequently it is found in roughly 50% of the infected infants.

The clinical consequences of conjunctival infection are well described. No problems related to gastrointestinal tract infection have yet been identified. In respect to the respiratory tract, two clinical states, asymptomatic infection and a syndrome of afebrile pneumonia, have been firmly linked to chlamydial infection of this site. There is evidence that additional respiratory illnesses, particularly nasopharyngitis, may also result from *C. trachomatis* respiratory infection.

Natally acquired chlamydial infections are usually symptomatic. Of 69 infected infants followed in various prospective studies, 44 (64%) developed conjunctivitis and 15 (22%) developed pneumonia; it seems likely that some of the 15% that escaped these illnesses had less characteristic symptomatology related to chlamydial infection.

The medical impact of these illnesses is significant. Almost all necessitate medical care. Although these infections respond well to systemic antichlamydial therapy, some infants with pneumonia need hospitalization, and occasional deaths from unexpected respiratory arrest have been observed. Additionally, accurate diagnosis and appropriate therapy are often not forthcoming, resulting in long and troublesome courses of illness.

In view of the frequency with which both chlamydial infection and illness occur in infants born of mothers with *C. trachomatis* infection, it seems desirable to prevent the natal transmission of this infection. This objective should be sought through the identification and treatment of infected mothers or prophylactic treatment of their infants or both.

Genital Mycoplasmal Infections

William M. McCormack

Mycoplasma hominis and *U. urealyticum* are common in the lower genital tract. They are acquired primarily through sexual contact. Although *U. urealyticum* is now accepted as a cause of some cases of NGU in men and *M. hominis* causes some cases of pyelonephritis in both men and women, most interest in the genital mycoplasmas has been focused on their role in genital infections in women.

Genital mycoplasmas have been isolated from the blood of about 10% of patients with fever after abortion and delivery. In one recent study utilizing serology, *M. hominis* was associated with 40 to 50% of fevers after vaginal delivery. *M. hominis* also causes some cases of pelvic inflammatory disease.

Several investigators have suggested that *U. urealyticum* might be an important cause of unexplained involuntary infertility. Several small controlled-treatment trials have not supported a causative role for ureaplasmas in infertility. Similarly, the association of infection with the genital mycoplasmas with habitual spontaneous abortion is based on uncontrolled studies in which women who had repeated spontaneous abortions were treated with broad-spectrum antibiotics and delivered normal full-term infants. This area is in need of well-controlled studies.

Pregnant women who are colonized with *U. urealyticum* give birth to infants who weigh significantly less than infants born to women who are not colonized. Colonization with *M. hominis* is also related to birth weight, although the association is less striking. Mycoplasmacidal antibody titer rises to *U. urealyticum* have also been associated with low birth weight. In a controlled treatment study, mycoplasma-colonized pregnant women who received erythromycin had fewer low-birth-weight infants than did women who received placebo.

Laboratory Diagnosis of Chlamydial and Mycoplasma Infections

Julius Schachter

Infections with *C. trachomatis* are best diagnosed by isolation of the agent in tissue culture systems. The most sensitive host system available appears to be cycloheximide-treated McCoy cells. Although chlamydial infections result in characteristic intracytoplasmic inclusions, cytological means of diagnosis are not recommended as a routine procedure because of problems of inadequate sampling and relatively poor sensitivity. Cytology is most useful for acute chlamydial conjunctivitis. Infection with *C. trachomatis* results in an abundant antibody response that is best measured by a microimmunofluorescent technique. Serological procedures, however, are not generally useful in diagnosis because the infections are often chronic and it is difficult to demonstrate rising antibody titers. In addition, there is a very high background prevalence rate of seropositive individuals among the sexually active population, and single-point titers are rarely useful. There is one exception: high levels of IgM antibody *C. trachomatis* found in infants with chlamydial pneumonia may be diagnostic.

Infections with *M. hominis* and *U. urealyticum* are also best diagnosed by isolation of the organism. Here the organisms can be cultured on artificial media and advantage may be taken of their distinct metabolic properties: *M. hominis* will preferentially utilize arginine, whereas *U. urealyticum* will metabolize urea. With appropriate pH indicators, the presence of the organism may be determined by pH change in selective media. Very high carrier rates make it difficult to interpret the significance of positive cultures when simple genital tract cultures are being obtained. Recovery of the organisms from normally sterile areas can be more significant. Serological procedures are available for measuring antibodies to these mycoplasms, but they have limited applications in diagnosis.

In Vitro Evaluation of Antimicrobials in NGU and Related Diseases

Geoffrey L. Ridgway

The susceptibility of *C. trachomatis* to various antimicrobial agents has proved useful in elucidating its microbiological characteristics and providing guidelines for treatment of associated diseases.

Early studies utilizing animal inoculation or embryonated hens' eggs were cumbersome and often provided discrepant results between different workers. Tetracyclines and erythromycin were, however, established to have high activity, whereas the aminoglycosides were shown to have no activity. This allowed, on the one hand, more rational therapy and, on the other hand, improved isolation techniques.

The perfection of cell culture techniques considerably simplified the in vitro study of antimicrobial activity against *C. trachomatis.* It became possible to assign an MIC for individual antimicrobials, and also an MBC, by the use of single- and multiple-passage techniques. The details of the methods used by different workers again vary and have been the subject of some controversy. An example is the timing of the addition of antimicrobials to infected cell cultures. Despite differences in technique, the overall results have been similar. Rifampin is the most active agent known against *C. trachomatis*, although resistance can be readily induced in vitro. The efficacy of tetracyclines and erythromycin is confirmed, and the high activity of newer compounds, for example, rosaramicin, has been demonstrated. The aminoglycosides and spectinomycin are inactive, along with vancomycin, metronidazole, and the more recent cephalosporin derivatives, sulfonamides, and chloramphenicol and its derivative thiamphenicol. These compounds are characterized by a large difference between MIC and MBC when a multiple passage is used. The possibility that they induce latency has been raised, and results of their therapeutic use have often proved disappointing.

The use of cell culture techniques for antimicrobial study allows direct vision by light microscopy of the morphological effect of the antimicrobial on *C. trachomatis*. This phenomenon is well illustrated with the penicillins.

There is now suggestive evidence of a role for *U. urealyticum* in the etiology of NGU. Reports on antimicrobial susceptibility are less well documented. The activity of tetracyclines (including the incidence of resistant forms), erythromycin, and the aminocyclitols is well known, along with the lack of activity of the sulfonamides and penicillin.

It is important to bear in mind that in vitro results give no more than an indication of clinical activity. The final arbiter remains the controlled clinical trial.

Clinical Management of NGU

J. David Oriel

The successful treatment of a sexually transmitted disease requires the elimination of its causal agent(s), the abolition of its symptoms and signs, and therapy for infected sex partners. In the case of NGU, the first of these can be only partially realized since its microbiology is not fully understood, but it is now possible to supplement clinical treatment evaluation by studying its effect on two common causal organisms, *C. trachomatis* and *U. urealyticum*.

The antimicrobials of choice are the tetracyclines. Tetracycline hydrochloride or oxytetracycline (250 to 500 mg every 6 h), minocycline (100 mg twice daily) and doxycycline (200 mg immediately followed by 100 mg once or twice daily) are all effective, but the duration of treatment is important. At least 1 week of therapy should be given, and if compliance is doubtful, 2 weeks is preferable; this has the added advantage of allowing adequate overlap with treatment of the partner. Clinical cure correlates well with the eradication of *C. trachomatis*, but less consistently with the eradication of *U. urealyticum*. When tetracyclines are contraindicated, erythromycin preparations should be given, e.g., erythromycin stearate, 500 mg twice daily for 2 weeks. Rosaramicin gives good results in the treatment of NGU and is effective against urethral chlamydial infections, but many patients develop gastrointestinal side effects.

Investigation of female sex partners is essential; one-third of these women are infected by *C. trachomatis*, and other relevant organisms such as *T. vaginalis* or *N. gonorrhoeae* may be present. Adequate treatment of female partners will reduce the possibility of reinfection of the male and of complications such as salpingitis. After clinical and routine microbiology examination, they should be treated with a full course of a tetracycline, or of erythromycin if they are pregnant or lactating.

Between 10 and 20% of men with NGU who are treated with a tetracycline either show incomplete resolution after therapy or relapse subsequently. In many cases this is due either to poor treatment compliance or to reinfection. In a few, the true cause of the urethritis may prove to be a trichomonal or herpetic infection. In some, however, the causes of treatment failure are obscure. Patients who give negative cultures for *C. trachomatis* and *U. urealyticum* before treatment appear to be particularly unresponsive to therapy. Whether tetracycline-resistant microbes are present in these patients, or whether host factors such as hyperimmune responses are involved, is not clear at present.

Complications of NGU

William R. Fair

The diagnosis of prostatitis is made by segmented lower urinary tract localization studies. The following specimens are collected: VB1, the first voided 10 ml of urine; VB2, the midstream bladder specimen; EPS, the expressed prostatic secretion; and VB3, the postprostatic massage urine specimen. In urethritis, the bacterial VB1 count exceeds the VB3 count, whereas in prostatitis the reverse is the case. By these means, prostatic infection in the presence of bacteriuria may be determined.

There are difficulties in documenting prostatitis due to organisms other than familiar bacteria. There are no quantitative culture data to implicate *C. trachomatis*, and in "nonbacterial" prostatitis there is a lack of the biochemical changes in the EPS which are present in chronic bacterial prostatitis, such as alterations in zinc levels, pH changes, and other markers.

Treatment of chronic prostatitis involves the choice of an appropriate antimicrobial agent with good prostatic penetration (minocycline has been shown to give high levels in prostatic tissue); the advisability of treatment of the patient's sexual partner should be considered in every case.

The etiology of acute epididymitis involves *C. trachomatis*, gram-negative pathogens, and other microorganisms. The symptoms include scrotal swelling pain, fever and malaise, and the signs of a tender indurated epididymis (particularly the globus minor) and a secondary hydrocele. Treatment is by the administration of tetracyclines, erythromycin, or other suitable antimicrobial drugs.

Urethral stricture is now most often due to trauma. Formerly, gonococcal infection was a common cause; NGU seldom leads to stricture formation. Treatment of urethral stricture is by dilation, internal urethrotomy, or open surgery.

Sexually Transmitted Diseases II

WILLIAM M. McCORMACK *Moderator*	*State Laboratory Institute* *Massachusetts Department of Public Health* *Jamaica Plain, Massachusetts 02130, U.S.A.*
JULIUS SCHACHTER *Moderator*	*University of California* *San Francisco, California 94143, U.S.A.*
RICHARD L. SWEET	*Department of Obstetrics and Gynecology* *San Francisco General Hospital* *San Francisco, California 94920, U.S.A.*
MICHAEL F. REIN	*Department of Medicine* *University of Virginia School of Medicine* *Charlottesville, Virginia 22908, U.S.A.*
EMILIANO PANCONESI	*Department of Dermatology* *University of Florence* *Florence, Italy*
J. DAVID ORIEL	*Department of Genito-Urinary Medicine* *University College Hospital* *London, England*
DANIEL C. WILLIAM	*New York, New York 10019, U.S.A.*
ROELAND A. COUTINHO	*Municipal Health Service* *Department of Infectious Diseases* *Amsterdam, The Netherlands*
FRANKLYN N. JUDSON	*Denver Department of Public Health* *Denver, Colorado 80206, U.S.A.*
GEORGE F. GRADY	*State Laboratory Institute* *Massachusetts Department of Public Health* *Jamaica Plain, Massachusetts 02130, U.S.A.*
ROBERTO CEVENINI	*Institute of Microbiology* *Bologna, Italy*

Clinical Epidemiology of Gonococcal Infection

William M. McCormack

The traditional view that infections with *Neisseria gonorrhoeae* are predominantly symptomatic in men and predominantly nonsymptomatic in women has arisen from studies conducted in sexually transmitted disease clinics which, by their nature, examine men with symptoms and women who do not have symptoms. Recent studies have shown that most men and women who are infected with *N. gonorrhoeae* develop symptoms as a result of that infection. These same studies have shown that a minority of patients develop nonsymptomatic gonococcal infection. Since these nonsymptomatically infected men and women are less likely to seek treatment, they have a much longer duration of infection than do their symptomatic counterparts. Nonsymptomatically infected men and women tend to accumulate so that at any given time most of the men and women in the population who are infected with *N. gonorrhoeae* have no symptoms.

Pelvic Inflammatory Disease

Richard L. Sweet

Coincident with the epidemic of sexually transmitted diseases, the incidence of pelvic inflammatory disease has risen sharply in recent years. Pelvic inflammatory disease is a major direct cause of infertility; in addition, it leads to ectopic pregnancies and chronic inflammatory residua requiring surgical intervention. This threat to the future fertility of women is rendered more serious by the difficulty of making a correct diagnosis and the likelihood that faulty diagnosis will result in inadequate treatment. The polymicrobial nature of pelvic inflammatory disease is not yet widely appreciated by clinicians. Pelvic inflammatory disease is caused not only by *N. gonorrhoeae*, but also by *Chlamydia trachomatis*, genital tract mycoplasmas, and mixed bacteria from the endogenous vaginal and cervical flora, especially anaerobes.

Diagnostic criteria include: (i) lower abdominal and pelvic pain; (ii) lower abdominal tenderness; (iii) elevation of erythrocyte sedimentation rate; (iv) adnexal inflammatory mass; and (v) presence of leukocytes and bacteria in the peritoneal fluid. Early diagnosis and prompt treatment appear to be crucial in preventing infertility. There are no data that prospectively evaluate the relative advantages of inpatient versus outpatient management of acute pelvic inflammatory disease. The recommendations of the Centers for Disease Control for outpatient treatment and the results of a multihospital collaborative study using these regimens were discussed at this symposium. Also, criteria for hospitalization and parenteral antibiotic therapy were presented.

Vaginitis

Michael F. Rein

Acute vaginitis encountered in the sexually transmitted disease clinic setting is usually trichomoniasis, vulvovaginal candidiasis, or nonspecific vaginitis.

Trichomoniasis is clearly sexually transmitted. Wet-mount examination misses about 30% of female cases, and diagnosis in men is difficult. Male carriage is usually asymptomatic and often self-limited, possibly by zinc in male genital secretions. *Trichomonas vaginalis* causes some cases of tetracycline-unresponsive nongonococcal urethritis. Systemic therapy is preferred, but organisms resistant to metronidazole are recognized with increasing frequency. Single-dose treatment with 2 g of metronidazole has proven effective in women; simultaneous treatment of male sexual partners is important.

The contribution of sexual transmission to vulvovaginal candidiasis is undefined, but the use of oral contraceptives and antimicrobial agents predisposes to symptomatic disease. Candidial balanitis is reported in up to 10% of male sexual partners. Newer imidazole antifungals seem superior to earlier treatments for vulvovaginal candidiasis, and boric acid powder is cheap and effective therapy. Prevention of recurrence remains a problem and is not improved by simultaneous treatment of a rectal focus.

Nonspecific vaginitis may result from a synergistic infection with *Gardnerella vaginalis* (formerly *Haemophilus vaginalis* or *Corynebacterium vaginale*) and anaerobic bacteria. The anaerobes elaborate diamines responsible for the characteristic fishy odor, and estimation of amine content in discharge may be useful diagnostically. Metronidazole therapy directed at the anaerobes may be therapeutically superior to ampicillin therapy directed at *G. vaginalis*, but this remains controversial.

Treatment of Syphilis

Emiliano Panconesi

Four decades of penicillin treatment of syphilis confirm the absolute priority of this drug in all stages of the disease. Various long-acting repository preparations, particularly benzathine penicillin G, are used in early and late syphilis, and even for prophylactic treatment, with satisfactory results. Treatment schedules, follow-up examinations, and indications for retreatment vary little from author to author and from country to country. Adverse reactions to penicillin, in particular the allergic ones, make alternative treatment with other antibiotics (tetracyclines, erythromycin, etc.) sometimes necessary.

Genital Warts

J. David Oriel

Human papillomaviruses (HPV) have not been propagated in tissue culture, so they cannot be studied by the procedures of classical virology. Recently, DNA hybridization techniques and restriction enzyme analysis have revealed that multiple strains of HPV exist. Analysis of anogenital wart tissue shows the presence of genome sequences related to HPV-1 and HPV-2, but there is at least one viral strain (HPV-7) which is unique to these lesions.

It is now accepted that genital warts are a sexually transmitted disease; other routes of infection are possible, but unusual. An association between maternal warts during pregnancy and the development of vulval warts and laryngeal papillomatosis in infants and young children has been shown. The epidemiology of anal warts in homosexual men is not well understood.

The flat condyloma, visible on colposcopy, is an HPV-containing lesion with a wartlike histology. It is a common condition which in the past may have been mistaken for dysplasia. Flat condylomas may regress spontaneously or develop into condylomata acuminata. A link between these lesions and some cases of cervical carcinoma has been suggested.

The clinical behavior of genital warts is influenced by the presence of normal cell-mediated immunity (hence their enlargement during pregnancy). The reported success of wart vaccines in therapy raises the question of how far conventional therapy with podophyllin or cautery depends on the release of viral antigenic material from the surface of genital warts into the deeper epidermal layers, where it is more likely to provoke an immune reaction.

Hepatitis and Other Sexually Transmitted Diseases in Gay Men and in Lesbians

Daniel C. William

The prevalence of most sexually transmitted diseases is disproportionately increased in gay men and paradoxically decreased in lesbian women. The spectrum of diseases seen in gay men includes a variety of enteric infections including hepatitis A, shigellosis, salmonellosis, *Campylobacter* enteritis, amebiasis, giardiasis, and enterobiasis as well as the more common sexually transmitted diseases. Hepatitis B is endemic in gay male populations. The patterns of sexual behavior are the major factors contributing to this unique epidemiology and pathology. Increased sexual activity explained by the unrestrained cultural expectation of maleness, the functional overlap during sex between the genitourinary and gastrointestinal systems, and anonymous sexual activity are all significant epidemiological components. Because the male genitalia can deeply inoculate many pathogens during intercourse, the risks of disease transmission via sex between men is multiplied.

Undetected asymptomatic carriers of sexually transmitted diseases significantly contribute to additional disease spread. Clinicians caring for sexually active homosexual men encounter several diagnostic obstacles. Identification of these patients is difficult because sexual preference is both inapparent and often actively concealed. Common sexually transmitted diseases may present with unusual manifestations. Syphilis, gonorrhea, herpes, and other sexually transmitted diseases have several syndromes infrequently considered in patients with oral or rectal disease. Still other patients presenting with signs and symptoms of the "new" enteric diseases may escape detection because the differential diagnosis of their symptoms excludes enteric pathogens in the absence of a sexual or an appropriate travel history. A detailed analysis of the epidemiology of hepatitis B underscores many of the characteristics and problems associated with sexual disease transmission within the gay male population.

Epidemiology of Sexually Transmitted Hepatitis B Infections in Heterosexuals

Franklyn N. Judson

An expanding epidemiological literature indicates that hepatitis B virus is maintained in human populations worldwide primarily by person-to-person transmission which occurs during intimate physical contact. Neither the specific types of contact nor their efficiencies in transmitting hepatitis B virus have been determined.

The evidence that hepatitis B virus is transmitted between heterosexuals as a result of sexual contact is indirect and incomplete and depends on definitions. In developed western countries, the highest attack rates for hepatitis B are found in sexually active young adults. Compared with "controls," prevalence rates of hepatitis B surface antigen (HBsAg) or its antibody or both are significantly higher in female prostitutes, in men and women with venereal diseases, and in spouses of patients with hepatitis B. Many investigators have reported chronologically related cases of hepatitis B in sexual partners; a few have prospectively followed susceptible spouse contacts for months and established subsequent attack rates of 18 to 32%. No study has determined what types of sexual contact lead to hepatitis B virus infection or the risk of infection from a single sexual encounter.

Testing of bodily fluids, secretions, and excretions for HBsAg has provided provocative results, not definitive answers. HBsAg is found in highest concentration in blood but also variably appears in saliva, semen, menstrual discharge, vaginal secretions, feces, urine, and tears. Although HBsAg-positive blood transmits infection to humans when given by mouth and injections of HBsAg-positive human saliva will transmit hepatitis B virus to gibbons or chimpanzees, the epidemiological importance of saliva and other secretions and excretions in transmitting hepatitis B virus during sexual contact is as yet unknown.

Hepatitis B Infections Among Male Homosexuals in The Netherlands

Roeland A. Coutinho

There are strong indications that hepatitis B can be transmitted by sexual contact, especially among male homosexuals. In 1980 and 1981, a study was done among 2,968 male homosexuals living in The Netherlands, mainly in Amsterdam. Blood samples were taken and tested for the presence of hepatitis B virus markers. Serological evidence of past or present hepatitis B infection was found in 60% of this group. This is 10 to 20 times higher than among Dutch blood donors of the same age group. From 316 male homosexuals, who initially had no hepatitis B markers, another blood sample was collected 2 to 20 months later. It was found that 36 persons had seroconverted. The annual attack rate of hepatitis B in this group was calculated at 28%.

Strategies for Prevention of Hepatitis B as a Sexually Transmitted Disease

George F. Grady

Hepatitis B can be acquired sexually through contact with two types of infective individuals, asymptomatic chronic HBsAg carriers (some of whom are infective) and acute cases (most of whom are infective). Geographic differences account for log order variations in carrier prevalence, e.g., 5 to 20% in parts of Asia and Africa, 0.5 to 2.0% in Japan, Central America, and Southern Europe, and 0.05 to 0.20% in Northwestern Europe, United States, and Canada. Exceptions to the low carrier rates are common in sexually promiscuous individuals, especially if they are male homosexuals. In these latter groups, acute hepatitis may be recognized more often than in endemic areas, where infection is acquired in childhood and is often asymptomatic. The design of prevention programs must be tailored to accommodate these differences while considering the cost and accessibility of immunization when educational campaigns alone would be insufficient.

Benefit-cost models can be developed to indicate when immunity testing (for susceptibility) would be worthwhile to target immunization campaigns more precisely and thus extend vaccine supplies. In endemic areas, susceptibility testing could be obviated if vaccine were available for all newborns, thus breaking the cycle (for female infants) of later transmission and (for male infants, principally) of hepatoma. By contrast, in areas where hepatitis B is sporadic, benefit-cost considerations may favor postexposure prophylaxis using hepatitis B immune globulin or vaccine or both. Sexually promiscuous individuals, as described above, should be tested routinely for absence of serological markers of present or past infection; vaccination of seronegatives should be pursued aggressively.

Chlamydial Infections in Italy

Roberto Cevenini

This report describes a 3-year study carried out to define the prevalence of genital infection with *C. trachomatis* in Italy. *C. trachomatis* was demonstrated in cell cultures in 96 of 300 (32%) men who had nongonococcal urethritis, whereas no isolations were obtained from 100 healthy volunteers matched for sex and age. All patients with chlamydial nongonococcal urethritis had serum antibody against *C. trachomatis*, with use of a single-antigen indirect immunofluorescence test, whereas only 54% of patients with nonchlamydial nongonococcal urethritis and 30% of healthy volunteers had serum antibody.

C. trachomatis was recovered from only 1 of 106 (0.9%) women seen in an obstetrical clinic for reasons other than genital tract infections. Among women who had glandular ectopia detected by colposcopy, *C. trachomatis* was isolated from 9 of 160 (5.6%). In the latter group of patients there was a significantly higher incidence of histological dysplasia in women who had both glandular ectopia and serum antibody against *C. trachomatis* than in women with glandular ectopia without such antibodies.

A seroepidemiological survey of a healthy population demonstrated the presence of antibody against *C. trachomatis* (detected by the indirect immunofluorescence test) in about 30% of subjects of both sexes.

Sexually Transmitted Infections and Cervical Atypia

Julius Schachter

It has long been known that cervical cancer is associated with several parameters of sexual activity. Risk factors include multiple sexual partners, early age of first coitus, history of venereal disease, multiple births, etc. For many years researchers have attempted to identify a sexually transmitted pathogen which is specifically associated with cervical atypia. Early studies found excess rates of syphilis, gonorrhea, and trichomoniasis among cervical cancer patients. More recently, a considerable body of evidence has linked herpes simplex virus (type 2) with cervical atypia. Seroepidemiological studies have found excess antibody levels among patients compared with controls, and there is other biological evidence, including oncogenesis by other herpesviruses in animals and humans and demonstration of herpes antigens or portions of the genome in transformed cells. One weakness of many of the studies on the association of herpes simplex virus with cervical atypia has been a failure to adequately control for sexual activity or to seek excess rates of other sexually transmitted pathogens. It is clear that herpes simplex virus is not the sole cause of cervical atypia because in some populations many patients have no antibody to this virus. In addition, only a small fraction of those exposed to herpes simplex virus develop atypia, indicating that, if it is a cause of atypia, atypia must be a rare outcome of exposure. A few studies have associated *C. trachomatis*, another sexually transmitted agent, with cervical atypia. If this infection were a cause it would be most important because it is responsive to antimicrobial therapy. The potential for interaction among sexually transmitted pathogens in inducing atypia has not been adequately considered.

New Trends in the Management of Tuberculosis

HELMUT KLEEBERG
Moderator
Tuberculosis Research Institute of the South African Medical Research Council
Pretoria, South Africa

CARLO GRASSI
Moderator
Clinica Tisiologica e Malattie dell'Università di Pavia
Istituto C. Forlanini
Pavia, Italy

ENNO FREERKSEN
Forschungsinstitut Borstel
Borstel, West Germany

MICHELE LUCCHESI
Istituto Policattedra di Tisiologia e Malattie dell'Apparato Respiratorio dell'Università di Roma
Rome, Italy

MASSIMO MATZEU
Istituto Policattedra di Tisiologia e Malattie dell'Apparato Respiratorio dell'Università di Roma
Rome, Italy

THOMAS MOULDING
The Institute for Respiratory and Immune Diseases and
University of Colorado Medical Center
Denver, Colorado 80220, U.S.A.

PIERRE CHAULET
Clinique de Pneumo-Phtisiologie A
Centre Hospitalier et Universitaire de Beni-Messous
Alger, Algeria

RICHARD URBANCZIK
University of Heidelberg
Heidelberg, West Germany
and
Schwarzwald-Sanatorium der BfA
Schömberg, West Germany

EDWARD GATNER
Medical University of Southern Africa
Pretoria, South Africa

RONALD ANDERSON
University of Pretoria
Pretoria, South Africa

Today the trend in tuberculosis (TB) therapy is away from long periods of treatment and towards short-course therapy lasting 6 to 9 months. Most regimens now consist of two phases: an initial, highly intensive phase lasting 2 or 3 months, followed by a continuation phase. Short-course therapy must include rifampin. Combinations of four and five drugs in the initial phase are not uncommon, there is a tendency to lower dosages, and some five or six of the older drugs (viomycin, kanamycin, capreomycin, *p*-aminosalicylic acid, cycloserine, and thiacetazone) are no longer being used. We encounter less toxicity today because we give lower doses and no longer use the more toxic drugs, and we speak of the eradication of TB by means of therapy alone. We now have a greater knowledge of the mechanisms of the various drugs and of their effect on dormant bacilli and on bacilli in the acid environment of cavities. We are moving away from judging by radiographic changes. We now use bacteriological sputum tests to measure the efficacy of drug regimens. In this year of the centenary of the discovery of the TB bacillus, the bacillus is once more in the forefront of our attention. We are closing TB hospitals, stopping the virtual imprisonment in sanatoria, and interfering as little as possible in the patient's life and work. We keep him in a general hospital, or we treat him at a clinic, at home, or at work, and we use intermittent regimens. We have discontinued long follow-up periods. We know of patients' poor compliance with prescribed drug intake, and we try to determine what rate of noncompliance a regimen can tolerate.

But what is new in the management of TB? To my mind it is doing active case finding rather than waiting passively for patients to come forward; keeping in contact with patients after their treatment has been concluded; evaluating treatment effectiveness in routine services; supervising treatment at clinics; planning new clinic infrastructures, such as integrating TB work into general services; controlling clinic personnel and not just trusting them to do a good job; motivating patients, nurses, and laboratory staff continuously; influencing community leaders; administering available funds prudently and not lavishing 70% of them on hospitals or spending huge amounts on one particular expensive drug. The TB doctor can no longer sit in his ward or office. He must apply himself to problems outside the hospital. And what are these problems? In less developed countries the greatest is the delay between gross lung destruction and diagnosis and treatment. On average this delay is 2 months, but in high-prevalence countries it is very often as long as 6 months. We admit to hospital people with grossly cavitated lungs who were working up to the end of the previous week. Incredibly, many of them do not feel unwell, and many do not even look ill, yet all of them have reported too late. Some of the reasons for the delay are lack of diagnostic facilities, fatalism, belief in traditional and herbal medicines, lack of communication between services and people, lack of education, and long distances between villages and clinics. Other major problems are patients' poor compliance with doctors' prescriptions, defaulting, and absconding from hospital or clinic. Again, the basic reasons are lack of understanding and lack of education.

We must generate in individuals and in communities a commitment to initiative and voluntary action. Nurses are generally more willing to enter the field of TB education. It is doctors, who should set an example, with whom the situation is most deplorable. Many of them shrug off the prospect of their own involvement in health education. The communication gap is the greatest constraining factor in the delivery of TB programs. In some areas TB services are neither acceptable nor utilized. Agencies wishing to control TB are faced with the lower classes' complacency and the upper classes' belief that TB has been eliminated. Health has different values and meanings for different people. For the poor the social situation has priority, and we cannot expect the breadwinner, or a mother with children, to remain in hospital for months on end. A good service that does not interfere too much in people's lives attracts them, and the best propaganda is total cure.

Modern clinical trials are done under optimum conditions by enthusiastic and committed doctors using selected, cooperative patients. Defaulters, absconders, and carriers of drug-resistant strains are excluded from these trials. However, it is unrealistic to apply the results of scientifically correct clinical trials to the practical situations in which routine services find themselves. The impressive results of such trials have given rise to a belief in wonder drugs and super-regimens, resulting in some clinicians becoming overconfident. In some countries space-age drug combinations have become available while the service infrastructure remains anchored to the middle ages. At the same time laboratories have often only just discovered the microscope, and patients still believe in cure by witchcraft after 3 months in hospital.

Wallace Fox speaks of three stages in modern investigation. The purely scientific stage is first. In the second stage regimens are tried out under less stringent conditions, but still on a limited scale. In the third stage effectiveness and acceptability are studied in a field campaign.

Once the disease has been diagnosed, we must select the number and kind of drugs to be used. In most countries this selection will be determined by the cost of the drugs. We must then decide whether the treatment is to be given in hospital, at a clinic, at home, or at work. A combination of hospitalization and outpatient treatment is the more usual in South Africa, as it is in most developed countries. There must be control over drug intake and some mechanism to detect adverse reactions. There must also be motivation of patients to prevent absconding and, if possible, laboratory tests to detect drug resistance and followup for 1 or 2 years to detect relapse. Standard 6-month schedules usually contain isoniazid (INH), rifampin, and pyrazinamide, with streptomycin in some countries and ethambutol in others as a fourth drug.

Chemotherapy and Eradication of TB

E. Freerksen

The idea that epidemics come and go in waves is not supported by the history of either TB or leprosy. Eradication is a goal that can be achieved by the complete curing of all carriers of infectious disease. What is important to determine is not the value of each drug but its effective use in an eradication program, and this is not a scientific task but a practical medical one. An eradication program must always fit into the sociological situation of the area for which it is designed. It is wrong to attach importance to the host factor or to so-called resistance and immunity factors. The control of TB demonstrates how these become increasingly irrelevant, at least as regards treatment. Standardization and simplification of practical applications are needed, and scientific findings should be taken into account. TB and leprosy have lost not only their terror for the public, but also their mystery. They are among the best known and most treatable of diseases. Their control programs do not need to await the development of new immunoprotective measures.

All of the anti-TB substances intended for use in humans must be investigated in humans. The best results are obtained by determining serum activity in humans. Eradication's only really useful tool is effective chemotherapy. Hospitalization must be considered a temporary measure. Mycobacterial therapy, or the treatment of TB and leprosy with the same drugs, is possible. The substances suitable for use on leprosy and TB outpatients are rifampin, INH, prothionamide, dapsone, and ethambutol.

In countries with compulsory notification at least 50% of cases are known at the start of any eradication program. These should be treated first, and then the results will encourage other patients to participate, the population will gain confidence in the procedure, and the government will realize that the procedure is successful. At some point an active search for unknown cases must be carried out. Relapses, like drug resistance, are due almost exclusively to deficient treatment. Only relapse control will provide conclusive evidence of the value of the treatment being given. Drugs can be taken daily in the presence of a reliable helper or at home, where a relative can be held responsible, or on the way to or from work. A weekly supply of drugs can be given to very reliable patients. In certain well-defined communities, pastors, social workers, teachers, and police officers can be trusted with the supervision and distribution of drugs. Cured patients also can supervise the intake of drugs.

New Trends in Intermittent Chemotherapy for TB

M. Lucchesi, M. Matzeu

Supported by in vitro and in vivo assays, the study of the intermittent therapy of pulmonary TB has aroused great interest among research workers all over the world for the past 20 years. The reasons are that costs of intermittent therapy are lower, it is easier to organize in less developed countries, and the drugs are better tolerated. Intermittent treatment poses some practical problems, the first of which is the choice of drugs. A combination of two or three drugs given twice a week for a minimum period of 6 months has been successfully used in highly developed countries. The combination was based on the tandem of rifampin and INH, to which is added either ethambutol or pyrazinamide. The less costly combination generally used in Africa and Asia consists of INH, streptomycin, and thiacetazone. The second problem is the question of the usefulness of a starting period of 3 to 4 weeks of continuous therapy. The experience of the Italian team has been that an initial continuous phase is preferable for patients with moderate to extensive lung pathology.

As regards single-drug dosage, it is our experience and that of other authors that high dosages are not necessary. Standard doses are preferable so as to avoid the toxic effects the drugs may have at high doses. An additional result of using intermittent therapy is that, when normal or slightly raised doses are given, there are fewer toxic side effects than with continuous regimens. Rifampin does not conform to this rule, for when it is given intermittently it causes allergic reactions which are sometimes serious, and these manifestations usually occur after the second month of therapy. Owing to this problem, we decided to substitute another drug for rifampin at the beginning of the third month of therapy. The immunological manifestations of rifampin worsen with the lengthening of the intervals between single doses, and they occur most frequently in elderly women. Intermittent therapy has proved to be especially useful and efficient in underdeveloped countries when ambulatory treatment is used. Intermittent therapy is easier to control, better tolerated, and less expensive. In countries with high economic and social levels, such as Italy, intermittent therapy can find useful application in controlled ambulatory treatment and in patients who do not tolerate anti-TB drugs well. Finally, we reported on a large-scale research project carried out by Giobbi in Milan, Italy.

The Supervision of Outpatient Chemotherapy

T. S. Moulding

Compliance with drug regimens remains the major problem in treating TB. Short-term chemotherapy offers only a partial solution. Completely supervised chemotherapy such as twice-weekly INH and streptomycin or three-times-weekly INH and rifampin is one solution, but it is not widely used because of expense to health agencies and inconvenience to patients, especially if they live any significant distance from the clinic. Most patients are treated with self-administered medication with considerable success, but there are many unnecessary failures due to noncompliance.

The medication monitor uses radioactive material and photographic film to record when medication is removed from a dispenser and to identify noncompliant patients. As a method of measuring compliance, it is much more accurate than pill counts or clinic-collected urines and much more practical than home-collected urines. When patients live at great distances from the clinic, the monitor permits the dispensing of several months' supply of medication, making TB treatment more convenient for the patients, while still maintaining a high degree of supervision over drug ingestion.

Among 122 patients taking chemotherapy for

tuberculosis in Denver, Colo., and selected as probably being reliable, 31% took less than 70% of their medication for 1 or more months. Income over $8,000 per year correlated with better medication consumption, but not sufficiently to fully separate reliable from unreliable patients. Nurses and physicians were only partially able to predict patient reliability. Cross-checking 150 urine samples collected on a surprise basis from 58 patients with film records found only two questionable instances where patients may have removed medication from the monitor without ingesting it. Among 13 unselected patients taking anti-TB chemotherapy in Malawi, Africa, 6 patients took less than 53% of their prescribed medication and 7 patients took more than 87%.

These data help to substantiate the thesis that the monitor is the most reasonable way to supervise self-administered treatment and make certain that most, if not all, unreliable patients are identified so they can be given special counselling to improve self-administered treatment or completely supervised treatment, if necessary.

A simple, inexpensive monitor for INH and thiacetazone and a film development system which can be used in the most primitive of conditions has been developed for use in developing countries. A monitor design utilizing digital watch computer chip technology to more accurately and more conveniently record the time of medication removal is being developed for use in technically advanced countries.

Toxicity of Modern TB Chemotherapy Regimens

P. Chaulet

The regimens used in the majority of Third World countries for 12 to 18 months were discussed. Treatment was either with streptomycin, INH, and thiacetazone during the intensive phase followed by INH and thiacetazone during the continuation phase, or the better-tolerated regimen consisting of INH, streptomycin, and ethambutol in the intensive phase followed by ethambutol and INH in the continuation phase. These regimens have a toxicity rate of 1 to 4%, and the rate is lower in regimens containing ethambutol than in those containing thiacetazone. Toxicity, cost, and overall effectiveness should be the main criteria when TB therapy regimens to be used in a national TB program are chosen. The short-course regimens lasting 6 to 9 months are those containing INH, rifampin, and ethambutol in the initial phase followed by INH and rifampin and those containing a combination of streptomycin, rifampin, INH, and pyrazinamide in the initial phase followed by INH and rifampin. The less costly combination consists of an initial phase of streptomycin, rifampin, INH, and pyrazinamide followed by INH and thiacetazone and also an initial regimen of INH, streptomycin, and pyrazinamide followed by twice-weekly streptomycin, INH, and pyrazinamide. The first two are used in industrialized countries and the last two are used in Third World countries. All four of these regimens have a toxicity rate of less than 1%. Temporary or permanent stoppage of drug intake is indicated in cases of cutaneous hypersensitivity, hepatitis, purpura, anemia, and nervous and renal reactions. These adverse reactions are due to either single drugs or combinations of drugs. To avoid the toxic effects of drugs or regimens, it is necessary to prescribe drug dosages according to the weight of a patient and to make a careful examination of each patient before treatment commences so as to detect those at risk of developing adverse reactions and to prescribe more appropriate treatment for them.

Influence of Drug Resistance on Today's Treatment Schedules

R. Urbanczik

Because of the enormous amount of information available, only two items were discussed: some newer thoughts on the mechanism of drug resistance in mycobacteria and the present position of susceptibility determination in the therapy and epidemiology of the disease. To illustrate the amazing complexity of the phenomenon of bactericidal activity and the rate and speed with which this activity is shown, certain laboratory conditions must be considered. The minimal active concentration is the lowest concentration causing decrease in bacterial numbers, the MIC is the lowest concentration preventing visible growth of bacteria, and the MLC or minimal lethal concentration is the lowest concentration causing irreversible decrease in bacterial numbers compared to the initial load.

Previously great importance was attached to the results of pretreatment susceptibility tests. Today a growing body of information seems to indicate, first, that there is at most a slender therapeutic benefit to be derived from adjusting a regimen on the basis of susceptibility tests carried out on pretreatment strains; second, that such tests may prove misleading if the results are not correct; and third, that the patient's compliance with the prescribed regimen may be more important for the overall success rate than the laboratory tests. However, a look at the results of several large short-course therapeutic trials indicates that both failure and relapse rates are higher among persons with initially resistant strains than among patients with susceptible strains. In three British Medical Research Council trials, the failure rates of patients with susceptible strains were between 10 and 14%, but those of patients with resistant strains were between 27 and 71%. Success rates were reduced, particularly in cases with initial INH resistance, wherea streptomycin resistance did not influence the rate of success. However, the addition of rifampin to regimens used in the treatment of initially drug-resistant patients seems to prevent failures and relapses. The question arises as to whether it would be good cost-benefit policy to give rifampin on a large scale for more than 2 months or whether it would be more economical to use simple laboratory tests to detect the initial INH resistance and to treat the selected group accordingly. According to the *World Atlas of Initial Drug Resistance*, three groups may be differentiated: those with low, intermediate, and high levels of initial drug resistance. A great deal of initial drug resistance is, in fact, undisclosed acquired resistance. The incidence of primary resistance in European countries and in the United States is below 5%, resistance to streptomycin being of the same order. True primary resistance may be due in part to the higher "natural" resistance of *Mycobacterium tuberculosis* and *M. africanum*. The blanket use of rifampin without preliminary laboratory tests poses the possible danger of selecting rifampin-resistant strains, particularly in patients with double resistance, for example to INH and streptomycin. It may be necessary to add ethambutol so such patients' regimens since pyrazinamide is a poor companion drug. A simplified standard test for INH susceptibility is advocated.

True acquired resistance rates rank among the best quality control indicators of adequate chemotherapy in a given country or territory. The examples of Venezuela and the German Federal Republic show that effective therapy will result in a declining trend of acquired resistance. Finally, the discontinuance of drug susceptibility testing of strains isolated before treatment is an emergency measure and should not be a desirable target. Standard tests can detect INH susceptibility accurately in relatively simple laboratories. Research on simplified tests for INH susceptibility, with the aim of decreasing the time factor, should be encouraged. Drug susceptibility testing is a must in retreatment cases and in diseases caused by mycobacteria other than *M. tuberculosis*.

Immune Responses and Immunostimulation in TB Therapy

E. M. S. Gatner, R. Anderson

Despite a reasonably extensive literature on cellular and humoral immune responses in TB disease, abnormalities tend to be secondary rather than predisposing to disease. No discrete immune deficiency or failure has been identified that would explain the progression from uninfected to infection with *M. tuberculosis* to TB disease. Investigation of humoral and cell-mediated immune responses in patients with TB has been ardently pursued by a plethora of researchers. Whereas the subject of immune function parameters has been topical for many years, the field of immunostimulation, or immunorestoration, is in its relative infancy and there is a need for these two fields to be condensed in the interest of eliminating TB. The levels of serum immunoglobulins found in TB patients tend to vary with the population under study, but the consensus of opinion is that there is a significant increase in serum IgG and IgA levels with no significant difference in the serum IgM concentrations. The numbers of circulating T-lymphocytes in TB patients have received attention, and there are reports of depressed numbers, normal numbers, and significantly elevated numbers. Several different mechanisms may be involved in the generation of the purified protein derivative-anergic condition in patients with pulmonary TB. The spontaneous recovery of tuberculin allergy in anergic TB patients makes the study of the use of immunostimulants exceedingly difficult. The precise nature of the defect(s) in cell-mediated immunity which leads from infection with *M. tuberculosis* to TB disease remains a mystery. The observation of defective neutrophil and monocyte chemotaxis and deficient purified protein derivative-induced lymphocyte proliferation prompted us to undertake a study of the effects of levamisole on patients with pulmonary TB. Parameters of cell-mediated immunity responded to levamisole stimulation much as expected. The overview of these trials would seem to be that the levamisole effect may be dependent on other powerful components of the antibiotic battery to be fully maintained. We have examined the effect of isoprodian on neutrophil chemotaxis in normal individuals and observed stimulation similar to that obtained with dapsone alone. There is evidence that TB disease occurs in a spectrum analogous to leprosy, and it would seem that if immunostimulants, as adjuncts to standard therapy, are to be of any value in the treatment of TB, they would most likely be applicable in the unreactive TB patients. The range of immunostimulants currently available tends to be indiscriminate in action and, as the target for the immunostimulant in TB disease is largely uncertain, the role of immune stimulants in TB therapy was discussed.

New Penicillins

WILLIAM L. HEWITT
Moderator
Department of Medicine
University of California School of Medicine
Center for the Health Sciences
Los Angeles, California 90024, U.S.A.

STEPHEN C. SCHIMPFF
Moderator
Section of Infection and Microbiological Research
Baltimore Cancer Research Center
Division of Infectious Diseases
University of Maryland School of Medicine
Baltimore, Maryland 21201, U.S.A.

HAROLD GAYA
Departments of Microbiology
National Heart and Chest Hospitals
Brompton Hospital
London SW3 6HP, England

HAROLD C. STANDIFORD
Division of Infectious Diseases
University of Maryland School of Medicine
Section of Infectious Diseases
Baltimore Veterans Administration Medical Center
Baltimore, Maryland 21218, U.S.A.

MARTIN FORBES
International Clinical Research
Lederle Laboratories
Pearl River, New York 10965, U.S.A.

JEAN KLASTERSKY
Institut Jules Bordet
Centre des Tumeurs de l'Université Libre de Bruxelles
1000 Brussels, Belgium

W. MICHAEL SCHELD
Department of Internal Medicine (Infectious Diseases) and Neurosurgery
University of Virginia School of Medicine
Charlottesville, Virginia 22908, U.S.A.

JOHN G. BARTLETT
Division of Infectious Diseases
Johns Hopkins Hospital
Baltimore, Maryland 21205, U.S.A.

DREW J. WINSTON
Division of Infectious Diseases
Department of Medicine
University of California School of Medicine
Center for the Health Sciences
Los Angeles, California 90024, U.S.A.

Susceptibility Studies with the New Penicillins

Harold Gaya

Since the original discovey of penicillin by Fleming and the subsequent isolation of the 6-aminopenicillanic acid nucleus, a multitude of semisynthetic penicillin derivatives have been synthesized. A few of the compounds have found a useful place in antimicrobial therapy, whereas the remainder have fallen by the wayside.

The earliest penicillins, benzylpenicillin and phenoxymethylpenicillin, demonstrate their major activity against gram-positive and -negative cocci but have relatively little effect on the majority of gram-negative bacilli. These penicillins are also inactivated by beta-lactamases. Thus, the aim in the development of the newer penicillins has been to broaden the spectrum of activity to include gram-negative bacilli and to improve beta-lactamase stability. Ampicillin was the first of the "broad-spectrum" penicillins with an activity against many gram-negative bacilli and, although it is inactive against *Pseudomonas aeruginosa* and is destroyed by beta-lactamase, it is still a very useful agent in clinical practice.

Some years later, in 1967, carbenicillin was introduced as the first carboxypenicillin, and this extended the ampicillin spectrum to include activity against *P. aeruginosa*. Although this drug's activity is not great, the high dosages used in clinical practice make it a useful antipseudomonas drug. In 1973, ticarcillin was introduced, with a spectrum of activity essentially similar to that of carbenicillin but approximately twice the antibacterial activity, allowing correspondingly lower doses of the antibiotic to be used.

More recently still, three *N*-acyl derivatives of ampicillin have become available—azlocillin, mezlocillin, and piperacillin.

Azlocillin (Bay 6905) is sodium 6-D-2-(2-oxo-imidazolidine-1-carboxamido)-2-phenyl-acetamido-penicillanate; mezlocillin (Bay 1353) is sodium 6-D-2-3-(methylsulfonyl)-2-oxo-imidazolodine-1-carboxamido-2-phenyl-acetamido-penicillanate; and piperacillin (T-1220) is sodium 6-D(−)-alpha-(4-ethyl-2,3-dioxo-1-piperazinyl-carbonylamino)-alpha-phenylacetimido-penicillanate. They all possess a broad spectrum of antibacterial activity, including potent antipseudomonal activity, which is summarized in Table 1 in comparison to the carboxypenicillins.

They all show good activity against penicillin-susceptible strains of *Staphylococcus aureus*, the various streptococcal species, beta-lactamase-negative *Neisseria gonorrhoeae*, *N. meningitidis*, beta-lactamase-negative *Haemophilus influenzae*, and most anaerobes, including many strains of *Bacteroides fragilis*. The differences between the agents are relatively small and of little clinical importance, especially as none of them would be the agent of first choice for therapy of infections caused by these bacteria.

Of much more interest is their activity against the enteric gram-negative bacilli, which is summarized in greater detail in Table 2. There are major differences in the values published in the literature for each of these compounds. Excluding methodology and inoculum size, it appears that most of the differences can be attributed to epidemiological variations between hospitals which is expressed in the beta-lactamase production of the bacterial strains in each culture collection. For example, ampicillin-resistant *Escherichia coli* and carbenicillin-resistant *P. aeruginosa* tend to be more resistant to the new penicillins than susceptible strains, a consequence of poor beta-lactamase stability (as compared with the newer cephalosporins).

For *E. coli*, piperacillin is about as active as mezlocillin, and these two are somewhat more active than the other three compounds. For *K. pneumoniae* mezlocillin is the most active of the penicillins, followed closely by piperacillin and then azlocillin. Carbenicillin and ticarcillin have

TABLE 1. *Activity of the newer penicillins against the major bacterial groups*

Organism	Activity[a]				
	Carbenicillin	Ticarcillin	Azlocillin	Mezlocillin	Piperacillin
Staphylococcus aureus (β-lac⁻)	+	+	+	+	+
S. aureus (β-lac⁺)	−	−	−	−	−
Streptococcus pyogenes	+	+	+	+	+
S. pneumoniae	+	+	+	+	+
Enterococcus	+	+	+	+	+
Neisseria gonorrhoeae (β-lac⁻)	+	+	+	+	+
N. gonorrhoeae (β-lac⁺)	−	−	−	−	−
N. meningitidis	+	+	+	+	+
Escherichia coli	+	+	+	+	+
Klebsiella	−	−	+	+	+
Proteus (indole −)	+	+	+	+	+
Proteus (indole +)	+	+	+	+	+
Enterobacter	−	−	−	−	−
Serratia marcescens	−	−	+	+	+
Pseudomonas aeruginosa	+	+	+	+	+
Haemophilus influenzae (β-lac⁻)	+	+	+	+	+
H. influenzae (β-lac⁺)	−	−	−	−	−
Bacteroides	+	+	+	+	+
Other anaerobes	+	+	+	+	+

[a] +, >75% of strains susceptible.

TABLE 2. *Representative median MICs (MIC_{50}) and concentrations inhibiting 90% of strains (MIC_{90})*

Organism	MIC_{50} (upper line) and MIC_{90} (lower line) in mg/liter				
	Carbenicillin	Ticarcillin	Azlocillin	Mezlocillin	Piperacillin
Escherichia coli	8 >256	4 >256	64 >256	4 128	2 >256
Klebsiella pneumoniae	>256 >256	>256 >256	32 >256	16 64	32 >256
Proteus mirabilis	0.5 128	0.5 64	4 128	1 64	0.5 64
Proteus spp. (indole +)	2 128	2 128	4 128	1 16	1 32
Enterobacter spp.	128 >256	128 >256	128 >256	16 >256	16 >256
Serratia marcescens	16 >256	8 >256	16 256	4 32	2 32
Pseudomonas aeruginosa	32 256	16 138	4 32	16 64	2 16

no useful activity against most klebsiellas. All the agents are highly active against *Proteus mirabilis*. Mezlocillin and piperacillin are the two most active compounds against indole-positive strains of *Proteus*, *Enterobacter* species, and *Serratia marcescens*. Piperacillin and azlocillin are more active than carbenicillin, ticarcillin, and mezlocillin against *P. aeruginosa*.

An inoculum effect on the MICs of all five compounds can be seen for most of the bacterial species tested. This effect is generally less obvious with non-beta-lactamase-producing strains, an increase in inoculum from 10^5 to 10^7 colony-forming units (CFU)/ml raising the MICs approximately twofold, whereas with beta-lactamase producers the difference may be 16-fold or more. Composition of culture medium and pH do not have large effects on MICs obtained with the new penicillins, although an alkaline pH produces lower values.

In summary, all five compounds, carbenicillin, ticarcillin, azlocillin, mezlocillin, and piperacillin, are highly active broad-spectrum penicillins. The differences between them are relatively minor, other than activity against *Klebsiella* for the new penicillins, when the massive doses possible with penicillins are considered, and they are all relatively unstable in the presence of beta-lactamase.

Pharmacokinetics and Synergy

Harold C. Standiford, Anne-Francoise Viollier, Marcia R. Moody, George L. Drusano

Antibiotics are frequently used in combination to treat patients with severe infections. In addition to providing broad antimicrobial coverage before identification of the infecting organisms, the combinations may produce a synergistic killing effect against specific pathogens. Delay in emergence of resistant strains is an additional potential but unproven benefit from antimicrobial combinations. Ticarcillin, because of its broad spectrum and known synergistic activity with aminoglycosides against *Pseudomonas* spp. and other potential pathogens, has been used frequently in this fashion. This discussion will compare the pharmacokinetic features of these newer broad-spectrum antipseudomonal penicillins, mezlocillin and piperacillin, with ticarcillin when used alone and in combination with the aminoglycoside antibiotic gentamicin. The serum bactericidal activity produced by these newer penicillin derivatives alone and in combination with gentamicin will also be discussed as well as the effects of one of these antipseudomonal penicillins in combination with a "third generation" cephalosporin, cefoperazone.

For serious infections in the compromised host, high doses of ticarcillin are frequently used in combination with an aminoglycoside such as gentamicin. We compared serum levels after 5-g infusions of mezlocillin and piperacillin with ticarcillin by giving the antibiotics alone or in combination with 80 mg of gentamicin to five volunteers in a crossover manner. For ticarcillin, blood levels immediately after this 30-min infusion were 450 μg/ml. Piperacillin achieved almost identical levels, whereas mezlocillin serum concentrations were 350 μg/ml immediately after the infusion. By 1 h, however, levels of ticarcillin were 181 μg/ml compared with 113 μg/ml for piperacillin and mezlocillin. By 6 h serum levels of all three agents were below 10 μg/ml. Mezlocillin and piperacillin fit well into a two-compartment pharmacokinetic mode, whereas ticarcillin fit poorly and could have been modeled in one or two compartments. For comparison, we chose a two-compartment model. There was a rapid distribution phase followed by a slower terminal elimination phase for the three antibiotics. The terminal half-lives of ticarcillin and piperacillin were almost identical at 1.40 h. This was longer than the half-life of mezlocillin, which was 1.12 h.

The volume of the central compartment for ticarcillin was 0.15 liter/kg or 10.5 liters in a 70-kg man. This value is almost identical to that obtained for piperacillin and explains the similarity of blood levels immediately after the 30-min infusion. The mezlocillin central compartment is 25% larger, partially accounting for the lower levels of this antibiotic at this time. The apparent volume of distribution in the body of ticarcillin is 0.21 liter/kg (or 14 liters in a 70-kg man) and compares to approximately 23 liters for mezlocillin and piperacillin. The total body clearance or the amount of blood cleared of the antibiotics per hour is fastest for mezlocillin (13.56 liters/h), intermediate for piperacillin (10.01 liters/h), and slowest for ticarcillin (7.08 liters/h).

Ticarcillin interacts with gentamicin, producing lower serum levels of the aminoglycoside. This reaction may be significant when the two agents are administered in the same container or when renal failure is present, which prolongs the time of contact between the two agents. When gentamicin was administered to the volunteers, levels of this antibiotic were significantly lower when administered with ticarcillin than when administered alone or with mezlocillin or piperacillin at most time periods. Some of this interaction occurred while the antibiotics were in the volunteers. Additionally, however, there was an interaction between the two drugs during the time required for processing the samples and measuring the antibiotics even though this was done in an optimal setting. Although this decrease in gentamicin concentration may have little significance in the clinical situation when renal failure is not present, it emphasizes the importance of the care of specimens once they are obtained from the patient so that significant errors in drug dosing are not made. This problem is minimized with the newer antipseudomonal agents.

The outcome of infections in patients with gram-negative sepsis in the compromised host has been shown to correlate with the degree of bactericidal activity produced in the serum by the antibiotics used for therapy. To compare the degree of bactericidal activity of the newer antipseudomonal penicillins with ticarcillin when administered alone or with gentamicin, we measured their killing effect immediately and 2 h after the antibiotic infusions against six strains each of *S. aureus*, *E. coli*, *Klebsiella*, and *P. aeruginosa*, the most common pathogens infecting cancer patients with granulocytopenia. Serum from the volunteers immediately after receiving ticarcillin failed to kill *Klebsiella*, at a dilution of 1:8, in the majority of the instances and frequently failed to kill *E. coli* and *P. aeruginosa*. Gentamicin alone failed to kill *P. aeruginosa*. The sera from volunteers receiving the ticarcillin-gentamicin combination, however, killed all the organisms including *S. aureus* at a dilution of 1:8 or greater 90% of the time. This high degree of serum bactericidal activity produced by the ticarcillin-gentamicin combination correlates well with the excellent clinical response obtained when this regimen is used for empiric antimicrobial therapy for fever in patients with granulocytopenia. In comparison, 2 h after the injection, serum from volunteers receiving piperacillin alone produced higher mean geometric bactericidal titers than the ticarcillin-gentamicin combination. The piperacillin-gentamicin combination was even more active. Sera from volunteers receiving mezlocillin alone produced a high degree of serum bactericidal activity against most of the organisms but not against *P. aeruginosa*. Gentamicin did not significantly increase the serum bactericidal activity of mezlocillin against this organism.

In our search for potentially less toxic antimicrobial combinations to use for sepsis in the granulocytopenic patient, the combination of mezlocillin and a new third-generation cephalosporin, cefoperazone, was evaluated. This new cephalosporin provides activity against *S. aureus* and also provides potential activity against *P. aeruginosa*. Preliminary in vitro data suggested a beneficial effect of this combination compared with each drug alone when tested against 40 strains of bacteria collected from the Institut Jules Bordet and the Baltimore Cancer Research Center. Three volunteers, therefore, were given 5 g of mezlocillin, 2 g of cefoperazone, and the two antibiotics in combination in a crossover manner. Serum from volunteers receiving the combination of antibiotics was more frequently bactericidal at 1 h after the infusion against *P. aeruginosa* and at 6 h against *E. coli*, *Klebsiella*, and *S. aureus*, suggesting that this combination warrants further preclinical investigation.

The newer antipseudomonal penicillins when compared with ticarcillin are highly active agents. Perhaps it is fair to say in regard to their pharmacokinetics that there are more similarities than there are differences. When they are used in combination with aminoglycosides the newer penicillins, like their predecessor ticarcillin, frequently show beneficial effects both by increasing their spectrum and enhancing their activity against specific bacteria. The high degree of bactericidal activity produced by piperacillin alone was particularly impressive and may permit single-agent therapy even for *Pseudomonas* once the organism is identified. The activity of the mezlocillin-cefoperazone combination appears encouraging as a potentially less toxic combination and deserves further careful preclinical evaluation. We are also currently evaluating the combination of piperacillin plus moxalactam in both preclinical and clinical trials.

Combinations of Beta-Lactam Antibiotics: Antibacterial Effects In Vitro and In Vivo

Martin Forbes, Nydia A. Kuck, Raymond T. Testa

The purposes of therapy with a combination of antibiotics are to provide an expanded spectrum of activity, exert synergistic antibacterial action, and eliminate resistant organisms or prevent their emergence. Many investigators have reported that the combination of aminoglycoside antibiotics with beta-lactam antibiotics shows in vitro synergy against a substantial proportion of gram-negative bacteria. Consequently, the use of aminoglycoside antibiotics in combination with beta-lactams, such as carbenicillin and ticarcillin, has become common practice in the treatment of gram-negative infection among severely ill or compromised patients. The newer penicillins, piperacillin, mezlocillin, and azlocillin, have also shown synergy with aminoglycosides and, if not synergy, at least no interference with the more active component of the combination.

With the development of expanded spectrum beta-lactam antibiotics, interest has focused on combinations of penicillins and cephalosporins. Since these antibiotics complement each other's activity, such combinations would have the advantages of broad-spectrum activity without the inherent potential of the oto- and nephrotoxicity of the aminoglycosides. Synergistic effects of combinations of various penicillins against a number of bacterial species were reported in early studies. More recently, several investigators have reported in vitro synergistic, indifferent or additive, as well as antagonistic effects with penicillin and cephalosporin combinations. The proportion of bacteria associated with the various effects varies with the drug combinations, antibiotic concentration, type of bacteria, and investigator. In general, combinations of cephalosporins and penicillins result in a moderate frequency of synergism.

The frequent reports of antagonism with combinations of beta-lactam antibiotics, however, are noteworthy. Cefoxitin has been shown to antagonize cefuroxime, cephaloridine, cephalothin, cephalexin, cephradine, cefazolin, cefamandole, cefotaxime, cefsulodin, and moxalactam, as well as penicillin, ampicillin, carbenicillin, ticarcillin, piperacillin, azlocillin, and mezlocillin. Antagonism has been reported for cefazolin combined with azlocillin, mezlocillin, or piperacillin, cefamandole combined with mezlocillin or piperacillin, cefotaxime combined with cefuroxime, moxalactam combined with carbenicillin, ticarcillin, or piperacillin, and cephalothin combined with pipercillin.

Of special interest is the frequency of antagonism reported for strains of *Enterobacter*, *Serratia*, indole-positive *Proteus*, and *Pseudomonas* since they are of major concern in the clinic. Our studies show a high rate of antagonism with these genera, particularly with combinations which include cefoxitin. The frequency of antagonism is less for combinations which include cefamandole, cephalothin, or cefotaxime. The antagonism appears to be a one-way interference. The more potent drug in the combination is rendered less effective in the presence of subinhibitory concentrations of the other antibiotic. With other types of bacteria we have observed mainly indifference and some synergy (Table 3).

To assess the clinical relevance of the synergistic and antagonistic effects of the combinations of beta-lactam antibiotics, we have tested them for activity against experimental infections in mice. Our results (Table 4) show that in vitro effects can be predictive of in vivo effects. Combinations of drugs that are synergistic in vitro also show synergism in mice. For example, cefoxitin and piperacillin were synergistic in vitro against *S. aureus*; in the in vivo tests the 50% effective dose of piperacillin for an infection produced by this organism was reduced more than 15-fold when this drug was administered along with a dose of cefoxitin, which by itself afforded no protection. Against infections produced with organisms associated with antagonistic effects, the doses of piperacillin or mezlocillin required for protection were increased when they were administered along with doses of the cephalosporins, which were ineffective when used alone. For example, the 50% effective dose of piperacillin was increased eightfold for the *Pseudomonas* infection when treatment included cefoxitin.

TABLE 3. *Combinations of beta-lactam antibiotics*[a]

Bacteria (10 strains each)	PIP + cefoxitin		PIP + cefamandole		PIP + cefotaxime		PIP + cephalothin		MEZ + cefoxitin		MEZ + cefamandole	
	% Synergy (S) or antagonism (A)											
	S	A	S	A	S	A	S	A	S	A	S	A
Pseudomonas	0	100	0	30	0	0	0	0	0	100	0	0
Serratia	0	100	0	80	10	10	0	90	0	100	0	60
Enterobacter	0	90	0	30	0	0	10	0	0	60	20	10
Proteus (indole +)	0	80	30	30	10	10	0	80	0	70	10	20
Klebsiella	10	0	10	0					10	0	10	0
Escherichia coli	20	0	0	0					10	0	0	0
Enterococcus	80	0	0	0	100	0			20	0	0	0
Staphylococcus	60	0	10	0	20	10			90	0	10	0

[a] PIP, Piperacillin; MEZ, mezlocillin.

TABLE 4. *Interaction of beta-lactam antibiotics: comparison of in vitro and in vivo antibacterial effects*

Organism	β-Lactam antibiotic combination	In vitro effect[a]	In vivo effect (fold change in ED_{50} of penicillin antibiotic)
Staphylococcus aureus	Cefoxitin + piperacillin	SYN	−15
Escherichia coli 311	Cefoxitin + piperacillin	ADD	−2
Pseudomonas aeruginosa	Cefoxitin + piperacillin	ANT	+8
	Cefoxitin + azlocillin	ANT	+3
	Cefamandole + piperacillin	ANT	+2
	Ampicillin + piperacillin	ANT	+3
Serratia marcescens	Cefoxitin + piperacillin	ANT	+4
	Cefoxitin + mezlocillin	ANT	+4
	Cefamandole + piperacillin	ANT	+2
	Cephalothin + piperacillin	ANT	+5
	Cephalothin + mezlocillin	ANT	+3
Enterobacter aerogenes	Cefoxitin + piperacillin	ANT	+4
Proteus morganii	Cefoxitin + piperacillin	ANT	+5
	Cefoxitin + mezlocillin	ANT	+5

[a] SYN, Synergy; ADD, additive; ANT, antagonistic.

Several mechanisms are postulated for the interaction between beta-lactam antibiotics. In cases of synergism one of the antibiotics may inhibit a beta-lactamase, thus protecting the other antibiotic from inactivation. Conversely, in cases of antagonism one of the antibiotics may induce a beta-lactamase that destroys the other antibiotic. Other suggested mechanisms involve competition of the antibiotics for the penicillin-binding proteins.

Implications of these studies are that combinations of beta-lactam antibiotics have therapeutic potential but that certain combinations, for instance, those including cefoxitin, should be avoided and that susceptibility tests should be conducted whenever possible.

Use of New Penicillins with Aminoglycosides: Investigation of Potential Synergy

Jean Klastersky

Azlocillin, mezlocillin, and piperacillin have been evaluated in severe gram-negative sepsis, especially when used in combination with other agents, namely, aminoglycosides. There are good reasons to associate azlocillin, mezlocillin, or piperacillin with other antimicrobials when therapy of severely compromised patients is to be undertaken. Recent reviews of the literature suggest that neutropenic patients will respond more often to a combination of two or three active antibiotics than to single-dose therapy. It appears clearly that beta-lactam combinations do not show an advantage over other combinations, especially those containing aminoglycosides. In fact, they may be antagonistic and should therefore be used cautiously in gram-negative infections, especially in neutropenic patients.

Azlocillin plus amikacin, cefotaxime plus amikacin, and azlocillin plus cefotaxime were compared in a recent preclinical study conducted by the European Organization for Research on the Treatment of Cancer (EORTC) International Antimicrobial Therapy Project Group. It was found that fractional inhibitory concentration indices greater than 2 (suggesting the presence of antagonism) were encountered with 24% of *P. mirabilis*, 60% of *Serratia* sp., 2% of *Klebsiella* sp., and 16% of *E. coli* tested with the cefotaxime-plus-azlocillin combination. In animal studies against *E. coli* and *Klebsiella pneumoniae*, cefotaxime plus amikacin and azlocillin plus amikacin were both significantly more effective than azlocillin plus cefotaxime. It is therefore unlikely that the newer penicillins, at least azlocillin, will be of great promise as a combination therapy with other beta-lactam antibiotics. The remainder of this section will consider the new penicillins in combination with aminoglycosides.

Combinations of various aminoglycosides (gentamicin, sisomicin, netilmicin, tobramycin, amikacin) with ticarcillin or carbenicillin usually result in a 60% rate of response in neutropenic patients when they are used as empirical therapy. No clear difference in clinical outcome has been detected between carbenicillin or ticarcillin or among the different aminoglycosides. Any of these combinations can therefore be used as controls for further studies of combinations of aminoglycosides with penicillins.

Few data are available so far about the clinical efficacy of combinations of the newer penicillins (azlocillin, mezlocillin, piperacillin) with aminoglycosides in the therapy of severe gram-negative bacillary sepsis. One study of piperacillin has been reported from the Baltimore Cancer Research Center, where 59 patients treated with amikacin and piperacillin led to 10 of 25 and 11 of 12 responses in microbiologically and clinically documented infections, respectively. All three infections caused by *P. aeruginosa* responded, as well as the one infection caused by a *Klebsiella* sp. The control combination of amikacin plus ticarcillin led to 11 of 20 and 8 of 14 favorable responses in microbiologically and clinically documented infections, respectively. Another similar study has been reported from the University of California at Los Angeles (UCLA), where 46 neutropenic patients were treated with piperacillin plus amikacin and 55 were treated with carbenicillin plus amikacin. The overall response was 76% in both groups for both documented and suspected infections, but there were four fatal *Klebsiella* septicemias among the patients who received carbenicillin plus amikacin. Thus, the experience with piperacillin combined with amikacin indicates an overall response rate similar to that with carboxypenicillin-aminoglycoside combinations.

At the Institut Jules Bordet, a comparative trial of ticarcillin plus sisomicin versus mezlocillin plus sisomicin in gram-negative bacillary bacteremia in non-neutropenic patients has been completed. Eleven of 14 patients responded favorably to ticarcillin plus sisomicin and 11 of 18 patients responded adequately to mezlocillin plus sisomicin. Mortality was equivalent in the two groups. Most of the failures were observed in infections caused by ticarcillin-resistant or mezlocillin-resistant organisms, most often *Klebsiella* sp.

There is likewise limited information on the efficacy of the azlocillin plus aminoglycoside combination. The EORTC International Antimicrobial Therapy Project Group undertook recently a preclinical trial including the combination of azlocillin plus amikacin. In vitro, the combination has been found frequently synergistic against *E. coli* and even more often against *P. aeruginosa*. Survival of *E. coli* and *K. pneumoniae* infections in mice was greater with azlocillin plus amikacin than with cefotaxime plus amikacin or azlocillin plus cefotaxime. Data in volunteers indicated that a satisfactory bactericidal activity in the serum could be obtained with the combination of azlocillin plus amikacin against *E. coli* and *K. pneumoniae* and was particularly high for *P. aeruginosa*. These data suggest that azlocillin plus amikacin might be a valuable regimen to be tested as an empiric therapy of presumed sepsis in neutropenic patients.

To date, the EORTC International Antimicrobial Therapy Project Group has treated empirically 30 neutropenic patients with azlocillin plus amikacin and 40 with ticarcillin and amikacin in a prospectively randomized controlled trial. Although this study is still in progress, a favorable response has been obtained in 8 of 15 documented infections among patients treated with azlocillin plus amikacin (4 of 6 microbiologically documented infections responded) and in 17 of 24 patients receiving the combination ticarcillin plus amikacin (9 of 12 of the microbiologically documented infections responded). It will be necessary to wait for the inclusion of more patients with microbiologically documented infections to fully evaluate this combination of azlocillin and amikacin.

It is likely that factors in addition to the timing and the nature of antimicrobial therapy are operative in determining the clinical response in severe infections of neutropenic patients with cancer. These include nonbacterial pathogens, inadequate antineoplastic therapy, prolonged marrow aplasia, and the underlying cancer itself. Therefore, it seems likely that the introduction of newer antibiotics will not alter in any impressive way the response rate which can be observed with the presently available regimens. On the other hand, the introduction of newer agents for empirical therapy of neutropenic patients might reduce the untoward effects associated with the presently used antibiotics. So far, however, there is no clear evidence that the newer drugs are associated with better tolerance than the carboxypenicillins.

It is recognized that this analysis (Table 5) only represents a partial experience as far as the clinical efficacy of the newer penicillins is concerned. It seems important that these new agents continue to be carefully evaluated in properly designed trials to provide us with a clear view of their potential importance in the antimicrobial armamentarium.

TABLE 5. *Summary of controlled studies in cancer patients with microbiologically and/or clinically demonstrated infections*

Combination	No. of favorable responses/total	
	New penicillin	Carbenicillin or ticarcillin
Piperacillin + amikacin	21/37[a]	19/34
	35/46[b]	42/55
Mezlocillin + sisomicin	16/24[c]	16/19
Azlocillin + amikacin	8/15[d]	17/24
Total	80/122 (66%)	94/132 (71%)

[a] Baltimore Cancer Research Center.
[b] University of California, Los Angeles.
[c] M. D. Anderson Tumor Cancer Center.
[d] EORTC (1981), study in progress.

Evaluation of New Penicillins in Experimental Animal Models of Infection

W. Michael Scheld

Despite widespread clinical trials, new penicillins have undergone little evaluation in discriminative animal models of infection, and most of the data are either unpublished or available only in abstract form. There are three main types of animal models used in experimental chemotherapy: basic screening (e.g., systemic mouse protection analysis), ex vivo, or discriminative. Because of the inherent difficulties with the first two types of models, and the more precise simulation of pathogenetic mechanisms by discriminative models, only the latter models are discussed here. Some of the newer penicillins have been studied in a few established animal models of infection, including osteomyelitis, pyelonephritis, endocarditis, meningitis, and intraabdominal abscess (for the latter, see below).

A new rabbit model of chronic *Pseudomonas* osteomyelitis was recently reported based on techniques utilized in a well-characterized model of staphylococcal osteomyelitis. Infection was established by direct inoculation of 2×10^7 CFU of *P. aeruginosa* plus sodium morrhuate into the tibia. Treatment was commenced 14 days after inoculation and continued for 14 or 28 days. Carbenicillin or sisomicin alone were ineffective in reducing the bacterial titer in the infected bone when compared with controls, despite serum levels approximating those found in humans. In contrast, treatment with both agents was significantly more effective than that with either agent alone. Azlocillin is currently under investigation in this model. The antibiotic concentrations in normal or diseased bone are similar to those achieved with carbenicillin.

Two rat models of experimental pyelonephritis have recently been utilized for the comparative evaluation of mezlocillin and azlocillin with other beta-lactam agents. In one model utilizing ureteral ligation and renal damage in rats, quantitative renal and urine cultures were performed 2 days after cessation of treatment. The two agents produced essentially equivalent decreases in bacterial titers of *E. coli* or *P. mirabilis*. In another rat model azlocillin was compared with cefulodin in experimental *P. aeruginosa* pyelonephritis. The mean $\log_{10}$ CFU per gram and number of positive kidneys/total number for each regimen were as follows: controls (no drug), 4.9, 12/12; azlocillin, 4.4, 9/10; and cefsulodin, 2.6, 1/12. Cefsulodin was significantly more effective than azlocillin in reducing intrarenal bacterial titers in this model.

Although multiple models of experimental endocarditis have been developed, the transcarotid polyethylene catheter-induced aortic valve trauma model in rabbits has been used extensively in the past decade. This model was used to compare cefsulodin with azlocillin in experimental *P. aeruginosa* endocarditis. The mean ± SD $\log_{10}$ CFU of *P. aeruginosa* per 0.1 g of vegetation on day 8 were as follows: controls, 6.4 ± 0.4; azlocillin, 5.8 ± 0.6; and cefsulodin, 2.6 ± 0.9. Cefsulodin was more active than azlocillin in this model of endocarditis, despite similar in vitro activity against the *P. aeruginosa* strain used.

Recently, we have developed a rabbit model of experimental *P. aeruginosa* meningitis. Meningitis was induced by the intracisternal inoculation of 10^7 CFU of *P. aeruginosa* and reliably simulated the human disease; all untreated animals died of meningitis within 4 days. All antibiotics were administered by continuous intravenous infusion over 8 h, beginning 16 h after inoculation. The mean change in bacterial titer after 8 h of therapy was chosen as the endpoint; these results are summarized in Table 6. In general, the best results with single agents (azlocillin and cefsulodin) were achieved when cerebrospinal fluid (CSF) antibiotic concentrations exceeded the MBC of the test strain by at least eightfold. Although aminoglycoside-azlocillin synergy was routinely observed in vitro for each of three aminoglycosides (gentamicin, tobramycin, and amikacin), an enhanced in vivo bactericidal effect was less predictable with combination therapy. Only the amikacin-azlocillin regimen reduced CSF bacterial titers significantly faster than azlocillin alone ($P < 0.02$). It is of interest that none of the regimens consistently produced a sterile CSF after 8 h; this may relate to the low metabolic activity of this organism in CSF (unpublished data), the poor activity of aminoglycosides at the low pH (mean = 7.02) of purulent CSF, or perhaps other factors. Studies on the most effective regimens are currently being expanded in our laboratory, as well as an assessment of the response to therapy of longer duration (16 to 24 h). In addition, a comparative evaluation of mezlocillin versus the currently recommended agent of choice is under investigation in experimental *S. pneumoniae*, *H. influenzae*, and *E. coli* meningitis.

Relative Efficacy of Piperacillin, Mezlocillin, and Carbenicillin Versus *Bacteroides fragilis* in a Mouse Model

J. G. Bartlett, G. J. Marien, M. Dezfulian

Piperacillin, mezlocillin, and carbenicillin were tested in a mouse model designed to examine antimicrobial penetration into abscesses and relative efficacy versus *B. fragilis*.

Abscess penetration studies. Mice were challenged with a subcutaneous injection of 0.25 ml containing 25% autoclaved cecal contents (sterile inocula) or 25% autoclaved cecal contents combined with $10^{7.2}$ *B. fragilis* strain ATCC 23745 (infected inocula). Antimicrobials were initiated 5 days after challenge, using doses of 600 to 800 mg/kg given at 8-h intervals for four doses. Pharmacokinetic properties were performed by determining antimicrobial levels in sera and abscess contents at 0, 10, 30, 60, and 120 min after the last dose. Both the sterile and infected inocula produced abscesses in this model; the difference between abscess levels of biological activity presumably reflects in vivo inactivation by *B. fragilis* beta-lactamase.

Results showed that all three penicillins penetrated into sterile abscesses to produce mean peak levels of 82 to 138 μg/ml. These levels represent 19 to 29% of peak mean serum concentrations. Comparison with other antimicrobials showed that all beta-lactam drugs tested (cephalothin, ampicillin, moxalactam, and cefoxitin) showed similar values for the ratio of abscess to serum concentrations; this ratio was 17% for chloramphenicol and 53% for clindamycin.

Mean peak levels (+1 SEM) of antimicrobials in abscesses infected with *B. fragilis* were 44 + 4 μg/ml for mezlocillin, 64 + 2 μg/ml for piperacillin, and 113 + 10 μg/ml for carbenicillin. Compared with levels in sterile abscesses, the mean peak levels were 46% for mezlocillin, 78% for piperacillin, and 82% for carbenicillin. By comparison, there was almost complete loss of cephalothin and ampicillin activity in abscesses infected with *B. fragilis*. Modest decreases of 10 to 25% were noted for moxalactam, cefoxitin, chloramphenicol, and clindamycin.

Efficacy versus *B. fragilis*. The same model was used except that the mice were challenged with 15 clinical isolates of *B. fragilis*, treatment was initiated at 1 h after challenge, and treatment was given at 8-h intervals for 5 days. Animals were sacrificed after treatment, abscesses were homogenized for quantitative culture, and results were expressed as the decrease in bacteria per lesion for treated animals compared with untreated controls. The mean decreases in counts for 15 strains of *B. fragilis* expressed as $\log_{10}$ + 1 SEM were 0.4 + 0.1 for mezlocillin, 1.0 + 0.3 for carbenicillin, and 2.6 + 0.6 for piperacillin. The results for carbenicillin and piperacillin are significantly different compared with untreated controls (*t* test of independent means). Comparative values for other drugs were 6.7 + 0.6 for metronidazole, 5.0 + 0.6 for clindamycin, 3.5 + 0.5 for cefoxitin, 1.6 + 0.5 for chloramphenicol, 0.4 + 0.2 for cephalothin, and 0.1 + 0.1 for ampicillin.

In summary, piperacillin, mezlocillin, and carbenicillin penetrate into experimentally induced abscesses to produce peak concentrations which are 19 to 29% of peak serum levels. These results are comparable to those achieved with other beta-lactam antimicrobials. These three penicillins showed modest decreases in levels of biological activity in abscesses infected with *B. fragilis* compared with sterile abscesses, presumably reflecting inactivation by beta-lactamase. In vivo efficacy versus *B. fragilis* showed significant activity for piperacillin and carbenicillin, but both drugs were somewhat inferior to other antimicrobials commonly advocated for infections involving this microbe.

TABLE 6. *Results of therapy in experimental Pseudomonas meningitis*

Drug	*n*	MBC (μg/ml)	CSF (μg/ml, mean)	Δ Bacterial titer after 8 h of therapy ($\log_{10}$ CFU/ml, mean ± SD)
Tobramycin	10	2	1.9	+0.15 ± 0.57
Gentamicin	6	4	6.7	+0.27 ± 0.38
Amikacin	6	4	13.2	+0.57 ± 0.22
Mezlocillin	10	32	23.7	−0.49 ± 0.44
Carbenicillin	10	64	6.7	−0.63 ± 0.87
Piperacillin	10	4	8.1	−0.91 ± 0.64
Ticarcillin	10	16	7.8	−1.09 ± 0.60
Cefsulodin	11	1	29.4	−1.47 ± 0.59
Azlocillin	9	4	30.0	−1.76 ± 0.71
Tobramycin/carbenicillin	4			−0.76 ± 0.50
Tobramycin/ticarcillin	6			−1.12 ± 0.78
Tobramycin/piperacillin	8			−1.40 ± 1.12
Tobramycin/cefsulodin	12			−1.47 ± 0.57
Tobramycin/azlocillin	11			−1.56 ± 0.65
Gentamicin/azlocillin	8			−1.68 ± 0.56
Amikacin/azlocillin	8			−2.64 ± 0.32

Clinical Studies of New Penicillins in Granulocytopenic Patients

Drew J. Winston

The broader activity of the new penicillins suggests the following clinical implications. First, the new penicillins might be useful as single agents for the empiric treatment of suspected gram-negative bacillary infections since their wide spectrum of antibacterial activity includes most gram-negative bacillary organisms commonly isolated from seriously ill patients. Presently, an aminoglycoside is usually required for the empiric treatment of these infections, but therapy with an extended spectrum beta-lactam antibiotic is more attractive because of potentially lesser toxicity. Second, the antimicrobial therapy of granulocytopenic patients generally includes a combination of an aminoglycoside plus carbenicillin or ticarcillin. However, such therapy is frequently complicated by hypokalemia and other fluid and electrolyte imbalances. The new penicillins, by virtue of their lower sodium content and lower dosage requirements, may have fewer of these disturbing side effects. Finally, *P. aeruginosa* and *Klebsiella* infections continue to have a relatively high mortality in granulocytopenic patients despite presently available antimicrobial therapy. The potential synergistic activity of the new penicillins and the aminoglycosides against *P. aeruginosa* and *Klebsiella* isolates might improve the outcome from these infections.

Table 7 summarizes the data from three trials of mezlocillin or piperacillin alone for the empiric treatment of infections in granulocytopenic patients (granulocyte count, <1,000/mm^3). The majority of these patients had acute leukemia. In the two studies of mezlocillin, the overall response rates were approximately 50% and were similar for both microbiologically documented and clinically suspected infections. Treatment was not infrequently associated with the isolation of mezlocillin-resistant organisms at the beginning, middle, or end of the mezlocillin therapy. Piperacillin used alone at the UCLA Center for the Health Sciences led to an initial favorable response in approximately 80% of patients even though most had persistent granulocytopenia. However, four patients subsequently developed bacteremic superinfections resistant to piperacillin while they were still receiving piperacillin. Thus, like single-agent therapy with mezlocillin, the use of piperacillin alone in granulocytopenic patients is limited by the possible emergence of resistant organisms during treatment. No trials of azlocillin used alone for these patients have been reported.

The side effects associated with the use of mezlocillin or piperacillin alone were relatively mild and infrequent. Pseudoproteinuria, asymptomatic transient rise in bilirubin, reversible hypokalemia, and diarrhea occurred in some patients, but no nephrotoxicity occurred in any of these trials.

Table 8 summarizes the results of three trials in which either piperacillin or mezlocillin was combined with an aminoglycoside and compared with carbenicillin or ticarcillin plus an aminoglycoside in the empiric treatment of febrile granulocytopenic patients (granulocyte count, <1,000/mm^3). Most of these patients also had acute leukemia. A similar comparative study utilizing azlocillin plus amikacin is under way with the EORTC group.

Both the UCLA and Baltimore studies com-

TABLE 7. *Single-agent therapy with mezlocillin or piperacillin in granulocytopenic patients*

Study	Antibiotic (dose)	Favorable response: Documented infection	Suspected infection	Total infections	Bacteremia	Comments
Baltimore Cancer Research Center	Mezlocillin (260–450 mg/kg per day)	11/21 (52)[a]	7/13 (54)	18/34 (53)	1/6 (17)	Seven of 23 pathogens isolated required ≥100 μg of mezlocillin per ml for inhibition; 18 patients colonized with mezlocillin-resistant organisms
M. D. Anderson	Mezlocillin (3 g every 4 h)	27/59 (46)	18/33 (55)	45/92 (49)	8/23 (35)	Nineteen of 54 pathogens isolated required ≥50 μg of mezlocillin per ml for inhibition
UCLA	Piperacillin (250–350 mg/kg per day)	7/9 (78)	8/10 (80)	15/19 (79)	6/8 (75)	Four bacteremic superinfections (*E. coli*, 2; *K. pneumoniae*, 1; *P. aeruginosa*, 1) resistant to piperacillin (MIC, >256 μg/ml)

[a] Number of favorable responses/number of cases evaluated for efficacy (percent).

pared amikacin plus piperacillin with either amikacin plus carbenicillin or amikacin plus ticarcillin. For all categories of infection, the results of therapy were somewhat better in the UCLA study whether amikacin plus carbenicillin or amikacin plus piperacillin was used. The reasons for the improved results in the UCLA patients are not readily apparent, although it is possible that more of the Baltimore patients had unfavorable prognostic factors (older age, terminal cancer, irreversible granulocytopenia) which influenced the effectiveness of the antimicrobial therapy. In the M.D. Anderson trial, tobramycin plus mezlocillin was compared with tobramycin plus ticarcillin. The tobramycin plus mezlocillin regimen was slightly less effective.

The enhanced activity of piperacillin and mezlocillin against *P. aeruginosa* and *Klebsiella* might be expected to improve the outcome from these infections. The best response rates for the treatment of *P. aeruginosa* and *Klebsiella* infections occurred when an aminoglycoside was paired with either piperacillin or mezlocillin. Indeed, if the results from all three trials are combined, the response rates of *P. aeruginosa* and *Klebsiella* infections to therapy including piperacillin or mezlocillin were 73% (8 of 11) and 75% (6 of 8), respectively, compared with 57% (4 of 7) and 46% (6 of 13), respectively, for carbenicillin or ticarcillin plus an aminoglycoside. The number of evaluable patients is extremely small, however, and further trials are needed to confirm these interesting trends.

Nephrotoxicity was uncommon in the three combination therapy studies. Despite the lower sodium content of piperacillin (1.98 meq/g) compared with ticarcillin (5.2 meq/g), the incidence of hypokalemia associated with piperacillin and ticarcillin was similar. On the other hand, the 27% incidence of piperacillin-related hypokalemia in the UCLA study was significantly less than the 46% incidence of carbenicillin-related hypokalemia.

Empiric antimicrobial therapy for the febrile, granulocytopenic patient has traditionally consisted of an aminoglycoside plus carbenicillin or ticarcillin. The results of studies using the new penicillins either as single-agent therapy or as part of combination antimicrobial regimens support the concept that broad-spectrum, frequently synergistic combinations are superior for these patients. Single-agent therapy in the granulocytopenic patient with mezlocillin or piperacillin is clearly hampered by the prospects of emergence of resistant organisms during treatment and cannot be recommended on a routine basis. On the other hand, regimens including an aminoglycoside with the mezlocillin or piperacillin are generally as effective as regimens consisting of an aminoglycoside plus carbenicillin or ticarcillin and also may be advantageous for certain *P. aeruginosa* and *Klebsiella* infections.

Clinical Evaluation of Mezlocillin and Piperacillin

Stephen C. Schimpff, William L. Hewitt

Miles Laboratories and Lederle Laboratories have evaluated 1,001 and 758 multiple-dose courses of mezlocillin and piperacillin, respectively. These were patients treated at multiple institutions by various investigators who followed standardized protocols. A course of the investigational agent (or a comparative regimen) was evaluable for clinical efficacy if the patient had received the antibiotic in the prescribed doses for at least 3 to 5 days, had a microbiologically documented infection with at least one pathogen susceptible to the study drug, and had not received any other presumably effective agent concurrently. Using these criteria, 546 courses of mezlocillin and 493 courses of piperacillin were evaluable for clinical efficacy. Both drugs were highly efficacious for susceptible organisms at a wide variety of infected sites. The complete resolution rate was 71% for mezlocillin and 69% for piperacillin, improvements having occurred in 18 and 22%, respectively, and failures in 11 and 8%, respectively. As a general rule, the bacteriological response was somewhat better than the clinical response, with complete elimination of the original pathogen(s) in 76% of the patients treated with either mezlocillin or piperacillin. The complete responses to mezlocillin (listed first) or piperacillin at the more common sites of infection were as follows: lower respiratory tract—63%, 66%; bacteremia—78%, 85%; skin and skin structure—59%, 58%; urinary tract—81%, 74%; intraabdominal—67%, 66%; female genital tract—87%, 82%; hepatobiliary tract—56% (piperacillin included in "intraabdominal"); bone and joint—56%, 57%.

Overall, the patient population was quite ill at the institution of antibiotic therapy. More than one-half of the patients who received either drug had serious underlying diseases and major damage to host defense mechanisms. As a result, it is not surprising that most patients who did not show a complete clinical response were among those patients with the most severe underlying diseases, structural abnormalities of anatomy, or impaired defense mechanisms. Indeed, in most cases a critical evaluation would suggest that failure of an infection to respond was in many cases not likely the result of inadequate antibiotic therapy.

Mezlocillin and piperacillin were compared with carbenicillin, ticarcillin, and, in a few cases, cefoxitin in prospective randomized trials. Again, patients entered into these studies usually had severe underlying diseases and serious infections. The response rates between the investigational agent and the comparative regimen were essentially equivalent. Unfortunately, there were insufficient numbers of infections caused by organisms of specific interest, such as *K. pneumoniae,* to reach a clinical judgment which would suggest superiority of the new penicillin to the carboxypenicillin. Nevertheless, the overall evaluation indicates that these agents are effective against the broad spectrum of gram-negative bacilli, including *E. coli, K. pneumoniae, P. aeruginosa, Serratia* species, *Enterobacter;* many gram-positive cocci, including *Streptococcus faecalis* and some infections caused by *S. aureus;* and many anaerobes, including *B. fragilis.*

As occurs with many of the semisynthetic penicillins, resistance to piperacillin or mezlocillin may develop rather rapidly, especially in patients in whom anatomic considerations (urinary stones, undrained abscesses, amputation stump abnormalities, etc.) preclude the likelihood of rapid eradication of the infecting organism. Superinfection occurred infrequently, although it was often caused by organisms normally susceptible to these agents such as *Klebsiella, Pseudomonas,* or *E. coli.* Some of these superinfecting organisms were found to be resistant to the agent used initially for therapy.

Adverse reactions were uncommon with piperacillin or mezlocilin just as they are with other semisynthetic penicillins. Drug fevers occurred occasionally, as did rashes. Drug-associated diarrhea, eosinophilia, and bilirubinemia have been noted, as have occasional cases of leukopenia and elevated liver enzymes. One of the most potentially serious side effects was the induction of hypokalemia.

It is reasonable to conclude that the new semisynthetic penicillins piperacillin and mezlocillin are clinically effective for the treatment of infections with susceptible organisms which usually include the majority of aerobic gram-negative rods, including *Klebsiella* and *Pseudomonas;* most anaerobic organisms, including *B. fragilis;* and many gram-positive cocci, including the enterococci. These new penicillins have the same safety characteristics as other broad-spectrum semisynthetic penicillins.

Summary

Stephen C. Schimpff, William L. Hewitt

The new penicillins, azlocillin, mezlocillin, and piperacillin, have an increased activity against many gram-negative bacilli, especially *Klebsiella, Pseudomonas,* and *Serratia,* when compared with the earlier carboxypenicillins. The new penicillins are generally highly synergistic when combined with aminoglycosides, but may be synergistic, indifferent, or antagonistic when combined with some cephalosporin-like compounds, especially cefoxitin. In vitro activity of these agents either singly or combined appears to correlate well with in vivo efficacy in animal models. The new penicillins are clinically effective for a very broad range of infections among hospitalized patients with only minimal adverse effects. Attention must be paid to the potential for infection by naturally resistant gram-negative bacilli such as some beta-lactamase-producing *E. coli* and for the rapid emergence of resistance during therapy. The granulocytopenic patient should only receive these agents in combination with another agent, such as an aminoglycoside, which will result in synergistic effects and, usually, a satisfactory response. Although the carboxypenicillins and the new penicillins have substantial similarities, it may be that piperacillin or mezlocillin or both will become the agents of choice among the broad-spectrum penicillins.

New Antimycotics

I. Systemic Treatment

HANS J. SCHOLER *Moderator*	*Hoffmann-La Roche & Company Ltd.* *Basel, Switzerland*
GUGLIELMO GARGANI *Moderator*	*Institute of Microbiology* *University of Florence* *Florence, Italy*
EDWARD DROUHET	*Institut Pasteur* *Paris, France*
RODNEY Y. CARTWRIGHT	*Public Health Laboratory* *St. Luke's Hospital* *Guilford, Surrey, U.K.*
DAVID A. STEVENS	*Institute for Medical Research* *San Jose, California 95128, U.S.A.*
ELSHEIKH MAHGOUB	*College of Medicine* *University of Riyadh* *Riyadh, Saudia Arabia*
MARIA ANNA VIVIANI	*Institute of Hygiene* *University of Milan* *Milan, Italy*
GERALD MEDOFF	*Washington University* *School of Medicine* *St. Louis, Missouri 63110, U.S.A.*

II. Topical Treatment

HARUKUNI URABE *Moderator*	*Faculty of Medicine* *Kyushu University* *Fukuoka, Japan*
EMILIANO PANCONESI *Moderator*	*Department of Dermatology* *University of Florence* *Florence, Italy*
OTTO MALE	*I. Universitäts-Hautsklinik* *Vienna, Austria*
E. DIFONZO	*Department of Dermatology* *University of Florence* *Florence, Italy*
GÜNTER STÜTTGEN	*Skin Department* *Free University of Berlin* *Rudolf-Virchow Hospital* *Berlin, Germany*
YVONNE M. CLAYTON	*Institute of Dermatology* *London, U.K.*

I. Systemic Treatment

Ketoconazole: a New Orally Active Antifungal Agent in Deep and Superficial Mycoses

Edouard Drouhet

The pharmacological history of several thousands of imidazole derivatives started after the discovery of the antibacterial and antifungal activity of benzimidazole by Weeley (1944), which later led to derivatives applied initially only topically on superficial mycoses. In 1968, with clotrimazole, a tritylimidazole, followed by miconazole and econazole (β-substituted 1-phenethylimidazole derivatives), a new generation of oral antifungal agents were applied in deep-seated mycoses, but in spite of their potent broad antifungal spectrum in vitro, the results in systemic mycoses were poor: clotrimazole induces microsomal enzymes in the liver, destroying the antifungal activities, and miconazole and econazole serum levels are disappointingly low for treatment of severe deep mycoses. All three imidazoles produce toxic side effects. Ketoconazole (Ktz), a new 1,3-dioxolanylmethylimidazole, is a very promising antifungal agent due to: (i) a broad antifungal spectrum effective against dermatophytes, yeasts (*Candida*, *Cryptococcus*, and *Torulopsis*), dimorphic systemic fungi (*Histoplasma*, *Blastomyces*, *Coccidioides*, and *Paracoccidioides*), and filamentous fungi (*Aspergillus*, *Phialophora*, etc.) without de novo resistance (the antifungal activity results principally from the inhibition of ergosterol synthesis of the fungal cellular membrane; the quantitative results for MICs varying between 0.002 and 10 μg/ml are dependent on inoculum size, culture medium, temperature of incubation, and growth phase, are less relevant than in vivo studies, and may be misleading); (ii) high effectiveness in all important superficial mycoses (candidosis, dermatophytosis, and pityriasis versicolor) and in predominant deep mycoses (systemic and granulomatous candidosis, histoplasmosis, coccidioidomycosis, paracoccidioidomycosis, blastomycosis, chromoblastomycosis, asgergillosis, etc.); (iii) ease of use due to oral administration once or twice daily, not necessitating hospitalization; (iv) good tolerance with a very low side effect profile and absence of organ toxicity even when given over long periods of time; (v) no liver enzyme induction and maintenance of adequate blood levels after prolonged treatment.

The evaluation of Ktz in superficial and deep mycoses is presented from the literature data from more than 1,500 patients treated in Europe and the Americas, most of them reported recently (1st International Symposium on Ketoconazole, Rev. Infect. Dis. **2**:519–692, 1980) and from personal data obtained in collaboration with B. Dupont and French clinicians and biologists. More than 150 cases of deep and superficial mycoses were studied with in vitro evaluation of MICs for the causal fungi, in vivo pharmacokinetic studies after oral administration, and clinical and mycological evaluation during several months to 1 to 2 years after treatment was stopped. Excellent results were obtained in six chronic mucocutaneous candidosis cases (*Candida albicans* granuloma unresponsive to classical antifungal therapy), with restoration of immunological disturbances; 15 cases of systemic candidosis including new aspects of heroin addicts with cutaneous, ocular, and osteoarticular localizations; 7 cases of *Histoplasma capsulatum* and *H. duboisii* histoplasmosis; 1 case of African blastomycosis (*Blastomyces dermatitidis*); 3 cases of mycetoma (2 due to *Petriellidium boydii*, 1 due to *Hendersenula toruloidea*); 2 cases of enthomophthorosis (*Conidiobolus coronata*, *Basidiobolus rananum*); 1 case of fungal arthritis due to a new hyphomycete resembling *P. boydii* and highly pathogenic for laboratory animals; 50 cases of dermatophytosis, including 38 cases of tinea capitis due to *Trichophyton violaceum* and *T. schoenleinii* and 25 cases of pityriasis versicolor and pityriasis capitis due to *Pityrosporum ovale*. Results obtained in sporotrichosis and chromblastomycosis were not as good. In one case of *Drechslera longirostrata* vertebral arthritis following a fungal endocarditis, cure was obtained only by association of oral Ktz and intravenous (i.v.) amphotericin B, each antifungal agent alone being ineffective. To ensure peak serum levels of >1 μg of Ktz per ml, the usual early dose of 2 × 200 mg was increased to 3 or 4 × 200 mg when necessary, without side effects.

Systemic Antifungals—Other New Agents

Rodney Y. Cartwright

Excluding flucytosine and Ktz, only a few new drugs against systemic fungal infections have been introduced in the past few years.

Miconazole. Miconazole is a β-substituted 1-phenethylimidazole derivative with a broad antifungal spectrum and a limited antibacterial activity. Its mode of action is similar to those of the other imidazoles, affecting the function of both internal and external cellular membranes. The results of animal testing and clinical trials have indicated that miconazole may be of value in treating patients with candidosis, cryptococcosis, coccidioidomycosis, and paracoccidioidomycosis. The results of a "monitored release" scheme in the United Kingdom provides evidence that i.v. miconazole is effective in treating patients with systemic candidosis. The majority of patients received the miconazole i.v., 600 mg three times daily, although bladder instillation, inhalation therapy, or local irrigations were also used in some patients. An overall response rate of 63% was recorded in *Candida* infections. Tolerance was good, with some reactions in 33%, usually of a minor nature and including: gastrointestinal disorders (nausea, vomiting, diarrhea), 16.5%; phlebitis at the infusion site, 11.5%; rash, 3.3%; cardiovascular disturbance, 2.5%; fever, 2.5%; sedation, 0.8%; flushing, 0.8%. Oral therapy has been used in paracoccidioidomysis but better results are obtained with i.v. therapy.

Coccidioidal infections have been treated by both the i.v. and intrathecal routes, and although favorable results have been reported even in patients not responding to amphotericin B, miconazole is not usually ranked as a first-line drug in this infection. Additional side effects were hyponatremia and, after intrathecal administration, arachnoiditis. Long therapy is necessary if miconazole therapy is to be successful.

Miconazole is a useful antifungal agent, especially in patients with candidosis, paracoccidioidomycosis, and coccidioidomycosis who do not respond to or are unable to tolerate first-line antifungals. Its use may also be considered in other systemic mycoses not responding to other therapy.

Econazole. Econazole has an antifungal spectrum similar to that of miconazole, although it has a greater in vitro activity agaisnt the *Aspergillus* species. It has been given i.v., intrathecally, by local instillation, and orally. There have not been sufficient reports to make recommendations on its use in systemic mycoses.

Amphotericin B methyl ester. Amphotericin B methyl ester has been studied in a bid to maintain the antifungal activity of amphotericin B but to increase its solubility and decrease its toxicity. Reduced activity was demonstrated in experimental mouse models against *Coccidioides immitis*, *H. capsulatum*, *B. dermatitidis*, *Cryptococcus neoformans*, and *Candida albicans.* Initial human studies have revealed an unexpected neurotoxicity.

Ambruticin. Ambruticin, a cyclopropylpyran acid, has a broad antifungal spectrum. Animal experiments showed it to be an effective oral drug against murine coccidioidomycosis, candidosis, and histoplasmosis and, in guinea pigs, *Trichophyton mentagrophytes* infections.

Carbohydrases. The alteration of cell walls to produce protoplasts is well known with the penicillins against bacteria. A mixture of carbohydrase enzymes was effective in curing mice experimentally infected with *Candida albicans* and *Aspergillus fumigatus.* They also enhanced subtherapeutic doses of amphotericin B.

There remains a need for more effective drugs against systemic fungal infections. As with all antimicrobial drugs, activity against the infecting organism is essential but the pathogenesis of fungal infections must be remembered when new antifungals are studied. The fungus is frequently difficult to reach from the bloodstream and long-term thereapy is usually necessary.

It is essential that toxicity and side effects do not prevent long-term therapy, and if possible, the drug should be effective after oral administration so that the time of hospitalization can be reduced.

Coccidioidomycosis: Focus on Ketoconazole in Skeletal Disease

David A. Stevens

Great interest has arisen with regard to the possibility of oral therapy with Ktz for coccidioidomycosis, the fungus disease that has been regarded as the most difficult to treat. My presentation discussed Ktz therapy in three manifestations of coccidioidomycosis. As the results with cutaneous coccidioidomycosis have been detailed elsewhere (R. L. Stiller et al., Pan Am. Health Organiz. Sci. Publ. **396:**375–381, 1980), as have the results with chronic pulmonary coccidioidomycosis (P. L. Williams, R. L. Stiller, and D. A. Stevens, this volume), the present discussion will summarize our results in bone and joint disease. These results have been tabulated by Paul L. Williams, Robert L. Stiller, and myself.

Thirteen patients (12 males, 1 female) with bone and joint coccidioidomycosis were treated with 200 to 600 mg of Ktz daily for at least 3 months (mean dose, 111 g; range, 54 to 214 g; mean, 388 days; range, 260 to 743 days). Their ancestry was as follows: eight whites, four blacks, one Filipino. The mean duration of skeletal disease preceding therapy was 65 months (range 2 to 300 months). Nine had failed previous amphotericin B therapy. Three also had extraskeletal disease (three soft tissue and one lymphatic). The involved areas were vertebrae (two), ribs (three), arms (four), hip/pelvis (three), legs (seven), and scapula/clavicle (four). Five had multiple osseous disease. Three had chronic intercurrent illnesses (one arteriosclerotic heart disease, one hypertension, one chronic renal failure, Potts disease, hypertension, and gout). Objective abnormalities and symptoms which could be followed were assigned points based on the parameter's usefulness in assessing disease status, in the form of a denominator; with improvement or resolution, points entered a numerator, as described elsewhere (Williams et al., this volume). A ratio of ≥ 0.5 was defined as major improvement; a ratio of <0.5 and >0 was defined as minor improvement. Improvement occurred in 12 (92%; 10 major, 2 minor). One did not improve after 273 days (108 g). Of those evaluable, 10 of 11 symptomatically improved, 4 of 6 became culture negative, 7 of 8 improved serologically, 8 of 10 improved or resolved scans or X rays, and 5 of 6 improved or resolved physical exam findings of inflammation, swelling, range of motion, or sinus drainage. There were no significant correlations between outcome and age, duration of illness, race, single versus multiple involvement, other dissemination sites, intercurrent illness, or total dose. There was a favorable trend relating therapy duration of >1 year and major improvement ($P = 0.07$). No serious toxicities occurred (one rash, one mild photophobia with normal ophthalmological exam, one menstrual irregularities). Therapy is planned for ≥12 months and 6 months after last evident activity; currently five have completed therapy. These data demonstrate that Ktz is associated with a favorable clinical response in >90% of patients with bone/joint coccidioidomycosis, and duration of therapy may be important in outcome.

Chemotherapy of Mycetoma

ElSheikh Mahgoub

The clinical syndrome of mycetoma, which produces the three signs of swelling, sinuses, and granules, is caused by a variety of aerobic actinomycetes (belonging to the bacteria) or fungi. The two forms are known as actinomycetoma and eumycetoma, respectively.

Actinomycetoma. The causative species of actinomycetoma are *Streptomyces somaliensis*, *Actinomadura madurae*, *A. pelletieri*, *Nocardia brasiliensis*, *N. caviae*, and, occasionally, *N. asteroides*. In tests in vitro, drug combinations were inhibitory at lower concentrations and on more strains of the above-mentioned species than were single drugs. This was particularly true for streptomycin plus co-trimoxazole (sulfamethoxazole-trimethoprim) versus co-trimoxazole or streptomycin alone and for sulfadoxine-pyrimethamine or rifampin plus streptomycin versus the single components. Streptomycin plus co-trimoxazole was more active than streptomycin plus dapsone.

The beneficial effect of combination therapy was confirmed by clinical trials we performed in the Sudan. Co-trimoxazole can be considered a combination in itself. Since mycetoma is a very chronic condition requiring treatment for 4 to 24 months, tolerance as well as activity of the drugs is of great importance.

Streptomycin (1 g, at first daily and later on alternate days) was fairly well tolerated. The same was true for co-trimoxazole (usually two tablets twice a day) with the exception of a few instances of reversible anemia or leukopenia or both. These hematological side effects were more pronounced with dapsone (100 mg twice a day).

Although co-trimoxazole is, generally, more effective, a few cases due to *S. somaliensis* and *A. madurae* only responded to dapsone. The use of rifampcin or sulfadoxine-pyrimethamine combined with streptomycin is reserved for cases which develop resistance to previous treatment.

Eumycetoma. Our experience with the treatment of eumycetoma is limited to cases caused by one species, *Madurella mycetomatis*, which are highly prevalent in the Sudan.

Although effective in vitro, clotrimazole administered orally proved to be inactive in the clinic. The same was true for i.v. miconazole. Griseofulvin, which is slightly active in vitro, was curative in only a few patients. Seven patients are currently under treatment with Ktz. Only two, who have now received the drug for 35 weeks, are showing some improvement.

It seems fair to say that, although a reasonable success has been obtained in the medical treatment of actinomycetomata, no effective drug is yet available for eumycetoma.

Chemotherapy of Cryptococcosis, Aspergillosis, and Candidosis

H. J. Scholer

Cryptococcosis. For the evaluation of antifungal drugs the central nervous system form of cryptococcosis offers unique advantages: diagnosis is unequivocal and, as a rule, not too difficult. Without effective antifungal treatment the disease is invariably fatal, and, therefore, any cure is a proof of efficacy of the drug(s) in question. Indeed, the follow-up of the patients must be long enough to exclude relapses.

In central nervous system cryptococcosis amphotericin B and, later, flucytosine provided formal proof of systemic antimycotic activity on their own, but it was also shown that they must no longer be used alone for this disease but rather only in combination. This combination (amphotericin B i.v. plus flucytosine orally) is considered the current "standard" for cryptococcosis versus which any new alternative drug(s) should be compared in controlled trials. As recently shown by Kerkering et al. (Ann. Intern. Med. **94**:611–616, 1981), pulmonary cryptococcosis must always be treated when it occurs in compromised hosts, whereas otherwise normal hosts do not need chemotherapy a priori.

Invasive aspergillosis. The natural history of this disease is extremely dependent on the underlying condition, e.g., with remission of leukemia and when grave neutropenia has been overcome, spontaneous recovery can occur even in the absence of antifungal chemotherapy. This may not be a frequent event; however, the "cure rates" must be considered with caution.

The published case reports of 88 patients with invasive aspergillosis receiving potentially effective antifungal chemotherapy suggest the following: amphotericin B appears to be definitely active, both alone and in combination with flucytosine (or, in a few cases, with rifampin); flucytosine alone is probably still active on its own but is clearly inferior. Although there is no statistical proof, we would favor the combination of amphotericin B plus flucytosine because it was synergistic or additive against aspergilli experimentally and proved clinically useful in cryptococcosis. For patients with grave neutropenia amphotericin B plus rifampin may be used as an alternative.

Candidosis. When we consider deep-seated candidosis from the point of view of chemotherapy, we are faced with many diseases rather than with a single entity. The conditions for evaluation of antifungal activity are quite good in a few rather rare forms, such as chronic mucocutaneous candidosis or candida osteoarthritis. In the more common forms, such as candida septicemia without evidence of hematogenous organ lesions, the conditions are difficult since the natural history is unpredictable. There are certainly good medical reasons for treating patients also suffering from "unreliable" forms; however, recovery is no proof of antifungal efficacy in these cases. Furthermore, efficacy found in a given form is not necessarily applicable to another form.

For example, flucytosine was highly active in osteoarthritis, meningitis, peritonitis, and urinary tract candidosis, but was disappointing in chronic mucocutaneous candidosis. On the other hand, Ktz was extremely effective in chronic mucocutaneous candidosis, whereas for several other forms the merits of this new drug still have to be established. For a number of forms, e.g., candida endophthalmitis, the combination of amphotericin B plus flucytosine is considered the current "standard," although the advantage versus amphotericin B alone has not been proven statistically. Controlled, comparative trials (particularly with miconazole) are urgently needed. Emphasis should also be put on new drug combinations, e.g., Ktz plus flucytosine.

Drug Activity on the Mycelial Phase of *Candida albicans*

G. Gargani

The test of drug susceptibility in vitro for dimorphic fungi may be misleading: a drug may be active on the saprophytic and not on the parasitic phase or vice versa.

Candida albicans offers a quite peculiar model: the mycelial phase is the pathogenic one, but the yeast phase also is found on the mucous membranes. We developed a culture of *C. albicans* on mammalian cells in a medium without animal serum; scanning electron microscopy demonstrated that, 6 h after the infection with *C. albicans*, thin filaments grew in strict connection with the surface of the animal cells (Vero line), after 12 h a fair mycelium was seen, and after 24 the mycelium started to damage the cell monolayer.

With optic microscopy the development of mycelium in very long filaments may be followed up to 3 or 4 days after infection, when the animal cells are completely destroyed.

In this experimental model we tested the activity of three drugs: 5-fluorocytosine (5-FC), econazole nitrate, and Ktz. The activity of 5-FC was that expected by titration in yeast morphology agar (0.18 to 3 μg/ml) but some serotype B strains were found to be resistant. Econazole was less active (0.78 to 12.5 μg/ml) than 5-FC, whereas Ktz was very active on some strains (0.04 μg/ml) but less active on others (12.5 μg/ml). No difference was seen between serotypes A and B.

When mycelium or yeast growth was recorded, the results were different for econazole nitrate and Ktz but not for 5-FC. No strains grew in the mycelial form in the presence of 0.78 μg of the imidazoles per ml, whereas 7 of 21 strains in the presence of Ktz and 10 of 21 strains in the presence of econazole nitrate, in doses over this level, grew in the yeast form.

Optic microscopy showed, in the presence of inhibiting quantities of Ktz and econazole, the development of a short mycelium after 24 h which later stopped increasing, whereas the cell monolayer was well preserved for up to 6 to 7 days of observation. Some strains changed to the yeast form after 24 to 48 h, which increased in the following days, with moderate damage of the cell monolayer. Scanning electron microscopy (one experiment) showed, 12 h after infection, and in the presence of Ktz or econazole nitrate, scanty thin filaments bound with the cell surface, quite similar to those seen in the controls (without the drugs) after 6 h.

The experiments reported suggest the growth of *C. albicans* in animal cells as a good experimental model, which partially mimics the condition on the mucous membrane and indicates that some *Candida* strains have the ability to escape the action of imidazole drugs changing from the mycelium to the yeast form.

There is also evidence for a working hypothesis that both econazole nitrate and Ktz have maximum activity on the initially growing mycelium.

(Paola Parronchi of my Institute collaborated in these experiments, and Giovanni Orlandini and Sandra Zecchi of the Institute of Human Anatomy collaborated in the scanning electron microscopy.)

Susceptibility Tests

Maria Anna Viviani

With the exception of 5-FC susceptibility testing, the standardization of which has afforded a great predictive value to the laboratory control of 5-FC therapy, the standardization and the routine performance of the in vitro activity of the other antifungal compounds to be used for systemic treatment has not yet been achieved.

The possibility of the emergence of resistance to polyenes or to imidazole drugs, supported by detection of amphotericin B resistance developing during treatment of yeasts infecting cancer patients (an 8% rate has been reported), strongly suggests that the test should be performed routinely for predicting the outcome of therapy. But problems affecting the standardization are many and varied and are related to the morphological complexity of the fungal cell, to the peculiar properties of the drugs, and to the difficulty in identifying the most reliable single methodology that would be optimum for all of the antifungals.

The composition of the culture medium is one of the most important factors to be considered: depending on the mode of action of the drug, antagonists and obfuscating agents have to be recognized and avoided. Taking into account its well-known mode of action, 5-FC in vitro activity is evaluated on yeast nitrogen base-glucose, which is free of purines and pyrimidines that would be taken into the fungal cell by cytosine permease instead of 5-FC. However, this medium is unsuitable for the in vitro testing of polyenes and imidazole derivatives, the antifungal activity of which seems primarily to take place through interaction with cell membrane molecules (ergosterols and unsaturated phospholipids, respectively). The divalent cations Mg^{2+} and Ca^{2+}, present in synthetic media, have been proven to compete with miconazole for the cell binding sites, as demonstrated with *C. albicans.* Furthermore, the acid pH of the medium is responsible for the in vitro impairment of imidazole activity, as we observed in a recent comparative study of the efficacy of four agar media differing in composition and pH: Casitone, pH 7.1; Sabouraud glucose, pH 5.6; yeast nitrogen base-glucose, pH 5.6; and the latter medium buffered at pH 7. Of the three imidazole drugs tested, Ktz appeared to be the most affected by the medium used, as we obtained, for *C. albicans*, MIC variations of >10,000-fold (e.g., MIC = 0.01 μg/ml on Casitone and >100 μg/ml on yeast nitrogen base-glucose, pH 5.6). This medium effect may explain the interlaboratory discrepancies of the in vitro tests and the complaints of in vitro inefficacy of this drug against *C. albicans.*

The choice of a liquid or solid medium is still a matter of great discussion. The weaker activity of the imidazoles in liquid media may be explained by slow precipitation of these agents in the broth due to their poor solubility in aqueous systems. This precipitation is obviously prevented when the compounds are suspended in agar. The neutral pH, optimum for their in vitro activity, would even enhance the precipitation.

Certainly further basic research is needed to reach the uniform test conditions which would allow a simultaneous evaluation of the activity of all antifungals and encourage the routine performance of the in vitro test in hospital laboratories.

Antifungal Agents of Choice

Gerald Medoff

I will attempt to give an overall clinical perspective of the advantages and disadvantages of each of the antifungal agents and indicate which are the most useful. I will then define the existing problems in antifungal therapy.

Amphotericin B. Amphotericin B is still the most desirable drug. It has a broad antifungal spectrum and manageable toxicity, and there are over 20 years of experience with this agent. There is a high level of success in therapy, and many of the treatment failures may be secondary to inadequacy of the host response to the infection rather than to the drug. The most important limitation to the use of the drug is its toxicity, predominantly to the kidney.

5-FC. It is clear that 5-FC has antifungal properties. However, a relatively narrow spectrum, limited to yeast, innate resistance of some strains of *Candida*, and rapid development of resistance in other organisms are problems which hamper its use. The toxicity of 5-FC is minimal and limited to bone marrow suppression and diarrhea. The former can be prevented by keeping blood levels below 100 μg/ml. In general, I do not recommend the use of 5-FC alone, but rather use it only in combination with amphotericin B to treat infections due to *Cryptococcus neoformans* and some *Candida* infections.

Miconazole. Miconazole has a broad antifungal spectrum on in vitro testing but clinical experience is minimal. Other disadvantages of the drug are a short half-life, requiring administration several times a day, and a variety of toxic reactions. One important toxicity that is not caused by miconazole is nephrotoxicity. I regard miconazole as a second-line drug to be used in patients intolerant to amphotericin B or in patients in whom it is important to avoid nephrotoxicity, such as the renal transplant patient.

Ktz. Ktz is an imidazole with good oral absorption, and therefore it may turn out to be a very useful agent for both systemic and superficial fungal infections. Thus far, its toxicity has been minimal and therapeutic results have been satisfactory. It is disconcerting that Ktz is only fungistatic in vitro, and this may limit its use in the treatment of opportunistic infections in immunocompromised hosts. There is not sufficient clinical experience with this drug to recommend it as a first-line agent at the present time.

Drug combinations. The only drug combination with demonstrated enhanced clinical effectiveness is amphotericin B plus 5-FC. A controlled clinical trial has shown this combination to be effective in the treatment of cryptococcal meningitis. Only uncontrolled data are available for other drug combinations used in treatment of other fungal infections.

Existing problems. Many of the problems in antifungal therapy relate to our ignorance about how the presently available agents work. It is not clear that present concepts of how they kill fungi are complete or even correct. In addition, many of these agents have important biological effects, besides toxicity, on the host. For example, we have shown that amphotericin B is a potent immunoadjuvant and has profound effects on lipoprotein composition. These biological effects on the host may play an important role in therapy. Understanding them may help us to design better predictive tests of clinical efficacy and also to use therapeutic regimens which are less toxic than the ones presently in use.

In addition to lack of information about mechanisms of action, we have very little data about appropriate doses and length of therapy with these agents in individual fungal infections. Should we be using maximally tolerated doses or lower doses which also have immunopotentiating capability? All of these questions can only be answered by basic and clinical research and good controlled clinical studies. To accomplish the latter, we need rapid specific and sensitive diagnostic tests for fungal infections other than cryptococcal meningitis. Early diagnosis will also allow initiation of therapy earlier, which will undoubtedly be beneficial in treating these patients with compromised host defense.

II. Topical Treatment

Naftifine

Otto Male

Most established synthetic antifungal agents can be assigned to one of two groups on structural grounds, the imidazoles or the thiocarbamates. Naftifine is the first member of a new class of synthetic antifungal agents, the allylamines, with the structure shown in Fig. 1: the free base is a colorless, viscous oil, which forms a stable, crystalline hydrochloride, readily soluble in water. Naftifine was first synthesized in the Wander laboratories in Berne, Switzerland: the specific antifungal activity of naftifine was observed during routine screening at the Sandoz Research Institute in Vienna. Naftifine is highly active in vitro against all pathogenic dermatophytes, with MICs in the range of 0.1 to 0.2 μg/ml as determined by serial dilution in Sabouraud dextrose broth (A. Georgopoulos, G. Petranyi, H. Mieth, and J. Drews, Antimicrob. Agents Chemother. **19**:386–389, 1981). Naftifine is moderately active against the pathogens of most common superficial yeast infections, with MICs in the range of 1.5 to ≥100 μg/ml.

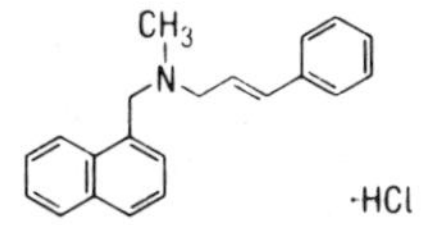

(E)–N–Methyl–N–(1–naphthylmethyl)–3–phenyl–2–propen–1–amine–hydrochloride

FIG. 1. *Structure of naftifine.*

The activity of naftifine in vivo was studied in the guinea pig trichophytosis model infection with *T. mentagrophytes* var. *quinckeanum*. Topical application of naftifine (formulated as a 1% cream) once daily for 7 consecutive days, beginning 48 h postinfection, resulted in a 100% myocological cure rate (G. Petranyi, A. Georgipoulos, and H. Mieth, Antimicrob. Agents Chemother. **19**:380–392, 1981).

Initial toxicological studies showed naftifine to have a very low toxic potential. Applied topically, or orally in doses of up to 4,000 mg/kg, it was not possible to determine LD_{50} values in any species. In chronic toxicity studies, application of up to 300 mg/kg to rats and of up to 200 mg/kg to monkeys for 6 months was well tolerated. Of the great number of additional studies required for the registration of a new drug, only a few of the most significant will be mentioned: naftifine showed no effects in reproduction studies designed to detect teratogenicity. In the Draize test for sensitization potential, naftifine was completely negative. Skin tolerance and eye irritation were investigated in New Zealand white rabbits: no abnormal effects of naftifine were detected.

To be effective, an antimycetic drug applied topically must be able to reach the deepest section of the hair follicles in concentrations sufficient to eliminate the pathogen in cases of deep trichophytosis. Radiographic studies with labeled compounds in guinea pig skin have shown naftifine to fulfill this requirement.

Naftifine is primarily fungicidal against both yeasts and dermatophytes. Unpublished studies on the mechanism of action have shown naftifine to act by inhibiting ergosterol biosynthesis.

Topical Antimycotics of the Imidazole Class

E. Panconesi, E. Difonzo

The topical antimycotics of the imidazole class (the less used imidazole derivatives chlormidazole and isoconazole, the most used clotrimazole, miconazole, econazole, and, finally, the incompletely studied biphonazole and tioconazole) have been examined. Their chemical and physiochemical properties, the very low MICs, modes of action (ultrastructural findings and biochemical effects), and so on have been referenced.

In vivo, the penetration, bioavailability, and antifungal action of the imidazole derivatives depend on various conditions such as interaction between the drug and the intact or lesioned cutaneous surface. Treatment with these drugs, which requires attention to the choice of the vehicle and form containing the active substance, results in rare, sporadic reports of intolerance, such as contact dermatitis (with the exception of chlormidazole).

Regarding clinical experimentation, an enormous amount of data is available, in particular, on clotrimazole, miconazole, and econazole, with extremely high percentages of success, often with short-term treatment.

However, not considering significant a global report based on diversified experimentation or evaluation criteria, the results of some sufficiently comparable case series (including personal experiences) have been shown in detail. For example, in tinea corporis, tinea pedis, tinea cruris, and mucocutaneous and vulvovaginal candidiasis the imidazole antifungal derivatives also give high percentages of success in double-blind studies. Tinea capitis, onychomycoses, granulomatous forms etc., require association with systemic treatment (e.g., griseofulvin, Ktz).

Bioavailability, Skin Penetration, and Permeation of Topical Antimycotics

Günter Stüttgen, Elke Bauer

The way in which topically applied antimycotics migrate into the target organ skin and, after having acted, their removal from that area and from the whole organism is a highly complex sequence of events. To clarify the terminology, the following processes are to be expected when a medical preparation is applied to the skin surface. *Liberation* describes the release rates of a substance from a vehicle. The movement of a drug into a layer of the skin is called *penetration*, whereas *permeation* means migration through one or more layers. *Resorption* is the process by which the drug reaches the blood and lymph vessels and by which it is removed from the local skin area of application. It may be distributed throughout the whole organism. *Absorption* represents the sum of the preceding processes.

The best topical drug is useless if the vehicle into which the drug is incorporated does not allow its release (Higuchi).

The problem of absorption is correlated with the structural state of the skin barrier, namely, the horny layer. Fungi that grow on the skin surface develop toxic and allergenic substances which may irritate the skin, especially the structure of the horny layer. The more the horny layer is damaged, the more the process of permeation takes place.

Our examination concerning the absolute concentration of an antimycotic drug in the different layers of the skin, which was achieved with labeled (^{3}H, ^{14}C) substances which were incorporated into an ointment or tincture to give a 1% concentration, is divided into two parts: (i) normal and damaged human skin in vivo and vitro; (ii) normal and damaged human nail in vitro. To obtain exact data about an antimycotic agent, it is necessary to compare the quantities (micrograms) found in the different layers of the skin (Fig. 2) with the antimycotic efficacy against the different types of fungi. The absolute quantity of the antifungal drugs in the horny layer and upper epidermis is obviously sufficient for the drugs isoconazole nitrate, dimethyl-morpholino-HCl, econazole, oxiconazole, clotrimazole, and also tolnaftate and nystatin. Their concentrations in killing different types of fungi were effective (Table 1). Obviously, it is not necessary to increased the influx rate of antimycotic agents by using salicyclic acid or dimethyl sulfoxide, which improve the penetration in the deeper horny layer if marked hyperkeratosis has taken place.

The clinical problem of topical treatment is deep mycosis and, not least, onychomycosis. In the examination of nails, we have used the same technique and the same procedure, putting the labeled drug on a 1-cm^2 surface of nail to obtain data about absorption. Obviously, a damlike effect of the deeper layers of the nail plate inhibits the steady outflow of the substance. A saturation of antimycotics takes place in this layer. The addition of dimethyl sulfoxide to the antimycotic increases the penetration rate (Table 2).

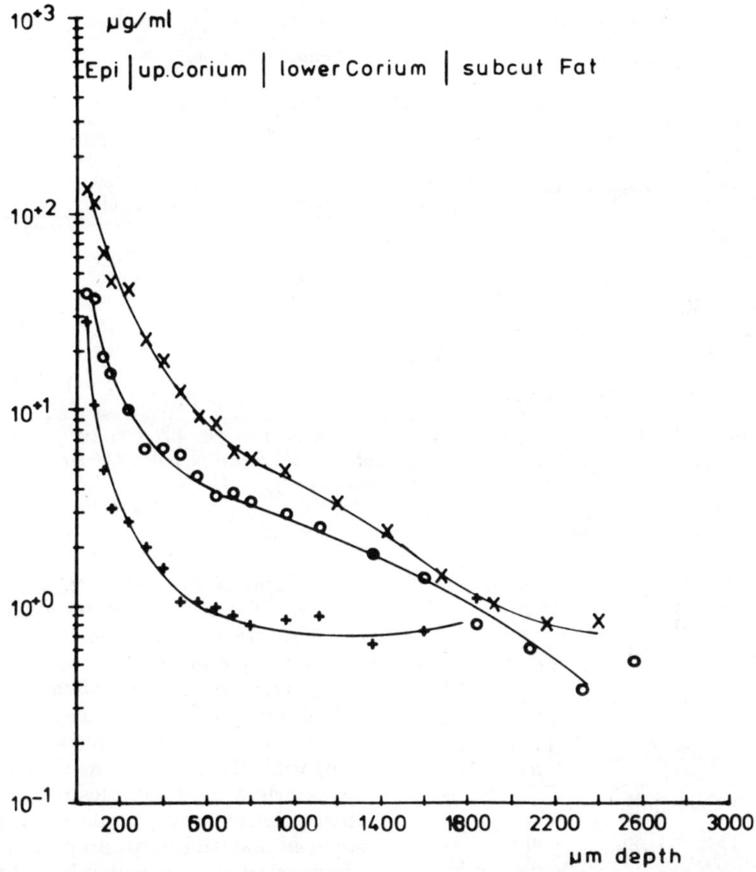

FIG. 2. *Penetration (after 1,000 min) into abdomen skin in vitro. Symbols: ×, oxiconazole ointment (1%); +, oxiconazole tincture (1%); ○, dimethyl-morpholino derivative tincture (0.5%).*

Concerning the comparison of tincture with ointment there is no doubt that antimycotics in tincture show a significantly higher uptake into the deeper layers of the nails. This is particularly true for the concentrations in the nail bed. According to our results, the problem encountered in the topical therapy of nail mycosis is not the transport or the permeability of the antimycotic agent, but rather the sporocidal concentration maintained there. The time factor, which includes renewal of the keratinocytes and the horny layers, including that of the nails, has to be respected.

Drugs of Choice

Yvonne M. Clayton

It is only in the last decade that the potential of the imidazole compounds as antifungal agents was realized and that other compounds with a similar broad spectrum of activity have become available for the treatment of dermatomycoses. The choice, therefore, of which antifungal compound to use is now greater and may be made from such agents as tolnaftate, clotrimazole, miconazole, econazole, haloprogin, tolciclate, and naftifine. The majority of these compounds are effective against dermatophyte and *Candida* infections and against pityriasis versicolor. Is one better than another?

One can try to determine this by in vitro susceptibility tests. However, as is very well known, the MIC of any compound varies with the strain of fungus, the size of the inoculum, state and composition of the medium, incubation temperature, and many other factors. Because of these variables, it is often meaningless to compare MICs obtained in different laboratories. Standardization of methods for the estimation of MICs of antifungal drugs is still awaited. Therefore, in vitro susceptibility determinations may not always be absolute guides to the efficacy of an antifungal compound and there may be a great deal of disparity between labo-

TABLE 1. *Permeation of different antimycotics into the skin layer after various exposure times*

Antimycotic	Permeation (μm/ml)									
	Horny layer (20 μm)		Epidermis (200 μm)		Upper corium (400 μm)		Deeper corium (800 μm)		Subcutis (1,200 μm)	
	100 min	300 min	100 min	300 min	100 min	300 min	100 min	300 min	100 min	1,000 min
Oxiconazole ointment, 1%	1,000	900	12	15	1	2	1	0.7	0.3	1.5
Tincture, 1%	3,000	2,500	4	4	1	0.5	0.2	0.3	0.07	0.8
Dimethyl-morpholino derivate ointment, 0.5%	800	2,000	10	14	2.5	6	2	5.5	0.1	1.0
Econazole ointment[a]	1,200		20	5			0.2	0.5	0.1[d]	
Isoconazole nitrate ointment, 1%[b]			10	9	8	5	0.8	1		
Clotrimazole[c]		1,000		30		0.5 (−40)				

[a] In vivo experiments (H. Schaefer and G. Stüttgen, Arzneim. Forsch. **26:** 432–435, 1976).
[b] U. Täuber, *in* H. Gartmann, Z. S. Itani, M. L. Langen, and F. Schröpl (ed.), *Dermatomykosen und ihre Therapie*, part 1, p. 21–36, 1980 (Excerpta Medica, Amsterdam).
[c] Bayer report, 1975.
[d] 0.61% of the dose recovered in urine.

TABLE 2. *Penetration of different antimycotics into the human nail after 1,000-min exposure time in vitro*

Antimycotic	Penetration (μg/ml)			
	Nail plate		Nail bed	
	Dorsal	Ventral	Upper layers	Deeper layers
Oxiconazole ointment	1,000	15	5	7[a]
Tincture	1,500	50	30	30
Dimethyl-morpholino derivate tincture	600	15	8	15[a]
Econazole ointment	1,000	10	10	12[a]

[a] Damlike effect.

ratory and clinical effectiveness. Final assessment of all new antifungal agents requires a study of their clinical effectiveness.

Many open and controlled comparative clinical studies have been carried out to try to determine whether one topical agent is likely to be more effective or more acceptable than another. Variations in the numbers of patients, type of infection, causative fungus, length of treatment, and different methods of assessing results make comparisons of such studies difficult. However, most studies show that the more recently introduced compounds with their broad spectra of activity are as efficient as other topical agents in current use. The broad spectrum of activity of the imidazoles and other compounds such as holoprogin makes them particularly suitable for use when facilities for laboratory mycological diagnosis are not readily available, since on clinical appearances alone it is sometimes difficult to differentiate between a dermatophyte infection, an infection caused by *Candida*, and the bacterial infection erythrasma—all of these conditions are susceptible to these compounds.

The development of resistance by fungi after topical application of these antifungal compounds has not yet been recorded. The majority of the topical agents now available are nonstaining, odorless, and practically free of any side effects. Patient acceptability of the preparation may well play an important part in ensuring that a compound is used correctly and regularly.

The site of the infection may also determine which antifungal agent should be used. For example, the intertriginous type of tinea pedis generally responds to topical therapy. However, the hyperkeratotic type of tinea pedis follows a more chronic course. It affects the soles, heels, and sides of the feet, and *Trichophyton rubrum* is the commonest cause of this variety of tinea pedis. Although there may be a partial response to topical therapy, since nails and other body sites are frequently involved as well, oral therapy is recommended. Oral therapy for lesions on the palms is also preferable to topical treatment, and topical therapy alone should not be used for cases of tinea barbae, capitis, or unguium. Until recently, griseofulvin was the only antifungal compound available for oral therapy, but now there is a choice between this antibiotic and the imidazole Ktz.

Ktz differs from griseofulvin in that it is effective not only against dermatophyte infections but also against *Candida* infections. It has been shown to be effective in the treatment of cases of vaginal candidosis, as have many other compounds, and there are probably more preparations marketed for this condition than for any other type of fungal infection. In addition to the polyene antibiotics and imidazoles, broad-spectrum antiseptics such as povidone iodine and chlordantoin are available. Many clinical trials have been pursued to determine whether one compound is more effective than another. These studies have shown that the imidazoles appear to give higher cure rates than the polyenes, but both the polyenes and imidazoles give significantly higher cure rates than povidone iodine and chlordantoin. The recommended durations of treatment by the various compounds is varied, ranging from 3 days (or less) for some imidazoles to 14 days for the polyenes. In the majority of patients, cure is readily achieved by the topical application of one of the imidazoles or polyenes for the recommended period of treatment. Some studies have shown that the shorter the course of treatment the more likely the patients are to complete it.

There is now a much wider choice of effective compounds available for the treatment of the majority of superficial fungal infections. The broader spectrum of activity of such topical compounds as the imidazoles is advantageous in many circumstances. Nevertheless, problems do remain. The successful eradication of dermatophytes from all cases of tinea unguium has still to be accomplished, and there is as yet no effective therapy for nondermatophyte infections of nails. The search for new and more effective antifungal agents should continue since skin and nail infections are still the commonest fungal diseases encountered in medical practice.

New Bacterial Vaccines

JEROME O. KLEIN
Moderator
Boston University School of Medicine
Boston City Hospital
Boston, Massachusetts 02118, U.S.A.

MARY P. GLODE
Moderator
University of Colorado
Health Sciences Center
School of Medicine
Denver, Colorado 80218, U.S.A.

CHRISTINE L. WILLIAMS
Lederle Laboratories
Pearl River, New York 10965, U.S.A.

DAVID H. SMITH
Department of Pediatrics
University of Rochester Medical Center
Rochester, New York 14642, U.S.A.

DONALD CRAVEN
Boston University School of Medicine
Boston City Hospital
Boston, Massachusetts 02118, U.S.A.

R. H. TIESJEMA
Rijksinstituut Voor de Volksgezondheid
Bilthoven, The Netherlands

P. HELENA MÄKELÄ
Central Public Health Laboratory
Helsinki, Finland

JØRGEN HENRICHSEN
Statens Seruminstitut
Copenhagen, Denmark

Infections caused by encapsulated bacteria remain a major threat to the health of young children throughout the world. Despite the development and licensure of a pneumococcal vaccine and meningococcal A and C vaccines, the population of children at highest risk for these bacterial infections remains unprotected. With the exception of meningococcus group A vaccine, the efficacy and immunogenicity of polysaccharide vaccines are limited in the most susceptible population, infants under 2 years of age. The presentations in this Symposium reviewed new information about the epidemiology and immunology of infections due to *Haemophilus influenzae* type b, *Neisseria meningitidis*, and *Streptococcus pneumoniae* in infants and children, the immunogenicity and protective efficacy of available polysaccharide vaccines in children, and results of current research efforts in development of new vaccines.

Epidemiology of *Haemophilus influenzae* Type b and Issues of Chemoprophylaxis

Mary P. Glode

It is now recognized that *Haemophilus influenzae* type b (HIB) causes a contagious disease of childhood. Young children who have been in intimate contact with an infant who develops HIB disease are at risk of both colonization and disease with HIB. This risk is greatest for close contacts less than age 2 years, where it approaches 2 to 3% in the month following exposure to an index case. Since nasopharyngeal carriage of HIB may persist for months in colonized individuals, the duration of risk of secondary disease is not clear.

What can be done to prevent secondary cases? Several authors have studied the efficacy of antimicrobial therapy in carriage eradication and prevention of secondary cases. We compared placebo with rifampin (20 mg/kg per day given in two divided doses) for eradication of HIB carriage in 396 contacts of 79 patients with proven invasive HIB disease. The overall carriage eradication rate with rifampin was 63.6% as compared to 23.9% for placebo recipients. However, in children less than 5 years of age, rifampin was not significantly better than placebo at eradication of HIB carriage.

Further studies are under way to assess the issues of dose and duration of prophylaxis, optimal drug, identification of contacts at risk for colonization or disease, method of administration (no suspension of rifampin currently available), cost, and risk/benefit analysis. Until these issues are resolved, the physician providing care for close contacts should be aware of the possibility of a secondary case, and all febrile or ill contacts should be evaluated for possible HIB disease, regardless of whether or not they received any chemoprophylaxis agents.

Safety and Immunogenicity of *Haemophilus influenzae* Type b PRP Vaccine with *Bordetella pertussis* Adjuvant in Infants

Christine L. Williams

Haemophilus influenzae type b is currently the leading cause of bacterial meningitis in the United States in children between 1 month and 10 years of age, with the greatest incidence between 4 and 9 months of age. Since antibody to the capsular polysaccharide polyribosyl-ribitol phosphate (PRP) correlates clinically with susceptibility to disease, PRP vaccine preparations have been extensively evaluated in pediatric field trials. PRP vaccine, though exhibiting immunogenicity in older children and consistently demonstrating a high margin of safety, has *not* proved to be immunogenic in children less than 1.5 to 2 years of age. This lack of antibody response to plain PRP vaccines in infants at highest risk for disease has stimulated further research into the use of various adjuvants of carrier proteins in an attempt to produce an effective vaccine for this target population. The present studies were designed to evaluate the safety and immunogenicity of a PRP vaccine utilizing an adjuvant of *Bordetella pertussis* cells. These trials were initiated in several sites in the United States and West Indies. Initial studies evaluated safety and immunogenicity in 2- to 6-year-old subjects and progressed to younger groups until the desired group, 2 to 3 months of age, was reached. The PRP + pertussis vaccine utilized consisted of a highly purified, high-molecular-weight PRP combined with *B. pertussis* cells, injected intramuscularly at a dose of 10 μg of PRP and 4 opacity units of *B. pertussis* per 0.5-ml dose.

Local and systemic reactions to immunization were as shown in Table 1.

Antibody response to one dose of PRP + pertussis vaccine was strongly age dependent, varying from 90% of 3- to 6-year-olds to 50% of 15- to 18-month-olds, 40% of 6- to 8-month-olds, and virtually none of the 2- to 3-month-old infants.

Multiple doses in infants under 1 year of age, however, produced a clear booster response. In four studies in which three doses of PRP + pertussis vaccine were administered to 2- to 3-month-old infants at 2-month intervals, approximately 50% responded with twofold or greater increases in antibody to PRP (Table 2).

These preliminary clinical studies indicate that the combined vaccine consisting of PRP complexed with *B. pertussis* was well tolerated and induced antibody response to PRP in infants.

Immunization for *Haemophilus influenzae* Type b

David H. Smith

Initial efforts in the development of a *Haemophilus influenzae* type b (HIB) vaccine indicated that antibody to the HIB capsule is bactericidal and protects against systemic HIB disease. The capsular substance of HIB, a polymer of ribitol, ribose, and phosphate (PRP), was purified in our laboratory and that of John Robbins (Bureau of Biologics, Food and Drug Administration) for use as a vaccine.

The kinetics of the antibody response in young adults differs from that to protein vaccines in that the response to PRP is not anamnestic and it persists for months to years after a single immunization. Furthermore, the responsiveness to the vaccine, in terms of percentage of persons responding and amount of antibody produced, is age related: young infants respond infrequently with low amounts of antibody, but children over 5 years of age have an adult-like response. Also noteworthy is the wide variation in the individual responses; the mean antibody response is associated with wide standard deviations.

The opportunity to use PRP as a control vaccine during a study of the efficacy of a group A meningococcal vaccine in Finland yielded important information: a single dose of PRP re-

TABLE 1. *Local and systemic reactions to immunization*

Vaccine	% of children showing:		
	24-h local reactions	24-h febrile reactions[a]	Other systemic reactions
DPT[b]	50	15	30
PRP + pertussis	30	8	15
PRP	10	3	5

[a] Temperature over 101°F (ca. 38.3°C).

[b] DPT, Diphtheria and tetanus toxoids combined with pertussis vaccine.

TABLE 2. *Booster response to multiple-dose vaccine*

Study	No. of patients	Investigator	No. (%) of responders[a]	No. (%) of nonresponders
I	20	D. King	18 (90)	2 (10)
II	11	D. King	5 (45)	6 (55)
III	21	D. Eitzman	11 (52)	10 (48)
IV	11	M. Glode	5 (45)	6 (55)
Totals	63		39 (62)	24 (38)

[a] Twofold increase in antibody to PRP.

duced systemic HIB disease in children older than 18 months of age by at least 90% for 2 or more years, but it had no effect in younger children.

Our laboratory questioned whether we could extend the infant's natural passive protection against HIB. We asked whether specific antibody could be increased enough to generate enough passively transferred antibody to protect infants until 18 months of age, when active immunization with PRP could be used. Results of a study in which women were immunized with PRP before becoming pregnant demonstrated the potential of this approach. The wide variation in antibody response to PRP was redocumented, and the pattern of antibody responses by arbitrarily defined groups of "low" and "high" responding women was analyzed. "High" responders produced a marked immunoglobulin G (IgG) antibody response in contrast to the "low" responders, who produced only a predominantly IgM antibody response. Neither the amount nor class distribution of antibody changed with repeat immunization of the lower responding women. When the maternal and infant titers of certain of the women were followed, "high" responding women were found to transmit levels of anti-PRP antibody sufficient to yield in the infants titers thought to be protective for 6 to 12 months; the infants of "low" responding women, however, recieved levels of anti-PRP antibody only minimally beyond those observed in healthy infants delivered from nonvaccinated mothers. Thus, this approach might be useful under certain circumstances, but it could not be universally successful.

Earlier, we had found that the anti-PRP antibody response following HIB disease exceeded that for immunization in children of similar ages. Reasoning that PRP exists in a different physical and chemical state in its purified form compared to that of the whole bacterium, Anderson in our laboratory has isolated and studied the vaccine potential of PRP-outer membrane complex. This complex is prepared in a form enriched for outer membrane proteins but with little lipopolysaccharide (endotoxin). Studies in rabbits revealed highly enhanced potency in raising anti-PRP antibody and anamnestic responsiveness. Studies in adult humans have found the vaccine to be immunogenic and nontoxic, and results in toddler-aged children appear promising.

The latest approach is the covalent linkage of capsular polysaccharide to specific proteins. Two distinct approaches are being followed. In Robbins' laboratory, intact PRP is coupled to a chemical linker which is then coupled to a protein. Anderson generates oligosaccharides which have terminal groups which can be covalently coupled to protein directly. The resulting products produce antibodies to the polysaccharide and the protein components, and, as expected, the anti-PRP antibodies are bactericidal in vitro and presumably protective. Anderson has employed an immunogenic, nontoxic diphtheria toxin (cross-reactive material) produced by a mutant diphtheria phage as the protein carrier and thereby arrives at a product that generates both anti-diphtheria toxin and anti-PRP antibodies.

Meningococcal Vaccines: Progress and Problems

Donald Craven

Endemic or epidemic disease caused by *Neisseria meningitidis* is usually manifest as bacteremia or cerebrospinal meningitis or both. Meningococcal disease can occur at any age, but children from 4 months to 2 years of age are most susceptible. Meningococci are classified into eight different serogroups based on chemically distinct capsular polysaccharide antigens. Serogroups A, B, and C account for more than 90% of meningococcal disease.

Group A and group C polysaccharide vaccines. Based on the early work of Kabat, Gotschlich et al. in 1969 prepared high-molecular-weight polysaccharide vaccines for protection against disease caused by meningococcal serogroups A and C. Both of these vaccines produced group-specific immunity, were of low toxicity, and subsequently had well-documented efficacy in controlling epidemic meningococcal disease. The development of these vaccines was particularly encouraging in light of increasing resistance of meningococci to sulfonamides, which were frequently used for chemoprophylaxis during outbreaks. Subsequent investigations demonstrated that poor antibody response to the polysaccharide vaccines occurred in children less than 2 years of age. Peltola et al. found that these children would respond to two doses (primary and booster) of group A polysaccharide. However, antibody levels were suppressed in children receiving two doses of group C polysaccharide. In addition, antibody levels of group C polysaccharide fell more rapidly than levels of antibody against group A. Thus, although group C polysaccharide would be quite effective in high-risk adult populations such as military recruits and in persons over 2 years of age during epidemics, an alternative vaccine should be considered for control of group C meningococcal disease in children less than 2 years of age.

Group B vaccines. Group B *N. meningitidis* is the leading cause of endemic meningococcal disease in the United States and has caused outbreaks in Europe and other parts of the world. In contrast to the group A and group C vaccines, group B vaccine has been a poor immunogen in both adults and children. Failure of purified high-molecular-weight group B polysaccharide to elicit antibody in humans has been attributed to: (i) its unstable structure in its purified state, (ii) its similarity to other sialic acid receptors on human cells, (iii) its rapid degradation by neuraminidases produced by many mammalian cells. Several alternative approaches to produce an effective vaccine against group B meningococci have included the use of outer membrane proteins, lipopolysaccharides, pili, and possibly IgA protease. To date, outer membrane protein vaccines have received the most attention. Epidemiological studies have suggested that certain protein serotypes are associated with disease (serotype 2) and are rarely found among carriers. Studies in guinea pigs and mice have suggested that purified serotype 2 protein vaccines are immunogenic and provide protection against challenge with encapsulated meningococci, but the same vaccines are poorly immunogenic in humans. Subsequent studies by Zollinger et al. with a combined group B polysaccharide type 2 protein complex (noncovalently bound) produced bactericidal antibody in small numbers of human volunteers, but this antibody was primarily IgM and of short duration. Subsequent studies have demonstrated that noncovalently bound group B polysaccharide type 2 protein in various ratios increases the antigenicity and immunogenicity of both components in human volunteers. Bactericidal antibodies directed against group B polysaccharide lasted for at least 6 weeks. Antibodies to the outer membrane proteins persisted longer but did not appear to have significant bactericidal activity. These studies demonstrated that antibodies elicited by the protein-polysaccharide complex vaccines may provide protection against group B meningococcal disease.

A group B polysaccharide type 2 protein complex vaccine prepared by Frasch et al. is being field tested in South Africa. Since this trial is being conducted in double-blind fashion and in the presence of group B type 2 meningococcal disease, the results should provide valuable information on the immunogenicity and efficacy of protein polysaccharide vaccines.

Current Developments in Meningococcal Polysaccharide Vaccines

R. H. Tiesjema

Purified vaccines against gram-negative bacteria in general, and against encapsulated meningococci in particular, can be considered to be those constituents of the cell envelope which come into direct contact with the host and to which natural, mostly bactericidal antibodies can be found. These antibodies are supposed to be acquired during asymptomatic carriage and, possibly, subclinical infection, caused by both encapsulated and non-encapsulated meningococci, or by contact with bacteria possessing identical or related cross-reacting antigens. The surface antigens that can be seen as potential vaccines are: pili, lipopolysaccharides (LPS), polysaccharide, and outer membrane proteins.

Pili are almost certainly responsible for the attachment of meningococci to host tissue. They appear to be present in greater number on non-groupable, non-encapsulated strains than on groupable, encapsulated strains. Antibodies against pili-associated antigen may prevent attachment, as is the case for gonococci, where much work has been done on the serology of pili and where pili are the prime candidate for a vaccine to prevent mucosal surface infections. However, no serotyping system based on the specificity of pili has yet been developed for meningococci, and it is not known whether antibodies to pili are bactericidal. Furthermore, eventual induction of local immunity in the oro- and nasopharynx, resulting in prevention of carriage of mainly non-encapsulated strains, is not the first aim of meningococcal vaccines, which have the primary objective of preventing disease by invading, encapsulated organisms. On a quantitative basis pili are not very attractive for large-scale vaccine production, especially since pili may be absent from strains subcultured in vitro. This makes pili an unlikely candidate for a vaccine to prevent meningococcal disease.

LPS exist in a wide variety of little or no cross-reacting serotypes. Natural antibody to LPS is bactericidal. LPS have intrinsic endotoxin activity and hence are, as such, unsuitable for use as a vaccine, but the polysaccharide part devoid of lipid A might have vaccine potential. LPS from meningococcal strains, at least when cultivated in vitro, lack the O-polysaccharide chain; the resulting low-molecular-weight core oligosaccharide when purified is less capable to induce antibody. Attempts to enhance the immunogenicity of LPS core oligosaccharide by coupling to protein, a method which has successfullly been applied to polysaccharide antigen, have been unsuccessful for LPS. All this makes LPS for the time being an unlikely vaccine candidate.

Capsular polysaccharide is the surface component most directly in contact with the host. The composition of the capsular polysaccharides includes small differences with large immunological consequences: groups B and C differ from each other only in the bond type between the repeating units; groups W135 and Y differ in the position of the —OH group on C-4 of lactose/glucose.

Vaccines against serogroups A and C have shown their effectiveness and safety both during epidemics and in field trials; protection is based on the induction of antibody with complement-dependent bactericidal activity. Vaccines composed of polysaccharides of serogroups 29E, W135, and Y are not yet in general use, but have successfully been tested in volunteers.

Purified polysaccharides, with a relatively simple repetitive structure (unlike protein vaccines such as tetanus toxoid), behave as thymus-independent antigens. No B-memory cells for polysaccharide are induced during primary or revaccination. After both injections only IgM antibodies are induced, with a secondary response similar to the primary one. For long-lasting vaccine-induced protection against invasive diseases caused by encapsulated bacteria a thymus-dependent response to polysaccharide antigens, resulting in more persistent IgG antibody, is desirable. This can be achieved by covalent coupling of polysaccharide to a thymus-dependent antigen, such as bovine serum albumin or tetanus toxoid. We have tested this conjugate in mice, which were revaccinated 10 weeks after primary immunization; a week after priming or revaccination with 0.5 μg of plain polysaccharide only a low IgM response was obtained and no IgG was found. Upon priming with the same amount of conjugated polysaccharide, the initial IgM response was higher, but more important is that IgG antibody was also induced and that revaccination resulted in boosting of both IgM and IgG antibody. Conjugation to protein carriers has also been tried for group B polysaccharide. In mice, however, the conjugates showed as little immunogenicity as the plain polysaccharides, that is to say, no immunogenicity at all: no IgM and no IgG response to the polysaccharide part.

Outer membrane proteins of meningococci can be divided among some 15 different serotypes, of which type 2 is the predominant one in cases caused by serogroup B and is also found frequently in cases caused by serogroups C, W135, and Y. Within serotype 2 three cross-reacting types, 2a, 2b, and 2c, can be discriminated. According to Frasch, antibodies to type 2 protein are bactericidal and are present in elevated concentrations in acute- and convalescent-phase sera.

Meningococcal and other polysaccharide vaccines behave as thymus-independent antigens and hence give insufficient immunological response in individuals without previous experience with the same antigen in a more native state. For this reason plain polysaccharide vaccines are mainly useful in epidemic situations, where short-lived enhanced antibody levels can also be of help. The response to polysaccharide antigens can be modified from thymus independent to thymus dependent by presenting the polysaccharide in a more native state, either by coupling to protein antigens or by incorporation into natural polysaccharide-protein complexes. There are some indications that the latter possibility might also be applicable to group B, although we are still far from a vaccine based on group B polysaccharide.

Clinical Studies with the Pneumococcal Vaccine in Infants and Children

P. Helena Mäkelä

Although severe pneumococcal infections are usually thought of as a problem of old age, the incidence of pneumococcal bacteremia and meningitis is in fact higher at 0 to 4 years of age: 18 per 100,000 in the first year of life and 6 per 100,000 in the years 1 to 4, representing nearly 20% of bacteremia at this age. The main pneumococcal problem in infants and children is, however, acute otitis media. Studies in both the United States and Finland have found attack rates close to 50% in the first 2 years of life, declining gradually towards school age. The main etiological agent isolated from the purulent aspirate from the middle ear is *S. pneumoniae* (40 to 60% of all cases): types 19, 6, 23, 3, and 14 accounted for 74% of otitis media in a recent survey in Finland.

We have studied the use of the currently available 14-valent vaccine (Merck Sharp & Dohme) in infants and children ranging from 3 months to 6 years of age. The vaccine was very well tolerated when given as a booster dose 6 months after the first dose (this was done to all those who were younger than 2 years when receiving their first dose of vaccine); we believe this to be correlated with the relatively lower serum antibody levels compared to adults. The antibody response measured by radioimmunoassay or enzyme-linked immunosorbent assay was variable; of the most common types, the response was uniformly good to type 3, also good but strongly age dependent to type 19F, and poorer to types 23F and especially to 6A. For the two last-mentioned types, IgM class predominated in the response. Serum IgA antibodies to all types were detectable after (but not before) vaccination in about half of the children.

In a controlled, randomized trial, we gave either the pneumococcal or a control (*H. influenzae* type b) vaccine to 827 children who were recovering from a previous attack of otitis media, and we followed the development of recurrent attacks. In the first 6 months after vaccination, ca. 25% of the children experienced one or more recurrent attacks of otitis media. Whereas the number of such attacks caused (on the basis of culture of middle ear fluid) by other agents than pneumococci was similar in both the pneumococcal and the control vaccine groups, the rate of attacks caused by pneumococci was significantly ($P < 0.01$) smaller in the recipients of pneumococcal vaccine than in the control-vaccinated children. The indicated protection was 50% in children vaccinated at 7 months to 6 years of age. The difference was mostly due to pneumococcal types present in the vaccine, with the exception of group 6: the protection against these types reached 67%. The vaccine effect appeared to be short-lived, mostly limited to the first 6 months after vaccination.

Protective ability correlated with the serum antibody response to the individual types; although the data are limited by the small number of cases caused by each type, types causing a predominantly IgG type response appeared to cause better protection. Infants 3 to 6 months old showed poor antibody responses to almost all types and showed no benefit from the vaccine.

Immunoprophylaxis of Pneumococcal Infections

Jørgen Henrichsen

The currently available pneumococcal vaccine consists of 14 (out of 83) highly purified pneumococcal capsular polysaccharides. The purified bacterial polysaccharides have been characterized as "T-cell independent" immunogens: they show no memory and no booster effect, and they are poorly immunogenic in children under the age of 1 year. Recent work with other bacterial polysaccharides (meningococcal and *Haemophilus influenzae* type b) indicates that such antigens may be rendered T-cell dependent by coupling to proteins, e.g., bovine serum albumin and hemocyanin as well as tetanus and diphtheria toxoids. Although tolerance is easily induced in animals, it has not been seen in humans.

Vaccine formulation depends on (i) the most prevalent types and (ii) optimum antibody response to the maximum number of types. The 14-valent vaccines in most places cover approximately 80% of the types most commonly isolated from serious infections, if the distribution of types within groups is not considered; otherwise the coverage is 10% lower. This is under study. Groups 6, 19, and 9 have already been examined. Type 6A will probably also protect against type 6B, whereas 19F apparently is not sufficiently cross-immunogenic to induce protection against 19A, which therefore might have to be included in an improved future vaccine. Type 9A cross-reacts more extensively with the other group 9 types than does type 9N, which is presently included in the vaccine.

A world-wide typing surveillance study is presently being carried out under auspices of the World Health Organization to collect the information necessary for making intelligent decisions about future vaccine composition on the basis of the prevalent types in cases as related to time and area. It is apparent that type 5, which is not included in the present vaccine, is among the commonest types in many places, e.g., France, Israel, and Africa. It seems likely that 20 to 25 types cover more than 90% of the isolates from serious infections in most parts of the world. Vaccines of higher valency are under trial to see whether they will provide equally good antibody responses. If not, two vaccines will probably be made available: a core vaccine of approximately 14 types, and one or more additional vaccines of up to 10 types to be given sometime later.

Vaccine efficacy was shown by MacLeod et al. in 1945 using a tetravalent vaccine given to military recruits. Recently, efficacy has been shown in studies in South African miners and in natives of Papua New Guinea. Recent studies of use of pneumococcal vaccine include the following observations. (i) Efficacy has not been decisively demonstrated in aged persons, who show somewhat reduced antibody responses. (ii) Studies in otitis media have been inconclusive. (iii) Considering the increased risk of acquiring pneumococcal infections and the few side reactions to vaccination in splenectomized individuals, vaccination is recommended in these cases but should not be relied upon as the only prophylactic measure. (iv) We vaccinated patients with Hodgkin's disease before splenectomy and treatment because they do not respond for sometimes several years after treatment and it seems reasonable to try to mount an antibody response earlier. (v) Revaccination with the present T-cell independent vaccine should not be considered for at least 5 years. Antibody determination might prove to be necessary in each individual in order to be able to decide whether revaccination is advisable.

Comparative Studies on the Bactericidal Activities of Tetracyclines, Chloramphenicol, and Other "Bacteriostatic" Antibiotics

MOHAMMAD BAKHTIAR AND SYDNEY SELWYN*

Department of Medical Microbiology, Westminster Medical School, University of London, London SW1P A2R, England

Although many tetracycline derivatives have been made available since the original compound, chlortetracycline, was isolated from *Streptomyces aureofaciens* in 1948, all the antibiotics of this group in clinical use possess remarkably similar antibacterial activity. In practical terms the only improvement achieved in more than 30 years of research has been the enhanced activity of newer derivatives, notably minocycline, against gram-positive cocci and some other bacteria such as meningococci. The major deficiencies of all hitherto available tetracyclines have been their relatively poor activity against members of the *Enterobacteriaceae* group and an essentially bacteriostatic mode of action.

With the recent development (R. Kirchlechner, W. Rogalski, E. Dingeldein, and H. Wahlig, Program Abstr. Intersci. Conf. Antimicrob. Agents Chemother., 17th, New York, abstr. no. 70, 1977) of a class of thiatetracyclines, striking improvements both in activity against gram-negative bacilli and in bactericidal effect have been observed in our preliminary studies (2). These aspects were investigated further for the thiatetracycline compound EMD 33 330 (structure as for doxycycline, but with a sulfur instead of a carbon atom at position 6 and deletion of the hydroxyl at position 5) in parallel with tetracyline, minocycline, and doxycycline. In addition, the studies were extended to chloramphenicol and erythromycin, both of which are generally believed to have merely bacteriostatic activity.

The investigations were carried out on 10 epidemiologically unrelated strains of each of the following bacteria, which were obtained from clinical infections: *Escherichia coli*, *Proteus* species (6 indole negative, 4 indole positive), *Klebsiella* species, *Staphylococcus aureus*, and *Streptococcus pyogenes*. MICs and MBCs were determined with bacterial inocula of approximately 10^5 colony-forming units per ml and parallel close-dilution series in Iso-Sensitest agar and broth (Oxoid Ltd.), except for *Proteus* spp., for which the solid medium was CLED (cysteine lactose electrolyte-deficient agar; Oxoid). Killing curves were then constructed with the same media and inoculum size, with antibiotic concentrations at the MIC, as well as at twice and five times the MIC. Viable counts were determined at 0.5-h intervals for 6 h, and finally after 24 h of incubation.

Against *Proteus* spp., MICs of thiatetracycline EMD 33 300 ranged from 0.1 to 5 μg/ml, and MBCs were between two and four times higher. Killing curves showed that the antibiotic achieved a 99.9% cidal effect within 30 min at five times the MIC (Fig. 1) and within 2 h at twice the MIC. Minocycline was considerably less active but was the most efficient of the remaining antibiotics, having MICs between 5 and 50 μg/ml, but MBCs were not reached at 100 μg/ml. In addition, minocycline at five times the MIC produced a fall in the viable count of 99% after 5 h. Doxycycline possessed about half the inhibitory activity of minocycline; moreover, it produced a decrease in viable count of less than one logarithm after 6 h (Fig. 1). In turn, tetracycline showed approximately 50% less bacteriostatic activity than doxycycline and gave a minimal decrease in viable count after 6 h. Erythromycin was even less active, and both it and chloramphenicol had no perceptible cidal effect at the concentration used.

In the case of *Klebsiella* spp., all the tetracyclines possessed similar MICs (2 to 10 μg/ml), but EMD 33 330 alone had MBCs which were in the same range. EMD 33 330 also reduced the viable count by over 99.9% (five logarithms) within 1 h at five times the MIC (Fig. 2) and within 2.5 h at twice the MIC, whereas with the other tetracyclines the count was reduced by only one logarithm after 6 h. Chloramphenicol possessed less inhibitory activity than the tetracyclines, and its cidal activity was only demonstrable at 10 times the MIC after 18 h. Erythromycin was without effect in concentrations up to 100 μg/ml.

The results for all the antibiotics were very similar against *E. coli*, EMD 33 330 again showing remarkable cidal activity. This unique effect was not, however seen against either *S. aureus* or *S. pyogenes*; all the tetracyclines at five times

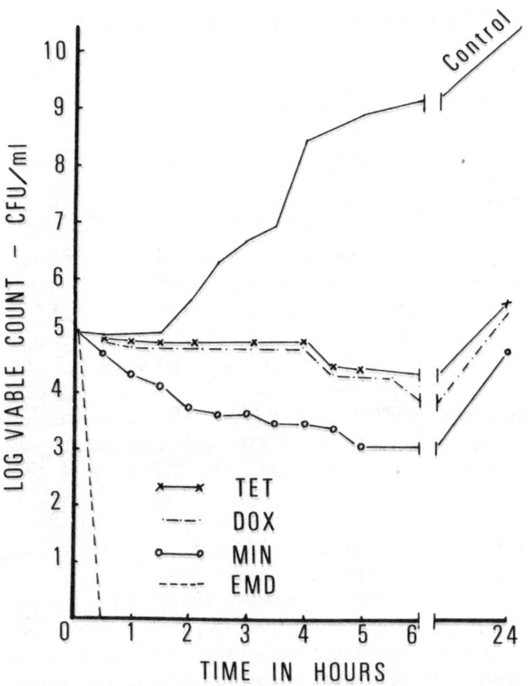

FIG. 1. *Tetracycline killing curves against Proteus mirabilis at five times the MIC in each case. TET, Tetracycline; DOX, doxycycline; MIN, minocycline; EMD, EMD 33 330.*

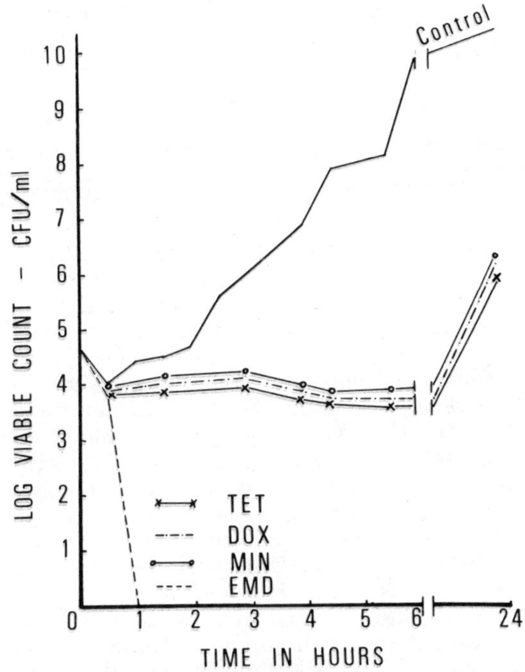

FIG. 2. *Tetracycline killing curves against Klebsiella aerogenes at five times the MIC in each case. Abbreviations as in Fig. 1.*

the MIC produced a decrease in viable count of about 1.7 log (98%) within 3 h. Chloramphenicol was slightly less active, but erythromycin was consistently the most active of the antibiotics against these gram-positive cocci in terms of MIC. Erythromycin's cidal effect was, however, relatively slow and limited.

The antibacterial effects of the antibiotics were also studied by both impediometry, by use of a Bactobridge (Lewis Williams & Co.), and turbidimetry, by use of a Biophotometer (Bonet-Maury). The Bactobridge provided the most detailed insight into the inhibitory action of the drugs from the earliest period of incubation, and it confirmed the remarkably rapid and powerful effect of EMD 33 330.

The customary generalization that tetracyclines have an exclusively bacteriostatic action is clearly misleading. Within therapeutic concentrations, a significant degree of cidal activity can be expected against susceptible gram-positive cocci, notably from minocycline. EMD 33 330 was, however, the only tetracycline with useful cidal activity against gram-negative bacilli within clinically achievable concentrations.

The cidal status of chloramphenicol is also controversial; although clinically significant bacterial killing is demonstrable against pneumococci, meningococci, and *Haemophilus influenzae*, this is not found against members of the *Enterobacteriaceae* (1). Erythromycin behaves similarly but with generally weaker cidal activity.

We thank E. Dingeldein and H. Wahlig of E. Merck for advice and for supplying EMD 33 330. We also thank A. Ur for advice on the Bactobridge, which was lent by Lewis Williams & Co.

1. **Rahal, J. J., Jr., and M. S. Simberkoff.** 1979. Bactericidal and bacteriostatic action of chloramphenicol against meningeal pathogens. Antimicrob. Agents Chemother. **16:**13–18.
2. **Teare, E. L., M. Bakhtiar, and S. Selwyn.** 1981. Comparative in vitro studies of a new thiatetracyline and three existing tetracyclines. Drugs Exp. Clin. Res. **7:** 307–311.

Comparative In Vitro Studies of 10 Antipseudomonal β-Lactam Antibiotics

SHEDDA AL-KHOURI, MOHAMMAD BAKHTIAR, AND SYDNEY SELWYN*

Department of Medical Microbiology, Westminster Medical School, University of London, London, SW1P A2R, England

Within the past 5 years, the pharmaceutical industry has made available for clinical use an embarrassingly rich choice of penicillins and, more recently, both cephalosporins and novel β-lactam compounds with activity against *Pseudomonas aeruginosa.* These antibiotics are to be particularly welcomed as safe alternatives to the relatively toxic aminoglycosides, but truly comparative data are urgently required to resolve the increasing confusion about the activities of these heterogeneous derivatives.

Comprehensive in vitro studies were therefore carried out in a strictly parallel manner on all the available anti-*Pseudomonas* β-lactam agents against 100 epidemiologically unrelated clinical isolates of *P. aeruginosa.* The antibiotics investigated were azlocillin, carbenicillin, cefotaxime, cefsulodin, ceftazidime, mezlocillin, moxalactam, piperacillin, ticarcillin, and a novel monocyclic β-lactam compound, monobactam SQ 26,776. In addition, the studies were extended to the aminoglycosides gentamicin, tobramycin, and amikacin, and to polymyxins B and E (colistin), to obtain comparative data on therapeutic indices across the whole range of systemic agents.

MICs and MBCs were determined in both Iso-Sensitest broth and agar (Oxoid Ltd.) with initial bacterial inocula of 10^5 colony-forming units per ml. Killing curves were constructed for each antibiotic against 10 representative strains; detailed information on the dynamics of antibacterial action was also derived from impediometry studies, performed with a Bactobridge (Lewis Williams & Co.), as well as by means of direct microscopic observations on morphological changes and turbidimetric studies performed with a Biophotometer (Bonet-Maury).

The highest inhibitory activity was possessed by piperacillin and ceftazidime, both of which had approximately 80% of their MICs falling below 5 μg/ml (Fig. 1). Cefsulodin, moxalactam, azlocillin, and SQ 26,776 were next in order of inhibitory activity, with approximately 80% of MICs below 15 μg/ml and 50% below 10 μg/ml. These were followed in descending order by cefotaxime, ticarcillin, mezlocillin, and carbenicillin with 80% cumulative inhibition at 30, 49, 78, and 90 μg/ml, respectively.

When five times the MIC of each antibiotic was added in parallel to fresh cultures that had received the relatively high inoculum level of 10^5 colony-forming units per ml, the most rapid bactericidal effects were observed with ceftazidime, moxalactam, and azlocillin. Each of them produced a 99.9% kill within 3 to 5 h, and usually no viable pseudomonads were detectable after a further 1 h. Cefsulodin, piperacillin, and SQ 26,776 took approximately 1 h longer to give the same bactericidal effect. The slowest cidal effect was generally produced by, in descending order, mezlocillin, ticarcillin, and carbenicillin. Cefotaxime often gave a biphasic result, with a relatively rapid kill to almost the 99.9% level, followed by slower subsequent activity, to achieve undetectable viable counts at about the same time as mezlocillin and azlocillin but before carbenicillin. Similar, but marginally slower cidal effects were obtained with twice the MIC.

Table 1 summarizes the results of one complete killing-curve experiment on a representative strain which did not produce significant amounts of β-lactamase. With five times the MIC, an apparently complete bacterial kill was achieved in 4 h by ceftazidime, azlocillin, and moxalactam; in 5 h by piperacillin, SQ 26,776, and cefsulodin; in 5.5 h by cefotaxime, mezlocillin, and ticarcillin; and finally in 6 h by carbenicillin.

Significant increases in MICs occurred with all the antibiotics when the inoculum size was raised by two or more logarithms, even in the case of nonproducers of β-lactamase. The increase ranged from 10- to 100-fold when the inoculum was changed from 10^4 to 10^8 colony-forming units per ml, and an even greater effect on MBCs was noted. This phenomenon has been widely recognized as a feature of the interaction of *P. aeruginosa* and carbenicillin, but it extends equally to ticarcillin and, to a lesser extent, to the acylureidopenicillins, as well as other anti-*Pseudomonas* β-lactam agents. The effect has, however, been reported to be minimal with the new derivative *N*-formimidoyl thienamycin (1). Preincubation of cultures for 2 h before addition of antibiotic is a convenient means of assessing the combined effect of inoculum increase and β-lactamase production. The influence of serum

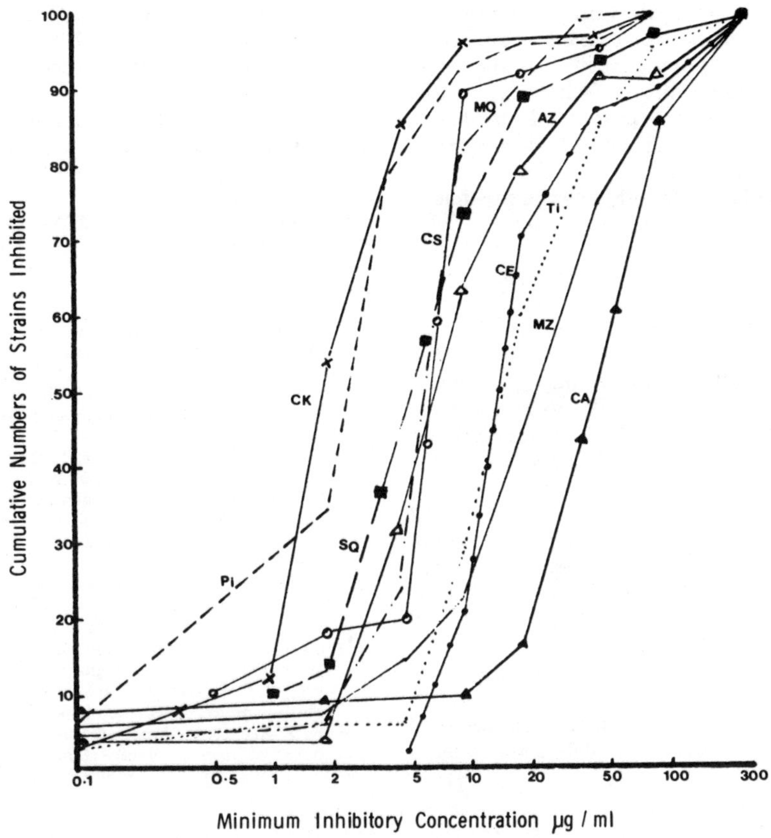

FIG. 1. *Cumulative MIC values for 10 β-lactam antibiotics against 100 strains of P. aeruginosa. Pi, Piperacillin; CK, ceftazidime; SQ, SQ 26,776; CS, cefsulodin; MO, moxalactam; AZ, azlocillin; CE, cefotaxime; Ti, ticarcillin; MZ, mezlocillin; CA, carbenicillin.*

TABLE 1. *Bactericidal effects of 10 β-lactam antibiotics on a representative strain of P. aeruginosa*[a]

Antibiotic	Log viable count (colony-forming units per ml)							
	0 h	0.5 h	1 h	2 h	3 h	4 h	5 h	6 h
Carbenicillin	4.8	4.2	4.2	3.4	2.8	2.8	1.8	0
Ticarcillin	4.8	4.8	4.6	4.5	3.0	2.2	1.5	0
Azlocillin	4.8	4.1	4.1	3.1	2.7	0	0	0
Mezlocillin	4.8	4.8	4.5	3.2	3.0	2.4	1.2	0
Piperacillin	4.8	4.5	4.5	4.0	3.4	2.5	0	0
Cefotaxime	4.8	4.2	3.8	2.2	1.8	1.8	1.5	0
Cefsulodin	4.8	4.8	4.5	3.8	2.1	1.8	0	0
Ceftazidime	4.8	4.5	4.2	4.0	2.2	0	0	0
Moxalactam	4.8	4.2	4.0	3.5	2.2	0	0	0
SQ 26,776	4.8	4.6	4.3	3.7	2.5	1.7	0	0
Control[b]	4.8	4.5	4.6	5.0	6.2	6.5	8.1	8.8

[a] Results of killing-curve studies.
[b] No antibiotic present.

protein binding can be readily observed in the same system (3), but with the antibiotics under review was found to produce a modest decrease of anti-*Pseudomonas* activity only with carbenicillin and ticarcillin.

Detailed observations on morphological changes, made by use of interference microscopy (Zeiss), confirmed our earlier finding that the production of spheroplasts relative to filaments is, for most β-lactam agents, sensitively dose dependent (3). In particular, no consistent differences were found between carboxypenicillins, acylureidopenicillins, or piperacillin in their ability to produce spheroplasts. When fully calibrated, the Biophotometer permitted automated monitoring of these changes under closely specified culture conditions.

The Bactobridge, however, was the most sensitive indicator of antibacterial action from within 10 min of setting up cultures. It clearly demonstrated the remarkably rapid inhibitory effect of piperacillin at relatively low concentrations, findings which are in keeping with the unusually high affinity of the drug for penicillin-binding proteins 1A and 3 of *P. aeruginosa* (2). The Bactobridge also revealed a very early antibacterial effect with SQ 26,776, a semisynthetic "monobactam" from *Chromobacterium violaceum* (4). This agent was selected for study from a group of novel monocyclic derivatives and possesses even greater activity against a wide range of otherwise antibiotic-resistant gram-negative bacilli, including *Enterobacter*, *Serratia*, and *Acinetobacter* species (unpublished data).

On a weight-for-weight basis, the three aminoglycosides and two polymyxins possessed between 3 and 10 times more anti-*Pseudomonas* activity than the six most active β-lactam agents (piperacillin, ceftazidime, cefsulodin, azlocillin, moxalactam, and SQ 26,776). However, when mean therapeutic indices were calculated from published toxicological and experimental chemotherapeutic data, all the β-lactam agents except mezlocillin and carbenicillin were superior to the aminoglycosides and polymyxins.

We thank A. Ur for advice on the use of the Bactobridge, which was lent by Lewis Williams & Co. R. B. Sykes, Squibb Research Institute, kindly supplied SQ 26,776.

1. **Hanslo, D., A. King, K. Shannon, C. Warren, and I. Phillips.** 1981. *N*-Formimidoyl thienamycin (MK 0787): *in-vitro* antibacterial activity and susceptibility to beta-lactamases compared with that of cefotaxime, moxalactam and other beta-lactam antibiotics. J. Antimicrob. Chemother. **7:**607–617.
2. **Mitsuhashi, S., Y. Fukuoka, T. Hayashi, N. Matsubara, T. Yasuda, and I. Saikawa.** 1978. Antibacterial activities of piperacillin, a new synthetic penicillin, p. 603–605. *In* W. Siegenthaler and R. Lüthy (ed.), Current chemotherapy, vol. 2. American Society for Microbiology, Washington, D.C.
3. **Selwyn, S.** 1980. The beta-lactam antibiotics: penicillins and cephalosporins in perspective, p. 57–62, 144–158. Hodder and Stoughton, London.
4. **Sykes, R. B., C. M. Cimarusti, D. P. Bonner, K. Bush, D. M. Floyd, N. H. Georgopapadakou, W. H. Koster, W. C. Liu, W. L. Parker, P. A. Principe, M. L. Rathnum, W. A. Slusarchyk, W. H. Trejo, and J. S. Wells.** 1981. Monocyclic β-lactam antibiotics produced by bacteria. Nature (London) **291:**489–490.

Chemical Composition of Outer Membranes from Nutrient-Depleted Cultures of *Pseudomonas Aeruginosa*

ROBERT M. COZENS* AND MICHAEL R. W. BROWN

Department of Pharmacy, University of Aston in Birmingham, Birmingham B4 7ET, United Kingdom

The cell envelope of gram-negative bacteria, particularly the outer membrane, is altered greatly with changes in the growth environment. These changes alter the response of the organism to antibacterial agents and body defense mechanisms. These observations have significant implications for the correlation of in vitro and in vivo activities of antibacterial agents.

The role of iron, and possibly other nutrients, in microbial infections suggests that the use of nutritionally defined cultures may be important in studies of antibacterial agents.

We used cultures of *Pseudomonas aeruginosa* NCTC 6750, grown to stationary phase, which had been induced by the depletion of one essential nutrient. Chemostat cultures limited by iron and magnesium at two different growth rates were also examined.

Protein and phospholipid analyses were undertaken on isolated outer membrane preparations obtained by sucrose density centrifugation of total membrane fractions. The assay methods used are well documented (1, 5, 6).

Total protein and lipid analyses are given in Table 1. It should be noted that the protein was markedly reduced in phosphate-limited cells. Iron-depleted cells and slow-growing iron-limited cells also showed a reduction in the protein content.

Whereas the total lipid (REL) varied markedly between cultures, the amount of phospholipid was relatively constant except for low contents in the fast-growing chemostat cultures. However, there was a big variation in the amounts of individual phospholipids. No general pattern occurred except that growing cells con-

TABLE 1. *Total protein and lipid content of the outer membrane of P. aeruginosa grown under various conditions*

Component	Cells depleted by							Chemostat cultures			
	O_2 nutrient broth	O_2 defined medium	Fe^{2+}	Mg^{2+}	Glucose	NH_4^+	PO_4^{3+}	Fe^{2+}, D = 0.055	Mg^{2+}, D = 0.055	Fe^{2+}, D = 0.25	Mg^{2+}, D = 0.25
Protein[a]	542	547	395	527	437	584	303	427	493	503	509
Total extractable lipid[a]	225	227	257	298	341	284	456	184	207	131	142
Phospholipid[a]	176	203	205	197	221	213	194	176	189	98	85
Diphosphatidyl glycerol[b]	31.5	66.7	74.2	58.2	56.3	65.2	45.3	56.6	42.7	43.8	38.3
Phosphatidyl ethanolamine[b]	24.1	15.2	9.3	21.2	24.4	17.3	10.3	15.2	31.2	34.2	38.0
Phosphatidyl glycerol[b]	ND	5.4	10.8	T	T	5.6	20.7	16.6	6.3	17.0	7.2
Unidentified phospholipid[b]	44.0	11.1	13.6	20.6	19.3	11.7	23.5	11.6	19.7	5.1	16.3

[a] Expressed as micrograms per milligram (dry weight) of outer membrane.
[b] Expressed as percentage of total phospholipid. T, Less than 2%; ND, none detected. Unidentified phospholipid (R_f = 0.32) was choline and ninhydrin negative.

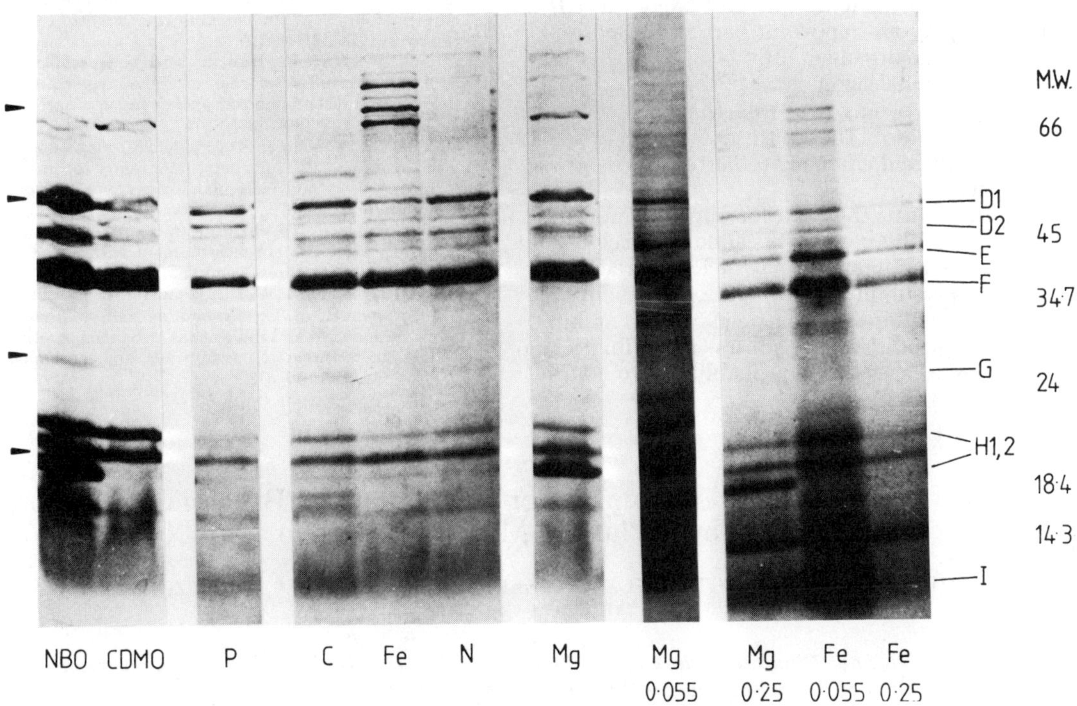

FIG. 1. *Sodium dodecyl sulfate-polyacrylamide gel electrophoresis profiles of outer membrane proteins from P. aeruginosa grown under various conditions. NBO, Oxygen depleted in nutrient broth; COMO, oxygen depleted in chemically defined medium; Fe, iron (ferrous) depleted; P, phosphate depleted; N, ammonium depleted; C, glucose depleted; Mg, magnesium depleted; Fe 0.055, Mg 0.055, Fe 0.25, and Mg 0.25, chemostat cultures limited by nutrient indicated and at dilution rate shown. Arrows indicate points of interest. Molecular weights given in kilodaltons.*

tained less phospholipid than stationary-phase or slow-growing cells.

Figure 1 shows sodium dodecyl sulfate-polyacrylamide gel electrophoresis profiles of the outer membrane proteins. Again, marked variation in the pattern was observed. The induction of proteins of about 70,000 daltons when cells are starved of iron is well known (4). The appearance of protein H1 when cells are starved of magnesium has also been reported (7). Protein

D1 has been shown to be induced when glucose is the carbon source (3). We have found that this protein is increased when cells become depleted of glucose. When glycerol replaced glucose as carbon source, this protein was not present in large amounts and was not increased when cells were depleted of glycerol (data not shown). Protein F (the major pore-forming protein) did not vary greatly with changes in growth conditions. Protein G was present in appreciable amounts in cultures depleted of glucose. No function has been assigned to this protein.

In addition to these observations, a closer examination of the data indicates that there may be other components (not assayed) associated with, or part of, the outer membrane which may vary when growth conditions are changed. These other components could be the antigenic polysaccharide side chain of the lipopolysaccharide or associated extracellular material which is known to be present around most bacterial cells and may play an important part in the pathogenicity of the organism (2).

The functional significance of these changes is not clear. It seems probable that the cell is adapting to obtain those nutrients which are in short supply and changing to better survive the starvation.

In interpreting the data for outer membrane composition, the possibility cannot be excluded that certain components may be lost or redistributed as a result of the preparation procedure.

There are differences between in vitro and in vivo susceptibilities of organisms to antibiotics, and in some cases this is probably due to adaptive changes in vivo. Similarly, it has been shown recently that clinical isolates have acquired resistance during therapy. This resistance was not due to the production of antibiotic-inactivating enzymes, but was probably due to an exclusion mechanism.

It would be interesting to see what effect sub-MICs of antibiotics would have on outer membrane composition in cells grown under various conditions, some of which may mimic the in vivo situation.

1. **Bligh, E. G., and W. J. Dyer.** 1959. A rapid method of total lipid extraction and purification. Can. J. Biochem. Physiol. **37**:911–917.
2. **Costerton, J. W., M. R. W. Brown, and J. M. Sturgess.** 1979. The cell envelope: its role in infection, p. 41–62. *In* R. G. Doggett (ed.), *Pseudomonas aeruginosa*: clinical manifestations of infection and current therapy. Academic Press, London.
3. **Hancock, R. E. W., and A. M. Carey.** 1980. Protein D1—a glucose inducible, pore-forming protein from the outer membrane of *Pseudomonas aeruginosa*. FEMS Microbiol. Lett. **8**:105–109.
4. **Hancock, R. E. W., K. Hantke, and V. Braun.** 1976. Iron transport in *Escherichia coli* K-12: involvement of the colicin B receptor and of a citrate inducible protein. J. Bacteriol. **127**:1370–1375.
5. **Kates, M.** 1972. Techniques of lipidology, p. 428–446. *In* T. S. Work and E. Work (ed.), Laboratory techniques in biochemistry and molecular biology, vol. 3. North Holland Publishing Co., Amsterdam.
6. **Lowry, O. H., N. J. Rosebrough, A. L. Farr, and R. J. Randall.** 1951. Protein measurement with the Folin phenol reagent. J. Biol. Chem. **193**:265–275.
7. **Nicas, T. I., and R. E. W. Hancock.** 1980. Outer membrane protein H1 of *Pseudomonas aeruginosa* involvement in adaptive and mutational resistance to ethylenediaminetetraacetate, polymyxin B, and gentamicin. J. Bacteriol. **143**:872–878.

Effect of Subinhibitory Antibiotic Concentrations on Bacterial Adhesion to Fibrin-Platelet Matrices In Vitro

W. MICHAEL SCHELD,* OTOKAR ZAK, KLAUS VOSBECK, LYDIA KLOETZLEN, AND MERLE A. SANDE

University of Virginia, Charlottesville, Virginia 22908, U.S.A.; Ciba-Geigy Limited, Basel, Switzerland; and San Francisco General Hospital, San Francisco, California 94110, U.S.A.*

Subinhibitory concentrations (sub-MICs) of many antibiotics have profound effects on the exposed bacteria, including a decreased growth rate, morphological alterations, enhanced leukocytic ingestion or killing, and reduced bacterial adhesion to epithelial cells in most systems (1). We have shown previously that adhesion of oral streptococci to nonbacterial thrombotic endocarditis (NBTE = the nidus for colonization in bacterial endocarditis) is important in the pathogenesis of this disease (3). The effect of sub-MICs on the adhesion of these strains to the constituents of NBTE (fibrin and platelets) is unknown but may be relevant to the prophylaxis or therapy of bacterial endocarditis.

The purposes of these studies were to determine the influence of sub-MICs on bacterial adhesion to the constituents of NBTE in vitro and to determine whether a reduced bacterial adhesion after exposure to sub-MICs of antibiotics correlates with a reduced propensity to produce endocarditis in vivo.

The in vitro studies utilized modifications of our previously described model of NBTE (3). An 18-h culture of the organism under study (*Streptococcus sanguis*, *S. faecalis*, or *Staphylococcus aureus*) was exposed to an antibiotic at various concentrations at 37°C for various periods of time. The organisms were washed (three times), resuspended in saline, filtered (8-μm membrane filter), diluted to $\simeq 10^3$ colony-forming units (CFU) per ml (verified by quantitative serial dilutions and pour plates in Trypticase soy agar), overlaid on a fibrin-platelet matrix in 65-mm tissue culture dishes (3), agitated for 15 min at 37°C, washed (three times) with saline, overlaid with Trypticase soy agar containing 5% defibrinated sheep blood, and counted after further incubation for 24 h at 37°C. The adherence ratio (AR) was defined as: AR = number of adherent organisms (CFU)/no. of organisms in initial inoculum (CFU). The AR was multiplied times 10^4 to facilitate comparisons. Various antibiotics were studied at one-fourth the MIC: penicillin, trimethoprim-sulfamethoxazole, rifampin, streptomycin, chloramphenicol, tetracycline, and vancomycin. Any dose dependence (vancomycin and *S. sanguis* or *S. faecalis* at 1/64, 1/32, 1/16, 1/8, and 1/4 the MIC) and effect of time of exposure (0.5, 1.0, 2.0, 3.0, 4.0, and 6.0 h at 1/4 the MIC) were also studied. Hydrophobic interaction chromatography was used to investigate any changes of sub-MICs (at 1/4 the MIC) on surface hydrophobicity of *S. sanguis* or *S. faecalis* (4).

The effect of sub-MICs on the development of endocarditis in vivo was assessed after catheter-induced aortic valve trauma (1-h catheterization) in New Zealand white rabbits (2). Two groups were studied at the same inoculum, 10^6 CFU, given intravenously: control *S. sanguis* and *S. sanguis* exposed to 1/4 the MIC of vancomycin for 4 h. Three days after inoculation, the animals were sacrificed, and the aortic valve vegetations were removed, weighed, homogenized, and quantitatively cultured on Trypticase soy agar-sheep blood pour plates.

The effect of sub-MICs of antibiotics (all at 1/4 the MIC) on adhesion of *S. sanguis* to the constituents of NBTE in vitro is shown in Table 1. Some agents, e.g., trimethoprim-sulfamethoxazole increased adhesion, but most decreased adhesion when compared with controls. The

TABLE 1. *Effect of sub-MICs (1/4 MIC) of antibiotics on adhesion of S. sanguis to fibrin-platelet matrices in vitro*

Drug	Adherence ratio (mean ± SD)[a]
None (controls)	643 ± 47
Penicillin	192 ± 60
Tetracycline	195 ± 46
Trimethoprim-sulfamethoxazole	1291 ± 81
Rifampin	543 ± 42
Streptomycin	293 ± 31
Chloramphenicol	221 ± 45
Vancomycin	113 ± 38

[a] All ratios have been multiplied times 10^4.

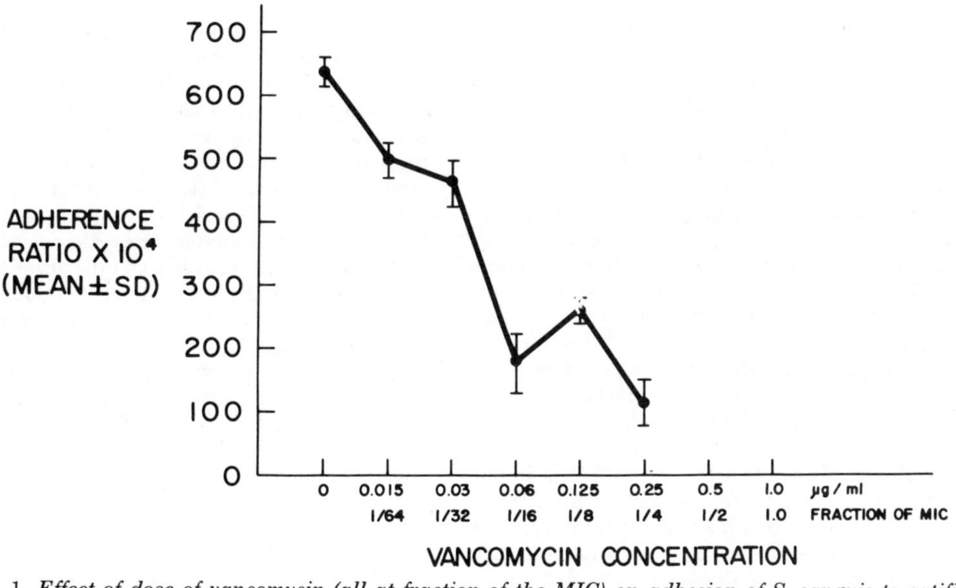

FIG. 1. *Effect of dose of vancomycin (all at fraction of the MIC) on adhesion of S. sanguis to artificial fibrin-platelet matrices in vitro.*

mean AR as a percentage of controls was as follows: penicillin, 30%; streptomycin, 45.6%; chloramphenicol, 34.4%; and vancomycin, 17.6% ($P < 0.01$ versus controls). Similar results were found with *S. faecalis* and *S. aureus*.

This effect was dose dependent (Fig. 1). For example, with vancomycin and *S. sanguis* the mean ARs, as a percentage of the control, were as follows: 1/64 MIC, 82.3%; 1/16 MIC, 44.6%; 1/4 MIC, 17.6%. Similar results were seen with penicillin or streptomycin and *S. sanguis*. The effect was dependent on time of exposure; a significant decrease was apparent after 1 h (69.3% of control, $P < 0.01$), and a maximum effect was observed after 4 to 6 h of incubation (17 to 32% of control, $P < 0.01$). There was no correlation between decreased bacterial adhesion and altered retention by hydrophobic interaction chromatography.

The reduced bacterial adhesion of *S. sanguis* after exposure to 1/4 the MIC of vancomycin directly correlated with a reduced ability to produce endocarditis in vivo. After injection of control *S. sanguis* (inoculum = $\log_{10}$ 6.178 CFU), 9 of 12 rabbits developed endocarditis versus only 3 of 12 with endocarditis after injection of vancomycin-exposed *S. sanguis* ($P = 0.05$, Fisher exact test).

The results may be relevant to the prophylaxis or therapy of endocarditis, in which sub-MICs of antibiotics may reduce adhesion of the gram-positive cocci at the mucosal surface or in the bloodstream to NBTE.

1. **Lorian, V.** 1980. Effect of subminimum inhibitory concentrations of antibiotics on bacteria, p. 342–408. *In* V. Lorian (ed.), Antibiotics in laboratory medicine.
2. **Scheld, W. M., J. H. Thomas, and M. A. Sande.** 1979. Influence of preformed antibody on experimental *Streptococcus sanguis* endocarditis. Infect. Immun. **25:**781–785.
3. **Scheld, W. M., J. A. Valone, and M. A. Sande.** 1978. Bacterial adherence in the pathogenesis of endocarditis: interaction of bacterial dextran, platelets, and fibrin. J. Clin. Invest. **61:**1394–1404.
4. **Smyth, C. J., P. Jonsson, E. Olsson, O. Soderlind, J. Rosengren, S. Hjerten, and T. Wadstrom.** 1978. Differences in hydrophobic surface characteristics of porcine enteropathogenic *Escherichia coli* with or without K88 antigen as revealed by hydrophobic interaction chromatography. Infect. Immun. **22:**462–472.

Sensitive and Rapid Microbiological Procedure for Assaying Antibiotics in Small Volumes

H. WAHLIG AND E. DINGELDEIN

Department of Medical Microbiology, E. Merck, Darmstadt, Federal Republic of Germany

Monitoring of serum concentrations after application of potentially toxic antibiotics is still indicated in severely ill patients because of the possibility of drug cumulation due to impaired renal function and to avoid toxic levels, as well as to ensure therapeutically effective concentrations. Various rapid methods such as enzymatic or radioimmunological procedures were developed to meet these requirements and to make dose adjustment possible during therapy. These techniques, however, require substantial expenditure on apparatus and cannot be carried out in every clinic.

A rapid and accurate high-temperature assay based on the conventional agar diffusion test has been developed in which *Bacillus stearothermophilus* is used as a test organism. Antibiotica-Agar No. 5, pH 8.0 (Merck, no. 5271) is inoculated with 5×10^5 colony-forming units per ml. Incubation is for 3 to 4 h at 62°C. Six-millimeter filter-paper discs can be used as drug reservoirs for standard and test fluids, and 10 to 20 μl of fluid gives sharp zones of inhibition of adequate size. As a result of the extreme sensitivity of the test strain, the high incubation temperature, and the short time of incubation, this method is suitable for several additional indications other than serum monitoring: (i) as a routine procedure for the evaluation of various antibiotics such as aminoglycosides, β-lactam antibiotics, lincomycin, clindamycin, or erythromycin; (ii) as bioassay of antibiotics even if only small volumes of test samples are available or if concentrations in the test fluids are low (determination in cerebrospinal fluid, in tissues, or tissue fluids, in pediatrics or in small laboratory animals); (iii) in preliminary investigations to check the trial plan; (iv) for estimation of the range of concentrations in samples in a pretrial to ensure an appropriate reading of the concentrations from the standard curve when no hint as to the concentration in the sample is available; and (v) in the evaluation of antibiotic concentrations in contaminated samples (urine, aqueous fecal sus-

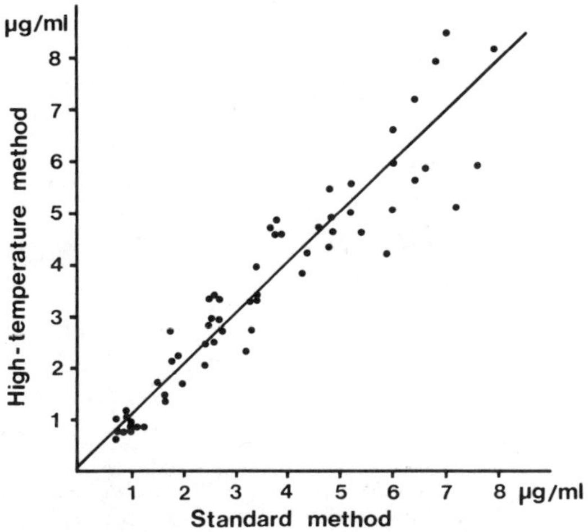

FIG. 1. *Correlation of concentrations assayed in high-temperature and standard methods.*

pension, pus) without aseptic conditions or sterilization of the test materials.

The following examples indicate the usefulness, accuracy, and applicability of the *B. stearothermophilus* assay.

Sixty serum samples from eight patients treated with gentamicin were tested by the high-temperature method and by a standard method using *B. subtilis*. Evaluation by the method of least error squares based on the linear regression equation $y = a + b \times x$ gave the following results: $y = 0.17 + 0.96 \times x$; SD, 0.665; correlation coefficient $r = 0.95$ (Fig. 1).

In a blind study, batches of 15 serum samples with known gentamicin concentrations (1, 4, and 8 μg/ml) were randomized and assayed by the high-temperature and standard methods. Mean values, SDs, and confidence limits demonstrated good agreement of the two procedures.

Standard curves of 17 different antibiotics were established by the high-temperature method. The results indicated that this method is most suitable for routine assays of aminoglycosides, β-lactam antibiotics, lincomycin, clindamycin, and erythromycin.

For evaluation of the pharmacokinetic parameters of cefazedone, capillary blood samples from 28 patients (6 neonates, 12 infants, 10 adults) were taken up to 6 h after an intravenous loading dose of 50 mg/kg of body weight and were assayed by the high-temperature method. The kinetics of cefazedone could be described by an open two-compartment model. There was a rapid distribution between the two compartments; however, the elimination constant was significantly lower in newborns (median: 0.339 h^{-1}) as compared with infants (1.00 h^{-1}) and adults (0.858 h^{-1}). Accordingly, the half-life was longer in neonates (3.3 h) than in infants (1.2 h) and adults (1.6 h), indicating reduced renal elimination in neonates.

The important advantage of this method which makes it most suitable for pharmacokinetic studies, particularly in small children, is the high sensitivity of *B. stearothermophilus*. Concentrations as small as 0.01 to 0.05 μg/ml can be measured, and small test samples of 10 to 20 μl are sufficient. Amounts of 40 μl of capillary blood can be easily withdrawn by puncture of the heel of newborns even if repeated sampling is required, and thus venipunctures can be avoided.

Paradoxical Effects in the Subinhibitory Activity of Fosfomycin

S. ENENKEL, U. CAMMAN,* AND W. STILLE

Zentrum der Inneren Medizin, J. W.-Goethe-Universität, Frankfurt am Main, West Germany

We investigated the activity of subinhibitory concentrations of fosfomycin in *Staphylococcus aureus* (eight strains) in comparison with β-lactam antibiotics, using the MS-2 Research System (Abbott Laboratories) and Mueller-Hinton broth. The subinhibitory activity of fosfomycin against *S. aureus* was found to differ markedly from that of β-lactam antibiotics. The minimal active concentration (MAC) of fosfomycin was 250 to 500 times lower than the MIC (Fig. 1, strain 9240: MIC > 200 μg/ml, MAC < 0.4 μg/ml), whereas the MAC of cefoperazone, for instance, is only 4 to 8 times lower than the MIC (strain 9240: MIC = 6.25 μg/ml, MAC = 1.6 μg/ml).

In *S. aureus* subinhibitory concentrations of fosfomycin led to paradoxical "double-peak" growth curves (Fig. 1). Low concentrations of fosfomycin (0.4, 0.8, 1.6, and 3.1 μg/ml = 0.2 to 1.5% of the MIC) led to gradual reduction of turbidity. With higher concentrations (6.25, 12.5, 25, and 50 μg/ml = 5 to 50% of the MIC) para-

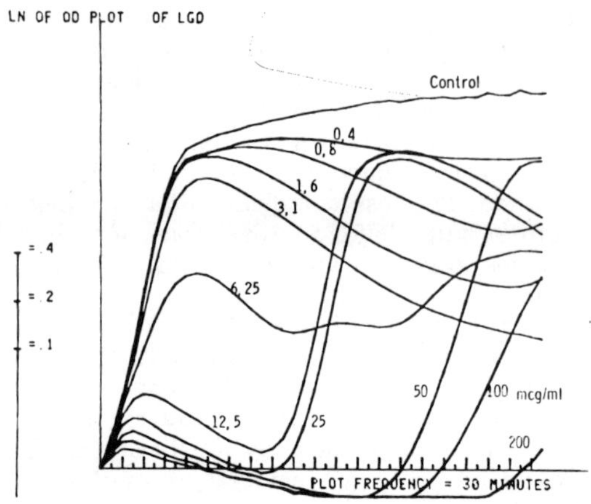

FIG. 1. *Subinhibitory activity of fosfomycin in S. aureus (9240). Inoculum: 10^6/ml. Mueller-Hinton broth.*

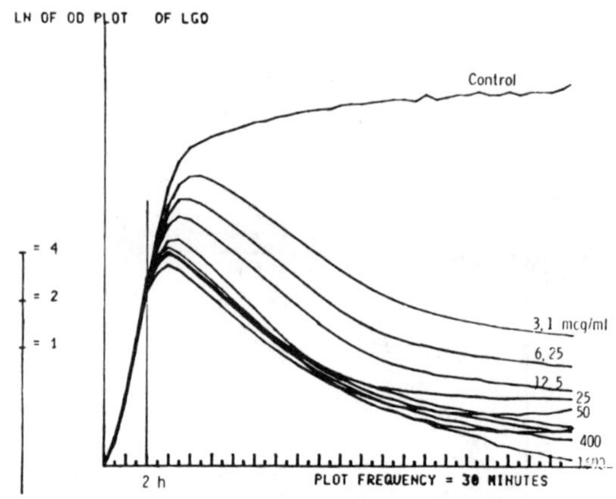

FIG. 2. *Growth inhibition of S. aureus (9240) by fosfomycin. Exposure: 2 h. Mueller-Hinton broth.*

doxical growth curves were observed: after an initial "up and down," a second rise was noticed with a subsequent second decline. Comparable growth curves cannot be demonstrated with other antibiotics.

High inocula (>10^4/ml) led to more pronounced paradoxical growth curves with fosfomycin. Using inocula below 10^5/ml, we only registered a delayed outgrowth of the strains.

The influence of fosfomycin on growing cultures of *S. aureus* depends on the exposure time. After exposure for 1 and 1.5 h, paradoxical growth curves could usually be demonstrated with fosfomycin. At times >2 h, after an initial rise of the curves a gradual decline could be observed (Fig. 2).

Paradoxical fosfomycin effects could also be demonstrated by turbidimetric analysis and cell count.

The in vitro activity of fosfomycin distinctly differs from that of other antibiotics. Our results confirm once more the position of fosfomycin as an abnormal antibiotic. In vitro results obtained with fosfomycin should be evaluated with great caution.

Comparative Bactericidal Effects of α-Carboxypenicillins (Carbenicillin and Ticarcillin) and Acylaminopenicillins (Apalcillin, Azlocillin, Mezlocillin, and Piperacillin) Against *Pseudomonas aeruginosa*

KEITH R. COMBER, KAREN E. GRIFFIN, ANTHONY R. WHITE, AND ROBERT SUTHERLAND*

Beecham Pharmaceuticals Research Division, Betchworth, Surrey, England

The broad-spectrum penicillins active against *Pseudomonas aeruginosa* fall into two classes: the α-carboxypenicillins, namely, carbenicillin and ticarcillin, and the acylaminopenicillins, that is, apalcillin together with the ureidopenicillin group comprised of azlocillin, mezlocillin, and piperacillin. The data reported here were derived from experiments designed to compare the bactericidal effects produced against *P. aeruginosa* by these two classes of penicillins. The tests included comparison of MIC and MBC values, turbidimetric measurement of bacteriolytic activity, determination of viable counts in tests against large and dilute inocula, studies of the morphological effects observed, and measurement of the β-lactamase activity of *P. aeruginosa* during the course of the bactericidal tests.

MICs and MBCs. Results in Table 1 show the MIC and MBC values of the six antipseudomonal penicillins against three typical strains of *P. aeruginosa*. The acylaminopenicillins were generally more active than the α-carboxypenicillins in the MIC tests against the test strains of *P. aeruginosa*, and the activity of the compounds (in descending order) was: apalcillin, pi-

TABLE 1. *MICs and MBCs of α-carboxypenicillins and acylaminopenicillins*

Penicillin	Concn (μg/ml) for *P. aeruginosa* strains					
	NCTC 10662		ATCC 27853		11	
	MIC[a]	MBC[b]	MIC	MBC	MIC	MBC
Ticarcillin	50	125	125	250	50	50
Carbenicillin	125	500	125	500	50	125
Azlocillin	25	5,000	25	>5,000	12.5	>5,000
Mezlocillin	50	>5,000	125	1,250	25	>5,000
Piperacillin	12.5	2,500	25	500	5.0	>5,000
Apalcillin	5.0	>5,000	12.5	1,250	5.0	>5,000

[a] Serial dilution in nutrient broth; inoculum, 1×10^5 to 4×10^5 cells per ml; MIC values read after 24 h at 37°C.

[b] A 0.01-ml amount subcultured onto Mueller-Hinton agar; MBC, <5 colonies (99.9% kill).

peracillin, azlocillin, mezlocillin, ticarcillin, and carbenicillin. However, the bactericidal activities of the compounds fell into a completely different order, and the α-carboxypenicillins were notably more effective than the acylaminopenicillins. Thus, the MBC values of carbenicillin and ticarcillin were only two- to fourfold higher than the MIC values, whereas the MBC values of azlocillin, mezlocillin, piperacillin, and apalcillin were usually in excess of 1,000 μg/ml.

The bacterial counts of the cultures in the serial-dilution tests with *P. aeruginosa* NCTC 10662 were measured after 24 h of incubation, i.e., when the MIC values were determined and when a loopful was subcultured for determination of MBCs. The results showed that the viable counts of the cultures grown in the presence of the acylaminopenicillins remained at or about the level of the starting inocula (10^4 to 10^5 cells per ml), at all concentrations above the MIC values (up to 250 μg/ml). In the case of the α-carboxypenicillins, the viable counts were low (10^2 to 10^3 cells per ml) at concentrations immediately above the MIC values.

Bacteriolytic studies. The comparative rates of lysis by azlocillin, piperacillin, and ticarcillin against the standard strain of *P. aeruginosa* NCTC 10662 were determined by nephelometry. The penicillins were added to a logarithmic-phase, shaken culture of the test organism when growth had become visible (bacterial count, approximately 2×10^8 to 5×10^8 cells per ml). The optical density of the shaken culture was measured at frequent intervals for a period of 6 h of incubation at 37°C. Azlocillin and piperacillin (2,500 μg/ml) had little effect on the growth of *P. aeruginosa* NCTC 10662 and caused little or no lysis, whereas ticarcillin (250 and 1,000 μg/ml) produced a rapid cessation of growth, followed by a fall in opacity.

Viable count studies. The bactericidal effects demonstrated in a test against a large inoculum (2×10^7 cells per ml) of a shaken culture of *P. aeruginosa* NCTC 10662 are shown in Fig. 1. In general, the acylaminopenicillins (2,500 μg/ml) failed to produce significant bactericidal effects, in contrast to the bactericidal activities of the α-carboxypenicillins. For instance, the viable counts of the cultures grown in the presence of the acylaminopenicillins stayed in the range of 10^7 to 10^8 cells per ml during the first 6 h of the test, after which further growth occurred, and at 24 h the counts of these cultures were close to that of the untreated control culture. Microbiological assay showed inactivation of the acylaminopenicillins during the tests, and no activity was measured at 24 h. Carbenicillin and ticarcillin, at lower concentrations (250 and 1,000 μg/ml), reduced the viable counts to about 10^6 cells per ml (90% kill) within 2 to 3 h, and at 24 h the counts had fallen to 10^4 to 10^5 cells per ml (99 to 99.9% kill). There was no significant loss of the α-carboxypenicillins during the course of the test.

In tests against a more dilute inoculum (5×10^5 cells per ml) of a shaken culture of *P. aeruginosa* NCTC 10662, the acylaminopenicillins produced greater bactericidal effects than against the large inoculum, causing a 90 to 95% reduction in the viable count at 6 h. By 24 h, however, there was an increase in the bacterial count, and

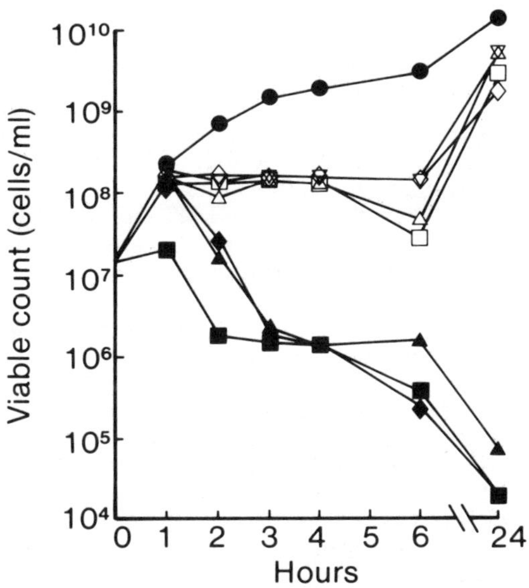

FIG. 1. *Comparative bactericidal activities of α-carboxypenicillins and acylaminopenicillins against a shaken culture of Pseudomonas aeruginosa NCTC 10662. Symbols: ●, control; ◆, ticarcillin (250 μg/ml); ■, ticarcillin (1,000 μg/ml); ▲, carbenicillin (1,000 μg/ml); ▽, apalcillin (2,500 μg/ml); △, azlocillin (2,500 μg/ml); □, mezlocillin (2,500 μg/ml); ◇, piperacillin (2,500 μg/ml).*

there was evidence of inactivation of the compounds (15 to 30%) by the bacteria. The α-carboxylpenicillins produced greater bactericidal effects than the acylaminopenicillins, reducing the count by 99% by 6 h, but there was some regrowth by 24 h in the cultures exposed to ticarcillin, although there was no inactivation of the compound.

Morphological effects. The effects of the penicillins on the morphology of *P. aeruginosa* NCTC 10662 during the course of the bactericidal tests against the large inoculum described above were followed by scanning electron microscopy. The acylaminopenicillins, at a concentration of 1,000 μg/ml, produced filamentous forms during the first 6 h of the test, but at 24 h, no compound was detected as a result of the β-lactamase activity of the organisms, and the cultures were comprised mainly of cells of normal bacillary shape together with a relatively small number of filamentous cells. In contrast, the α-carboxypenicillins caused the rapid formation of spheroplasts which lysed readily, so that from 3 h onwards the microscopical fields contained mainly cell debris.

Conclusions. The data presented here confirm that there are substantial differences in the bactericidal effects produced by the two classes of broad-spectrum penicillins active against *P. aeruginosa*. The poor activity of the acylaminopenicillins in MBC tests against *P. aeruginosa* is well known and contrasts with the bactericidal activities of the α-carboxypenicillins. The discrepancy between the MIC and MBC values of ureidopenicillins has been attributed to the presence of resistant cells (2, 3) or to instability to the β-lactamase produced by *P. aeruginosa* (1). In the tests against the large inocula, the relative lack of bactericidal activity of the acylaminopenicillins is presumably due to the formation of filaments which lyse slowly, in contrast to the rapid lytic effects produced by the α-carboxypenicillins as a result of the formation of spheroplasts. In these tests, the β-lactamase activity of *P. aeruginosa* against the acylaminopenicillins also clearly played a part, although this was not the obvious explanation for the regrowth that occurred in the tests against the dilute inocula.

1. **Basker, M. J., R. A. Edmondson, and R. Sutherland.** 1979. Comparative antibacterial activity of azlocillin, mezlocillin, carbenicillin and ticarcillin, and relative stabilities to beta-lactamases of *Pseudomonas aeruginosa* and *Klebsiella aerogenes*. Infection **7**:67–73.
2. **Bodey, G. P., and T. Pan.** 1977. Mezlocillin: in vitro studies of a new broad-spectrum penicillin. Antimicrob. Agents Chemother. **11**:74–79.
3. **Sanders, C. C., and W. E. Sanders, Jr.** 1975. BL-P1654: a bacteriostatic penicillin? Antimicrob. Agents Chemother. **7**:435–440.

In Vitro Activity of Rosoxacin Against Aerobic Isolates

K. LIEBERMEISTER,* I. BRAVENY, K. MACHKA, AND T. KAMMERMEIER

Institute of Medical Microbiology, Technical University of Munich, D-8000 Munich 80, Federal Republic of Germany

Since the introduction of nalidixic acid in 1962, similar drugs, such as pipemidic acid, piromidic acid, oxolinic acid, and miloxacin have been described. Rosoxacin, 1-ethyl-1,4-dihydro-4-oxo-7(-4 pyridyl)-3 quinoline carboxylic acid, is a new broad-spectrum pyridyl quinoline derivative. O'Connor et al. (2) recently reported the high antibacterial activity of rosoxacin against most gram-negative pathogens and staphylococci. We have already demonstrated (1) a high degree of susceptibility of *Neisseria gonorrhoeae* strains to rosoxacin.

The purpose of our study was to evaluate the activity of rosoxacin compared with nalidixic acid, pipemidic acid, and gentamicin against gram-negative bacilli and gram-positive cocci. A total of 479 strains freshly isolated from urine, sputum, and various other sources were investigated. Only one strain per species from the same patient was included in the study. The MIC was determined by the microdilution method; the medium used was Mueller-Hinton broth with 0.002% phenol red.

The results of the susceptibility tests are summarized in Table 1. Rosoxacin was highly effective against *Enterobacteriaceae*; all strains of *Escherichia coli*, *Klebsiella* spp., *Proteus* spp., *Enterobacter* spp., and *Serratia* spp. were susceptible to a concentration of 8 mg/liter or less. The same concentration of rosoxacin inhibited 98% of *Staphylococcus aureus* strains. *Pseudomonas aeruginosa* was moderately susceptible: 71% of the strains were inhibited at a concentration of 8 mg/liter or less. Rosoxacin proved to be more active against all strains than pipemidic acid and nalidixic acid. Cross-resistance could not be established between rosoxacin and ampicillin or gentamicin. Of 324 strains resistant to ampicillin (MIC, >8 mg/liter), 306 were susceptible to rosoxacin at concentrations of 8 mg/liter or less. Of 115 strains resistant to gentamicin, 98 were susceptible to rosoxacin (MIC, 8 mg/liter or less).

We also examined the effects of the inoculum

TABLE 1. *Comparative activity of rosoxacin, nalidixic acid, pipemidic acid, gentamicin, and ampicillin against aerobic isolates*

Bacteria (no. of isolates)	Drug[a]	Cumulative % inhibition (MICs in mg/liter)										
		0.25	0.5	1	2	4	8	16	32	64	128	256
Staphylococcus aureus (60)	RO		18	82	90	90	98	98	100			
	NA								25	45	63	100
	PA							10	55	85	90	100
	GE	52	82	87	87	87	88	97	98	98	98	100
	AM	10	17	23	30	32	35	45	58	67	77	100
Streptococcus faecalis (30)	RO						80	93	97	100		
	NA											100
	PA										7	100
	AM	3	7	7	100							
Escherichia coli (66)	RO	53	95	99	100							
	NA			11	58	97	100					
	PA			27	100							
	GE	6	51	79	95	100						
	AM				11	53	62	64	65	70	70	100
Proteus mirabilis (60)	RO	7	70	95	97	98	100					
	NA			2	6	82	93	97	98	98	98	100
	PA				85	97	97	98	98	98	100	
	GE	2	38	70	92	98	98	98	100			
	AM		2	38	82	85	87	87	87	87	88	100
Indole-positive *Proteus* spp. (47)	RO	13	83	94	98	100						
	NA			2	40	89	96	96	100			
	PA			47	98	98	98	100				
	GE	17	64	87	92	96	100					
Klebsiella spp. (61)	RO	3	51	84	89	93	100					
	NA			2	15	79	84	93	95	97	98	100
	PA			12	67	85	90	95	98	100		
	GE	31	59	71	75	80	89	97	98	100		
Enterobacter spp. (40)	RO	25	93	98	98	100						
	NA				8	55	90	93	98	98	100	
	PA		5	20	65	85	95	98	100			
	GE	33	63	70	70	75	98	100				
Citrobacter spp. (31)	RO	10	48	84	97	97	97	100				
	NA				29	68	87	94	94	94	100	
	PA			32	61	94	94	94	97	100		
	GE	48	84	87	90	94	97	100				
Serratia spp. (24)	RO	21	58	88	96	100						
	NA			4	42	75	92	92	100			
	PA			13	46	67	83	92	96	100		
	GE	13	42	46	50	50	63	79	88	92	96	100
Pseudomonas aeruginosa (60)	RO	2	3	3	10	42	72	90	92	93	100	
	PA					17	57	82	88	95	100	
	GE	25	58	70	72	73	78	78	83	93	98	100

[a] RO, Rosoxacin; NA, nalidixic acid; PA, pipemidic acid; GE, gentamicin; AM, ampicillin.

size and the differences between MICs and MBCs. The inoculum in the test had a significant effect at a concentration of 10^7 colony-forming units (CFU)/ml. The mean MIC of rosoxacin for *Staphylococcus aureus* was 0.4 mg/liter with an inoculum of 10^5 CFU/ml, 0.8 mg/liter with an inoculum of 10^6 CFU/ml, and 3.8 mg/liter with an inoculum of 10^7 CFU/ml. The mean MIC of rosoxacin for 28 strains of *Enterobacteriaceae* was 0.6 mg/liter with an inoculum of 10^5 CFU/ml and 1.6 mg/liter with an inoculum of 10^7 CFU/ml. There was only a very small difference between MICs and MBCs of rosoxacin.

In conclusion, we found rosoxacin to be the most active of the drugs tested against *Enterobacteriaceae*. Rosoxacin was as effective as gentamicin against *Staphylococcus aureus*. Clinical studies should show whether rosoxacin is of value in the treatment of infections caused by these organisms.

1. **Braveny, I., and K. Machka.** 1980. In vitro activity of rosoxacin (Win 35 213) against Neisseria gonorrhoeae. Drug Res. (II) **9**:1476–1478.

2. **O'Connor, J. R., R. A. Dobson, P. E. Came, and R. B. Wagner.** 1980. Rosoxacin, a new synthetic agent for the treatment of systemic gram-negative infections, p. 440–442. *In* J. D. Nelson and C. Grassi (ed.), Current chemotherapy and infectious disease. American Society for Microbiology, Washington, D.C.

Lasting Effects of P2 Components of Pristinamycin on *Staphylococcus aureus*

SOLANGE BERTEAUX AND DANIEL H. BOUANCHAUD*

Rhône-Poulenc, Centre Nicolas Grillet, 94400 Vitry, France

The streptogramin family of antibiotics includes drugs that are mixtures of two or more compounds (5, 10). These compounds can be placed in two major groups: group A=M=II (cyclic peptolides) and group B=S=I (hexadepsipeptides). Mixtures of A+B components display a strong synergic activity on most gram-positive and on some gram-negative bacteria. For instance, MICs of pristinamycin are 0.5 to 1 μg/ml for most *Staphylococcus aureus* strains.

Until 1975, the percentage of resistant strains (likely chromosomal mutants) was lower than 1% (3), and it has been demonstrated that resistance to related drugs (such as erythromycin and lincomycin) does not affect pristinamycin activity (4). First cases of plasmid-mediated resistance were described in 1977 (2, 6), but no large-scale epidemic of R plasmids or transposons has so far been described (7), and the percentage of resistant strains in hospital environments is lower than 3% (S. Kernbaum, personal communication).

On the other hand, some aspects of in vivo activity of pristinamycin remain partially unexplained. For instance, it has been shown that the A=M=II/B=S=I ratio is close to ¼ in "natural" antibiotic (8), but pharmacological studies have demonstrated that absorption, serum protein binding, catabolism, and excretion are different for each pristinamycin component (1, 11). Dramatic changes of the A=M=II/B=S=I ratio in vivo made it somewhat difficult to correlate therapeutic activity with data obtained in vitro.

For these reasons, it was of interest to study in vitro the kinetics of action of A=M=II and B=S=I compounds, and the effects on bactericidal kinetics of changes in the ratio of pristinamycin components. In this study, representative compounds of the B=S=I group will be referred to as "P1," and representative compounds of the A=M=II group will be referred to as "P2" (P1, 27,404 RP; P2, 12,536 RP).

An *S. aureus* (Smith strain) inoculum in mid-log phase was adjusted to 10^7 cells/ml and submitted to various concentrations of P1+P2 (20%+80% or 80%+20%), and of P1 or P2 alone. After 0.5, 1, and 3 h in nutrient broth at 37°C, bactericidal activity was estimated from the number of surviving cells in colony-forming units (CFU). Aliquots of cultures were harvested on Swinnex membranes (Millipore), washed twice, resuspended, and carefully vortexed in ice-cold NaCl 0.3 N, then diluted and plated on tryptic soy agar. After 48 h at 37°C, the number of colonies was determined with an automatic Artek 880 colony counter (Fig. 1). Our results demonstrated that: (i) P1 has no activity at 5 μg/ml; (ii) that P2 is bactericidal at 5 μg/ml; (iii) that the P1+P2 mixture (20%+80%), very similar to natural pristinamycin, has bactericidal activity at 0.50 μg/ml; and (iv) that the P1+P2 mixture (80%+20%), in which P1 and P2 relative concentrations are similar to those observed in serum,

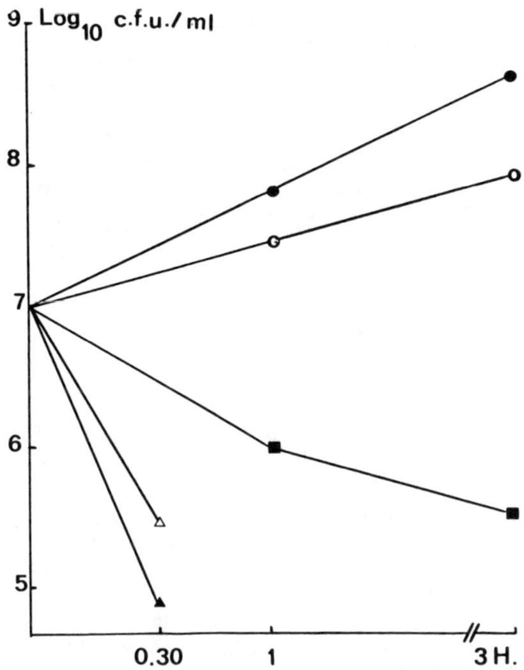

FIG. 1. *Bactericidal activity of P1, P2, and P1+P2 in nutrient broth on S. aureus. Symbols:* (●) *control;* (○) *P1 (5 μg/ml);* (■) *P2 (5 μg/ml);* (▲) *P1+P2, ratio 20/80 (0.5 μg/ml);* (△) *P1+P2, ratio 80/20 (0.5 μg/ml).*

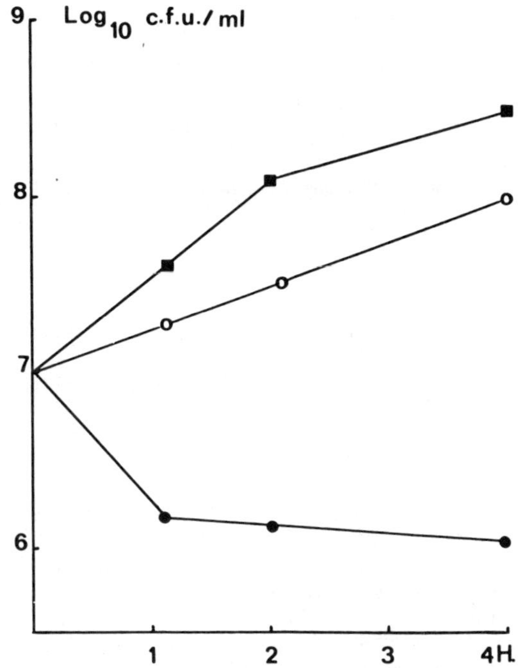

FIG. 2. *Alteration of cell viability upon incubation with pristinamycin components. Symbols:* (■) *control;* (○) *cells submitted to P1 then incubated in P2;* (●) *cells submitted to P2 then incubated in P1 (see text).*

has also a strong bactericidal activity ($-1.5 \log_{10}$ in 0.5 h at 0.50 μg/ml). Bactericidal activity of pristinamycin appears to be not strictly dependent on P1/P2 ratio, as previously demonstrated for bacteriostatic activity (1). These phenomena are likely to occur in vivo, and support the hypothesis that variations of P1 and P2 relative concentrations may not affect pristinamycin therapeutic activity.

To dissociate the respective activity of P1 and P2, cells were sequentially incubated with: (i) P1 (5 μg/ml, 0.5 h) and harvested, washed, and incubated with P2 (0.25 μg/ml, 4 h), or (ii) P2 (1 μg/ml, 0.5 h) then P1 (1 μg/ml, 4 h) (Fig. 2). Bactericidal kinetics were determined as described above. It can be seen that the P1-P2 treatment does not affect cell viability, but that the P2-P1 treatment results in loss of viability (0 to 1 h), then in bacteriostasis (1 to 4 h). These findings indicate that P2 action persists upon its removal, and strongly synergizes P1, which has no activity at 1 μg/ml (see Fig. 1). Differences between P1-P2 and P2-P1 sequential treatments might be explained by complex binding equilibrium between I and II compounds and their bacterial ribosomal targets (M. L. Capmau, J. Abbé, E. Vindimian, and F. Le Goffic, personal communication; 9). In conclusion, our results may in part explain the bactericidal effect of pristinamycin in vivo, in spite of the short half-life and low concentration of P2.

We thank F. Bénazet for helpful comments, and C. Godefroy, M. Lacueil, and J. Thomas for expert technical assistance.

1. **Bénazet, F., and M. Dubost.** 1967. Etude biologique de la pristinamycine: activité *in vitro*, activité chez l'animal de laboratoire, circulation, métabolisme, p. 97–109. *In* Séminaire international consacré à l'antibiothérapie antistaphylococcique par la pristinamycine. Specia, Paris.
2. **Bouanchaud, D. H., J. M. Fouace, and G. Bieth.** 1977. Physical studies of a *Staphylococcus aureus* plasmid mediating resistance to streptogramins, lincosamins and aminoglycosides. Ann. Microbiol. (Inst. Pasteur). **128:** 431–437.
3. **Buré, A. M., J. L. Witchitz, and M. J. Hornstein.** 1975. Choix d'une antibiothérapie antistaphylococcique bactéricide. Med. Mal. Infect. **5:**156–163.
4. **Chabbert, Y. A., and J. Baudens.** 1967. La pristinamycine et ses relations avec les macrolides et la lincomycine, p. 49–59. *In* Séminaire international consacré à l'antibiothérapie antistaphylococcique par la pristinamycine. Specia, Paris.
5. **Cocito, C.** 1979. Antibiotics of the virginiamycin family, inhibitors which contain synergistic components. Microbiol. Rev. **43:**145–198.
6. **Dublanchet, A., C. J. Soussy, F. Squinazi, and J. Duval.** 1977. Résistance de *Staphylococcus aureus* aux

streptogramines. Ann. Microbiol. (Inst. Pasteur). **128:** 277–287.

7. **El Solh, N., J. M. Fouace, Z. Shalita, D. H. Bouanchaud, R. P. Novick, and Y. A. Chabbert.** 1980. Epidemiological and structural studies of *Staphylococcus aureus* R plasmids mediating resistance to tobramycin and streptogramin. Plasmids **4:**117–120.
8. **Jollès, G., B. Terlain, and J. P. Thomas.** 1965. Metabolic investigations on pristinamycin. Nature (London) **207:**199–200.
9. **Parfait, R., and C. Cocito.** 1980. Lasting damage to bacterial ribosomes by reversibly bound virginiamycin M. Proc. Natl. Acad. Sci. U.S.A. **77:**5492–5496.
10. **Vasquez, D.** 1975. The streptogramin family of antibiotics, p. 520–534. *In* J. W. Corcoran and F. E. Hahn (ed.), Antibiotics III: mechanism of action of antimicrobial and antitumor agents. Springer-Verlag, Berlin.
11. **Videau, D., and V. Roiron.** 1965. Titrages et taux sanguins de la pristinamycine chez l'homme. Presse Med. **37:**2101–2103.

Adhesion of *Escherichia coli* to Tissue Culture Cells

ALAN D. ELBEIN AND KLAUS VOSBECK*

Research Department, Pharmaceuticals Division, CIBA-GEIGY Limited, Basel, Switzerland

The adhesion of bacteria to mammalian cells involves receptor molecules on the mammalian cell surface which are recognized by the specific bacterium and to which the bacterium binds. To understand the mechanism of adhesion of *Escherichia coli* SS142 to Intestine 407 cells, an attempt was made to isolate and identify the specific receptor of the Intestine 407 cells. The presence of the receptor or the recognition molecule was determined by an inhibition assay (2). That is, if the receptor molecule was present in a solution, it should bind to *E. coli* SS142 and prevent the bacteria from binding to the Intestine 407 cell monolayers.

A membrane preparation from Intestine 407 cells inhibited the adhesion of *E. coli* SS142 to the Intestine 407 cells, and this inhibition increased when increasing amounts of membranes were mixed with the bacteria. On the other hand, membranes from CHO cells, a cell line to which *E. coli* SS142 does not bind, had no effect on the adhesion. The Intestine 407 membranes were extracted with chloroform and chloroform-methanol to remove glycolipids and other lipids, and these lipids were separated into individual components by thin-layer chromatography. None of the lipid bands eluted from the thin-layer plates showed any activity when tested over a range of concentrations. The membrane residue remaining after lipid extraction was digested exhaustively with pronase to obtain a glycopeptide fraction, and this material was separated into the high-mannose glycopeptide and the complex glycopeptide on a column of Bio-Gel P-4. Neither of these purified glycopeptides inhibited the adhesion of *E. coli* SS142 when tested over a range of concentrations. However, the high-mannose-type glycopeptides did inhibit the adhesion of *E. coli* B-886, a bacterium whose binding is sensitive to α-methylmannoside (1). Thus, the receptor for *E. coli* SS142 either is not a glycoprotein or a glycolipid or is present in these membranes in concentrations too low to allow them to be easily isolated.

We also tested the effect of various enzymes to see whether they would alter the receptor and therefore affect bacterial binding. Thus, the enzymes were used to treat the cell monolayers directly and also the isolated cell membranes. Among the enzymes tested were neuraminidase, α- and β-galactosidase, α-mannosidase, and endoglucosaminidases H and D. In some cases, the enzyme treatment showed an inhibitory effect on binding, but this was attributed to the fact that some of these enzyme preparations contained protease activity, which disrupted the Intestine 407 cell monolayers. This resulted in an artifactual inhibition. Therefore, we concluded that the tested glycosidases had no effect on adhesion.

We also tested a variety of different sugars and other compounds to see whether they would affect bacterial adhesion. Among the sugars tested were simple sugars such as *N*-acetylglucosamine, *N*-acetylgalactosamine, sialic acid, α-methylmannoside, and so on. These monosaccharides were all inactive over a wide range of concentrations. Also inactive were various polyanions such as heparin, polysaccharides such as yeast mannan, proteins such as serum albumin, and so on. However, we did find that certain oligosaccharides which had terminal α-galactosyl residues were inhibitors of *E. coli* SS142 binding. Thus, melibiose, a disaccharide of α-galactose linked to glucose, and raffinose, a disaccharide of α-galactose linked to sucrose, were inhibitors of this reaction. Although 100 mM concentrations or higher of these saccharides were required for inhibition, the inhibition increased with increasing concentrations, raffinose being a better inhibitor than melibiose. Stachyose, a tetrasaccharide containing a terminal α-galactose, was about equal to raffinose. Lactose, a disaccharide having a β-galactose residue attached to glucose, was also inhibitory but considerably less effective than melibiose. Maltose showed no inhibition and, in fact, was somewhat stimulatory. Thus, these studies suggest that α-galactosides could be involved in the recognition of *E. coli* SS142. The fact that high concentrations of these simple galactosides were required for inhibition may indicate that the recognition site involves a larger molecular structure than an α-galactose residue.

Since the recognition site appeared to involve more than an α-galactose residue, we decided to determine whether any hydrophobic interactions could be involved in this bacterial recognition and adhesion system. In collaboration with Richard Huang at the Institute of Virology, Giessen, West Germany, we tested a number of synthetic galactose-containing lipids which he had synthesized chemically. These included such compounds as melibiosyl-phytol (α-galactoside), lactosyl-phytol (β-galactoside), lactosyl-oleate, and lactosyl-cholesterol, as well as various natural glycolipids. We found that melibiosyl-phytol was a fairly effective inhibitor of adhesion, blocking adhesion by 60% at concentrations of 0.5 to 1 mg/ml, whereas the lactosyl-phytol was not a good inhibitor at these concentrations. The lactosyl-oleate was found to inhibit this reaction, but this inhibition was due to the fact that this compound was a detergent and removed the Intestine 407 cells from the plates. Therefore, the activity of this material did not appear to be associated with any recognition activity.

Based on the studies described here, it appears likely that the recognition and adhesion site on the Intestine 407 cells to which *E. coli* SS142 binds involves an α-galactosyl residue. Although it is not certain to what type of molecule the α-galactose is attached, it may be that membrane-bound glycolipids are the site of attachment. It will obviously be necessary to isolate and characterize this molecule before its role can be definitely established.

1. **Jann, K., G. Schmidt, E. Blumenstock, and K. Vosbeck.** 1981. Adhesion of *Escherichia coli* to mammalian and yeast cells: role of piliation and surface hydrophobicity. Infect. Immun. **32**:484–489.
2. **Vosbeck, K., H. Handschin, E. B. Menge, and O. Zak.** 1979. Effects of subminimal inhibitory concentrations of antibiotics on adhesiveness of *Escherichia coli in vitro*. Rev. Infect. Dis. **1**:845–851.

Bacterial Adhesion to Tissue Culture Cells and Hemagglutination

HELMUT METT* AND KLAUS VOSBECK

Pharmaceuticals Division, CIBA-GEIGY Limited, Basel, Switzerland

It has previously been shown by Vosbeck et al. (2) that *Escherichia coli* SS142, a strain originally derived from a pyelonephritic patient, binds specifically to Intestine 407 cells, a human epithelioid cell line. Furthermore, Jann et al. (1) demonstrated that these bacteria interact with human erythrocytes, leading to mannose-resistant hemagglutination. It was of interest to determine whether hemagglutination by *E. coli* SS142 was likewise specific and whether the mechanism of bacterial adhesion to cell monolayers, on one hand, and to erythrocytes, on the other hand, was different. We therefore investigated the correlation between the interaction of the bacteria with these two eucaryotic cell types.

Hemagglutinating activity was assayed in microtiter plates by incubation of serial twofold dilutions of a bacterial suspension (or solubilized adhesin; see below) together with a freshly prepared suspension of human erythrocytes (final concentration, 0.3%) in phosphate-buffered saline containing calcium and magnesium. Adhesion of radiolabeled bacteria to Intestine 407 cell monolayers was assayed essentially as described previously (2).

Hemagglutinating activity of *E. coli* SS142 appeared to be rather specific, since only erythrocytes from humans, sheep, and pigs were agglutinated, but not erythrocytes from cows, horses, guinea pigs, rabbits, rats, or mice. A high degree of specificity was also observed with respect to adhesion of bacteria to various tissue culture cells (1). *E. coli* SS142 adhered only to Intestine 407 cells, and not to Vero cells, porcine kidney (PK_1) cells, feline embryo cells, or primary cultures of rat kidney cells.

Human erythrocyte membranes (ghosts) inhibited both cell monolayer adhesion and hemagglutinating activity of *E. coli* SS142 (Table 1). Various extracts obtained from erythrocyte

TABLE 1. *Inhibition of E. coli SS142 adhesion to erythrocytes and Intestine 407 cells by erythrocyte membrane fractions*

Erythrocyte membrane fraction added to the assay	Hemagglutinating activity (% of control)	Adhesion to monolayers (% of control)
Control (no inhibitor added)	100	100
Intact erythrocyte ghosts	15	62
Ultrasonic membrane vesicles	23	93
Chloroform-methanol-soluble membrane extract	12	102

ghosts by sonication or organic solvent extraction inhibited hemagglutination, but did not affect the adhesion of bacteria to Intestine 407 cell monolayers.

A comparative investigation of hemagglutinating and cell-binding activity of *E. coli* SS142 was done by subjecting the bacteria to various treatments (Table 2). Strong shearing forces (repeated treatment with an ultramixer) reduced both the hemagglutinating activity of the bacteria and their adhesiveness in the monolayer adhesion assay. The bacteria remained viable, indicating that this treatment did not cause gross damage to the cells. Sedimenting the bacteria (1 h at 27,000 × *g*), which had been subjected to shearing forces, yielded a cell-free extract which showed high hemagglutinating activity (soluble adhesin). The hemagglutinating activity of intact bacteria and of soluble adhesin was destroyed by proteolytic enzyme treatment and by fixation with glutaraldehyde (Table 2).

We conclude that similar structures on the bacterial surface may be involved in hemagglutinating activity and in their capacity to bind to Intestine 407 cells. These structures appear to involve a protein(s), since their activity is lost upon proteolytic digestion. They may resemble fimbria-like bacterial appendices. The mechanism of binding of the bacteria to cell monolayers seems to differ from the mechanism of hemagglutination. We assume that multiple sites (and possibly multiple steps) are involved in the tissue culture cell-binding mechanism, whereas only few sites may be required on the erythrocytes for hemagglutination.

TABLE 2. *Effects of various pretreatments of E. coli SS142 and of soluble adhesin on hemagglutination and on adhesion to Intestine 407 monolayer cells*

Pretreatment	Hemagglutination (% of control)	Monolayer adhesion (% of control)
Bacteria		
Untreated control	100	100
Shearing force (ultramixer)		
3 times 30 s	38	52
10 times 30 s	13	45
Glutaraldehyde fixation	4	10
Proteases		
Pronase	3	10
Trypsin	69	ND[a]
Papain	100	ND
Soluble adhesin		
Untreated control	100	ND
Glutaraldehyde fixation	0	ND
Proteases		
Pronase	0	ND
Trypsin	3	ND
Papain	100	ND

[a] ND, Not determined.

1. **Jann, K., G. Schmidt, E. Blumenstock, and K. Vosbeck.** 1981. Adhesion of *Escherichia coli* to mammalian and yeast cells: role of piliation and surface hydrophobicity. Infect. Immun. **32:**484–489.
2. **Vosbeck, K., H. Handschin, E. B. Menge, and O. Zak.** 1979. Effects of subminimal inhibitory concentrations of antibiotics on adhesiveness of *Escherichia coli in vitro.* Rev. Infect. Dis. **1:**845–851.

In Vitro Antibacterial Activity of the Iron Chelator Deferoxamine

B. S. VAN ASBECK,* J. H. MARCELIS, H. VAN KATS, J. J. M. MARX, AND J. VERHOEF

Departments of Internal Medicine and Bacteriology, University Hospital, Utrecht, The Netherlands*

Patients with iron overload often suffer from recurrent infections (4). It has been shown that an increase in the availability of iron in the tissues of the host, such as in thalassemia and primary hemochromatosis, decreases the resistance to infections. This may be a result of two circumstances. Iron may affect host resistance by protecting bacteria from destruction by polymorphonuclear leukocytes. On the other hand, iron enhances the virulence of bacteria such as *Mycobacteria*, *Listeria*, *Yersiniae*, *Staphylococci*, *Clostridia*, several *Enterobacteriae*, and *Gonococci*, giving support to the view that excess of available iron puts humans at increased risk of infection by even moderately pathogenic bacteria.

Deferoxamine (Desferal, DF) is a specific iron chelator for clinical use. Since simultaneous administration of ascorbic acid leads to a marked increase in urinary excretion of iron, excess body iron is often treated with the combination of DF and vitamin C (DF + vit C).

Recently, Lee et al. (2) showed that the increase in susceptibility to infection by iron in rats with *Escherichia coli* peritonitis was nullified by DF. However, an enhanced susceptibility of iron-loaded, DF-treated mice to *Salmonella* infection was observed by Jones et al. (1). Therefore, we investigated the effect of DF on bacterial growth in vitro.

DF and DF + vit C were tested by growing 41 strains in nutrient broth, with or without DF or DF + vit C, for 48 h at 37°C. Growth was studied by measuring the absorbance at 660 nm with an automated turbidimeter and expressed as Klett units. The effect of DF was assessed by adding various concentrations of DF (0 to 200 μg/ml) or DF + vit C (0 to 400 μg/ml) to the culture medium. Ferric citrate was used for the iron supply. Significance of the results was assessed with the one-sided Wilcoxon test ($P < 0.05$, significant).

A dose-response effect of DF or DF + vit C was observed for the susceptible strains. In most cases, growth inhibition was limited to 6 to 24 h, but an increase of this time was observed when DF or DF + vit C was added repeatedly. DF had a significant antibacterial activity ($P < 0.05$) (Fig. 1). However, when vit C was added the inhibitory effect of DF was greatly enhanced ($P < 0.001$). Vit C alone had no significant effect on bacterial growth.

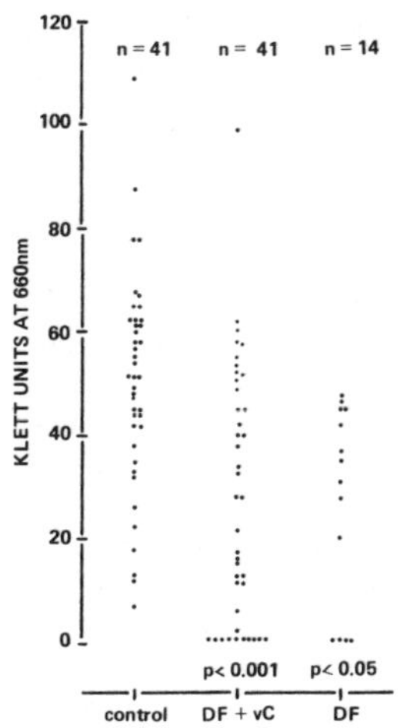

FIG. 1. *Influence of DF (200 μg/ml) + vit C (100 μg/ml) and DF (200 μg/ml) on 41 and 14 strains, respectively, after 8 h of incubation compared with controls.*

After 8 h of incubation, DF + vit C had a significant inhibitory effect on the growth of *Staphylococcus aureus* (five strains; $P < 0.05$), *Staphylococcus epidermidis* (five strains; $P < 0.005$), *E. coli* (six strains; $P < 0.05$), *Klebsiella pneumoniae* (five strains; $P < 0.05$), and *Proteus mirabilis* (four strains; $P < 0.025$). Furthermore, two *Providencia* and *Neiseria meningitidis* strains and one *Salmonella typhi* and one *Alcaligenes faecalis* strain were strongly inhibited. The inhibition of seven *Pseudomonas aeruginosa* and three *Enterobacter* strains was not significant, whereas one strain of each showed an increase in growth in the presence of DF + vit C.

Iron is essential for bacterial growth because it is involved in a number of mitochondrial components (3). In its natural state, however, iron is virtually unavailable. To overcome this problem, bacteria produce chelators, which seek out iron in the environment and return it to the microorganisms. Therefore, the antibacterial activity of DF may be due to competition between DF and bacterial iron-chelating substances. Indeed, when DF was saturated with iron, the inhibitory effect on bacterial growth was virtually nullified (Fig. 2). Ferric citrate had no significant effect on the control cultures. Enhancement of the antibacterial activity of DF by vit C might be a

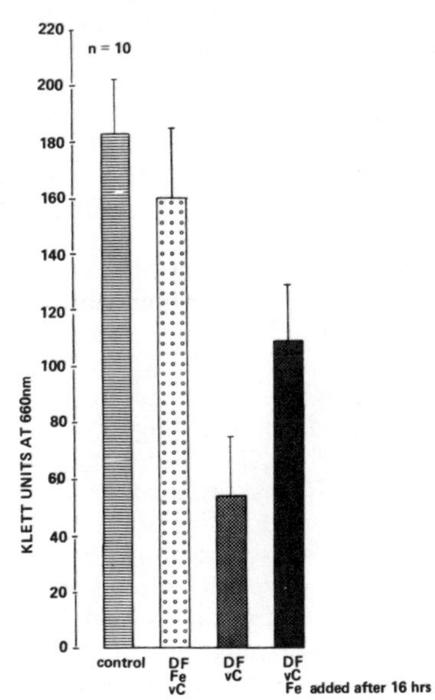

FIG. 2. *Influence of iron on the inhibiting effect of DF (200 μg/ml) + vit C (100 μg/ml) on the growth of 10 susceptible strains after 36 h of incubation. DF was 100% saturated with iron before it was added to the culture medium and after 16 h of incubation.*

result of reduction of ferric iron to the more soluble ferrous iron, in which state it is available for chelating substances.

Our data suggest that DF has antibacterial activity due to limitation of iron available to the microorganism and that vit C enhances this property. This observation is of clinical relevance, since the combination of DF + vit C is widely used in patients with iron overload, and these patients are more susceptible to infections.

1. **Jones, R. L., C. M. Peterson, R. W. Grady, T. Kumbaraci, A. Cerami, and J. H. Graziano.** 1977. Effects of iron chelators and iron overload on Salmonella infection. Nature (London) **267**:63–65.
2. **Lee, J. T. Jr., D. H. Ahrenholz, R. D. Nelson, and R. L. Simmons.** 1979. Mechanisms of the adjuvant effect of hemoglobin in experimental peritonitis. V. The significance of the coordinated iron component. Surgery **86:** 41–48.
3. **Light, P. A., and R. A. Clegg.** 1974. Metabolism in iron limited growth, p. 35–64. *In* J. B. Neilands (ed.), Microbial iron metabolism. A comprehensive treatise. Academic Press, Inc., New York.
4. **Weinberg, E. D.** 1978. Iron and infection. Microbiol. Rev. **42**:45–66.

Differing Bactericidal Activities of Ticarcillin and Azlocillin in Liquid and Solid Media

W. BRUMFITT AND J. M. T. HAMILTON-MILLER*

Department of Medical Microbiology, Royal Free Hospital (University of London), London NW3, England

Several members of the ureidopenicillins (e.g., mezlocillin, azlocillin, and piperacillin) are now available for therapeutic use. This group of antibiotics, which may be regarded as substituted ampicillins (5), combine the desirable properties of ampicillin and of carbenicillin: thus, they are highly active against both *Streptococcus faecalis* and *Pseudomonas aeruginosa*. However, some reports have suggested that the bactericidal activity of the ureidopenicillins may be poor, or even totally lacking (4), whereas others (1) have not found this deficiency. To clarify this situation we have carried out a comparative study of the bacteriostatic and bactericidal activities of azlocillin and of ticarcillin against *P. aeruginosa*.

Methods. Eighty-two strains of *P. aeruginosa* isolated from clinical material were tested. All were susceptible both to azlocillin and to ticarcillin.

MIC and MBC were determined in both solid and liquid media. (i) Doubling dilutions of antibiotic were made in Iso-Sensitest agar and 1-μl suspensions of the test organisms containing 10^4, 10^5, or 10^6 colony-forming units (CFU) were inoculated. MICs were read after overnight incubation. MBCs were determined by replicating (using velvet pads) from plates originally inoculated with 10^6 CFU onto blood plates. Eighty-two strains were tested on the solid medium. (ii) Antibiotic dilutions were also made in tubes containing 1 ml of Iso-Sensitest broth, which was inoculated with 10^5 organisms, and incubated overnight at 37°C, after which MIC was read. MBC was determined by subculturing to blood agar 5 μl from each tube in which no visible growth had occurred. Nine strains were tested in this way.

Cultures which had been exposed to various antibiotic concentrations were stained with methylene blue and examined at a magnification of ×1,200.

Killing experiments were carried out by adding 10^5 CFU of the test strain per ml to five 250-ml flasks (swirled at 100 rev/min), each containing 100 ml of Iso-Sensitest broth with the addition of various concentrations of azlocillin or ticarcillin, representing a control, 0.5× MIC, 1× MIC, 2× MIC, and 4× MIC for each test strain. Flasks were incubated at 37°C, and 0.1-ml samples were removed at intervals for viable counting on agar containing penicillinase (Wellcome) to neutralize residual antibiotic. Four strains were tested, and mean values of viable counts taken at 2, 4, 6, and 8 h were plotted to construct the killing curve.

Results. On the solid medium, geometric mean MICs of ticarcillin were 34, 40.5, and 45.4 μg/ml for the inocula of 10^4, 10^5, and 10^6 CFU, respectively. For azlocillin the corresponding figures were 5.7, 8.7, and 10.9 μg/ml. MBCs were 54.4 μg/ml for ticarcillin and 15.5 μg/ml for azlocillin (Table 1). Thus, for both antibiotics MBC was not in excess of double the MIC.

In the liquid medium, the geometric mean MIC of ticarcillin was 40 μg/ml and of azlocillin was 6.3 μg/ml—very similar to the figures obtained in the solid medium. However, MBC for ticarcillin was 118 μg/ml (3× MIC), and azlocillin failed to sterilize the cultures under these conditions (MBC > 1,024 μg/ml).

Bacteria which had been grown in the pres-

TABLE 1. *Antibacterial activities of azlocillin and ticarcillin on solid medium*

Inoculum size (CFU)	Antibiotic	No. of strains tested	No. of strains showing indicated MIC (μg/ml)								
			1	2	4	8	16	32	64	128	256
10^4	Ticarcillin	81	1			11	14	26	10	19	
10^5	Ticarcillin	82	1			3	12	35	11	20	
10^6	Ticarcillin	81				3	10	28	23	17	
10^4	Azlocillin	81	1	7	34	28	11				
10^5	Azlocillin	82	1	6	16	32	19	7	1		
10^6	Azlocillin	80		3	12	30	27	1	3		4
			No. of strains showing indicated MBC (μg/ml)								
10^6	Ticarcillin	81				2	9	23	20	26	1
10^6	Azlocillin	80		2	6	25	27	8	5	3	3 (1 > 1,024)

ence of 0.5× MIC of either antibiotic, in either liquid or solid medium, had grossly abnormal morphology: all organisms visible after staining were in the form of long filaments.

The results of killing experiments are shown in Fig. 1. It is clear that concentrations of either ticarcillin or azlocillin which are in excess of their respective MIC are bactericidal. Ticarcillin appears to act slightly faster.

Discussion. Our results show that changing experimental conditions may have a decisive effect on the apparent bactericidal activity of these antipseudomonal compounds. A somewhat similar situation exists with another β-lactam antibiotic, mecillinam (3). In a solid medium for both azlocillin and ticarcillin, MBC < 2× MIC, whereas in the same medium in a liquid form, MBC for ticarcillin is 3× MIC, and azlocillin failed to sterilize cultures. However, the results of killing curves show clearly that both antibiotics kill bacteria in a progressive manner at concentrations in excess of MIC. The morphological reaction of *P. aeruginosa* is filamentation, a consequence of the fact that both antibiotics bind preferentially to penicillin-binding protein-3 (2). We did not find a significant inoculum-size effect with either antibiotic.

It is dangerous to extrapolate from in vitro findings to clinical conditions. In patients with normal defense mechanisms there is no evidence that a bactericidal antibiotic is therapeutically superior to a bacteriostatic compound, except under special and unusual circumstances. Thus, our experimental results give no reason to believe that there will be any differences between ticarcillin and azlocillin in terms of clinical efficacy. A controlled clinical trial is the only way to settle such questions.

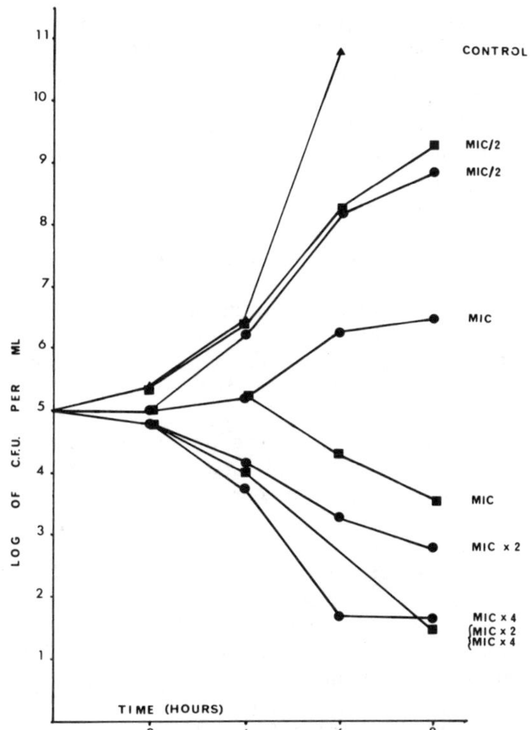

FIG. 1. *Killing of P. aeruginosa by ticarcillin (■) or azlocillin (●) in Iso-Sensitest broth. Each point is the mean of four different strains.*

1. **Coppens, L., and J. Klastersky.** 1979. Comparative study of anti-pseudomonas activity of azlocillin, mezlocillin, and ticarcillin. Antimicrob. Agents Chemother. **15**:396–399.
2. **Curtis, N. A. C., D. Orr, G. W. Ross, and M. G. Boulton.** 1979. Competition of β-lactam antibiotics for the penicillin-binding proteins of *Pseudomonas aeruginosa, Enterobacter cloacae, Klebsiella aerogenes, Proteus rettgeri*, and *Escherichia coli*: comparison with antibacterial activity and effects upon bacterial morphology. Antimicrob. Agents Chemother. **16**:323–328.
3. **Reeves, D. F.** 1977. Antibacterial activity of mecillinam. J. Antimicrob. Chemother. **3** (Suppl. B):5–11.
4. **Sanders, C. C., and W. E. Sanders.** 1975. BL-P1654: a bacteriostatic penicillin? Antimicrob. Agents Chemother. **7**:435–440.
5. **Wise, R.** 1977. Substituted ampicillins. J. Antimicrob. Chemother. **3**:289–290.

Comparison of the Activity of Four Aminoglycosides, Using Sensitive Techniques at Sub-Bactericidal Concentrations

LEONARD SCHRIRE, ROY G. ROBINSON, RICHARD G. DOEHRING,* AND HENDRIK J. KOORNHOF

South African Institute for Medical Research, Johannesburg, Republic of South Africa

To compare the activity of gentamicin, tobramycin, amikacin and netilmicin against a range of clinical isolates of gram-negative bacilli, MIC and MBC were measured by conventional broth microdilution techniques, with overnight incubation. The effect of different exposure times on selected organisms was then noted, using a series of antibiotic concentrations above and below the MBC, with an endpoint represented by a growth of 10% or less of the number of colony-forming units (CFU) in an antibiotic-free control culture. This was used as the criterion for the minimum antibiotic concentration (MAC). For short antibiotic exposure periods (before a 10-fold increase in the growth of the control culture has occurred), this is determined predominantly by bactericidal effects, whereas as exposure times increase the relative contributions of bactericidal and inhibitory effects cannot be separated. The MAC thus determined will become equivalent to the MAC "inhibition" as defined by Lorian for a 5.5-h period (1).

A 90% reduction of the potential bacterial population in a clinical infection may significantly affect the disease process where the antibiotic concentration exceeds the MAC (2, 3).

MAC estimations of this type are based on counting survivors, i.e., relatively resistant bacterial cells in the inoculum that have continued to multiply in the particular antibiotic concentration, usually at a reduced rate, as well as those cells that have been inhibited from multiplying but are still viable on subculture. The 90% reduction in potential CFU compared with the control culture thus reflects a slower overall growth rate. The longer the exposure time, the more difficult it becomes to assess the antibiotic effect, because selective pressure favors the more resistant cells, which multiply and constitute an increasing proportion of the survivors. We therefore limited our experiments to exposure times of 1, 2, 4, and 6 h, which could yield information of clinical relevance within the usual aminoglycoside dosing intervals of 8 h.

A further measure of the activity of an antibiotic can be shown by the MBC/MAC ratio for a particular organism. The two measurements are based on different test criteria and they bear no direct relationship to each other, the MBC being a constant, whereas the MAC is time dependent. A large ratio indicates an increased spread of bactericidal activity between the MBC and the MAC, which could be advantageous in clinical use (2). The ratio, however, appears to be independent of the absolute MBC values in comparing one drug with another. By adding the dimension of exposure time, changes in the ratio can be related to the pharmacokinetics of aminoglycoside therapy.

Table 1 illustrates the influence of exposure time on the MAC of each of the four aminoglycosides, with *Klebsiella pneumoniae* as the test organism. The results, also expressed as the MBC/MAC ratio, indicate a progressive increase in activity up to 4 h, i.e., a falling MAC, therefore a rising MBC/MAC ratio, and a tendency to reach a plateau at that point. Similar trends were observed with *Escherichia coli*, *Pseudomonas aeruginosa*, and *Serratia marcescens*.

Comparing the effects of each drug, netilmicin showed the highest activity against *K. pneumoniae* in terms of having the lowest MAC and MBC, and, in addition, it had the highest MBC/MAC ratio for the first 2 h. Different patterns emerged with the other test organisms; e.g., gentamicin had the lowest MAC and MBC, with the highest ratio for the first 2 h, when tested against *S. marcescens*. In contrasting two antibiotics of equal MBC, it seems reasonable to suppose that the one with the highest MBC/MAC ratio will produce a clinically useful effect at a lower tissue concentration.

The increased activity over a 6-h period may partially compensate for the fall in tissue levels following the postdosage peak.

We have also explored the comparison of these related antibiotics by using gentamicin as an arbitrary reference standard (unity) and calculating an activity range index (ARI) for the MBC/MAC ratios of each of the other drugs.

Table 2 summarizes our findings and demonstrates the degree to which each drug's MBC/MAC ratio at each time differs from that of gentamicin. It will be noted that the ARI appears to be independent of the exposure time, so that a single (mean) index may be regarded as a specific characteristic of each antibiotic-organ-

TABLE 1. *Klebsiella pneumoniae: MAC in milligram per liter (geometric mean of five strains) with MBC/MAC ratios, at different exposure times*[a]

Exposure time (h)	Gentamicin		Tobramycin		Amikacin		Netilmicin	
	MAC	MBC/MAC	MAC	MBC/MAC	MAC	MBC/MAC	MAC	MBC/MAC
1	2.77	0.31	1.36	0.34	2.08	0.25	0.54	0.46
2	0.90	0.94	0.48	0.98	0.72	0.74	0.19	1.31
4	0.60	1.42	0.24	1.95	0.39	1.36	0.14	1.78
6	0.60	1.42	0.24	1.95	0.39	1.36	0.13	1.92

[a] Gentamicin: MBC, 0.85 (range, 0.23 to 6.32); tobramycin: MBC, 0.47 (range, 0.19 to 1.05); amikacin: MBC, 0.53 (range, 0.20 to 1.05); netilmicin: MBC, 0.25 (range, 0.11 to 0.39).

TABLE 2. *ARI relative to gentamicin for four organisms at different exposure times*

Drug	Exposure time (h)	ARI: *Klebsiella pneumoniae*	*Pseudomonas aeruginosa*	*Escherichia coli*	*Serratia marcescens*
Tobramycin	1	1.12	0.87	1.03	0.92
	2	1.04	0.79	1.12	0.76
	4	1.35	0.95	0.67	1.07
	6	1.35	0.94	0.93	1.10
Arithmetic mean		1.22	0.89	0.94	0.96
Standard deviation		0.16	0.07	0.19	0.16
Amikacin	1	0.83	1.18	1.10	0.65
	2	0.78	1.20	0.94	0.56
	4	0.93	1.17	0.78	1.07
	6	0.93	1.26	0.93	1.10
Arithmetic mean		0.87	1.20	0.94	0.85
Standard deviation		0.08	0.04	0.13	0.28
Netilmicin	1	1.50	1.89	3.47	0.75
	2	1.34	1.90	2.38	0.71
	4	1.23	1.67	2.10	1.01
	6	1.35	1.79	1.97	1.20
Arithmetic mean		1.36	1.81	2.48	0.92
Standard deviation		0.11	0.10	0.68	0.23

ism relationship. Further studies will be needed to determine the general applicability of this concept.

A separate series of experiments was carried out, based on membrane transfer techniques, with agar containing different antibiotic concentrations. This was done to measure the concentration required to kill 90% (or more) of the CFU in the inoculum over different exposure periods. This approach has the merit of segregating the progeny of individual bacterial cells in the inoculum, thus giving a more direct measurement of the proportion of cells killed over each period and at each antibiotic concentration. By contrast, liquid medium techniques result in a bias toward the progeny of the more resistant cells, thus making it very difficult to separate the inhibitory from the bactericidal effects.

The results, for six strains of *K. pneumoniae* tested, tended to parallel those obtained by the broth technique, the MBC/MAC ratio rising with increasing exposure time. However, as might be expected, due to a time lag for diffusion across the membrane, these ratios were in all cases lower, and more slowly rising, than the broth results, and had not reached a plateau by 6 h.

Unexpectedly, the ranking of the four drugs in terms of ARI was altered using this technique, netilmicin now showing the lowest ARI. This is most probably a reflection of the relative diffusibility of the four drugs, and further studies will be required to investigate its relevance.

At present it would seem preferable to accept the results of the broth technique as being the more clearly defined and less influenced by poorly characterized factors.

1. **Lorian, V.** 1975. Some effects of subinhibitory concentrations of antibiotics on bacteria. Bull. N.Y. Acad. Med. **51:**1046–1055.
2. **Lorian, V.** 1980. Effects of subminimum inhibitory con-

centrations of antibiotics on bacteria, p. 342–408. *In* V. Lorian (ed.), Antibiotics in laboratory medicine. The Williams & Wilkins Co., Baltimore.

3. **Lyman, I. R., J. G. Tenery, and R. P. Basson.** 1970. Correlation between decrease in bacterial load and rate of wound healing. Surg. Gynaecol. Obstet. **130:**616–621.

New In Vitro Device for Examining the Response of Bacteria to Changing Drug Concentrations

DAVID GREENWOOD* AND HELEN TUPPER

Department of Microbiology, University Hospital, Queen's Medical Centre, Nottingham NG7 2UH, England

The laboratory investigation of the response of bacteria to antibiotics has been carried out traditionally in conditions in which the drug concentration does not change, except in the special circumstance in which bacteria are able to inactivate the antibiotic. Some workers have curtailed the exposure period to study antibacterial effects which persist after the antibiotic has been removed (4), but this still does not parallel the situation existing in treatment in which the concentration of drug rises as it is absorbed and falls again as it is eliminated.

To investigate these circumstances, a number of workers have devised models in which serum profiles of antibiotics can be simulated (1, 3, 5–7). In several of these models a single pulse of the antibacterial agent is added to the system (simulating an intravenous bolus injection), and the antibiotic is progressively diluted out at the required rate. A disadvantage of dilution methods is that bacteria are concomitantly diluted together with the drug. Models described by Al-Asadi et al. (1) and Shah (7) overcome this problem by interposing filters in the system.

The purpose of the present communication is to describe a new model in which simulated serum profiles of virtually any description can be achieved very simply, without diluting the bacteria.

Design of the model. An exploded diagram of the model is shown in Fig. 1. The system consists essentially of two small chambers separated by a 0.45-μm-pore-size cellulose acetate filter membrane. In use, both chambers are completely filled with broth and the top chamber is seeded with bacteria. A flow of broth through the device is maintained by a peristaltic pump; a magnetic stirrer paddle rotates on the surface of the membrane to prevent blockage of the pores. A flow rate of at least 1 ml/min can be reliably maintained for prolonged periods even in the presence of a fully grown bacterial culture. Bacterial growth in the upper chamber of the model is monitored continuously using a high-intensity red light-emitting diode and a matched phototransistor aligned on opposite sides of the chamber.

Drug profiles. Changes in concentration of antibiotic entering the growth chamber are achieved using a commercially available gradient former (MixoGrad; Gilson Medical Electronics). This device arranges for two fluids to be mixed in a continuously changing ratio according to a prearranged profile. By using antibiotic-containing and antibiotic-free broth, a changing antibiotic concentration, passed into the growth chamber by the peristaltic pump, can be achieved.

Since the drug profile provided by the gradient former is reflected in the inflow of broth entering the growth chamber, allowance must be made for dilution there in calculating the concentration to which the bacteria are exposed. The simplest way of obtaining the desired concentration in the growth chamber is to arrange for the drug concentration in the inflow to change abruptly at intervals, corresponding to the period during which the volume of fluid in the model is completely changed. Thus, if the concentration of antibiotic entering the system changes from 0 to 50 μg/ml, a gradual build-up of antibiotic will occur in the growth chamber; if the flow rate is 1 ml/min and the model holds 48 ml, the concentration will rise to 50 μg/ml over a 48-min period. If the concentration in the inflow is then reduced to 25 μg/ml, the concentration to which the bacteria are exposed will decline to that value over the next 48 min.

The precise shapes of the exposure curves obtained by this method do not conform exactly to those obtained in vivo, but concentrations of cephalosporins measured (by high-pressure liquid chromatography) at appropriate intervals in the outflow of the system and in the growth chamber itself indicate that exposure profiles can be achieved that correspond closely with in vivo serum profiles.

The model in use. Pilot studies with the

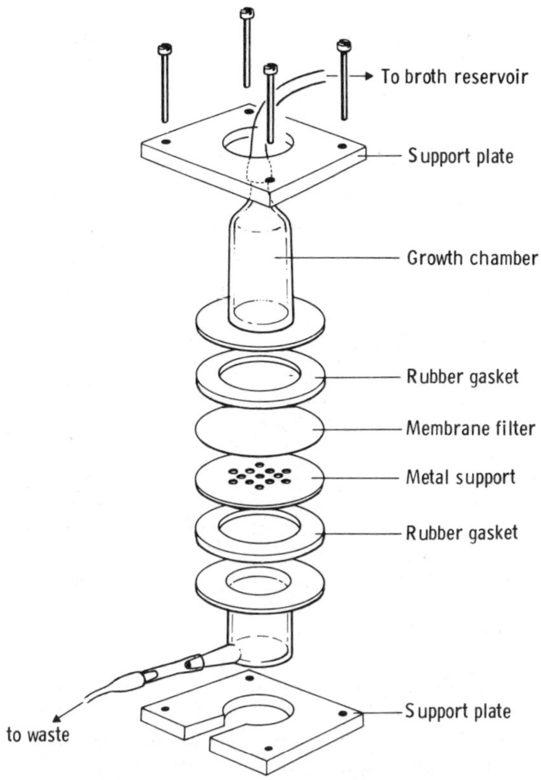

FIG. 1. *Diagrammatic representation of the model. In use, a magnetic stirrer below the device activates a Teflon-coated paddle situated on the filter membrane to prevent blockage by bacteria.*

flow-through system confirmed that the model can be used successfully with a wide variety of organisms, including *Escherichia coli*, *Staphylococcus aureus*, and *Pseudomonas aeruginosa*. Difficulties have sometimes been experienced with bacteria that produce abundant gas (this has been a particular problem with *P. aeruginosa* in nitrate broth), and it will be necessary to incorporate some kind of venting system to accommodate this type of organism.

Experimentally, the model has been used to verify the results obtained in our earlier model, in which the emergence of low-level aminoglycoside resistance was studied under conditions of transient drug exposure (1, 2). More recently, aspects of the response of *E. coli* to cephalosporins have been investigated.

Figure 2 shows the response of an ampicillin-susceptible strain of *E. coli* (MIC of ampicillin, 4 μg/ml; MIC of cephalothin, 8 μg/ml; MIC of cefotiam, 0.5 μg/ml) to a changing concentration of cephalothin which achieved a peak concentration of 50 μg/ml after 1 h and declined to 0 over a further 5 h. A deviation from normal growth

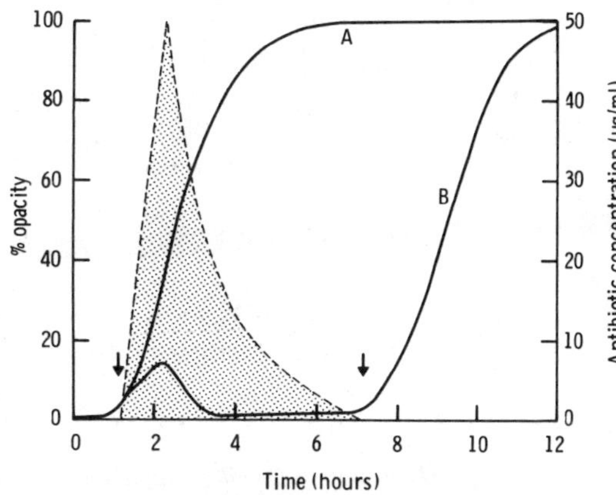

FIG. 2. *Continuous opacity records obtained in the model with an ampicillin-susceptible strain of E. coli. A, Normal growth curve; B, exposure to cephalothin commenced at first arrow and stopped at second arrow. The concentration of cephalothin achieved in the growth chamber is indicated by the stippled area.*

was observed as the antibiotic concentration rose to an inhibitory level and lysis ensued once the peak concentration was reached. Bacterial growth resumed as the cephalothin concentration fell.

In similar experiments in which a peak concentration of 10 μg of cephalothin per ml was achieved after 1 h, a transient fall in opacity was observed with recovery after about 1 h, but identical 6-h exposure profiles achieving peak concentrations of 10 μg of ampicillin per ml or 10 μg of cefotiam per ml suppressed growth for several hours beyond the period of exposure.

When an ampicillin-resistant *E. coli* strain was tested (MIC of ampicillin, >500 μg/ml; MIC of cephalothin, 16 μg/ml; MIC of cefotiam, 0.5 μg/ml) using a 6-h exposure profile with a peak of 50 μg/ml after 1 h, ampicillin and cephalothin had little or no effect on bacterial growth, but cefotiam suppressed growth of this strain for approximately 5 h beyond the period of drug exposure.

These findings will be reported in full elsewhere.

1. **Al-Asadi, M. J. S., D. Greenwood, and F. O'Grady.** 1979. In vitro model simulating the form of exposure of bacteria to antimicrobial drugs encountered in infection. Antimicrob. Agents Chemother. **16:**77–80.
2. **Al-Asadi, M. J. S., K. Towner, and D. Greenwood.** 1981. Acquired cross resistance to aminoglycosides in gentamicin-sensitive and gentamicin-resistant strains of enterobacteria. J. Med. Microbiol. **14:**171–183.
3. **Bergan, T., I. B. Carlsen, and J. E. Fuglesang.** 1980. An in vitro model for monitoring bacterial responses to antibiotic agents under simulated in vivo conditions. Infection **8** (Suppl. 1)**:**S96–S102.
4. **Bundtzen, R. W., A. U. Gerber, D. L. Cohn, and W. A. Craig.** 1981. Postantibiotic suppression of bacterial

growth. Rev. Infect. Dis. **3**:28–37.

5. **Grasso, S., G. Meinardi, I. de Carneri, and V. Tamassia.** 1978. New in vitro model to study the effect of antibiotic concentration and rate of elimination on antibacterial activity. Antimicrob. Agents Chemother. **13**: 570–576.
6. **Nishida, M., T. Murakawa, T. Kamimura, and N. Okada.** 1978. Bactericidal activity of cephalosporins in an in vitro model simulating serum levels. Antimicrob. Agents Chemother. **14**:6–12.
7. **Shah, P. M.** 1980. An improved method to study antibacterial activity of antibiotics in an in vitro model simulating serum levels. Meth. Find. Exp. Clin. Pharmacol. **2**:171–176.

Antibiotic Susceptibilities of Strains of Different Coagulase Types of *Staphylococcus aureus* Isolated from Pyodermas

SATOSHI DEKIO* AND KENTARO ONIMURA

Department of Dermatology and Department of Clinical Microbiology, Hiroshima Hospital of Japanese National Railways, Futabanosato 3-1-36, Hiroshima 730, Japan*

Coagulase of *Staphylococcus aureus* has been shown to be typed in eight types by the differences of its antigenicity (3, 4). We have already reported that all of the strains of *S. aureus* isolated from lesions of pyodermas could be typed in eight types by coagulase typing and that relationships were obviously present between coagulase types and diagnoses of original dermatoses (1). In this study, relationships between coagulase types and antibiograms of *S. aureus* from pyodermas were investigated.

Four hundred and seventy-one strains of *S. aureus* isolated from the lesions of various pyodermas seen at Department of Dermatology, Hiroshima Hospital of Japanese National Railways, in the period from January 1978 to December 1980 were investigated. Coagulase typing was carried out by inhibition of coagulase-induced rabbit plasma coagulation by rabbit antisera to eight antigenically different types of coagulase (3, 4). Coagulase type was defined as the type for which the anticoagulase inhibited coagulation, with the confirmation that none of the other anticoagulases inhibited coagulation. Antibiotic susceptibilities were examined by disk diffusion method (2). Bacteria of susceptibilities of (+++) and (++) to an antibiotic were determined to be susceptible, and those of (+) and (−) to be resistant, to the drug. The antibiotics tested were ampicillin, cephalexin, erythromycin, tetracycline, chloramphenicol, clindamycin, and gentamicin.

All of the strains studied could be typed in eight types, type I to VIII, by coagulase typing, and the same relationships between coagulase types and diagnoses of pyodermas as previously reported (1) were present. The numbers of strains of each coagulase type were as follows: type I, 76; type II, 30; type III, 51; type IV, 82; type V, 179; type VI, 8; type VII, 41; and type VIII, 4. Few or no strains resistant to cephalexin were seen in the strains of any coagulase types. Chloramphenicol-resistant strains composed 18.3% of the strains of type IV, and few or no chloramphenicol-resistant strains were present in the strains of the other coagulase types. Gentamicin-resistant strains composed 11.8 and 12.5% of the strains of type III and VI, respectively. Tetracycline-resistant strains composed 62.2 and 14.0% of the strains of type IV and V, respectively. The strains resistant to ampicillin, erythromycin, and clindamycin were of many coagulase types. The ampicillin-resistant strains constituted 10.0 and 17.3% of the strains of type II and V, and 31.4, 25.0, and 26.8% of those of type III, VI, and VII, respectively. Erythromycin-resistant strains composed 13.7 and 12.5% of the strains of type III and VI, 40.0% of those of type II, and 56.6, 62.2, and 54.2% of those of type I, IV, and V. The clindamycin-resistant strains composed 10.0 and 21.2% of the strains of type II and V, and 39.5 and 45.1% of those of type I and IV, respectively. These results indicate apparently that the antibiograms were specific to coagulase types in *S. aureus* derived from pyodermas.

Coagulase is bacteriologically the most important product in many substances produced by *S. aureus*. Therefore, coagulase typing is, in a sense, a more fundamental method for typing *S. aureus* than other methods such as phage typing and serological typing. On the other hand, most of the antibiotic resistance genes of *S. aureus* have been shown to be located in plasmids, which have been studied widely in the field of molecular genetics. Little interest, however, has been taken in the relationships between coagulase and antibiotic resistance. The present study has shown that relationships were obviously present between coagulase types and antibiograms, which strongly suggests that specific compatibility-incompatibility relationships are present between coagulase genes of different coagulase types and different antibiotic resistance genes.

1. **Dekio, S., and K. Onimura.** 1981. Coagulase types of coagulase-positive *Staphylococci* from bacterial skin infections. J. Dermatol. **8:**223–228.
2. **Dekio, S., K. Takagaki, R. Yamasaki, K. Hamanaka, S. Ikeda, and K. Onimura.** 1981. *Staphylococci* isolated from pyodermas and their sensitivities to antibiotics. J. Dermatol. **8:**215–221.
3. **Ushioda, H., T. Terayama, S. Sakai, and H. Zen-yoji.** 1975. Simplified method for the coagulase typing of *Staphylococcus aureus* and its application to routine works. Annu. Rep. Tokyo Metr. Res. Lab. Pub. Health **26:**1–6.
4. **Ushioda, H., T. Terayama, M. Shingaki, S. Sakai, and H. Zen-yoji.** 1976. Identification of a new antigenic type of staphylococcal coagulase, coagulase type VIII. Annu. Rep. Tokyo Metr. Res. Lab. Pub. Health **27:**1–4.

Antibacterial Efficacy of Cephalosporins Predicted from Conventional Susceptibility Testing in Comparison with In Vivo Results

ECKHARD SCHULZ,* KLAUS SACK, AND REINHARD MARRE

Klinik f. Innere Medizin and Institut f. Medizinische Mikrobiologie, Medizinische Hochschule, Lübeck, Federal Republic of Germany*

The therapeutic concept with β-lactam antibiotics depends on in vitro susceptibility testing which is based on the MIC in relationship to the antibiotic serum levels measured in the middle between two applications ($\tau/2$; 2). The validity of this therapeutic regime is often questioned because it has been derived from a theoretical concept which does not always correspond to clinical observation and which has hardly been experimentally demonstrated. For this reason we compared the antibacterial efficacy predicted from conventional susceptibility testing to the actual therapeutic results of a cephacetrile and cefotaxime treatment on *Escherichia coli* pyelonephritis in rats.

The MICs (1) of cephacetrile and cefotaxime for the *E. coli* strain O2:1:4 were determined in Mueller-Hinton broth (MHB), which is required for the $\tau/2$-rule, and additionally in human plasma ultrafiltrate (PUF), a natural body fluid.

Cefotaxime is characterized by a much lower MIC in MHB (0.125 mg/liter) than cephacetrile (8 mg/liter). In PUF the MIC of cephacetrile increases to 64 mg/liter, whereas the cefotaxime activity remains unimpaired. Serum levels were measured after intramuscular application of 25, 150, or 1,200 mg of cephacetrile per kg and 5, 25, or 150 mg of cefotaxime per kg. Additionally, the not-protein-bound serum concentrations were evaluated (3). From these concentration-time curves the time periods were calculated during which the serum concentrations reach or exceed the MIC up to the breakpoint. Twice the length of this period after the $\tau/2$-rule should correspond to the period of effective tissue concentrations (2). This would mean that a dose of 150 mg of cefotaxime per kg should be effective for 12 h and 150 mg of cephacetrile per kg for 4 h.

The validity of the time-dependent antibacterial activity of cephacetrile and cefotaxime, which is theoretically expected, was examined in the following in vivo model (Tables 1 and 2) (4). After transurethral instillation of an *E. coli* (strain O2:1:4) suspension into the bladder of female rats, the ensuing pyelonephritis was treated 36 h later with single doses of 25, 150, or 1,200 mg of cephacetrile or 5, 25, or 150 mg of cefotaxime per kg intramuscularly. At 3, 6, 12,

TABLE 1. *Comparison of the antibacterial efficacy predicted from in vitro testing after the $\tau/2$-convention with the actual therapeutic results on E. coli pyelonephritis in rats 3, 6, 12, and 24 h after intramuscular (i.m.) application of 25, 150, or 1,200 mg of cephacetrile per kg*

Antibiotic	Dose (mg/kg) i.m.	Period of antibacterial efficacy							
		3 h		6 h		12 h		24 h	
		in vitro	in vivo	in vitro	in vivo	in vitro	in vivo	in vitro	in vivo
Cephacetril	25	-	-	-	+	-	+	-	-
Cephacetril	150	+	-	-	+	-	+	-	-
Cephacetril	1200	+	+	+	+	-	+	-	+

TABLE 2. *Comparison of the antibacterial efficacy predicted from in vitro testing after the τ/2-convention with the actual therapeutic results on E. coli pyelonephritis in rats 6, 12, and 24 h after intramuscular (i.m.) application of 5, 25, or 150 mg of cefotaxime per kg*

Antibiotic	Dose (mg/kg) i.m.	Period of antibacterial efficacy					
		6 h		12 h		24 h	
		in vitro	in vivo	in vitro	in vivo	in vitro	in vivo
Cefotaxim	5	–	–	–	+	–	+
Cefotaxim	25	+	–	–	+	–	+
Cefotaxim	150	+	+	+	+	–	+

and 24 h after cephacetrile application and 6, 12, and 24 h after cefotaxime treatment, the therapeutic results were evaluated by a quantitative bacteriological analysis of the infected kidneys. In the case of cefotaxime the 3-h period was not examined, because at this time point the kidneys contained high antibiotic concentrations vitiating the viable count.

If the above-represented periods of antibacterial efficacy of cephacetrile predicted from in vitro testing after the τ/2-convention are compared to the actually demonstrated therapeutic results with cephacetrile on the *E. coli* pyelonephritis for the chosen observation periods, considerable discrepancies are revealed (Table 1). These discrepancies become even more evident if the MIC is done with PUF instead of MHB or if the not-protein-bound antibiotic concentrations in the serum are taken into account.

Comparing the predicted and experimentally obtained results of cefotaxime in relation to their periods of therapeutic efficacy, it is again obvious that a reduction of the renal bacteria content is detected after a longer period and persists much longer than was expected from theoretical considerations.

The main reasons for the differences between in vitro and in vivo results seem to be due to the fact that the in vivo speed of the antibacterial action in the presence of effective antibiotic concentrations is overestimated in the theoretical model. Furthermore, the exposure period of the bacteria to the antibiotic, which is postulated to be necessary for an antibacterial effect, from a theoretical point of view is longer than actually necessary, since in vivo a therapeutic efficacy may at first occur or continue after complete excretion of the drug.

This work was supported by the Deutsche Forschungsgemeinschaft, Bad Godesberg, Federal Republic of Germany.

1. **Ericsson, H. M., and J. C. Sherris.** 1971. Antibiotic sensitivity testing. Report of an international collobor-ative study. Acta Pathol. Microbiol. Scand. Suppl. B **217**:1–90.
2. **Naumann, P.** 1975. Cephalosporin-Antibiotika aus der Sicht des Mikrobiologen. Ein Vergleich der antibakteriellen und pharmakokinetischen Eigenschaften. Int. J. Clin. Pharmacol. **11**:85–92.
3. **Paschen, K., W. Bautz, and J. Bohner.** 1976. Anaerobe Serumultrafiltration-eine neue Methode zur Bestimmung der Eiweißbindung von Pharmaka unter physiologischen Bedingungen. Arzneim.-Forsch./Drug Res. **26**:2137–2141.
4. **Schulz, E., K. Sack, and W. Henkel.** 1980. Therapeutic studies in acute and chronic urinary tract infection in rats, p. 6–29. *In* H. Losse, A. W. Asscher, and A. E. Lison (ed.), Pyelonephritis, vol. 4. Thieme, Stuttgart.

Dose-Activity Relationship of Cephalosporins In Vitro and In Vivo

ECKHARD SCHULZ,* REINHARD MARRE, AND KLAUS SACK

Klinik für Innere Medizin and Institut für Medizinische Mikrobiologie, Medizinische Hochschule, 24 Lübeck, Federal Republic of Germany*

In the treatment of bacterial infections, different dosages of β-lactam antibiotics are usually proposed. For example, treatment with 2.25 g of cefuroxime or 3 to 4 g of cefoxitin per day is recommended for uncomplicated bacterial infections with susceptible strains, whereas severe infections or moderately susceptible strains should be treated with 4.5 to 6 g of cefuroxime or 6 to 12 g of cefoxitin per day. Such therapeutic recommendations give the impression that a proven dose-activity relationship in vivo or increased therapeutic safety for the patient due to higher cephalosporin doses exists.

In reality, this concept is based on theoretical considerations which have not been clinically verified and which have been insufficiently investigated in vivo. For this reason we compared the concentration-activity relationships of cefuroxime and cefoxitin in vitro and in vivo.

In vitro cultures of *Escherichia coli* strain O2:1:4 in human plasma ultrafiltrate (2) in the logarithmic phase of growth were exposed to various antibiotic concentrations (4 to 120 mg/liter), which corresponded to the serum levels after application of the intermediate doses used in the in vivo experiment. When the numbers of colony-forming units, determined by the viable count method, were plotted as a function of time on a semilogarithmic scale, the initial slopes of the resulting killing curves (which represent the speed of the bactericidal antibiotic effect) were defined in terms of the kill rate constants, thus giving a measure of the bactericidal activity of the antibiotic as a function of its concentration (1).

The kinetic in vitro setup was, as far as possible, transferred to an experimental organ infection (3). After transurethral instillation of an *E. coli* suspension (strain O2:1:4) into the bladder of female rats, the ensuing pyelonephritis was treated 36 h later with a single dose of 25, 150, or 1,200 mg of cefuroxime or cefoxitin per kg, followed by a quantitative bacteriological analysis of the infected kidneys 3, 6, 12, and 24 h after intramuscular application of the drug. Whereas the maximal bactericidal efficacy of cefuroxime in vitro was reached at the MIC (4 mg/liter) and 30-fold higher concentrations had no additional effect, with cefoxitin concentrations from 16 to 60 mg/liter, increasing kill rates were obtained. Maximum bactericidal cefoxitin activity ranged from 60 to 120 mg/liter, and was more intensive than that of cefuroxime.

With *E. coli* pyelonephritis, 3 h after application of 25, 150, and 1,200 mg of cefuroxime per kg a bactericidal effect was still absent in comparison with the control. Only after 6 and 12 h did significantly decreased renal bacteria numbers result with all three doses. However, in agreement with the in vitro results, there was no significant difference among the three doses.

TABLE 1. *Dose-activity relationships of cefuroxime and cefoxitin evaluated from bactericidal kinetics in E. coli cultures in vitro and from therapeutic results in E. coli pyelonephritis in rats*

Cephalosporin	Dose - activity relationship	
	in vitro	in vivo
Cefuroxime	o	o
Cefoxitin	+	+

After application of 25, 150, and 1,200 mg of cefoxitin per kg at each time point and as early as 3 h in comparison with the control, a significant therapeutic efficacy against the *E. coli* pyelonephritis was obvious. In correspondence with the concentration-activity relationship of cefoxitin in vitro after 12 h, the 1,200 mg dose was significantly more effective than the 25-mg/kg dose, and after 24 h, 150 mg of cefoxitin per kg resulted in a significant reduction of the renal bacteria content compared with the 25-mg/kg dose.

In summary (Table 1), for cefuroxime, a positive dose-activity relationship was not detectable either in vitro or in vivo, whereas for cefoxitin, a concentration-dependent increase in bactericidal activity in vitro corresponded to a positive dose-efficacy correlation in vivo. From a clinical point of view these results confirm that commonly proposed antibacterial treatment with different β-lactam antibiotic dosages should be critically considered.

This work was supported by the Deutsche Forschungsgemeinschaft, Bad Godesberg, Federal Republic of Germany.

1. **Garrett, E. R., and C. M. Wong.** 1973. Kinetics and mechanisms of drug action on microorganisms XVII: bactericidal effects of penicillin, kanamycin, and rifampicin with and without organism pretreatment with bacteriostatic chloramphenicol, tetracycline, and novobiocin. J. Pharm. Sci. **62:**1666–1673.
2. **Helm, E. B., and W. Stille.** 1978. Resistenzbestimmungen von Antibiotika in Körperflüssigkeiten. Immun. Infect. **6:**217–222.
3. **Schulz, E., K. Sack, and W. Henkel.** 1980. Therapeutic studies in acute and chronic urinary tract infection in rats, p. 26–29. *In* H. Losse, A. W. Asscher, and A. E. Lison (ed.) Pyelonephritis, vol. 4. Thieme Verlag, Stuttgart.

Pseudomonas aeruginosa: Differences in Antibiotic Susceptibility, Enzymatic Activity, and Antigenicity Associated with Segregating Colonial Morphotypes

DANIEL J. SHEEHAN, J. MICHAEL JANDA, AND EDWARD J. BOTTONE*

Department of Microbiology, The Mount Sinai Hospital, New York, New York 10029, U.S.A.

The dissociation of *Pseudomonas aeruginosa* strains into different colonial morphotypes was first observed over 50 years ago, and more recently by Gaby (1) and Zierdt and Schmidt (4). The latter investigators reported that 77 of 115 (66%) primary cultures of *P. aeruginosa* on blood agar displayed colonial heterogeneity and attributed this phenotypic variation to a refluxing lysogenic phage in the bacterium. Although these 77 isolates showed biochemical identity, they were shown to be different by phage typing.

Seale et al. (2) and Thomassen and colleagues (3) focused their attention on colonial variants of *P. aeruginosa* arising from sputum cultures of cystic fibrosis patients. These authors attributed their observations to the possibility of coinfection by multiple strains of *P. aeruginosa* or by a single strain displaying morphologic heterogeneity.

In our laboratory, we encountered 11 dissociating strains of *P. aeruginosa* from nine patients (Table 1). Patients 2 and 4 had identical isolates obtained from the same or different body sites. None of these nine subjects had cystic fibrosis but presented, instead, with a variety of illnesses.

The 11 *P. aeruginosa* isolates each rendered two to three different colonial morphotypes. These were selected by plating 100-fold dilutions of each isolate from primary cultures onto dialyzed brain heart infusion-skim milk agar, which enhanced the visualization of different colonial morphotypes and their degrees of proteolytic activity. In addition to proteolytic activity, the colonial morphotypes could be distinguished by colonial pigmentation, size, shape, texture, and degree of spreading. The majority of the isolated colonial morphotypes maintained their morphologic integrity on numerous subcultures. The colonial segregants differed, however, in their antibiotic susceptibility (resistance to gentamicin, carbenicillin, chloramphenicol, and tetracycline), presence or absence of exoenzymes (lecithinase, gelatinase, and elastase), degree of proteolytic activity, pigmentation, biochemical profiles, and antigenicity.

Three colonial morphotypes arising from a single urinary isolate exhibited differences in enzymatic properties and antibiotic susceptibility patterns (Table 2). The smooth morphotype showed a marked degree of proteolysis (caseinase activity), was gelatinase and elastase positive, and susceptible to colymycin but moderately resistant to chloramphenicol (Bauer and Kirby). The other colonial morphotypes differed significantly in exoenzyme activity and carbenicillin susceptibility. Similar differences were noted among the colonial morphotypes of the other 10 *P. aeruginosa* isolates.

Serological analysis of eight of nine strains and their 23 colonial dissociants revealed antigenic identity among the colonial morphotypes of seven strains. Only one sputum isolate (patient 4) displayed serological nonidentity among three colonial segregants; two were serotype 11, and one was nontypable. The nontypable morphotype was also distinct on the basis of its antibiogram being resistant to tetracycline and chloramphenicol and moderately resistant to carbenicillin.

To advance the hypothesis that *P. aeruginosa* undergoes in vivo dissociation with the emergence of a single morphotype, we monitored the urinary isolates of *P. aeruginosa* from a single patient over a 1-month period.

Initially, in February, while the patient was not receiving any form of antibiotic therapy, four morphotypes were isolated. Each of these was identical serologically (serotype 11) but showed differences in degree of proteolytic activity. On the basis of MICs, each morphotype was found to be resistant to gentamicin, carbenicillin, and tetracycline. The carbenicillin MIC of the composite original isolate was 100 μg/ml. Over the next 3-week period, the number of colonial morphotypes recoverable from the primary urinary isolate decreased to two, with no concomitant change in the carbenicillin MIC. On 1 March, a urine culture from this patient revealed only a single morphotype of *P. aeruginosa* which now showed a carbenicillin MIC of 800 μg/ml. Evidence that this morphotype was indeed derived from the original parental strain comes from its serological identity to the original strain and constancy of exoenzyme production and antimicrobial susceptibility to agents other than carbenicillin.

The results of this study indicate that multiple varieties of *P. aeruginosa* can be recovered from single primary cultures originating from non-

TABLE 1. *Epidemiological factors associated with patients harboring multiple morphotypes of Pseudomonas aeruginosa*[a]

Patient	Sex (age)	Underlying diagnosis	Source	No. of morphotypes	Serotype	Antibiogram differences	
						Major	Minor
1	M (75)	Hemiparesis	Urine	2	1	0	0
2	F (33)	Metastatic cancer	Ulcer	2	3	0	0
			Ulcer	3	3	0	1
3	M (26)	ESRD	Wound	2	11	0	1
4	M (76)	Cancer of larynx	Wound	2	11	0	0
			Sputum	3	11[b]	1	2
5	F (74)	CVA	Sputum	2	NA	0	0
6	M (46)	Renal failure	Sputum	2	12	0	0
7	F (60)	Histocytic lymphoma	Wound	3	NA	1	1
8	F (76)	COPD	Urine	2	11	2	1
9	—	Urinary tract	Urine	2	11	0	0

[a] Abbreviations: ESRD, end stage renal disease; CVA, cerebral vascular accident; COPD, chronic obstructive pulmonary disease; NA, nonagglutinable.
[b] One of these three morphotypes was nontypable.

TABLE 2. *Exoenzyme variation and antimicrobial susceptibility differences among three different colonial morphotypes from a single urinary isolate*

Variety	Morphology[a]	Proteolysis[b] (mm)	Gelatinase	Elastase	Antibiogram[c]		
					Co	C	Cb
GR15A	Smooth	4.6	+	+	S	MR	
GR15B	Rough	1.1	–	–	S		
GR15C	Smooth	3.2	+	–	S		S

[a] Morphology determined on blood agar plate.
[b] Caseinase activity of reisolated (pure) varieties.
[c] Co, Colymycin; C, chloramphenicol; Cb, carbenicillin; S, susceptible; MR, moderately resistant.

cystic fibrosis patients with a frequency somewhere in excess of 10%.

Many of the phenotypically different colony derivatives also differed in extracellular enzyme production and in antimicrobial susceptibility after in vitro isolation. Enzymatic differences were noted in elastase activity, degree of overall proteolysis, and gelatinase, lecithinase, and lipase production. Since several of these enzymes have been extensively implicated in the pathogenicity of *P. aeruginosa*, the observation that colonial dissociants vary in their enzymatic expression is of considerable importance. In vivo dissociation with concomitant changes in enzymatic properties might greatly enhance the potential invasiveness (virulence) of a given segregant strain. Alternatively, the loss of a given property might signify self-attenuation by a strain. Changes in antimicrobial sensitivity could dramatically affect the outcome of chemotherapy and in part afford an explanation for the failure of drug treatment in cases where one would have anticipated a therapeutic response.

Still speculative is whether other changes associated with colonial dissociation, such as enzyme production and antimicrobial susceptibility, might also occur in vivo, thereby altering pathogenicity or even enhancing virulence. Testimony to in vivo dissociation and perhaps even selection was evident in the one case presented. Most of the colonial variants appear to represent dissociation of a single strain rather than coinfection with different *P. aeruginosa* strains. Still to be correlated more precisely with virulence are the phenotypic changes associated with colonial dissociants. This question is being addressed presently in our laboratory through animal experimentation with each morphotype.

1. **Gaby, W. L.** 1946. A study of the dissociative behavior of *Pseudomonas aeruginosa*. J. Bacteriol. **51:**217–234.
2. **Seale, T. W., H. Thirkill, M. Tarpay, M. Flux, and O. M. Rennert.** 1979. Serotypes and antibiotic susceptibilities of *Pseudomonas aeruginosa* isolates from single sputa of cystic fibrosis patients. J. Clin. Microbiol. **9:** 72–78.
3. **Thomassen, M. J., C. A. Demko, B. Boxerbaum, R. C. Stern, and P. J. Kuchenbrod.** 1979. Multiple isolates of *Pseudomonas aeruginosa* with differing antimicrobial susceptibility patterns from patients with cystic fibrosis. J. Infect. Dis. **140:**873–880.
4. **Zierdt, C. H., and P. J. Schmidt.** 1964. Dissociation in *Pseudomonas aeruginosa*. J. Bacteriol. **87:**1003–1010.

Susceptibility of *Legionella pneumophila* and Other *Legionella* Species to Various Antibiotics

C. H. CHANG,* A. SAITO, M. NAKATOMI, K. IZUMIKAWA, Y. SHIGENO, AND K. HARA

Second Department of Internal Medicine, Nagasaki University School of Medicine, Nagasaki, Japan

Recently, studies regarding whether the type of medium used affects the MIC (minimal inhibitory concentration) of antimicrobial agents against *Legionella pneumophila* have been reported (1, 4). However, the comparison of activity of various antimicrobial agents against *L. pneumophila* and other species of *Legionella* in the two different media, BCYE and BYE agar, have still not been undertaken. The present study was performed to determine and to compare the in vitro antibacterial activity of antimicrobial agents in these two media and to find the effect of the medium and the inoculum size on the susceptibility of Legionaires disease bacteria to various antimicrobial agents.

Two media were utilized for the study: BCYE agar and BYE agar. BCYE agar was made in the conventional way, whereas BYE agar was prepared with a different method. In BYE agar, activated charcoal was not added to the medium, and therefore yeast extract was sterilized, not by autoclaving, but through filtration, the same as L-cystein hydrochloride and ferric pyrophosphate. In both media, the indicated concentration of tested antibiotics was then added for the susceptibility tests.

Strains used for the tests were standard strains stocked in our laboratory and strains isolated from clinical specimens and from the environment. Ten stock strains obtained from the Centers for Disease Control in Atlanta and Wadsworth Medical Center in Los Angeles were used. These were *L. pneumophila*, serogroup I-VI, *L. micdadei*, *L. bozemanii*, and *L. dumofii*. In addition, a total of 11 clinical strains of *L. pneumophila*, 10 of which were isolated in Los Angeles and 1 of which was isolated in our clinic, as well as 4 strains of *L. pneumophila* isolated from the cooling-tower water in Nagasaki city were investigated.

Susceptibility tests were performed by the agar dilution method with a Steer's replicator. To determine the effect of inoculum size on the MIC, two inoculum sizes, 10^6 and 10^4 CFU per spot, for all strains were used.

The results of in vitro susceptibility tests for 22 strains of *L. pneumophila* on BCYE and BYE agar with a final inoculum of 10^6 and 10^4 CFU per spot are shown in Tables 1 and 2. With BCYE agar, the MIC was read after 48 h of incubation. Rifampin showed the greatest activity of all antibiotics. The MICs of erythromycin (EM), gentamicin, minocycline (MINO), amikacin, and chloramphenicol (CP) were also low. The activity against the strains was in decreasing order of rifampin (RFP), EM, gentamicin, MINO, amikacin, and CP, respectively. For the beta-lactam antibiotics, the strains showed various degrees of susceptibility, but all strains were considered to be susceptible to ampicillin, piperacillin, cefoxitin, moxalactam (6095S, oxy-cephem), and cefotaxime. Among the beta-lactam antibiotics, cefoxitin was the most active agent, whereas commonly used beta-lactam antibiotics, such as cefazolin (CEZ), showed no activity. The greater activity of newer beta-lactam antibiotics reflected their resistance to beta-lactamase produced by *L. pneumophila*.

Strains studied on BYE agar showed a slower growth than those on BCYE agar. The MIC was read 72 h after incubation.

The MICs obtained from BYE agar showed susceptibility patterns similar to those studied on BCYE agar with lower values. The difference between the MICs of BCYE and BYE agar was as follows: on BCYE agar, RFP gave an MIC of 0.0125 μg/ml, whereas on BYE agar, the MIC was 0.0062 μg/ml; the MIC of EM was 0.1 μg/ml on BCYE agar, whereas on BYE agar, the MIC was 0.05 μg/ml. CP, MINO, the aminoglycosides, and the beta-lactam antibiotics showed similar results. In general, MIC values of strains grown on BYE agar were one to two dilutions lower than those studied on BCYE agar. For all of the antibiotics, the larger inoculum yielded an MIC one to two dilutions higher than the lower inoculum on both media.

In regard to the strains of other species of *Legionella*, the results of antimicrobial susceptibility tested on BCYE and BYE agar exhibited different susceptibility patterns. Significant differences among the MICs of *L. pneumophila* and *L. micdadei*, *L. bozemanii*, and *L. dumofii* were noted. The MICs of *L. micdadei*, *L. bozemanii*, and *L. dumofii* were lower than those of *L. pneumophila*, and except for tests with CEZ, the antibiotics tested were very active against *L. micdadei*, *L. bozemanii*, and *L. dumofii*. CEZ was active against *L. micdadei* and was active when tested with a lower inoculum size against

TABLE 1. *Susceptibility of L. pneumophila to antibiotics on BCYE agar*[a]

Antimicrobial agent[b]	Inoculum size (CPU/ml)	No. of strains susceptible at an MIC (μg/ml) of:														
		≦0.0062	≦0.0125	0.025	0.05	0.10	0.20	0.39	0.78	1.56	3.13	6.25	12.5	25	50	100
EM	10^6						12	10*[c]								
	10^4				6	7	9									
RFP	10^6		2	18	2	*										
	10^4	2	19	1												
CP	10^6									21	1	*				
	10^4							7	6	9	*					
MINO	10^6								5	17*						
	10^4						1*	19	2							
GM	10^6					*		11	9	2						
	10^4				*		10	9	3							
AMK	10^6							*	13	6	3					
	10^4					*		9	10	3						
AMPC	10^6						3	5	2*	7	4	1				
	10^4			1		5	2*	11	3							
PIPC	10^6						7	1	1	1*	3	9				
	10^4				2	5	3	4*		4	4					
CEZ	10^6							*					1	4	5	12
	10^4				*								7	6	8	1
CFX	10^6					7	13	2				*				
	10^4				7	15		*								
6059S	10^6							1	3	3	5	10	*			
	10^4					1	3	2	4	11	1*					
CTX	10^6							7	14	1		*				
	10^4				5	1	15	1		*						

[a] Twenty-two strains incubated for 48 h.

[b] GM, Gentamicin; AMK, amikacin; AMPC, ampicillin; PIPC, piperacillin; CFZ, cefoxitin; 6059S, moxalactam, oxy-cephem; CTX, cefotaxime.

[c] MICs against *Staphylococcus aureus* 209 p.

L. bozemanii and *L. dumofii*. Testing with the higher inoculum led to a significant increase of the MIC, and a higher MIC on BCYE agar than on BYE agar was also observed. These results in our study were similar to those of Hebert et al. (2), and the difference between the MICs of *L. pneumophila* and other species of *Legionella* toward CEZ might be best explained by the production of beta-lactamase by *L. pneumophila*. *L. bozemanii* and *L. dumofii* were not susceptible to CEZ when tested with a higher inoculum size. This might suggest their variable production of beta-lactamase.

To determine the difference between stock strains and clinical and environmental strains of *L. pneumophila*, the results of susceptibility tests of three groups of strains were compared. Both on BCYE and BYE agar the MICs of most antibiotics against environmental strains were lower than those against stock and clinical strains. EM, RFP, CP, MINO, and the aminoglycosides showed higher MICs against stock strains than against clinical strains, whereas the MICs of beta-lactam antibiotics against stock strains were lower. The reverse was noted in clinical strains. Although the interpretation of these results was difficult, Edelstein (1) contributed the findings to the medium adaptation of the stock strains and suggested that the sole use of stock strains for susceptibility testing might

TABLE 2. *Susceptibility of L. pneumophila to antibiotics on BYE agar*[a]

Antimicrobial agent[b]	Inoculum size (CFU/ml)	No. of strains susceptible at an MIC (μg/ml) of:														
		≦0.0062	≦0.0125	0.025	0.05	0.10	0.20	0.39	0.78	1.56	3.13	6.25	12.5	25	50	100
EM	10^6					13	4	5								
	10^4	4	2	3	6	5	3									
RFP	10^6	22														
	10^4	22														
CP	10^6	1			1	2	3	4	10	1						
	10^4	4					11	7								
MINO	10^6						7	15								
	10^4			2		8	12									
GM	10^6						4	12	5	1						
	10^4				4	5	4	7	2							
AMK	10^6								17	4	1					
	10^4			5	2	1	2	4	4	4						
AMPC	10^6			2		4	2		4	9	1					
	10^4			7	1	2		8	4							
PIPC	10^6				4	3	2	2	2	5	2	2				
	10^4				6	3	5	2	6							
CEZ	10^6												4	2	9	7
	10^4											1	6	2	9	3
CFX	10^6					3	7	11	1							
	10^4		11			1	9	1								
6059S	10^6						4		4	2	5	6	1			
	10^4		6				3	2	3	5	2	1				
CTX	10^6		1		5	1	4	3	7	1						
	10^4		6	1	2	2	5	5	1							

[a] Twenty-two strains incubated for 72 h.
[b] GM, Gentamicin; AMK, amikacin; AMPC, ampicillin; PIPC, piperacillin; CFX, cefoxitin; 6059S, moxalactam, oxy-cephem; CTX, cefotaxime.

be inadequate. Further studies were needed to reveal this mechanism.

Higher MIC values obtained when BCYE agar was used for susceptibility testing indicated that the antimicrobial agents might be inactivated by activated charcoal. To investigate the influence of activated charcoal toward antimicrobial agents, two different concentrations, 100 and 10 μg/ml, of the 16 antimicrobial agents were added to the activated charcoal-containing medium, and the activities of antimicrobial agents in the medium were measured by the bioassay method. The values of activity when tested at concentrations of 100 and 10 μg/ml were as follows: ampicillin, 10.5, 3.8; piperacillin, 50, 5.0; CEZ, 10, 0; cefoxitin, 6, 0; cefotaxime, 20, 4.0; moxalactam, 46, 2.0; EM, 100, 5.0; RFP, 60, 3.6; lincomycin, 80, 3.2; MINO, 6, 0.8; doxycycline, 10, 0; CP, 30, 0; gentamicin, 38, 5.2; amikacin, 60, 1.9; sulfamethoxazole, 29, 1.3; trimethoprim, 20, 0. The decrease of activity by activated charcoal was markedly observed in ampicillin, CEZ, cefoxitin, doxycycline, and MINO, whereas the effect on EM, RFP, lincomycin, and amikacin was minimal.

In conclusion, the in vitro susceptibility tests performed on BCYE agar exhibited higher MICs than did those on BYE agar. This was due to the inactivation of antimicrobial agents when BCYE agar with activated charcoal was used, an observation which our study substantiates. Since BCYE agar recently became the standard culture medium for *L. pneumophila* (3), and the susceptibility tests of antimicrobial agents might be performed on it, the effect of activated charcoal in BCYE agar made the results of the tests inaccurate. For this reason, a medium without activated charcoal was considered to be needed; we therefore prepared a new medium, BYE agar, for susceptibility tests and compared it with BCYE agar. We found that, although strains grew late (72 h on BYE agar versus 48 h on BCYE agar), the new medium gave good results which make it the most ideal medium for susceptibility testing to date. Our suggestion for future research is to develop a faster growth medium without activated charcoal, as the previously stated culture required 72 h of incubation when BYE agar was used. A faster-growing medium would enable a more accurate MIC reading.

1. **Edelstein, P. H., and R. D. Meyer.** Susceptibility of *Legionella pneumophila* to twenty antimicrobial agents. 1980. Antimicrob. Agents Chemother. **18:**403–408.
2. **Hebert, G. A., C. W. Moss, L. K. McDougal, F. M. Bozeman, R. M. McKinney, and D. J. Brenner.** 1980. The Rickettsia-like organisms Tatlock (1943) and Heba (1959): bacteria phenotypically similar to but genetically distinct from Legionella pneumophila and the WIGA bacterium. Ann. Intern. Med. **92:**45–52.
3. **Pasculle, A. W., et al.** 1980. Pittsburgh pneumonia agents: direct isolation from human lung tissue. J. Infect. Dis. **141:**727–732.
4. **Pohlod, D., L. Saravolatz, E. Quinn, and M. Somerville.** 1980. O. Legionnaires and other pulmonary infections: susceptibility of *Legionella pneumophila* to 17 antimicrobial agents, p. 997–998. *In* J. D. Nelson and C. Grassi (ed.), Current chemotherapy and infectious disease, vol. 2. American Society for Microbiology, Washington, D.C.

In Vitro Mechanisms of Nitroimidazole Cytotoxicity

DAVID I. EDWARDS,* RICHARD J. KNOX, IRENA M. SKOLIMOWSKI, AND RICHARD C. KNIGHT

Chemotherapy Research Unit, North East London Polytechnic, London E15 4LZ, England

Hypoxic cells are more resistant to ionizing radiation than well-oxygenated ones, and their presence in human tumors may lead to the failure of radiotherapy. In addition to their ability as radiosensitizers, nitroimidazole drugs are selectively cytotoxic to hypoxic cells. The basis of structure-activity relationships in the development of such drugs is a linear positive correlation of the type, $-\log C = b_0 + b_1 E$, where B_0 and b_1 are constants, C is the drug concentration required to cause a specific biological effect, and E is the electron affinity of the drug usually expressed as the one-electron redox potential E_7^1. The equation indicates that the more electron affinic the drug (i.e., the more positive its E_7^1 value), the greater its radiosensitization and cytotoxicity; this has been well documented for mammalian cells (1, 2). In anaerobic microorganisms, however, the correlation of electron affinity and cytotoxicity is a negative one; that is, the less electron affinic the drug, the greater its cytotoxicity (A. Reynolds, J. Antimicrob. Chemother., in press).

To clarify the interaction of reduced nitroimidazoles with their target (DNA), we have electrolytically reduced a number of nitroimidazoles at constant potentials in the presence of DNA (see Table 1 for details) and measured the relative damage induced in DNA (3–5, 9). The damage is related to DNA base composition (10) and is associated specifically with the release of thymidine phosphates (6; R. J. Knox et al., Biochem. Pharmacol., in press). Such a system may therefore be used to investigate structure-activity correlations of reduced nitroimidazoles at the DNA target.

In general, each drug was reduced under N_2 at potentials shown in Table 1 in the presence of *Escherichia coli* DNA at a drug/nucleotide ratio of 1:1, as previously described (3–5, 9). Samples were removed before and after reduction, which was measured as the loss of absorbance at the wavelength of maximal absorbance and zero current. DNA damage was measured as the amount of [^{14}C]thymidine release determined after 18 h of dialysis against water.

Table 1 summarizes the results obtained with 10 nitroimidazoles reduced in the presence of *E. coli* DNA. The results were fitted to a Hansch-type plot (Fig. 1), which yields a linear negative correlation described by the equation, $-\log C = -0.003\ E_7^1 - 1.4$ ($r = 0.70$), where C is the drug/nucleotide ratio required to produce a 10% release of thymidine from DNA. This equation is similar to that obtained in *Bacteroides fragilis,* where cytotoxicity was measured as the MBC (Reynolds, in press).

An alternative mode of reduction was carried out on four drugs, covering the half-wave potential ($E_{1/2}$) range of −272 to 475 mV; these were reduced at −500 mV for 24 h and DNA damage was measured as labeled thymidine release. This

TABLE 1. *Redox values of and damage produced by reduced nitroimidazoles*

No.	Drug	$E_{\frac{1}{2}}{}^{a}$ (mV)	$E_7{}^{1b}$ (mV)	Damage[c]	Log[1]/C^d	Reduction potential (mV)
1	Benznidazole	−200	−380	2.7	−0.569	−700
2	Misonidazole	−272	−389	5.0	−0.301	−800
3	Nimorazole	−345	−457	4.1	−0.393	−850
4	Ornidazole	−345	−467	7.4	−0.131	−850
5	Tinidazole	−340	−464	12.7	0.104	−850
6	Azomycin	−375	−418	6.0	−0.222	−900
7	Metronidazole	−382	−486	9.5	−0.022	−900
8	Dimetridazole	−388	−475	10.4	0.017	−900
9	8609 RP	−475	−550	10.3	0.013	−1,000
10	4(5)-Nitroimidazole	−540	−527	7.5	−0.125	−1,000

[a] Polarographic half-wave potential measured against a standard Ag/AgCl reference electrode at pH 7.0.
[b] One-electron redox potential measured against the normal hydrogen electrode.
[c] Damage measured as the percent release of [^{14}C]thymidine from DNA.
[d] C is the drug/nucleotide ratio calculated to produce a 10% release of thymidine from DNA.

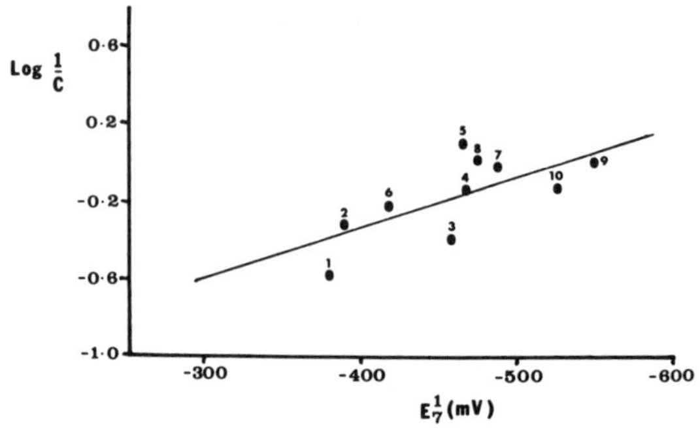

FIG. 1. *Correlation between DNA damage and electron affinity for 10 nitroimidazoles. C is the drug/nucleotide ratio which produces a 10% release of thymidine from DNA, and $E_7{}^1$ is the one-electron redox potential relative to the normal hydrogen electrode.*

experiment was designed to model the weak redox system corresponding to those in hypoxic cells. The results of such reductions when plotted graphically show a linear positive correlation between the log of DNA damage, measured as the percent thymidine release, and the electron affinity ($E_7{}^1$), which is described by the equation, $-\log C = 0.011\ E_7{}^1 + 4.47$ ($r = 0.97$). The correlation is very similar to those obtained for electron affinity and cytotoxicity in hypoxic cells (7, 8). This latter result, however, arises as a consequence of the rate of drug reduction and thus the amount of drug reduced. If the log of the amount of drug reduced per unit time (C) is plotted against $E_7{}^1$, an almost identical correlation to the previous one is obtained, described by the equation, $-\log C = 0.011\ E_7{}^1 + 5.84$ ($r = 0.96$).

These results establish that structure-activity correlations of nitroimidazole-induced cytotoxicity and electron affinity is related to the amount of drug reduced and thus depends upon the endpoint chosen to assess the cytotoxic effect of the drug. If complete drug reduction occurs, the negative correlation obtained is very similar to that found for anaerobic bacteria. If a unit time scale for reduction is considered, a positive correlation is found similar to that found for cytotoxicity in hypoxic cells (7, 8). Since the mechanism of cytotoxicity is identical in all cell types, viz., DNA damage (3–6, 9, 10), it is apparent that the positive correlation arises as a consequence of the different reduction rate of each drug which itself is a direct function of the drugs' relative electron affinity.

The differences in cytotoxicity of nitroimidazoles arise because those drugs which are cytotoxically potent in anaerobes are relatively less effective in hypoxic mammalian cells in which weak redox systems predominate. At the molecular level the mechanism of cytotoxicity in hypoxic mammalian cells, anaerobic bacteria, and protozoa is identical, with greater cytotoxicity being shown by nitroimidazole drugs of low electron affinity.

We thank the Cancer Research Campaign, the Medical Research Council, and Roche Products Ltd. for financial support.

1. **Adams, G. E., E. D. Clarke, I. R. Flockhart, R. S. Jacobs, D. S. Sehmi, I. J. Stratford, P. Wardman, and M. E. Watts.** 1979. Structure-activity relationships in the development of hypoxic cell radiosensitizers. I. Sensitization efficiency. Int. J. Radiat. Biol. **35:**133–150.
2. **Adams, G. E., E. D. Clarke, P. Gray, R. S. Jacobs, I. J. Stratford, P. Wardman, and M. E. Watts.** 1979. Structure-activity relationships in the development of hypoxic cell radiosensitizers. II. Cytotoxicity and therapeutic ratio. Int. J. Radiat. Biol. **35:**151–160.
3. **Edwards, D. I., D. A. Rowley, R. J. Knox, I. M. Skolimowski, and R. C. Knight.** 1980. Nature of DNA damage induced by electrolytically reduced nitroimidazole drugs, p. 561–563. J. D. Nelson and C. Grassi. (ed.), Current chemotherapy and infectious dis-

ease, vol. 1. American Society for Microbiology, Washington, D.C.
4. **Knight, R. C., D. A. Rowley, I. M. Skolimowski, and D. I. Edwards.** 1979. Mechanism of action of nitroimidazole antimicrobial and antitumour radiosensitizing drugs. Effect of reduced misonidazole on DNA. Int. J. Radiat. Biol. **36:**367–377.
5. **Knight, R. C., I. M. Skolimowski, and D. I. Edwards.** 1978. The interaction of reduced metronidazole with DNA. Biochem. Pharmacol. **27:**2089–2093.
6. **Knox, R. J., R. C. Knight, and D. I. Edwards.** 1980. Mechanism of action of misonidazole. International Research Communications System J. Med. Sci. **8:**190.
7. **Olive, P. L.** 1979. Inhibition of DNA synthesis of nitroheterocycles. I. Correlation with half-wave reduction potential. Br. J. Cancer **40:**89–93.
8. **Olive, P. L.** 1980. Mechanisms of the *in vitro* toxicity of nitroheterocycles including Flagyl and misonidazole, p. 39–44. *In* L. W. Brady (ed.) Radiation sensitizers. Masson Publishing, New York.
9. **Rowley, D. A., R. C. Knight, I. M. Skolimowski, and D. I. Edwards.** 1979. The effects of nitroheterocyclic drugs on DNA: an *in vitro* model of cytotoxicity. Biochem. Pharmacol. **28:**3009–3013.
10. **Rowley, D. A., R. C. Knight, I. M. Skolimowski, and D. I. Edwards.** 1980. The relationship between misonidazole cytotoxicity and base composition of DNA. Biochem. Pharmacol. **29:**2095–2098.

Interaction of Chloramphenicol with Intestinal Bacteria: Comparison with Thiamphenicol

GIANFRANCO MARCA,* ENRICO ALBINI, AND LUIGI BONANOMI

Research Laboratories, Zambon Farmaceutici S.p.A., Bresso (Milan), Italy

One of the metabolic pathways which chloramphenicol (CAP) undergoes is the reduction of the nitro group performed by the nitro-reductases present in the tissues and particularly in the intestinal microflora of the host (1).

The substitution of the nitro group in the *para* position of the aromatic ring of CAP with a methylsulfonyl moiety, as in the CAP analog thiamphenicol (TAP), should significantly modify the biological reactivity of the molecule (2).

To verify and quantitate this difference, we studied the in vitro decay of the activity of the two molecules when incubated with intestinal bacteria. Rat cecal content was used, after dilution with brain heart infusion broth, up to a concentration of about 1×10^8 to 5×10^8 bacteria per ml. This preparation was incubated at 37°C, with either CAP or TAP at a final concentration of 100 μg/ml, all of the operations described taking place under strict anaerobic conditions. At fixed times up to 6 h after addition of the drug, a known volume of the incubating mixture was drawn, and the residual antibacterial activity was measured by microbiological assay, employing an agar diffusion method with *Pasteurella multocida* NCTC 10722 as the indicator strain.

Thin-layer chromatography and gas-liquid chromatography analyses were also performed after extraction with ethyl-acetate to detect both the unmodified drugs and possible metabolites (i.e., acetyl and nitro-reduction derivatives). Results are shown in Fig. 1, where the residual activity is plotted against time. As can be seen, CAP is rapidly inactivated by the rat cecal microflora, whereas the activity of TAP shows no significant change.

In fact, after the first hour of incubation at 37°C, more than 50% of CAP was inactivated, and at the end of 6 h, the inactivated fraction was almost 100%. In contrast, the inactivated fraction of TAP was only 9% after 6 h of incubation under the same conditions.

The thin-layer chromatography analysis, which is quite sensitive in revealing the presence of acetylated metabolites, did not show the formation of any such compound. The enzymatic esterification of the hydroxy groups in the lateral chain is a well-known mechanism whereby resistant bacteria inactivate these antibiotics, both

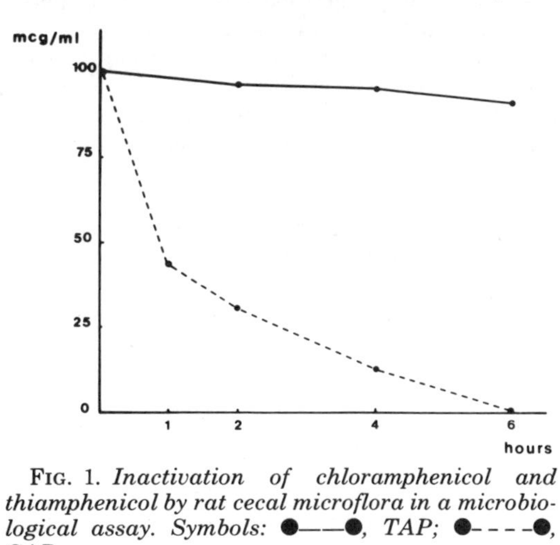

FIG. 1. *Inactivation of chloramphenicol and thiamphenicol by rat cecal microflora in a microbiological assay. Symbols:* ●——●, *TAP;* ●- - - -●, *CAP.*

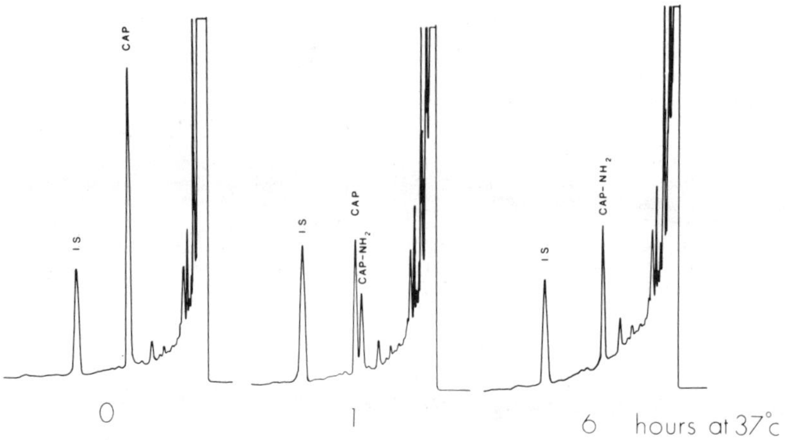

FIG. 2. *Detection of chloramphenicol and its aminophenyl derivative by gas-liquid chromatography. CAP-NH_2, Aminophenyl derivative; I.S., internal standard.*

of which are equally susceptible substrates for the acetyl transferase (3). The absence of acetylated metabolites indicated that, in one case, inactivation took place through another enzymatic pathway.

The gas-liquid chromatography analysis revealed the formation of the aryl amino derivative of CAP (see Fig. 2), whose formation involved the loss of antibacterial activity. On the contrary, TAP, after 6 h of incubation at 37°C, was found to be present only as the original unmodified molecule.

It should be noted that the nitroreduction of CAP is not an actual mechanism of resistance for facultative anaerobic bacteria, because in these microorganisms, it takes a much longer time than that required for the acetylation process to be completed. This is not true for the cecal rat microflora, which mainly consists of anaerobic bacteria (5). In this case, CAP nitroreduction, however slower than the acetylation process, is rapid enough to be of possible practical meaning.

The nitroreduction may, then, explain some therapeutic failures of CAP, seen in patients suffering from infections caused by anaerobic bacteria (4).

Last but not least, the possibility is real that, during the nitroreduction of CAP, some reactive intermediates are formed (nitroso and hydroxylamino derivatives), which are known to be cytotoxic (6). Because of their transient nature, the compounds are not detected with the usual techniques.

In contrast, TAP, lacking a nitro group, retains antibacterial activity in the presence of nitroreductase-producing bacteria, and it cannot possibly form toxic intermediates due to partial nitroreduction.

1. **Glazko, A. J.** 1966. Identification of chloramphenicol metabolites and some factors affecting metabolic disposition. Antimicrob. Agents Chemother. **1966:**655–665.
2. **Manyan, D. R., G. K. Arimura, and A. A. Yunis.** 1975. Comparative metabolic effects of chloramphenicol analogues. Mol. Pharmacol. **11:**520–527.
3. **Shaw, W. V.** 1975. Chloramphenicol acetyltransferase from chloramphenicol-resistant bacteria. Methods Enzymol. **43:**737–755.
4. **Thadepalli, H., S. L. Gorbach, and J. G. Bartlett.** 1977. Apparent failure of chloramphenicol in the treatment of anaerobic infections. Curr. Ther. Res. Clin. Exp. **22:** 421–426.
5. **Wheeler, L. A., F. B. Soderberg, and P. Goldman.** 1975. The relationship between nitro group reduction and the intestinal microflora. J. Pharmacol. Exp. Ther. **194:** 135–144.
6. **Yunis, A. A., A. M. Miller, Z. S. Corbett, and G. K. Arimura.** 1980. Nitroso-chloramphenicol: possible mediator in chloramphenicol-induced aplastic anemia. J. Lab. Clin. Med. **96:**36–46.

Epidemiology and Antimicrobial Susceptibility of *Pseudomonas aeruginosa* in a Large Metropolitan General Hospital

P. M. SOUTHERN,* S. S. SOUTHERN, S. K. WILLIAMS, AND I. PHILLIPS

University of Texas Health Science Center, Dallas, Texas 75235, U.S.A., and St. Thomas's Hospital Medical School, London, United Kingdom

All isolates of *Pseudomonas aeruginosa* from patients in St. Thomas's Hospital were collected during the period July through December 1980. In addition, several environmental strains of *P. aeruginosa* were collected from hospital sources. All organisms were tested in vitro for susceptibility to the following antimicrobial agents: amikacin, azlocillin, carbenicillin, cefotaxime, cefsulodin, colistin, gentamicin, moxalactam, ticarcillin, and tobramycin. Testing was done by an agar dilution method similar to that described by Washington and Sutter (4). The organisms were serotyped by the method recommended by the subcommittee on *Pseudomonadaceae* of the International Committee on Systematic Bacteriology (Difco antisera). Sensitivity to the bactericidal activity of serum and susceptibility to phagocytosis by polymorphonuclear leukocytes were performed by the methods of Young and Armstrong (5). Each isolate was also tested for production of extracellular protease, lecithinase, and elastase (1–3). In addition, patients' clinical courses were followed to ascertain the source and clinical significance of the *P. aeruginosa* strains isolated, as well as the eventual outcome of therapy.

Three hundred twenty-five isolates of *P. aeruginosa* were obtained from 185 patients and several environmental sources as follows: wounds and abscesses, 83; urine, 77; sputum, 43; ear, 33; blood, 19; endotracheal aspirates, 11; ulcers, 11; intravenous catheters, 7; and miscellaneous, 41. By clinical criteria, the organisms were deemed to be significant or probably significant in 82 instances, not or probably not significant in 98, possibly significant in 70, of unknown significance in 66, and irrelevant (not from human sources) in 9 instances. Of the 185 patients studied, 12 died (6.5%), with infection due to *P. aeruginosa* a major contributing factor in at least 8 individuals. All 7 patients with bacteremia due to *P. aeruginosa* died.

A summary of the antimicrobial susceptibility testing results appears in Table 1. Colistin, amikacin, tobramycin, and cefsulodin, in that order, were the most efficacious agents. No isolates were inhibited by clinically relevant concentrations of moxalactam. Gentamicin inhibited only 76.2% of isolates at achievable serum concentrations.

Results of enzyme activity of the isolates are shown in Table 2. Only nine organisms failed to produce protease, and only three failed to produce protease, lecithinase, or elastase. The latter three strains were all of different serotypes.

Only 75 of 316 organisms were susceptible to the bactericidal activity of normal human serum, and only 37 of 225 isolates were susceptible to phagocytosis by human polymorphonuclear leukocytes.

Serotype 3 was most prevalent (75), followed by serotypes 2, 11, and 12 (35 each), and serotypes 6 and 4 (26 and 24, respectively). There were no organisms in serotypes 8, 9, 15, or 16, and there were only single isolates of serotypes 3–5, 6–10, 7–8, and 11–12. Fourteen strains were untypable. Persons dying with *P. aeruginosa* bacteremia were infected by organisms of serotypes 1 through 5 and serotypes 11 and 12. The infecting organism in one such patient was traced to a water bath used to warm frozen

TABLE 1. *Antimicrobial susceptibility of 325 strains of P. aeruginosa from St. Thomas's Hospital*

Agent	Percent susceptible	Median MIC (μg/ml)
Amikacin	90.7	8
Azlocillin	60.9	32
Carbenicillin	73.8	128
Cefotaxime	69.2	16
Cefsulodin	89.9	4
Colistin	93.6	4
Gentamicin	76.2	8
Moxalactam	0	64
Ticarcillin	82.6	64
Tobramycin	90.7	2

TABLE 2. *Enzyme activity of P. aeruginosa from St. Thomas's Hospital*

Enzyme	No. positive	No. negative
Protease	312	9
Lecithinase	41	280
Elastase	262	59
None	—	3
All three enzymes	37	—

plasma being used during an open heart procedure. It was of the same serotype (type 2) and antibiogram, as well as of the same pyocine type (J. Cooper, A. King, and M. Casewell, personal communication).

Infections due to *P. aeruginosa* continue to be extremely important, especially in patients hospitalized with serious underlying disorders. New strategies for management must be sought continually. Antimicrobial agents are important adjuncts in such therapy, but mortality and morbidity in serious *Pseudomonas* disease remain unacceptably high.

1. **Holder, I. A., and C. G. Haidaris.** 1979. Experimental studies of the pathogenesis of infections due to *Pseudomonas aeruginosa*: extracellular protease and elastase as in vivo virulence factors. Can. J. Microbiol. **25:** 593–599.
2. **Sokol, P. A., D. E. Ohman, and B. H. Iglewski.** 1979. A more sensitive plate assay for detection of protease production by *Pseudomonas aeruginosa*. J. Clin. Microbiol. **9:**538–540.
3. **Southern, P. M., Y. E. Todar, and D. A. Morton.** 1979. Bacteremia due to *Pseudomonas aeruginosa*: can we predict survivors?, p. 85–95. *In* D. N. Gilbert and J. P. Sanford (ed.), Infectious diseases: current topics, vol. 1. Grune and Stratton, Inc., New York.
4. **Washington, J. A., II, and V. L. Sutter.** 1980. Dilution susceptibility test: agar and macro-broth dilution procedures, p. 453–458. *In* E. H. Lennette, A. Balows, W. L. Hausler, Jr., and J. P. Truant (ed.), Manual of clinical microbiology, 3rd ed. American Society for Microbiology, Washington, D.C.
5. **Young, L. S., and D. Armstrong.** 1972. Human immunity to *Pseudomonas aeruginosa*. I. In-vitro interaction of bacteria, polymorphonuclear leukocytes, and serum factors. J. Infect. Dis. **126:**257–276.

Antibacterial Activity of Ten Antibiotics Against 261 Strains of *Pseudomonas aeruginosa*

A. G. PARADELIS, N. A. GRANITSAS, V. FIDANI, AND Y. TSELENTIS

Department of Experimental Pharmacology, Medical Faculty, Aristotelian University of Thessaloniki, Thessaloniki, Greece

Before 1969, there were only a few antimicrobial agents for clinical use against serious infections caused by *Pseudomonas aeruginosa*. Subsequently, gentamicin and carbenicillin were introduced into therapy as drugs of choice for pseudomonal infections. Because of the rapidly increasing resistance of *P. aeruginosa* to carbenicillin and gentamicin (3), in the last several years there has been a dramatic increase of antimicrobial agents with promising activity against carbenicillin- or gentamicin-resistant strains of *P. aeruginosa*.

Despite a number of sensitivity studies published dealing with the in vitro activity of each of the individual antimicrobial agents, there are no available sensitivity studies with *P. aeruginosa* which compare the old and new antimicrobial agents with significant antipseudomonal activity.

This study was carried out to compare, under the same experimental conditions, the in vitro antibacterial activity of 10 old and new antibiotics against 261 strains of *P. aeruginosa* isolated from hospitalized patients and against 1 control strain of *P. aeruginosa*, ATCC 27853. The strains of *P. aeruginosa* were identified in accordance with *Cowan and Steel's Manual for the Identification of Medical Bacteria* (1).

Standard powders of the following 10 antimicrobial agents were used: carbenicillin, ticarcillin, azlocillin, amikacin, dibekacin, gentamicin, sisomicin, tobramycin, cefsulodin, and cefotaxime. All antibiotic solutions were prepared fresh on the day used.

MICs were determined by using a serial dilution method of antibiotic assay in Müeller-Hinton broth. The inoculum of the tested strains was adjusted turbidimetrically to contain approximately 10^5 colony-forming units per ml. A medium control with no antibiotic added was provided for each strain tested to assure viability, and medium controls with no antibiotic and no organism were also used to assure sterility of the medium. The MICs were expressed as the lowest concentrations of antibiotic that totally inhibited visible growth after incubation for 24 h at 37°C. Cumulative percent inhibitions, MIC_{50} and MIC_{90}, were determined for each antibiotic.

The results of this study are presented in Table 1. Among the β-lactam-type antibiotics, cefsulodin was the most active compound against *P. aeruginosa*. Inhibitory concentrations ranged between 4.5 and 45 μg/ml, with inhibition of 50 and 90% of the strains occurring at 6 and 12 μg/ml, respectively. Nevertheless, strains of *P. aeruginosa* with high-level resistance to cefsulodin have already been isolated in this coun-

TABLE 1. *Comparative in vitro activities of 10 antibiotics against 261 strains of P. aeruginosa*

Antibiotic	MIC (μg/ml)		
	MIC_{50}	MIC_{90}	Range
Carbenicillin	61	≥250	16.0–≥250.0
Ticarcillin	31	≥125	8.0–≥125.0
Azlocillin	12	55	4.5–70.0
Amikacin	8	50	2.5–60.0
Dibekacin	1.5	6	0.5–9.5
Gentamicin	2.5	55	1.0–≥100.0
Sisomicin	1.5	12	0.5–25.0
Tobramycin	1.5	8	0.5–20.0
Cefsulodin	6	12	4.5–45.0
Cefotaxime	25	60	12.0–80.0

try (A. G. Paradelis, J. Papapanagitou, W. Zurukzoglou, and J. Tselentis, Abstr. Annu. Meet. Am. Soc. Microbiol. 1981, A53, p. 9). Azlocillin and cefotaxime were found to be less active, with inhibition of 50% of the tested strains occurring at 12 and 25 μg/ml, respectively.

Dibekacin, among five aminoglycoside antibiotics, was the most active against the 261 strains of *P. aeruginosa*. Inhibitory concentrations ranged between 0.5 and 9.5 μg/ml, with inhibition of 50 and 90% of the strains occurring at 1.5 and 6 μg/ml. Most of the tested strains of *P. aeruginosa* were susceptible to tobramycin, sisomicin, and gentamicin, with inhibition of 50% at 1.5, 1.5, and 2.5 μg/ml, whereas the inhibition of 50% of the strains with amikacin had occurred at 8 μg/ml. These results are in agreement with previous findings concerning the in vitro antibacterial activity of dibekacin and gentamicin against 200 strains of *P. aeruginosa* (3), although recently other investigators (using different methodology) found dibekacin to be slightly more active than gentamicin against 35 strains of *P. aeruginosa* (2).

We conclude that, of the β-lactam-type antibiotics, cefsulodin exerts the greatest activity against *P. aeruginosa* followed by azlocillin and cefotaxime. Of the aminoglycoside antibiotics, tobramycin, sisomicin, gentamicin, and amikacin do not differ greatly from each other as far as antipseudomonal activity is concerned, whereas dibekacin was found to display the greatest activity against *P. aeruginosa* of all the antibiotics tested.

1. **Cowan, S. T.** 1975. Cowan and Steel's manual for the identification of medical bacteria. Cambridge University Press, New York.
2. **Hill, C. D., G. W. Counts, and M. Turck.** 1981. In vitro comparison of dibekacin and gentamicin activities. Antimicrob. Agents Chemother. **19:**190–192.
3. **Paradelis, A. G., J. Douboyas, G. Stathopoulos, A. Grigoriadou, C. Triantaphyllidis, and J. Papapanagiotou.** 1978. In vitro comparison of kanamycin, kanendomycin, gentamicin, amikacin, sisomisin, and dibekacin against 200 strains of *Pseudomonas aeruginosa*. Antimicrob. Agents Chemother. **14:**514–515.

Susceptibility of 77 Clinical Isolates from Meningitis to Nine Antimicrobials

J. AZNAR, E. MUÑOZ, AND M. C. GARCIA IGLESIAS

Department of Microbiology, Medical School, University of Seville, Seville-9, Spain

The in vitro activity of nine antimicrobials, penicillin, ampicillin, chloramphenicol, cefuroxime, cefotaxime, cefoperazone, moxalactam, thienamycin, and co-trimoxazole, against 77 clinical isolates (61 *Neisseria meningitidis* [57 group B and 5 group A], 9 *Streptococcus pneumoniae*, and 7 *Haemophilus influenzae* [5 β-lactamase producers]) from patients with meningitis were tested.

The MICs and MBCs were determined by the agar dilution method on Mueller-Hinton agar for *N. meningitidis* isolates and on Mueller-Hinton agar supplemented with Fildes (5%) for *H. influenzae* and *S. pneumoniae*. The inoculum for *N. meningitidis* was 10^4 colony-forming units/ml, and two different inoculum sizes (10^4 and 10^6 colony-forming units/ml) were used for the latter two groups.

The MIC_{90} and MBC_{90} of the nine antimicrobials for the three different bacterial groups are summarized in Table 1.

***N. meningitidis*.** All antibiotics were active against *N. meningitidis* (MIC_{90} and MBC_{90}, 0.01 to 0.16 μg/ml), except chloramphenicol (2.5 μg/ml). The most inhibitory and most bactericidal were moxalactam, penicillin, ampicillin, and cefotaxime.

***S. pneumoniae*.** With a light inoculum, all antibiotics were active against *S. pneumoniae* with MIC_{90} and MBC_{90} ranging from 0.0025 to 1.25 μg/ml (5 μg/ml for chloramphenicol); they showed slight inoculum-dependent decreases in

TABLE 1. *Strains inhibited and killed (MIC_{90} and MBC_{90} in micrograms per milliliter)*

Antibiotic	*N. meningitidis*		*S. pneumoniae*				*H. influenzae*			
			10^4 CFU/ml		10^6 CFU/ml		10^4 CFU/ml		10^6 CFU/ml	
	MIC_{90}	MBC_{90}	MIC_{90}	MBC_{90}	MIC_{90}	MBC_{90}	MIC_{90}	MBC_{90}	MIC_{90}	MBC_{90}
Penicillin	0.02	0.04	0.0025	0.04	0.0025	0.04	>20	>20	>20	>20
Ampicillin	0.04	0.08	0.01	0.02	0.04	0.04	>20	>20	>20	>20
Cefuroxime	0.16	0.16	0.005	0.08	1.25	1.25	0.64	20	0.64	20
Moxalactam	0.01	0.01	0.0025	0.01	1.25	1.25	0.08	0.08	0.32	1.25
Cefotaxime	0.04	0.04	0.005	0.01	0.005	0.005	0.08	0.08	0.16	1.25
Cefoperazone	0.08	0.16	0.0025	0.0025	0.08	0.08	0.32	>20	0.64	>20
Thienamycin	0.08	0.16	0.01	0.01	0.04	0.08	2.5	10	10	>20
Chloramphenicol	2.5	2.5	5	5	5	10	10	>20	10	>20
Co-trimoxazole	>0.8–16	>0.8–16	0.2–4	0.2–4	0.2–4	0.2–4	0.8–16	>0.8–16	>0.8–16	>0.8–16

[a] CFU, Colony-forming units. Inoculum size.

their inhibitory and bactericidal activities, with the exception of cefotaxime. Those most affected by the inoculum size, a fourfold increase in the MIC_{90} and MBC_{90}, were cefoperazone, cefuroxime, and moxalactam.

H. influenzae. The MIC_{90} for *H. influenzae* with a light inoculum was 0.08 to 2.5 μg/ml, except penicillin and ampicillin, which showed no activity against all five β-lactamase-producing *H. influenzae* isolates (MIC_{90}, >20 μg/ml for both). Chloramphenicol showed poor activity against all five strains (MIC_{90} and MBC_{90}, 10 μg/ml).

Penicillin and ampicillin were not affected by the inoculum size against non-β-lactamase-producing *H. influenzae*, ampicillin (MIC and MBC, 0.32 μg/ml) being more active than penicillin (MIC and MBC, 5 μg/ml). There was no difference in susceptibility between the β-lactamase producer and -nonproducer strains of *H. influenzae* among the remaining antibiotics. Cefotaxime, moxalactam, cefoperazone, and cefuroxime showed the greatest inhibitory activity against all strains of *H. influenzae*, the only bactericidal compounds being cefotaxime and moxalactam (MBC_{90}, 0.08 μg/ml for both). The MBC_{90}'s were higher than 20 μg/ml for all of the remaining antibiotics.

All antibiotics showed slight inoculum-dependent decreases in their inhibitory activity, but not as pronounced as described previously (2). The effect of the inoculum size on the MBC could not be evaluated as all these values were higher than the highest concentrations (20 μg/ml) used. Only moxalactam and cefotaxime, at a heavy inoculum, showed bactericidal activity (MBC_{90}, 1.25 μg/ml for both), corroborating data published previously (2).

The formation of osmotically stable spheroplasts (1, 3) induced by cell wall-active antibiotics and the high osmolality of the medium used could explain the high MBC we found, in disagreement with Bulger and Washington (2), because when plating for determination of MBC in antibiotic-free medium, reversion to vegetative *H. influenzae* is effected.

Co-trimoxazole showed good activity against *S. pneumoniae* (MIC_{90} and MBC_{90}, 0.2/3 μg/ml) and none against *N. meningitidis* and *H. influenzae* (MIC_{90} and MBC_{90}, >0.8 to 16 μg/ml).

All antibiotics showed good, and similar, inhibitory and bactericidal activities against *N. meningitidis* and *S. pneumoniae*, although chloramphenicol, cefuroxime, and moxalactam showed marked inoculum-dependent decreases in inhibitory and bactericidal activity when tested against *S. pneumoniae*.

1. **Bottone, E. J., A. Bradman, and S. S. Schneierson.** 1976. Spheroplasts of *Haemophilus influenzae* induced by cell wall-active antibiotics and their effect upon the interpretation of susceptibility tests. Antimicrob. Agents Chemother. **9:**327–333.

2. **Bulger, R. R., and J. A. Washington II.** 1980. Effect of inoculum size and β-lactamase production on in vitro activity of new cephalosporins against *Haemophilus influenzae* species. Antimicrob. Agents Chemother. **17:** 393–396.

3. **Klein, R. D., and G. H. Luginbuhl.** 1977. Ampicillin-induced morphological alterations of *Haemophilus influenzae* type b. Antimicrob. Agents Chemother. **11:** 559–562.

In Vitro Susceptibility of *Pseudomonas aeruginosa*

P. VAN DER AUWERA,* A. ALEWAETERS, AND F. SCHUYTENEER

Hôpital Civil de Charleroi, Charleroi, Belgium

Hôpital Civil in Charleroi, Belgium, is a 600-bed community hospital. *Pseudomonas aeruginosa* is a major pathogen in intensive care and cancer units. This organism is also responsible for superinfections of indwelling catheters and surgical wounds. From October 1978, all strains of *P. aeruginosa* from clinical specimens were collected for epidemiological purposes. Only one strain for each patient was included in the collection. We studied the susceptibilities of two samples from this collection to evaluate (i) the MICs of old and new antipseudomonal drugs and (ii) the kind of aminoglycoside-degrading enzymes occurring, using the disk susceptibility pattern (1).

MIC. A total of 150 strains were randomly selected for MIC determination. Three strains were rejected for close relatedness of pyocinotype, lysotype, and serotype, suggesting the same strain. The agar dilution method was used with a multipoint inoculator on Mueller-Hinton agar. The inoculum size was 10^4 colony-forming units per spot. The following antibiotics were used: aminoglycosides—gentamicin, tobramycin, amikacin, and netilmicin; penicillins—carbenicillin, ticarcillin, and piperacillin; cephalosporins—cefsulodin and moxalactam.

TABLE 1. *MIC determination for 147 randomly selected strains of P. aeruginosa*

Drug	MIC_{50} (μg/ml)	MIC_{90} (μg/ml)
Tobramycin	1	4
Cefsulodin	1.5	8
Gentamicin	2	8
Piperacillin	4	12
Amikacin	4	12
Netilmicin	6	16
Moxalactam	8	64
Ticarcillin	8	32
Carbenicillin	64	128

Disk susceptibility testing. A total of 350 strains were randomly selected for disk susceptibility testing; 15 strains were rejected for close relatedness of pyocinotype, lysotype, and serotype, suggesting the same strain. The Kirby-Bauer method was used with Isosensitest (Oxoid) agar. The following aminoglycosides were tested (micrograms per disk): kanamycin (30), amikacin (30), netilmicin (30), gentamicin (10), sisomicin (10), tobramycin (10), paromomycin (30), lividomycin (60), and streptomycin (10).

Results. (i) MIC. Tobramycin was the best aminoglycoside against *P. aeruginosa* (Table 1). Cefsulodin was two to three dilutions better than moxalactam. Ticarcillin was two to three dilutions better than carbenicillin. Gentamicin and cefsulodin showed the same activity. Amikacin and piperacillin showed the same activity. Moxalactam and ticarcillin were equally effective against 90% of the strains.

(ii) Aminoglycoside disk susceptibility pattern (Tables 2 and 3). A total of 84% of the strains were resistant to streptomycin (Table 2); this might be due to APH(3″), APH(6), ANT(3″), or ANT(9), which act only on streptomycin or spectinomycin. A total of 3.6% of the strains were susceptible to all of the aminogly-

TABLE 2. *Disk susceptibility patterns of 335 randomly selected strains of P. aeruginosa to aminoglycosides*

	Kanamycin	Amikacin	Tobramycin	Gentamicin	Sisomicin	Netilmicin	Paromomycin	Lividomycin	Streptomycin	No. of strains	% of strains
(1)[a]	R	S	S	S	S	S	R	R	S	1	0.3
								R	R	69	20.6
								S	R	181	54
								S	S	40	11.9
	S	S	S	S	S	S	S	S	S	12	3.6
(2)[b]	R	S	R	R	R	R/S	R/S	R/S	R/S	21	6.3
(3)[c]	Unusual phenotypes									11	3.3

[a] Probably APH(3′) enzyme. Streptomycin resistance may be due to one of the following enzymes: APH(3″), APH(6), ANT(3″), or ANT(9).

[b] Probably AAC(3) enzyme. Of these strains, four were resistant to moxalactam (19%) and four were resistant to cefsulodin (19%).

[c] Eight strains were resistant to amikacin.

TABLE 3. *Unusual disk susceptibility patterns of 11 strains of P. aeruginosa to aminoglycosides*

Kanamycin	Amikacin	Tobra-mycin	Genta-micin	Sisomicin	Netilmi-cin	Paromo-mycin	Livido-mycin	Streptomycin
R	R	S	R	S	S	R	R	R
R	R	R	R	R	R	R	R	R (3 strains)
R	R	S	S	R	R	R	R	R
R	R	R	S	R	R	R	R	R
R	R	R	S	S	R	R	R	R
R	R	S	R	S	R	R	R	R
R	S	R	R	R	R	R	S	R (3 strains)

cosides tested. A total of 6.3% of the strains showed a pattern of resistance that suggested an AAC(3) enzyme, and 3.3% of the strains showed an unusual pattern of resistance, including amikacin resistance in eight strains (2.4%). Nineteen percent of the strains with the AAC(3) phenotype were resistant to moxalactam or cefsulodin, or both.

1. **Davies, J.** 1980. Aminoglycoside-aminocyclitol antibiotics and their modifying enzymes, p. 474–489. *In* V. Lorian (ed.), Antibiotics in laboratory medicine. The Williams & Wilkins Co., Baltimore.

Comparative Study of Susceptibility to Antibiotics of *Staphylococcus aureus* Strains Isolated from School Children

V. LEPOSAVIĆ,* L. SAVIĆEVIĆ, M. JOVANOVIĆ, O. N. BERGER-JEKIĆ, AND S. JANOŠEVIĆ

Institute of Microbiology and Immunology, School of Medicine, Belgrade, Yugoslavia

As Williams states, although staphylococcal infections have been studied in detail, they are still interesting with regard to the variations of biotypes in various environments and periods of time. Heavy staphylococcal infections represent an important diagnostic and therapeutic problem because their agents are often resistant to antibiotics and hemotherapeutics. Jensen and Lassen (6) have shown that the ability of staphylococci to acquire resistance even during short-time treatment, as well as the fast evolution of infection, clearly explains certain difficulties experienced in the course of treatment. Infections caused by strains of staphylococci resistant to penicillin represent an additional problem in everyday practice, because these microorganisms are generally resistant to some other antibiotics too, as shown by Goldie et al. (5).

Djurišić et al. (3), Krajinović (8), Marić (11), Skalova (12), and Jensen et al. (7) have shown that the percentage of urban carriers with pathogenic staphylococci (PS) in the upper respiratory tract is between 30 and 70%, whereas lately there has been a tendency for rural carriers to increase in number, as shown by Leposavić et al. (9).

To improve the prevention of staphylococcal infections, a detailed investigation of carriers was undertaken among the pupils in the isolated rural area of Montenegro, Yugoslavia. The aims of the investigation were as follows: (i) to determine the number (percentage) of carriers with PS in the upper respiratory tract; (ii) to determine the susceptibility of isolated strains to a number of antibiotics belonging to the beta-lactam group, macrolides, and aminoglycosides, which are frequently used in the treatment of staphylococcal infections; (iii) to analyze statistically the frequency of occurrence of the strains susceptible to penicillin, ampicillin, and carbenicillin, tested by the diffusion and dilution methods; and (iv) to determine the phage groups to which the isolated strains of staphylococci belong and establish the phage type predominant in the above-mentioned rural area.

The investigation covered 412 school children from ages 6 to 15 years. Positive results were found with 158, or 38.3%, of the total. The isolated strains of staphylococci were tested by the coagulase test. The coagulase-positive staphylococci, i.e., 193 strains, were tested for susceptibility according to various groups of antibiotics, using the diffusion (13) and agar dilution antibiogram methods, as described by Ericsson and Sherris (4). A standard strain of *Staphylococcus aureus* ATCC 2593 was also included (2). The following antibiotics were used: penicillin G, ampicillin, carbenicillin, methicillin, cefazolin, erythromycin, lincomycin, clindamycin, gentamicin, and tobramycin. Phage typing of the iso-

TABLE 1. *Susceptibility of 193 strains of S. aureus to the beta-lactam group of antibiotics*

Assay method	Penicillin		Ampicillin		Carbenicillin		Methicillin		Cefazolin	
	No.	%	No.	%	No.	%	No.	%	No.	%
Diffusion										
Susceptible	31	16.6	31	16.6	77	39.9	193	100	193	100
Resistant	162	83.4	162	83.4	116	60.1	0	0	0	0
Agar dilution										
Susceptible	28	14.5	28	14.5	28	14.5	193	100	103	100
Resistant	165	85.5	165	85.5	165	85.5	0	0	0	0

TABLE 2. *Susceptibility of 193 S. aureus strains to 10 antibiotics*

Antibiotics	Susceptibility at given MIC (μg/ml)																			
	0.04		0.09		0.19		0.39		0.78		1.56		3.12		6.25		12.5		50	
	No.	%	No.	%	No.	%	No.	%	No.	%	No.	%	No.	%	No.	%	No.	%	No.	%
Penicillin			12	6.2	16	8.3	6	3.1	39	20.2	59	30.6	35	18.1	20	10.4	6	3.1		
Ampicillin	1	0.5	5	2.6	22	11.4	6	3.1	55	28.5	61	31.6	31	16.1	9	4.7	1	0.5	2	1.0
Carbenicillin									28	14.5	3	1.6	90	46.6	72	37.3				
Methicillin											77	39.9	116	60.1						
Cefazolin					8	4.1	137	71	37	19.2	11	5.7								
Erythromycin			21	10.9	145	75.1	26	13.5	1	0.5										
Lincomycin					3	1.6	34	17.6	139	72	5	2.6	12	6.2						
Clindamycin	1	0.5	187	96.9	2	1			1	0.5	1	0.5	1	0.5						
Gentamicin			6	3.1	51	26.4	90	46.6	31	16.1	12	6.2	3	1.56						
Tobramycin			2	1	62	32.1	95	49.2	23	11.9	8	4.2	3	1.6						

lated PS strains was performed by the standard method at the Reference Laboratory for Phage Typing in Zagreb (1, 14, 15).

Table 1 shows the susceptibility of the 193 PS strains to the group of beta-lactam antibiotics. It can be clearly seen that 165, or 85.5%, of the isolated strains were resistant to penicillin, ampicillin, and carbenicillin, whereas 100% of them were susceptible to methicillin and cefazolin. The results obtained suggest that a high percentage of the isolated strains were resistant to the beta-lactam group of antibiotics affected by beta-lactamase (penicillin, ampicillin, and carbenicillin).

Table 2 shows the MIC ranges for the 193 *S. aureus* strains. Ampicillin showed the widest range, from 0.04 to 50.0 μg/ml. Similar values were obtained for penicillin. The MIC range for carbenicillin was from 0.78 to 6.25 μg/ml, whereas all of the susceptible strains had the same MIC value, 0.78 μg/ml. The susceptibility to gentamicin and tobramycin showed the identical MIC range, from 0.09 to 3.12 μg/ml. Maliwan et al. (10) have also shown that susceptibility to gentamicin is followed by susceptibility to tobramycin.

Analysis of the results obtained showed that 38.3% of 412 school children were carriers of PS strains colonized in the upper respiratory tract. A total of 85.5% of 193 PS strains were resistant to penicillin, ampicillin, and carbenicillin, but 100% were susceptible to methicillin and cefazolin. All of the PS strains investigated were susceptible to the antibiotics used, which belong to the group of macrolides and aminoglycosides. There were no significant differences in the frequency of isolation of strains susceptible to penicillin, ampicillin, and carbenicillin ($\chi^2 = 1.55$; df $= 2$; $P = 0.05$). Most of the isolated PS strains belonged to phage group II (42.5%), whereas there was no predominance of any phage type.

1. **Blair, J. E., and R. E. O. Williams.** 1961. Phage typing of staphylococci. Bull. W.H.O. **24:**771–784.
2. **Coyle, M. B., M. F. Lampe, C. L. Aitkin, P. Feigl, and J. C. Sherris.** 1976. Reproducibility of control strains for antibiotic susceptibility testing. Antimicrob. Agents Chemother. **10:**436–440.
3. **Djurišić, M., Z. Vukčević, J. Tomić, J. Marić, and V. Šćepan.** 1966. Nalaz Staphylococcus pyogenes-a kod bolesnika i osoblja bolničkih ustanova, kod gradskog i seoskog stanovništva i njegova osetljivost prema raznim antibioticima. Glas Srpske akademije nauka i umetnosti CCLXVII, **19:**11–19.
4. **Ericsson, H. M., and J. C. Sherris.** 1971. Antibiotic sensitivity testing. Acta Pathol. Microbiol. Scand. Sect. B **217**(Suppl.):1–90.
5. **Goldie, D. J., V. G. Alder, and W. A. Gillespie.** 1971. Changes in the drug resistance of Staphylococcus aureus in a non-hospital population during a 20-year period. J. Clin. Pathol. **24:**44–47.
6. **Jensen, K., and C. A. Lassen.** 1964. Fulminating staphylococcal infections treated with Fucidin and penicillin or semisynthetic penicillin. Ann. Intern. Med. **60:**790–798.

7. **Jensen, O., K. Rosendal, P. Bulow, V. Faber, and E. K. Riewerts.** 1969. Changing staphylococci and staphylococcal infections. N. Engl. J. Med. **281**:627–635.
8. **Krajinović, S.** 1964. Neki današnji epidemiološki i bakteriološki problemi intrahospitalnih infekcija. Preventivna Medicina, Rijeka, **7**:289–312.
9. **Leposavić, V., O. Berger-Jekić, L. Savićević, and M. Jovanović.** 1981. A bacteriological study of the action of the beta-lactam group antibiotics on Staphylococcus aureus. Staphylococci and staphylococcal infection. Zentrabl. Bakteriol. Parasitenkd. Infektionskr. Hyg. **10**(Suppl.)**3**:777–780.
10. **Maliwan, N., H. G. Grieble, and T. J. Bird.** 1975. *Pseudomonas aeruginosa*: surveillance of resistance to gentamicin and transfer of aminoglycoside R factor. Antimicrob. Agents Chemother. **8**:415–420.
11. **Marić, R.** 1972. Osetljivost stafilokoka na antibiotike u gradske i seoske dece. Antibiotici i antibiotska terapija, Zagreb, 57–61.
12. **Skalova, R.** 1973. Hospitalne infekcije u Jugoslaviji. Hospitalne infekcije, Zagreb, 20–27.
13. **W.H.O. Tech. Rep. Ser. (BS) 1129**:5–25, 1976.
14. **Williams, R. E. O.** 1963. Subcommittee on phage typing of staphylococci. Int. Bull. Bacteriol. Nomencl. Taxon. **13**:119.
15. **Williams, R. E. O., and J. E. Rippon.** 1952. Bacteriophage typing of Staphylococcus aureus. J. Hyg. **50**:320–353.

Distribution of Labeled Antibiotics in Normal and Infected Rat Brain: an Autoradiographic Study

H. KOURTOPOULOS,* S. E. HOLM, AND B. WINBLAD

Departments of Neurosurgery, Clinical Bacteriology, and Clinical Pathology, University Hospital, Umeå, Sweden*

Since abscesses in the central nervous system can appear in any area of the brain, the drugs used for therapy should reach adequate antimicrobial concentrations in the white as well as the gray matter. Cohen et al. (1) showed by autoradiography that some drugs penetrate into gray matter more rapidly than into white matter. White matter has very few perforating vessels since most of the small perforating vessels with a diameter of 50 to 60 μm supply solely the cerebral cortex and never penetrate deep into the white matter (7). Because of the hypovascularity of the white matter and a more frequent occurrence of brain abscesses at the junction between gray and white matter (4), it is important to define the pattern of distribution of antibiotics throughout the brain.

The aim of this investigation was to study the distribution characteristics of labeled antibiotics in the central nervous system by using autoradiography in healthy animals and in animals with experimentally induced brain abscesses. Since it is well known that various antibiotics differ widely in their ability to penetrate the central nervous system, we chose to study the distribution of ^{35}S-labeled benzylpenicillin in the normal and infected rat brain, and to compare these results with those obtained with ^{14}C-labeled cefuroxime.

Fifteen Spraque-Dawley rats weighing 200 g were used. Abscesses were produced in 10 of the animals. After narcotizing them with intraperitoneal pentobarbital, the top of the head was shaved and a 15-mm midline scalp incision was made under aseptic precautions. A 2-mm burr hole was made, 2 mm behind the coronar suture and 4 mm lateral to the midline. A microliter needle was positioned above the burr hole and could be slowly lowered stereotactically 2.5 mm into the brain under simultaneous microscopic control. For the infection, 1 μl of a freshly washed suspension of *Bacteroides fragilis* containing 10^8 colony-forming units per ml was injected during a period of 30 min, thus avoiding spread and pressure-volume effects on the parenchyma. After an additional 5 min, the needle was slowly withdrawn.

All noninfected animals were injected intravenously with ^{35}S-labeled penicillin.

Four days after bacterial inoculation in the brain, 5 of 10 infected animals were injected with ^{35}S-labeled penicillin and 5 were injected with ^{14}C-labeled cefuroxime. Fifteen minutes after the antibiotic injection, all rats were killed; the brains were removed immediately, transferred into a sodium carboxymethyl cellulose embedding medium, and frozen by hexane cooled with dry ice, by the technique of whole-body autoradiography originally described by Ullberg (10, 11).

Macroscopic examinations of the uninfected rat brains served as controls. Examination of the infected brains in most cases revealed the presence of swelling (9 of 10), midline shift, and localized superficial discoloration of the injected hemisphere.

The autoradiographs were examined for evaluation of the activity in the section. In the control series that received only ^{35}S-labeled penicillin, radioactivity was mainly found in the pial vessels, with variable dispersion in the subarachnoid space and choroid plexus. No activity was seen in deeper cortical layers or white matter. In the infected animals, the distribution of the two labeled antibiotics used in this experiment was markedly different. The autoradiographs of the rats injected with ^{35}S-penicillin exhibited a diffuse scattered radioactivity in the subarachnoid space and pial vessels similar to the findings in the normal rat brain autoradiography. Activity was also seen in the superficial cortex layers although abscess formation was seen macroscopically in this region. On the other hand, radioactivity was clearly seen in the autoradiographs of the rats injected with ^{14}C-cefuroxime, not only in the surrounding subarachnoidal space and pial vessels but also in the surrounding and in a well-defined intracerebral abscess.

Several factors have been shown to influence the penetration of antibiotics into the cerebrospinal fluid and brain tissue (3, 6, 8). These factors include not only molecular size of the antibiotic, degree of binding to serum proteins, degree of lipophilicity, and ionization at the pH of the blood, cerebrospinal fluid, and brain, but also cerebral blood flow and general permeability of cerebral blood vessels (2, 6). Although the vascular pattern and penetration of an antibiotic through the blood-brain barrier is significantly altered in cases of infection, our clinical knowledge mainly relates to cases with superficial parenchymatous infections such as meningitides or ventriculitides. Since cerebral abscesses are considerably more frequent at the junction between gray and white matter (4) and since, as a result of their excentric growth, most of them appear in the deeper areas of the white matter, the sparse capillary supply found there (9) will strongly limit the antibiotic penetration to the surrounding tissue and also inside the abscess cavity. In our material from healthy animals, penicillin was mainly detected in the pial vessels. No activity was found in the deeper layers of gray or white matter.

Hassler and Forsgren (5) in their series of experimentally induced brain abscesses in rabbits found that the vascular reaction around cerebral abscesses was very weak, the newly formed vessels being thinner and more sparsely distributed compared with abscesses in other body sites. It therefore seems likely that antibiotics such as benzylpenicillin, with poor penetration into the brain and especially in the deep white matter, where abscess formation is common, will be insufficient in the light of our present findings for the treatment of brain abscesses. On the other hand, even though vascularity is sparse in the white matter, antibiotics such as

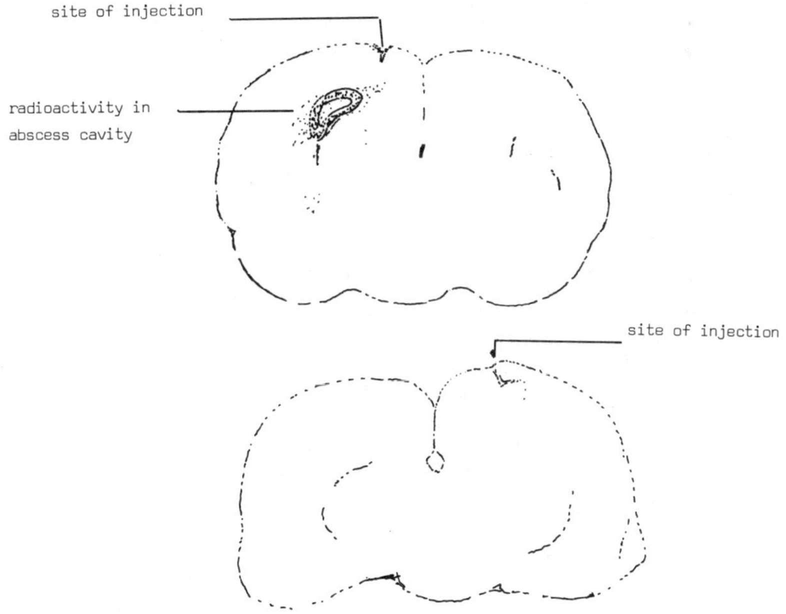

FIG. 1. *Distribution of ^{14}C-labeled cefuroxime (top) and ^{35}S-labeled penicillin (bottom) in experimentally induced abscess in the rat brain 5 min after injection. In the lower drawing, radioactivity is visible only at the site of injection. Note the enlargement of the hemisphere due to edema.*

cefuroxime will penetrate more readily, as found in our experiment.

It should be added that the amount of ^{35}S-penicillin and ^{14}C-cefuroxime, however, was only qualitatively examined. It seems to us that this type of experimental analysis can produce useful information, as can be seen in Fig. 1 when the radioactive region is isolated or of large size relative to the resolution. In cases where more detailed information is required, quantitative measurements must be undertaken, e.g., for comparison between two antibiotics with almost equal penetration capacity or different concentration gradients.

These preliminary findings on experimentally induced brain abscesses in the rat show that this animal model together with autoradiographic techniques provides an easy method for visualization of brain abscesses and for study of the penetration of different labeled antibiotics into the normal and infected brain.

1. **Cohen, E. N., K. L. Chow, and L. Mathers.** 1972. Autoradiographic distribution of volatile anaesthetics within the brain. Anaesthesiology **37**:324.
2. **Crone, C.** 1965. The permeability of brain capillaries to non-electrolytes. Acta Physiol Scand. **64**:407.
3. **Davson, H.** 1967. Physiology of the cerebrospinal fluid. Little, Brown & Co., Boston.
4. **Greenfield, J. B.** 1963. Neuropathology, p. 138–156. The Williams & Wilkins Co., Baltimore.
5. **Hassler, O., and A. Forsgren.** 1964. Experimental abscesses in brain and subcutis. A microangiographic study in the rabbit. Acta Pathol. **62**:59–67.
6. **Norrby, R.** 1978. A review of the penetration of antibiotics into CSF and its clinical significance. Scand. J. Infect. Dis. **14**:296–309.
7. **Raimondi, J. A., and C. Di Rocco.** 1979. The physiopathogenetic basis for the angiographic diagnosis of bacterial infections of the brain and its coverings in children. II. Cerebritis and brain abscess. Child's Brain **5**:398–407.
8. **Schanker, L.** 1965. Passage of drugs into and out of the central nervous system. Antimicrob. Agents Chemother. **5**:1044.
9. **Stehbens, E. W.** 1972. Pathology of cerebral blood vessels, p. 60–76. C. V. Mosby Co., St Louis.
10. **Ullberg, S.** 1954. Studies on the distribution and fate of ^{35}S-labeled benzylpenicillin in the body. Acta Radiol. Suppl., p. 1–110.
11. **Ullberg, S.** 1977. Technique of whole body autoradiography. Sci. Tools.

Effect of Dosing Regimens on the Activity of Antimicrobial Agents in an In Vivo Model

ANDREAS U. GERBER,* ROBERT W. BUNDTZEN, AND WILLIAM A. CRAIG

Departments of Medicine, William S. Middleton Memorial Veterans Administration Hospital and University of Wisconsin, Madison, Wisconsin 53706, U.S.A.

The relationship between drug dose and corresponding antimicrobial activity has been well documented for most current antibiotics. In contrast, little is known about the impact of the dosing interval and its duration on the efficacy of these drugs. Experimental models both in vitro and in vivo needed for studying this question have not yet been well established. An animal model for such investigations requires that the pharmacokinetics of the drug and the corresponding antimicrobial effect can be easily and accurately quantitated at the same time and in the same animal. In such an attempt we evaluated a mouse thigh model (2, 3) for studying the effect of two different dosing intervals of penicillin G on two clinical isolates of a very susceptible organism (*Streptococcus pneumoniae*). We chose the mouse thigh model because the thigh can be removed intact quite easily and the number of bacteria can be quantitated by plating serial dilutions of thigh homogenate onto agar. Furthermore, antibiotic concentrations in the interstitial fluid of muscle have been shown to parallel the fluctuations in levels observed in serum (4). Leukopenic mice were used to examine more directly the effect of the antibiotic on the infecting microorganism.

Approximately 10^6 colony-forming units of *S. pneumoniae* were injected into the thigh muscle of mice made leukopenic by two previous injections of cyclophosphamide. One hour later, treatment was started with subcutaneous injections of penicillin G containing a tracer amount of radiolabeled (^{14}C) drug. The two dosing regimens chosen were 2 μg/g every 4 h versus 0.5 μg/g given hourly. Thus, identical total doses resulted after 4 (and 8) h. At various time intervals blood was drawn from the retroorbital sinus for determination of penicillin levels (three mice per sampling point). At intervals of 1 to 2 h, groups of three mice were sacrificed and the thigh muscles were removed and homogenized in iced saline. The numbers of colony-forming units per thigh were calculated after plating serial 10-fold dilutions of 10% thigh homogenates onto blood agar plates.

Figure 1 shows the penicillin kinetics in blood and the antimicrobial effect in thighs for the two treatment regimens. As expected, peak penicillin concentrations in blood were four times higher after the dose of 2 μg/g than those observed after injections of 0.5 μg/g. However, the total area under the penicillin concentration-versus-time curve calculated from 0 to 5 h by the trapezoidal method was similar in both groups (68.3 and 69.9 μg.h/ml for the treatments every 4 h and every 1 h, respectively). Drug levels in total thigh tissue (determined in 10% homogenates) were approximately 26% of the simultaneous blood level and paralleled the fluctuations in antibiotic concentration observed in blood.

The maximal bactericidal effect of a single penicillin G dose of 2 μg/g was observed at 1 h after injection; regrowth of the test organisms started 2 to 3 h after injection. In contrast, the hourly injections of the smaller dose were less effective during the first 2 h after treatment was started. However, by 4 h, the hourly regimen proved to be significantly more effective. By this time, it had reduced the number of viable organisms to less than 1% of the initial inoculum. Regrowth of the test organisms occurred by 3 h after the last injection of penicillin.

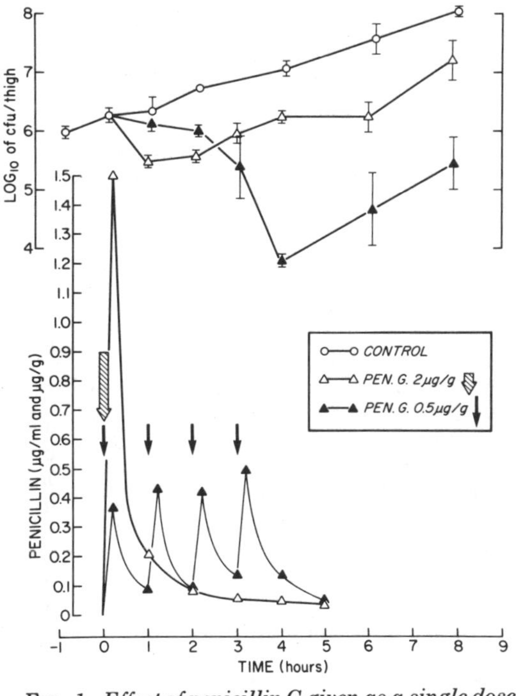

FIG. 1. *Effect of penicillin G given as a single dose (2 μg/ml) or four divided doses (0.5 μg/g) 1 h apart on S. pneumonia (clinical isolate VA 1562). Drug kinetics and drug effect were determined in the very same mice. Peak blood concentrations were obtained 10 min after drug injections. Each point represents the mean value for three mice (geometric mean ± 1 SD for colony-forming units).*

Figure 2 shows a similar experiment performed with another clinical isolate as the test organism. Treatment was started 2 h after the injection of bacteria. The treatment regimens were the same as in Fig. 1, but their duration was expanded to 8 h. Clearly, the treatment failure of the injections every 4 h was due to significant bacterial regrowth, occurring after the penicillin blood level had fallen below the MIC. On the other hand, despite fourfold smaller individual doses, the hourly treatment regimen did not allow for bacterial regrowth and resulted in almost complete eradication of the test organisms from mouse thighs by 8 h.

Our studies demonstrate the usefulness of the mouse thigh model for studying the activity of antimicrobials in vivo. The results obtained are not simply endpoints such as survival or death. Rather, bacterial growth and kill curves can be easily and reproducibly obtained in vivo, and the kinetics of the drug can be correlated with the antimicrobial effect. Thus, although it is not a natural infection, we consider this model a useful tool for studying the impact of the dosing interval on the antimicrobial efficacy of a drug.

In this model a low dose of penicillin G proved to give much higher bactericidal activity in vivo against *S. pneumoniae* when given hourly in small doses than when given in larger doses every 4 h. A major difference between these dosage regimens was the length of time tissue levels were above the MIC, being much longer for the multiple small doses. We expected that the postantibiotic persistent effect (1, 5) would prevent regrowth of bacteria when levels fell below the MIC, especially with the dosing every 4 h. However, the tissue levels obtained were

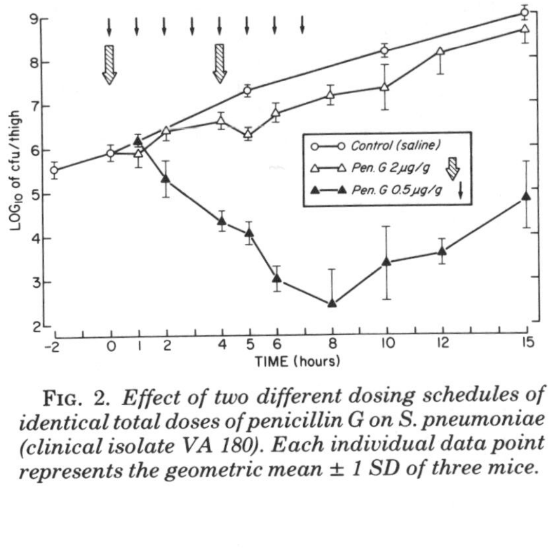

FIG. 2. *Effect of two different dosing schedules of identical total doses of penicillin G on S. pneumoniae (clinical isolate VA 180). Each individual data point represents the geometric mean ± 1 SD of three mice.*

not much above the MIC, and this may explain why a prolonged postantibiotic effect was not obtained with this treatment regimen. Hence, further studies are needed looking at higher total doses of penicillin to determine whether the penicillin concentration needs to be maintained above the MIC at all times to inhibit regrowth and to exert maximal bactericidal efficacy against *S. pneumoniae* in vivo.

1. **Bundtzen, R. W., A. U. Gerber, D. Cohn, and W. A. Craig.** 1981. Post-antibiotic suppression of bacterial growth. Rev. Infect. Dis. **3**:28–37.
2. **Gerber, A. U., and W. A. Craig.** 1981. Growth kinetics of respiratory pathogens after short exposures to ampicillin and erythromycin *in vitro*. J. Antimicrob. Chemother. (in press).
3. **Hunter, P. A., G. N. Rolinson, and D. A. Witting.** 1976. Effect of carbenicillin on Pseudomonas infection, p. 289–294. *In* J. D. Williams and A. M. Geddes (ed.), Chemotherapy, vol. 2. Proceedings of the 9th International Congress of Chemotherapy. Plenum Press, New York.
4. **Kunst, M. V., and H. Mattie.** 1978. Cefazolin and cefradine: relationship between serum concentrations and tissue contents in mice. Infection **6**:166–170.
5. **McDonald, P. J., W. A. Craig, and C. M. Kunin.** 1977. Persistent effects of antibiotics on *Staphylococcus aureus* after exposure for limited periods of time. J. Infect. Dis. **135**:217–223.

Efficacy of Fosfomycin with and Without Glucose 6-Phosphate in Experimental Infection

MANFRED L. ROTTER,* ALEXANDER HIRSCHL, AND GEROLD STANEK

Hygiene-Institute of the University, Vienna, Austria

With certain bacterial species the antimicrobial efficacy of fosfomycin is considerably enhanced in vitro by the presence of hexose 6-phosphates (H-6-P) such as glucose 6-phosphate (G-6-P) (1, 2, 5). This phenomenon is thought to be based on improved transportation of fosfomycin into the bacterial cell by activation of a second transport system across the barrier of the bacterial cell membrane. In addition to the activity of the usual carrier, the α-glycerolphosphate (α-GP) transport system, this mechanism leads to much higher intracellular concentrations of the antibiotic (2, 5). In contrast to the constitutive α-GP system, it is known to be an inducible enzymatic system in cells of *Staphylococcus aureus* and of *Enterobacteriaceae* excepting those of *Proteus* and *Providencia* species (2, 4). Resistant mutants of these inducible bacteria lacking the α-GP system regain full susceptibility to fosfomycin when the H-6-P transport system is activated by the presence of an H-6-P (2).

As reported by Kahan et al. (2) and by our group (4), the antimicrobial efficacy of fosfomycin was considerably increased in vivo also by G-6-P in chemotherapy of mice that were infected experimentally with *Escherichia coli* and *Salmonella typhimurium*, respectively. In the latter case the ED_{50} was reduced to one-thirteenth when G-6-P was added to the solution of fosfomycin at a dose of 50 mg per kg of body weight (4).

This investigation was undertaken to elucidate (i) the influence of G-6-P on the ED_{50} of fosfomycin in chemotherapy of mice experimentally infected with bacterial species or strains possessing or not possessing the H-6-P system, (ii) blood levels of G-6-P in dogs after subcutaneous or intravenous administration, and (iii) effect of duration that inducible bacterial cells are in contact with G-6-P on the MIC of fosfomycin.

Inbred male mice (strain G. P., NIH) weighing 20 ± 2 g were infected with either of two bacterial strains possessing an inducible H-6-P transport system (*Klebsiella oxytoca*, *K. aerogenes* II) or with either a strain of *Proteus mirabilis* or a mutant of *K. aerogenes* (strain I) not possessing an inducible H-6-P system. All bacterial strains had been held in liquid nitrogen, and after one subculture they were suspended in isotonic saline containing 2.5% (wt/vol) gastric mucin. The mice were infected by injecting 0.5 ml of this suspension into the peritoneal cavity. The infectious dose was adapted to cause death in at least 95% of untreated mice within 48 h (10^3 to 10^7 colony-forming units per animal). Groups of 10 infected animals each were then treated 1 and 6 h after infection by subcutaneous administration of 0.1 ml of a solution in distilled water of either fosfomycin (sodium salt) in various concentrations ($\log_2$ steps) or fosfomycin plus G-6-P (disodium salt, 100 mg/kg of body weight). As controls, infected mice received either a solution of G-6-P alone or distilled water only. The ED_{50} was calculated by probit analysis. Differences were tested for significance by the method of Spearman and Karber. Usually, MICs were assessed by the agar dilution technique using Mueller-Hinton agar (35°C for 24 h). When necessary, the MIC was sometimes assessed in Mueller-Hinton broth incubated for 48 h.

Blood levels of G-6-P were determined in dogs (beagles) weighing 16 to 20 kg after subcutaneous (neck) or intravenous (foreleg) injection of a solution of 100 mg of G-6-P disodium salt per kg of body weight. Venous samples were collected at various intervals up to 4 h. Immediately after a blood specimen was drawn, it was deproteinized. Later, the concentrations of G-6-P were determined as described by Lang and Michal (3).

The effect of duration of contact of an inducible bacterial strain with G-6-P on the MIC of fosfomycin was assessed in vitro with a strain of *K. oxytoca*. In principle, the MIC was measured in a broth dilution test by adding to cultures in logarithmic growth either fosfomycin at various concentrations or fosfomycin plus G-6-P, or distilled water as a control. The concentration of G-6-P was always 25 mg/liter. At the end of the scheduled contact periods, G-6-P dehydrogenase, NADP, and $MgCl_2$ were added to inactivate G-6-P if present.

The results demonstrated that G-6-P did not influence the ED_{50} of fosfomycin in infections due to organisms that lack an H-6-P transport system (*P. mirabilis* and *K. aerogenes* I); the MIC in vitro also remained unchanged by the presence of G-6-P (Table 1). With the two other strains possessing an inducible H-6-P system (*K. oxytoca* and *K. aerogenes* II), the presence of G-6-P not only reduced the MIC but also the ED_{50} values significantly (Table 1).

Subcutaneous administration in dogs resulted in maximum blood levels of G-6-P of 7.7 to 13.5 mg/liter after 30 to 45 min. Concentrations of 10 mg/liter have been demonstrable for 40 to 50 min, and concentrations of 5 mg/liter, for 45 to 70 min.

TABLE 1. *MICs of fosfomycin[a] without or with addition of G-6-P[b] in agar dilution tests and ED_{50} of fosfomycin[c] without or with G-6-P[d] 24 h after infection*

Infecting organism	MIC (mg/liter)		ED_{50} of fosfomycin (mg/kg of body weight)	
	G-6-P absent	G-6-P present	G-6-P absent	G-6-P present
P. mirabilis	1	1	5.4	6.6
K. aerogenes I	64	64	28.8	29.9
K. oxytoca	64	1	12.0	3.7[e]
K. aerogenes II	512	32	1,810.0	194.0[e]

[a] Pure substance, milligrams per liter.
[b] Disodium salt, 25 mg/liter.
[c] Pure substance, milligrams per kilogram of body weight.
[d] Disodium salt, 2 × 100 mg/kg of body weight.
[e] Significant (2 $P < 0.05$).

Intravenous injection of G-6-P led to maximum blood concentrations of 89.5 to 113 mg/liter after 5 min. Levels of ≥10 mg/liter have been observed for 27 to 32 min and ≥5 mg/liter for 45 to 70 min.

The MIC of *K. oxytoca* in the broth dilution test was 128 mg/liter (Fig. 1). Presence of G-6-P for 15 min lowered the MIC to 64 mg/liter. The MIC was reduced to 16 mg/liter by 60-min contact and to 8 mg/liter by 120-min contact. For the full induction on the H-6-P transport system, 480 min (= 8 h) was required, resulting in an MIC of 2 mg/liter.

Since the addition of G-6-P to solutions of fosfomycin improves the therapeutic effect only in infections due to pathogens possessing an inducible H-6-P transport system, it is inferred that this augmentation of the antimicrobial effect in vivo is based on the same mechanism as in vitro.

As a result of fast enzymatic alteration, G-6-P is available in the body at low concentrations only, in spite of its continuous formation by the glucose metabolism. If administered parenterally in sufficient quantity (100 mg/kg of body weight), however, blood levels of ≥5 mg/liter can be obtained for a while. This concentration is known to induce the H-6-P transport system, at least in vitro (1). The length of period that G-6-P must be in contact with the bacterial cell for induction was shown to range from 15 min to 8 h (Fig. 1). Thus, blood levels of 5 mg/liter and

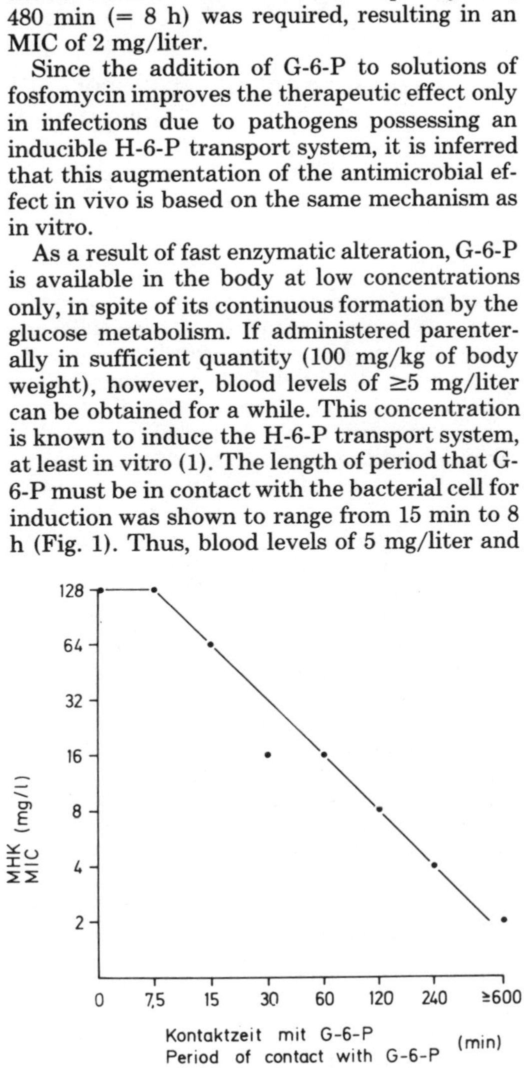

FIG. 1. *Influence of the period of contact with G-6-P (25 mg/liter) on the MIC of fosfomycin with a strain of K. oxytoca.*

above for at least 45 min may be expected to reduce the MIC to one-sixth in vivo. If they persist for 120 min, the MIC can be lowered to one sixteenth. G-6-P can be given to produce sufficient concentrations in the blood over an adequate time to boost the therapeutic effect of fosfomycin in infections due to staphylococci and most members of the *Enterobacteriaceae* family. To our knowledge, the combined usage of fosfomycin and G-6-P has never been tried in humans. Clinical studies are therefore required. As G-6-P is nontoxic, we regard such studies as justifiable when therapeutic use of fosfomycin is indicated.

1. **Goto, S.** 1977. Fosfomycin, antimicrobial activity in vitro and in vivo. Chemotherapy (Basel) **23**(Suppl. 1):63–74.
2. **Kahan, F. M., J. S. Kahan, P. J. Cassidy, and H. Kropp.** 1974. The mechanism of action of fosfomycin (phosphonomycin). Ann. N.Y. Acad. Sci **235**:364–386.
3. **Lang, G., and G. Michal.** 1974. D-Glucose-6-Phosphat und D-Fructose-6-Phosphat, p. 1283–1287. *In* H. U. Bergmeyer (ed.), Methoden der enzymatischen Analyse, vol. 1. Verlag Chemie, Weinheim.
4. **Rotter, M., A. Hirschl, and G. Stanek.** 1980. Enhancement of efficacy of fosfomycin in experimental infection by the addition of glucose-6-phosphate. Drugs Exp. Clin. Res. **6**:325–327.
5. **Woodruff, H. B., J. M. Mata, S. Hernandez, S. Mochales, A. Rodriguez, E. O. Stapley, H. Wallick, A. K. Miller, and D. Hendlin.** 1977. Fosfomycin: laboratory studies. Chemotherapy (Basel) **23**(Suppl. 1):1–22.

Experimental Staphylococcal Endocarditis: Single and Combined Antibiotic Therapy with Cloxacillin and Fosfomycin

M. V. DE VICENTE, T. OLAY, AND A. RODRÍGUEZ

Instituto de Farmacología Española, Madrid, Spain

Staphylococcus aureus is one of the most common organisms causing infective endocarditis. Staphylococcal endocarditis is a serious disease with a high mortality due to the virulence of *S. aureus*. Few clinical isolates of *Staphylococcus* are susceptible to penicillin G, and for this reason, the alternatives for treatment are penicillinase-resistant penicillins and vancomycin (4).

As fosfomycin is a very active antibiotic against *S. aureus*, including the penicillin- and methicillin-resistant strains (3), the purpose of this investigation was to study the effectiveness of cloxacillin, fosfomycin, and their combination in the treatment of experimental endocarditis induced by a penicillin-resistant *S. aureus* strain.

Endocarditis was established in white New Zealand rabbits by the techniques of Garrison and Freedman (1). After intravenous administration of 10 mg of Ketolar per kg, a polyethylene catheter was inserted through the right carotid artery into the left ventricle. It was clamped and tied to the carotid and left in place. The infection was produced by a strain of *S. aureus* (1019) 48 h after catheter placement. An inoculum of 1 ml containing an average of 1.3×10^6 colony-forming units (CFU) was injected into the marginal ear vein. The MICs were 0.5 μg/ml for cloxacillin and 32 μg/ml for fosfomycin. The susceptibility at critical MIC levels of cloxacillin and fosfomycin was studied for 32 clinical isolates of *S. aureus*. Sixty-five percent of the strains were susceptible to cloxacillin at 0.5 μg/ml, and 100% were susceptible to fosfomycin at 64 μg/ml.

An interaction test of the combination of cloxacillin plus fosfomycin against these 32 strains was made by the checkerboard method. Interaction was classified as synergistic or partially synergistic when fractional inhibitory concentration indices were less than or equal to 0.5 or less than or equal to 0.75, respectively (2). Fifty-six percent of the strains showed synergism and 41% showed partial synergism, with a total of 97%. The fractional inhibitory concentration index against the strain used to produce endocarditis was 0.5. Time-kill curves of cloxacillin at 0.25 μg/ml and fosfomycin at 16 μg/ml and their combination were performed in Mueller-Hinton broth against the test organism (Fig. 1). After 24 h, the combination of fosfomycin and cloxacillin produced a remarkable decrease of 5 to 6 logs in the number of viable CFU compared with each antibiotic alone.

Previous blood cultures were done 18 h after infection. Only those animals demonstrating bacteremia were used for the study. Therapy was begun immediately after the blood was taken for culture. The doses used were 75 mg of cloxacillin per kg and 100 mg of fosfomycin per kg, both administered intramuscularly twice daily during 3 or 5 days separately or in combination. Inoculated control animals were left untreated.

To determine the concentration of antibiotic in serum and vegetations, a group of animals, not included in the therapeutic trials, received an intramuscular injection of either cloxacillin or fosfomycin twice daily. After 3 days, blood was drawn from the ear vein and vegetations were removed from the heart. Antibiotic concentrations were determined by a diffusion plate method using *Sarcina lutea* ATCC 9341 for cloxacillin and *Proteus vulgaris* ATCC 21100 for fosfomycin. The mean peak serum antibiotic concentrations ± SD were 133.5 ± 29 μg/ml at 30 min for fosfomycin and 42.9 ± 18.2 μg/ml at 1 h for cloxacillin. Antibiotic concentrations achieved in vegetations after 1 h were 62.6 ± 23 μg/ml for fosfomycin and 12.9 ± 3.4 μg/ml for cloxacillin.

To evaluate the infection, any animal dying after three doses of antibiotic was considered in the study. Four or six days after infection and 16 h after the last dose, surviving animals, both treated and untreated, were sacrificed and blood cultures were made. The hearts were removed and the vegetations were excised and weighed. After homogenization, the number of CFU was determined by serial dilution in plates. Student's *t* test was used to determine statistically significant differences in the mean $\log_{10}$ ± SD of the

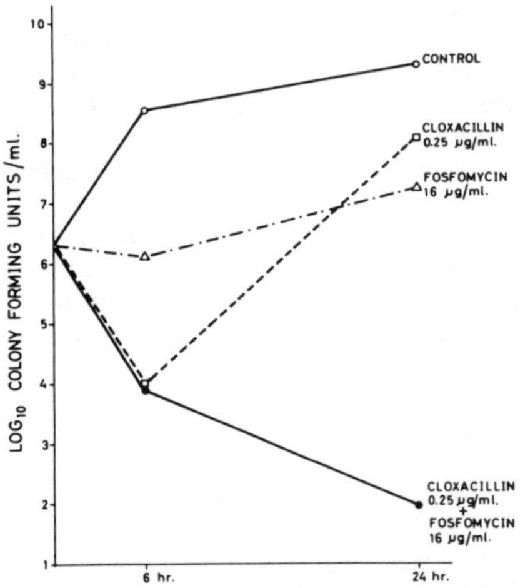

FIG. 1. *Killing curves of cloxacillin, fosfomycin, and their combination against the test strain.*

number of bacteria recovered per gram of cardiac vegetation.

The results are summarized in Table 1. The mortality rate in untreated controls was 94%, and 68% died 48 h after infection. After 3 days of therapy, the mortality rate was very low for antibiotics administered alone and no animals died with the combination. In the group treated with the combination all blood cultures were sterile. When the CFU per gram of vegetation in the combination group is compared with the other groups, significantly fewer bacteria were recovered from animals treated with the combination than from untreated controls, and from those treated with fosfomycin; a difference that was not statistically significant was found with the cloxacillin group.

After 5 days of antibiotic treatment, the mortality rate increased in the groups treated with the antibiotics alone, and 1 rabbit of 15 died in the combination group, being the only one with positive hemoculture. The mean $\log_{10}$ of CFU in the vegetations were 8.66, 7.93, and 4.96 for rabbits treated with fosfomycin, cloxacillin, and the combination. There was a significant reduction in the number of CFU of *S. aureus* per gram of vegetations in rabbits treated with the combination in comparison with rabbits given either fosfomycin or cloxacillin.

MIC determinations for fosfomycin and cloxacillin were performed on colonies recovered from the vegetations of rabbits in all groups. In the group treated with fosfomycin alone during the period of 5 days, resistant strains emerged, but no evidence of resistance was found in the combination groups.

In summary, the in vitro synergism results obtained in the study with the combination of cloxacillin and fosfomycin have a good correlation with the in vivo results, as the combination of the two antibiotics produced a greater reduction in the number of *Staphylococcus* cells cultured from the vegetations than the administration of the antibiotics separately, and no evidence of fosfomycin-resistant mutants was ob-

TABLE 1. *Summary of results of experimental endocarditis therapy in rabbits*

Antibiotic	No. of animals	Mortality	Blood cultures		Vegetations	
			Positive	Mean $\log_{10}$ CFU/ml (±SD)	Mean $\log_{10}$ CFU/ml (±SD)	*P* vs. combination
None	16	15 (93.7%)	16	4.24 (0.93)	9.80 (0.96)	<0.001
Fosfomycin (3 days)	6	1 (16.6%)	5	3.70 (1.51)	9.25 (1.32)	<0.005
Cloxacillin (3 days)	5	1 (20.0%)	5	3.02 (0.98)	7.77 (1.32)	NS[a]
Combination (3 days)	7	0	0	—	6.13 (1.04)	—
Fosfomycin (5 days)	11	8 (72.0%)	7	4.66 (0.42)	8.66 (1.58)	<0.001
Cloxacillin (5 days)	8	2 (25.0%)	5	2.93 (0.93)	7.93 (1.11)	<0.005
Combination (5 days)	15	1 (6.6%)	1	1.69	4.96 (1.99)	—

[a] Not significant, $P > 0.05$.

served in the combination groups. This study suggests the possibility, therefore, of finding a new alternative for the treatment of human endocarditis caused by penicillin-resistant *S. aureus*, but further studies are necessary to confirm these results.

1. **Garrison, P. K., and L. R. Freedman.** 1970. Experimental endocarditis. I. Yale J. Biol. Med. **42:**294–310.

2. **Neu, H. C.** 1976. Synergy of mecillinam, a beta-amidinopenicillanic acid derivative, combined with beta-lactam antibiotics. Antimicrob. Agents Chemother. **10:**535–542.

3. **Peters, G., F. Schumacher-Perdreau, and G. Pulverer.** 1980. Vergleich der Staphylokokken -und Mikrokokken-Virksamkeit von Fosfomycin, Oxacillin und Penicillin G. Dtsch. Med. Wochenschr. **105:**1541–1543.

4. **Sande, M. A., and W. M. Scheld.** 1980. Combination antibiotic therapy of bacterial endocarditis. Ann. Intern. Med. **92:**390–395.

Efficacy of Antimicrobial Therapy in Experimental Listeriosis in Normal Mice and Mice with Impaired T Cell-Mediated Immune Response

IRMA A. J. M. BAKKER-WOUDENBERG, WILLEM B. VAN LEEUWEN, AND MARC F. MICHEL

Department of Clinical Microbiology and Antimicrobial Therapy, Erasmus University, Rotterdam, The Netherlands

The purpose of this study was to investigate the importance of intact host defense mechanisms for successful antimicrobial therapy. The critical role of T cell-mediated immunity in relation to antimicrobial therapy of intracellular *Listeria* infection was studied in normal mice and thymusless nude mice. Nude mice were used for these experiments because antibacterial resistance to the facultative intracellular bacterium *L. monocytogenes* depends on development of cellular immunity, induced specifically by a T cell-mediated reaction. Nude mice lack T cells, and the antimicrobial therapy alone is responsible for killing the intracellular bacteria, whereas in normal mice killing of the bacteria is the combined effect of the curative action of the antibiotic and the activity of the cellular defenses of the host.

Experimental infections were produced by intravenous injections of mice with suspensions of *L. monocytogenes* type 4b cells. The severity of the infection was measured in terms of the number of viable *Listeria* cells recovered from the spleen, liver, and blood at different intervals after inoculation. Normal mice developed short-term listeriosis, the course of which depended upon numbers of bacteria inoculated. An inoculum of 5×10^5 *Listeria* cells was lethal for normal mice within 48 to 72 h. At 36 h, blood contained 380 colony-forming units per ml. Inoculation of 10^5 *Listeria* cells resulted in a progressive increase in bacterial populations of the spleen and liver followed by decreases in number. By day 16, spleens and livers were sterile. The blood was sterile throughout the observation period. With inoculation of 5×10^4 *Listeria* cells, normal mice recovered quickly within 10 days. Nude mice showed a chronic infection independent of the inoculum; they did not recover from the infection, but they did not die. They were able to restrain bacterial populations, but were not able to effectively terminate the *Listeria* infection. Blood was always sterile. Ten days after inoculation *Listeria* were also cultured from lung, kidney, heart, and central nervous system. The course of *Listeria* infection in nude mice in relation to their defect in host defense mechanisms corresponds to the clinical experience that infection with opportunistic pathogens such as *L. monocytogenes* may occur in patients with defects in their cell-mediated immune mechanisms as a consequence of malignancies, such as lymphomas and leukemias, or immunosuppressive treatment (3).

The MICs of the antibiotics tested for the *Listeria* isolate used in this study were as follows: ampicillin, 0.16 μg/ml; rifampin, 0.04 μg/ml; DL 473, 0.01 μg/ml; and gentamicin, 0.16 μg/ml. Administration of 5 mg of ampicillin every 12 h for eight doses subcutaneously was the minimal effective therapy for normal mice, sterilizing spleen, liver, and blood of normal mice inoculated with 5×10^5 *Listeria* cells by day 14. In normal mice inoculated with 10^5 *Listeria* cells the same ampicillin treatment sterilized spleen, liver, and blood by day 6.

These ampicillin treatment schedules that were adequate to cure normal mice were without effect on the course of disease in nude mice. During antibiotic treatment, bacteria recovered from the spleens and livers decreased initially but increased again as soon as ampicillin treatment was terminated in nude mice inoculated with 5×10^5 or 1×10^5 *Listeria* cells. We investigated to what extent the antimicrobial response in nude mice could be improved by intensifying the antibiotic treatment. Increasing the daily dose of ampicillin to 10, 25, or 50 mg, decreasing the interval between doses from 12 to 8 h, and increasing the number of doses from 8 to 32, effected only a marginal improvement in results. Some intensive treatment schedules effected temporary sterilization of spleen and liver and also of lung, kidney, heart, and central nervous system; however, these organs were again culture positive 5 days after the last dose of ampicillin. In nude mice infected with 10^5 *Listeria* cells, administration of 25 mg of ampicillin every 12 h for 32 doses appeared to be fully curative.

Peak concentrations of ampicillin in sera of normal mice and nude mice after subcutaneous administration of 5- and 25-mg doses were 180 μg/ml with the 5-mg dose and 550 μg/ml with the 25-mg dose. Concentrations in excess of 0.16 μg/ml, the MIC for the *Listeria* isolate used in this study, were present for about 4 and 5 h at the respective doses.

From these experiments we may conclude that the reduced efficacy of ampicillin in nude mice was due to impaired host defense mechanisms. Lack of cellular immunity cannot or can hardly be compensated by intensification of the ampicillin treatment schedule. Since the bacteria isolated from nude mice treated with high doses of ampicillin had retained their susceptibility to ampicillin, the failure of ampicillin treatment is due either to inability of the drug to reach the bacteria in their intracellular location because of lack of penetrating capacity or to the low metabolic activity of the intraleukocytic bacteria in nude mice. In vitro studies suggest that ampicillin might penetrate poorly into cells (1). Besides, it must be realized that ampicillin has a short half-life in mice and that the inhibitory levels were present in serum for only part of the dosage interval, with active multiplication and repopulation occurring in the drug-free interval.

To test these aspects of failure of ampicillin therapy we applied another antimicrobial drug, rifampin, which—compared with ampicillin—is more capable of penetrating into host cells (2) and has a longer half-life in mice (6 h and 25 min for rifampin and ampicillin, respectively). Low doses of rifampin, 0.024 and 0.012 mg, respectively, administered every 24 h for four doses, were adequate to cure normal mice inoculated with 5×10^5 and 1×10^5 *Listeria* cells. These doses were without effect on the course of disease in nude mice. Even administration of 0.96 mg of rifampin every 24 h for 16 doses was not fully curative. DL 473, a derivative of rifampin which has a long serum half-life in mice (20 h), effected sterilization of spleens and livers of nude mice infected with 10^5 *Listeria* cells only when administered for eight doses of 0.12 mg every 48 h.

In summary, we may conclude that lack of cell-mediated immune functions cannot or can hardly be compensated by intensive treatment schedules with long-term effective serum concentrations of an antimicrobial drug which is capable of penetrating into host cells. Low metabolic activity of the bacteria located within cells whose intracellular killing mechanisms fail to function may account for this failure of antimicrobial therapy.

1. **Brown, K. N., and A. Percival.** 1978. Penetration of antimicrobials into tissue culture cells and leukocytes. Scand. J. Infect. Dis. Suppl. **14**:251–260.
2. **Easmon, C. S. F.** 1979. The effect of antibiotics on the intracellular survival of *Staphylococcus aureus* in vitro. Br. J. Exp. Pathol. **60**:24–80.
3. **Nieman, R. E., and B. Lorber.** 1980. Listeriosis in adults: a changing pattern. Report of eight cases and review of the literature, 1968–1978. Rev. Infect. Dis. **2**:207–227.

4-Aminopyrazolo(3,4-*d*)Pyrimidine in the Treatment of Experimental Acute Chagas' Disease

JOSÉ L. AVILA,* EDGAR MUÑOZ, ANGELA AVILA, AND HÉCTOR MONZÓN

Instituto Nacional de Dermatología, Apartado 4043, Caracas 1010A, Venezuela

The successful use of allopurinol [4-hydroxypyrazolo(3,4-*d*)pyrimidine (HPP)] has recently been demonstrated in the treatment of experimental acute Chagas' disease (1). According to the in vitro experiments of Marr et al. (6), the selective toxicity of this drug toward *Trypanosoma cruzi* has been attributed to their unique ability to convert HPP-ribose-5′-PO_4 to 4-aminopyrazolo(3,4-*d*)pyrimidine ribonucleotide (APP-ribose-5′-PO_4), which is converted to the triphosphate and incorporated into RNA. These analogs of adenine nucleotides are not detected in the uninfected tissues of the mammals that also form HPP-ribose-5′-PO_4 (7).

In this paper, instead of using the parasitic amination of HPP to APP to obtain a trypanostatic effect, we have directly administered very low doses of APP to chagasic mice, thus obtaining a clear therapeutic effect.

In vitro experiments. *T. cruzi* was grown in a fetal calf serum-containing liquid medium at 28°C as described previously (5). Fresh media were inoculated with 0.5×10^6 cells per ml. After 10 days of culture, *T. cruzi* epimastigotes grown in the media supplemented with APP at 1, 5, and 10 μg/ml were harvested by centrifugation and inoculated in fresh media, and their growth was estimated as described (5). It was found that all eight strains of *T. cruzi* tested (seven Venezuelan strains and one Brazilian strain) were similarly affected for a given drug concentration, a 75% inhibitory dose (ID_{75}) (a dose producing more than 75% inhibition compared with control growth) of 0.5 μg/ml, thus suggesting a broad spectrum of action of APP. Similar results have been found for HPP (2). However, lower concentrations of APP were inhibitory. Attempts to subculture *T. cruzi* epimastigotes grown at APP concentrations of 5 and 10 μg/ml were successful, thus suggesting a trypanostatic effect similar to that previously reported for HPP (2). It is noteworthy that APP 2′-deoxyriboside (0 to 100 μg/ml) was without effect as a trypanostatic drug. This latter result is similar to that found for HPP-ribose and HPP-ribose monophosphate (6).

In vivo experiments. The Ya strain of *T. cruzi* was maintained by serial syringe passages of infected blood in mice. Inbred C57BL/6J and outbred NMRI-IVIC mice, each weighing 18 to 20 g, were inoculated intraperitoneally with 1×10^5 bloodstream forms. In all experiments, treatment started 3 days after inoculation. Daily records of mortality were kept throughout the experimental period. In all mice, tail blood was microscopically examined for living flagellates as described (4), over a period of 50 days beginning 3 days after inoculation; animals showing at least 10 consecutive direct negative examinations were submitted to subinoculation experiments. These were carried out as previously described (2). In both mice strains, parasitemia was maximal (about 1×10^6 to 3×10^6 parasites per ml) at about day 7, with 95 to 99% of the animals dying at about 20 days postinoculation. When mice were treated twice daily with APP (0.25 to 1 mg/kg of body weight per day for only 10 days), a significant therapeutic effect was immediately seen at all doses. The minimal dose that protected all animals was 0.25 mg/kg. The treatment was characterized by a marked fall in parasitemia and increased survival time in the APP group compared with that of the control mice (Table 1). Parasitemia (direct counts) remained persistently negative for more than 320 days after treatment. Furthermore, subinoculation to susceptible mice disclosed no parasites in the several tissues studied (heart, liver, spleen) (Table 2), suggesting that the tissue parasite levels are too low to be detected even by this highly sensitive method as was found for HPP (2). Similar results were obtained by histological studies. Surviving untreated animals showed abundant *T. cruzi* nests only in liver, spleen, and heart. As a recent paper has shown in chagasic mice, independently of the parasitemia pattern or level and strain origin, there are marked differences in the sensitivity to HPP between several *T. cruzi* strains (3). These results suggested

TABLE 1. *Effects of APP treatment on the course of infection with Trypanosoma cruzi in mice*

Daily APP dose (mg/kg of body wt)[a]	Effect		
	Parasitemia (10^6/ml)[b]	Mean survival time (days)	No. dead
0	1.43	14	20
0.125	0.73	80[c]	2
0.250	0.41	300[d]	0
0.500	0.35	300[d]	0
1.000	0.19	300[d]	0

[a] APP was given divided into two daily doses at 3 days after infection because of the short APP half-life (about 6 h) (9). There was a total of 20 animals.

[b] Determined 7 days after intraperitoneal inoculation.

[c] $P < 0.005$.

[d] $P < 0.001$.

TABLE 2. *Percentage of T. cruzi-infected C57BL/6J recipient mice subinoculated with several tissues (whole blood or homogenates) obtained from APP-treated chagasic mice at different times after treatment initation*

Days after APP treatment initiation[b]	% Infected recipient mice inoculated with:[a]				
	Heart	Blood	Liver	Spleen	Skeletal muscle
10	10	25	10	20	0
50	0	5	0	5	0
100	0	0	0	0	0
150	0	0	0	0	0

[a] Each group was divided into pools of about four mice which were killed, and their pooled tissues were subinoculated, after homogenization, into five unexposed mice. Subinoculated mice were checked for parasitemia, using direct methods at 15 and 21 days after intraperitoneal inoculation.

[b] APP given at a dose of 1 mg/kg of body weight per day.

to us the possibility that similar in vivo differences could exist for APP. Preliminary results have shown that indeed this is the case, as there is no correlation between HPP or APP regarding in vivo resistance or sensitivity to treatment (Avila et al., unpublished data).

The optimal doses (0.25 mg/kg per day) found in vivo for APP in the successful treatment of Chagas' disease is about 150- to 300-fold lower than that reported as optimal for HPP (2). Furthermore, this dose is about 40- to 100-fold lower than LD_{50} reported for APP-treated mice (8, 9) and quite similar to that reported as nontoxic in human studies (9).

In conclusion, this paper provides further evidence for the ability of pyrazolopyrimidines to control *T. cruzi* infection in vivo. The lack of toxicity of APP at antichagasic doses (no difference being found between controls and mice treated with 1 mg of APP per kg in parameters such as body weight increase, blood cell counts, prothrombin time, serum cholesterol, triglycerides, or alkaline phosphatase or in the hepatic total lipids) and the clear protective effects in acute *T. cruzi* infections of mice suggest that this drug may be useful against Chagas' disease.

This research was supported by a grant from CONICIT (SAL-8).

1. **Avila, J. L., and A. Avila.** 1980. Allopurinol in the treatment of experimental acute Chagas' disease, p. 1121–1123. *In* J. D. Nelson and C. Grassi (ed.), Current chemotherapy and infectious disease. American Society of Microbiology, Washington, D.C.
2. **Avila, J. L., and A. Avila.** 1981. *Trypanosoma cruzi*: allopurinol in the treatment of mice with experimental acute Chagas' disease. Exp. Parasitol. **51**:204–208.
3. **Avila, J. L., A. Avila, and E. Muñoz.** 1981. Effect of allopurinol on different strains of *Trypanosoma cruzi*. Am. J. Trop. Med. Hyg. **30**:795–800.
4. **Avila, J. L., A. Bretaña, and A. Avila.** 1979. Chemotherapy with ethidium bromide-DNA complex in established Chagas' disease. Am. J. Trop. Med. Hyg. **28**:456–460.
5. **Avila, J. L., A. Bretaña, M. A. Casanova, A. Avila, and F. Rodriguez.** 1979. *Trypanosoma cruzi*: defined medium for continuous cultivation of virulent parasites. Exp. Parasitol. **48**:27–35.
6. **Marr, J. J., R. L. Berens, and D. J. Nelson.** 1978. Antitrypanosomal effect of allopurinol: conversion *in vivo* to aminopyrazolopyrimidine nucleotides by *Trypanosoma cruzi*. Science **201**:1018–1020.
7. **Nelson, D. J., J. L. Buggé, H. C. Krasny, and G. B. Elion.** 1973. Formation of nucleotides of [6-^{14}C]allopurinol and [6-^{14}C]oxipurinol in rat tissues and effects on uridine nucleotide pools. Biochem. Pharmacol. **22**: 2003–2022.
8. **Scholler, J., F. S. Philips, and S. S. Sternberg.** 1956. Production of fatty livers by 4-aminopyrazolo(3,4-d)pyrimidine. Toxicological and pathological studies. Proc. Soc. Exp. Biol. Med. **93**:398–402.
9. **Shaw, R. K., R. N. Shulman, J. D. Davidson, D. P. Rall, and E. Frei.** 1960. Studies with the experimental antitumor agent 4-aminopyrazolo(3,4-d)pyrimidine. Cancer **13**:482–489.

Nomograms for Prediction of Infusion Parameters to Achieve Steady-State Serum Concentrations of Antibiotics

ZDENĚK MODR,* IVO JANKŮ, VLASTIMIL KREBS, AND KAREL KVOŘÁČEK

Institute for Clinical and Experimental Medicine and Institute of Pharmacology, Czechoslovak Academy of Sciences, Prague, Czechoslovakia*

Using pharmacokinetic principles of drug administration by continuous intravenous (i.v.) infusion, the physician can estimate an appropriate infusion rate of a drug to achieve a desired steady-state serum concentration (1). However, this method takes four to five biological half-lives to create a steady-state serum concentration of a drug. Thus, in cases where the desired serum concentration is to be achieved as quickly as possible, it is necessary to use a loading dose of a drug. The loading dose can be administered either by i.v. bolus injection or by short-term i.v. infusion. For prediction of all needed infusion parameters, we have constructed several nomograms. The goal of this study was a practical examination of these nomograms, using two antibiotics as model drugs.

The first nomogram (Fig. 1) enables a rapid estimation of both the initial loading dose necessary to achieve the desired therapeutic concentration of drug and the i.v. infusion rate necessary to maintain steady-state serum concentration. This nomogram reflects graphically the relationship between the following pharmacokinetic data: the value of the initial loading dose (D_i), which is given by multiplication of the desired therapeutic serum concentrations (C_{ther}) and volume of distribution (V_d), and the infusion rate (R_{cont}), which is given by multiplication of the desired therapeutic serum concentration (C_{ther}) by the volume of distribution and the elimination rate constant (K_e). Use of a two-compartment model of drug pharmacokinetics requires the use of $V_{d\,(\text{area})}$ for the value of the

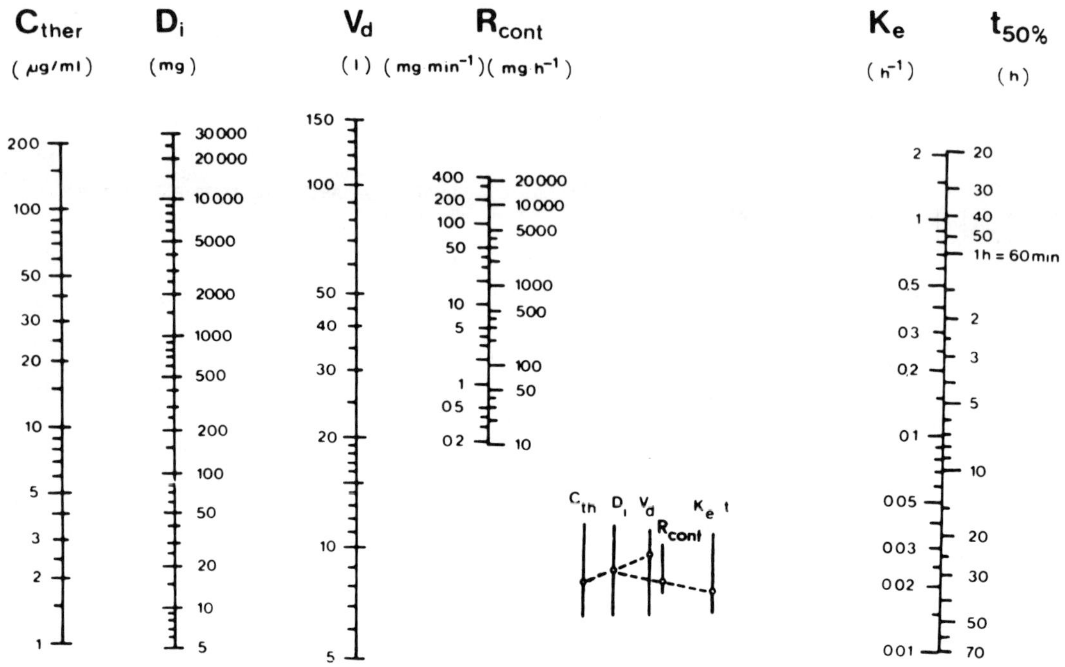

FIG. 1. *Nomogram for estimation of an initial loading dose (D_i) and an infusion rate (R_{cont}) to achieve a desired therapeutic steady-state serum concentration.*

volume of distribution and of β for the value of the elimination rate constant, whereas using a one-compartmental model requires the use of parameters V_d and K_e, respectively. The other nomograms (not presented here) are used for estimation of other parameters (data for i.v. solution preparation, number of drops per time, etc.). The validity of the nomograms was examined by using two antibiotics administered by i.v. infusion.

For the ampicillin study, 10 volunteers (five males and 5 females) with the following parameters were examined (mean values are given): age, 40.6 years; weight, 71.7 kg; height, 170.3 cm. The desired serum concentration was 10 mg/liter. The pharmacokinetic parameters used were: $V_{d\,(\text{area})}$, 18 liters; $t_{1/2\beta}$, 53 min. The corresponding values estimated by nomogram were: D_i, 180 mg/min; R_{cont}, 150 mg/h. Time intervals of the blood sampling were as follows: 5, 20, 30, 40, and 60 min after the start of infusion and 10 min after the end of infusion. The bioassay of antibiotic was performed by a microbiological diffusion cup plate method, using *Sarcina lutea* ATCC 9341.

For the study with mezlocillin, seven volunteers (four males and three females) with the following parameters were examined (mean values are given): age, 37.9 years; weight, 71.0 kg; height, 173.9 cm. The desired steady-state serum concentration of mezlocillin was 100 mg/liter. The following pharmacokinetic parameters were used: $V_{d\,(\text{area})}$, 16 liters; $t_{1/2\beta}$, 51 min. The predicted values were: D_i, 1.6 g/5 min; R_{cont}, 1.3 g/h. Time intervals for blood sampling were as follows: 5 min after the initial dose, 5, 15, 30, 45, and 60 min after the start of infusion, and 5, 15, 30, 60, and 120 min postinfusion. Blood levels of mezlocillin were determined by the microbiolog-

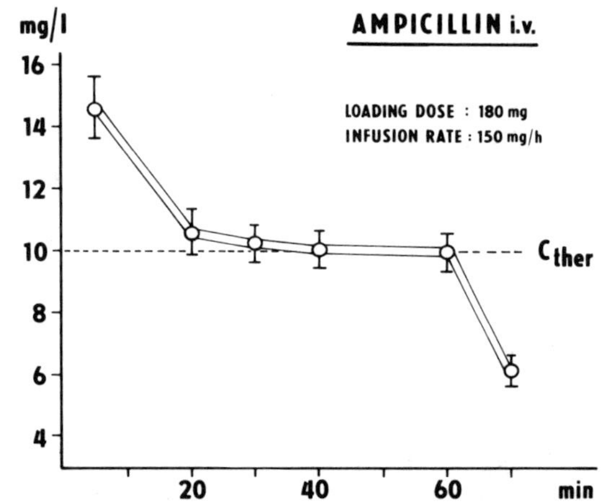

FIG. 2. *Determined serum concentrations of ampicillin administered by i.v. infusion; infusion parameters were estimated with nomograms.*

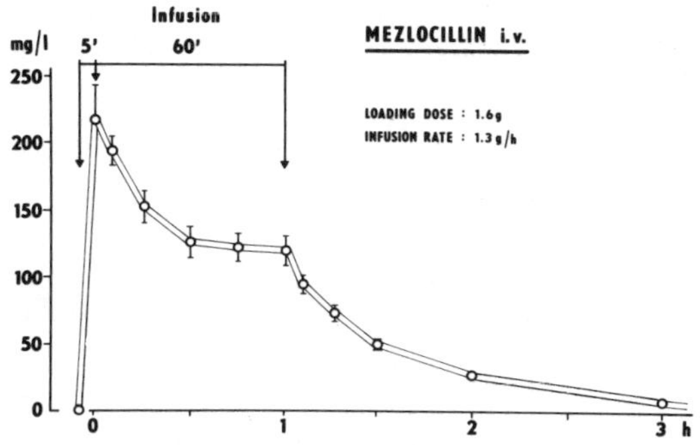

FIG. 3. *Determined serum concentrations of mezlocillin administered by i.v. infusion; infusion parameters were estimated with nomograms.*

ical diffusion cup plate method, using *Bacillus subtilis* 6633.

In the study with ampicillin, the steady-state serum concentration was reached at 20 min after the start of infusion, and the desired concentrations were successfully maintained throughout the infusion (Fig. 2); the determined serum concentrations were identical with the desired predicted drug serum concentrations. In the study with mezlocillin (Fig. 3), the steady-state serum concentrations were achieved only 30 min after the start of infusion; the actually determined serum concentrations were close to the desired serum concentrations (100 mg/liter). The higher initial serum concentrations of both antibiotics found after administration of the initial loading dose (before the steady state was achieved) could be explained by physiological dynamics of the process of drug distribution after administration into the central compartment. The actually determined drug serum concentrations were, however, also influenced by the validity of the pharmacokinetic parameters and constants used.

The practical examination of our nomograms proved that they could be used in clinical practice as a simple and useful device for estimating parameters for i.v. infusion. By using these nomograms, sufficient values of an initial loading dose and infusion rate needed to achieve the desired steady-state serum concentrations of ampicillin and mezlocillin were estimated.

1. **Mitenko, P. A., and R. I. Ogilvie.** 1972. Rapidly achieved plasma concentrations plateaus with observations on theophylline kinetics. Clin. Pharmacol. Ther. **13:**329–335.

Relationship Between Method of Administration and Cerebrospinal Fluid Penetration of Antibiotics

T. HARUTA,* Y. KOBAYASHI, AND Y. MORIKAWA

Kobe Central Municipal Hospital, Kobe Sakuramachi Hospital, Tokyo

In the treatment of purulent meningitis, the intravenous route is the usual method of administration of antibiotics. However, there are two different methods of intravenous administration of drugs, that is, bolus injection and intravenous drip infusion, and there are still few publications available that provide decisive data concerning which of these methods results in better penetration of the drug into the cerebrospinal fluid (CSF). Accordingly, we established experimental staphylococcal meningitis in rabbits and then administered three antibiotics, ampicillin, cefotaxime, and 6059S, at a dosage level of 100 mg/kg by both the bolus injection method and the 1-h intravenous drip infusion method. We then carried out a pharmacological investigation of the effects of these methods on the penetration of these antibiotics into the CSF.

Purulent meningitis was induced in albino rabbits weighing 1.5 to 2.5 kg by intracisternal inoculation of 0.5 ml of a *Staphylococcus aureus* FDA 209P suspension containing 10^8 colony-forming units per ml. These animals were divided into groups and used in the experiment 24 h after inoculation. After the bolus intravenous injection or 1-h intravenous drip infusion samples of blood were obtained from an ear vein and CSF samples were obtained by cisternal puncture. These samples were collected at intervals of 15 min during the first 2 h and then at 30-min intervals during the 3rd hour.

Antibiotic concentrations were measured by the paper disk bioassay method. The indicator strains used were *Bacillus subtilis* ATCC 6633 for ampicillin, *Micrococcus luteus* ATCC 9341 for cefotaxime, and *Escherichia coli* 7437 for 6059S. The standard curves were prepared by using a pH 7.0, 0.67 M phosphate buffer for the dilutions.

The values measured for each sampling time

TABLE 1. *Comparison of penetration rate of various antibiotics to CSF of rabbits with S. aureus meningitis when 100 mg/kg was administered as bolus injection and as 1-h intravenous drip infusion*

Antibiotic	Method of administration[a]	No. of rabbits	C_{max} in CSF ± SE (μg/ml)	t_{max} in CSF (min)	C_{max} CSF/serum (%)	AUC in CSF (μg. h/ml)	AUC CSF/serum (μg. h/ml) up to 3 h (%)	$t_{1/2}$ in CSF (min)	$t_{1/2}$ CSF/serum
Ampicillin	BI	5	19.3 ± 7.87	30	7.04	851	11.1	29.9	1.28
	DI	5	7.24 ± 2.52	60	4.83	556	5.5	48.1	1.85
Cefotaxime	BI	9	9.35 ± 3.35	15	9.17	744	15.4	74.4	1.74
	DI	10	3.84 ± 0.71	75	5.33	416	7.8	75.9	2.29
6059S	BI	10	12.5 ± 1.06	60	4.94	1,520	11.8	121	3.06
	DI	13	13.4 ± 1.71	60	5.80	1,573	9.5	127	3.29

[a] BI, Bolus injection; DI, drip infusion for 1 h.

were averaged for the animals in each of the administration groups, and these median values were plotted. From these curves, the maximum concentration (C_{max}), the time required to achieve the maximum concentration (t_{max}), the ratio of the maximum concentration in the CSF to the maximum concentration in the serum (C_{max} CSF/serum), the area under the curve (AUC), the ratio of AUC for the CSF to AUC for the serum (AUC CSF/serum), the half-life ($t_{1/2}$), and the ratio of the half-life of the drug in the CSF to the half-life in the serum ($t_{1/2}$ CSF/serum) were calculated. The AUC CSF/serum value was considered to represent the degree of penetration of the antibiotic into the CSF (1).

The results (Table 1) show that the bolus intravenous injection of ampicillin and cefotaxime gave values larger than those for the intravenous drip infusion in terms of C_{max} in the CSF, C_{max} CSF/serum, AUC for the CSF, and the penetration rate.

In the case of 6095S, the drip infusion method gave somewhat larger values for C_{max} in the CSF and C_{max} CSF/serum, whereas the AUC for the CSF was about the same for the two administration methods, and the penetration rate was larger in the case of the bolus injection. However, none of these differences was statistically significant.

It is not clear why there apeared to be an administration method-dependent difference in the CSF penetration of ampicillin and cefotaxime compared with 6059S. However, as regards whether bolus injection or drip infusion is more advantageous in clinical terms, it is reasonable to think that there may at least be some difference, depending on the MIC of the causative bacterium. A comparison was thus made of the two methods with regard to the shift in the relative CSF concentration, using the median MIC values of *Haemophilus influenzae* as the reference level.

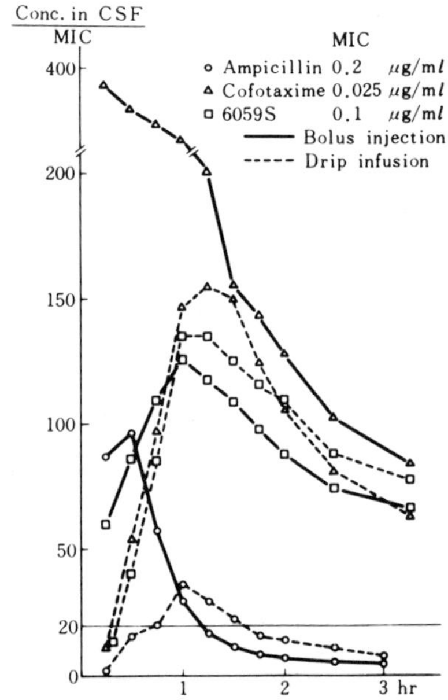

FIG. 1. *Shifts in ratios of antibiotic concentrations in CSF to median MIC of H. influenzae isolates.*

Let us assume that a concentration 20 times higher than the median MIC for each bacterium will guarantee that the relative antibiotic concentration in the CSF is an effective level. In the case of ampicillin (median MIC = 0.2 μg/ml),

AUC for the time interval showing CSF concentrations 20 or more times higher than the MIC was clearly larger after the bolus intravenous injection compared with the drip infusion, and the length of time for which this "effective" concentration was maintained was longer. With cefotaxime (median MIC = 0.025 μg/ml), there was little difference between the two administration methods in terms of the length of time for which the high CSF concentration was maintained, but AUC for the time interval showing concentrations 20 or more times higher than the median MIC was much larger in the case of the bolus intravenous injection. With 6059S (median MIC = 0.1 μg/ml) as well, there was no large difference between the two administration methods in terms of either AUC for the time interval showing concentrations 20 or more times higher than the median MIC or the length of time for which the high CSF concentration was maintained (Fig. 1). In other words, on the basis of these findings, when the relative antibiotic concentration in the CSF is low, it appears that administration of the antibiotic is more effective by intravenous bolus injection than by intravenous drip infusion. Conversely, when the relative antibiotic concentration in the CSF is high, the drug will be clinically efficacious regardless of the intravenous administration method used. However, when the same dosage is administered, the drip infusion method yields a lower effective concentration in the CSF and therefore includes some degree of waste. In addition, from the viewpoint of the prevention of side effects, it is possible to lower the administered dosage in the case of bolus intravenous injections. These considerations lead to the conclusion that, in fact, the bolus injection method is more advantageous in this situation.

1. **Morikawa, Y.** 1981. Comparative pharmacokinetics of ampicillin and carbenicillin in the cerebrospinal fluid of rabbits with staphylococcal meningitis, with reference to half-lives and areas under the curve. Jpn. J. Antibiot. **34:**211–218.

Bioavailability of Oral Antibiotics in Geriatric Patients

ROBERT SCHÄFER, GÜNTHER WITKOWSKI, GERT HÖFFKEN, PETER KOEPPE, AND HARTMUT LODE

Medical Department of the Klinikum Steglitz, Freie Universität Berlin, and Institute of Biology, Technische Universität Berlin, 1000 Berlin 45, West Germany*

Few data exist on the bioavailability of oral antibiotics in elderly patients. For this reason the pharmacokinetic parameter of the bioavailability of two frequently prescribed oral antibiotis (amoxicillin [AM] and cephalexin [CEX]) was determined in normal subjects, in people more than 70 years old, and in elderly patients with an insufficiency of the right heart. These two chemotherapeutic agents were chosen because of the middle-grade bioavailability (approximately 50 to 70%) of AM and the very good bioavailability (approximately 90 to 95%) of CEX (3, 4).

In a comparative study with 10 healthy (5 males and 5 females; age, 32.3 ± 7.2 years; weight, 67.4 ± 12.8 kg) and 9 elderly (6 males and 3 females; age, 77.1 ± 6.2 years; weight, 53.2 ± 7.5 kg) volunteers, the pharmacological parameters were determined after a single oral fasting dose of 500 mg of AM. The same experimental design was chosen for CEX (1,000 mg) with 10 healthy subjects (5 males and 5 females; age, 28.8 ± 6.3 years; weights, 66.5 ± 11.7 kg), 6 elderly persons (4 males and 2 females; age, 74.8 ± 5.0 years; weight, 61.6 ± 9.9 kg), and 8 elderly patients with cardiac insufficiency (3 males and 5 females; age, 74.0 ± 7.8 years; weight 71.8 ± 11.8 kg). The serum concentrations were determined at the following times: before and 15, 30, 45, 60, 90, 120, 180, 240, 380, and 480 min after application. The serum concentrations were determined by an agar diffusion test (cup plate method [1] in a modification of the method of Reeves and Bywater [5]). The test strains for AM were *Sarcina lutea* ATCC 9341 and ATCC 8340 (lower detection limit, 0.03 mg/liter). Those for CEX were *Bacillus subtilis* ATCC 6633 and *S. lutea* 9341 (lower detection limit, 0.6 mg/liter). All values were recalculated for a body weight of 70 kg. The calculations of the pharmacokinetic parameters (Table 1) were based on the assumption of an open two-compartment model.

The mean values of the individual AM serum peak concentrations were 7.5 ± 2.0 mg/liter in normal subjects and 10.0 ± 2.8 mg/liter in the elderly. The mean values of the maximal serum concentrations (y_{max}) were reached after 77 min

TABLE 1. *Mean pharmacokinetic parameters*

	$t_{50\%\ inv.}\left(\frac{\ln 2}{k_\alpha}\right)$ [min]	y_{max} [mg / l]	x_{max} [min]	$t_{50\%\ el.}$ [min]	AUC [h mg / l]
AMOXICILLIN					
young volunteers (n=10)	29,6	6,5	77	69	19,5
elderly volunteers (n=9)	40,4	7,9	99	95	33,2
CEPHALEXIN					
young volunteers (n=10)	11,2	25,6	66	61	58,1
elderly volunteers (n=6)	11,6	25,8	74	90	88,4
elderly patients (n=8) with cardiac ins.	11,0	33,8	67	116	124,9

(normal subjects) and after 99 min (elderly subjects) and were 6.5 and 7.9 mg/liter, respectively. The mean elimination half-life ($t_{1/2el}$) was calculated to be 69 and 95 min. Also, the area under the curve (AUC) was lower in the young subjects (19.5 mg.h/liter) than in the older subjects (33.2 mg.h/liter). The invasion constant, k_α, of the young subjects was greater than that of the older ones, so that the quotient $\ln 2/k_\alpha$ (invasion half-life) was 30 min in the first and 40 min in the second group. Figure 1 shows clearly the difference in AUC, maximal serum peak concentrations, duration (x_{max}), and delayed elimination in older people. This must be due mainly to the decrease in the glomerular filtrate in old kidneys, in spite of nonsignificant differences in the serum creatinine (83 ± 26 versus 76 ± 18 μmol/liter).

The mean values of the CEX serum peak concentrations were nearly identical in normal subjects and in older healthy ones (35.2 ± 9.2 and 33.2 ± 6.3 mg/liter, respectively). Only the older patients with an insufficiency of the right heart showed a tendency toward a higher level, with a value of 43.3 ± 12.7 mg/liter. The values of y_{max} were also nearly identical (25.6 and 25.8 mg/liter, respectively); only in the patients with cardiac insufficiency was y_{max} increased (33.8 mg/liter). x_{max} was 66 min in normal subjects, 74 min in older subjects, and 67 min in patients with cardiac insufficiency. The values of the quotient $\ln 2/k_\alpha$ showed the same tendencies (11.2, 11.6, and 11.0 min). The elimination half-life was 61 min (normal subjects), 90 min (older subjects), and 116 (older subjects with cardiac insufficiency) min. The AUC was 58.1, 88.4, and 124.9 mg.h/liter.

Based on these values, the following conclusion can be formulated. The pharmacokinetic parameters (AUC, y_{max}) indicate a moderately elevated bioavailability of AM and CEX in elderly people. This is even more valid in cases of an additional cardiac insufficiency, as could be

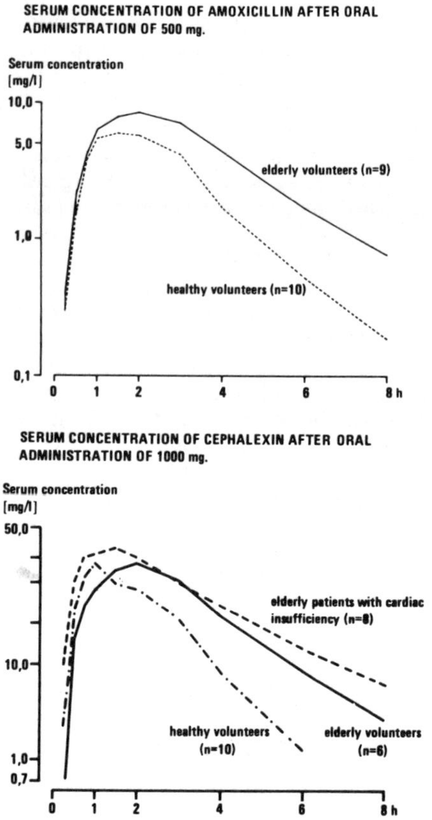

FIG. 1. *Serum concentrations after oral administration of AM (500 mg) and CEX (1,000 mg).*

shown in the example of CEX. To explain this increased bioavailability, one must consider the slowed-down elimination of the substances due to the age-dependent reduced glomerular filtrate (2). Therapy of an infection with AM or CEX in elderly people with or without insufficiency of the right heart should be given at normal dosages.

1. **Bennett, J. V., J. L. Brodie, E. J. Benner, and W. M. M. Kirby.** 1966. Simplified, accurate method for antibiotica assay of clinical specimens. Appl. Microbiol. **14:** 170–177.
2. **Kampmann, J. P., and J. E. Mølholm Hansen.** 1979. Renal excretion of drugs, p. 77–87. *In* J. Crooks and J. H. Stevenson (ed.), Drugs and the elderly. The MacMillan Press Ltd., London.
3. **Lode, H., P. Janisch, G. Küpper, and H. Weuta.** 1974. Comparative clinical pharmacology of three ampicillins and amoxicillin administered orally. J. Infect. Dis. **129:** 156–168.
4. **Lode, H., R. Stahlmann, and P. Koeppe.** 1979. Comparative pharmacokinetics of cephalexin, cefaclor, cefadroxil, and CGP9000. Antimicrob. Agents Chemother. **16:**1–6.
5. **Reeves, D. S., and M. J. Bywater.** 1976. Assay of antimicrobial agents, p. 21–78. *In* J. D. Louvois (ed.), Selected topics in clinical bacteriology. Tindall, London.

Antibiotic Levels in Plasma and Peritoneal Fluid After Administration of Amoxicillin, Ampicillin, and Bacampicillin During Pelvic Inflammatory Disease

MATHIAS ONSRUD,* TOM BERGAN, AND HALVARD GJØNNAESS

Aker Hospital, Oslo, Norway

The clinical effect of an antibiotic depends on the concentrations obtained at the site of infection and on the susceptibility of the infectious agent. Adequate concentrations within an infected locus are related to both the peak plasma level and the area under the concentration-time curve (AUC) (1).

Ampicillin is incompletely absorbed after oral administration. Amoxicillin and bacampicillin have improved absorption and consequently result in less diarrhea. These aminopenicillins are frequently used in the treatment of pelvic inflammatory disease. We have, in patients with this disease, studied the plasma and peritoneal fluid concentrations after single oral doses of these three antibiotics.

Fifteen patients (aged 17 to 41 years) with laparoscopically verified pelvic inflammatory disease had thin polyethylene catheters inserted through the abdominal wall into the pouch of Douglas for sampling of peritoneal fluid. At hourly intervals, peritoneal fluid and capillary blood were collected. Five patients each received an oral dose of 0.5 g of ampicillin or amoxicillin or 0.8 g of bacampicillin (approximately equimolar doses). The tablets (provided by Astra Läkemedel AB, Södertälje, Sweden) were given 18 to 20 h after laparoscopy and after more than 8 h of fasting. Care was taken to include patients with approximately the same body weight and the same degree of visual pelvic inflammatory changes in each of the treatment groups. Ampicillin and amoxicillin were both assayed by the method of Jalling et al. (2), using standard disks produced by AB Biodisk, Stockholm. Pharmacokinetic estimations for each patient were carried out with the computer program AUTOAN 2/NONLIN of Sedman and Wagner/Metzler (3). The open, first-order, one-compartment model was found the best fit, as evidenced by nonlinear regression coefficients.

The median peak plasma concentration was obtained 1 h after ampicillin and bacampicillin administration and 2 h after amoxicillin administration (Fig. 1). The highest median peak plasma level was observed after administration of bacampicillin, being nearly twice that obtained after ingestion of ampicillin. The amoxicillin peak was between the two. Bacampicillin showed a higher rate of absorption (k_A = 2.19 ± 0.39 h^{-1}) and a shorter plasma half-life ($t_{1/2p}$ = 0.88 ± 0.14 h) than amoxicillin (k_A = 1.39 ± 0.45 h^{-1}; $t_{1/2p}$ = 1.28 ± 0.18 h). The plasma AUCs were, however, similar for amoxicillin and bacampicillin (25.13 ± 3.22 and 21.55 ± 6.75 mg·h/liter), whereas that of ampicillin was significantly smaller (13.59 ± 4.12 mg.h/liter; $P < 0.01$, Wilcoxon rank sum test). The relative bioavailability of bacampicillin was 1.59 of that observed after oral ampicillin.

In peritoneal fluid, the median peak concentrations were found 2 h after ingestion of ampicillin and bacampicillin and 3 h after ingestion of amoxicillin (Fig. 1). The median peak levels were similar after bacampicillin and amoxicillin and significantly higher than that observed after ampicillin (P = 0.03). The rate of invasion into peritoneal fluid was lower for amoxicillin (k_I = 0.73 ± 0.12 h^{-1}) than for bacampicillin (k_I = 1.65 ± 0.19 h^{-1}). The peritoneal fluid half-life was longer for amoxicillin ($t_{1/2pf}$ = 1.41 ± 0.20 h) than for bacampicillin ($t_{1/2pf}$ = 1.04 ± 0.17 h). Still, the AUC for amoxicillin was similar to that obtained after dosage with bacampicillin (25.85 ± 2.04 and 24.78 ± 3.32 mg.h/liter) and significantly greater than the AUC after dosage with classical ampicillin (10.68 ± 2.30 mg.h/liter; P = 0.01). The peritoneal fluid AUC for ampicillin was only 43% of that observed after an approximately equimolar dosage of bacampicillin.

Both for plasma and peritoneal fluid concentrations, the interindividual variations were less for bacampicillin than for the other drugs. The k_I/k_A ratios of 0.53 for amoxicillin and 0.76 for bacampicillin together with a higher k_I value of the latter agent indicate a more rapid penetration after bacampicillin. But the ratios between plasma AUC and peritoneal fluid AUC were similar for amoxicillin and bacampicillin (0.89 and 0.87, respectively). It is therefore unlikely that one of the agents is superior to the other. The slightly more prolonged duration of amoxicillin might, however, be of clinical importance. Our study shows that 0.5 g of ampicillin orally results in a therapeutic level in the peritoneal fluid for 4 to 5 h, whereas equimolar doses of amoxicillin or bacampicillin prolong this period to 5 to 8 h. This circumstance and the observa-

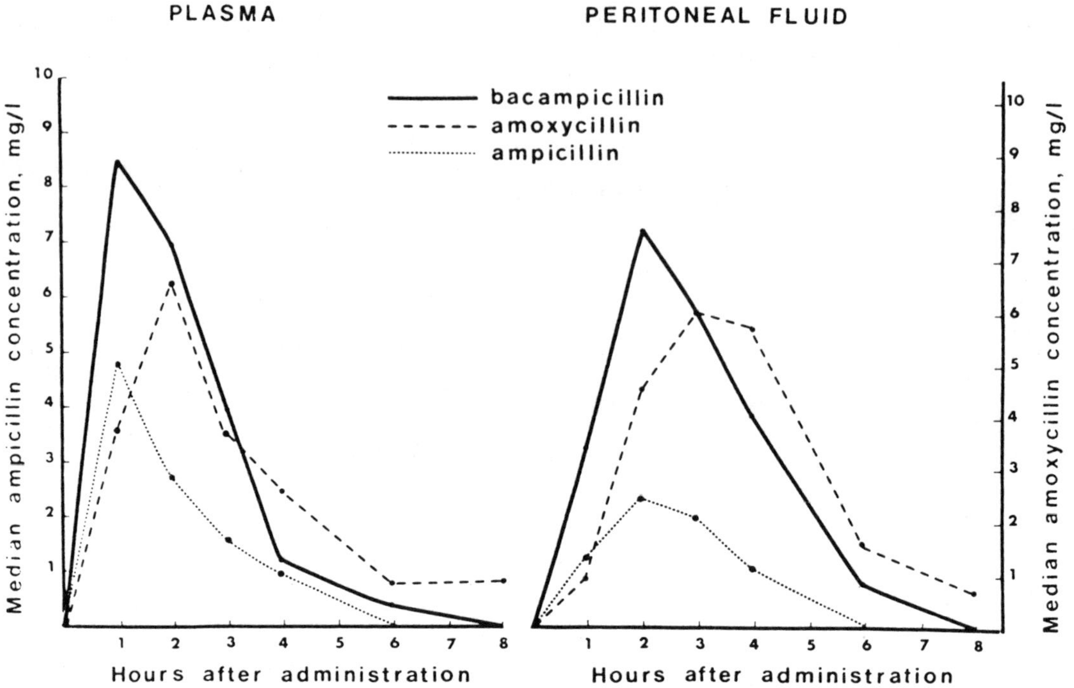

FIG. 1. *Median plasma and peritoneal fluid concentration after single oral administration of approximately equimolar doses of amoxicillin (0.5 g), ampicillin (0.5 g), and bacampicillin (0.8 g). Bacampicillin appears as ampicillin after absorption, whereas amoxicillin is absorbed and is antibacterically active as such. The amoxicillin curves have therefore been drawn on a scale equimolar to ampicillin in reference to the left ordinate and in milligrams per liter on the right axis.*

tion that classical ampicillin tablets are associated with a higher frequency of diarrhea indicate that one of the newer drugs is preferable for oral treatment; ampicillin should now be reserved for parenteral administration.

1. **Bergan, T.** 1978. Kinetics of tissue penetration. Are high plasma peak concentrations or sustained levels preferable for effective antibiotic therapy ? Scand. J. Infect. Dis. **14**:36–46.
2. **Jalling, B., A.-S. Malmberg, A. Lindman, and L. O. Boréns.** 1972. Evaluation of a micromethod for detection of antibiotic concentration in plasma. Eur. J. Clin. Pharmacol. **4**:150–156.
3. **Wagner, J. G.** 1975. Fundamentals of clinical pharmacokinetics. Drug Intelligence Publications Inc., Hamilton, Ill.

Rate Constants of Acetylation and Deacetylation of Some Sulfonamide Derivatives

TOM B. VREE,* CHIEL A. HEKSTER, MARGRIET BAAKMAN, ITA BAARS, TOM JANSSEN, MARIJN OOSTERBAAN, EMIEL TERMOND, AND MARIAN TIJHUIS

Department of Clinical Pharmacy, St. Radboud Hospital, University of Nijmegen, Nijmegen, The Netherlands

Sulfonamides are eliminated from the body by metabolism and renal excretion. The metabolic pathway is predominantly by acetylation to form N_4-acetylsulfonamide derivatives. The acetylation process elicits an unexplained phenomenon of a "high" or "low" yield of acetylation, or "fast" and "slow" acetylators, depending on the genetic type of the patient. In addition, some sulfonamides are acetylated in an unimodal way, e.g., sulfamethoxazole and sulfametrole, and some are hardly acetylated or not at all, e.g., sulfamethizole and sulfaethidole (4). So it seems that the substituent at the N_1 atom influences the yield of acetylation.

The renal excretion of sulfonamides, as the counterpart of metabolism in the overall elimination, shows different mechanisms for parent drug and metabolite. The parent drug is excreted by means of glomerular filtration minus tubular reabsorption (except when the N_1 substituent has a sulfur atom at two atomic bonds from the N_1 atom, e.g., sulfamethizole, sulfaethidole, and sulfathiazole [10]). As soon as the parent drug is acetylated into the metabolite N_4-acetylsulfonamide, this metabolite is excreted predominantly by active tubular secretion (10). A limiting factor in the elimination may be the degree of protein binding of the compounds and the resulting free concentration of the drug and its metabolite in plasma, from which they are metabolized and excreted. The overall scheme of elimination of sulfonamides is given in Fig. 1.

The different rate constants in the scheme of Fig. 1 are influenced by the following variables. (i) The structure of the substituent at the N_1 atom determines the pK_a value and the degree of protein binding (1–3, 6, 7). The pK_a value and lipid solubility determine the degree of tubular reabsorption. (ii) The acetyl substituent at the N_4 atom determines the elimination by renal excretion by means of active tubular secretion (10). From the protein binding of the metabolites, the true renal clearance value of each metabolite can be established.

The protein binding of sulfonamides and their corresponding metabolites can be measured in each plasma sample of volunteers or patients by means of Ultrafree filters (Worthington Biochemicals Corp.) high-pressure liquid chromatography analysis (8). The average percentage protein binding obtained of at least eight plasma samples is used for the calculations.

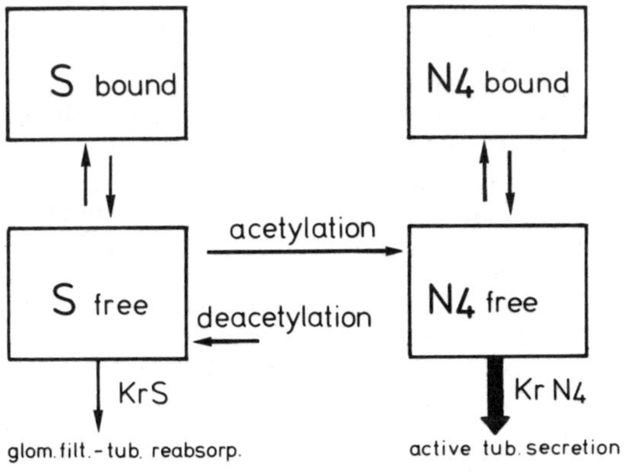

FIG. 1. *Flow scheme of protein binding, renal clearance, and acetylation-deacetylation reactions of sulfonamides.*

TABLE 1. *Rate constants of acetylation (K_{12}) and deacetylation (K_{21}) of some sulfonamide derivatives*

Compound	K_{12} acetylation (h^{-1})	K_{21} deacetylation (h^{-1})	K_{12}/K_{21} acetylation index
Sulfadiazine	0.0645	0.3040	0.2
Sulfamerazine	0.3605	2.0530	0.2
Sulfadimidine	0.8900	0.3950	2.0
Sulfisomidine	1.933	2.875	0.66
Sulfamethoxazole	0.3075	0.7567	0.40
Sulfamethizole	0.0918	3.8749	0.025

The renal clearance values (apparent and true) of parent drug and metabolite can be calculated from the renal excretion rate during each urine sample collection period and the corresponding average plasma concentration. Over an elimination time period of 60 to 100 h, 30 to 40 urine samples and renal clearance values can be obtained. The average renal clearance ± SD is used for the calculations. So from the scheme in Fig. 1, the unknown variables are still the rate of acetylation and deacetylation.

Deacetylation can be demonstrated when N_4-acetylsulfonamide derivatives are ingested by volunteers (4). In cases in which volunteers are unable to show a measurable degree of deacetylation, such as with N_4-acetylsulfamethoxazole and N_4-acetylsulfametrole, patients with severely impaired kidney function and corresponding lack of elimination of N_4-acetylsulfamethoxazole show deacetylation to a visible extent (9, 11). The existence of a deacetylation-acetylation equilibrium has recently been demonstrated by the ingestion of N_4-trideuteroacetylsulfamerazine. The trideuteroacetyl group is removed in the human body and replaced by a normal acetyl group derived from acetyl coenzyme A and *N*-acetyl-transferase (T. B. Vree, M. W. Tijhuis, M. Baakman, and Y. A. Hekster, submitted for publication).

The above-mentioned observations justify the model shown in Fig. 1. The rates of acetylation and deacetylation can be calculated for every individual by means of the NON-LIN program, obtained by the courtesy of C. M. Metzler (5). When the measured values of protein binding, renal clearance, half-lives, and distribution volumes are substituted, values as summarized in Table 1 are obtained.

1. **Anton, A. H.** 1960. The relation between the binding of sulfonamides to albumin and their antibacterial efficacy. J. Pharmacol. Exp. Ther. **129:**282–290.
2. **Bell, P. H., and R. O. Roblin.** 1942. Studies in chemotherapy. J. Am. Chem. Soc. **64:**2905–2917.
3. **Despopoulos, A.** 1965. A definition of substrate specific-

ity in renal transport of organic anions. J. Theor. Biol. 8:163–192.
4. **Hekster, Y. A., and T. B. Vree.** 1981. Clinical pharmacokinetics of sulphonamides and their N_4-acetyl derivatives. Antibiot. Chemother. 1–94.
5. **Metzler, C. M., G. L. Elfring, and A. J. McEwen.** 1976. A users manual for NONLIN and associated programs. Research biostatistics. The Upjohn Co., Kalamazoo, Mich.
6. **Seydel, J. K.** 1968. Sulfonamides, structure-activity relationship, a mode of action. J. Pharm. Sci. **57**:1455–1478.
7. **Struller, T.** 1968. Progress in sulfonamide research. Prog. Drug Res. **12**:389–457.
8. **Vree, T. B., Y. A. Hekster, A. M. Baars, J. E. Damsma, and E. van der Kleijn.** 1978. Determination of trimethoprim and sulfamethoxazole in body fluids of man by means of HPLC. J. Chromatogr. Biomed. Appl. **146**: 103–112.
9. **Vree, T. B., Y. A. Hekster, J. E. Damsma, R. van Dalen, J. C. M. Hafkenscheid, and W. T. Friesen.** 1981. Renal excretion of sulfamethoxazole and its metabolite N_4-acetylsulfamethoxazole in patients with impaired kidney function. Ther. Drug Monit. **3**:129–135.
10. **Vree, T. B., Y. A. Hekster, J. E. Damsma, M. Tijhuis, and W. T. Friesen.** 1981. Pharmacokinetics and mechanism of renal excretion of short acting sulfonamides and N_4-acetylsulfonamide derivatives in man. Structural requirements of sulfonamides for active tubular secretion. Eur. J. Clin. Pharmacol. **20**:283–292.
11. **Vree, T. B., Y. A. Hekster, and E. van der Kleijn.** 1981. Significance of apparent half lives of a metabolite which has a higher elimination rate than its parent drug. Drug. Intell. Clin. Pharmacol., in press.

Biochemical and Pharmacological Studies on KB-1585, a New Orally Well-Absorbed Ester of Ampicillin

GORO TSUKAMOTO,* TAKASHI NOSE, AKIRA SUZUKI, AND ISAMU UTSUMI

Pharmaceutical Research Center, Kanebo, Ltd., Osaka 534, Japan

Ampicillin (ABPC) has been established as a practical drug for treatment of various infections, but it is poorly absorbed orally and one of the side effects is diarrhea. Activated double esters, pivampicillin, bacampicillin (BAPC), and talampicillin (TAPC), have been developed as prodrugs to improve absorption. However, they are not without gastrointestinal side effects (1).

KB-1585, (5-methyl-2-oxo-1,3-dioxolen-4-yl)-methyl D-α-aminobenzylpenicillinate hydrochloride, is a new hydrolyzable ABPC ester which differs chemically from the conventional ones. This paper compares biochemical and pharmacological data for KB-1585 with those for the prodrugs TAPC and BAPC.

Serum level in rats. The three drugs were administered in single oral doses of 100 mg/kg (of ABPC equivalent) each to three male albino rats. Concentrations of free ABPC in the serum were determined by microbiological assay. A disk plate method was used, and *Bacillus subtilis* ATCC 6633 was used as the test organism. Serum ABPC levels for KB-1585 were similar to those for BAPC, but less than those for TAPC.

Plasma level in dogs. Single oral doses (20 mg of ABPC equivalent per kg) of KB-1585 and TAPC were given 1 week apart to three starved male beagle dogs. ABPC peak levels for KB-1585 at 1 h were four times greater than those for TAPC (13.4 ± 3.3 and 3.3 ± 1.5 mg/liter, respectively).

Table 1 shows hydrolysis in 0.1 M phosphate buffer (pH 7.4), rat intestine homogenate, and plasmas of rats, dogs, and humans. The results show that the stability of KB-1585 in intestine homogenate is superior to those of TAPC and BAPC. The stability in gastric fluid of these compounds is well recognized. Hence, KB-1585 is relatively stable in the gastrointestinal tract. KB-1585 was easily hydrolyzed in rat, dog, and human plasma, whereas hydrolysis of TAPC and BAPC demonstrated differences among species.

Metabolism of KB-1585 in rat liver preparation. Livers excised from male rats were homogenized with an equal volume of 0.1 M phosphate buffer (pH 7.4). The supernatant obtained by centrifugation of the homogenate was used as the reaction medium. A reaction mixture containing KB-1585 and a cofactor (reduced nicotinamide adenine dinucleotide [NADH] or NADPH) was added to the reaction medium and incubated at 37°C. The metabolites were identified by high-pressure liquid chromatography and gas chromatography-mass spectroscopy, and change of the product distribution was monitored by mass fragmentography. KB-1585 was rapidly hydrolyzed to ampicillin and diacetyl (2), which was further metabolized to 2,3-butanediol via acetoin. The metabolic pathway of KB-1585 is shown in Fig. 1. Cleavage of the terminal carbonate bond possibly initiates the reaction.

Acute toxicity. Solutions of the prodrugs in distilled water were administered to male mice. The LD_{50}'s (milligrams per kilogram, intrave-

TABLE 1. *Hydrolysis of KB-1585, TAPC, and BAPC in 0.1 M phosphate buffer, rat intestine homogenate, and plasma of rats, dogs, and humans*

Medium	Rate constant (min^{-1})		
	KB-1585	TAPC	BAPC
0.1 M phosphate buffer (pH 7.4)	0.014 (49.5)[a]	0.037 (18.7)	0.003 (231.0)
1% Rat intestine homogenate in 0.1 M phosphate buffer	0.022 (31.5)	0.515 (1.3)	0.515 (1.3)
1% Rat plasma in 0.1 M phosphate buffer	0.151 (4.6)	0.188 (3.7)	0.197 (3.5)
1% Dog plasma in 0.1 M phosphate buffer	0.128 (5.4)	0.045 (15.4)	0.003 (231.0)
1% Human plasma in 0.1 M phosphate buffer	0.174 (4.0)	0.094 (7.4)	0.005 (138.6)

[a] The number in parentheses is the half-life (minutes).

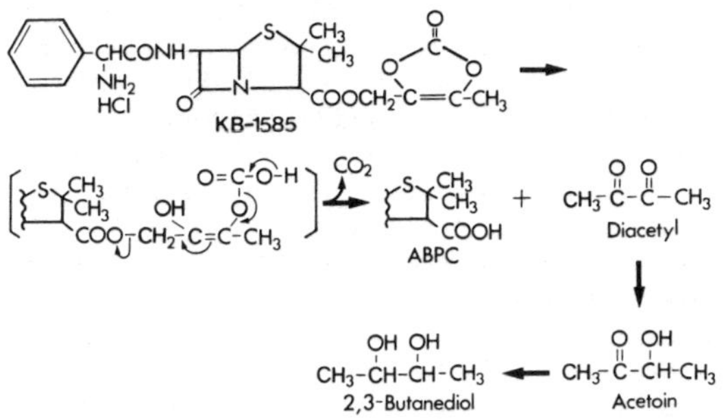

FIG. 1. *Metabolic pathways of KB-1585.*

nously, intraperitoneally, and orally, respectively) were as follows: KB-1585—711, 1,403, and >7,000; TAPC—590, not tested, and >4,000; BAPC—141, 713, and 3,200. Acute toxicity of KB-1585 was also determined in Sprague-Dawley rats. The LD_{50}'s (milligrams per kilogram, intravenously, intraperitoneally, and orally, respectively) were as follows: male—870, 4,362, and >10,000; female—838, 4,441, and >10,000. No difference was observed between sexes.

Three-month subacute toxicity in rats. Subacute toxicity after oral administration (625 to 5,000 mg/kg per day) was examined in Sprague-Dawley rats for 90 successive days. There were no deaths. Feces became soft, but no diarrhea was observed. Loss of body weight was observed in the group of male rats given the highest dose, whereas an increase was observed in female rats. There were no abnormalities in hematological and urinary parameters. Ophthalmological findings were normal. Biochemical analyses showed an increase in the albumin/globulin ratio bearing a decrease of total protein, a lowering of the Ca^{2+} concentration, and an increase of inorganic phosphorus. Although enlargement of cecum and weight gain of the adrenal glands, liver, and kidneys were observed at autopsy, histopathological findings demonstrated minor changes, such as swelling in centrilobular hepatocytes and the adrenal cortex. The increases in weight of the adrenal gland, liver, and kidneys were considered adaptive changes due to excessive dosing.

Summary. (i) KB-1585 has a new type of promoiety. (ii) Plasma ABPC levels after KB-1585 administration in dogs were four times greater than with TAPC. (iii) KB-1585 is stable in rat intestine homogenate. This suggests that gastrointestinal side effects can be reduced. In plasma, the rate of hydrolysis is faster and shows no difference among species. Thus, side effects in the liver are not anticipated. (iv) Since diacetyl is contained in some foods, these metabolites are considered to be safe. (v) Toxicity is low. From these results, we believe KB-1585 to be a more useful and safer prodrug of ABPC than the others.

A comparative pharmacokinetic study of KB-1585 and TAPC is reported elsewhere in this volume (C. L. Affoo, F. Moosdeen, B. N. Singleton, J. D. Williams, and S. Yamake, this volume).

1. **Bergan, T.** 1978. Antibiotics and chemotherapy, p. 61–63. *In* H. Schönfeld, R. W. Brochman, and F. E. Hahn (ed.), Monographs in penicillins, vol. 25. S. Karger, Basel.
2. **Gabriel, M. A., H. Jabara, and U. S. A. al-Khalidi.** 1971. Metabolism of acetoin in mammalian liver slices and extracts: interconversion with butane-2,3-diol and biacetyl. Biochem. J. **124**:793–800.

Single-Dose Tinidazole Intravenously: Pharmacokinetic and Clinical Studies

KARL-ERIK GIERCKSKY* AND ARTHUR REVHAUG

Regionsykehuset, University of Tromsø, Norway

Tinidazole is a synthetic nitroimidazole derivative with the same in vitro antimicrobial properties as metronidazole. It has a more pronounced lipid solubility and, given orally, a longer half-life than metronidazole. Using a recently developed gas chromatographic assay that allows measurements of concentrations of tinidazole in tissue to a lower limit of 50 ng/g, serum and tissue concentrations of tinidazole after a single intravenous infusion were studied.

Fifteen patients undergoing elective gastrointestinal surgery were given 1,500 mg of tinidazole intravenously 2 h before the start of the operation. Blood samples were drawn before infusion and 2, 8, 24, 48, and 96 h after infusion. Another blood sample was drawn immediately before tissue specimens were removed. Types of tissue specimens varied according to type of surgical procedure. Immediately after removal, the tissue specimens were gently dried with a sponge to remove blood contamination and frozen. Serum, urine, bile, and tissue samples were frozen immediately at −20°C until they were analyzed.

A selective gas chromatographic assay with internal standardization which allows measurements of tinidazole concentrations in tissue to a lower limit of 50 ng/g was used for all samples. The method has recently been thoroughly described by Laufen et al. (1). The serum and urine samples were processed in portions of 1 ml. The tissue specimens were homogenized with an Ultra-Turrax without any additives. The homogenates were divided into portions of 0.4 to 1.0 g in such way that at least two analyses could be carried out on each specimen.

The mean tinidazole concentration in serum 2 h after the end of infusion was 36 μg/ml. Tissue concentrations above MIC levels for *Bacteroides fragilis* were usually observed for 48 h (Fig. 1). The mean half-life, calculated from a nonlinear regression analysis of all data pairs, was 16 h. Tinidazole was detected in all tissue samples containing values above MIC levels for *B. fragilis.* We observed a tendency for the tissues originating from the gastrointestinal tract (and muscle) to contain more tinidazole than the liver, oment, subcutis, and epiploic fat samples (Fig. 2).

A total of 234 consecutive patients between 14 and 80 years old undergoing elective colonic and rectal surgery were randomly allocated to either a single-dose or 5-day prophylactic regimen. There were no significant differences in age, sex, diagnosis, or surgical procedures between the two groups. Patients were excluded from the study if they had received any antibiotic during the 10 days preceding the operation, had known hematological disorders, or were uremic. Enemas were given on each of the three evenings before surgical treatment, and the patients were given only a fluid diet after the enema regimen was begun.

The patients were given either 1,600 mg of tinidazole and 400 mg of doxycycline intravenously in the morning starting 1 to 2 h before the operation or 800 mg of tinidazole and 200 mg of doxycycline daily for 5 days. In the group given antimicrobial agents for 5 days, the first dose was always given before the operation. The infusion of antimicrobial agents was administered by the nurse in charge. The clinical evaluations were done by the medical staff according to the study protocol. Appropriate bacteriological specimens were taken and examined for anaerobic as well as aerobic microorganisms according to the clinical situation.

The patients were evaluated clinically, and all wounds and perineal areas were inspected on day 3, 7, 15, and 30 after the operation. Patients who had left the hospital before the last control either came back to the surgical outpatient department or were examined by their own doctor. Wound sepsis was defined as the presence of pus in the incision or a discharge with positive bacteriological culture. Perineal sepsis was defined as discharge of pus from the perineal wound or drain channel. Abdominal or pelvic abscess was defined as either a spontaneous discharge from a palpable mass or collection of pus requiring surgical drainage.

Fourteen patients given 5 days of prophylaxis developed a total of 16 infectious complications, whereas 6 patients given single-dose prophylaxis developed 9 such complications. Six patients given prophylactic treatment for 5 days developed wound infections, whereas none of the pa-

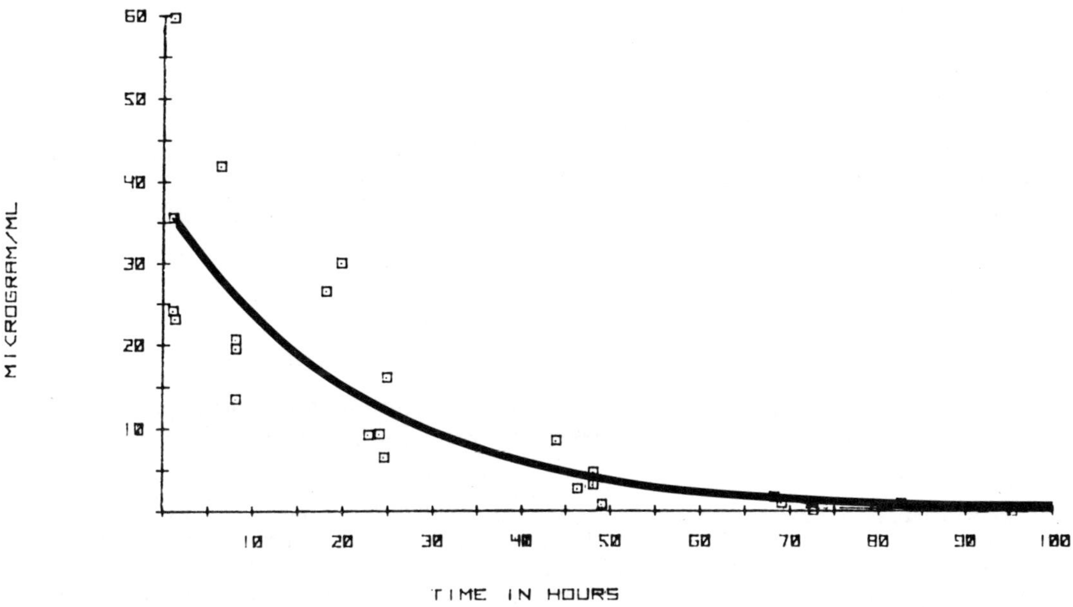

FIG. 1. *Concentrations of tinidazole in serum after infusion of 1,500 mg.*

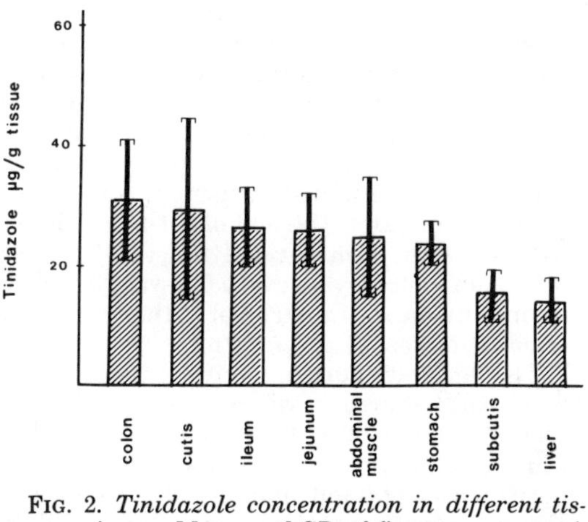

FIG. 2. *Tinidazole concentration in different tissue specimens. Mean and SD of five or more specimens.*

tients given only single-dose treatment developed wound infection. Three patients in both groups developed an intraabdominal abscess; two patients receiving 5 days of prophylaxis and one patient in the single-dose group developed a perineal abscess. Anastomotic dehiscence was demonstrated in eight patients, 3 given 5 days of prophylaxis and 5 given single-dose prophylaxis. Two patients developed septicemia; both had received 5 days of antimicrobial prophylaxis. Uncomplicated lower urinary tract infections was seen postoperatively in four patients given 5 days of prophylaxis versus six given a single dose. Clinical signs of pneumonia were demonstrated in five patients receiving 5 days of prophylaxis and in four patients receiving single-dose prophylaxis. Frequency of wound infection was the only significant difference in infectious complications ($P < 0.05$) between the two groups.

The powerful effects of nitroimidazoles against pathogenic human anaerobes have been explored clinically for only a few years. Of the different nitroimidazoles, metronidazole is the compound most widely used. There is no convincing difference in activity against human anaerobes between the various nitroimidazoles; only in pharmacokinetic properties does there seem to be a significant difference which could be of practical importance in some clinical situations. We have demonstrated that another nitroimidazole, tinidazole, will provide values well above MICs in serum, bowel wall, subcutaneous tissue, bile, and muscle tissue for more than 24 h after a single infusion of 1.5 g. Tinidazole, therefore, seems to have a very suitable pharmacokinetic profile for testing the single-dose hypothesis.

In spite of the fact that agents active against only anaerobes are capable of a substantial reduction of postoperative wound infections, we still believe that *Escherichia coli* and other aerobes do play an important part in the total picture of infectious complications. Gram-negative aerobic septicemia is still a dreaded complication of bowel surgery. Doxycycline is reasonably active against coliforms. Its side effects are few and mild, and it has a pharmacokinetic profile very similar to that of tinidazole. Doxycycline does not initiate a catabolic state or produce azotemia and therefore differs considerably from other tetracyclines.

In conclusion, our results indicate that a single preoperative dose of tinidazole and doxycycline is a simple and effective prophylaxis against infectious complications after elective colorectal surgery.

1. **Laufen, H., F. Scharpf, and G. Bartsch.** 1979. Selective gas chromatographic assay of tinidazole in tissue and plasma. J. Chromatogr. **163**:217–220.

Vancomycin Pharmacokinetics

KENT CROSSLEY* AND JOHN ROTSCHAFER

St. Paul-Ramsey Medical Center, St. Paul, Minnesota 55101, and The Medical School and College of Pharmacy, University of Minnesota, Minneapolis, Minnesota 55455, U.S.A.

Vancomycin is a bactericidal antistaphylococcal antibiotic made available for clinical use in 1956. The drug has been widely used in the United States only in recent years, as infections caused by methicillin-resistant staphylococci have become more frequent. Because this drug was not commonly used until very recently, there is only limited information available about its pharmacokinetics. We report here some selected aspects of our recent studies of the pharmacokinetics of vancomycin.

These studies were conducted in a group of 28 adult patients being treated with vancomycin for staphylococcal infection. The patients ranged in age from 18 to 80 years. Twenty-one of the 28 were being treated for burn wound infection. Twenty-three of the 28 had normal renal function.

All of the patients were studied after receiving a dose of 250 or 500 mg of vancomycin delivered over 1 h by an infusion pump. A trough level just before the infusion and 11 postinfusion levels (collected every 15 min for the 1st hour and then at 1.5, 2, 3, 4, 6, 8, and 10 h) were collected. The sera were frozen at −70°C until serum vancomycin concentrations were determined by an agar diffusion technique or by radioimmunoassay.

Data were analyzed by means of a standard two-compartment pharmacokinetic model (2). A biexponential equation describing this model was used to analyze these data, and the standard hybrid coefficients (A, B, α, β) were derived from this equation. A and B were corrected for infusion rate, infusion time, and predose serum concentration. The distribution half-life ($t_{1/2}\alpha$), elimination half-life ($t_{1/2}\beta$), central compartment volume (V_c), distribution volume ($V_{d\beta}$), and vancomycin clearance were calculated by standard methods (2). Analysis by means of a Pearson correlation table was done with all appropriate variable pairs. Pharmacokinetic parameters were grouped for burned and nonburned patients and examined for significant differences ($P < 0.05$) between these two populations.

A summary of the results of this study is presented in Table 1. Vancomycin half-life, rate of elimination, distribution volume, and clearance varied substantially between patients. Even in the 23 patients with normal renal function, the terminal half-life ($t_{1/2}\beta$) ranged from 2.7 to 13.3 (mean, 5.82) h. The mean peak serum concentration (determined by using specimens collected 15 min after the end of a 1-h infusion) in patients with normal renal function receiving 500 mg of vancomycin every 6 h was 30.2 ± 11.4 μg/ml; the mean trough level in the same group of patients was 5.1 ± 3.7 μg/ml.

The variables burn/nonburn or percentage of body surface area burn were not significantly related to any of the pharmacokinetic variables. Pharmacokinetic parameters observed in burned patients and nonburned patients were also not significantly different ($P > 0.05$). The observed correlation between vancomycin clearance and creatinine clearance ($r = 0.45$) indicated that only 22% of the variance (r^2) in vancomycin clearance could be explained on the basis of creatinine clearance (Fig. 1).

Most of the available studies of the pharmacokinetics of vancomycin were conducted in the mid-1950s. These studies indicated that vancomycin's half-life was between 4 and 6 h and that the drug was eliminated almost entirely by a renal mechanism. Clinical evidence suggested that ototoxicity seemed to correlate with elevated vancomycin serum levels. On the basis of these observations, the manufacturer of vancomycin has recommended a dosage of 500 mg every 6 h or 1 g every 12 h for an adult.

TABLE 1. *Vancomycin subject characteristics and pharmacokinetic parameters*[a]

Reference	Age (yr)	Body wt (kg)	Creatinine clearance (ml/min)	Vancomycin clearance (ml/min)	V_c (liters)	$V_{d\beta}$ (liters)	$t_{1/2}\alpha$ (h)	$t_{1/2}\beta$ (h)
Present study (n = 28 patients)	43.1 ± 18 (18–80)	71.1 ± 13 (55–107)	142.6 ± 79 (5–282)	73.0 ± 35 (13–184)	9.0 ± 4 (1–20)	39.3 ± 25 (14–111)	0.5 ± 0.3 (0.2–1.2)	6.0 ± 3 (3–13)
1 (n = 8 normal adults)	—[b] —	— —	— —	132.1 ± 21 (115–165)	— —	76.7 ± 14 (66–98)	— —	6.7 ± 1 (5–9)
3 (n = 4 normal adults)	36.3 ± 3.9 (32–40)	68.6 ± 9.3 (57–80)	119.3 ± 12.5 (106–132)	81.2 ± 10 (74–96)	7.7 ± 0.6 (7.4–8.4)	60.8 ± 15.5 (39–72)	0.12 ± 0.01 (0.1–0.13)	8.9 ± 2.9 (5–11)

[a] All values are mean ± SD, with range given in parentheses.
[b] —, Not stated or could not be calculated from the published data.

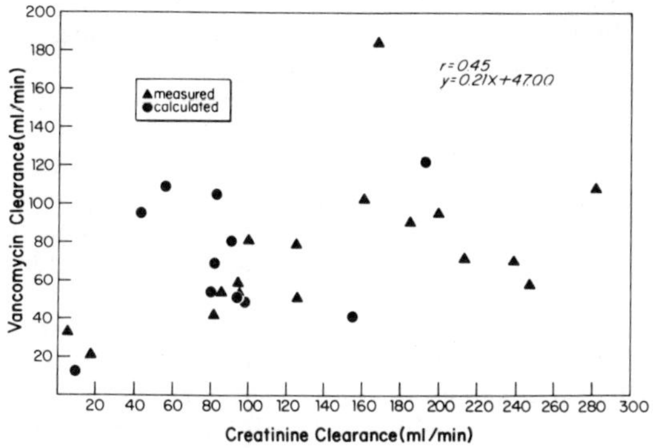

FIG. 1. *Vancomycin clearance versus creatinine clearance.*

Data from this study indicate that some individuals may have unnecessarily high peak serum levels after a dosage of 500 mg of vancomycin. Our measured peak levels followed a 1-h infusion of vancomycin. It would be expected that the peaks would be substantially higher if shorter infusion periods were used. On the basis of these observations, we would recommend infusing the drug over a minimum period of 1 h.

In adult patients with normal renal function, an initial regimen of 6.5 to 8 mg of vancomycin per kg given every 6 to 12 h will provide therapeutic serum concentrations. Longer dosage intervals may be required in older patients or in patients with compromised renal function. Adjustments in dose and dosage interval should be based on trough and peak serum vancomycin concentrations obtained 24 h after starting therapy and periodically during treatment. The prolonged distribution phase of vancomycin adds complexity and potential error when adjusting dosages.

Comparison of our data with results of other studies is difficult because of differences in study methods and in data analysis and reporting. In contrast to reports of Moellering et al. (4) and Nielsen et al. (5), we found a rather poor correlation between creatinine clearance and vancomycin clearance. The high values (0.23 to 6.6) we observed for the ratio of vancomycin clearance to creatinine clearance in patients with compromised renal function suggest that a nonrenal mechanism for vancomycin elimination may partially explain our findings. Further evidence for a significant nonrenal route of elimination includes (i) the positive intercept in the plot of vancomycin clearance versus creatinine clearance (Fig. 1) and (ii) the observation that four of five patients in this study with abnormal renal function had a normal terminal half-life.

Preliminary studies in rabbits and in patients receiving vancomycin suggest that a significant amount of vancomycin is eliminated by a biliary route. Additional studies are needed to define the role of hepatic and gastrointestinal mechanisms of vancomycin elimination.

1. **Geraci, J. E., F. R. Heilman, D. R. Nichols, W. E. Wellman, and G. T. Ross.** 1956. Some laboratory and clinical experiences with a new antibiotic, vancomycin. Proc. Staff Meet. Mayo Clin. **31:**564–582.
2. **Greenblatt, D. J., and J. Koch-Weser.** 1975. Clinical pharmacokinetics. N. Engl. J. Med. **293:**702–705, 964-970.
3. **Krogstad, D. J., R. C. Moellering, Jr., and D. J. Greenblatt.**. 1980. Single-dose kinetics of intravenous vancomycin. J. Clin. Pathol. **20:**197–201.
4. **Moellering, R. C., D. J. Krogstad, and D. J. Greenblatt.** 1981. Vancomycin therapy in patients with impaired renal function: a nomogram for dosage. Ann. Intern. Med. **94:**343–346.
5. **Nielsen, H. E., H. E. Hansen, B. Korsager, and P. E. Skov.** 1975. Renal excretion of vancomycin in kidney disease. Acta Med. Scand. **197:**261–264.

Effective Instillation of Antibiotics

KENJI NISHIZUKA

Department of Ophthalmology, Suibara-go Hospital, Suibara-machi, Niigata, Japan

The optimum dosages of antiobiotic preparations are generally prescribed for instillation treatment of eye infections. There are very few studies, however, on the relation between instillation method and chemotherapeutic effect. The following experiments were conducted to determine the instillation method best suited to the particular characteristics of two drugs, gentamicin and sulbenicillin.

Method. A 10% solution of NaOH was used to produce corrosion on the corneas of white rabbits. Solutions of 0.3% gentamicin and 1% sulbenicillin were instilled once, five times at 5-min intervals, or 12 times at hourly intervals, after which the infiltration concentrations in the tissues of the cornea were measured, using the thin-layer cup method with *Bacillus subtilis* ATCC 6633. *Psuedomonas aeruginosa* was then introduced to cause keratitis, the above solutions were instilled six times at 5-min intervals morning and evening or 12 times at hourly intervals, and a comparison of the effects of treatment on each group was made. Each group received the same daily dosage. In addition, a control group received instillations of a normal saline solution.

Results. Infiltration concentrations in the tissues of the cornea are shown in Table 1. Hourly instillations produced almost constant concentrations, whereas instillations at 5-min intervals demonstrated markedly high peak values. The results of experimental treatment are shown in Fig. 1. The most effective method of treatment was evidenced in the group which received six instillations of gentamicin solution at 5-min intervals in the morning and evening. This method was clearly superior to hourly instillation. In the groups that received sulbenicillin, hourly instillations proved most effective.

Discussion. The experiments conducted by Eagle et al. (1) on dosages and intervals between doses of antibiotic substances are well known. Since then, Nishino et al. (3) have reported that

TABLE 1. *Antibiotic[a] concentrations (micrograms per gram) in corneal tissues by instillation method*

Group I: Single instillation

Time		10 minutes	30 minutes	60 minutes	2 hours	4 hours	6 hours
Eye lotion	0.3% GM solution	5.65	6.47	3.75	1.18	0.025	0
	1% SBPC solution	33.9	43.8	33.6	10.4	1.83	0.79

Group II: Five instillations at 5-minute intervals

Time		10 minutes	1 hour	4 hours	8 hours	12 hours
Eye lotion	0.3% GM solution	62.0	55.0	7.28	0.69	0.50
	1% SBPC solution	216.4	140.0	31.9	1.26	0

Group III: Instillations every hour 12 times a day

Hours after first administration		1 hour	4 hours	8 hours	12 hours	14 hours	19 hours	23 hours
Eye lotion	0.3% GM solution	3.75	3.94	8.31	5.35		0.16	0.006
	1% SBPC solution	33.6	35.0	36.0	40.6	13.0	0	0

[a] GM, Gentamicin; SBPC, sulbenicillin.

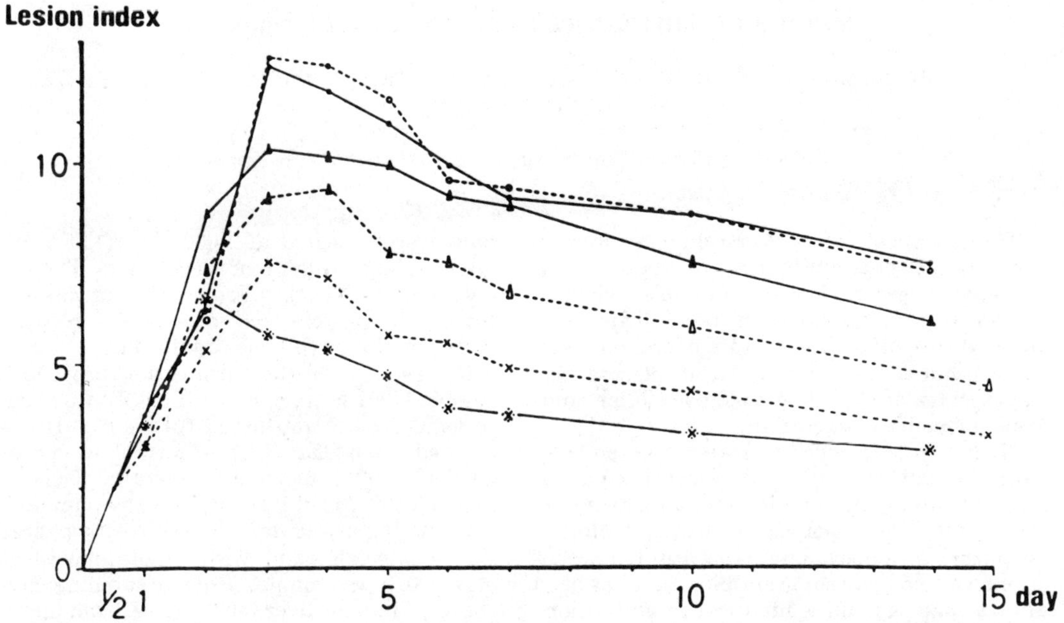

FIG. 1. *Changes in lesion indices. Symbols: ○, instillation of physiological sodium chloride solution every hour 12 times per day; ●, six instillations of physiological sodium chloride solution at 5-min intervals in the morning and evening; △, instillation of 1% sulbenicillin every hour 12 times per day; ▲, six instillations of 1% sulbenicillin at 5-min intervals in the morning and evening; X, instillation of 0.3% gentamicin every hour 12 times per day; ·Ẋ·, six instillations of 0.3% gentamicin at 5-min intervals in the morning and evening.*

even if the dosage of sulbenicillin or gentamicin is kept constant, its effect on *P. aeruginosa* varies, depending on the interval between the doses. In the experimental treatments which I conducted, hourly instillation of sulbenicillin produced results far superior to instillation at 5-min intervals, but it is my impression that treatment of *Pseudomonas* keratitis by sulbenicillin is not completely effective.

The effectiveness of gentamicin in the treatment of *Pseudomonas* keratitis is widely recognized. Francis et al. (2), have reported on its topical, subconjuctival, and intramuscular ocular penetration. Instillation doses are generally considered to be less effective in the treatment of severe keratitis than are subconjuctival, intravenous, and intramuscular injections and other forms of systemic administration. My experiments indicate, however, that concentrated instillation methods, such as six instillations at 5-min intervals, produce results that compare favorably with other forms of systemic administration, such as intravenous and intramuscular injections.

1. **Eagle, H., et al.** 1950. The bacterial action of PC in vivo. Ann. Intern. Med. **33**:544–571.
2. **Francis, P., et al.** 1967. Ocular penetration and tolerance of gentamicin. Am. J. Opthalmol. **64**:42.
3. **Nishino, T., et al.** 1977. Experimental studies on administration of chemotherapeutic agents. The Saishin-Igaku **32**:1491–1496.

Binding of Antibiotics to Human Liver Ligandin

TAKASHI KOMATSU,* HAJIME NISHIYA, KOICHIRO IWATA, MICHIO WATANABE, AND OTOHIKO KUNII

Institute of Medical Science, University of Tokyo, Tokyo, Japan

The extents of biliary excretion of antibiotics are various; some antibiotics are known to be excreted in great amounts into bile, whereas others are known to be excreted little. The mechanisms of biliary excretion are not well known, but uptake of drugs from plasma into hepatocytes and binding to intracellular components might be important.

"Ligandin" is a specific protein isolated from rat or human liver which may serve as an intracellular binding protein. It binds to several organic anions or drugs, e.g., bilirubin, sulfobromophthalein, indocyanine green, azo-dye carcinogens, steroids, and some antibiotics. It has been shown that ligandin is identical to glutathione (GSH) *S*-transferase. Many studies suggest that ligandin may be an important determinant in the uptake of these organic anions or drugs from plasma into bile and their retention and flux.

We have purified ligandin from human liver and studied the characteristics of its binding to several antibiotics in comparison with serum albumin.

Materials and methods. The human liver GSH *S*-transferases (anionic GSH *S*-transferase and cationic GSH *S*-transferase [ligandin]) were purified, as described by Awasthi et al. (1), from a liver which was collected at autopsy from the victim of a disease unrelated to liver disorders who had not been treated with any drug. Human serum albumin was a gift from Calbiochem (fraction V, lot 803212). GSH *S*-transferase activities of the protein were determined by measuring the conjugation of 1-chloro-2,4-dinitrobenzene with GSH as described by Habig et al. (3).

The binding of antibiotics to ligandin, anionic GSH *S*-transferase, and albumin were measured by a modification of the Penefsky method (5). [^{14}C]cefotetan (YM 09330, Yamanouchi Seiyaku Co.), [^{14}C]benzylpenicillin, [^{14}C]chloramphenicol, [^{14}C]cefazolin, and [^{3}H]gentamicin were used. The reaction mixtures contained 5 μl of antibiotics at various concentrations and 5 nmol of proteins in 50 μl of 10 mM potassium phosphate buffer, pH 7.4, and were incubated at 37°C for 2 h. The reaction mixtures were applied to the top of the centrifuge column which was previously packed with Sephadex G-25 into a disposable 1-ml plastic syringe, and centrifugations were repeated at 1,000 rpm (150 × *g*, 2 min), adding 50 μl of buffer each time. Then the radioactivity of each collected effluent was measured. The protein concentrations were determined by the method of Bradford (2).

Results. After the purification procedures, anionic GSH *S*-transferase (pI 4.7 to 5.4) and cationic GSH *S*-transferase (pI 8.6 to 9.1) were isolated. Each GSH *S*-transferase showed a single peak, with a molecular weight of 45,000, on Sephadex G-75 gel filtration, and sodium dodecyl sulfate-polyacrylamide gel electrophoresis showed a single band, with a molecular weight of 23,000. It was composed of two subunits. From 860 g of human liver, 46.3 mg of ligandin was isolated, and the specific activity was 17.56 U/mg of protein. Final recovery of ligandin was 4.6%.

In preliminary experiments on the binding of antibiotics to the protein by the centrifuge column method, the protein-bound drugs were eluted in three centrifugations and free drugs were eluted later. So the free and protein-bound drugs could be separated.

According to this procedure, the bindings of the drugs to ligandins, anionic GSH *S*-transferase, and albumin were determined and the dissociation constants (K_d values) were evaluated by Scatchard plots (Table 1). Cefotetan bound to ligandin to the greatest extent, followed by benzylpenicillin, cefazolin, and chloramphenicol. Gentamicin bound little. The extents of binding of these antibiotics to anionic GSH *S*-transferase were similar to those observed for ligandin, but the K_d values for cefazolin, chloramphenicol, and gentamicin could not be determined. The K_d values for albumin with cefotetan and benzylpenicillin were greater than those for ligandin and anionic GSH *S*-transferase.

From Scatchard plots, the numbers of antibiotic binding sites on ligandin, anionic GSH *S*-transferase, and albumin were determined (Table 2). The numbers of antiobiotic binding sites on albumin were greater than those on ligandin and anionic GSH *S*-transferase. The numbers of binding sites of cefotetan and benzylpenicillin were greater than those of cefazolin, chloramphenicol, and gentamicin.

Discussion. Kornguth et al. (4) reported the

TABLE 1. *K_d values for cationic or anionic GSH S-transferases and for albumin by the centrifuge column procedure*

Ligand	K_d (mM)		
	GSH *S*-transferases		Albumin (mM)
	Cationic	Anionic	
Cefotetan	8.3	13.6	11.2
Benzylpenicillin	17.3	27.1	29
Cefazolin	13.1		13.7
Chloramphenicol	>100		27.3
Gentamicin	124.7		

TABLE 2. *Numbers of binding sites on cationic and anionic GSH S-transferases and on albumin, obtained by Scatchard plots at sufficiently high drug concentration*

Antibiotic	Antibiotic mol/protein (mol)		
	GSH *S*-transferase		Albumin
	Cationic	Anionic	
Cefotetan	2.6	2.7	11.7
Benzylpenicillin	2.4	2.32	16.5
Cefazolin	0.41		0.7
Chloramphenicol		0.014	0.34
Gentamicin	0.06	0.046	

binding of several antibiotics to rat liver ligandin. They suggested that ligandin might be important in uptake and transport of antibiotics, as well as other ligands, in the liver. In the human liver, binding of antibiotics to ligandin has not been well documented.

This study demonstrated that not only ligandin but also anionic GSH *S*-transferase had binding activity for the antiobiotics. It was shown that cefotetan was bound to the greatest extent to both cationic (ligandin) and anionic GSH *S*-transferases, followed by benzylpenicillin, cefazolin, and chloramphenicol, and gentamicin was bound little.

Moreover, it has been known that in humans, cefotetan is excreted into the bile extensively, cefazolin and chloramphenicol are excreted to a lesser extent, and gentamicin is excreted little. These facts suggest that the extents of binding of the antibiotics to the liver GSH *S*-transferases may be correlated with the extents of biliary excretion.

Other studies (6) showed that the K_d of ligandin for bilirubin was 8 to 160 nM, and the K_d for indocyanine green was 20 mM. Comparing these data with those of this study, it is suggested that the binding of antibiotics to ligandin is not so tight as that of bilirubin or indocyanine green.

It is said that the flux of antibiotics across the plasma membranes into hepatocytes depends not only on the number of binding sites on the carrier proteins but also on the concentrations of the carriers in each component. So the fact that albumin has more binding sites for the antibiotics than does ligandin does not always mean that the antibiotics have difficulties in transport from plasma into hepatocytes, because both cationic and anionic GSH *S*-transferases are abundant in the human liver. The fact that the K_d of ligandin for cefotetan or benzylpenicillin was not greater than that of albumin may imply that ligandin has a greater affinity for the antibiotics than does albumin.

In conclusion, this study suggests that the human liver GSH *S*-transferases might have an important role in the transport of antibiotics from plasma into bile.

1. **Awasthi, Y. C., D. Dao, and R. P. Saneto.** 1980. Interrelationship between anionic and cationic forms of glutathione S-transferases of human liver. Biochem. J. **191:**1–10.
2. **Bradford, M. M.** 1976. A rapid and sensitive method for the quantitation of microgram quantities of protein utilizing the principle of protein-dye binding. Anal. Biochem. **72:**248–254.
3. **Habig, W. H., M. J. Pabst, and W. B. Jacoby.** 1974. Glutathione S-transferases. The first enzymatic step in mercapturic acid formation. J. Biol. Chem. **249:**7130–7139.
4. **Kornguth, M. I., R. A. Monson, and C. M. Kunin.** 1974. Binding of antibiotics to a soluble protein from rat liver. J. Infect. Dis. **129:**552–558.
5. **Penefsky, H. S.** 1977. Reversible binding of Pi by beef heart mitochondrial adenosine triphosphatase. J. Biol. Chem. **252:**2891–2899.
6. **Simons, P. C., and D. L. Vander Jagt.** 1980. Bilirubin binding to human liver ligandin (glutathione S-transferases). J. Biol. Chem. **255:**4740–4744.

Distribution of Antibiotics in Liver-Damaged Animals

K. MAEHARA,* H. OKUBO, Y. OKAMOTO, AND Y. UEDA

First Department of Internal Medicine, Kansai Medical University, Osaka, Japan

The liver and kidneys are the most important organs affecting the metabolism and kinetics of drugs, not excepting antibiotics, in the body. Drugs are metabolized chiefly in the liver, whose damage may cause abnormalities in their absorbtion, metabolism, and excretion; thus, liver damage may influence the in vivo effectiveness of antibiotics and the incidence of their side effects. In this respect, the kinetics of antibiotics in the bodies of liver-damaged patients deserve to be studied. In 1975, a general assembly of the Japanese Society of Chemotherapy held a symposium entitled "Chemotherapy Under Hepatic Damage." On that occasion, Y. Okamoto reported that, in cirrhotic patients, the serum concentration and urinary excretion of antibiotics, such as cefazolin (CEZ), josamycin, and gentamicin (GM), are different from those of healthy volunteers. Since then, we have studied antibiotic distribution in experimentally liver-damaged animals by using the bioassay method and performing micro-autoradiography of their livers with labeled antibiotics.

Liver damage was produced in rats by pretreatment with carbon tetrachloride (CCl_4), galactosamine, or α-naphthylisothiocyanate (ANIT) and was followed by GM (100 mg/kg intramuscularly), CEZ (100 mg/kg intramuscularly), or carbenicillin (100 mg/kg intramuscular), whose distributions in the body were examined.

For the micro-autoradiography studies, [^{3}H]GM (200 μCi/mouse), [^{14}C]CEZ (5 μCi/mouse), and [^{14}C]benzylpenicillin (10 μCi/mouse) were given to mice pretreated with CCl_4 or ANIT.

The micro-autoradiography technique was as follows. The labeled livers were frozen as soon as possible after removal, and frozen sections were made on a cryostat. The following procedures were carried out in a darkroom under a safelight: the frozen sections are picked up on a cold glass slide covered with radiosensitive film; after 6 weeks of exposure in the freezer, the sections are fixed, the films are processed, and the sections are stained.

Antibiotic distribution in rats. Carbenicillin concentrations were lower in the galactosamine-, ANIT-, and acutely CCl_4-damaged livers than in the controls. The blood levels in the GalN- or ANIT-damaged rats were slightly higher than in the normal rats. Like the carbenicillin concentrations, the CEZ levels were lower than in the normal livers (Fig. 1), but in the kidneys and blood, the CEZ levels were not remarkably different from those of the controls. In contrast, GM was found to accumulate and stay in the damaged livers, especially in those pretreated with galactosamine or ANIT (Fig. 2). This behavior of GM was in marked contrast to those of carbenicillin and CEZ. The renal levels of GM were higher in the ANIT-damaged rats than in the controls, whereas the blood levels were similar in both the experimental and the control animals. These data led us to carry out micro-autoradiography studies on the livers by using labeled antibiotics.

Liver micro-autoradiographic findings in mice. Thirty minutes after [^{14}C]benzylpenicillin administration, in damaged livers a reduction in [^{14}C]benzylpenicillin could be seen. In the hepatic cell region, the amounts of scattered grains were similar in both normal and damaged livers. Sixty minutes after administration, in normal livers the grains in the bile ducts were decreased. In CCl_4-damaged livers, the grains in the bile ducts were increased. Thirty minutes after [^{14}C]CEZ administration, grains could be seen mainly in the portal veins of both control and ANIT-damaged livers. In normal livers, but not in ANIT-damaged livers, grains were accumulated in the bile duct. Sixty minutes after [^{14}C]CEZ injection, normal livers displayed isotope grains only in the bile duct, whereas ANIT-damaged livers presented a huge accumulation of grains in the bile duct. In the case of micro-autoradiographs taken 60 min after [^{3}H]GM injection, in control livers [^{3}H]GM grains were found only in the Glisson's capsule, whereas in the CCl_4-damaged livers a marked accumulation of grains was found in the fatty degenerated hepatic cell area. One hundred twenty minutes after [^{3}H]GM injection, only a few grains remained in normal livers, whereas an abundance remained in the CCl_4-damaged livers.

These findings on antibiotic distributions in liver-damaged rats, as well as the results obtained by micro-autoradiographic studies on the livers, suggest that, although all the antibiotics examined were overwhelmingly excreted through the kidneys without becoming metabolized, GM differed in kinetics in the damaged

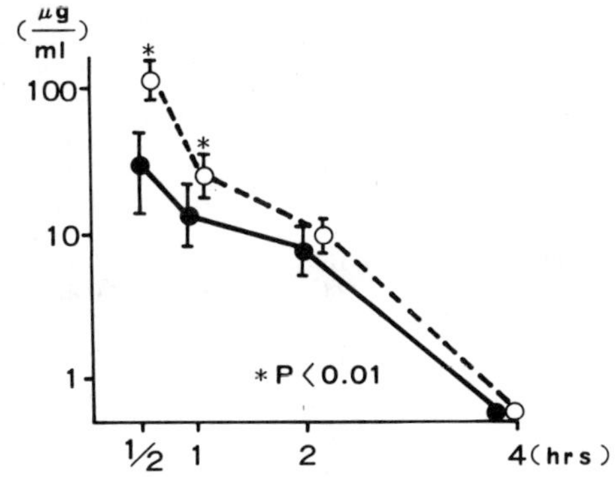

FIG. 1. *CEZ levels in galactosamine-damaged* (●) *and normal* (○) *livers.*

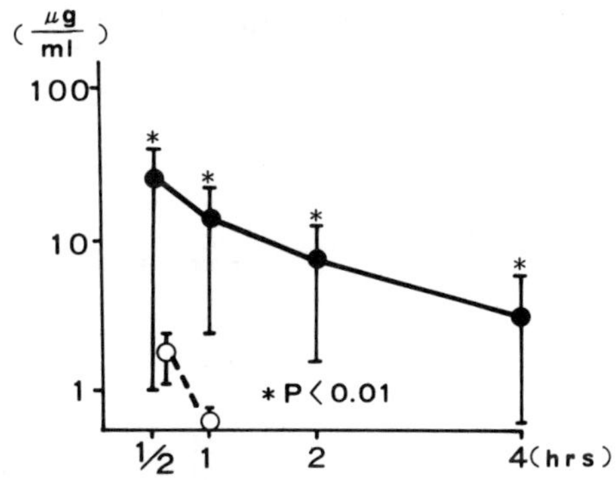

FIG. 2. *GM levels in galactosamine-damaged* (●) *and normal* (○) *livers.*

livers from carbenicillin, or benzylpenicillin insofar as GM was the only one which accumulated in the damaged livers. In 1977, Habermann (1) reported that GM accumulation in the kidneys is closely comparable with that known for polypeptides, such as aprotinin, and proposed a hypothesis that aminoglycosides are handled by the proximal tubule cells in a manner similar to that for polypeptides, i.e., by binding to the brush border, endocytotic uptake, and ultimate intralysosomal accumulation. In another study (2), Just and Habermann found the inhibitory effect of several aminoglycoside antibiotics upon polypeptides binding to isolated renal brush border membranes. If the supposed blood-liver barrier mechanism is broken in the experimentally damaged liver, GM may gain access to lysosomes of the damaged liver cells, and, as Just and Habermann supposed in the kidneys, it may accumulate there and stay longer than other kinds of antibiotics. Although these findings need further studies for interpretation in the clinical field, they may at least warn against the careless administration of aminoglycosides to liver-damaged patients, even if not so imperatively as with regard to patients with renal failure.

1. **Habermann, E.** 1977. Transmembranal and intracellular transport of pharmacologically active proteins and polypeptides. Naunyn-Schmiedeberg's Arch. Pharmacol. **297** (Suppl. 1):S11–S14.
2. **Just, M., and E. Habermann.** 1975. The renal handling of biologically active peptides. Contrib. Nephrol. **1:**62–68.

Penetration of Four β-Lactam Antibiotics with Antipseudomonal Activity into Human Aqueous Humor

H. GIAMARELLOU,* E. KAVOUKLIS, M. GRAMMATIKOU, AND G. K. DAIKOS

First Department of Propedeutic Medicine, Athens University School of Medicine, King Paul's Hospital, Athens 609, Greece

Pseudomonas aeruginosa eye infections constitute a major nosocomial threat. Although studies referring to intraocular penetration of antibiotics in humans are few, many studies have been carried out in rabbit eyes. However, this species differs from humans because of the size of the eye in relation to the body, absence of pigment, and size of vascularity (1). On the other hand, systemically administered "old" antibiotics penetrate very poorly into the various eye compartments because of various blood-ocular barriers which require specific antibiotic properties, such as lipid solubility, low protein binding, and low degree of ionization. It has been estimated that about 10% and 1% of the peak serum level of an antibiotic are detected in the aqueous humor and the vitreous, respectively (1). Only trimethoprim, chloramphenicol, and fusidic acid, which are more lipid-soluble antibiotics, exhibit adequate penetration. However, the latter antibiotics do not have antipseudomonal activity, whereas carbenicillin and gen-

TABLE 1. *Cefoperazone and moxalactam penetration into the human aqueous humor*

Agent	Patient-sex	Age (yr)	Time after the last dose (h)	Blood level (μg/ml)	Aqueous humor level (μg/ml)
Cefoperazone	1-M	66	2	48	3.6
	2-F	80	4	40	1.6
	3-F	70	4	55	1.7
	4-F	85	4	24	3
	5-M	77	4	16	3.4
	6-F	58	5	24	0.4
	7-M	69	5	24	1.1
	8-M	77	7	11	2.8
Moxalactam	1-F	68	3	31.5	3.3
	2-M	64	3.5	25	2.4
	3-M	45	4	24	2.5
	4-M	70	4.30	27.5	3.0
	5-F	90	5	22.5	9.5
	6-F	70	5	NA[a]	>10[b]
	7-M	70	5	137.5	18[b]
	8-M	50	5.5	19.0	2.5

[a] Not available.
[b] Patient with diabetes and renal insufficiency.

TABLE 2. *Cefsulodin and ceftazidime penetration into the human aqueous humor*

Agent	Patient-sex	Age (yr)	Time after the last dose (h)	Blood level (μg/ml)	Aqueous humor level (μg/ml)
Cefsulodin	1-F	90	3	75	6.5
	2-F	60	3	36	9
	3-M	70	3	43.5	8.5
	4-F	58	4	12	1.8
	5-M	65	4	16	2.4
	6-F	76	5	8	2
	7-M[a]	82	5	NA[b]	6.5
Ceftazidime	1-F	73	2	35	1.3
	2-F	78	2.5	28	1.2
	3-M	73	3	25	2.5
	4-M	80	3	100	7.0[a]
	5-M	81	3	105	7.5[a]
	6-F	78	4	28	2.1
	7-M	80	4	25	3.0
	8-F	65	5	19	2.0
	9-M	88	5	12	3.3
	10-F	55	6	7.0	3.2

[a] Patient with renal insufficiency.
[b] Not available.

tamicin penetration into the aqueous humor when given parenterally is inadequate to cover *Pseudomonas* strains (2, 4). On the other hand, the ever-increasing resistance of *P. aeruginosa* to gentamicin and carbenicillin, particularly in the nosocomial environment, prompts the eye kinetic studies of new antibiotics with antipseudomonal activity.

In the present study 33 patients who were going to undergo elective cataract extraction were given four new β-lactam antibiotics with antipseudomonal activity at the following dosages: (i) cefoperazone (8 patients), 2 g every 12 h, 0.5-h infusion; (ii) cefsulodin (7 patients), 2 g every 8 h, 0.5-h infusion; (iii) moxalactam (8 patients), 2 g every 8 h, 0.5-h infusion; and (iv) ceftazidime (10 patients), 1 g every 8 h intramuscularly. Aqueous humor samples derived through direct puncture of the anterior chamber before cataract extraction, with simultaneous blood samples, were obtained at various timing intervals after at least three doses of the tested antibiotics. Serum and aqueous humor levels were measured by an agar diffusion assay with the proper microorganisms.

Pharmacokinetic results are shown in Tables 1 and 2. Taking into account that the MIC_{50} of cefoperazone and moxalactam against *P. aerugi-*

nosa strains was found to be ≤6 μg/ml (3), whereas only 20% of the strains were inhibited at a concentration of ≤3 μg/ml, it should be concluded that for both antibiotics MIC determination is required before deciding which is the proper antibiotic. However, when moxalactam was administered (patients 6 and 7, Table 1), higher blood levels also created higher levels in the aqueous humor, exceeding 10 μg/ml. This observation indicated that moxalactam is probably passively transported into the aqueous humor, and therefore a higher daily dose than the conventional treatment schedule should be administered in *P. aeruginosa* eye infections.

Cefsulodin and ceftazidime kinetic results were very promising. Cefsulodin, 3 h after a 2-g dose, created levels ranging between 6.5 and 9 μg/ml, whereas an MIC_{50} of ≤3 μg/ml was found, and ≤4.5 μg/ml inhibited almost 80% of the strains (3). Compared with the other antibiotics studied, ceftazidime aqueous humor levels were the most stable, being constantly above 2 μg/ml; unexpected high blood levels in two patients because of underlying renal insufficiency (patients 4 and 5, Table 2) were also followed by a higher aqueous humor concentration of ceftazidime. Considering that the MIC_{50} of ceftazidime against *P. aeruginosa* strains was found to be ≤1.5 μg/ml, and that ≤3 μg/ml inhibited 80% of the tested strains, it is clear that ceftazidime should be the antibiotic of choice when dealing with *P. aeruginosa* eye infections. However, it should be kept in mind that, as a result of their broad spectrum of activity and their very low MICs against the *Enterobacteriaceae* family (3), aqueous humor levels of cefoperazone, moxalactam, and ceftazidime are more than adequate therapeutically to cover eye infections caused by *Enterobacteriaceae*.

1. **Barza, M.** 1980. Intraocular penetration of antibiotics, p. 40–41. *In* J. D. Nelson and C. Grassi (ed.), Current chemotherapy and infectious disease, vol. 1. American Society for Microbiology, Washington, D.C.
2. **Barza, M., J. Baum, B. Birkby, and L. Weinstein.** 1973. Intraocular penetration of carbenicillin in the rabbit. Am. J. Ophthalmol. **75:**307–313.
3. **Giamarellou, H., A. Avlami, V. Matsakas, J. Kosmidis, and G. K. Daikos.** 1981. In vitro studies with Ceftazidime. J. Antimicrob. Chemother. **8:**(Suppl.).
4. **Litwack, D. K., T. T. Pett, and B. L. Johanson.** 1969. Penetration of gentamicin administered intramuscularly and subconjunctivally into aqueous humor. Arch. Ophthalmol. **82:**687–693.

Pregnancy and Anaerobic Infections: Which Chemotherapeutic? A Study of Kinetics Through the Amniotic Fluid

H. GIAMARELLOU,* G. PETRIKKOS, J. GAZIS, A. ATSAKLIS, K. TSATSIADIS, D. KASKARELIS, AND G. K. DAIKOS

First Department of Propedeutic Medicine, Athens University School of Medicine, King Paul's Hospital, Athens, 609, Greece, and First Department of Obstetrics and Gynaecology, Athens University School of Medicine, Alexandra Maternity Hospital, Athens, 611, Greece*

An efficient antibiotic for use in obstetrical infections must be safe for the fetus, and it should achieve therapeutic concentrations in amniotic fluid. To date, as far as we know, it has been reported that methicillin, cephaloridine, cephacetrile, ampicillin, amoxicillin, erythromycin, clindamycin, gentamicin, cephradine, cefoxitin, thiamphenicol, and co-trimoxazole are effectively concentrated in maternal and neonatal cord serum as well as in amniotic fluid (1, 2), whereas cefuroxime and azlocillin concentrations in amniotic fluid have been found inadequate to inhibit both aerobes and anaerobes (H. Giamarellou et al., 2nd Mediterranean Congress of Chemotherapy, Nice, France, 1980, abstr. 146).

There is, however, a paucity of information on the pharmacokinetics of the new chemotherapeutics in pregnancy. On the other hand, the major pathogens implicated in intrauterine infections are the anaerobes, particularly *Bacteroides fragilis* strains, which are not susceptible to most of the above-mentioned antibiotics.

The purpose of the present report, which is part of a series of studies, is to evaluate the pharmacokinetics through the amniotic fluid of six chemotherapeutics with proven in vitro and in vivo activity against anaerobes, namely, cefoxitin, clindamycin, metronidazole, ornidazole, and tinidazole, as well as ceftriaxone (Ro 13-9904), a new broad-spectrum third-generation cephalosporin (4).

Forty-one pregnant women with mean age of gestation of 20.2 (±1.8) weeks whose fetuses were suffering from Cooley's disease, as proved by electrophoresis of fetal blood samples obtained by antenatal embryoscopy, have been included in this report. All studied chemotherapeutics had been preadministered 24 h before labor induction by amniocentesis and intrauterine infusion of prostaglandin F2a, on the following schedules: (i) cefoxitin at a dose of 2 g every 8 h as a 30-min infusion in nine women with a mean age of gestation of 20.5 (±1.6) weeks; (ii) ceftriaxone at a dose of 1.5 g every 24 h as a 30-min infusion in nine women with a mean age of gestation of 21.2 (±1.6) weeks; (iii) clindamycin at a dose of 600 mg every 8 h as a 30-min infusion in seven women with a mean age of gestation of 19.2 (±1.2) weeks; (iv) metronidazole at a dose of 500 mg rectally every 8 h in six women with a mean age of gestation of 20.3 (±1.4) weeks; (v) ornidazole at a dose of 500 mg every 12 h as a 30-min infusion in six patients with a mean age of gestation of 19.5 (±3.0) weeks; (vi) tinidazole at a dose of 1 g rectally every 12 h in four patients with a mean age of gestation of 19.5 (±0.5) weeks. Before F2a infusion and during the amniocentesis, amniotic fluid and mother's blood samples were collected simultaneously at various time intervals.

Ornidazole and ceftriaxone levels were measured by the high-pressure liquid chromatography method; metronidazole and trinidazole levels, by the Ralph and Kirby method (5); and clindamycin and cefoxitin levels, by applying the standard agar well diffusion method with *Sarcina lutea* and *Bacillus subtilis* spores (1904E), respectively.

Kinetic results are shown in Fig. 1 and 2. In four women who were to undergo cesarean section, Bergogne-Berezin et al. (1) detected amniotic fluid levels of cefoxitin ranging between 2.7 and 7.6 μg/ml, levels very similar to those found in the present study. However, the observed levels are adequate to inhibit only 50% of the *Enterobacteriaceae* and *B. fragilis* strains (3).

Ceftriaxone achieved rather constant amniotic fluid levels ranging between 2.2 and 8.2 μg/ml. Although these levels inhibited more than 80% of the *Enterobacteriaceae* organisms, they are very low to cover successfully most of the anaerobic infections (4).

Amniotic fluid levels of clindamycin ranged between 0.6 and 2.0 μg/ml, levels equal to or above the required MICs for most of the anaerobic species. However, it should be noted that mothers' serum levels of clindamycin were found to be one-third lower than the expected concentrations. In contrast, no difference in the serum kinetic behavior of the other chemotherapeutics

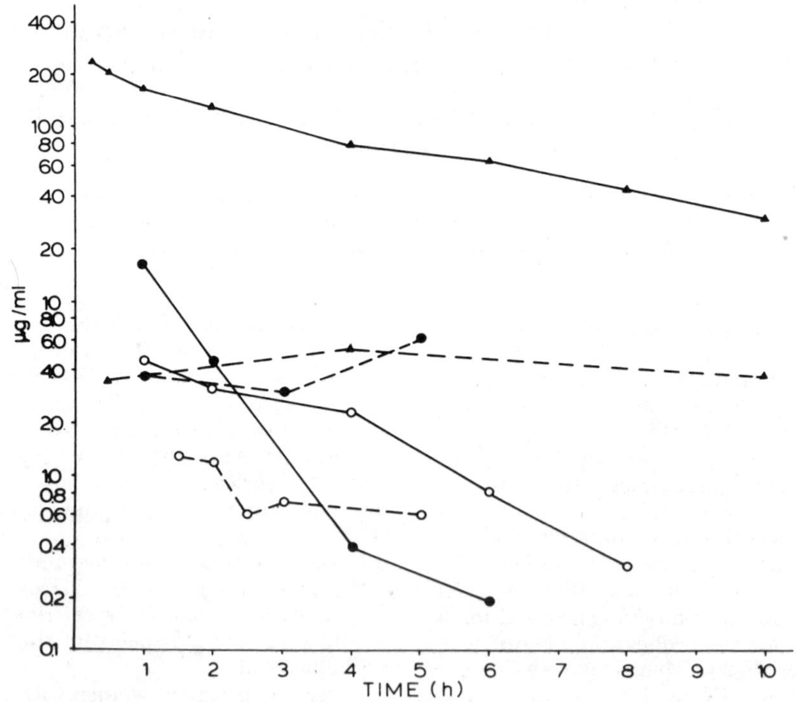

FIG. 1. *Serum (▲——▲) and amniotic fluid (▲---▲) levels of ceftriaxone compared with serum (●——●) and amniotic fluid (●---●) levels of cefoxitin and serum (○——○) and amniotic fluid (○---○) levels of clindamycin.*

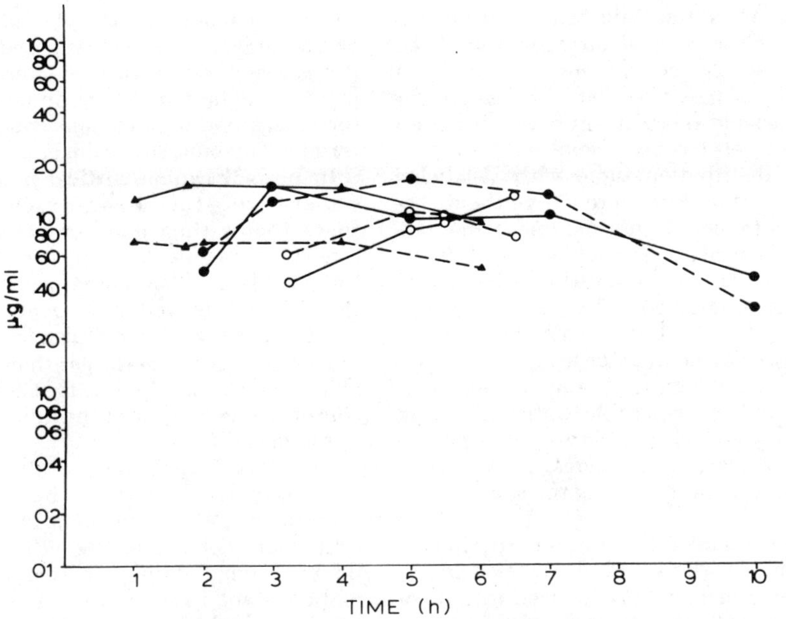

FIG. 2. *Serum (●——●) and amniotic fluid (●---●) levels of metronidazole compared with serum (▲——▲) and amniotic fluid (▲---▲) levels of ornidazole and serum (○——○) and amniotic fluid (○---○) levels of tinidazole.*

studied was observed. Probably clindamycin turnover is faster during pregnancy than in the normal host.

The three nitroimidazole compounds, as shown in Fig. 2, all cross the placenta and were concentrated in the amniotic fluid at 4 to 10 times above the required levels for killing *B. fragilis* strains.

Although from the reported study the kinetic behavior of nitroimidazoles through the amniotic fluid was the most advantageous, in the presence of intrauterine infections the possibility of fetal mutagenicity should always be kept in mind whenever administering nitroimidazole compounds therapeutically.

1. **Bergogne-Berezin, E., N. Lambert-Zechovsky, and J. L. Rouvillois.** 1979. Étude du passage transplacentaire des bêta-lactamines. J. Gynecol. Obstet. Biol. Reprod. **8**:359–364.
2. **Craft, J., and T. C. Forster.** 1978. Materno-fetal cephradine transfer in pregnancy. Antimicrob. Agents Chemother. **14**:924–926.
3. **Giamarellou, H., A. Avlami, V. Matsakas, J. Kosmidis, and G. K. Daikos.** 1981. In vitro studies with ceftazidime. J. Antimicrob. Chemother. **8**(Suppl.).
4. **Giamarellou, H., B. Poulopoulos, A. Katsabas, G. Petrikkos, M. Papapetropoulou, and G. K. Daikos.** 1981. Antibacterial activity of Ro13-9904 and preliminary experience in gonorrhoea and chronic urinary tract infections. Chemotherapy (Basel) **27**(Suppl. 1):70–74.
5. **Ralph, E. D., and W. M. M. Kirby.** 1975. Bioassay of metronidazole with either anaerobic or aerobic incubation. J. Infect. Dis. **132**:587–592.

Osseous Pharmacokinetics of Gentamicin in Normal and Osteomyelitic Bone

WILLIAM R. QUINLAN AND ROBERT H. FITZGERALD, JR.*

Mayo Clinic and Mayo Foundation, Rochester, Minnesota 55901, U.S.A.

Peak and trough levels of gentamicin in serum have proved to be of clinical value in monitoring therapy for the prevention of iatrogenic complications. However, the relationship of the serum concentration to the gentamicin concentration at the primary site of drug-microorganism interaction—the interstitial fluid space—in normal and osteomyelitic cortical bone has not been defined. When gentamicin concentrations in bone have been measured with bioassay techniques, a variable relationship between serum and osseous levels has been reported.

Volume of distribution studies with ^{3}H-labeled gentamicin were performed to define the distribution of gentamicin in normal and osteomyelitic canine cortical bone. The volume of distribution is a virtual volume in which the virtual concentration is assumed to be the same as that in the reference space but in which the cortical concentration may be more or less.

The relative sizes of the plasma, extracellular, interstitial, and exchangeable water spaces in normal and osteomyelitic bone were determined with ^{99m}Tc-labeled erythrocytes, [^{14}C]sucrose, and water of desiccation during the same experiments.

Since the volume of distribution experiments were performed with isotopically labeled gentamicin, the serum and bone concentrations of gentamicin could be quantitated with an isotope assay. When this information was combined with the volume of distribution of gentamicin and the size of the various fluid spaces, it was possible to determine the concentration of gentamicin in the interstitial fluid space of normal and osteomyelitic bone.

TABLE 1. *Volume of distribution of gentamicin in normal and osteomyelitic canine cortical bone*

Condition	No.	Mean volume of distribution (ml/ml of bone)	Exchangeable water space
Normal	13	0.2558 ± 0.1063	0.2515 ± 0.0197
Osteomyelitis			
Subacute	6	0.5019 ± 0.1629	0.4540 ± 0.0917
Acute	7	1.5663 ± 0.7557	0.4996 ± 0.0806

The calculated interstitial fluid concentration of gentamicin could be compared with simultaneous serum concentrations determined by high-pressure liquid chromatographic assay and isotope assay and with osseous concentrations determined by bioassay and isotope assay.

In normal canine cortical bone, gentamicin was distributed in the entire exchangeable water space; that is, the volume of distribution of gentamicin was equivalent to the water of desiccation (Table 1). A similar relationship existed in subacute osteomyelitis. In acute osteomyelitis, however, the volume of distribution of gentamicin was three times larger than the exchangeable water space, a finding that suggests concentration in one or more of the fluid compartments of osteomyelitic bone.

The interstitial fluid concentrations of gentamicin, calculated from the volume of distribution experiments, were equivalent to the serum concentrations determined by either high-pressure liquid chromatography or isotope assay in normal bone and in subacute and acute osteomyelitic bone (Table 2). Osseous concentrations, determined by either bioassay or isotope assay, were variable. There was no apparent relationship to serum concentrations.

In steady-state conditions, the serum level accurately reflects the interstitial fluid concentrations of gentamicin. In contrast, osseous concentrations have no relationship to either interstitial fluid or serum concentrations. Thus, serum concentrations can be used to accurately monitor gentamicin concentrations at the primary site of drug-microorganism interaction—the interstitial fluid space—in patients with osteomyelitis.

This investigation was supported in part by Public Health Service research grant AM-26928 from the National Institutes of Health.

TABLE 2. *Gentamicin concentrations in normal and osteomyelitic canine cortical bone*[a]

Condition	No.	Mean gentamicin concn: ISF (μg/ml)	Serum (μg/ml): HPLCA	Serum (μg/ml): IA	Bone (μg/g): BA	Bone (μg/g): IA
Normal	13	4.7 ± 1.6	5.5 ± 1.7	5.0 ± 1.7	—	1.75 ± 0.45
Osteomyelitis						
Subacute (1.5 mg/kg)	6	5.75 ± 1.16	6.1 ± 1.6	5.8 ± 1.7	8.8 ± 5.3	2.2 ± 1.0
Acute (1.0 mg/kg)	7	2.64 ± 0.68	3.85 ± 1.48	4.35 ± 2.58	3.93 ± 1.97	4.89 ± 4.10

[a] ISF, Interstitial fluid; HPLCA, high-pressure liquid chromatographic assay; IA, isotope assay; BA, bioassay.

Elimination of Gentamicin and Cephalosporins Is Influenced by Kinetic Interactions

ARIS POLYZOS,* JOHN KOSMIDIS, JOHN ALEXOPOULOS, AND GEORGE K. DAIKOS

First Department of Propedeutic Medicine, Athens University School of Medicine, King Paul's Hospital, Athens, Greece

Nephrotoxicity of aminoglycosides is a danger borne in mind by all clinicians and drastically reduces the prescribing of these agents. It does, however, occur in everyday practice and often also leads to ototoxicity. The effect of hypotension and shock, as well as that of the infection itself, and concomitant administration of diuretics and cephalosporins have been incriminated as precipitating or potentiating factors. The subject of nephrotoxic interaction between aminoglycosides and cephalosporins was reviewed by Marsh (3). Concomitant use of aminoglycosides and cephalosporins, especially that of gentamicin (GENT) and cephalothin (CFT), was reported as particularly nephrotoxic in various case reports and clinical trials. However, animal experiments failed to demonstrate nephrotoxic synergy between aminoglycosides and cephalosporins; on the contrary, a protective effect was noted when the cephalosporin was administered simultaneously with the aminoglycoside, but not when a certain time interval separated the administrations. On the other hand, in a carefully controlled prospective clinical study in patients suffering from mild infections, no potentiation of nor protection from nephrotoxicity was detected with the simultaneous administration of GENT and CFT (1).

Since trapping of GENT inside the tubular cells is considered as a possible mechanism for nephrotoxicity, pharmacokinetic interactions with cephalosporins, leading to an increase or decrease of such trapping, may be responsible for alterations of the toxicity potential. We decided to investigate, therefore, the elimination kinetics of GENT and two cephalosporins, cephaloridine (CRD) and CFT, given alone and in combination.

Eighteen healthy male volunteers aged 22 to 35 years and weighing from 65 to 85 kg, all with creatinine clearances above 90 ml/min, participated in the study. Each volunteer was studied in three phases, separated by intervals of at least 5 days. In one phase the volunteers received a single dose of GENT alone, in a second phase they received the cephalosporin alone, and in a third phase GENT and the cephalosporin were given simultaneously. The order of the three phases was different for each volunteer and was determined by using random numbers. Nine volunteers received the following regimens in the three phases: (i) 80 mg of GENT intramuscularly, (ii) 500 mg (6 volunteers) or 1 g (3 volunteers) of CRD intramuscularly, and (iii) i and ii simultaneously. The remaining nine received: (i) 80 mg of GENT intravenously, (ii) 1 g (6 volunteers) or 2 g (3 volunteers) of CFT intravenously, and (iii) i and ii simultaneously.

After administration of the antibiotics, serial specimens of blood and urine were collected, and antibiotic concentrations were measured by microbiological well plate methods as follows. GENT was assayed using a strain of *Bacillus subtilis* when given alone and a multiresistant strain of *Staphylococcus albus* in the presence of CRD or CFT. CRD and CFT were assayed using a strain of *S. aureus*. When GENT was also present in the specimen, it was inactivated by addition of 0.6% liquoid in the agar.

The results are presented in Tables 1 and 2. The serum terminal half-life of CRD was slightly shortened by simultaneous administration of GENT, resulting in lower CRD levels, especially after the first 2 h. Total urinary recovery increased from 74.3% to 80.6% after a 500-mg dose and from 68.8% to 83.1% after a 1-g dose. Excretion of CRD was shifted to earlier urine collection periods.

With CFT, serum levels became higher with simultaneous administration of GENT until 2 to 3 h after the dose but later approached and equaled those of CFT given alone. The half-life at β phase was prolonged from 20.2 min to 42.0 min with a 1-g dose, but was not altered at the 2-g dose. On the other hand, the half-life at γ phase was shortened from 61 to 54 min at the 1-g dose and from 72 to 51 min at the 2-g dose. Total urinary recovery decreased from 33.1 to 22.2% of the 1-g dose and from 31.2 to 29.0% of the 2-g dose with a considerable shift to later collections.

The half-life of GENT was prolonged by the simultaneous administration of either cephalosporin at all dosages. The most pronounced effect was observed with 1 g of CFT, which prolonged the half-life of GENT from 92.5 to 160.5 min. On all occasions levels of GENT were higher when a cephalosporin had also been ad-

TABLE 1. *Serum concentrations of CRD, CFT, and GENT given alone or in combination in healthy volunteers*

Treatment	Mean concn (mg/liter) at the indicated times (h or min)									Half-life (min)	
	5	15	30	1	2	3	4	6	8	β	γ
CRD (500 mg) alone			32	30	14.9		6.2	2.9	1.32	108.5	
With GENT			25	30	18.7		5.2	2.7	0.96	90.3	
CRD (1 g) alone			45	48	27		11.2	5.0	2.05	94.5	
With GENT			45	42	24		8.5	3.2	1.10	81.0	
CFT (1 g) alone	61	19	8.1	2.1	0.42	0.26	0.13	<0.1		20.2	61
With GENT	72	25	10	3.1	0.75	0.32	0.14	<0.1		42.0	54
CFT (2 g) alone	102	31	11	4.8	1.10	0.62	0.35	0.1		27.0	72
With GENT	102	33	17	7.4	1.45	0.62	0.27	<0.1		27.0	51
GENT alone			6.2	4.9	4.3		2.0	0.9	0.43	130	
With CRD (500 mg)			5.4	4.8	3.9		2.3	1.2	0.66	148	
GENT alone			3.3	4.0	3.1		1.6	0.75	0.38	122	
With CRD (1 g)			3.2	4.2	3.4		1.8	1.02	0.54	139	
GENT alone	10.4	6.8	3.3	2.4	1.5	0.87	0.53	0.22		92.5	
With CFT (1 g)	10.8	6.9	3.6	2.6	2.0	1.5	1.17	0.78		160.5	
GENT alone	10.0	6.2	2.8	2.0	1.2	0.74	0.45	0.18		91	
With CFT (2 g)	11.0	6.4	3.1	2.7	2.1	1.35	0.96	0.43		105	

TABLE 2. *Urinary recovery of CRD, CFT, and GENT given alone or in combination in healthy volunteers*

Treatment	Mean recovery (mg) at the indicated time intervals (h)				Total recovery (% of dose)
	0–2	2–4	4–6	6–8	
CRD (500 mg) alone	202	116	48	5.6	74.3
With GENT	201	145	52	5.1	80.6
CRD (1 g) alone	240	195	160	93	68.8
With GENT	488	238	73	32	83.1
CFT (1 g) alone	324	6.2	0.8		33.1
With GENT	206	14.6	1.4		22.2
CFT (2 g) alone	602	20.5	1.4		31.2
With GENT	542	27.0	10.2		29.0
GENT alone	31.6	21.4	4.7	1.8	73.1
With CRD (500 mg)	26.4	22.1	8.1	2.8	76.7
GENT alone	25.3	18.7	5.6	4.1	67.1
With CRD (1 g)	23.2	24.4	12.2	10.4	87.8
GENT alone	47.2	9.4	3.3		74.9
With CFT (1 g)	38.4	17.7	7.7		79.7
GENT alone	52.8	10.0	3.1		82.4
With CFT (2 g)	47.2	12.2	6.0		81.8

ministered and sometimes were substantially higher. Differences were more pronounced with CFT. Total urinary recovery of GENT was not significantly affected, except when 1 g of CRD was also given, which caused an increase of GENT recovery from 67.1 to 87.8% of the dose. On all occasions GENT excretion was shifted to later collections.

The above results indicate that urinary excretion of CRD is enhanced by simultaneous GENT, whereas that of CFT is probably delayed. Excretion of desacetyl-CFT is also enhanced, as shown by the shortening of the half-life in γ phase of CFT-like activity in serum. Activity at this phase is known to be mainly due to this metabolite. This finding confirms the similarity in the kinetic behavior of desacetyl-CFT with that of CRD but not CFT (2). Excretion of GENT is delayed by both cephalosporins.

Kinetic interactions between GENT and cephalosporins therefore seem to exist. Their significance is, however, far from clear. Could delay in excretion of GENT mean trapping inside tubular cells, causing nephrotoxicity? Total urinary recovery of GENT is, however, not diminished, but rather is increased. Could that mean the opposite? Is excessive concentration of GENT in tubular lumen, which is observed at the 0- to 2-h period, avoided by delay in GENT excretion, with a protective effect as a result? Until the whole subject of potentiation versus protection from GENT nephrotoxicity by the cephalosporins is completely clarified, these questions cannot be answered with certainty.

Further studies are indicated, involving administration of the drugs on different schedules and dosages. Protection from toxicity seems to depend on simultaneity of administration, and kinetic interactions between cephalosporins and furosemide are influenced by differences in administration times (2).

1. **Giamarellou, H., C. Metzikoff, S. Papachristophorou, A. S. Dontas, and G. K. Daikos.** 1979. Prospective comparative evaluation of gentamicin or gentamicin plus cephalothin, in the production of nephrotoxicity in man. J. Antimicrob. Chemother. **5**:581–590.
2. **Kosmidis, J., A. Polyzos, and G. K. Daikos.** 1980. Pharmacokinetic interactions between cephalosporins and furosemide are influenced by administration time relationships, p. 673–675. *In* J. D. Nelson and C. Grassi (ed.), Current chemotherapy and infectious disease. American Society for Microbiology, Washington, D.C.
3. **Marsh, F. P.** 1978. Do cephalosporins potentiate or antagonize aminoglycoside nephrotoxicity? J. Antimicrob. Chemother. **4**:103–106.

Penetration of Doxycycline Through Respiratory Mucosa: a Study Using Secretory Otitis Media as a Model

LENNART SUNDBERG,* TONY EDÉN, AND STEFAN ERNSTSON

Department of ENT, Central Hospital, S-37185 Karlskrona, and Clinical Bacteriological Laboratory, Central Hospital, S-29185 Kristianstad, Sweden*

Since its introduction about 20 years ago, doxycycline has proved to be an effective antibiotic in the management of bacterial diseases. In sinusitis, for example, doxycycline penetrates the secretions to attain levels well above the MICs for the common pathogens (2). The emergence of β-lactamase–producing strains of *Branhamella catarrhalis* and *Haemophilus influenzae* in respiratory tract infections (3, 4) has enhanced the interest in evaluating alternatives to the established β-lactam antibiotics.

Secretory otitis media is a suitable model for studying antibiotic penetration of an inflamed respiratory mucosa, and the results should be valid for any area lined with a respiratory epithelium (5). In the present investigation, this method was used to study the penetration of doxycycline.

The study consisted of 57 patients with long-standing secretory otitis media, 28 males and 29 females, with a mean age of 30 years (range, 8 to 81 years). Tablets of doxycycline (Idocyklin) were given in a dosage of 200 mg initially followed by 100 mg every 24th hour. At different times during the treatment, i.e., after 3, 12, 24, 36, 48, and 120 h, myringotomy was performed, and the middle ear secretion was aspirated. Blood samples were drawn simultaneously. The same procedure was done 24 and 36 h after the last dose.

The concentration of doxycycline in middle ear secretions and in plasma was determined by means of an agar well diffusion method, the principles of which were described in an earlier corresponding study on the penetration of erythromycin (5).

The results presented in Fig. 1 are all mean values. The concentration of doxycycline in middle ear secretions was 1.0 mg/liter 3 h after the first dose. A level of 2.5 mg/liter, a value comparable to the initial peak in plasma, was reached 10 h later. During the continued course of treatment, the concentration in secretions ranged between 1.8 and 2.8 mg/liter. The elimination of doxycycline from secretions was slower than from plasma, and 24 and 36 h after the last dose the concentration in secretions was still 1.0 and 0.6 mg/liter, respectively.

The results show that an adequate level of doxycycline is obtained already after 3 h. The MICs for the common pathogens are surpassed by a wide margin. It should be observed that the pathogens are mainly present in the secretions covering the respiratory mucosa and that an adequate concentration in secretions denotes a still better level in the respiratory mucosa (2). The rapid penetration of doxycycline to the middle ear secretions is in contrast to the somewhat slower penetration of erythromycin demonstrated in a corresponding study (5).

The slow elimination of doxycycline from secretions as compared with plasma—a therapeutic level in secretions still being present 24 h after the last dose—implies small fluctuations of the concentration during the course of treatment. It is also obvious that one dose a day should be sufficient to obtain satisfactory levels in the secretions of an inflamed respiratory mucosa.

There seems to be an increasing number of failures in the treatment of respiratory tract infections with β-lactam antibiotics. This might

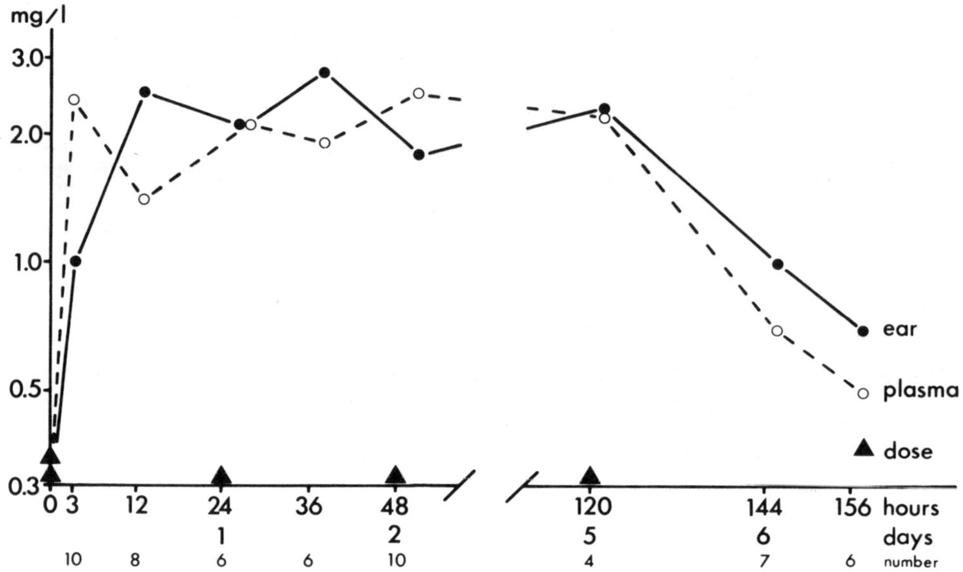

FIG. 1. *Doxycycline concentration in middle ear secretions and in plasma of patients with secretory otitis media. All values are means of several determinations.*

be due to β-lactamase-producing strains of *B. catarrhalis* and *H. influenzae* (3, 4). Furthermore, β-lactamase-producing nonpathogenic saprophytes have been isolated in cultures from adenoid tissue (1). An enzymatic inactivation of penicillin may in these cases be a contributing factor to failures.

When evaluating alternatives to penicillins in the management of respiratory tract infections, the penetration characteristics through an inflamed respiratory mucosa and the stability to β-lactamase should be taken into consideration. In these respects doxycycline can be looked upon as an attractive alternative.

In conclusion, in the secretions of an inflamed respiratory mucosa, the concentration of doxycycline 3 h after the first dose was well above the MICs for the common respiratory pathogens. The concentration remained at a therapeutic level until 24 h after the last dose.

1. **Brook, I.** 1981. Aerobic and anaerobic bacteriology of adenoids in children: a comparison between patients with adenotonsillitis and adenoid hypertrophy. Laryngoscope **91:**377–382.
2. **Eneroth, C. M., C. Lundberg, and B. Wretlind.** 1975. Antibiotic concentrations in maxillary sinus secretions and in the sinus mucosa. Chemotherapy (Basel) **21**(Suppl. 1)**:**1–7.
3. **Kamme, C.** 1980. Penicillinresistent Branhamella catarrhalis. Frekvens och lämplig terapi. Lakartidningen 77, **51:**4858–4859.
4. **Schwartz, R., W. Rodriguez, W. Khan, and S. Ross.** 1978. The increasing incidence of ampicillin-resistant *Haemophilus influenzae*. J. Am. Med. Assoc. **239:**320–323.
5. **Sundberg, L., T. Edén, S. Ernstson, and R. Pahlitzsch.** 1979. Penetration of erythromycin through respiratory mucosa. A study using secretory otitis media as a model. Acta Oto-Laryngol. Suppl. **365:**1–17.

Pharmacokinetics of Pipemidic Acid in Normal Subjects and Patients with Impaired Renal Function

G. GUNDLACH,* P. BRÜHL, T. KÖHLER, AND C. KRASEMANN

Department of Biochemistry, University of Giessen, Giessen, and Departments of Urology and Medical Microbiology and Immunology, University of Bonn, Bonn, Federal Republic of Germany*

Pipemidic acid (Deblaston, Dr. Madaus & Co., Cologne, Federal Republic of Germany) is a synthetic substance with antibacterial activity, especially against gram-negative bacteria in urinary tract infections. Within 24 h, an average of 56% of the substance is excreted in a microbiologically active form in the urine, with a concentration maximum between 165 and 970 μg/ml after a single oral administration (400 mg). These urinary levels are already reached within 4 h after medication. The fluorometric determination of the concentration of active substance in the serum in 10 test subjects with normal kidney function revealed maximum values of 0.5 to 4.0 μg/ml after a single administration, with a half-life of 3 h (Fig. 1). Under medication with normal doses (400 mg twice a day) over 3 days, no increase in the serum concentration could be detected. In the urine, the maximum concentration was reached 2 to 4 (up to 6) h after pipemidic acid medication (single dose of 400 mg). On average, it was 400 μg/ml, and 12 h after application of the active substance it was still higher than 100 μg/ml (Fig. 2) (1, 4).

Since the rates of resistance to pipemidic acid are relatively low, the significance of this substance with regard to its chemotherapeutic application in urinary tract infections with renal insufficiency must be taken into account. We have therefore carried out comparative determinations of the concentration with the microbiological and fluorometric level in the same patients with renal impairment during treatment for several days with normal dosage (400 mg twice a day).

The microbiological concentration was determined in the agar diffusion test, in which the biologically active substance was detected by determining the diameters of inhibitory areolae (2). The fluorometric investigation was carried out by use of a Perkin-Elmer fluorometer with a modification of the method described by Montay et al. (7) and Leverge et al. (5). For this, the property of pipemidic acid to absorb light and to reemit it with another, longer wavelength was used.

For calculation of the pharmacokinetic parameters of pipemidic acid from serum concentration and from the amounts excreted in the urine, an open two-compartment model was chosen. The estimation of the model parameters (minimization of the quadratic distances between measurement values and model function) was performed simultaneously by means of the direct search technique of Hooke and Jeeves (3).

Under continuous medication with normal dosage in patients 5, 6, and 7 with highly restricted kidney function (serum creatinine, 2.2,

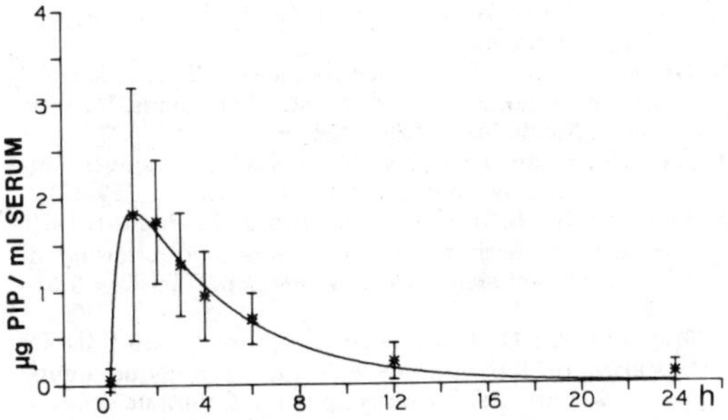

FIG. 1. *Serum concentration of pipemidic acid (PIP) after a single oral dose of 400 mg (fluorometric method, open two-compartment model). Results of the total assessment (mean values ± SD).*

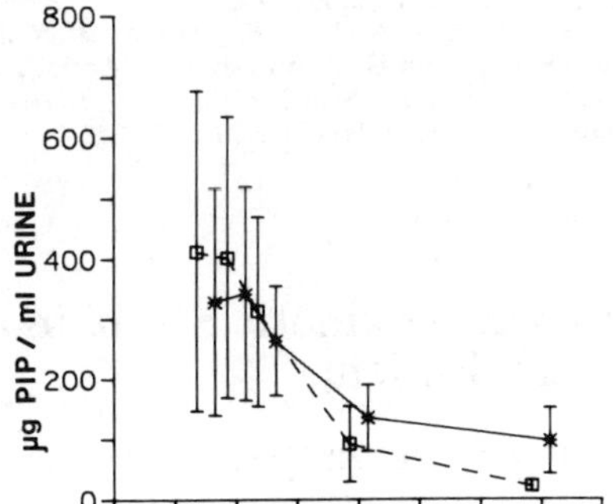

FIG. 2. *Urine concentration of pipemidic acid (PIP) after single oral dose of 400 mg. Dashed line: microbiological method. Solid line: fluorometric method. Results of the total assessment (mean values ± SD).*

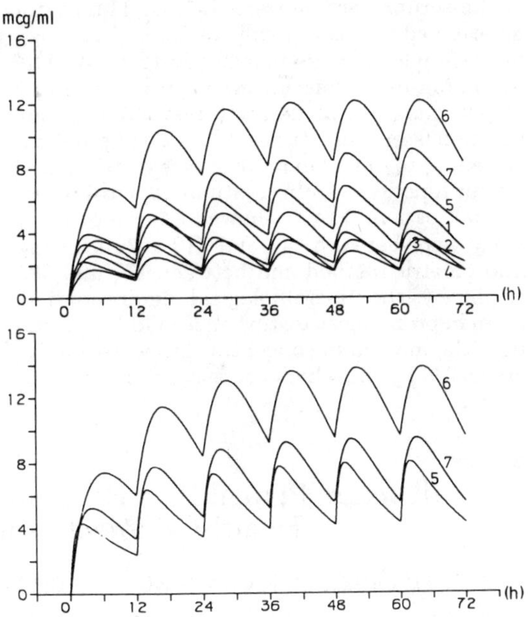

FIG. 3. *Serum concentration of pipemidic acid after standard dosage for 3 days (400 mg twice a day) in 10 patients with slightly (patients 1 to 4) and severely (patients 5 to 7) impaired renal function. Top: fluorometric method. Bottom: microbiological method.*

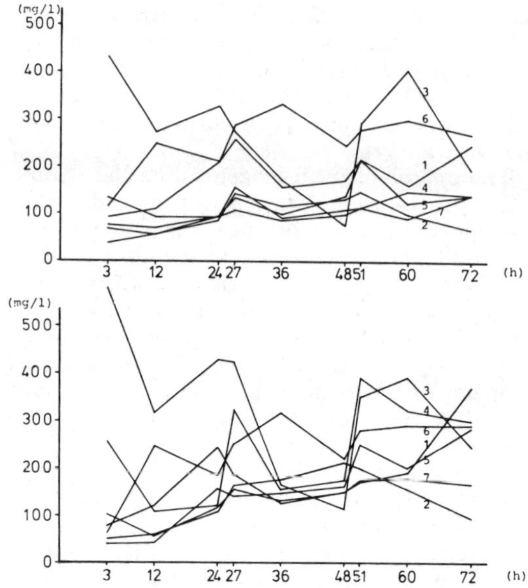

FIG. 4. *Urine concentration of pipemidic acid after standard dosage for 3 days (400 mg twice a day) in 10 patients with slightly (patients 1 to 4) and severely (patients 5 to 7) impaired renal function. Top: fluorometric method. Bottom: microbiological method.*

2.4, and 4.8 mg/100 ml), concentration maxima in the serum were between 7.4 and 11.5 μg/ml determined fluorometrically or 8.6 and 12.8 μg/ml determined microbiologically (Fig. 3). The maximum urine concentrations in this therapy of patients with moderately restricted kidney function (serum creatinine, 1.7 to 2.0 mg/100 ml; patients 1 to 4) and in more severe restriction of kidney function (serum creatinine, 2.2 to 4.8 mg/100 ml; patient 5 to 7) showed a large overlap. They were between 141 and 413 μg/ml by the fluorometric method and between 177 and 580 μg/ml by the microbiological determination. Even in pronounced disturbance of kidney function, the maximum concentrations were, on average, 230 μg/ml, which corresponds to a therapeutically optimal concentration with a constant dosage interval of a constant normal dosage (Fig. 4). Despite a reduction of the absolute urine level in restricted kidney function, the concentrations required for therapy are thus fully reached. On the other hand, under normal dosage medication for 3 days, an elevation of the serum concentration to 2.6 to 12.8 μg/ml was found, which was of therapeutic interest. We were able to observe an equilibrium between pipemidic acid intake and elimination on roughly the third day. Even in pronounced renal insufficiency, the concentrations of active substance in the serum did not rise to values at which a large increase of side effects was to be expected despite normal dosage treatment. According to investigations of Meyrier et al. (6), this might be expected at concentrations of active substance in excess of 20 μg/ml.

1. **Brühl, P., G. Gundlach, C. Krasemann, and T. Köhler.** 1981. Untersuchungen zur Pharmakokinetik der Pipemidsäure; Serum und Urinspiegel bei normaler Nierenfunktion. Hyg. Med. **6**, in press.
2. **Grove, D. C., and W. A. Randall.** 1955. Assay methods of antibiotics. A laboratory manual. Medical Encyclopedia, New York.
3. **Hooke, R., and T. A. Jeeves.** 1961. "Direct search" solution of numerical and statistical problems. J. Assoc. Comp. Mach. **8:**212–229.
4. **Lajudie, P. de.** 1974. L'acide pipémidique, nouvel antibactérien de synthèse. J. Pharmacol. Clin. **1:**155–171.
5. **Leverge, R., L. R. Guesnier, and J. L. Sachot.** 1979. Pharmacokinetic study of pipemidic acid following intravenous infusion in man. Drugs Exp. Clin. Res. **5:**31–52.
6. **Meyrier, A., O. Kourilsky, G. Montay, and R. Le Verge.** 1979. Utilisation de l'acide pipémidique comme antibiotique chez l'insuffisant rénal. Cinétique des concentrations sériques et urinaires. Pharmacol. Exp. **27:** 181–188.
7. **Montay, G., M. Vigouroux, F. Roquet, and M. Reynier.** 1977. Dosage spectrofluorimétrique de l'acide pipémidique dans les liquides biologiques. Absorption dig. et élimination urinaire chez le Rat, le Lapin, le Chien et l'Homme. Therapie **32:**553–561.
8. **Peters, G., H. Freiesleben, R. Marre, H. Metz, H. Tannenberg, and G. Pulverer.** 1979. Antibakterielle In-Vitro-Wirksamkeit von Pipemidsäure und Nalidixinsäure. Dtsch. Med. Wochenschr. **104:**946–948.

Sulbactam Pivoxil Plus Bacampicillin: Pharmacokinetic Study in Healthy Subjects and in Uremic Patients

J. P. FILLASTRE,* C. CHARUEL, J. NACHBAUR, A. LEROY, C. REVERT, AND G. PORTOS

Groupe de Physiopathologie Tissulaire, Université de Rouen, Rouen, and Centre de Recherche Pfizer, Amboise, France

In both gram-positive and gram-negative bacteria, production of β-lactamase contributes to the resistance to β-lactam antibiotics. It seems very useful to find an agent whose sole purpose is to irreversibly inhibit these β-lactamase enzymes. Such an agent would be used in conjunction with existing β-lactam antibiotics to afford activity against otherwise resistant bacteria. Sulbactam pivoxil is the pivaloyloxymethyl ester of sulbactam, a penicillanic acid sulfone which is an irreversible inhibitor of the hydrolysis of penicillinases and cephalosporinases produced by many gram-positive and gram-negative aerobic and anaerobic species (1). Combination of sulbactam pivoxil with ampicillin results in a marked lowering of the MIC of both agents in ampicillin-resistant organisms where the resistance is mediated by β-lactamase production. An association of sulbactam pivoxil plus bacampicillin has just entered clinical studies. It appeared necessary to know the pharmacokinetics of this association in uremic patients with different degrees of renal insufficiency compared to normal subjects.

A single oral dose of sulbactam pivoxil (376 mg) formulated with 400 mg of bacampicillin in a single tablet (equivalent to 250 mg of sulbactam and 278 mg of ampicillin) was given to 6 subjects with normal hepatic and renal function (group 1) and to 22 uremic patients. The 22 uremic patients were divided into four groups: group 2, 5 patients with creatinine clearance of 30 to 80 ml/min per 1.73 m^2; group 3, 7 patients with creatinine clearance of 10 to 29 ml/min per 1.73 m^2; group 4, 4 patients with creatinine clearance below 10 ml/min per 1.73 m^2; group 5, 6 patients with a very poor renal function, who were being treated by hemodialysis. Patients in group 5 were studied between and during a hemodialysis session.

After an overnight fast, each subject voided his bladder and drank 300 ml of water. A blood sample was taken, and the subject immediately swallowed one tablet. Blood samples (10 ml) were taken at 0.5, 1, 2, 3, 4, 6, 8, and 10 h (groups 1 and 2) and at 24 and 32 h (groups 3, 4, and 5). Total urine was collected over four periods up to 24 h. All serum and urine samples were immediately frozen and stored at −20°C until assayed.

For sulbactam, *Escherichia coli* (E273) was used as test organism. For ampicillin, *Sarcina lutea* (ATCC 9341) was the test organism, and a gelose antibiotic medium (Difco no. 11) was used. The pharmacokinetic data were fitted by computer to a one-compartment open model, assuming first-order absorption and elimination rate constants.

In normal subjects, the peak serum concentration of ampicillin was obtained at 1 to 2 h after administration, with a mean of 3.5 ± 1.8 mg/liter. The mean area under the curve was 7.0 ± 2.9 mg.h/liter. When fitted to a one-compartment open model, the mean elimination half-life was 1.18 ± 0.42 h. Urine excretion of ampicillin was variable: 17.2 to 54.1% of the dose in 24 h. Maximum excretion occurred in urine samples collected between 0 and 4 h after administration. Peak serum concentrations of sulbactam in normal subjects were obtained at 1 to 4 h and were of the same order of magnitude as those of ampicillin. Areas under the curve were 16 and 19 mg.h/liter, and half-lives were 1.79 and 2.66 h in two subjects in whom it was possible to calculate these values. Urinary excretion of sulbactam was maximal at 0.4 h and accounted for 36.6 to 81.9% of the dose in 24 h.

In uremic patients in groups 2, 3, and 4, peak serum concentrations of ampicillin were attained later (2 to 6 h; mean, 3 h) and were higher (between 8.3 and 9.9 mg/liter). An increase of areas under the curves was constantly observed. Half-lives of ampicillin for all five groups were as follows: group 1 (n = 6), 1.18 ± 0.42 h; group 2 (n = 5), 2.57 ± 0.74 h; group 3 (n = 5), 4.84 ± 2.65 h; group 4 (n = 4), 8.85 ± 3.37 h; group 5 (n = 6), 10.00 ± 3.91 h. Urinary excretion of ampicillin in uremic patients was delayed relative to that in normal subjects, and in severely uremic patients (groups 4 and 5) it was markedly reduced to ca. 8 to 19% of the dose in 24 h.

Peak serum concentrations of sulbactam were also obtained later in uremic patients (between 3.3 and 4.2 h after the dose) and were 6.9 ± 1.2 (group 2), 9.1 ± 4.0 (group 3), 9.0 ± 0.7 (group 4), and 10.4 ± 2.4 mg/liter (group 5). Areas under the curves increased markedly in uremic patients. Half-lives of sulbactam for all five groups were as follows: group 1 (n = 2), 2.23 h; group 2 (n = 4), 2.03 ± 0.35 h; group 3 (n = 7), 5.58 ± 1.82 h; group 4 (n = 4), 6.56 ± 1.11 h; group 5 (n = 6), 9.88 ± 3.17 h. Urinary excretion of sulbactam was considerably decreased in patients with severe renal insufficiency. Hemodialysis tended to restore normal values for both ampicillin and sulbactam.

Our results show that for both compounds, sulbactam and ampicillin, peak concentrations were higher and were attained later in uremic patients, particularly when creatinine clearance was less than 30 ml/min. Areas under the curve increased markedly, and urinary elimination decreased, being only 10 to 15% of the dose in the patients with severe renal impairment. It is important to note that sulbactam pivoxil and bacampicillin administered concurrently had similar pharmacokinetic properties which were modified in an analogous manner in patients with renal failure. From these preliminary results obtained after a single oral dose, we can conclude that the usually recommended twice daily administration of sulbactam pivoxil plus bacampicillin needs no modification in patients with creatinine clearance of >30 ml/min. For patients with more severe renal insufficiency, particularly those with a creatinine clearance below 10 ml/min, one tablet a day should maintain satisfactory serum concentrations. For patients treated by hemodialysis, the dose should be given after the dialysis.

We thank G. Croix, I. Lagelle, and G. Bailly for excellent technical assistance.

1. **English, A. R., J. A. Retsema, A. E. Girard, J. E. Lynch, and W. E. Barth.** 1978. CP-45,899, a beta-lactamase inhibitor that extends the antibacterial spectrum of beta-lactams: initial bacteriological characterization. Antimicrob. Agents Chemother. **14**:414–419.

Comparison of Sensititre with the Proposed Reference Method for Susceptibility Testing of Anaerobic Bacteria

ELIZABETH T. HOUANG* AND NERGISH DESAI

Department of Medical Microbiology, The London Hospital Medical College, Whitechapel, London E1 2AD, England

Sensititre is a commercially produced microtiter tray for the determination of MICs. Its wells are already dosed with dried antibiotics so as to give serial dilutions. It is stable at room temperature for 12 months. Potentially, it represents a convenient and efficient method for susceptibility testing in a routine clinical laboratory. We therefore compared Sensititre with the recently proposed reference method for the susceptibility testing of anaerobes (6).

The study was carried out in two parts: (i) comparison of Sensititre with the proposed method for susceptibility testing of anaerobes and (ii) reproducibility of results by Sensititre using the quality control strains.

Ninety-five strains of anaerobes were used, including 29 of *Bacteroides fragilis*, 12 of other *Bacteroides* species, 17 of *Clostridium perfringens*, 21 of other *Clostridium* species, and 16 gram-positive anaerobic cocci. The four strains used for quality control were *B. thetaiotaomicron* ATCC 29741, *B. fragilis* ATCC 25285, *B. fragilis* NTCC 9343, and *C. perfringens* ATCC 13124. The Sensititres were supplied by the manufacturer. The antibiotics used included chloramphenicol (64 mg/liter), clindamycin (64 mg/liter), erythromycin (64 mg/liter), penicillin (32 mg/liter), metronidazole (64 mg/liter), cefoxitin (128 mg/liter), carbenicillin (256 mg/liter), and cephalexin (128 mg/liter) in 11 twofold dilutions.

The inoculum was prepared by suspending 48-h growth on blood agar plates (Oxoid Ltd.) into Robertson's cooked meat broth which was allowed to incubate for 48 h. Dilutions in Wilkins-Chalgren broth (GIBCO Diagnostics) supplemented with hemin and vitamin K_1, at 5 and 0.5 mg/liter, respectively, were made so that the final dilutions for inoculation contained 5×10^5 to 5×10^6 colony-forming units of test organism per ml. The Sensititre trays were inoculated with 100 μl per well inside the anaerobic chamber. The Wilkins-Chalgren agar for the reference method was made up as reported (7) with the use of the same batch of supplemented Wilkins-Chalgren broth used for the Sensititres. Similar inocula of test organisms were applied to the antibiotic-containing plates with a Steers replicator inside the anaerobic chamber. The size of the inocula was checked by doing a viable colony count after the inoculation of the plates or Sensititre. Each of the 95 organisms was tested in duplicate by both methods. After 48 h of incubation in the anaerobic chamber, the MICs for each strain by both methods were determined.

Sensititre was used to obtain the MIC of each of the four quality control strains on 20 separate occasions as described above.

The duplicate results were identical or only different by 1 well in all tests. The results were

TABLE 1. *Percentage distribution of discrepancies, discrepancies after subtraction, and significant discrepancies according to antibiotics (95 tests for each antibiotic)*

Antibiotic	Discrepancies	Discrepancies after subtraction	Significant discrepancies
Penicillin	2.1	0	0
Clindamycin	14.7	10.5	1
Metronidazole	26.3	7.4	0
Chloramphenicol	1	1	0
Cefoxitin	3.2	3.2	1
Erythromycin	7.4	4.2	3
Carbenicillin	20	9.5	0
Cephalexin	11.2	11.2	6

TABLE 2. *Percentage distribution of (1) discrepancies, (2) discrepancies after subtracting, and (3) significant discrepancies according to anaerobic species*

Organism	No. tested	Test	Penicillin	Clindamycin	Metronidazole	Chloramphenicol	Cefoxitin	Erythromycin	Carbenicillin	Cephalexin
Gram-positive cocci	16	1	—[a]	19	13	—	—	13	50	19
		2	—	6	13	—	—	—	13	19
		3	—	—	—	—	—	—	—	6
Bacteroides species	41	1	—	15	2	2	7	12	17	7
		2	—	12	2	2	7	10	17	7
		3	—	—	—	—	—	7	—	7
Clostridium species	38	1	5	13	58	—	—	—	11	13
		2	—	11	11	—	—	—	—	13
		3	—	5	—	—	—	—	—	5

[a] No discrepancy.

analyzed as the number of discrepancies between the two methods. A discrepancy was defined as a difference of more than twofold between the two methods. A significant discrepancy was one that indicated a change in the susceptibility status from susceptible to resistant or vice versa. The MIC breakpoints above which the organisms were considered to be resistant are as follows (mg/liter): penicillin, 2; clindamycin, 4; metronidazole, 8; chloramphenicol, 16; cefoxitin, 16; erythromycin, 4; carbenicillin, 32; and cephalexin, 4. The number of discrepancies after subtracting results of MICs in the extremely susceptible range (≤0.5 mg/liter) by Sensititre was also considered.

Of the 760 pairs of results, there were 82 (10.8%) discrepancies, 45 discrepancies after subtraction (5.9%), and 12 significant discrepancies (1.6%). The number of discrepancies varied with the antibiotic and the types of bacteria.

Table 1 shows the percentage distribution of discrepancies according to antibiotics. Clindamycin, metronidazole, carbenicillin, erythromycin, and cephalexin showed relatively high discrepancies. However, with the exception of erythromycin and cephalexin, significant discrepancy was ≤1% for all other antibiotics. With metronidazole and cephalexin, the discrepancies resulted from the higher MICs obtained by Sensititre, whereas the reverse was the case with erythromycin.

Table 2 shows the distribution of discrepancies according to species of anaerobes. Cephalexin showed a high degree of significant discrepancy with all three groups of organisms.

Erythromycin and clindamycin gave 7 of 80 and 2 of 80 results, respectively, of greater than 1 well difference from the mode MICs of the four quality control strains for these two antibiotics. All the other antibiotics gave consistent results of equal to or less than 1 well difference from the mode MICs.

Reeves and others (2) have compared Sensititre with the standard agar dilution method for aerobic bacteria. They found that nearly 90% of results obtained by the two methods were ≤1 $\log_2$ dilution different. Using anaerobic bacteria, we obtained a similar rate of agreement. Our results also broadly agree with those obtained by Rosenblatt et al. (3), who compared the microdilution and broth disk methods with agar dilution using Wilkins-Chalgren medium. We have also chosen to compare the results primarily on the basis of significant discrepancies between the two methods (3). It could be argued that the total number of discrepancies, i.e., any result differing by more than 1 $\log_2$ dilution from the reference result, should also be considered.

Nevertheless, the results of our study indicate that, for all of the antibiotics tested with the exception of erythromycin and cephalexin, significant discrepancy occurred at ≤1% by Sensititre when compared with the reference method. Therefore, in a routine laboratory, Sensititre is a convenient method for the susceptibility testing of anaerobes. It would accurately reflect the in vitro pattern of susceptibility or resistance as related to the anticipated serum levels. The problem of testing the susceptibility of anaerobes to erythromycin and lincomycin has been studied by many workers (1, 4, 5). Hansen et al. showed that incubation in an atmosphere of 5% CO_2 (GasPak, BBL Microbiology Systems) resulted in a discrepancy of pH in the media of 0.2 to 0.4. The pH change did not adversely affect the growth of anaerobes, but it reduced the activity of erythromycin (1). Erythromycin gave a relatively high rate of significant discrepancies as well as the least consistent results, together with clindamycin, in the reproducibility study. The pH of the medium in the wells or agar after incubation was not monitored. The exact concentration of CO_2 in the anaerobic chamber might have varied from time to time as mixed gases (85% N_2, 10% CO_2, and 5% H_2) as well as pure N_2 gas were used. Furthermore, the character of the change in pH as a result of incubation in an anaerobic chamber may be different in the case of broth in the Sensititre wells from that in agar.

The high rate of discrepancy with metronidazole occurred mainly with *Clostridium* species (*C. sporogenes*, *C. bifermentans*) other than *C. perfringens*. It was noted during the study that the endpoint was particularly difficult to ascertain for these strains. Rosenblatt et al. also found a significant discrepancy rate of 6% with cephalothin (3). However, neither cephalothin nor cephalexin is generally used to treat anaerobic infections. They would, therefore, not present problems in the routine clinical laboratory.

1. **Hansen, S. L., P. Swomley, and J. Drusano.** 1981. Effect of carbon dioxide and pH on susceptibility of *Bacteroides fragilis* group to erythromycin. Antimicrob. Agents Chemother. **19**:335–336.
2. **Reeves, D. S., A. Holt, M. J. Bywater, R. Wise, M. N. Logan, J. M. Andrews, and J. M. Broughall.** 1980. Comparison of Sensititre dried microtitration trays with a standard agar method for determination of minimal inhibitory concentrations of antimicrobial agents. Antimicrob. Agents Chemother. **18**:844–852.
3. **Rosenblatt, J. E., P. R. Murray, A. C. Sonnenwirth, and J. L. Joyce.** 1979. Comparison of anaerobic susceptibility results obtained by different methods. Antimicrob. Agents Chemother. **15**:351–355.
4. **Rosenblatt, J. E., and F. Schoenknecht.** 1972. Effect of several components of anaerobic incubation on antibiotic susceptibility test results. Antimicrob. Agents Chemother. **1**:433–440.
5. **Stalons, D. R., C. Thornsberry, and V. R. Powell, Jr.** 1974. Effect of culture medium and carbon dioxide concentration encountered in clinical specimens. Appl. Microbiol. **27**:1098–1104.
6. **Sutter, V. L., A. L. Barry, T. D. Wilkins, and R. J. Zabransky.** 1979. Collaborative evaluation of a proposed reference dilution method of susceptibility testing of anaerobic bacteria. Antimicrob. Agents Chemother. **16**:495–502.
7. **Wilkins, T. D., and S. Chalgren.** 1976. Media for use in antibiotic susceptibility testing of anaerobic bacteria. Antimicrob. Agents Chemother. **10**:926–928.

In Vitro Antimicrobial Susceptibility of Anaerobic Bacteria

M. G. MENOZZI,* R. ALOE, A. CAVALLI, AND G. C. SCHITO

Institute of Microbiology, University of Parma, Parma 43100, and Institute of Microbiology, University of Genoa, Medical Schools, Genoa 16100, Italy

Several reports have indicated that a significant number of anaerobic bacteria, isolated from clinical sources, show an unpredictable pattern of susceptibility to various antimicrobial agents. This is particularly true for *Bacteroides fragilis*, which is often resistant to several drugs, including beta-lactam antibiotics, erythromycin, tetracycline, and aminoglycosides.

The purpose of the present study was to examine the in vitro activity of drugs currently in use for therapy of anaerobic infections. We also wished to determine the activity of new agents against anaerobic bacteria recently isolated from clinical sources in our medical center.

Two hundred thirty-eight anaerobic microorganisms were tested for susceptibility to 19 antimicrobial agents, 11 of which were beta-lactam antibiotics. MICs were determined by agar dilution, using brain heart infusion agar supplemented with vitamin K and hemin. A final inoculum of 10^4 to 10^5 colony-forming units/ml was obtained by a multipoint inoculator (Denley).

Ninety percent of 129 strains of the *B. fragilis* group were susceptible to metronidazole, rifampin, chloramphenicol, clindamycin, and lincomycin. Erythromycin was active only against 50% of the tested strains. Resistance to tetracycline and to kanamicin was found in 60 and 100%, respectively, of our isolates (Table 1).

With few exceptions, these drugs were about equally active against 30 isolates of *Clostridium* sp. (17 *C. perfringens* and 13 other species), 41 strains of the *Peptococcus*/*Peptostreptococcus* group, 7 isolates of *Fusobacterium* sp., 14 strains of *B. melaninogenicus*, 13 isolates of *Propionibacterium* sp., and 4 isolates of *Veillonella* sp. Tetracycline was more active against the *Peptococcus*/*Peptostreptococcus* group and *B. melaninogenicus* (75% MIC of ≤4 μg/ml). Metronidazole, on the contrary, was ineffective against 6% of the *Peptococcus*/*Peptostreptococcus* group (MIC of ≥128 μg/ml) and against all strains of *Propionibacterium* sp. (MIC of ≥64 μg/ml).

We also investigated the activity of various beta-lactam antibiotics against these same microorganisms. Cefoxitin, moxalactam, and cefoperazone were the most active drugs against 129 clinical isolates of *B. fragilis*. The results with the penicillins were similar. In fact, ampicillin showed the same level of activity as carbenicillin,

TABLE 1. *Activities of eight antibiotics against 129 clinical isolates of B. fragilis group*[a]

Antibiotic	MIC (μg/ml)			
	Range	To inhibit 50% of organisms	To inhibit 75% of organisms	To inhibit 90% of organisms
Clindamycin	<0.1->128	0.1	2	8
Lincomycin	<0.1->128	2	4	16
Erythromycin	<0.1->128	2	8	32
Rifampin	<0.1->128	0.1	1	2
Metronidazole	<0.1-64	0.5	1	2
Chloramphenicol	<0.1->128	4	4	8
Tetracycline	<0.1->128	8	32	64
Kanamycin	32->128	>128		

[a] Includes 107 isolates of *B. fragilis,* 10 isolates of *B. thetaiotaomicron,* 6 isolates of *B. ovatus,* and 2 isolates of *B. distasonis.*

TABLE 2. *Comparative activities of beta-lactam antibiotics against 129 clinical isolates of B. fragilis group*[a]

Antibiotic	MIC (μg/ml)			
	Range	To inhibit 50% of organisms	To inhibit 75% of organisms	To inhibit 90% of organisms
Cephalothin	0.5->128	64	128	>128
Cephaloridine	1->128	64	128	>128
Cefazolin	1->128	128	>128	
Cefoxitin	0.5->128	8	32	64
Cefotaxime	0.5->128	32	64	128
Cefuroxime	0.5->128	64	128	>128
Moxalactam	<0.1->128	1	8	32
Cefoperazone	0.5->128	4	16	64
Penicillin	1->128	32	64	>128
Ampicillin	2->128	16	32	64
Carbenicillin	0.5-128	16	32	64

a result which has been reported by several other investigators (6, 9). The conventional cephalosporins had disappointing activity against *B. fragilis.* This group of drugs included cephalothin, cephaloridine, cefotaxime, and cefuroxime (Table 2).

Niney percent of *Clostridia* were susceptible to beta-lactam antibiotics, and only a few strains were resistant to moxalactam and cephalothin (MIC of ≥64 μg/ml and ≥128 μg/ml, respectively).

These drugs were very active against the *Peptococcus/Peptostreptococcus* group. However, we could find some strains among this group resistant to several of the different cephalosporins with MICs in the range of 32 to 128 μg/ml.

The activity of penicillin, ampicillin, and cephalosporins was generally good against *Propionibacterium* and *Veillonella* spp. (90% MIC of ≤4 μg/ml). Cephalothin and cephaloridine among the beta-lactam antibiotics had relatively poor activity against many *B. melaninogenicus* strains (MIC of ≤8 μg/ml). All of the beta-lactam drugs were somewhat less effective against *Fusobacterium* spp. (MIC of ≥4 μg/ml), although we studied only five organisms in this group.

Our results indicate that chloramphenicol, clindamycin, and metronidazole are still of great value in the management of anaerobic infections in our hospital, and these findings are in agreement with those of several authors (3, 6, 9).

An interesting observation was the incidence of isolates resistant to clindamycin, defined as an MIC of ≥8.0 μg/ml. Five percent of our clinically isolated *B. fragilis* strains were resistant to clindamycin, and two of them showed an MIC of greater than 2,000 μg/ml. *Clostridium* and *Peptococcus/Peptostreptococcus* strains were also resistant to this agent. This incidence of clindamycin resistance is more or less similar to the results of other workers (2, 5, 9). As expected, the strains were also resistant to lincomycin and erythromycin.

Four percent of *Clostridium* strains and only 2% of the *B. fragilis* group were resistant to chloramphenicol, with MICs of 16 μg/ml. We do not know whether the resistance is related to enzymatic degradation of chloramphenicol, as reported by Britz and Wilkinson (1).

With regard to metronidazole, we found six strains belonging to the *B. fragilis* group that showed a high level of resistance (MIC ≥32 μg/

ml). These strains were all isolated from clinical specimens. We also found metronidazole-resistant strains among *Clostridium* spp. (4%) and the *Peptococcus/Peptostreptococcus* group (6%). All the *Propionibacterium* spp. tested (13 isolates) had an MIC of 64 μg/ml. These interesting findings on metronidazole resistance agree with recent reports from other institutions (1, 2, 4, 9).

The *B. fragilis* group showed the expected high percentage of resistant strains to penicillin.

Moxalactam, cefoxitin, cefotaxime, and cefoperazone, in that order, were the most active beta-lactam antibiotics against all of the anaerobic species tested. Nevertheless, we found some strains of *B. fragilis* and *Clostridia* with high MICs (≥64 μg/ml).

Our observation of a high incidence of resistance among anaerobic bacteria may reflect the situation in a large medical center with extensive use of antibiotics and many compromised patients. This situation leads easily to the emergence of resistance among microorganisms. It therefore seems advisable to perform susceptibility tests on anaerobic bacteria in order to ensure the correct choice of antibacterial agents.

1. **Britz, M. L., and R. G. Wilkinson.** 1979. Isolation and properties of metronidazole-resistant mutants of *Bacteroides fragilis.* Antimicrob. Agents Chemother. **16:** 19–27.
2. **Brown, W. J., and P. E. Waatti.** 1980. Susceptibility testing of clinically isolated anaerobic bacteria by an agar dilution technique. Antimicrob. Agents Chemother. **17:**629–635.
3. **Phillips, I.** 1974. Antibiotic sensitivity of non-sporing anaerobes, p. 37–58. *In* I. Phillips and M. Sussmann (ed.), Infection with non-sporing anaerobes. Churchill Livingstone, Edinburgh.
4. **Rotimi, V. O., B. I. Duerden, V. Ede, and A. E. MacKinnon.** 1979. Metronidazole-resistant *Bacteroides* from untreated patient. Lancet **i:**833.
5. **Salaski, J. S., R. Black, F. P. Tally, and J. W. Kislak.** 1976. *Bacteroides fragilis* resistant to the administration of clindamycin. Am. J. Med. **60:**426–428.
6. **Sutter, V. L., and S. M. Finegold.** 1976. Susceptibility of anaerobic bacteria to 23 antimicrobial agents. Antimicrob. Agents Chemother. **10:**736–752.
7. **Tally, F. P., B. R. Goldin, N. Sullivan, J. Johnston, and S. L. Gorbach.** 1978. Antimicrobial activity of metronidazole in anaerobic bacteria. Antimicrob. Agents Chemother. **13:**460–465.
8. **Trestman, I., D. Kaye, and M. E. Levison.** 1979. Activity of semisynthetic penicillins and synergism with mecillinam against *Bacteroides* species. Antimicrob. Agents Chemother. **16:**283–286.
9. **Tytgat, F.** 1980. Activité de sept antibiotiques sur *Bacteroides fragilis.* Ann. Microbiol. (Paris) **131A:**39–44.

Growth Curves of *Bacteroides fragilis, Bacteroides thetaiotaomicron* and *Bacteroides vulgatus* Submitted to Six Antibiotics

E. YOURASSOWSKY,* M. P. VAN DER LINDEN, M. J. LISMONT, AND F. CROKAERT

Department of Microbiology, Brugmann University Hospital, Brussels, Belgium

A collaborative study by a Working Group for Development of Standard Methods for Susceptibility Testing of Anaerobic Bacteria (3) has recommended the agar dilution method as reference. *Bacteroides fragilis* ATCC 25285, *B. thetaiotaomicron* ATCC 29742. and *B. vulgatus* ATCC 29327 may be used as reference strains with a well-defined susceptibility to six major antibiotics. On the other hand, the broth elution disk method has been of considerable value for the clinical laboratory (2–4). An automatic machine for susceptibility testing such as MS-2 is based on the broth elution disk method. The antibiotic effects on *Bacteroides* growth curves were evaluated to define: (i) the correlation between the known MICs of reference strains and absence of growth in broth, (ii) rapid reading performance, and (iii) minimum antibiotic concentration (MAC) (1) measurement on growth curves.

The MS-2 system (Abbott Laboratories) was used for the growth curve study. The whole culture is manipulated in an anaerobic chamber (Forma Scientific). Each strain was streaked on an agar plate (Columbia horse blood agar supplemented with menadione, 5 μg/ml). Portions of five or more colonies were inoculated in Schaedler broth (BBL Microbiology Systems). After overnight incubation, turbidity was adjusted with clear Schaedler broth to 0.5 on the McFarland scale and then diluted 10 times in Schaedler broth (200 ml). The colony-forming unit in these cultures was approximately 10^7/ml. The multichamber cuvette (transfer cuvette MS-2) was prepared as follows. The disks were prepared in our laboratory to obtain final concentrations from 120 to 0.25 μg/ml of broth (the volume of each chamber of the multichamber cuvette being 0.8 ml). Disks were sealed to the bottom of the appropriate cuvette chamber by using the loader-sealer unit. This bottom was coated with a quick-setting ethylacetate varnish. The cartridges thus prepared were placed in the anaerobic chamber and remained inside for 12 h

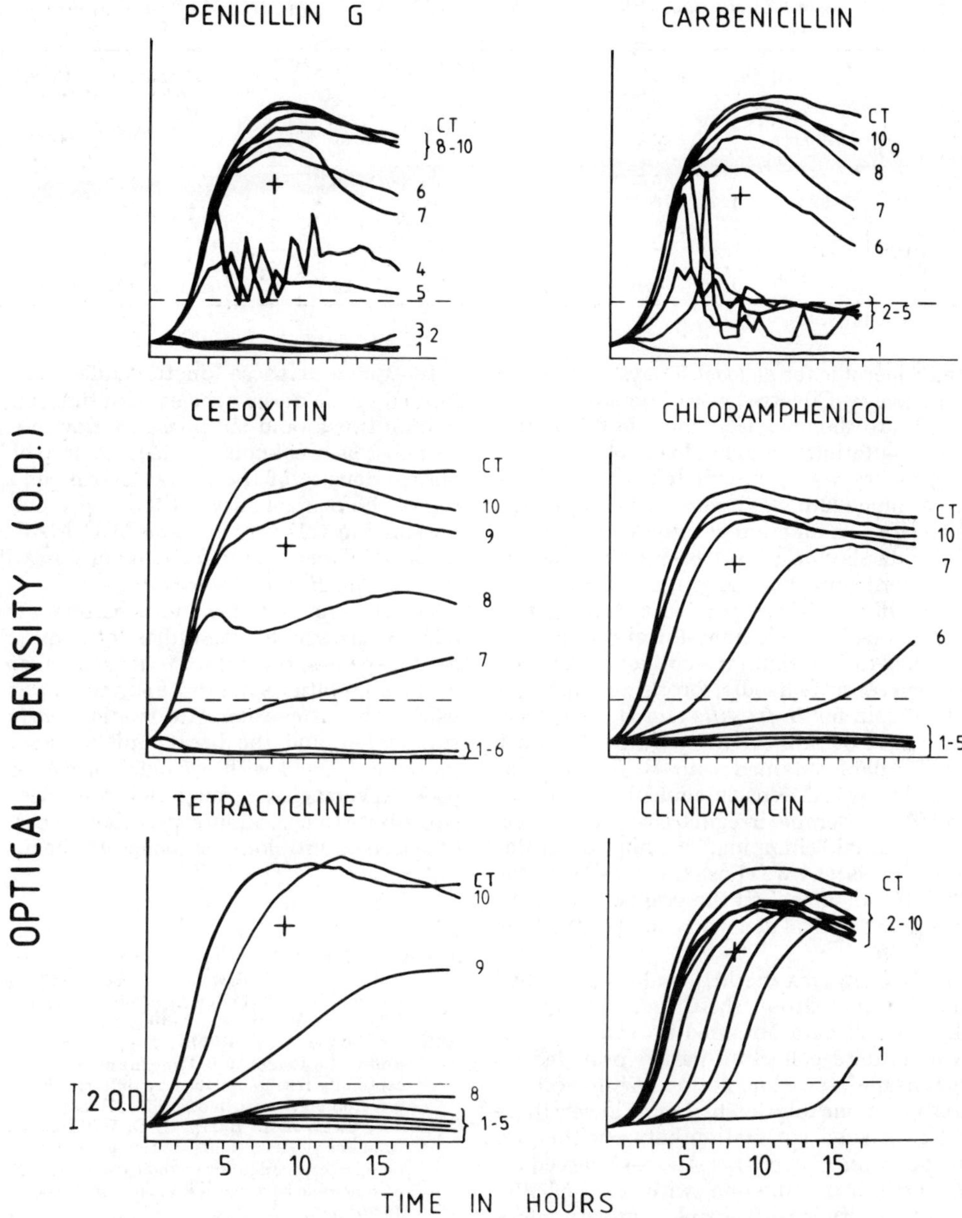

FIG. 1. *Growth curves of B. fragilis for different antibiotic concentrations. Numbers refer to concentrations expressed in micrograms per milliliter: 1:120; 2:60; 3:30; 4:15; 5:8; 6:4; 7:2; 8:1; 9:0.5; 10:0.25 (except for clindamycin, for which a twofold dilution began at 0.25 to 0.001). The crosses represent a drop of log 0.4 from the top of the control curve. Dotted lines represent log 0.2, chosen as breakpoint for the growth inhibitory activity.*

before use. After adjusting the turbidity of the bacterial suspension, 16 ml was introduced in the upper part of the multichamber cuvette. The transfer from the upper chamber to the lower chamber was realized in the interchange by a fall of −20 in. (50.8 cm) of mercury followed by introduction of nitrogen (88% N_2, 7% CO_2, and 5% H_2) at normal pressure into the interchange. This cycle was carried out at least twice. Finally, the cartridge was replaced in the anaerobic chamber and stopped (the adequate stopper was completely sealed with Plasticine). Testing with reduced methylene blue confirmed that the multichamber cuvette prepared in this way re-

TABLE 1. *MIC (μg/ml) by the agar dilution method and MIC, MAC, and MIC/MAC ratio by growth curve study*

Drug	*B. fragilis* ATCC 2585				*B. thetaiotaomicron* ATCC 29742				*B. vulgatus* ATCC 29327			
	Agar[a]	Growth curve	MAC	MIC/MAC	Agar	Growth curve	MAC	MIC/MAC	Agar	Growth curve	MAC	MIC/MAC
Penicillin G	32	30	15.6	2	32	30	15	2	0.5	0.5	—	—
Carbenicillin	32	8	8	1	32	15	15	1	0.125	0.5	0.25	2
Cefoxitin	8	4	1	4	16	8	4	2	1	1	1	1
Chloramphenicol	4	8	2	4	8	8	4	2	4	1	1	1
Tetracycline	0.25	1	0.5	2	16	30	8	4	8	15	4	4
Clindamycin	1	0.25	0.025	10	4	2	0.25	10	0.031	0.06	0.015	4

[a] Sutter et al. (3).

mained anaerobic for at least 5 days in an ordinary incubator. Cuvettes were immediately introduced into the analytical module (35°C and continual agitation throughout the test). Optical density values were immediately collected on magnetic tape (22-h maximum). The graph (optical density as a function of time) was obtained from the display of a Tectronix 4006-1 instrument as hard copy. On the graph, a drop of 0.4 in optical density corresponded approximately to a fall of one $\log_{10}$ in colony-forming units.

The generation time (calculated from the growth curve) in Schaedler broth was approximately 30 min for *B. fragilis* and *B. thetaiotaomicron,* and 60 min for *B. vulgatus.* Figure 1 shows the data obtained with *B. fragilis.* An increase in optical density could be seen, followed by considerable irregularity in the graphs due to bacterial "clumping," leading to heterogeneity. This is why we chose the breakpoint for the "inhibitory effect" on the graphs at a maximum of 0.2 in optical density related to the base line.

Table 1 compares the MIC values published by the Working Group (MIC agar, incubation for 488 h) and data obtained in broth in 22 h (maximum data collection period provided on magnetic tape). If we had not taken into account a variation of one dilution higher or lower, there would be a good correlation between the two methods. Three discrepancies were observed for *B. fragilis*: a major one with carbenicillin (strains susceptible to 8 μg/ml in growth curve and 32 μg in agar) and two minor ones with tetracycline and clindamycin (strains remained susceptible by both methods).

Inasmuch as these kinetic studies were performed on bacterial species with different generation times (and lag phase in growth curve), we chose as breakpoint for MAC a drop of 0.4 in optical density of the curve determined at the top of the control curve. Table 1 presents data obtained in this way and the MIC/MAC ratio. This ratio was higher for clindamycin with *B. fragilis* and *B. thetaiotaomicron.*

Despite the fact that multichamber cuvettes allowed growth curve studies for some *Bacteroides* species, the actual routine configuration of the apparatus is not quite suitable for routine work without caution. Automatic transfer was suppressed, and the breakpoint for anaerobes must be defined with a single charge for each disk. Nevertheless, growth curve studies might contribute to a good interpretation of the mode of action of antibiotics on anaerobic bacteria.

1. **Lorian, V.** 1980. Effect of subminimum inhibitory concentrations of antibiotics on bacteria, p. 342–408. *In* V. Lorian (ed.), Antibiotics in laboratory medicine. The Williams & Wilkins Co., Baltimore.
2. **Rosenblatt, J. E., P. R. Murray, A. C. Sonnenwirth, and J. L. Joyce.** 1979. Comparison of anaerobic susceptibility results obtained by different methods. Antimicrob. Agents Chemother. **15:**351–355.
3. **Sutter, V. L., A. L. Barry, T. D. Wilkins, and R. J. Zabransky.** 1979. Collaborative evaluation of a proposed reference dilution method of susceptibility testing of anaerobic bacteria. Antimicrob. Agents Chemother. **16:**495–502.
4. **Thornsberry, C., T. L. Gavan, and E. H. Gerlach.** 1977. Cumitech 6, New developments in antimicrobial agent susceptibility testing. Coordinating ed., John C. Sherris. American Society for Microbiology, Washington, D.C.

Susceptibility Profile of the *Bacteroides fragilis* Group and Clostridium Against 19 Cephalosporins

J. E. GARCÍA-SÁNCHEZ,* A. C. GÓMEZ-GARCÍA, M. C. SÁENZ, AND J. A. GARCÍA-RODRIGUEZ

Department of Microbiology, Faculty of Medicine, University of Salamanca, Salamanca, Spain

The *Bacteroides fragilis* group and clostridia are clinically the most important among anaerobic bacteria, because they are easily found in clinical samples and the *B. fragilis* group is also the most resistant to antibiotics. It is, therefore, important to know the activity of antimicrobial agents against this group of organisms.

The vertiginous discovery of new cephalosporins makes it difficult to bring the knowledge concerning their antimicrobial activity up to date. We have studied the susceptibility of the *B. fragilis* group and clostridia to 19 cephalosporins and related antibiotics: cephalothin, cephapirin, cephacetrile, cephaloridine, cefazolin, cephaloglycin, cephalexin, cephradine, cefaclor, cefadroxil, cefamandole, cefuroxine, cefsulodin, cefoperazone, cefotaxime, ceftriaxone, cefoxitin, cefmetazole, and moxalactam. Thirty-four strains of the *B. fragilis* group and 30 strains of clostridia recently isolated from clinical specimens were tested. Twenty of these strains belonged to the species *B. fragilis*, 10 strains to *B. thetaiotaomicron*, 3 strains to *B. vulgatus*, 1 strain to *B. distasonis*, 14 strains to *C. perfringens*, and 16 to *Clostridium* sp.

All 64 strains were characterized by the biochemical methods of Holdeman et al. (1) and the gas chromatographic method of Sutter et al. (3). The MIC was obtained by using twofold serial dilutions of the antimicrobial agents into solid medium without blood, as described by Wilkins and Chalgren (4). The inoculum, an overnight culture in brucella broth, was adjusted to the 0.5 McFarland (nephelometer) standard with Wilkins and Chalgren broth and then applied to the surface of the plate with a Steers

TABLE 1. *Susceptibility[a] of B. fragilis group and clostridia to β-lactamase–sensitive cephalosporins*

Drug	Organism	Range		MIC_{50}	MIC_{75}	MIC_{90}
		Low	High			
Cephalothin	*B. fragilis* group	16	≥256	128	128	≥256
	Clostridium	0.5	64	1	2	8
Cephapirin	*B. fragilis* group	16	≥256	64	128	≥256
	Clostridium	≤0.125	8	0.5	1	4
Cephacetrile	*B. fragilis* group	4	≥256	64	128	≥256
	Clostridium	0.5	16	1	2	4
Cephaloridine	*B. fragilis* group	8	≥256	64	128	≥256
	Clostridium	0.25	16	0.5	1	16
Cefazolin	*B. fragilis* group	4	≥256	32	64	≥256
	Clostridium	≤0.125	2	0.5	1	1
Cephaloglycin	*B. fragilis* group	64	≥256	≥256	≥256	≥256
	Clostridium	0.5	128	8	16	16
Cephalexin	*B. fragilis* group	16	≥256	64	64	128
	Clostridium	1	8	2	4	4
Cephradine	*B. fragilis* group	8	≥256	32	64	128
	Clostridium	0.25	32	4	8	8
Cefaclor	*B. fragilis* group	8	≥256	≥256	≥256	≥256
	Clostridium	≤0.125	32	2	4	16
Cefadroxil	*B. fragilis* group	8	≥256	64	64	128
	Clostridium	1	16	2	4	8

[a] Micrograms per milliliter.

TABLE 2. *Susceptibility[a] of B. fragilis group to β-lactamase–resistant cephalosporins, cephamicins, and moxalactam*

Drug	Organism	Range		MIC_{50}	MIC_{75}	MIC_{90}
		Low	High			
Cefamandole	*B. fragilis* group	4	≥256	64	≥256	≥256
	Clostridium	≤0.125	32	4	8	16
Cefuroxime	*B. fragilis* group	8	≥256	64	128	≥256
	Clostridium	≤0.125	32	0.5	1	4
Cefsulodin	*B. fragilis* group	8	≥256	64	≥256	≥256
	Clostridium	2	64	16	32	32
Cefoperazone	*B. fragilis* group	8	≥256	32	64	≥256
	Clostridium	0.25	4	1	2	2
Cefotaxime	*B. fragilis* group	≤0.125	≥256	16	64	128
	Clostridium	≤0.125	16	2	4	16
Ceftriaxone	*B. fragilis* group	4	≥256	64	128	≥256
	Clostridium	≤0.125	8	2	2	4
Cefoxitin	*B. fragilis* group	2	32	8	16	16
	Clostridium	0.25	64	1	1	8
Cefmetazole	*B. fragilis* group	4	64	16	32	32
	Clostridium	≤0.125	16	0.25	1	2
Moxalactam	*B. fragilis* group	0.25	16	4	8	16
	Clostridium	≤0.125	4	0.5	1	2

[a] Micrograms per milliliter.

replicator (2). Incubation was carried out by the GasPak (BBL Microbiology Systems) method, and the MIC was recorded as the minimal amount of chemotherapeutic agent which did not allow visible growth after 48 h of incubation at 35°C.

The activity of β-lactamase–sensitive cephalosporins, parenteral as well as oral, can be seen in Table 1. All members of this group of antimicrobial agents showed little activity against the *B. fragilis* group, because they required a high concentration to inhibit 90% of our strains (128 μg/ml, 256 μg/ml, or more). Cefazolin showed the highest activity within this group, with a range between 4 and 256 μg/ml or more, and an MIC_{50} of 32 μg/ml. Among the oral cephalosporins, the less active ones were cephaloglycin and cefaclor, with an MIC_{50} of 256 μg/ml or higher. Against clostridia, all β-lactamase–sensitive cephalosporins showed excellent activity, with an MIC_{90} of 16 μg/ml; the most active was cefazolin, with an MIC_{90} of 1 μg/ml.

Table 2 shows the activity of β-lactamase–resistant cephalosporins and also cephamycins and moxalactam.

Cefamandole is considered a powerful drug against gram-negative anaerobic facultative bacilli. Compared with the first cephalosporins (cephalothin, cephapirin, etc.), it is not more active against the *B. fragilis* group. In our experience, concentrations of 256 μg/ml or higher were required to inhibit 90% of the strains tested. Similar characteristics were presented by cefuroxime, and for this reason these two drugs should not be considered useful in the treatment of infections from which the *B. fragilis* group is isolated.

Similar results occurred with cefsulodin and cefoperazone, which showed a range of activity between 8 and 256 μg/ml.

Cefotaxime and ceftriaxone are slightly more active than the previously mentioned antibiotics. Though they are clearly β-lactamase resistant, they required higher concentrations to be active. (Cefotaxime showed an MIC_{50} of 16 μg/ml and an MIC_{90} of 128 μg/ml.)

The drugs currently active against the *B. fragilis* group are cephamycins and oxacefems. Ninety percent of the strains were inhibited by cefoxitin, cefmetazole, and moxalactam at 16, 32, and 16 μg/ml, respectively. In a general sense, moxalactam clearly surpasses the cephamycins. The activity of these drugs makes it necessary to restate the therapy of anaerobic infections in which the *B. fragilis* group participates, since they are the anaerobic bacteria most resistant and most frequently isolated.

The clostridia have an adequate susceptibility to these drugs. Their activity ranged between 0.125 and 64 μg/ml. Ninety percent of the strains were inhibited at concentrations between 1 and 16 μg/ml except with cefsulodin, which required 32 μg/ml. The most active antimicrobial agents were cefoperazone, cefmetazole, and moxalactam, with an MIC_{90} of 2 μg/ml.

No significant differences were found between the various species of the *B. fragilis* group and clostridia, except for *B. thetaiotaomicron*. All 10 strains of *B. thetaiotaomicron* studied showed a high resistance to cephalosporins. Their MICs ranged between 32 and 256 μg/ml or higher.

Cephamycins and moxalactam showed high activity. The MIC of cefoxitin ranged from 2 to 32 μg/ml, that of cefmetazole from 4 to 64 μg/ml, and that of moxalactam from 0.25 to 16 μg/ml.

1. **Holdeman, L. V., E. P. Cato, and W. E. C. Moore (ed.).** 1977. Anaerobe laboratory manual, 4th ed. Anaerobe Laboratory, Virginia Polytechnic Institute and State University, Blacksburg.
2. **Steers, E., E. L. Foltz, B. D. Gravez, and J. Riden.** 1959. An inocula replicating apparatus for routine testing of bacterial susceptibility to antibiotics. Antibiot. Chemother. (Basel) **9**:307–311
3. **Sutter, V. L., D. M. Citron, and S. M. Finegold.** 1980. Wadsworth anaerobe bacteriology manual, 3rd ed. C. V. Mosby Co., St. Louis.
4. **Wilkins, T. D., and S. Chalgren.** 1976. Medium for use in antibiotic susceptibility testing of anaerobic bacteria. Antimicrob. Agents Chemother. **10**:926–928.

Comparison of the In Vitro Activities of Ceftizoxime, Cefoperazone, Cefoxitin, Cefamandole, and Clindamycin Against *Bacteroides fragilis* Group Organisms

PETER N. R. HESELTINE* AND MARIA D. APPLEMAN

University of Southern California, Los Angeles, California 90033, U.S.A.

Therapy of infections caused by organisms in the *Bacteroides fragilis* group has most often included chloramphenicol or clindamycin. More recently, carbenicillin, cefoxitin, and metronidazole have also been reported as being efficacious. All of these compounds have limited spectra of antibacterial action and are most notably deficient of in vitro activity against many nosocomial pathogens, including *Pseudomonas*, *Serratia*, and *Enterobacter* species. Thus, the therapy of mixed infections has required combinations of antibiotics which together are active against anaerobic and aerobic pathogens.

Early studies indicate that two new cephalosporins, cefoperazone and ceftizoxime, have excellent in vitro activities against facultative and obligate aerobic gram-negative pathogens. This report addresses the activity of these new drugs against *B. fragilis* group organisms. Sporadic resistance to commonly used antibiotics among the *B. fragilis* group is well recognized although the clinical significance of this is ill defined. For these reasons, we chose to examine the activity of ceftizoxime and cefoperazone against clinical isolates of the *B. fragilis* group known to have moderate or high-level resistance to clindamycin, cefoxitin, and cefamandole. This last drug, though not considered a primary choice for anaerobic infections, is widely used in the United States in surgical patients.

All organisms were identified as members of the *B. fragilis* group by biochemical and fermentative analyses. Using the nomenclature proposed by Johnson in 1978 (1), we selected 62 isolates of *B. distasonis*, *B. fragilis*, *B. thetaiotaomicron*, *B. vulgatus*, and *B. ovatus* from clinical specimens in two large hospitals on the basis of their resistance to cefoxitin, clindamycin, or cefamandole, or to more than one of these.

Five of the strains which were highly resistant to cefamandole (MIC > 256 μg/ml) and moderately resistant to cefoxitin (MIC = 32 μg/ml) did not degrade the Glaxo chromogenic cephalosporin as did all other strains. In addition, these five strains grew in the presence of 256 μg of cefamandole per ml without destruction of the β-lactam ring of this drug, as measured by high-pressure liquid chromatography. The exact mechanism of resistance in these strains remains undetermined, but we believe it to be different from that usually encountered.

The MICs of cefoperazone, ceftizoxime, clindamycin, cefamandole, and cefoxitin for the 62 isolates were determined by an agar dilution method. Purity of the inocula was confirmed by colonial morphology on blood agar plates. Inocula of 10^5 organisms in the rapid phase of growth were delivered with a Steers replicator. The test medium was freshly prepared, but not prereduced, brucella agar supplemented with sheep erythrocytes and vitamin K and containing a known concentration of the antibiotic. Incubation was performed in anaerobic GasPak jars (BBL Microbiology Systems) at 37°C for 48 h.

An endpoint was interpreted as no growth, a light haze, or fewer than three colonies. All antibiotics were tested concurrently with appropriate control organisms. Susceptibility tests were performed in triplicate. Resistance was defined for clindamycin as an MIC of ≥8 μg/ml and for cefoxitin, cefamandole, cefoperazone, and ceftizoxime as an MIC of ≥32 μg/ml. Moderate resistance to clindamycin was defined as an MIC of 4 μg/ml. The lower limits of these values represent approximately 50% of the achievable human serum levels after 1 h at customary doses. Statistical significance of the results was examined by matched pair analysis (McNemar test). In this test, for any given isolate the MICs of each drug were converted into susceptible or resistant, based on the aforementioned definitions. A matrix of pairs was then developed, and the difference for any two drugs was compared.

Examining these differences in activity of each drug against individual species, we found that ceftizoxime was significantly more active than cefoperazone or cefamandole, but not different from clindamycin or cefoxitin against *B. fragilis*.

Ceftizoxime was significantly more active than cefoperazone, cefamandole, or cefoxitin against *B. distasonis* but not different from clindamycin. Ceftizoxime was also significantly more active against *B. thetaiotaomicron* than cefoperazone and cefamandole but not different from cefoxitin or clindamycin. No differences were noted for *B. vulgatus* and *B. ovatus*.

We also analyzed the activity of the two drugs against the isolates on the basis of their resistance to clindamycin, cefoxitin, and cefamandole. Ceftizoxime was significantly more active than cefoperazone or cefamandole, but not different from cefoxitin against *Bacteroides* species moderately or highly resistant to clindamycin. Ceftizoxime was significantly more active than cefoperazone and cefamandole against isolates resistant to cefoxitin and showed a trend of greater activity than clindamycin.

Finally, though no statistically significant differences were seen, no resistance was seen to ceftizoxime among the five strains with an unusual mechanism of resistance to cefamandole, whereas several strains were resistant to cefoxitin and cefoperazone.

These data indicate that ceftizoxime was more active than cefoperazone against resistant *B. distasonis*, *B. fragilis*, and *B. thetaiotaomicron*. Ceftizoxime was significantly more active than cefoperazone against *Bacteroides* with moderate resistance to cefoxitin. Ceftizoxime was more active than cefoperazone but not different from cefoxitin against *Bacteroides* with moderate or high-level resistance to clindamycin. Based on these findings and the reported in vitro activity of ceftizoxime against resistant nosocomial pathogens, we conclude that this compound is worthy of clinical trial in the therapy of mixed infections, including those caused by pathogens likely to be resistant to clindamycin, cefoxitin, or gentamicin.

1. **Johnson, J. L.** 1978. Taxonomy of the *Bacteroides*. I. Deoxyribonucleic acid homologies among *B. fragilis* and other saccharolytic bacterial species. Int. J. Syst. Bacteriol. **28**:245–256.

Quantitation of the Effect of Anti-Anaerobic Drugs in *Bacteroides fragilis* Infection in Mice

B. A. C. DIJKMANS* AND H. MATTIE

Department of Infectious Diseases, University Hospital, Leiden, The Netherlands

Assessment of the efficacy of antimicrobial agents in vivo requires suitable animal models of infection (2). Recently, several attempts have been made to develop a pure *Bacteroides fragilis* infection in animals, but with only partial success. Because in the clinical situation anaerobes are usually found in combination with aerobes at the site of infection, use was later made of an infection model in which *B. fragilis* was combined with an aerobic microorganism (3). Having developed an experimental *B. fragilis* infection in a thigh lesion model in mice, we were able to study the relative efficacy of anti-anaerobic drugs.

Inoculation of 10^8 to 2×10^8 colony-forming units (CFU) of *B. fragilis* into a thigh muscle did not result in outgrowth of this microorganism up to 48 h after inoculation, i.e., the time at which the animals were killed. The infected thigh was then removed and homogenized, dilutions of the thigh homogenate were incubated for 48 h in a GasPak jar (BBL Microbiology Systems), and *B. fragilis* was counted as CFU. Co-inoculation of *B. fragilis* with *Escherichia coli* (10^6 to 2×10^6) resulted in a significantly ($P < 0.005$) higher number of *B. fragilis* CFU 24 h after inoculation, but the values obtained 6 h after inoculation with and without *E. coli* did not differ significantly (Fig. 1). The number of *E. coli* CFU after combined inoculation differed significantly ($P < 0.005$) from the values for the single inoculum of *E. coli*, not only after 24 h but also after 6 h ($P < 0.005$) (Fig. 2).

In this infection model the inhibition of the growth of the injected *B. fragilis* by metronidazole and tinidazole could be measured quantitatively. Mice were inoculated with a mixture of 10^8 to 2×10^8 CFU of *B. fragilis* and 10^6 to 2×10^6 CFU of *E. coli*. Six hours later, metronidazole or tinidazole was administered subcutaneously as a single dose (2.5, 5, or 10 mg/kg of body weight), and 18 h after drug administration the animals were killed and the number of viable microorganisms was counted as CFU. The potency ratio, defined as the relative efficacy of metronidazole and tinidazole against *B. fragilis* (2), was calculated according to standard bioassay procedures. In four experiments the potency ratio was 1.02 in favor of tinidazole. Because the

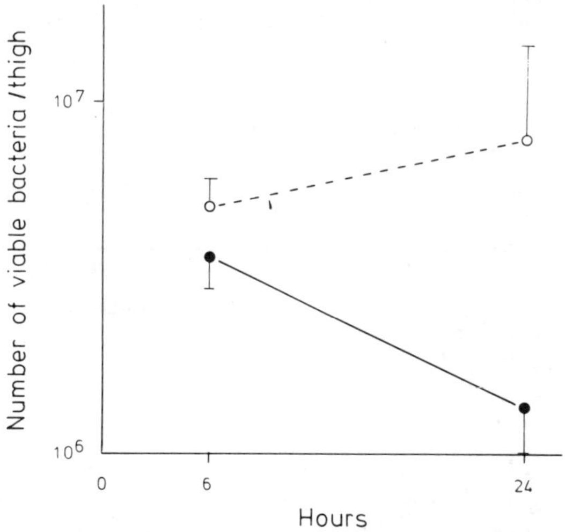

FIG. 1. *Numbers of viable B. fragilis CFU recovered from homogenate of an infected mouse thigh. The animals were killed 6 and 24 h after inoculation with 10^8 to 2×10^8 CFU of B. fragilis or a mixture of 10^8 to 2×10^8 CFU of B. fragilis and 10^6 to 2×10^6 CFU of E. coli. Each point represents the mean value of 12 mice given B. fragilis alone (●) or together with E. coli (○).*

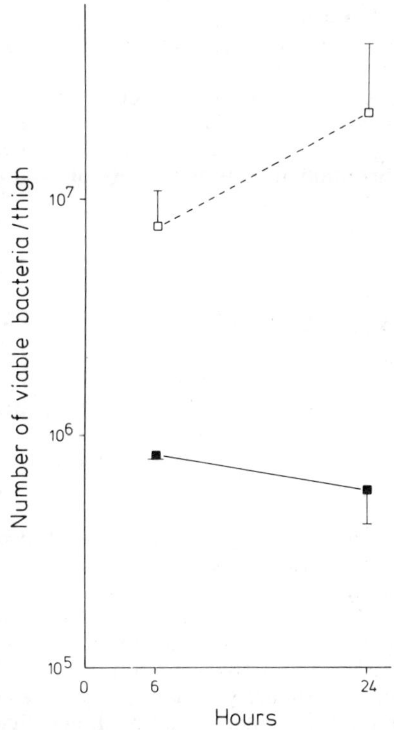

FIG. 2. *Numbers of viable E. coli CFU recovered from homogenate of an infected mouse thigh. The animals were killed 6 and 24 h after inoculation of 10^6 to 2×10^6 CFU of E. coli or a mixture of 10^8 to 2×10^8 CFU of B. fragilis and 10^6 to 2×10^6 CFU of E. coli. Each point represents the mean value of 12 mice given E. coli alone (■) or together with B. fragilis (□).*

variability of the bioassay was large and the accuracy was therefore rather limited, the role of *E. coli* in this variability was analyzed by multiple regression analysis, which showed a highly significant covariation of the log numbers of CFU of *B. fragilis* and *E. coli* in each of the dosage groups ($P < 0.005$). After correction for this source of variability, the potency ratio of metronidazole to tinidazole was virtually unchanged (mean of 1.06 in favor of tinidazole), although the accuracy of the calculation was much higher. The similarity of the potency ratio according to both calculations reflects the finding that the average number of *E. coli* CFU was similar in all treatment groups. These findings made in vivo appeared to be inconsistent with the in vitro results, since the colony counts at 24 h indicated that metronidazole was almost twice as effective. It is conceivable that different pharmacokinetics are responsible for this apparent discrepancy between in vitro and in vivo results.

Thus, co-inoculation of *B. fragilis* and *E. coli*

is essential for outgrowth of *B. fragilis*. This finding supports the concept of bacterial synergy described in the literature (1).

The thigh lesion model described here permits quantitative study of the activity of antibiotics in *B. fragilis* infections, as illustrated by the results obtained with metronidazole and tinidazole.

1. **Editorial.** 1980. Synergy in mixed aerobic/anaerobic infections. Lancet **i**:405–406.
2. **Kunst, M. W., and H. Mattie.** 1978. Cefazolin and cephradine: relationship between antibacterial activity in vitro and in experimentally infected mice. J. Infect. Dis. **137**:391–402.
3. **Onderdonk, A. B., D. L. Kasper, B. J. Mansheim, T. J. Louie, S. L. Gorbach, and J. G. Bartlett.** 1979. Experimental animal models for anaerobic infections. Rev. Infect. Dis. **1**:291–301.

Activity of Nimorazole in Subcutaneous Infection with *Bacteroides fragilis* in Mice

GISELLA MONTI* AND IVO DE CARNERI

Farmitalia Carlo Erba R. & S., Milan, Italy

Considered at first as typical antiprotozoal drugs, the nitroimidazoles have proven during the last decade to be active also on numerous procaryotic (facultative and obligate) anaerobes. Wise et al. (2) found that nimorazole exerts in vitro a marked activity on *Bacteroides*. In this study, we compared in vivo in mice the activity of nimorazole, chloramphenicol, cefoxitin, and clindamycin against *Bacteroides fragilis* VPI 9032, taking into account the inoculum size.

Infection was induced by inoculating the bacterial suspension into subcutaneous metal chambers. Assessment was based on a count of the live bacterial cells 24 h after drug treatment. We used the following method: a coiled cylindrical metal chamber 1.5 cm long and 0.5 cm in diam-

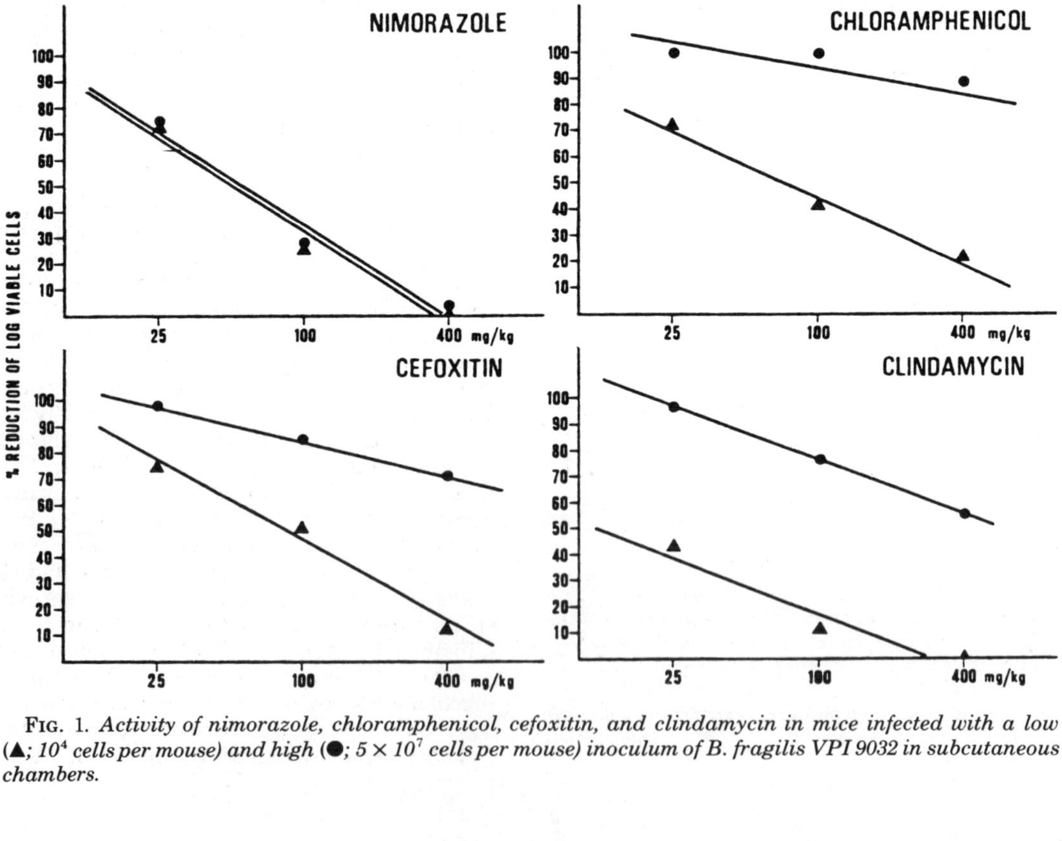

FIG. 1. *Activity of nimorazole, chloramphenicol, cefoxitin, and clindamycin in mice infected with a low (▲; 10^4 cells per mouse) and high (●; 5×10^7 cells per mouse) inoculum of B. fragilis VPI 9032 in subcutaneous chambers.*

TABLE 1. *Activity of nimorazole, chloramphenicol, cefoxitin, and clindamycin in mice against B. fragilis infection in subcutaneous chambers*

Drug	ED_{50}[a] (mg/kg per treatment)	
	Mice infected with low inoculum	Mice infected with high inoculum
Nimorazole	50	53
Chloramphenicol	75	>400
Cefoxitin	90	>400
Clindamycin	12	550

[a] Dose required to reduce by 50% the log number of bacteria present in the nontreated mice (controls); treatment was given at both 0 and 6 h postchallenge.

eter was inserted subcutaneously on the back of albino male Iva:NMRI (specific pathogen free) mice weighing 20 g; 5 days later, infection was induced by injecting the bacterial suspension, in a volume of 0.05 ml per chamber, directly into the liquid accumulated in the chamber. The infecting suspension was obtained by cultivating *B. fragilis* VPI 9032 for 40 h at 37°C under anaerobic conditions (GasPak anaerobic system) in chopped-meat broth (1) and diluting as needed with the same broth without meat.

For this experiment, 130 mice were infected with 10^4 cells per mouse (low inoculum), and 130 were infected with 5×10^7 cells per mouse (high inoculum). Immediately after infection and again 6 h later, the drugs were administered. Nimorazole, chloramphenicol, and clindamycin were given orally in a 1% Methocel suspension, and cefoxitin was injected subcutaneously in saline solution. The volume administered was 0.25 ml, giving doses of 400, 100, and 25 mg/kg to groups of 10 mice per dose. Antimicrobial activity was checked 24 h later in a sample (0.1 ml) of the fluid taken by an insulin syringe from the subcutaneous chamber. Using the Oxford sampler micropipetting system, samples were diluted serially 1:100 with saline, and a drop (0.05 ml) of each dilution was plated on selective agar.

After 40 h of incubation at 37°C under anaerobic conditions, a count was made of the live cells (Fig. 1 and Table 1). The mean log numbers of cells for each dose were compared with the mean for nontreated controls. From the percentage values thus obtained, a dose-effect curve is constructed on a graph and the ED_{50} is obtained; in this case, the ED_{50} was the dose required to reduce by 50% the log number of bacteria present in the nontreated controls.

It may be concluded that in mice infected with *B. fragilis* VPI 9032 in subcutaneous chambers, nimorazole was active at around 50 mg/kg per treatment. It was not influenced by the size of the bacterial inoculum: the ED_{50} was virtually the same for a 5,000-fold concentration. The other three drugs were appreciably affected by the inoculum size.

Chloramphenicol and cefoxitin were active at 75 and 90 mg/kg per treatment, respectively, on the low inoculum, but had virtually no effect on the more concentrated one. The ED_{50} for clindamycin was 12 mg/kg per treatment with the 10^4 inoculum, but rose to 550 mg/kg per treatment for 5×10^7 cells.

1. **Holdeman, L., and W. E. C. Moore (ed.).** 1973. Anaerobe laboratory manual, 2nd ed. Virginia Polytechnic Institute and State University, Blacksburg.
2. **Wise, R., J. M. Andrews, and K. A. Bedford.** 1977. The activity of four antimicrobial agents, including three nitroimidazole compounds, against *Bacteroides* sp. Chemotherapy **23:**19–24.

In Vitro, In Vivo Experimental and Clinical Evaluation of Doxycycline Hyclate: Comparison with Penicillin Therapy for Anaerobic Lung Infections

HARAGOPAL THADEPALLI,* VINOD K. DHAWAN, VINH T. BACH, AND DON W. KANNANGARA

Division of Infectious Diseases, Department of Internal Medicine, Charles R. Drew Postgraduate Medical School, Los Angeles, California 90059, U.S.A.

Penicillin is considered the antibiotic of choice for anaerobic lung infections. From July 1974 to June 1979, 124 patients with anaerobic lung infections were treated with various antibiotics. During this period 44 patients with lung abscess, 34 with aspiration pneumonia, 31 with empyema, and 15 with necrotizing pneumonia were treated. Among them 68 had mixed aerobic/

anaerobic infections and 56 had exclusively anaerobic bacteria. The anaerobic isolates included 78 strains of *Bacteroides* including 21 isolates of *B. fragilis*, 42 strains of *Peptococcus*, 35 of *Peptostreptococcus*, 23 of *Eubacterium*, 17 of *clostridium*, 16 of *Fusobacterium*, and 16 isolates of *Actinomyces* and other bacteria. There were 10 different species of *Bacteroides*. In vitro, penicillin at 8 μg/ml inhibited nearly 82% of all anaerobes except *B. fragilis*; only 59% of this species were susceptible to it. Carbenicillin and ticarcillin inhibited >80% of the isolates at 32 μg/ml. Cefoxitin at 8 μg/ml also inhibited >80%. Clindamycin was effective against nearly 90% of all isolates except clostridia (67%). Doxycycline inhibited nearly 77% of all anaerobes and 74% of *B. fragilis* at 5 μg/ml.

Thirty-four patients were treated with 200 to 300 mg a day of intravenous (i.v.) doxycycline (Pfizer Inc.) given in two divided doses; 28 were treated with i.v. clindamycin, 600 to 800 mg four times a day; 19 patients received penicillin in a dose of 5×10^6 U four times a day; 18 patients received carbenicillin i.v. in 5 g four times a day; 13 patients also received i.v. ticarcillin in the same dose schedule; and i.v. cefoxitin was given in 3 g four times a day to 12 patients. The therapeutic response was graded as good if there was clinical and roentgenographic improvement after a minimum course of 7 to 10 days of therapy. Absence of such an improvement or worsening was called a failure. Therapy was successful in 30 of 34 (88%) treated with doxycycline, 26 of 28 (93%) on clindamycin, 11 of 19 (58%) on penicillin, 16 of 18 (89%) on carbenicillin, 9 of 13 (69%) on ticarcillin, and 10 of 12 (83%) on cefoxitin. The difference noted in the superior efficacy of clindamycin or doxycycline over penicillin was statistically significant ($P < 0.01$). Seven of eight patients that failed on penicillin had susceptible bacteria but one had resistant organisms.

Experimental model. Transtracheal inoculation of an overnight growth of a mixture of *Peptococcus morbillorum*, *B. fragilis*, *E. lentum*, and *F. nucleatum* consistently produced lung abscess in white male New Zealand rabbits (1). All isolates used in our experiments were susceptible to all the antibiotics used in this study. The *B. fragilis* isolate was susceptible to penicillin at 4 μg/ml, carbenicillin at 4 μg/ml, chloramphenicol at 1 μg/ml, cefoxitin at 8 μg/ml, clindamycin at 0.5 μg/ml, and doxycycline at 4 μg/ml.

None of the eight animals used as controls received any antibiotics. They developed pneumonia during the first week and lung abscess during the second week after the inoculation and died within 3 to 12 weeks.

Evaluation of treatment. One week after the transtracheal inoculation, 14 animals were treated with procaine penicillin (300,000 U every 12 h intramuscularly); 9 received carbenicillin, 1 g every 12 h i.v.; 8 received chloramphenicol, 100 mg every 12 h i.v.; 8 received clindamycin, 45 mg every 12 h i.v.; and 8 received doxycycline, 20 mg every 12 h i.v. The antibiotic treatment was stopped after 2 weeks and autopsy was done 1 week later. The penicillin level 1 h after the stated dosage was 8 μg/ml in the serum and 10 μg/g in the lung tissue. Correspondingly, the lung tissue and serum levels were 40 and 128 for carbenicillin, 12 and 8 for chloramphenicol, and 8 and 12 for cefoxitin. Both clindamycin and doxycycline levels were higher in the lung—34 and 4 and 29 and 11 for clindamycin and doxycycline, respectively. The success rates on antibiotic therapy as evidenced by negative lung cultures were 6 of 14 (43%) on penicillin, 6 of 9 (67%) on carbenicillin, 7 of 8 (88%) on chloramphenicol, 8 of 9 (89%) on clindamycin, and 7 of 8 (88%) on doxycycline. The superior efficacy of chloramphenicol, clindamycin, and doxycycline over penicillin was again significant ($P = 0.02$).

Chemoprophylaxis. Immediately after transtracheal inoculation, antibiotic therapy was started in the above doses and continued for two more days. All eight controls developed pneumonia and later lung abscess. None of the animals treated with procaine penicillin, chloramphenicol, or doxycycline was protected, whereas cefoxitin protected two of eight (25%) animals and both clindamycin and carbenicillin protected seven of eight (88%) animals each. Clindamycin therapy afforded better prophylaxis than penicillin that was statistically significant ($P = 0.01$).

Modern chemotherapeutic agents appear to be more effective than penicillin in the treatment of anaerobic infections. It is conceivable that penicillin may have given good results had therapy continued longer, but carbenicillin, cefoxitin, doxycycline, and clindamycin showed therapeutic response within the same period.

Clinical evaluation may be subject to investigator bias. We therefore designed the animal model to study whether this was the case. In our hospital, *B. fragilis* was isolated in 21 of 124 (16.9%) patients and therefore was not uncommon. Our experimental studies confirm our clinical observation that clindamycin and doxycycline are superior to penicillin in the treatment of anaerobic lung infections.

1. **Kannangara, D. W., H. Thadepalli, V. T. Bach, and D. Webb.** 1981. Animal model for anaerobic lung abscess. Infect. Immun. **31**:592–597.

Factors Affecting the Susceptibility of *Campylobacter jejuni* to Metronidazole

GORDON RICH,* SEAN McDERMOTT, JULIET PITT, AND WALTER WOODS

Institute of Medical and Veterinary Science and South Australian Institute of Technology, Adelaide, South Australia*

Almost all anaerobic bacteria are susceptible to metronidazole, and it has been suggested that metronidazole has exclusive activity against anaerobic organisms. *Campylobacter* species are true microaerophilic organisms, optimal growth occurring at oxygen concentrations below atmospheric and growth under strict anaerobic conditions being very poor. Therefore, *Campylobacter* species might be expected to be resistant to metronidazole. However, when tested in optimal atmospheric conditions, only 44% of our strains were resistant to metronidazole (Met^r).

Milne et al. (3) reported that variation in atmosphere altered the susceptibility of *Clostridium* species to metronidazole and suggested that the same might apply to *Campylobacter* species. We examined 10 metronidazole-susceptible (Met^s) strains and 10 Met^r strains of *Campylobacter* in a variety of atmospheres and performed disk susceptibility tests to metronidazole. There was no significant variation in zone size in the various oxygen concentrations (Table 1). However, in anaerobic conditions one of the resistant strains gave a zone 24 mm in diameter, and five gave zones between 8 and 16 mm.

The MIC for two susceptible and five resistant strains was determined in cysteine-HCl broth in 10% CO_2 and in anaerobic conditions (Table 2). Only two strains grew anaerobically, and in these conditions MICs were 0.25 mg/liter. For the two susceptible strains the MIC was 1 mg/liter at 24 h, but at 48 h the MICs for these strains had increased considerably, and after 7 days, growth was detectable in the broth containing 50 mg/liter. These strains subcultured from the 7-day 50-mg/liter metronidazole medium were resistant on disk testing. The control broths (metronidazole-free) yielded organisms still susceptible by disk tests. The "newly resistant" strains from the 50-mg/liter broth remained resistant after 18 passages in metronidazole-free medium.

Ten Met^s *Campylobacter* isolates were sequentially subcultured at 48-h intervals onto blood agar plates containing 0.5, 2.5, 5, 7.5, and 15 mg of metronidazole per liter and were incubated in optimal atmospheric conditions. Eight strains grew on these increasing concentrations, and the resultant isolates were resistant by disk testing, both in optimal growth conditions and in anaerobic conditions. These original Met^s strains remained susceptible when not exposed to metronidazole.

Fluctuation experiments showed a variance ratio of 3.5 and a probability of <1% that identical populations were being sampled; this suggests that preexisting Met^r cells were being selected. However, the very high frequency of Met^r colonies found could be due to a background of cells that survive long enough for metronidazole to cause mutations, including mutation to Met^r. The latter was confirmed by replica-plating experiments which showed that some Met^r clones were superimposed, indicating preexisting resistance, whereas others were in random positions, indicating new mutants.

With *Campylobacter* sp. we did *not* see the gradual effect shown by Milne et al. (3) with clostridia as the O_2 content of the atmosphere increased. (We were able to confirm their findings.) The only effect that we demonstrated was that 6 of 10 resistant strains of *Campylobacter* showed some susceptibility to metronidazole when grown in anaerobic conditions.

In summary, not all strains are susceptible to metronidazole under strict anaerobic conditions and, conversely, many strains are susceptible in the presence of oxygen. This confirms doubts that metronidazole action depends solely on interference with electron transfer. The fact that newly resistant strains remain resistant despite repeated subculture makes it unlikely that the resistance is due to enzyme induction. It is possible that metronidazole may induce mutants resistant to itself, but why do they not appear in anaerobes such as *Bacteroides*? Metronidazole is bactericidal to anaerobes, the activity being due to a reduced metabolite, but it is not bactericidal to facultative anaerobes. It is mutagenic to *Salmonella*, and this is also through a reduced metabolite. This would indicate that the DNA synthesis of *Salmonella* is not as sensitive to the metabolite as that of anaerobes or the reduced metabolite is different.

The analogous drug nitrofurantoin also requires reduction to become bactericidal and mutagenic. This drug is active against both aerobes and anaerobes. The Met^r strains of *Bacteroides* produced and examined by Britz and Wilkinson

TABLE 1. *Effect of atmosphere on metronidazole susceptibility of Campylobacter (10 Met^r and 10 Met^s strains)*

Result	O_2 (%)[a]				
	18[b]	10	5	2.5	0 (an)[c]
Susceptible strains					
Zone <14 mm	2	7	6	4	10
Zone >14 mm	3	3	4	6	0
Resistant strains					
Zone zero	8	10	10	10	4
Zone <14 mm	0	0	0	0	4
Zone >14 mm	0	0	0	0	2

[a] All in combination with 10% CO_2.
[b] Seven strains failed to grow in 18% O_2.
[c] Anaerobic.

TABLE 2. *MICs of metronidazole (milligrams per liter) for Campylobacter and Clostridium (in broths)*[a]

Organism	10% CO_2			Anaerobic
	24 h	48 h	7 days	48 h
Campylobacter 1052	50	50	>50	NG
Campylobacter 820	50	50	>50	NG
Campylobacter 863	1	5	>50	NG
Campylobacter 866	10	10	20	<0.25
Campylobacter 842	NR	>50	>50	NG
Campylobacter 862	50	50	50	<0.25
Campylobacter 493	1	50	50	NG
Clostridium tertium	50	50	50	5
C. perfringens	<0.25	NT	NT	5

[a] NT, Not tested; NR, not recordable; NG, no growth.

(1) simultaneously became resistant to nitrofurantoin. This presumably is due to loss of the reduction system. In contrast, both the wild and the laboratory-produced Met^r strains of *Campylobacter* were susceptible to nitrofurantoin. Six of the wild resistant strains we examined showed evidence of susceptibility to metronidazole in a strict anaerobic atmosphere, indicating that some reaction had occurred. Similarly, Rosenkrantz and Speck (4) found that a "nitroreductase-deficient" strain of *Salmonella typhimurium* (TA 100 FRI) also reduced metronidazole when grown anaerobically.

To explain these observations, we suggest that there are at least three nitroreduction systems. Type 1 is a protein receptor of the ferredoxin type which produces a bactericidal metabolite from metronidazole and nitrofurantoin. Type 2 produces a bactericidal metabolite from nitrofurantoin and a mutagenic metabolite from metronidazole. Type 3 is a reduction system active only in anaerobic conditions which produces both bactericidal and mutagenic end products (or a single product with both properties).

Applying the hypothesis, we suggest the following.

(i) Campylobacter species have both type 1 and type 2 systems, and having type 2 reduction the organism is exposed to the mutagenic metabolite and may mutate to lose its type 1 enzyme. The selective pressure of metronidazole rapidly produces an entirely resistant population. As the type 2 system is still active, it is still susceptible to nitrofurantoin.

(ii) *Bacteroides* species possess only type 1, and thus they are susceptible and mutation is very rare before the organisms are killed. When the type 1 system is lost (e.g., Britz strains), the organism becomes resistant to both metronidazole and nitrofurantoin.

(iii) The gram-negative facultative anaerobes discussed by Ingham et al. (2) would be expected to have only type 3. Thus, a mutagenic end product enhances the selection of Met^r variants, explaining why isolates from patients taking metronidazole were resistant to this effect. Jackson (personal communication) demonstrated that the phenomenon is only temporary (24 h or so) in vitro. The exposure to metronidazole leads to the loss of the type 3 system and cessation of production of the bactericidal metabolite.

(iv) In the less demanding anaerobes such as *C. tertium*, we suggest that only type 1 is present. This is supported by our finding that nitrofurantoin susceptibility is reduced (in the same way as metronidazole susceptibility) in aerobic conditions (unpublished data). Presumably, these organisms switch off the ferredoxin-linked pathway when they grow in the presence of oxygen.

1. **Britz, M. L., and R. G. Wilkinson.** 1979. Isolation and properties of metronidazole-resistant mutants of *Bacteroides fragilis*. Antimicrob. Agents Chemother. **16:** 19–27.
2. **Ingham, H. R., C. J. Hall, P. R. Sisson, D. Tharagonnet, and J. B. Selkon.** 1980. Activity of metronidazole against facultative anaerobic bacteria. J. Antimicrob. Chemother. **6:**343–347.
3. **Milne, S. E., E. J. Stokes, and P. Waterworth.** 1978. Incomplete anaerobiosis as a cause of metronidazole resistance. J. Clin. Pathol. **31:**933–935.
4. **Rosenkranz, H. S., and W. T. Speck.** 1975. Mutagenicity of metronidazole: activation by mammalian liver microsomes. Biochem. Biophys. Res. Commun. **66:**520–525.

Possible Mechanisms of Resistance of Anaerobes to Nitroimidazoles

D. A. ROWLEY* AND D. I. EDWARDS

Chemotherapy Research Unit, North East London Polytechnic, London, England

Nitroimidazoles are selectively toxic to anaerobic organisms and are preferentially taken up by susceptible cells due to passive diffusion along a concentration gradient which is continuously regenerated by intracellular reductive metabolism (3). An obvious way in which cells could increase their resistance to these drugs would be to reduce the level of this uptake. Mechanisms by which this may be achieved have been investigated.

Uptake of ^{14}C-labeled misonidazole was measured in two strains of the anaerobic bacterium *Bacteroides fragilis*, 122020 and 122023, having MICs against this drug of 25.5 and 16.5 μg/ml, respectively. The rate and level of uptake were found to increase linearly with misonidazole concentration, were unaffected by the presence of closely related compounds in the incubation medium, and were greatly reduced in the presence of traces of oxygen. All of these observations provide confirmation of the proposed mechanism for nitroimidazole uptake. The rate of uptake was also found to be greater in the strain having the lowest MIC for misonidazole (Fig. 1).

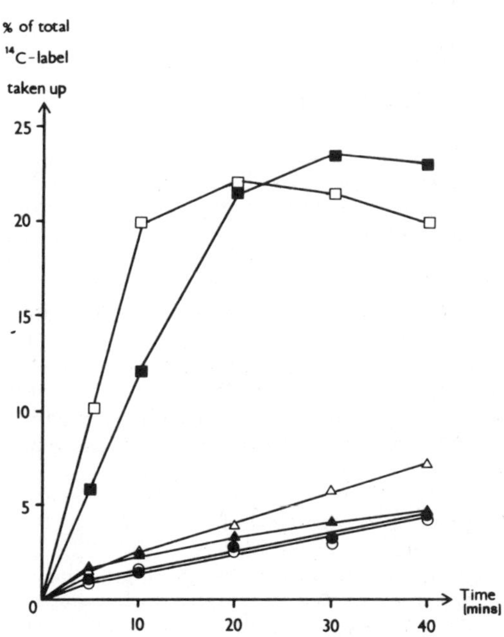

FIG. 1. *Uptake of ^{14}C-labeled misonidazole by E. coli and B. fragilis. Uptake was measured in two strains of E. coli, DC0 (circles) and DC2 (triangles), under aerobic (solid symbols) and anaerobic (open symbols) conditions and in two strains of B. fragilis, 122020 (solid squares) and 122023 (open squares) under anaerobic conditions only.*

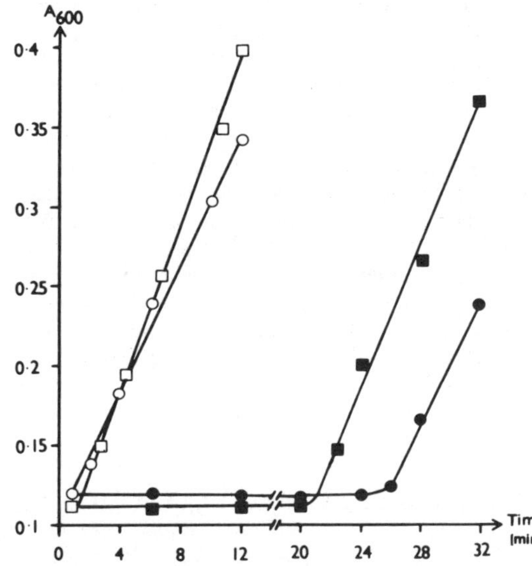

FIG. 2. *Pyruvate dehydrogenase activity in cell lysates of B. fragilis. Activity was measured by the appearance of reduced methyl viologen with an absorption maximum at 600 nm. Two strains of B. fragilis were used, 122020 (circles) and 122023 (squares). Solid symbols refer to experiments in which 1 μmol of misonidazole was added to the incubation mixture.*

Previous workers (1) have shown that artificially induced mutants of *B. fragilis*, showing increased resistance to metronidazole, have a reduced level of pyruvate dehydrogenase, one of the major sites of nitroimidazole reduction in these cells. Pyruvate dehydrogenase activity was measured in anaerobic cell lysates of the two *B. fragilis* strains used in this study. Crude lysates were added to pyruvate and coenzyme A in sealed vessels filled with nitrogen. Enzyme activity was assayed at 37°C by measuring reduction of methyl viologen, which results in the appearance of a blue chromophore with an absorption maximum at 600 nm. The results (Fig. 2) show that activity was highest in *B. fragilis* strain

122023, which had the lower MIC for misonidazole, indicating that the level of this enzyme is an important factor in determining the susceptibility of these organisms to nitroimidazoles.

Uptake of [^{14}C]misonidazole was also investigated in two strains of the facultative organism *Escherichia coli*. One of the strains used (DC2), a mutant of the other (DC0), showed increased permeability and susceptibility to penicillins (2). Under aerobic conditions, uptake was low and similar in both strains. In an anaerobic environment, the internal redox conditions of the cells become more negative, facilitating reduction of nitroimidazoles, and a much higher rate of uptake would be expected. The results obtained (Fig. 1) show that this is the case with the permeability mutant DC2. In the parent strain, however, the rate of uptake showed only a slight increase over aerobiosis, indicating that permeability plays an important role in governing uptake of nitroimidazoles in this organism. MIC determinations for the two strains under anaerobic conditions confirmed the increased susceptibility of the mutant strain, which had an MIC of 50 μg/ml, compared with 250 μg/ml for the parent.

The results presented in this study indicate two possible ways in which cells may decrease the uptake of and consequent susceptibility to nitroimidazole drugs.

1. **Britz, M. L., and R. G. Wilkinson.** 1979. Isolation and properties of metronidazole-resistant mutants of *Bacteroides fragilis*. Antimicrob. Agents Chemother. **16:** 19–27.
2. **Curtis, N. A. C., C. Brown, M. Boxall, and M. G. Boulton.** 1979. Inhibition of *Escherichia coli* K-12 by β-lactam antibiotics with poor antibacterial activity: interaction of permeability and intrinsic activity against penicillin-binding proteins. Antimicrob. Agents Chemother. **15:**332–336.
3. **Ings, R. M. J., J. A. McFadzean, and W. E. Ormerod.** 1974. The mode of action of metronidazole in Trichomonas vaginalis and other micro-organisms. Biochem. Pharmacol. **23:**1421–1429.

Effects of Antibiotic, Antifungal, and Antiviral Drugs on Neutrophil Function

LIONEL A. MANDELL

McMaster University, Hamilton, Ontario, Canada

The bulk of the literature on antibiotic agents deals with the effects of these drugs on various microorganisms. The effects of these drugs on the host has received much less attention. The polymorphonuclear leukocyte (PMN), because of its ability to ingest and kill bacteria, serves as our first line of defense against infection, and an understanding of drug effects on these cells is not only desirable but necessary if optimal use of antibiotics is to be made. Many of the studies have attempted to examine these effects by using various cell types and concentrations of drugs that are often not within the therapeutic range. In addition, studies of phagocytic function in particular have often been carried out with techniques that do not allow adequate distinction between simple attachment to the surface of the cell and true ingestion, thereby making any conclusions about the effects on phagocytosis questionable.

With these considerations in mind, we have studied the effects of various antibacterial, antiviral, and antifungal drugs on the phagocytic and microbicidal activity of the human PMN. The concentrations of the drugs used have included values that are well within the acceptable therapeutic range as well as a value that is well above this range. By choosing three such values, we felt that we would be able to demonstrate any dose-response effect if one, in fact, exists. The method used to study phagocytosis was that described by Stossel, which measures the uptake of diisodecyl phthalate Oil Red O particles (1). The technique is very quantitative as well as sensitive and allows for accurate measurement of true ingestion. The nitroblue tetrazolium (NBT) reduction test was used to measure bactericidal activity.

The PMNs were separated from blood by differential centrifugation, and viability was then tested by trypan blue exclusion. The cells were then incubated with the particular concentration of a specified drug under investigation at 37°C for 30 min and were then washed to remove any drug. This step was particularly important since, by washing the cells before incubating them with the particles, any effect on phagocytosis or NBT reduction would be due solely to the interaction of drug with the PMN since the particles did not come in contact with the drug at any point. In a separate step, the diisodecyl phthalate Oil Red O particles were prepared and then stabilized with *Escherichia coli* lipopolysaccharide. The particles were then opsonized by adding to them an equal volume of fresh serum and incubating at 37°C for 30 min. The opsonized particles were then added to the washed PMNs to initiate the phagocytic process. At the end of three specified times, the reaction was stopped, nonphagocytosed particles were separated, and the Oil Red O was extracted from the PMNs and read spectrophotometrically. By use of a predetermined formula, the optical density was converted to milligrams of phthalate per 10^7 cells. For the bactericidal assay, NBT was added to tubes containing standardized amounts of particles and PMN. By a method similar to that used for the Oil Red O, the formazan was extracted from the PMN and the optical density was determined. A formula allowed final results to be expressed as micrograms of formazan per 10^7 cells. A number of controls were carried out to ensure the validity of the assay and included temperature, presence or absence of PMNs, alteration of particle-to-cell ratios, and PMNs from a patient with chronic granulomatous disease.

For each drug tested, the data from a single outcome measure formed a classic randomized block design, with the blocking factor being blood sample and the treatment factor being dose level. When analyzing our data three statistical questions were of primary interest. First, is there any evidence to suggest that the phagocytic or bactericidal activity was different between the treatment groups? Second, is there any evidence to suggest that the average therapeutic response is different from the control, and finally, is there any evidence to suggest a dose response relationship between the drug-treated groups? The first question was tested by using the F statistic in the analysis of variance technique, and the second two questions were investigated with the technique of linear contrast.

We found that drug effects were limited to phagocytosis since microbicidal activity of the PMN as measured by the NBT test was unaltered. Certain drugs stimulated phagocytosis, and in certain cases a dose response was evident. Interestingly, enhancement of particle ingestion was not limited to any one particular class of drug. Examination of our results allowed us to conclude the following. (i) The following drugs potentiate phagocytosis: antibacterial—erythromycin, chloramphenicol, penicillin G, cephalothin, vancomycin, and tetracycline; antiviral—adenine arabinoside; antifungal—5-fluorocytosine. (ii) The effect is due to drug influence on the cell and not the ingested particle. (iii) The effect is not related to basic modes of action of the drugs. (iv) No effect on NBT reduction is seen.

Investigations are currently under way in our laboratory to determine why certain drugs are capable of stimulating phagocytosis. One possibility is that those agents that potentiate the endocytic process somehow enhance calcium movement into the cell.

1. **Stossel, T. P.** 1973. Evaluation of opsonic and leukocyte function with a spectrophotometric test in patients with infection and with phagocytic disorders. Blood **42:**121–130.

Correction of Polymorphonuclear Leukocyte Chemotaxis Defects with Trimethoprim-Sulfamethoxazole

A. DE LA CRUZ, J. OLESKE,* J. LA BRAICO, R. COOPER, D. FISHMAN, A. MINNEFOR, R. LIN, AND R. GARCIA

Department of Pediatrics, College of Medicine & Dentistry of New Jersey, New Jersey Medical School, and Saint Michael's Medical Center, Newark, New Jersey, 07102, and Hoffmann-La Roche Inc., Nutley, New Jersey 07110, U.S.A.*

Chemotaxis (CT), the directed movement of leukocytes towards a chemotactic agent, is an important function of our defense mechanism against pyogenic infections. During the past decade many studies have investigated CT and its central role in host defense (4). Several classes of drugs have been shown to modulate host defense responses, including antibiotics (1). Martin et al. (2) reported the inhibitory effects of tetracyclines on leukocyte migration. Subsequent studies have investigated the in vitro effect of several antibiotics on CT (1). Based on the clinical observation that compromised patients, especially those with polymorphonuclear leukocyte (PML) defects, improved more dramatically on trimethoprim-sulfamethoxazole (TMP/SMZ) than should be expected on its antimicrobial effects alone, we studied the effects of TMP/SMZ on PML-CT.

This study examined the in vitro effects of

TABLE 1. *In vivo effects of TMP/SMZ on PML-CT*

Patient no.	No. of cells that migrated toward CT			
	Pre-TMP/SMZ	On TMP/SMZ	Off TMP/SMZ	On TMP/SMZ
1	64	280	120	279
2	169	295	185	202
3	96	222	62	197
4	23	157	ND[a]	ND
5	19	82	ND	ND
6	218	263	ND	ND
7	36	86	ND	ND
8	29	331	ND	ND

[a] ND, Not determined.

TABLE 2. *In vitro effects of TMP/SMZ on PML-CT*

Patient no.[a]	No. of cells that migrated toward CT	
	PML incubated without TMP/SMZ	PML incubated with 10× TMP/SMZ
1 (P)	64	297
2 (P)	29	305
3 (C)	374	410
4 (C)	187	205
5 (C)	295	347
6 (C)	182	280
7 (C)	307	352
8 (C)	256	352

[a] P, Patients with CT defect; C, normal control subjects.

TMP/SMZ on six normal individuals and two patients with PML-CT defects as well as the in vivo effects of TMP/SMZ on eight patients with known PML-CT defects. Our PML-CT assay was a modification of the method reported by Nelson et al. (3). In brief, 5 ml of 0.75% agarose in medium 199 supplemented with 10% fetal calf serum was placed in 60-mm-diameter plastic petri dishes. Six sets of three wells each, 2 mm in diameter and 2 mm apart, were made in the agarose plates; Zymogen-activated serum was put in the outer well, washed PMLs at 5×10^7/ml were placed in the center well, and saline was placed in the inner well as a control. For both in vitro and in vivo studies, PMLs were separated by dextran sedimentation followed by density centrifugation over Ficoll-Hypaque. For in vitro studies the separated PMLs were first incubated for 30 min with various concentrations of TMP/SMZ (10×, 25×, 100× peak serum concentrations) before the cells were placed in the agarose wells. The CT assay plates were then incubated at 37°C for 3 h in 5% CO_2. After Formalin fixation and safranin staining, the plates were examined under a 10× objective lens with a 10 by 10 mm grid. The total number of cells migrating in a path 1 mm wide between the center well and the outer (chemotactic factor) well and the center well and the inner (control) well were determined.

Eight patients with PML-CT defects (six with hyper IgE syndrome, one with Behc'et's syndrome, and one with recurrent pulmonary abscess) were studied before and 5 days after starting Bactrim (Hoffmann-La Roche) at standard doses by mouth during an acute infectious episode. All patients had an excellent clinical response to therapy and all had substantial improvement in PML-CT while on treatment (Table 1). PML-CT returned to pretreatment levels in these patients after therapy was discontinued. In three of our patients a repeat course of Bactrim was again associated with improvement in both clinical parameters and PML-CT.

In vitro experiments in six normal individuals and in two patients with PML-CT defects demonstrated that a normal individual's PMLs do not show a significant increase in PML-CT after incubation with TMP/SMZ. This is in contrast to the substantial increase in PML-CT in two patients with PML-CT defects when their PMLs were preincubated with TMP/SMZ (Table 2).

These preliminary data support previous observation that drugs, in particular, antibiotics, may affect host response to infections. TMP/SMZ substantially improves PML-CT in patients with chemotactic defects and accounts in part for the efficacy of this antimicrobial in such patients. Continued research is needed to define the effects of antimicrobial agents on both inflammatory and immune responses in normal as well as in compromised individuals. Both inhibition and enhancement of host defenses by antimicrobials need to be delineated. An understanding of such effects will allow for a more rational application of presently available antimicrobials and will give direction to development of antimicrobials that have both specific antimicrobial action and positive effects on host defense systems.

1. **Forsgren, A., and D. Schmeling.** 1977. Effects of antibiotics on chemotaxis of human leukocytes. Antimicrob. Agents Chemother. **11:**580–584.
2. **Martin, R. R., G. Warr, H. Yeager, R. Couch, and V. Knight.** 1974. Effect of tetracycline on chemotaxis. J. Infect. Dis. **129:**110–116.
3. **Nelson, R. D., P. Quie, and R. L. Simmons.** 1975. Chemotaxis under agarose: a new and simple method for measuring chemotaxis and spontaneous migration of human polymorphonuclear leukocytes and monocytes. J. Immunol. **115:**1650–1656.
4. **NIH Conference.** 1980. Disorders of phagocyte chemotaxis. Ann. Infect. Med. **92:**520–538.

Polymorphonuclear Leukocyte Adherence in Patients with Sepsis

FRANK R. VENEZIO* AND JOHN P. PHAIR

Northwestern University Medical School, Chicago, Illinois, U.S.A.

During septic shock, it is postulated that the interaction of activated C5 with polymorphonuclear leukocytes (PMN) results in sequestration of aggregated neutrophils in pulmonary capillaries (1). This mechanism may be partially responsible for the adult respiratory distress syndrome (ARDS) (2). Results of this study demonstrate that PMN adhesiveness is increased in whole blood obtained from patients with bacteremia, and indirect evidence indicates that this altered adherence is plasma (complement) mediated.

All patients studied were clinically septic and had documented bacteremia. Three groups of patients were evaluated. Group I consisted of septic patients studied at the time blood cultures were obtained. Group II patients had been treated for bacteremia for 24 h with appropriate antibiotics before being studied. Group III patients were assayed at the time "septic shock" was recognized and 4 and 8 h later. Shock was defined as systolic blood pressure of <90 mmHg (ca. 12 kPa) with evidence of inadequate tissue perfusion. Four group III patients were restudied before hospital discharge.

Adherence of PMN was determined by using a whole-blood assay described by MacGregor et al. (3). To determine the role of humoral factors in altered adherence, type O donor PMN were suspended in Hanks balanced salt solution plus 25% patients' plasma, nonautologous plasma, or normal plasma incubated with 2 mg of zymosan per ml for 30 min at 37°C to activate the alternate pathway of complement. One milliliter of the PMN-plasma suspension was added to each of three columns. Adherence values were calculated by determining the number of PMN in the effluent and the percentage of PMN retained by the fiber. The adherence value represents the average retention using three columns. Results were compared by using Student's two-sample *t* test.

In group I, five patients had infections caused by gram-negative bacilli and five had infections caused by gram-positive cocci. One patient with serious burns died of enterococcal sepsis despite appropriate therapy. Four patients in group II had bacteremia due to gram-negative bacilli and six had bacteremia due to gram-positive cocci. Two patients died, one with pneumococcal peritonitis and a second with *Pseudomonas aeruginosa* bacteremia following aortic graft placement. Thirteen patients (group III) presented in shock. Ten were infected with aerobic gram-negative bacilli, two had polymicrobial bacteremia, and one grew *Clostridium perfringens* in blood cultures. Four group III patients were treated with corticosteroids. A total of five patients in shock died; one had been treated with corticosteroids. ARDS developed in two patients; neither had received corticosteroids.

The mean PMN adherence, using the whole-blood assay in the three groups of patients, were as follows: group I, 70.9 ± 4.9%; group II, 79.2 ± 8.6%; group III patients at the onset of shock, 91.1 ± 8.5%. Adherence values in all three groups differed significantly from one another at $P < 0.01$. Mean adherence in concomitantly studied controls was 72.1 ± 2.8%, which differed significantly from patients in groups II and III ($P < 0.01$). PMN adherence in group III patients was also measured 4 and 8 h after the onset of shock (Fig. 1). Four patients received methylprednisolone (30 mg/kg) within 1 h of identifying the shock state. Initial mean adherence values before steroid therapy did not differ significantly from that noted in untreated patients: 90.8 ± 8.9% versus 85.4 ± 13.3% ($P > 0.2$). At 4 h, a significant decrease in mean PMN adherence was demonstrable when the four patients treated with corticosteroids (61.0 ± 18.8%) were compared with the nine untreated patients (92.1 ± 7.7%, $P < 0.001$). By 8 h, the eight surviving patients not receiving corticosteroids had a mean adherence value of 90.0% ± 7.6; in contrast, mean adherence in the three surviving corticosteroid-treated patients was 65.0 ± 20.0% ($P < 0.005$).

Retention by nylon of normal PMN suspended in plasma obtained from non-corticosteroid-treated patients at 0, 4, and 8 h was augmented significantly compared with that induced by control plasma but less than that of cells suspended in zymosan (Fig. 2). The initial plasma obtained from corticosteroid-treated patients also induced greater retention of PMN than did control plasma. After treatment with corticosteroids, plasma obtained from these patients at 4 and 8 h no longer induced significant augmentation of PMN retention. Mean adherence values induced by plasma from patients studied at discharge were as follows: control, 20.9 ± 4.4%; convalescent, 20.1 ± 1.9%; and zymosan, 59.6 ± 4.6%. Mean adherence of PMN in

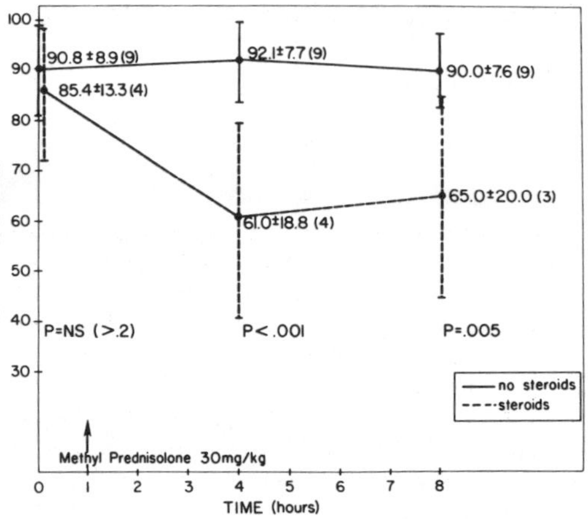

FIG. 1. *Adherence of PMN to nylon columns in patients with bacteremic shock as measured by the whole-blood assay. Numbers in parentheses indicate the numbers of patients studied in each group at each time interval. Patients were studied when shock was recognized and 4 and 8 h later. Methylprednisolone (30 mg/kg) was administered intravenously to the treatment group within 1 h of identifying the shock state. Mean adherence of concomitantly studied controls was 72.1 ± 2.8%. NS, Not significant.*

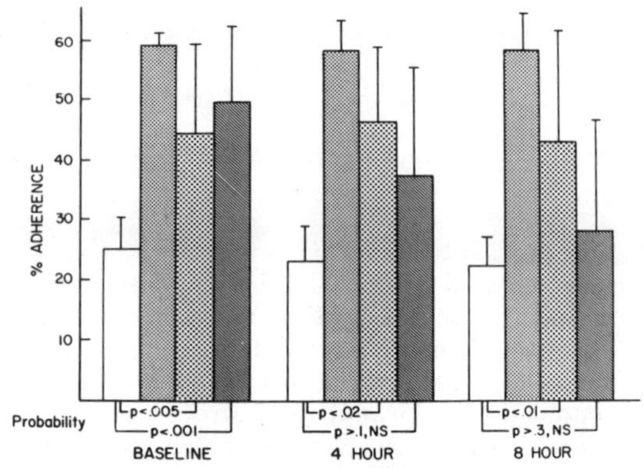

FIG. 2. *Retention by nylon columns of normal donor PMN suspended in various plasmas: control plasma (open columns), zymosan-activated plasma (small dots), plasma from patients not receiving corticosteroids (large dots), and corticosteroid-treated patients (dashed lines). Adherence was measured at the onset of shock (base line) and 4 and 8 h later. NS, Not significant.*

convalescent plasma when compared with control plasma did not differ ($P > 0.3$), but both were significantly lower than that induced by zymosan ($P < 0.0001$). Adherence values were not altered by the species of infecting organisms. Gram-positive bacteremia induced a mean PMN adherence of 81.1 ± 13.2%; gram-negative bacteria induced a mean adherence of 82.8 ± 22.4% ($P > 0.3$, not significant).

Retention of PMN by nylon columns as measured by using the whole-blood assay is augmented in patients with bacteremic shock; this enhancement is plasma mediated. The augmenting factor in plasma is probably activated C5, which has been shown to be elevated in patients with shock (2). It has been postulated that ARDS occurs as a result of selective leukocyte adherence to pulmonary capillary endothelium induced by complement activation (1). PMN retention and the plasma-mediated augmenting effect was significantly decreased 4 and 8 h after patients had received corticosteroids. Four of nine patients with bacteremic shock who did not receive corticosteroids died, including two who developed ARDS. Four patients received corticosteroids; one died early and none developed ARDS. This series is too small and the patients were not prospectively randomized to receive corticosteroids; thus, no conclusions as to the clinical efficacy of corticosteroids can be made. However, PMN adherence with the whole-blood assay is a simple, indirect measure of complement activation which prospectively may identify "septic" patients at risk of developing shock and ARDS.

1. **Goldblum, S. E., W. P. Reed, R. L. Sopher, and D. L. Palmer.** 1981. Pneumococcus-induced granulocytopenia and pulmonary leukocstasis in rabbits. J. Lab. Clin. Med. **97**:278–290.
2. **Hammerschmidt, D. E., L. E. Hudson, L. J. Weaver, P. R. Craddock, and H. S. Jacob.** 1980. Association of complement activation and elevated plasma C5a with adult respiratory distress syndrome. Lancet **i**:947–949.
3. **MacGregor, R. R., P. J. Spagnuolo, and A. L. Lentnek.** 1974. Inhibition of granulocyte adherence by ethanol, prednisone, and aspirin measured with an assay system. N. Engl. J. Med. **291**:642–646.

Local Effect of Penicillin Drugs on the Mucociliary Activity in Vitro

N. G. TOREMALM* AND K. JOSEFSSON

Department of Otolaryngology, University of Lund, Malmö General Hospital, S-214 01 Malmö, Sweden

Many drugs have obvious clinical side effects, some severe and others moderate. An unknown number produce only subclinical manifestations. It is necessary to try to identify such effects and, if possible, to analyze their possible pathogenetic significance. This can be done by using different experimental models. In the case of side effects of penicillin, neurotoxicity studies have been used for many years. A special type comprises the ototoxicity studies (for example, of aminoglycosides), which have been frequently described. The questions we want to call attention to are as follows: Has penicillin an inhibitory effect upon the mucociliary function of the respiratory mucosa? If so, do the different types of penicillins differ in this respect? Is there any reliable explanation for such toxic effects on the mucociliary function?

As early as 1945, Proetz (2) demonstrated that local application of 5,000 IU of benzylpenicillin per ml had a pronounced inhibitory effect on mucociliary activity. Since then, very few studies have been done to verify this interesting observation with objective experimental techniques.

In our laboratory, we are using a standardized method for indirect recording of the mucociliary function via light reflex variations on the mucous membrane surface due to wave movements in the secretion layer. Rabbit trachea specimens are placed in an experimental chamber at 37°C and at a relative humidity above 90% in the surrounding air. The surface light reflections are converted to electrical signals via a photodiode mounted on one of the microscope oculars and then recorded continuously (3).

During previous pilot studies on the effect of bacterial toxins on mucociliary activity, we became interested in the possible effect of antibiotics. In preliminary in vitro studies, we found a ciliostatic effect by benzylpenicillin in a 1% isotonic, neutral solution. However, corresponding experiments with kanamycin and gentamicin had no influence on the mucociliary function in vitro. This was confusing if a comparison is made of the serious effects produced by aminoglycosides on the inner ear hair cells, which are similar in structure to the cilia of the respiratory tract. We have now tested a series of different penicillins, classified according to their hydrophobic reactions, which are characterized by their partition coefficients or solubility gradient between octanol and water.

The effect of penicillin G on the mucociliary activity in vitro in the rabbit trachea was as follows: A 0.1% solution had no effect, a 1% solution had a moderate effect, but a 2% solution gave a total inhibition of the mucociliary activity within 3 h. In the penicillin V group there was a total ciliestasis already within 1.5 h with a 1% solution.

The effect of cloxacillin on the mucociliary activity was a very fast and severe inhibition on exposure to a 0.1% solution. The formula $T = \text{const}/t_{50} \cdot C$ demonstrates our calculation formula for the mucociliary toxicity index, where t_{50} is the time in minutes indicating 50% reduction of the mucociliary wave movements, C is the penicillin concentration in mmoles/liter, and const is equal to 10^4.

A comparison between the partition coefficient along the x-axis and the mucociliary tox-

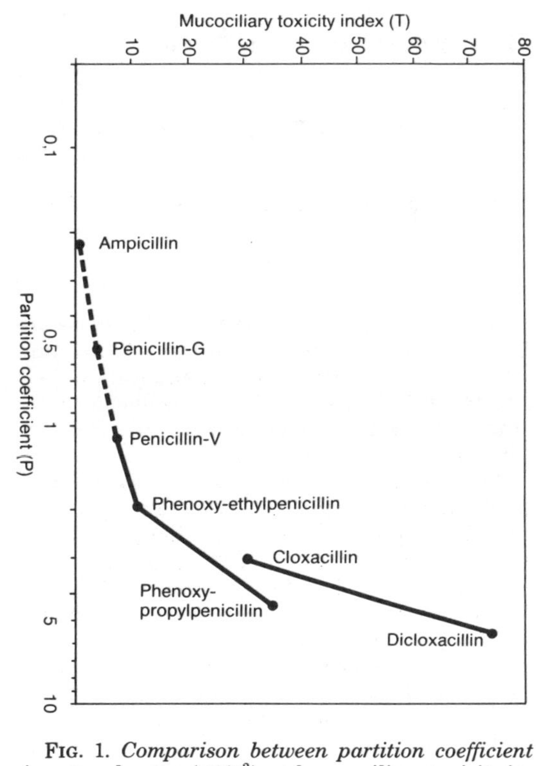

FIG. 1. *Comparison between partition coefficient in octanol-water (×10^{-2}) and mucociliary toxicity index of different penicillins.*

icity index along the *y*-axis for the different penicillins appears in Fig. 1. Ampicillin had no effect, whereas dicloxacillin, which has a rather high hydrophobic character, showed the highest degree of ciliary toxicity. A similar grading is described for neurotoxicity according to Weihrauch et al. (5). These authors also described a close relationship between the neurotoxic effect of the drugs and their lipophilicity. The inhibition of the mucociliary function in our experiments followed the same pattern. The penicillin G group was less cilietoxic than the penicillin V group, which in turn was less toxic than cloxacillin (Toremalm et al., to be published).

Our preliminary conclusions from these results are either that the penicillins interfere with lipoproteins of the cell membrane of ciliated cells, producing a true toxic effect on the cilia, or that the penicillins influence the release of viscous secretions, implying only a secondary retardation of the movements of the cilia within the secretion layer. This problem is still of theoretical and toxicological interest even without any certain clinical significance. Ordinary doses of penicillins seem not to decrease the transportation of secretion according to clinical studies published by Vinther and Elbrønd (4). However, Forsgren and Schmeling (1) have found that certain antibiotics have an inhibitory effect on leukocyte chemotaxis, and our findings regarding mucociliary activity may have the same background, but the true nature of the effects of penicillin and other antibiotics on various biological organs and functions is not yet properly understood.

1. **Forsgren, A., and D. Schmeling.** 1977. Effect of antibiotics on chemotaxis of human polymorphonuclear leucocytes. Antimicrob. Agents Chemother. **11:**580–584.
2. **Proetz, A. W.** 1945. Cilia and penicillin. Ann. Otol. **54:** 94–95.
3. **Reimer, Å., C. H. Håkanson, U. Mercke, and N. G. Toremalm.** 1977. The mucociliary activity of the upper respiratory tract. I. A method for use in experimental studies on human material. Acta Otolaryngol. **83:**491–497.
4. **Vinther, B., and O. Elbrønd.** 1978. Nasal mucociliary function during penicillin treatment. Acta Otolaryngol. **86:**132–134.
5. **Weihrauch, T. R., D. Höffler, and J. Krieglstein.** 1976. Significance of the hydrophobic character of penicillins for their neurotoxicity, p. 644–648. *In* J. D. Williams and A. M. Geddes (eds.), Chemotherapy 4. Pharmacology of antibiotics. Plenum Press, New York.

Antitumor and Antibacterial Activity of Dextran LU-122 and Its Effect on Macrophage Activity

S. M. NAVASHIN, M. E. PREOBRAZHENSKAYA, I. P. FOMINA, T. G. TERENTYEVA, A. N. LOBUSEVA, A. B. SOKOLOV, AND E. L. ROZENFELD

National Research Institute of Antibiotics, Institute of Biological and Medical Chemistry of the Academy of Medical Sciences of the USSR, Moscow, USSR

Dextran LU-122 containing 1,2-glycoside bonds in the branching points (one branching point per four anhydroglucose residues) was isolated from the culture fluid of *Leuconostoc dextranicum*. Its activity in various biological systems was studied earlier (1).

The protective effect of LU-122 was studied in albino mice with sepsis. The mice were inoculated intraperitoneally with 2 LD_{50} of *Escherichia coli* per mouse. LU-122 was administered intraperitoneally 24, 48, 72, and 96 h before inoculation. The dextran doses were 5, 10, 20, 40, 80, and 160 mg/kg. The antitumor effect of LU-122 was estimated on models of ascitic sarcoma 37 and solid sarcoma 180 tumors. The drug was administered intraperitoneally in a single dose 24 h before tumor implantation and on days 1, 2, 3, and 4 of implantation or repeatedly on days 1 to 9 and on days 2, 4, 6, and 8 of implantation.

The phagocytosis indices were studied on days 1, 3, 5, and 10 of the intraperitoneal administration of dextran in a single dose of 10 mg/kg to the intact mice and mice with sarcoma 180 tumors. Phagocytosis activity as a percentage of the phagocytosing macrophages was calculated, and the phagocytic index was measured by the number of phagocytosed *Staphylococcus aureus* 209P cells.

It was found that the protective effect of LU-122 in the mice with experimental sepsis caused by *E. coli* was evident when the drug was administered in a dose of 10 to 40 mg/kg 48 and 72 h before inoculation, the survival rate being 28% for the 20-mg/kg dose and 48% per cent for the 10-mg/kg dose. The maximum effect was observed when LU-122 was administered 72 h before inoculation. The changes in the administration schedule with respect to the administration time and dose did not result in any increase of the protective effect of LU-122.

In the experiments with the intact animals it was shown that even 24 h after polysaccharide administration the phagocytosis activity and phagocytic index increased by 46 and 64%, respectively, compared with the control. In 3 days these values increased 3- to 3.6-fold compared with the control and correlated with the highest level of the drug protective effect in the mice with sepsis caused by *E. coli* (the maximum effect was observed on day 3) (Fig. 1).

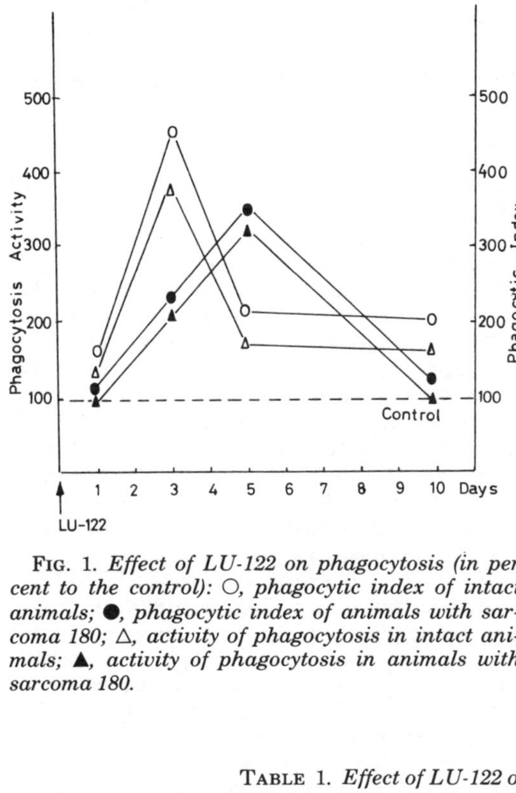

FIG. 1. *Effect of LU-122 on phagocytosis (in per cent to the control): ○, phagocytic index of intact animals; ●, phagocytic index of animals with sarcoma 180; △, activity of phagocytosis in intact animals; ▲, activity of phagocytosis in animals with sarcoma 180.*

A pronounced antitumor effect of LU-122 was observed with respect to ascitic sarcoma 37 (tumor growth inhibition, 92%). The effect on sarcoma 180 was medium (tumor growth inhibition, 53%) (Table 1). Dependence of the polysaccharide activity on the dose and treatment schedule was shown. A single dose of LU-122 at 10 mg/kg on day 4 of tumor implantation, as well as its repeated use, was optimal.

The use of the polysaccharide in a single dose before and on day 1, 2, or 3 of implantation was not effective. No antitumor effect was observed upon intravenous administration of LU-122 according to the schedule optimal for the intraperitoneal administration.

Study of the phagocytic indices after administration of dextran to mice with sarcoma 180 showed that the activity of the peritoneal macrophages significantly increased (Fig. 1) from the first days of drug administration. By day 5 it reached the maximum level. During this period the phagocytic index and phagocytosis activity increased 3.5- and 3.3-fold, respectively, compared with the control.

Therefore, the effect of LU-122 evident from an increase in the activity of the peritoneal macrophages in the animals with sarcoma 180 was somewhat retarded in time compared with that in the intact animals. The highest levels of the effect (up to 333 to 352% with respect to the activity of phagocytosis and phagocytic index) were observed on days 7 to 12 of tumor development.

The studies showed that LU-122 was slightly

TABLE 1. *Effect of LU-122 on development of mouse sarcoma*

Administration route	Administration scheme	LU-122 single dose (mg/kg)	Tumor growth inhibition (%)	
			Sarcoma 37	Sarcoma 180
Intraperitoneal	Once, 24 h before inoculation	5.0–20.0	0	0
	On day:			
	1	5.0–40.0	0	0
	2	5.0–40.0	0	0
	3	5.0–40.0	18	21
	4	5.0	54	
		10.0	92	53
		40.0		49
	Days 2, 4, 6, and 8	5.0	47	31
	Day 1–9	10.0	82	45
Intravenous	Days 2, 4, 6, and 8	5.0–15.0	0–26	0–35

active in protection of mice with sepsis caused by *E. coli*, markedly active with respect to ascitic sarcoma 37, and moderately active with respect to solid sarcoma 180. The maximum phagocytic activity of LU-122 coincided in time with the highest level of its antibacterial and antitumor activities.

1. **Preobrazhenskaya, M. E., E. I. Rosenfeld, and L. Kandra.** 1978. Studies on some biologically active dextrans. Carbohydr. Res. **66:**213–223.

Alveolar Macrophages Function in Chronic Respiratory Diseases

TOMOAKI ISHIKAWA,* SHIGERU ITAKURA, SOICHI NAGATA, YUTAKA NODA, SHIGEO IBUKI, MARI SHIBATA, HISAKAZU TAI, TETSUO SATO, SHIGEYUKI TSUIKI, AND MASAHARU HORIGUCHI

Department of Internal Medicine and Division of Nephrology, 3rd Hospital, Jikei University, School of Medicine, Komae shi, Tokyo, Japan

Immunological characteristics of alveolar macrophages obtained from patients with chronic respiratory infection (CRI) were compared with those from patients with neoplasma and from healthy subjects. Phagocytic functions determined with human immunoglobulin A (IgA)-coated beads from CRI were almost the same as those in the other samples. The nitroblue tetrazolium (NBT) reducing activity score of macrophages from CRI was slightly higher than that of the other samples. However, the cytotoxicity test with anti-human leukocyte locus A-DR (anti-HLA-DR) antibody containing Ia antigen and complement showed a significantly higher killing rate in macrophages from CRI than in other samples.

It has been shown that the onset of CRI by bacteria is mainly due to rupturing of the mucous barrier in the bronchi. One of the factors in the development of symptoms by bacterial infection is the effect of the local immune response such as macrophage function and secretory IgA. The infiltration of macrophages in the bronchi is evident, especially in patients with CRI. In this study, characteristics of alveolar macrophages from those patients were examined by the NBT reduction test, phagocytic function, and expression of surface antigen.

Ten patients with CRI, five patients with lung neoplasma, and five healthy subjects were selected as donors of macrophages. The cells, taken from bronchial washing with a bronchoscope, were incubated to collect glass-adherent cells. The adherent cells were stained with alpha-naphthyl butyrate to detect esterase specific for macrophages and monocytes. From 80 to 85% of the adherent cells were shown to be positive for esterase.

In the NBT reduction test, 50 μl of 0.2% NBT and 50 μl of 10^6 macrophages per ml was expressed as the score calculated from the data of 100 cells.

To determine the phagocytic activity of macrophages, 50 μl of a human IgA-coated bead suspension (Bio-Rad Laboratories) was added to 50 μl of a 10^6/ml macrophage suspension and incubated at 37°C for 30 min. The number of macrophages ingesting the beads was counted under the microscope.

For the cytotoxicity test with anti-HLA-DR antibody, macrophages were incubated with anti-HLA-DR antibody (New England Nuclear Corp.) and low TOX-H rabbit complement. Viability of the cells was determined by the trypan blue dye exclusion test.

In the group of specimens with CRI, the NBT score was 229 to 356. Taking 278 as the mean and comparing it with the neoplasma group's mean of 240 and control group's mean of 218, the figure represents a high numerical value.

In the immunobead phagocytic index, the CRI group was 92.5%, the neoplasma group was 89.0%, and the control group was 88.5%. The CRI group was numerically a little high, but it cannot be clearly deducted from the 92.5% figure that it was on the increase.

In the experiment with the macrophage population containing the Ia antigen, the percentage of alveolar macrophages killed by anti-HLA-DR antibody and complement was less than 2% in the neoplasma group and the healthy group (Fig. 1). However, the value for the CRI group was 8.7%, which was a significantly higher value than for the other groups.

It is already known that during CRI neutrophilic leukocytes, macrophages, and lymphocytes pathologically infiltrate. When they infiltrate the bronchial tissue, local inflammation arises and quick recovery is generally seen, but many points concerning the function of the re-

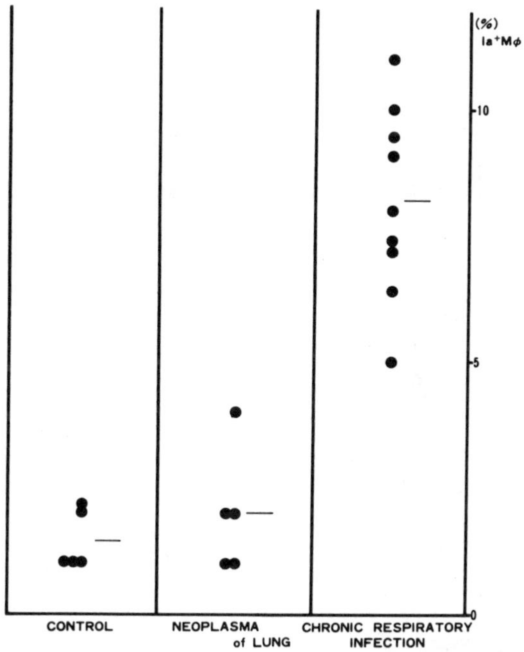

FIG. 1. *Macrophages with immunoaccessory antigen receptor (Ia⁺Mφ).*

leased macrophages and lymphocytes have not yet been clarified. In this experiment, it has been shown through the staining of esterase that released lung macrophages are derived from monocytes (3). Also, concerning the function of macrophages, the NBT score for the chronic respiratory infection specimens was numerically higher than the score for the other groups. This shows that, depending on the infection, superoxide activity in the cell is activated (2). However, conclusions on phagocytosis cannot be drawn from the tests conducted on the three groups, and cell activation can be considered irrelevant to phagocytosis.

Macrophages have the function of transmitting antigen information, referred to as accessory cell activity. S. Muramatsu and others have reported that macrophages that have accessory cell activity have Ia antigen (1). In the above experiment, the Ia-positive percentage of normal adults was 2% or less, but in the case of CRI the numerical value was clearly high. This fact shows that released macrophages not only contain local biodefense mechanisms for phagocytosis, bactericides, etc., but also are mediated for T-cells and B-cells and an immunological mechanism against the spread of infection throughout the entire body.

We conducted the experiments on the function of local macrophages from an immunological standpoint. However, in future experiments, the phase of infectious illness, the presence or absence of various antibiotics, changes in the mucous barrier of infected areas, and effects of aging need to be taken into consideration.

1. **Hedes, R. J., G. B. Ahman, K. S. Hatcock, H. B. Dickler, and A. Singer.** 1978. Cellular and genetic control of antibody responses in vitro. J. Immunol. **121:** 1501–1509.
2. **Hocking, W. G., and D. W. Golde.** 1979. The pulmonary-alveolar macrophages in the normal steady state. J. Exp. Med. **149:**1504–1518.
3. **Van Furth, R., Z. A. Cohn, J. G. Hirsch, J. H. Humphrey, W. G. Spector, and H. L. Langevoort.** 1972. The mononuclear phagocyte system: a new classification of macrophages, monocytes and precursor cells. Bull. W.H.O. **46:**845–852.

Interaction of Piliated *Escherichia coli* with Phagocytes

K. JANN,* B. JANN, AND E. BLUMENSTOCK

Max-Planck-Institut für Immunobiologie, D-78 Freiburg, West Germany

Bacterial pili (or fimbriae) mediate adherence of bacteria to the surface of eukaryotic cells. If this adherence can be inhibited by α-mannosides, it is termed mannose sensitive (MS); otherwise, it is termed mannose resistant (MR). The term MR applies to pili which may be structurally or functionally different. MS pili mediate adherence to many epithelial cells (including tissue culture cells) and also to phagocytes. MR pili cause adherence to mainly uroepithelial, buccal, or intestinal epithelial cells (1a, 2). Most *Escherichia coli* strains causing urinary tract or enteric infections exhibit MR pili, which play a role in the infective process. It was therefore of interest to know whether phagocytes also have receptors for MR pili. To evaluate the situation in a nonimmune host, the adherence of *E. coli* with MS or MR pili to rat peritoneal macrophages and to human peripheral polymorphonuclear granulocytes was tested

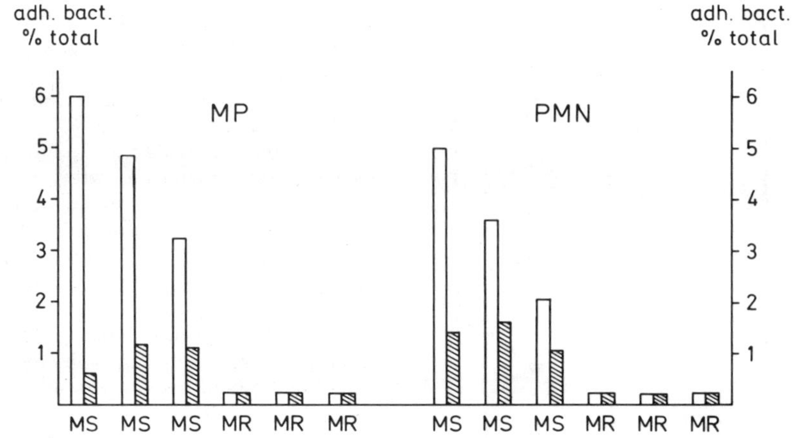

FIG. 1. *Adherence of E. coli with MS or MR pili to phagocytes in the absence (□) or presence (▨) of 50 mM α-methylmannoside. Abbreviations: PM, rat peritoneal macrophages; PMN, human peripheral polymorphonuclear granulocytes.*

in the absence of antibodies. The adherence was monitored with radiolabeled *E. coli* and also by measuring the chemiluminescence which accompanies the adherence of particles and bacteria (3).

The bacteria (*E. coli* isolated from urine, feces, or blood) were cultivated before the tests by three daily passages in static culture in Merck standard broth and then grown in the same medium for 18 h with or without [^{14}C]acetate, according to the test used. To repress the formation of pili, the bacteria were grown at 20°C (pilus-restrictive temperature) instead of 37°C. In all experiments, 10^8 bacteria were added to monolayers of about 10^6 phagocytes. The phagocytes were cultivated in the absence of serum, and the bacteria were not opsonized (i.e., not treated with antiserum). For measurement of chemiluminescence, the phagocytes were cultivated in Packard vials. Adherence of radioactive bacteria was measured after 40 min, and chemiluminescence was measured continuously for 60 min in a scintillation counter at 37°C in the off coincidence mode.

As measured by radioactivity, *E. coli* with MS pili exhibited MS adherence to the phagocytes, and *E. coli* with MR pili did not adhere at all (Fig. 1). In the same fashion, chemiluminescence was observed with the phagocytes only after contact with *E. coli* exhibiting MS pili. Bacteria with MR pili did not induce chemiluminescence (Fig. 2).

In parallel experiments, we found that more than 95% of the adherent *E. coli* were killed by the phagocytes within 40 min. Thus, nonimmune adherence of *E. coli* to phagocytes results in the elimination of the bacteria.

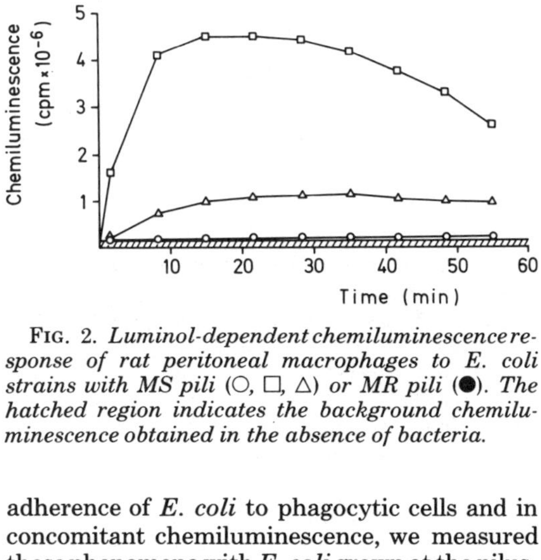

FIG. 2. *Luminol-dependent chemiluminescence response of rat peritoneal macrophages to E. coli strains with MS pili (○, □, △) or MR pili (●). The hatched region indicates the background chemiluminescence obtained in the absence of bacteria.*

Since MS pili seemed to play a role in the adherence of *E. coli* to phagocytic cells and in concomitant chemiluminescence, we measured these phenomena with *E. coli* grown at the pilus-restrictive temperature of 20°C. In some cases, neither adherence nor chemiluminescence was observed; in others, both were exhibited to the same extent as with piliated bacteria. Thus, piliation is not the only means of adherence, which can presumably also be mediated by cell wall adhesins (1).

The results indicate that plasma membranes of phagocytes contain receptors for bacterial MS pili (or MS cell wall adhesins) but do not contain or express receptors for bacterial MR pili. Because MR pili of pathogenic *E. coli* mediate adherence to epithelial cells but not to phagocytes, these bacteria are able to start mucous membrane-borne infections and to escape phagocytosis in the absence of antibodies (i.e., in the preimmune state of the host at the onset of infection). Thus, MR pili are bacterial assets for pathogenicity.

1. **Blumenstock, E., and K. Jann.** 1982. Adhesion of piliated *Escherichia coli* strains to phagocytes: differences between bacteria with mannose-sensitive pili and those with mannose-resistant pili. Infect. Immun. **35:** 264–269.
1a. **Duguid, J. P., and D. C. Old.** 1980. Adhesive properties of Enterobacteriaceae, p. 185–217. *In* E. H. Beachey (ed.), Receptors and recognition, vol. B6, Bacterial adherence. Chapman and Hall, London.
2. **Jann, K., B. Jann, G. Schmidt, and K. Vosbeck.** 1981. Adhesion of *Escherichia coli* to mammalian and yeast cells: role of pilation and hydrophobicity. Infect. Immun. **32:**484–489.
3. **Nelson, R. D., E. L. Mills, R. L. Simmins, and P. R. Quie.** 1976. Chemiluminescence response of phagocytizing human monocytes. Infect. Immun. **14:**129–134.

Effect of Antiteichoic Acid Antibody on the Adherence to Damaged Heart Valves of Bacterial Cells Grown in Subinhibitory Concentrations of Penicillin

CARLOS H. RAMIREZ-RONDA,* ZELMA FUXENCH-CHIESA, AND RAMON A. RAMIREZ-RONDA

Infectious Disease Program, University of Puerto Rico School of Medicine and Veterans Administration Medical Center; Departments of Research and Medicine, Veterans Administration Medical Center, and Department of Medicine, University of Puerto Rico School of Medicine, San Juan 00936 Puerto Rico, U.S.A.*

Gram-positive cocci adhere well to normal heart valves in vitro, whereas aerobic gram-negative bacilli do not adhere well with the exception of *Pseudomonas aeruginosa* (2). The ability of a given bacterial strain to adhere to a specific surface is one important factor in determining localization of infection caused by the specific bacterial strain. This adhering ability contributes to the pathogenicity of that organism (1). The adherence of gram-positive cocci to damaged heart valves, valves covered with fibrin and platelets, is five times greater than the adherence to normal valves (7). This increased adherence has been demonstrated with glucan-producing strains like *Streptococcus sanguis* and glucan-negative strains like *Enterococcus* and *Staphylococcus* (10). The production of glucans by glucan-positive strains is partially responsible for the adherence of such strains. The increased adherence of glucan-negative strains depends on factors other than glucan production. The adherence of *S. sanguis*, a glucan-positive strain, to damaged heart valves is dependent on dextrans of high molecular weight, including commercial dextran T-2000 and glucans from *S. sanguis* and *S. mutans* (6). This adherence can be partially interfered with by the use of low-molecular-weight dextrans (7). The adherence of glucan-negative strains to damaged heart valves can be blocked by the addition of exogenous crude extracts of teichoic acids and by purified teichoic acids (9). Preincubation of damaged heart valves with exogenous purified teichoic acids and preexposure of *S. sanguis*, *S. mutans*, *Enterococcus*, *S. aureus*, and *S. epidermidis* to rabbit antiteichoic acid serum (ATAS) interfered with adherence of these strains, resulting in a decreased adherence (9). The binding of certain bacteria to epithelial cells has been shown to be mediated by a group of heterogenous substances, ligands, that are present on the surface of the organisms and are capable of recognizing specific determinants, receptors, on the membranes of epithelial cells (3). The data from previous studies suggest that teichoic acids may be a ligand for gram-positive cocci adherence.

Growth of microorganisms in subinhibitory concentrations (SIC) of antibiotics has been demonstrated to alter their morphological characteristics (4). Growth of gram-positive cocci in SIC of antibiotics decreases the adherence to damaged heart valves (8) and suppresses the bacterial adherence of *Escherichia coli* to epithelial cells (5). The supernatant of bacterial cells grown in SIC of antibiotics has been found to have teichoic acids.

A study was designed to determine the role of teichoic acids in the inhibition of adherence found when the bacteria are grown in SIC of antibiotics and to determine the effect of ATAS on such adherence inhibition, looking specifically at penicillin and two glucan-negative strains of gram-positive cocci, *S. aureus* CR-100 and *Enterococcus* KG-3. We also wanted to explore the possible role of teichoic acids as ligands in the adherence.

The bacterial strains used were recovered from patients with endocarditis, were serum resistant, and had the following MIC for penicillin: *S. aureus*, 0.0625 μg/ml; and *Enterococcus*, 4 μg/ml. The bacteria were kept lyophilized and were reconstituted fresh for the experiments. Bacterial cells from overnight cultures were grown to log phase; they were then subcultured into a growth medium containing a concentration of penicillin equal to one-eighth the MIC of the organisms and grown for 4 h. After this growth period, the bacterial cell suspension was standardized as previously described (2, 6, 7). Experiments were carried out with the antibiotic-grown bacterial suspension or with a collection of the treated cells suspended in different adherence media, such as phosphate-buffered saline (PBS), fresh growth medium, fresh growth medium with penicillin, or rabbit serum as defined in the tables. Adherence was also carried by using the supernatant of the growth medium with SIC of penicillin. Before use, the supernatant was centrifuged three times and passed through a 0.45-μm membrane filter. In this medium, adherence was determined with fresh bacterial cells and treated bacterial cells and after addition of various concentrations of ATAS to the adherence medium.

Adherence was determined as previously described (2, 6, 7), using circular canine heart valve sections of 2-mm diameter. Valve damage was produced in dogs by placement of a catheter in the left ventricle for 18 h as previously described (2, 6, 7). The adherence ratio was the number of cells that adhered to the valve sections over the number of cells in the standardized bacterial suspension.

ATAS was prepared by immunizing New Zealand white rabbits with purified teichoic acids dissolved in 0.25 ml of solvent plus an equal volume of Freund complete adjuvant. Immunization was repeated serially for 8 to 12 weeks. Antibody was quantitated by double diffusion in agar against purified teichoic acids; the titers ranged from 1:8 to 1:64, with a median of 1:16.

Table 1 shows the effect of growth in SIC of penicillin on the two study strains. Adherence

TABLE 1. *Effect of growth of S. aureus and Enterococcus in SIC of penicillin (one-eighth MIC for 4 h) on the adherence to damaged canine heart valves*[a]

Condition	Adherence ratio (×10⁵) (mean ± SEM)	
	S. aureus	*Enterococcus*
Control	2,900 ± 180	5,400 ± 280
SIC growth		
Adherence in growth medium	690 ± 80	1,290 ± 192
Adherence in PBS	1,095 ± 186	2,041 ± 280
Adherence in fresh penicillin	1,108 ± 174	2,076 ± 271

[a] A minimum of four experiments were conducted under each experimental condition.

decreased threefold when the bacterial cells were grown in SIC. When the adherence medium was other than the original supernatant (PBS, fresh growth medium with penicillin), the adherence was slightly decreased.

When ATAS was mixed at various concentrations with the supernatant of the bacterial cells grown in SIC of penicillin, the adherence blocking ability of the supernatant was decreased and adherence was partially restored. ATAS neutralized the free or liberated teichoic acids present in the supernatant released from the bacterial cells. This effect (Table 2) was maximal at an ATAS dilution of 1:10 and was similar for both study strains.

Preexposure of bacterial cells to ATAS decreased the adherence of these cells; ATAS apparently blocked the teichoic acids in the surface

TABLE 2. *Effect of the supernatant of bacterial cells grown in SIC of penicillin (one-eighth MIC for 4 h) on the adherence of fresh bacterial cells to damaged heart valves and modification of the effect by rabbit ATAS*[a]

Condition	Adherence ratio (×10⁵) (mean ± SEM)	
	S. aureus	*Enterococcus*
Control	2,900 ± 180	5,400 ± 280
SIC growth		
No antiserum	690 ± 80	1,290 ± 192
ATAS, 1:1	2,164 ± 172	3,826 ± 186
ATAS, 1:5	2,401 ± 178	3,960 ± 176
ATAS, 1:10	2,289 ± 149	3,919 ± 200
ATAS, 1:20	2,060 ± 161	3,624 ± 202
ATAS, 1:40	1,840 ± 78	3,433 ± 192
Fresh cells		
No antiserum	1,399 ± 174	2,701 ± 280
ATAS, 1:1	2,501 ± 181	3,809 ± 300
ATAS, 1:5	2,662 ± 179	4,101 ± 293
ATAS, 1:10	2,600 ± 194	4,005 ± 273
ATAS, 1:20	2,132 ± 183	3,404 ± 206
ATAS, 1:40	1,699 ± 181	3,001 ± 302

[a] See Table 1.

TABLE 3. *Effect of preexposure of bacterial cells, damaged heart valves and supernatant of cells grown in STC of bacteria to rabbit ATAS (antibody titer, 1:32)*

Condition	Adherence ratio (×10⁵) (mean ± SEM)	
	S. aureus CR-100	*Enterococcus* KG-3
Control	2,900 ± 1800	5,400 ± 280
Growth in SIC	690 ± 80	1,290 ± 192
Preexposure to ATAS		
Bacterial cells	750 ± 93	1,084 ± 176
Heart valves	2,810 ± 176	5,390 ± 299
Supernatant	2,600 ± 194	4,005 ± 273

or cell wall of the bacteria. Preexposure of the damaged valve sections to ATAS had no demonstrable effect on adherence. The data suggest that teichoic acids may be the ligands and that the receptors are in the damaged valve (Table 3).

Teichoic acids present in the bacterial cell wall of the study strains are one of the mediators of adherence of these organisms to damaged heart valves. Growth of the bacterial cells in SIC of antibiotics causes release of teichoic acids to the growth medium, and these "free ligands" bind to the receptor sites in the damaged valve, blocking adherence of the bacterial cell. Teichoic acids appear to be a ligand in the adherence of gram-positive cocci to damaged heart valves.

1. **Gibbons, R. J.** 1977. Adherence of bacteria to host tissue, p. 395–406. *In* D. Schlessinger (ed.), Microbiology—1977. American Society for Microbiology, Washington, D.C.
2. **Gould, K., C. H. Ramirez-Ronda, R. K. Holmes, and J. P. Sanford.** 1975. Adherence of bacteria to heart valves *in vitro*. J. Clin. Invest. **56**:1364–1370.
3. **Jones, G. S.** 1978. The attachment of bacteria to the surface of animal cells, p. 139–176. *In* J. L. Reissing (ed.), Receptors and recognition, series B, vol. 3, Microbial interaction. Chapman and Hall, London.
4. **Lorian, V., M. Koike, O. Zak, U. Zanon, L. Sabath, G. Grassi, and W. Stille.** 1978. Effects of subinhibitory concentrations of antibiotics on bacteria, p. 72–78. *In* W. Siegenthale and R. Luthy (ed.), Current chemotherapy. American Society for Microbiology, Washington, D.C.
5. **Ofek, I., E. H. Beachey, B. I. Eisenstein, et al.** 1979. Suppression of bacterial adherence by subminimal inhibitory concentrations of β-lactam and aminoglycoside antibiotics. Rev. Infect. Dis. **1**:832–837.
6. **Ramirez-Ronda, C. H.** 1978. Adherence of glucan-positive and glucan-negative streptococcal strains to normal and damaged heart valves. J. Clin. Invest. **62**:805–814.
7. **Ramirez-Ronda, C. H.** 1980. Effects of molecular weight of dextran on the adherence of *Streptococcus sanguis* to damaged heart valves. Infect. Immun. **29**:1–7.
8. **Ramirez-Ronda, C. H., and J. Gutierrez.** 1980. Decreased adherence of *S. sanguis* to damaged heart valves by subinhibitory concentrations of penicillin *in vitro*. Clin. Res. **28**:377A.
9. **Ramirez-Ronda, C. H., J. Gutierrez, and R. H. Bermudez.** 1980. Effects of teichoic acids on adherence of *S. sanguis*, *S. mutans* and Enterococci to damaged heart valves *in vitro*. Clin. Res. **28**:377A.
10. **Sheld, W. M., J. A. Valone, and M. A. Sande.** 1978. Bacterial adherence in the pathogenesis of endocarditis. Interaction of bacterial dextran, platelets and fibrin. J. Clin. Invest. **61**:1394–1400.

Kinetics of Adhesion of *Escherichia coli* SS142 to Intestine 407 Tissue Culture Cells

KLAUS VOSBECK* AND HELMUT METT

Pharmaceuticals Division, Research Department, CIBA-GEIGY Limited, Basel, Switzerland

We have developed an in vitro assay technique for measuring bacterial adhesion that is sufficiently accurate and reproducible to determine the kinetics of bacterial adhesion (1). The assay measures the binding of radiolabeled bacteria to monolayers of the human epithelioid tissue culture cell line Intestine 407 (ATCC CCL6). A comparative study of the adhesiveness of more than 30 *Escherichia coli* strains in several different assay systems (adhesion to different tissue culture cells, adhesion to urinary tract epithelial cells, hemagglutinating capacity, and hydrophobic interaction chromatography) showed that strains found to be adhesive by other techniques frequently also adhered to Intestine 407 cells. This assay was therefore judged to measure biologically relevant adhesive properties of bacteria. The interaction of *E. coli* SS142 with Intestine 407 cells was investigated in more detail.

E. coli SS142 was found to adhere specifically to Intestine 407 cells. Adhesion was linear with time for at least 90 min under the conditions used. Bacterial binding was also linear with increasing bacterial concentration up to 10^9 bacteria per monolayer when incubation times of less than 40 min were used. Saturation of adhesion was observed at higher bacterial numbers or at prolonged incubation times. Within the range of linear conditions, a constant rate of bacterial adhesion of approximately 4%/h of the total added radioactivity was observed. These binding characteristics, including the low apparent rate of bacterial adhesion, are in good agreement with adhesion characteristics in different assay systems reported by other investigators.

The relatively low rate of bacterial adhesion might be due to the presence of bacterial subpopulations with different adhesiveness. To test this hypothesis, we added a radiolabeled bacterial suspension to Intestine 407 cell monolayers and allowed the bacteria to adhere for 20 min. Thereafter, unbound bacteria were collected, transferred to fresh monolayers, and again allowed to adhere for 20 min. This procedure was repeated six times. Bacterial adhesion expressed as the percentage of radioactivity bound after each transfer to fresh monolayers was found to be constant throughout the experiment (Fig. 1). This result, together with the linearity of the assay with time, is strong evidence against the presence of stable bacterial subpopulations differing in their adhesiveness, since such a heterogeneity of the bacteria would have resulted in decreasing adhesiveness in this experiment.

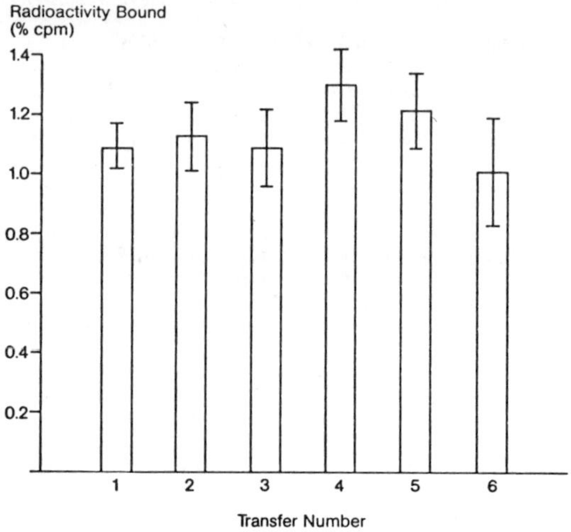

FIG. 1. *Homogeneity of bacterial suspension. A suspension of radiolabeled E. coli SS142 was allowed to adhere to Intestine 407 monolayers for 20 min. The unbound bacteria were collected, transferred to fresh monolayers, and again allowed to adhere for 20 min. This process was repeated six times. The percentage of radioactivity bound to the monolayers was determined after each transfer.*

TABLE 1. *Irreversibility of E. coli SS142 adhesion to Intestine 407 monolayers*[a]

Incubation time[b] (min)	No. of *E. coli* SS142 cells[c] ($\times 10^6$): Remaining bound to monolayer	Released into buffer
0	4.2	0.72
20	4.4	0.74
40	4.3	0.73
60	4.3	0.77

[a] During the initial incubation, 5×10^8 *E. coli* SS142 (5.9×10^{-4} cpm per bacterium) were allowed to adhere to Intestine 407 monolayers. Unbound bacteria were then removed, and the radioactivity associated with the cell monolayers, as well as the radioactivity in the buffer, was monitored.

[b] Time after removal of unbound bacteria.

[c] Calculated from radioactivity measurements.

A low rate of bacterial adhesion might also be due to reversible binding of bacteria to cell monolayers. We found, however, that adhesion of *E. coli* SS142 to Intestine 407 cells was essentially irreversible. A radiolabeled bacterial suspension was added to cell monolayers, and the bacteria were allowed to adhere. Thereafter, unbound bacteria were removed by washing, and buffer without bacteria was added to the monolayers. The radioactivity associated with the monolayers, as well as the radioactivity in the buffer, was monitored at intervals during 60 min. During this time neither a decrease of the cell-associated radioactivity nor an increase of the radioactivity in the buffer could be detected, indicating the irreversibility of bacterial binding (Table 1). It should be mentioned that *E. coli* SS142 did not multiply under the conditions of this experiment. The irreversibility of bacterial adhesion was not due to cellular engulfment of bacteria, as shown by transmission electron microscopy. More than 200 bacteria attached to Intestine 407 cells in a 40-min incubation were randomly checked by transmission electron microscopy. None of them was located inside an Intestine 407 cell. Rather, the bacteria were seen in close contact with many microvilli, suggesting multiple binding and consequent irreversible microvillar entanglement of bacteria. Bacteria entangled in a meshwork of microvilli could also be observed by scanning electron microscopy. The rate-limiting step in adhesion may be a comparatively slow cellular process, such as formation of microvilli. Since adhesion is irreversible, it may be highly effective in mediating colonization even though it proceeds at a slow rate.

The assistance of C. Brücher and J. Suter (CIBA-GEIGY Limited, Pharmaceuticals Division, Basel, Switzerland) in preparing the electron microscopic preparations is gratefully acknowledged.

1. **Vosbeck, K., H. Handschin, E. B. Menge, and O. Zak.** 1979. Effects of subminimal inhibitory concentrations of antibiotics on adhesiveness of *Escherichia coli* in vitro. Rev. Infect. Dis. **1**:845–851.

Effect of Treatment with Subinhibitory Concentrations of Antibiotics and In Vivo Fate of Bacteria in the Mouse

ZSUZSANNA PUSZTAI-MARKOS AND F. PRANADA

Department of Medical Microbiology, RWTH Aachen, 5100 Aachen, West Germany

In a recent study (Zs. Pusztai-Markos, F. Pranada, and C. Leimbrock, Chemotherapy, in press) we found that the filamentous form of a serum-resistant *Escherichia coli* strain (isolated from a patient with chronic pyelonephritis; the strain showed a high mouse virulence after intraperitoneal [i.p.] administration; LD_{50}, 5×10^5 to 5×10^6) which developed under in vitro exposure to a sub-MIC of moxalactam showed a higher resistance against host defense than the nontreated bacteria. Significantly diminished lethality and a longer-lasting persistence in the peritoneal cavity of the mouse were found after i.p. infection. To exclude the suggestion that the enhanced virulence was due only to the separation of filaments into several normal virulent bacilli, the course of experimental infection with normal virulent bacteria was investigated in mice under treatment with subtherapeutic doses of the antibiotic. For evaluation of differences in the degree of virulence, which are not pronounced, the estimation of the lethal effect did not seem to be suitable. LD_{50} defines only the lethal effect but gives no information about the severity of the infectious process when not leading to death. Therefore, we estimated the peritoneal clearance 4 h after i.p. infection as a measure of macrophage function, and we found that in animals treated with repeated doses of 10 to 15 μg of moxalactam per kg a significantly smaller elimination rate of bacteria took place in the peritoneal cavity than in animals injected with saline.

The present study was designed to reinvestigate this phenomenon in respect to other antibiotics and, furthermore, in respect to other serum-resistant and serum-susceptible *E. coli* bacteria.

Male mice of the outbred line NMRI weighing 14 to 16 g were treated subcutaneously 6 and 2 h before and 2, and in the case of the longer-lasting experiments also 6 and 10, h after infection with different doses of antibiotics (0.2, 2, and 20 μg per mouse); control animals were given saline. We compared the in vivo effect of moxalactam (compound LY 127935, lot no. CT-4765-OP), cefamandole (Mandokef, lot no. AXPOD 53), ampicillin (Pen-Bristol, lot no. 2283), and fosfomycin (Fosfocin, lot no. 725843). Each of them was active in vitro against the serum-resistant *E. coli* strain. MICs were as follows (g/liter): moxalactam, 0.125; cefamandole, 1; ampicillin, 4; and fosfomycin, 2. We found a significantly diminished peritoneal clearance only in the case of moxalactam under in vivo treatment. The other antibiotics exhibited neither positive nor negative effects although given in higher concentration, at least under these experimental conditions.

With regard to the survival of bacteria in the spleen, i.e., under the longer-lasting follow-up of the experimentally induced infection, a more pronounced influence of the antibiotic treatment was observable (Fig. 1). Depending on the concentration, either a significant increase of colony-forming units (CFU) in comparison with the control, i.e., an enhancement of virulence and a diminished host defense, or a decrease of CFU, i.e., a therapeutic effect, could be demonstrated. This effect seems to be the result of a complex mechanism controlled by the antibiotic on the one hand and by the infecting microorganism on the other. In the case of the antibiotic, its mechanism of action and the actual in vitro activity may play a crucial role. From the point of view of the microbes, the ratio of the number of injected bacteria to the dose of the antibiotic has to be considered and in this connection also their virulence, which mainly depends on the cell wall structure, especially in the case of gram-negative bacilli. It is well known that the cell wall structure is decisive for serum susceptibility and for resistance to phagocytosis and that the synthesis of the cell surface components depends on the growth environment (2) and the multiplication rate (3).

Therefore, we investigated in a further series of experiments the effect of moxalactam treatment on the in vivo fate of a serum-sensitive *E. coli* strain (ATCC 25922; MIC of moxalactam, 0.125 g/liter). The mouse virulence of the serum-sensitive *E. coli* strain was low in contrast to the highly virulent serum-resistant strain. No significant differences were observed between control and treated animals evaluated with viable count either in the peritoneal lavage or in the spleen, although several experiments were carried out with different infecting doses. Similarly, no effect was demonstrated when higher doses of moxalactam were given. On the other hand,

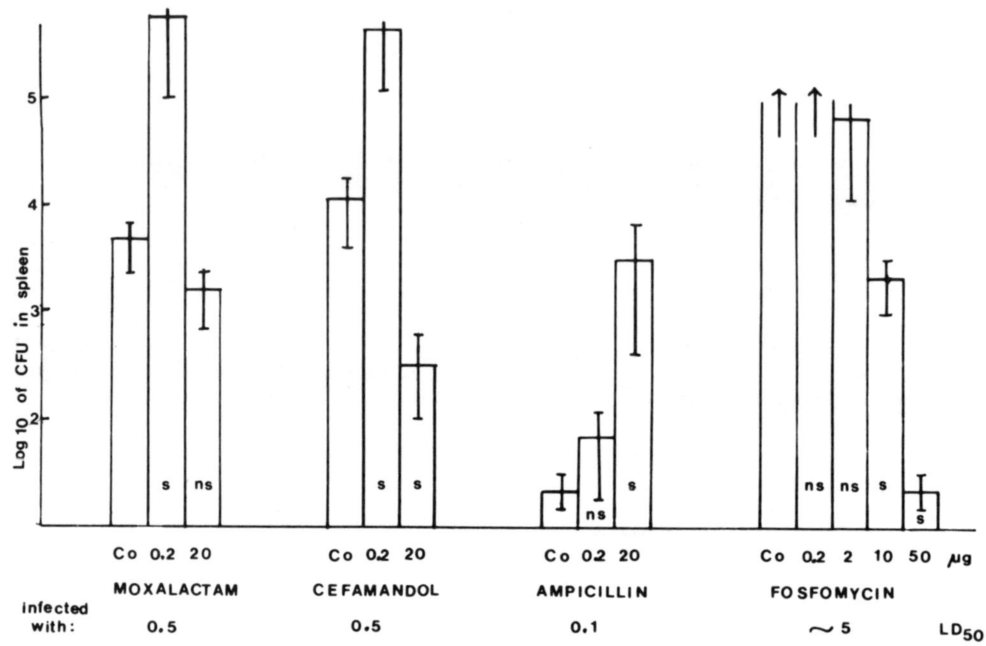

FIG. 1. *In vivo fate of the serum-resistant E. coli strain in mice. Mice were treated subcutaneously with antibiotics 6 and 2 h before and 2, 6, and 10 h after infection with 10^6 bacteria i.p. CFU in the spleen were determined 18 h later. Control animals were treated with saline. Mean ± 1 SD; statistical comparison of groups was established by t test.*

we could reproduce our findings with a further serum-resistant *E. coli* strain (O55:B4) in respect to a diminished in vivo elimination rate under antibiotic treatment.

This different behavior of the serum-resistant and the serum-susceptible strains suggests that the antibiotic effect is due to differences in the surface structures. Cell wall synthesis, and in this connection serum resistance, depends, among other things, on the degree of the actual state of cell division. The rate of cell multiplication can be influenced by culture conditions. In an attempt to prove the correlation between the actual surface of bacteria and the in vivo effect of moxalactam, we subcultured the serum-resistant *E. coli* strain in different ways to induce populations with different cell surfaces. Bacterial cells obtained were investigated to determine their serum susceptibility as well as their fate in vivo in animals treated with moxalactam. Bacteria grown for 2 h in a fluid medium (Iso-Sensitest broth) lost their serum resistance (99% bactericidal effect in 2 h), but bacteria of 18-h agar cultures (diagnostic sensitivity test agar) were nearly fully resistant (15% bactericidal effect), and bacteria grown for 18 h in Iso-Sensitest broth multiplied even in the presence of fresh human serum. This effect was reproducible with several *E. coli* strains showing different degrees of serum resistance. In accordance with this, distinct differences were registered in vivo (Fig. 2). The effect corresponds to the sequences in serum sensitivity: serum-sensitive bacteria induced higher CFU values in the spleen, and, correspondingly, the relative enhancement of CFU in animals treated with antibiotic was more pronounced.

This finding is seemingly in contrast to the supposition that serum-resistant organisms are more virulent. Many reports about experimentally induced infections with gram-negative bacteria in mice and in other animals suggested that serum bactericidal activity may be important as a host defense mechanism, but they were by no means conclusive. Several workers have not found support for this concept. In this context, we have to consider that the basis of serum resistance in gram-negative bacteria has not been defined with any certainty. It appears that no single factor, such as the amount or structure of lipopolysaccharide or other surface antigens, is responsible. It seems likely that under certain in vitro or in vivo influences phenotypic changes can take place but for different reasons. Probably such alterations are also inducible by antibiotics, especially by β-lactam compounds. Several publications have confirmed this assumption by experiments in vitro (see 1).

Summarizing our results, we suggest that such phenotypic conversions, in principle inducible in all bacteria, can result in a change of resistance against host defense mechanisms in a positive as

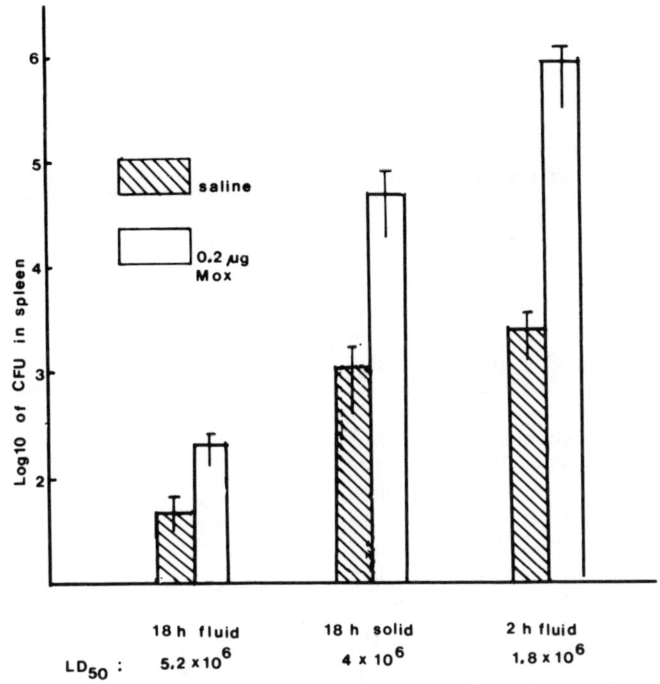

FIG. 2. *Influence of culture conditions on the in vivo fate of the serum-resistant E. coli strain in mice. Animals were treated with 0.2 µg of moxalactam (10 to 12 µg/kg of body weight). For details see Fig. 1 and text.*

well as in a negative manner. In this respect, antibiotics probably belong to the important group of triggering substances. One can presume that the effect of antibiotics in modifying the cell wall structure is most pronounced in rapidly multiplying microorganisms. Therefore, under experimental conditions this phenomenon can be accomplished more easily with virulent or serum-resistant bacteria.

1. **Lorian, V.** 1980. Effects of subminimum inhibitory concentration of antibiotics on bacteria, p. 342–408. *In* V. Lorian (ed.), Antibiotics in laboratory medicine. The Williams & Wilkins Co., Baltimore.
2. **Taylor, P. W., P. Messner, and R. Parton.** 1981. Effect of the growth environment on cell-envelope components of Escherichia coli in relation to sensitivity to human serum. J. Med. Microbiol. **14**:9–19.
3. **Waisbren, B. A., and I. Brown.** 1964. Effect of wide spectrum antibiotics on bactericidal activity of human serum in vitro and in vivo. Am. J. Med. Sci. **248**:56–62.

Enhancement of Resistance to Experimental Infections by Immunomodulating Lipopeptides

FRANÇOIS FLOC'H, JEAN BOUCHAUDON, AURELIO ZERIAL, GEORGES H. WERNER,* DANIELE MIGLIORE-SAMOUR, AND PIERRE JOLLES

Centre Nicolas Grillet, Rhône-Poulenc Recherches et Développement, 94400 Vitry-sur-Seine, and Laboratoire des Protéines, Université de Paris V, 75270 Paris, France*

Our group has described (8) the immunopotentiating activities of a microbial tetrapeptide chemically coupled with lauric acid and of a synthetic derivative, N^2-[N-(N-lauroyl-L-alanyl)-γ-D-glutamyl]N^6-(glycyl)DD,LL 2,6-diaminopimelamic acid, which is hereinafter referred to as lauroyltetrapeptide (LTP). Comparison of the in vitro and in vivo immunomodulating activities of LTP with those of the muramyl dipeptide (MDP; N-acetylmuramyl-L-alanyl-D-isoglutamine) (4) revealed many similarities but some notable differences: both compounds stimulated macrophages and exerted adjuvant effects in a number of animal models but, overall, LTP was less active than MDP in augmenting antibody production but more active in potentiating delayed-type hypersensitivity reactions. In this paper, we focus our attention on the enhancing activities of LTP and of some synthetic analogs on resistance of mice to experimental infections. The latter models included intravenous (i.v.) challenge of adult CD-1 mice with *Listeria monocytogenes* (strain EGD), intramuscular challenge of adult OF-1 mice with *Klebsiella pneumoniae* (type 2, strain IP 7823), intraperitoneal (i.p.) challenge of adult OF-1 mice with murine hepatitis virus (MHV, Friend-Braunsteiner strain), and i.v. challenge of adult OF-1 mice with *Candida albicans* (strain isolated from a human case).

In all four models, the challenge inoculum was of such size as to produce 85 to 100% mortality in less than 10 days in control mice. Treatments with MDP, LTP, and lipopeptide analogs were performed by the i.p., i.v., or subcutaneous (s.c.) routes, usually 1 day before infectious challenge (one single treatment, using graded doses of the test compound).

Table 1 summarizes the results of four experiments performed with LTP in mice infected with *L. monocytogenes*: i.p., i.v., s.c., and also oral treatments with the compound exerted significant enhancing effects on the resistance of the animals to this infection. Our own data (6) and those of others (1, 2) indicate that MDP exerts little or no effect on the infection of mice with this intracellular bacterium. When multiple i.p. treatments with LTP were performed (i.e., 14, 11, 7, 3, and 1 day before infectious challenge), protection was obtained with smaller doses (0.2 or 0.1 mg/kg) than in the case of a single treatment.

Table 2 gives the results of a comparative test of LTP and MDP in mice infected with *K. pneumoniae*. Both compounds exerted a marked enhancing effect on resistance, LTP giving higher rates of protection than MDP.

With respect to i.v. infection of mice with *C. albicans*, s.c. treatments with 0.5 and 2.5 mg of MDP per kg 3 days and 1 day before challenge increased the survival time of the animals, as already reported by others (5), whereas LTP was ineffective in this system, in which polymorphonuclear leukocytes play a key role in natural resistance (3). The *N*-palmitoyl analog of LTP, however, exerted at 0.5 mg/kg a significant resistance-enhancing effect against this infection.

In six experiments out of 10, i.p. treatment with LTP 1 day before i.p. inoculation of MHV increased significantly (P = 0.02 to 0.05) the average survival time of the infected mice; the effective dose varied, however, between 0.3 and 10 mg/kg i.p. from one experiment to another. MDP was without effect in this experimental system. It is known that experimental viral infections respond less well than bacterial infections to chemically defined low-molecular-weight immunomodulators (7).

Many analogs of LTP have been synthesized in our laboratories and examined for their in vitro and in vivo immunomodulating activities (including enhancement of resistance against infections). Among these analogs are lipodipeptides and lipotripeptides containing no diaminopimelic acid as well as lipotetra- and pentapeptides in which diaminopimelic acid is replaced with L-lysine. We report here salient data concerning their activities on infections.

Of the lipodipeptides tested, *N*-palmitoyl-L-alanyl-D-glutamic acid exerted at 10 mg/kg i.p. (1 day before challenge) a significant protective effect in mice infected with *L. monocytogenes*

TABLE 1. *Effect of pretreatment with LTP on i.v. infection of mice with L. monocytogenes*

Expt	LTP dose (mg/kg) and route	Timing of treatment (day)	Surviving mice on day +10	P value
1	None (controls)	—[a]	1/20	
	10, i.p.	−1	6/10	≤0.02
	3, i.p.	−1	7/10	≤0.02
2	None	—	1/15	
	2, i.p.	−1	6/15	≤0.006
	0.4, i.p.	−1	5/14	≤0.01
	0.1, i.p.	−1	2/15	NS[b]
3	None	—	4/30	
	2, i.p.	−1	6/15	≤0.004
	2, i.p.	−2	6/15	≤0.015
	2, s.c.	−2	6/15	≤0.04
	2, i.v.	−2	8/15	≤0.001
4	None	—	1/10	
	50, orally[c]	−2	4/10	≤0.01
	10, orally	−2	1/10	NS

[a] Controls were treated with saline.
[b] NS, Not significant.
[c] Compound was dissolved in soybean oil.

TABLE 2. *Effect of pretreatment with LTP or MDP on intramuscular infection of mice with K. pneumoniae*

Compound	Dose (mg/kg) and route	Timing of single treatment (days)	Surviving mice on day +10	P value
None (controls		—[a]	4/30	
LTP	2.5, i.v.	−1	14/15	≤0.001
LTP	0.5, i.v.	−1	6/15	≤0.004
MDP	2.5, i.v.	−1	10/15	≤0.001
MDP	0.5, i.v.	−1	3/15	≤0.01

[a] Controls were treated with saline.

but was inactive on infections with *C. albicans* and MHV. Two s.c. treatments (days −3 and −1) with this compound at 2.5 mg/kg enhanced resistance against *K. pneumoniae*. On the other hand, *N*-behenoyl-L-alanyl-D-glutamic acid was active (at 2.5 mg/kg i.v. or s.c.) against *K. pneumoniae* but inactive against *L. monocytogenes*, *C. albicans*, and MHV.

Two lipotripeptides exhibited some resistance-enhancing activities. $N\alpha$-[*N*-(lauroyl-L-alanyl)-γ-D-glutamyl]-L-lysine was active at 30 mg/kg i.p. against *L. monocytogenes* but ineffective against the other infections, whereas $N\alpha$-[*N*-(*N*-palmitoyl-L-alanyl)-γ-D-glutamyl]-L-lysine bromohydrate was active at 0.5 and 0.1 mg/kg s.c. against *K. pneumoniae*, slightly active at 10 mg/kg i.p. against *L. monocytogenes*, and inactive against the two other infections.

The lipopentapeptide $N\alpha$-[*N*-(*N*-lauroyl-L-alanyl)-γ-D-glutamyl]$N\xi$-(glycyl)-L-lysyl-D-alanine and the lipotetrapeptide $N\alpha$-[*N*-(*N*-lauroyl-L-alanyl)-γ-D-glutamyl]$N\xi$-(glycyl)-L-lysine exerted discrete protective effects in mice infected with *L. monocytogenes* but were inactive against the other infections.

In conclusion, nonspecific resistance-enhancing activities of immunopotentiating agents such as our lipopeptides may vary to a considerable extent, in their intensity and also in their spectrum, with their chemical configuration and the nature of the fatty acid chain, independently from the other in vitro and in vivo immunomodulating activities which they may exert. In this family of compounds, nonspecific antiinfectious activity was maximal when the molecules contained diaminopimelic acid.

1. **Finger, H., and C. H. Wirsing von König.** 1980. Failure of synthetic muramyldipeptide to increase antibacterial resistance. Infect. Immun. **27**:288–291.
2. **Humphres, R. C., P. R. Henika, R. W. Ferraresi, and J. L. Krahenbuhl.** 1980. Effects of treatments with muramyldipeptide and certain of its analogs on resistance to *Listeria monocytogenes* in mice. Infect. Immun. **29**:462–466.
3. **Hurtrel, B., P. H. Lagrange, and J. C. Michel.** 1980. Systemic candidiasis in mice. II. Main role of polymorphonuclear leukocytes in resistance to infection. Ann. Immunol. (Inst. Pasteur) **131C**:105–118.
4. **Lederer, E.** 1980. Synthetic immunostimulants derived from the bacterial cell wall. J. Med. Chem. **23**:819–825.
5. **Matthews, T. R., and E. B. Fraser-Smith.** 1980. Protective effect of muramyl-dipeptide and analogs against *Pseudomonas aeruginosa* and *Candida albicans* infections of mice, p. 1734–1735. *In* J. D. Nelson and C. Grassi (ed.), Current chemotherapy and infectious disease. American Society for Microbiology, Washington, D.C.
6. **Migliore-Samour, D., J. Bouchaudon, F. Floc'h, A. Zerial, L. Ninet, G. H. Werner, and P. Jollès.** 1980. A short lipopeptide, representative of a new family of immunological adjuvants devoid of sugar. Life Sci. **26**: 883–888.
7. **Werner, G. H.** 1979. Immunopotentiating agents with antiviral activity. Pharmacol. Ther. **6**:235–273.
8. **Werner, G. H., F. Floc'h, A. Zerial, J. Bouchaudon, L. Ninet, D. Migliore-Samour, and P. Jollès.** 1980. Immunopotentiating activities of a microbial tetrapeptide after coupling with lauric acid, p. 1728–1730. *In* J. D. Nelson and C. Grassi (ed.), Current chemotherapy and infectious disease. American Society for Microbiology, Washington, D.C.

Bacteriological Activities of New Cephalosporins with Regard to the Phagocytosis of Human Polymorphonuclear Leukocytes

K. HIROMATSU, T. TAKASHIMA, K. TABUKI, AND T. NISHIMURA*

Department of Pediatrics, Osaka Medical College, Osaka, Japan

To evaluate the properties of new cephalosporins under conditions more closely approximating in vivo those previously used for conventional cephalosporins, effects on human polymorphonuclear leukocyte (PMN) phagocytosis, which plays an important role in the nonspecific prophylaxis of infection, were investigated.

The new cephalosporins tested were cefotaxime, ceftizoxime, cefuroxime, and 6059S (moxalactam). Cefazolin was selected as a conventional cephalosporin. The organisms tested were beta-lactamase–elaborating and -non-elaborating *Escherichia coli* and *Klebsiella pneumoniae* and beta-lactamase–elaborating *Proteus vulgaris*, *Enterobacter cloacae*, and *Staphylococcus aureus* (phage type, 80/81). The bactericidal activity of the aforementioned antibiotics alone and their bactericidal activities in the presence of human PMNs were determined and used to derive the relative bactericidal potentiation coefficient K by the formula: $K = [(\log c/b) - (\log c/a)] = (\log a/b)$, where a = bactericidal activity for the organism plus antibiotic, b = bactericidal activity for the organism plus antibiotic plus PMN, c = bactericidal activity for the organism, and d = bactericidal activity for the organism plus PMN.

In the case of both beta-lactamase–elaborat-

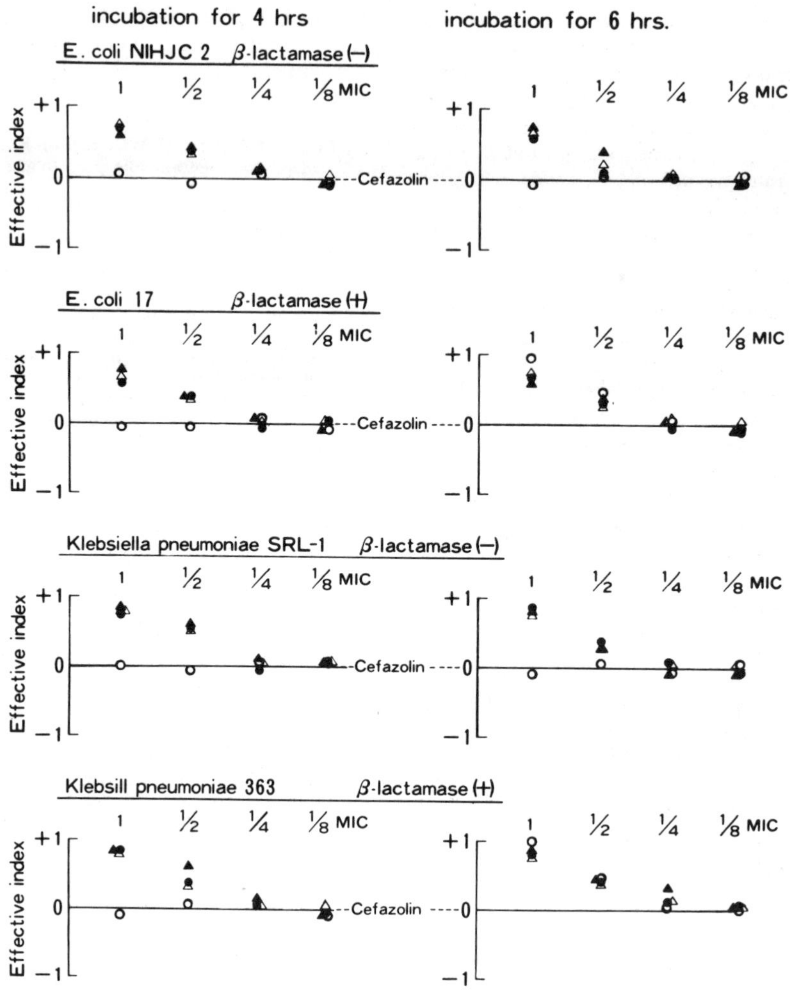

FIG. 1. *Comparison of phagocytosis of Escherichia coli by human PMNs in the presence of cefotaxime* (●), *ceftizoxime* (▲), *moxalactam* (△), *cefuroxime* (○), *and cefazolin.*

ing and -non-elaborating *Escherichia coli*, the addition of the MIC or one-half of the MIC of the new cephalosporins produced a higher bactericidal potentiation coefficient than did cefazolin. Likewise, in terms of PMN phagocytosis, the new cephalosporins apparently caused greater damage to the test organism. However, for cefuroxime, beta-lactamase–non-elaborating strains did not exhibit any difference in bactericidal potentiation coefficient compared with cefazolin. After 6 h of culturing beta-lactamase–elaborating strains, the bactericidal potentiation coefficient was increased. A similar tendency was observed for *K. pneumoniae*. This tendency became more distinct when strong beta-lactamase–elaborating strains of *P. vulgaris* and *Enterobacter cloacae* were used (Fig. 1).

To investigate how the properties of the above new cephalosporins are displayed in the therapy of a so-called compromised host, the time of leukopenia was estimated at a PMN/bacteria ratio raised from the conventional 1:1 to 1:100, and a culture period of at least 6 h was provided. When *P. vulgaris* 9, a beta-lactamase–elaborating strain, was used as the test organism, the bactericidal potentiation coefficients, with cefazolin as the control, at the MIC and one-half of the MIC, averaged 1.61 and 1.15 for cefotaxime, 1.61 and 1.09 for ceftizoxime, and 1.56 and 1.06 for moxalactam, respectively. In contrast to the results obtained for a PMN/bacteria ratio of 1:1, namely, average values of 0.78 and 0.6 for cefotaxime, 0.78 and 0.5 for ceftizoxime, and 0.8 and 0.6 for moxalactam, drug activity was distinctly enhanced. Similar studies with PMNs from patients under steroid therapy were done,

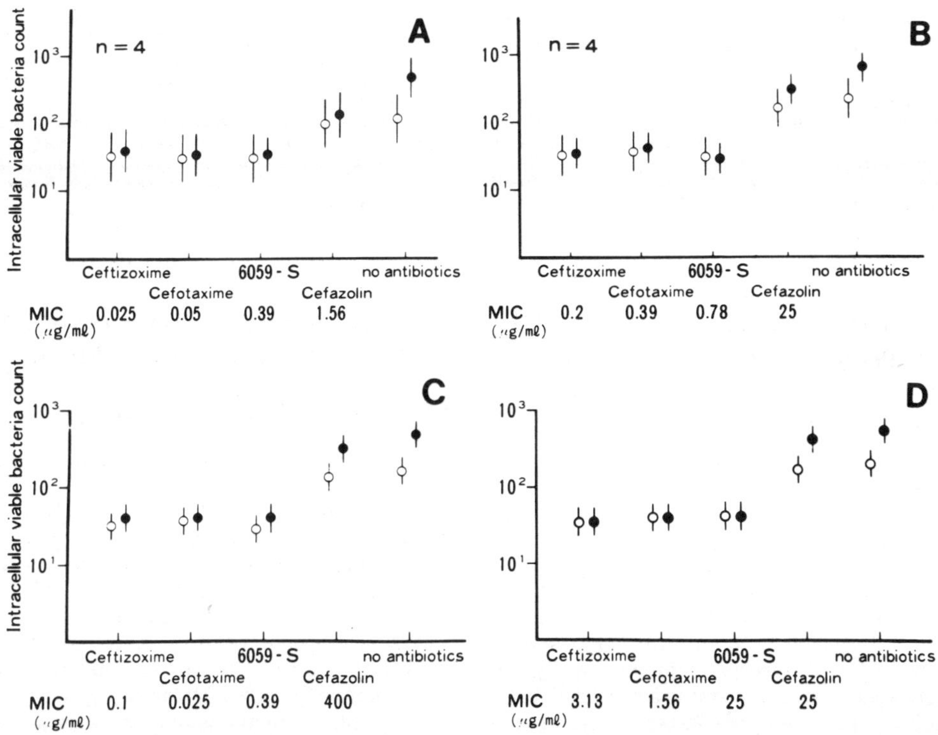

FIG. 2. *Comparison of intracellular killing of organisms pretreated with antibiotics by human PMNs. Beta-lactamase Escherichia coli NIH JC 2 (A), beta-lactamase-positive Escherichia coli 17 (B), beta-lactamase-positive P. vulgaris 9 (C) and Enterobacter cloacae 91 (D) were pretreated for 30 min with the MIC of antibiotics and incubated for 2 h. Symbols: ●, patient treated with steroid hormone; ○, healthy volunteer.*

and the results were compared with those obtained with PMNs from healthy subjects. The bactericidal potentiation coefficient was higher for PMNs from patients treated with steroids.

Next, to investigate the bactericidal process after the bacteria damaged by antibiotics are intaken by PMNs, the bacteria were pretreated for 30 min in 1 MIC of antibiotics, the antibiotic was removed, and the bacteria were allowed to be phagocytosed by the PMNs. After culturing for 2 h, the number of viable bacteria in the PMNs was investigated, using PMNs from steroid-treated patients and healthy subjects. In the case of beta-lactamase–non-elaborating *Escherichia coli* not undergoing antibiotic treatment, the number of viable bacteria in PMNs of healthy volunteers and patients treated with steroids was higher than that in the case of bacteria undergoing antibiotic treatment. This was particularly marked for PMNs for patients treated with steroids. However, after pretreatment with the new cephalosporins, there was almost no difference between the number of viable bacteria in PMNs of healthy volunteers and patients receiving steroid treatment. In comparison to cefazolin pretreatment, the viable bacteria count in the PMNs was distinctly lower (Fig. 2). In the case of beta-lactamase–elaborating *Escherichia coli*, there was no difference between the viable bacteria count of patients receiving steroids and that of healthy volunteers, even for cefazolin. After treatment with the new cephalosporins, the results were similar to those obtained with beta-lactamase–non-elaborating strains. Similar tests using *P. vulgaris* 9 and *Enterobacter cloacae* 91, strains with pronounced beta-lactamase activity, did not reveal any difference with antibiotic-pretreated bacteria, even cefazolin-pretreated bacteria, with regard to the viable bacteria count in PMNs of patients receiving steroids and those of healthy subjects. However, after pretreatment with new cephalosporins, the viable bacteria count was low for both types of PMNs, and there was no difference between the viable bacteria count in PMNs of patients receiving steroids and healthy subjects.

The above results from an investigation of the phagocytic bactericidal effects of human PMNs showed that the antibacterial activities of cefotaxime, ceftizoxime, cefuroxime, and moxalactam were superior to that of cefazolin against gram-negative rods but lower than known cephalosporins against gram-positive organisms (*S. aureus*).

1. **Chabbert, Y. A., and A. J. Luts.** 1978. HR 756, the *syn* isomer of a new methoxyimino cephalosporin with unusual antibacterial activity. Antimicrob. Agents Chemother. **14**:749–754.
2. **Cynthia, H., et al.** 1976. Cefuroxime—a new cephalosporin antibiotic. J. Antibiot. **29**:29–37.
3. **Kojo, H., M. Nishida, S. Goto, and S. Kuwahara.** 1979. Antibacterial activity of ceftizoxime (FK 749), a new cephalosporin, against cephalosporin-resistant bacteria, and its stability to β-lactamase. Antimicrob. Agents Chemother. **16**:549–553.
4. **Yoshida, T., S. Matsuura, M. Mayama, Y. Kameda, and S. Kuwahara.** 1980. Moxalactam (6059-S), a novel 1-oxa-β-lactam with an expanded antibacterial spectrum: laboratory evaluation. Antimicrob. Agents Chemother. **17**:302–312.

Reconstitution of a Functional Tn*3*-like Transposon from a *Neisseria gonorrhoeae* Plasmid Sequence Specifying β-Lactamase Synthesis

OLIVIER FAYET, YVETTE FROMENT, AND JEAN C. PIFFARETTI*

Department of Microbiology, School of Medicine, University of Geneva, 1205 Geneva, Switzerland

Since 1976, *Neisseria gonorrhoeae* strains highly resistant to penicillins (Amp^r) have been isolated throughout the world. These strains produce a plasmid-encoded β-lactamase, similar to the TEM-1 enzyme commonly found among members of the *Enterobacteriaceae* family (5). The gonococcal Amp^r plasmids are either 7.4 or 5.1 kilobases (kb) long, the latter plasmid being probably a deletion derivative of the former (6). Further studies have shown that the gonococcal β-lactamase gene is carried by a DNA sequence homologous to about 40% of the Tn*3*-like transposons. These are 5.0-kb-long transposable DNA elements flanked by two 38-base-pair inverted repeat sequences (IR-L and IR-R) necessary for the transposition process (see Fig. 1); they encode three proteins: a transposase (gene *tnpA*), a regulatory protein (gene *tnpR*), and the β-lactamase (gene *bla*) (2). Heteroduplex analysis confirmed that the gonococcal Amp^r homology region is 1.6 kb long and demonstrated its relatedness with the right part of the Tn*3*-like transposons (see Fig. 1), including the *Bam*HI cleavage site (3; this laboratory). From such observations, it was suggested that the gonococcal Amp^r sequence had originated from Tn*3*-like transposons (commonly found among enteric bacteria) by deletion. In this paper, we give strong evidence supporting this hypothesis by demonstrating that the gonococcal Amp^r sequence has retained an intact and functional portion of the Tn*3*-like transposons (from the *Bam*HI site within *tnpR* to the IR-R sequence included). This was done by reconstructing an active transposon by in vitro recombination. The principle of this reconstitution is diagrammed in Fig. 1. We attempted to link the 2.4-kb *bla*-containing *Bam*HI fragment from pPJ102 (a gonococcal Amp^r plasmid isolated in Geneva) to the *Bam*HI-*Eco*RI 6.8-kb fragment of pPJ3b which carries the left part of Tn*2301* (pPJ3b is a resistance plasmid isolated from an *Escherichia coli* clinical isolate; it carries Tn*2301*, which is a Tn*3*-like transposon [4]).

To supply an *Eco*RI–*Bam*HI linker and to provide an efficient replication unit for the recombinant plasmid, we used the large 4.8-kb *Eco*RI–*Bam*HI fragment of pMB9 (1). The three plasmids were digested with the endonucleases *Bam*HI and *Eco*RI, and the appropriate fragments were purified by agarose gel electrophoresis, ligated, and transformed into *E. coli* C600. Amp^r colonies were obtained, and 48 of them were analyzed for their plasmid content. Five had the expected fragment composition, and one, pPJ109, was further analyzed by Southern hybridization experiments to ensure that its three endonuclease fragments were derived from the expected sources.

Transposition of Amp^r from plasmid pPJ109 onto bacteriophage λ DNA was assayed by infecting, at 37°C, *E. coli* C600 (pPJ109) cultures with phage λ*c*I857*b*515*b*519*Sam*7 (λbb) at a multiplicity of five phages per bacterium. The infected cultures were incubated for 210 min at 37°C and lysed by the addition of chloroform. Phages were titrated, and the frequency of infective particles able to transduce Amp^r (i.e., having inserted an Amp^r transposon into their DNA) was measured by infecting *E. coli* C600 and selecting at 30°C for Amp^r lysogens on nutrient agar containing ampicillin.

Using these conditions, we found that Amp^r could transpose from pPJ109 onto λbb DNA

[1] Present address: Centre de Biochimie et Genétique Cellulaires du CNRS, 31077 Toulouse, France.

[2] Present address: Istituto Cantonale Batteriologico, 6904 Lugano, Switzerland.

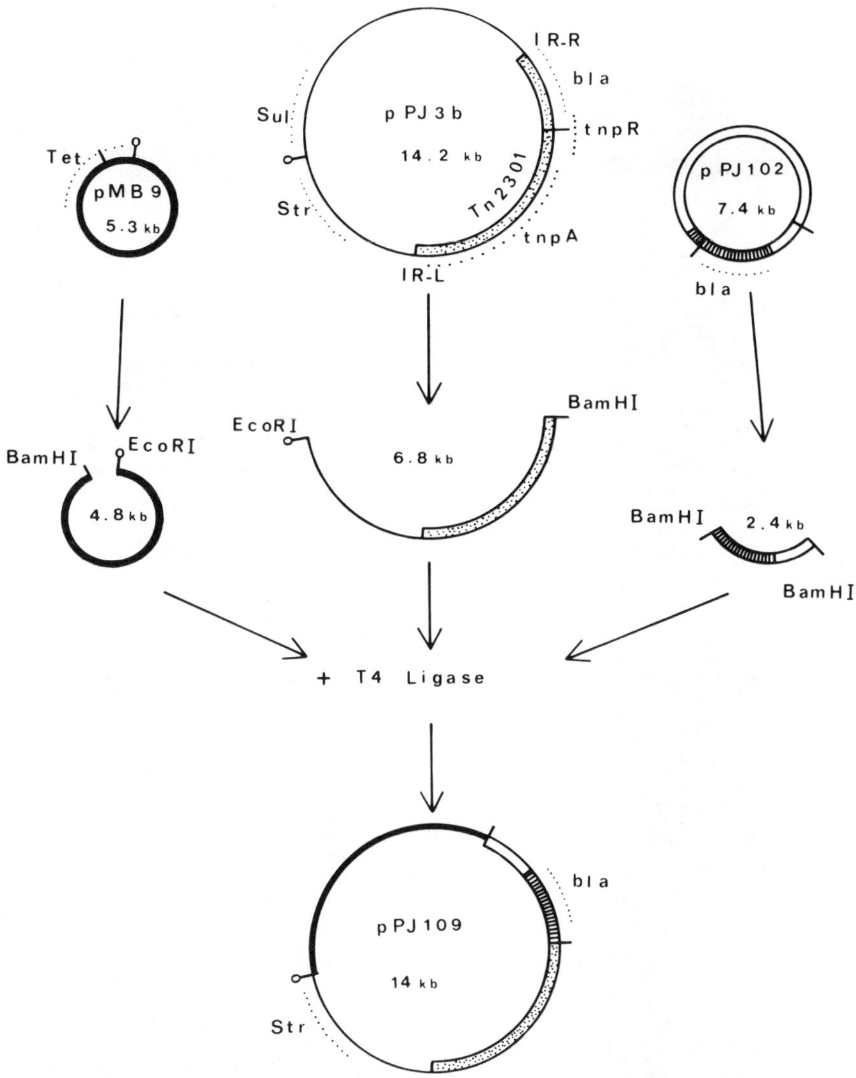

FIG. 1. *Construction of a recombinant plasmid by the addition of the 4.8-kb EcoRI-BamHI fragment of pMB9, the 6.8-kb EcoRI-BamHI fragment of pPJ3b, and the 2.4-kb BamHI fragment of pPJ102. Tn2301 is a Tn3-like transposon (4).*

with a frequency of 1.7×10^{-7}. This is similar to the 2.0×10^{-7} value obtained for the control experiment with plasmid pPJ3b (which carries Tn*2301*) as a transposon donor. Amp^r lysogenic colonies obtained after infection of *E. coli* C600 with phage λbb grown on strains harboring pPJ109 were then purified and used to prepare phage stocks. Their Amp^r transducing activity was found to be very high, up to 100% for single lysogens. This is what is expected for true transposition events.

The presence of a 5-kb insertion (the length of a Tn*3*-like transposon) in the DNA of λbb is demonstrated here for one of these high-frequency transducing phage lysates, by use of *Eco*RI endonuclease restriction analysis. Figure 2 shows that the 5.6-kb *Eco*RI fragment of λbb (slot 1) has disappeared and has been replaced by a novel 10.6-kb fragment in the λbb transducing DNA (slot 2), i.e., by a fragment enlarged by 5.0 kb. This clearly indicates that the gonococcal plasmids do contain, in addition to the *bla* gene, an IR-R flanking sequence, since the presence of such a sequence is necessary for transposition (2). They must also contain an intact right part of a *tnpR* gene, since inactiva-

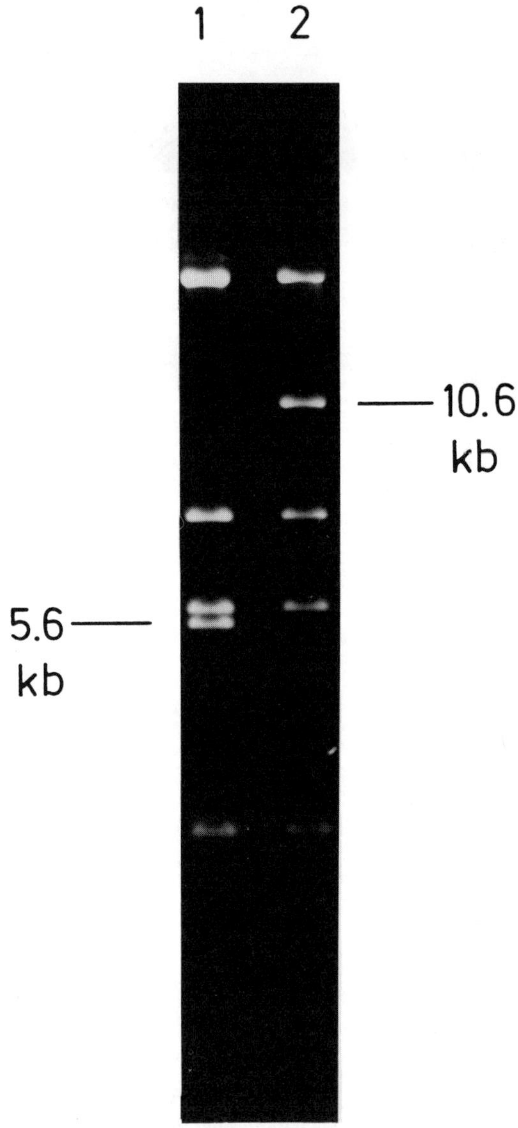

FIG. 2. *Agarose gel electrophoresis of the DNAs digested with EcoRI of λbb (slot 1) and λbb which has received the Amp^r transposon from pPJ109 (slot 2).*

tion of this gene would have resulted in higher transposition frequency (2). Thus, the hypothesis that gonococcal Amp^r plasmids have evolved from a plasmid which contained an entire Tn*3*-like transposon by a deletion event that removed the left side of the transposable element is clearly supported.

The presence of part of a Tn*3*-like transposon, the base composition, and the ability to replicate in *E. coli* suggest an enteric origin for the Amp^r gonococcal plasmids. This would imply the transfer of genetic material between *N. gonorrhoeae* and other bacterial species. The finding of similar plasmids in Amp^r *Haemophilus influenzae* strains supports this hypothesis. Among the possible mechanisms for such transfer are conjugation and transformation, both of which have been shown to occur in the gonococcus. However, additional epidemiological and genetic studies are required to clarify the origin of the gonococcal Amp^r plasmids.

This work was supported by a grant (3.258-77) from the Swiss National Science Foundation to J.C.P.

1. **Bolivar, F., R. L. Rodriguez, M. C. Betlach, and H. W. Boyer.** 1977. Construction and characterization of new cloning vehicles. I. Ampicillin-resistant derivatives of the plasmid pMB9. Gene **2:**75–93.
2. **Heffron, F., B. J. McCarthy, H. Ohtsubo, and E. Ohtsubo.** 1979. DNA sequence analysis of the transposon Tn*3*: three genes and three sites involved in transposition of Tn*3*. Cell **18:**1153–1163.
3. **Laufs, R., P. M. Kaulfers, G. Jahn, and U. Teschner.** 1979. Molecular characterization of a small *Haemophilus influenzae* plasmid specifying β-lactamase and its relationship to R factors from *Neisseria gonorrhoeae.* J. Gen. Microbiol. **111:**223–231.
4. **Piffaretti, J. C., and Y. Froment.** 1981. Analysis of the plasmid content of an *E. coli* clinical isolate: characterization of pPJ3a, pPJ3b, and of the transposon Tn*2301.* FEMS Microbiol. Lett. **10:**169–174.
5. **Roberts, M., L. P. Elwell, and S. Falkow.** 1977. Molecular characterization of two beta-lactamase-specifying plasmids isolated from *Neisseria gonorrhoeae.* J. Bacteriol. **131:**557–563.
6. **Sox, T. E., W. Mohammed, and P. F. Sparling.** 1979. Transformation-derived *Neisseria gonorrhoeae* plasmids with altered structure and function. J. Bacteriol. **138:**510–518.

R-Plasmid from a Clinical Isolate, *Pseudomonas putida* KPS45

MEGUMI KONO, KOJI O'HARA, KIYOSHI MAKINO, HAJIME HAMASHIMA, AND MASANORI SASATSU

Tokyo College of Pharmacy, 1432-1, Horinouchi, Hachioji, Tokyo 192-03, Japan

In the past few years, a large number of R-plasmids have been reported in *Pseudomonas aeruginosa* (3). Recently, an R-plasmid coding for tetracycline (TC) and ampicillin resistance in *P. cepacia* was reported by Williams et al. (5) in 1979. A naturally occurring recombinant plasmid between a degradation plasmid and an R-plasmid coding for resistance to streptomycin (SM) and sulfonamide was also isolated from *Pseudomonas* spp. by Yano and Nishi (6). This paper deals with a transferable R-plasmid coding for resistance to SM and kanamycin (KM) of a clinical isolate, *P. putida* KPS45. This strain was isolated from a patient suffering from urinary tract infection.

The MIC of SM for KPS45 was 800 μg/ml. This strain has also been found to have SM-inactivating ability. Conjugal transfer of the SM resistance of KPS45 to various species of gram-negative rods was examined. Recipient strains used were all marked with rifampin (RFP) resistance. Mating was carried out at 37 or 30°C by the plate mating method (4) or the filter mating method (1). Transconjugants were selected on the plate containing RFP-SM or RFP-KM. Results of conjugal transfer of SM resistance in KPS45 to the drug-susceptible recipients are shown in Table 1. Bacteria developed on the selection plate were all resistant to SM, with an MIC of more than 100 μg/ml, and could inactivate SM. This implies that the SM resistance of KPS45 was introduced into *P. aeruginosa*, *P. fluorescens*, *P. putida*, *Escherichia coli*, *Shigella flexneri*, *Salmonella typhi*, and *Serratia marcescens.* As can be seen in Table 1, transconjugants were also highly resistant to KM. This suggests that the donor strain KPS45 had KM resistance as well as SM resistance, even though the MIC of KM for the strain was relatively low at 25 μg/ml. Resistance to SM or KM could not be introduced into *Proteus vulgaris*, *P. mirabilis*, *P. rettgeri*, and *P. morganii* by conjugation. Secondary intraspecific transfer of the SM/KM resistance was examined, and it was found that the drug resistance of the transconjugant obtained from *P. aeruginosa* 2704RFP *met*$^-$, *his*$^-$ by mating with KPS45, and the transconjugant obtained from *E. coli* K-12 W3110RFP by mating with KPS45, could be introduced into the second recipients *P. aeruginosa* KPS47RFP and *E. coli* ML1410, respectively (data not shown). From the data described above, it was confirmed that a transferable R-plasmid coding for SM and KM resistance was present in KPS45. The detection of R-plasmids from KPS45 and the transconjugants obtained from the strains (Table 1) by mating with KPS45 was carried out. When agarose gel electrophoresis of the cleared lysate was applied, plasmid DNA was not detected from KPS45. However, when the method of Hansen and Olsen (2) was used for the isolation of plasmid DNA, a plasmid DNA band was found by agarose gel electrophoresis from KPS45 and three transconjugants, as shown in Table 1. Plasmid DNA recovered from the agarose gel plate was examined in an electron microscope, and the molecular weight of the plasmid was estimated. As can be seen in Table 2, R-plasmids from KPS45 and the three transconjugants obtained from *P. aeruginosa* 2704-RFP, *P. aeruginosa* KPS47RFP, and *E. coli* W1895HfrC RFP were found to have the same size, and the DNA was estimated at 52 megadaltons. This plasmid was designated as pTP450.

Plasmid pTP450 obtained from KPS45 was digested with the restriction endonuclease *Eco*RI followed by agarose gel electrophoresis. Although the data are not shown here, 18 fragments having various sizes (13.5, 11.0, 6.8, 3.4, 2.9, 2.9, 2.1, 1.6, 1.6, 1.4, 1.3, 1.05, 0.80, 0.80, 0.66,

TABLE 1. *Transfer of SM and KM resistance of P. putida KPS45*

Strains used							Transconjugants			
Strain no.	MIC (μg/ml)				Mating[a]	Selected by[b]	MIC (μg/ml)		SM inactivation	Plasmid
	TC	CP	SM	KM			SM	KM		
P. putida KPS45	12.5	50	800	25						
P. aeruginosa 2704RFP *met*$^-$, *his*$^-$	25	50	50	25	37°P	RFP/SM	800	200	+	+
P. aeruginosa KPS47RFP	50	100	50	100	37°P	RFP/SM	800	400	+	+
P. fluorescens 1070RFP	6.3	50	3.2	0.8	30°F	RFP/SM	800	800	+	NT[c]
P. putida 581RFP	25	400	50	1.6	30°F	RFP/KM	>800	>800	+	NT
E. coli K-12 W3110RFP	12.5	6.3	6.3	6.3	37°F	RFP/SM	100	100	+	−
E. coli K-12 W1895HfrC RFP	12.5	<3.2	<3.2	<3.2	37°F	RFP/SM	100	400	+	+
S. flexneri TCP290RFP	12.5	3.2	3.2	3.2	37°F	RFP/SM	200	400	+	NT
S. typhi 901RFP	12.5	6.3	50	6.3	37°F	RFP/KM	400	>1600	+	−
S. marcescens TCP2951RFP	50	25	25	<3.2	37°F	RFP/KM	400	>1600	+	−

[a] See text.
[b] RFP, 100 μg/ml, and SM, 400 μg/ml, for *Pseudomonas* strains; RFP, 100 μg/ml, and SM, 25 μg/ml (or KM, 50 μg/ml), for the others.
[c] NT, Not tested.

TABLE 2. *Plasmids isolated from KPS45 and transconjugants resistant to SM and KM*

Bacteria	Plasmid DNA isolated		
	No. of molecules measured	Contour length ± SSD[a] (μm)	Molecular wt[b]
KPS45	20	25.3 ± 1.3	$52.4 \pm 2.7 \times 10^6$
Transconjugants from			
P. aeruginosa 2704RFP	12	25.5 ± 1.3	$52.8 \pm 2.7 \times 10^6$
P. aeruginosa KPS47RFP	10	25.4 ± 1.8	$52.6 \pm 3.7 \times 10^6$
E. coli K12W1895 HfrC RFP	10	25.1 ± 1.0	$52.0 \pm 2.1 \times 10^6$

[a] Sample SD.
[b] The molecular weight of plasmid DNA was estimated by using a factor of $2.04 \pm 0.04 \times 10^6/\mu m$.

0.50, 0.28, and 0.26 megadaltons) were observed. The total molecular weight of the DNA fragments was 52.8×10^6, which corresponded to the molecular weight estimated by electron microscopy. To analyze the genetic nature of pTP450, we attempted the introduction of the plasmid into *E. coli* by transformation. In this experiment, a much smaller plasmid than pTP450 was also expected to be obtained. A sample of DNA for the transformation was used after digestion with *Eco*RI followed by ligation with T4 ligase. *E. coli* C was used as the recipient. Eight transformants were obtained from the selection plate, which was a Drigalski agar plate containing 25 μg of SM per ml. From the representative transformant, designated TF4, a 13.0-megadalton plasmid was detected. This corresponded to the size of the largest DNA fragment obtained by *Eco*RI digestion of pTP450. The plasmid, designated pTP451, was stable in the new host after 10 successive subcultures in a drug-free medium. Strain TF4 required MICs of more than 400 μg/ml for both SM and KM and possessed SM-inactivating ability. From the results, it was concluded that SM- and KM-resistant genes are present in the 13-megadalton region within the 52 megadaltons of the original plasmid pTP450.

In the presence of the crude extract from KPS45, [γ-^{32}P]ATP was clearly shown to be incorporated into the SM molecule. This indicated that the mechanism of SM inactivation by KPS45 was due to phosphorylating enzyme activity. Further details of the mechanism of the resistance of KPS45 to SM and KM will be published in another report.

1. **Bryan, L. E., H. M. Van Den Elzen, and J. T. Tseng.** 1972. Transferable drug resistance in *Pseudomonas aeruginosa*. Antimicrob. Agents Chemother. **1**:22–29.
2. **Hansen, J. B., and R. H. Olsen.** 1978. Isolation of large bacterial plasmids and characterization of P2 incompatibility group plasmids pMG1 and pMG5. J. Bacteriol. **135**:227–238.
3. **Jacoby, G. A.** 1979. Plasmids of *Pseudomonas aeruginosa*, p. 271–309. *In* R. G. Doggett (ed.), *Pseudomonas aeruginosa*. Academic Press, Inc., New York.
4. **Kono, M., and K. O'Hara.** 1975. Prevalence of R factors in *Pseudomonas aeruginosa*. J. Gen. Microbiol. **91**: 191–194.
5. **Williams, J. A., J. P. Yeggy, C. C. Fields, and A. J. Markovetz.** 1979. Resistance plasmids in *Pseudomonas cepacia* 4G9. J. Bacteriol. **140**:1017–1022.
6. **Yano, K., and T. Nishi.** 1980. pKJ1, a naturally occurring conjugative plasmid coding for toluene degradation and resistance to streptomycin and sulfonamides. J. Bacteriol. **143**:552–560.

Influence of Plasmid-Mediated Aminoglycoside-Modifying Enzymes on the Bactericidal Action of Aminoglycosides

S. S. CHUNG, H. B. DRUGEON, J. WITCHITZ, AND A. L. COURTIEU

Laboratoire de Bactériologie A, CHU, Hôtel-Dieu, Nantes, France

The extensive use of aminoglycoside antibiotics despite their toxicity is based on their bactericidal activity. In a previous paper (2), we compared the bactericidal activity of principal molecules of aminoglycosides on *Escherichia coli* ATCC 25922, demonstrating good activity of sisomicin and gentamicin and less activity of tobramycin.

The plasmid-mediated resistance results from the production of enzymes that modify the antibiotic molecule. Certain aminoglycoside antibiotics have the site for the enzymatic reaction without the diminution of their bacteriostatic activity.

In this work we have studied whether the presence of a site for enzymes influences the

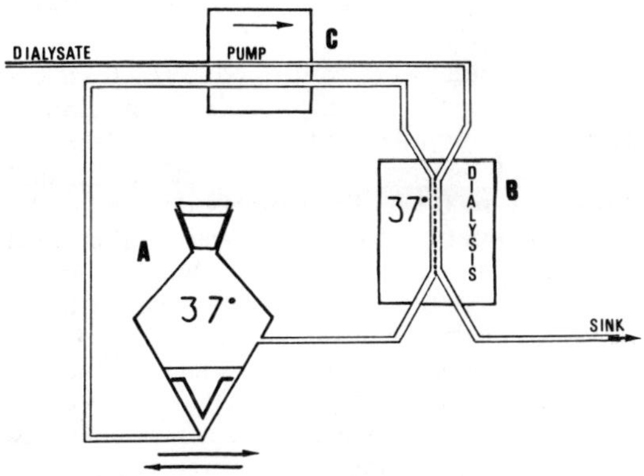

FIG. 1. *Dynamic model used.*

bactericidal activity of aminoglycosides. Six aminoglycoside antibiotics (amikacin, tobramycin, gentamicin, sisomicin, and dibekacin) were studied in five strains of *E. coli* K-12 carrying plasmids and two susceptible strains of *E. coli* K-12 as controls. The plasmid-mediated enzymes studied were AAC(6′)-I·R5, ANT(2″)·Rip 55, AAC(3)-I·Rip 135, and AAC(3)-II·Rip 176.

The bactericidal activity was studied in a static model (1) using 0.5, 1, 1.5, 2, and 3 times the MIC as antibiotic concentrations. The surviving bacteria were counted each hour during 7 h. From bactericidal kinetics the minimal bactericidal times (MBTs) were calculated. MBT is the time required for antibiotic to decrease the initial population to 0.01% survival of bacteria. This value can be extrapolated (1).

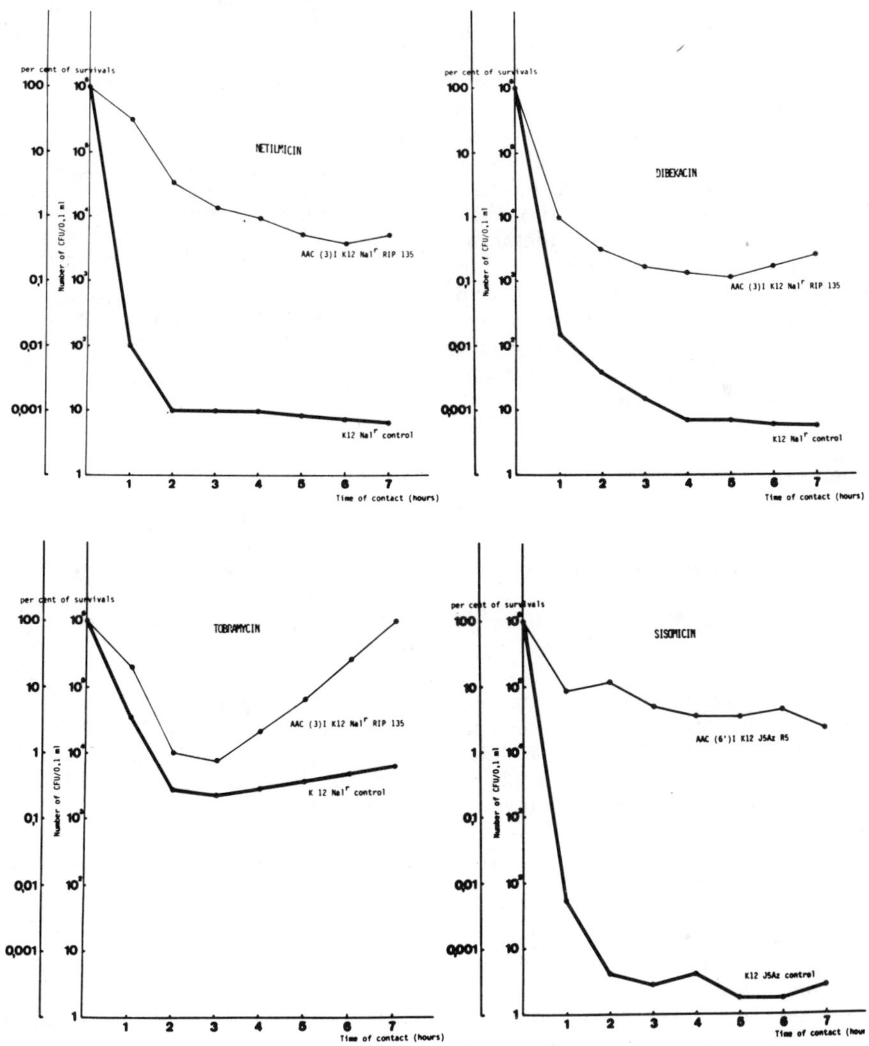

FIG. 2. *Killing curves in the dynamic model.*

The bactericidal activity of these aminoglycosides was also studied in a dynamic model simulating the serum pharmacokinetics of antibiotic (3). For this dynamic model we used the apparatus represented in Fig. 1. The decreasing concentrations of antibiotic were realized by dialysis. The half-life obtained was a linear function of volume *V* of Mueller-Hinton broth in the reaction circuit.

The surviving bacteria were counted each hour during 7 h. The concentrations of antibiotic were checked by dosage using the agar diffusion method. The comparison of results was limited to the antibiotics possessing the target of the enzyme and sensitive to the modification without augmentation of MIC. We also studied the activity of gentamicin and sisomicin against AAC(6′)-I, amikacin against ANT(2″), AAC(3)-I, and AAC(3)-II, netilmicin against ANT(2″) and AAC(3)-I, and tobramycin and dibekacin against AAC(3)-I.

In a static model, AAC(3)-I brought an important diminution of the bactericidal effect of netilmicin, dibekacin, and tobramycin. For the first molecule the MBT could not be obtained even at three times the MIC. For the two others the MBT was almost 24 h at three times the MIC. AAC(6′)-I decreased the bactericidal activity of sisomicin but not that of gentamicin. This difference could be explained by the fact that gentamicin is a complex of three molecules and that gentamicin C_1 does not have the enzymatic site for this enzyme. The activity of netilmicin was not modified by ANT(2″), and that of amikacin was not modified by ANT(2″), AAC(3)-I, and AAC(3)-II.

These results were confirmed in the dynamic model (Fig. 2). With AAC(3)-I, netilmicin brought the population to slightly less than 1% survival of bacteria at the seventh hour, and dibekacin, to 0.1%. Tobramycin decreased the initial population to 1% survival at the third hour, but a secondary growth was observed, leading to 100% survival at the seventh hour. These three molecules have an activity that is bacteriostatic rather than bactericidal. This was the same for sisomicin with AAC(6′)-I. We observed a little more than 1% survival at the seventh hour. Amikacin and gentamicin did not have the modification of their bactericidal activity. Their killing curves were identical with strains carrying plasmid and the controls.

In summary, netilmicin, tobramycin, and dibekacin showed only bacteriostatic activity on the strain possessing AAC(3)-I. Sisomicin had the same effect on the strain with AAC(6′)-I. Amikacin and gentamicin always showed bactericidal activity.

1. **Drugeon, H. B., and A. L. Courtieu.** 1979. Comparaison des pouvoirs bactéricides de 4 aminosides: amikacine, gentamicine, kanamycine et tobramycine. Ann. Microbiol. (Paris) **130A:**331–343.
2. **Drugeon, H. B., S. S. Chung, B. Maurisset, and A. L. Courtieu.** 1980. Activité bactéricide des aminosides, p. 37–57. *In* Journées de réanimation de l'Hôpital Claude-Bernard 1980. Librairie Arnette, Paris.
3. **Drugeon, H. B, B. Maurisset, and A. L. Courtieu.** 1979. Bactéricidie des aminosides dans un système statique et dans un modèle dynamique. Nouv. Presse Med. **8:**3403–3407.

R Factors in Clinical Isolates of *Bacteroides*

RUFINO JIMÉNEZ, JOSÉ C. PALOMARES,* AND EVELIO J. PEREA

Department of Microbiology, Medical School, University of Seville, Seville, Spain

Bacteroides, an obligate anaerobic gram-negative bacillus, is the predominant microorganism of the fecal microflora and is frequently isolated from other sites from healthy persons as well as from numerous infections; clinical isolates are usually resistant to several drugs.

We studied 60 *Bacteroides* strains (38 *B. fragilis*, 8 *B. vulgatus*, 6 *B. ovatus*, 5 *B. distasonis*, and 3 *B. thetaiotaomicron*) isolated from clinical specimens for the presence of plasmids, and, when isolated, their transmissibility and relationship with antibiotic resistance.

MICs were determined as described previously (1). The following antibiotics were used: cephalothin (CF), cefadroxil, cefoxitin (CX), cefuroxime, cefoperazone (T-1551), cefsulodin, moxalactam, cefotaxime (CTX), metronidazole, erythromycin, cefamandole, carbenicillin, chloramphenicol, cefaclor, tetracycline (TC), and clindamycin.

The presence of plasmids in the strains was detected by using agarose gel electrophoresis of purified DNA, as previously described (5). To determine the transferability of the plasmids detected, the filter-mating method, described by Breffort et al. (2), was used. Two different recipient strains were used in these experiments: *B. fragilis* TM4000 and *Escherichia coli* K-12 E711.

Electrophoresis was carried out on all the

strains. The results of the strains that showed any DNA band are expressed in Table 1. Only nine strains showed plasmids by this method, and the size of such plasmids ranged from 4.0 to 20.0 megadaltons (Mdal). All these strains were used as donors in filter-mating experiments, with both *B. fragilis* TM4000 and *E. coli* K-12 E711 as recipients. Only four strains showed transferability of part of their antibiotic resistance pattern (Table 2).

Drug-resistant transconjugants of *B. fragilis* A107 and *E. coli* K-12 E711 and *B. vulgatus* A182 and *E. coli* K-12 E711 matings contained a plasmid with a size of approximately 5.0 Mdal and showed resistance to ampicillin (AM), CTX, and CF. We were unable, by this method, to transfer these plasmids to *B. fragilis* TM4000 used as receptor. Transconjugants of *B. fragilis* A108 and *B. fragilis* TM4000 and *B. fragilis* A140 and *B. fragilis* TM4000 matings contained a plasmid of approximately 4.0 Mdal and showed resistance to TC. We were unable to transfer these plasmids to *E. coli* K-12 E711. The other five strains with plasmids of 4.0 Mdal (four strains) and 20.0 Mdal (one strain) did not transfer antibiotic resistance to the recipient strains.

TABLE 1. *Plasmids detected in 60 Bacteroides spp. clinical isolates*

Strain	Antibiotic resistance pattern[a]	Plasmid (Mdal)
B. fragilis A 108	CL, CAR, CTX, AM, CF, TC, EM	4.8
B. fragilis A 140	CL, CAR, CTX, AM, CF, TC, EM	4.8
B. fragilis A 107	CL, MTZ, CTX, AM, CF, EM	5.0
B. ovatus A 182	CL, MTZ, CTX, AM, CF, EM	5.0
B. fragilis A 138	CTX, AM, CF	20.0
B. vulgatus A 159	CTX, AM, CF	4.0
B. fragilis A 167	CTX, AM, CF	4.0
B. fragilis A 169	CTX, AM, CF	4.0
B. fragilis A 176	CTX, AM, CF	4.0

[a] Antibiotics tested: clindamycin (CL), carbenicillin (CAR), cefotaxime (CTX), ampicillin (AM), cephalothin (CF), tetracycline (TC), erythromycin (EM), and metronidazole (MTZ).

The presence of plasmids in *Bacteroides* has been well documented (3, 4, 6–8), with different patterns of resistance or with different cryptic plasmids. In this study, we have found four different plasmids in *Bacteroides* spp. with a size of 4.0, 4.8, 5.0, and 20.0 Mdal, respectively. Usually plasmids with a size of 4.0 or 5.0 Mdal are nontransferable because the number of genes needed (over 20) for that process is very high, and they required a bigger autotransferable plasmid than that which promotes the cotransference of the small one (8).

Nevertheless, the transconjugant we obtained, showing resistance to TC, or to CTX, AM, and CF, had the same plasmids as the donor strains, and we have not been able to detect any other plasmid of bigger size in such strains. No conjugation with donor-cell filtrates or chloroform-treated donor-cell supernatants has been detected, which argues against transduction, though the possibility of transformation still remains.

The plasmid that confers resistance to β-lactam antibiotics (CTX, AM, and CF) codes for the production of β-lactamase that has also been demonstrated in the transcipients of *E. coli* K-12 which did not produce it before the mating process. These data suggest that there are two types of plasmids, one of them conferring β-lactamase production (resistance to CTX, AM, and CF) with a size of 5.0 Mdal and the other conferring resistance to TC alone of 4.2 Mdal. The mechanisms of plasmid transfer still remain to be clarified, possibly by conjugation.

1. **Borobio, M. V., J. Aznar, R. Jiménez, F. Garcia, and E. J. Perea.** 1980. Comparative "in vitro" activity of 1-oxa-β-lactam (LY 127935) and cefoperazone with other β-lactam antibiotics against anaerobic bacteria. Antimicrob. Agents Chemother. **17:**129–131.
2. **Breffort, G., M. Magot, H. Ionesco, and M. Sebald.** 1977. Characterization and transferability of *Clostridium perfringens* plasmids. Plasmid **1:**52–66.
3. **Guiney, D. G., and C. E. Davis.** 1975. Isolation of plasmid deoxyribonucleic acid from two strains of *Bacteroides*. J. Bacteriol. **124:**503–510.

TABLE 2. *Transfer of antibiotic[a] resistance from B. fragilis and B. vulgatus to B. fragilis TM 4000 and to E. coli K-12 E 711*

Donor strain	Recipient strain	Selected markers	Plasmids in transcipients	Unselected markers
B. fragilis A 107	*E. coli* K-12 E 711[b]	AM^r, aerobic growth	5.0	CTX, CF
B. vulgatus A 182	*E. coli* K-12 E 711	AM^r, aerobic growth	5.0	CTX, CF
B. fragilis A 108	*B. fragilis* TM 4000[c]	TC^r, RA^r	4.8	
B. fragilis A 140	*B. fragilis* TM 4000	TC^r, RA^r	4.8	

[a] Antibiotics tested: ampicillin (AM), tetracycline (TC), rifampin (RA), cefotaxime (CTX), cephalothin (CF), clindamycin (CL), metronidazole (MTZ), erythromycin (EM), carbenicillin (CAR), and nalidixic acid (NA).

[b] *E. coli* K-12 E 711 is resistant to CL, MTZ, EM, and NA.

[c] *B. fragilis* TM 4000 is resistant to CL, CAR, CTX, AM, CF, and RA.

4. **Guiney, D. G., and C. E. Davis.** 1978. Identification of a conjugative R plasmid in *Bacteroides ochraceus* capable of transfer to *Escherichia coli*. Nature (London) **274**:181–182.
5. **Palomares, J. C., and E. J. Perea.** 1979. R plasmid ecology in *Salmonella* in human gut. *In* S. Mitsuhashi, L. Rosival, and V. Krcmery (ed.), Fourth International Symposium on Antibiotic Resistance. Springer-Verlag, Vienna.
6. **Privitera, G., A. Dublanchet, and M. Sebald.** 1979. Transfer of multiple antibiotic resistance between subspecies of *Bacteroides fragilis*. J. Infect. Dis. **139**:97–101.
7. **Tally, F. P., D. R. Snydman, S. L. Gorbach, and M. H. Malamy.** 1979. Plasmid mediated, transferable resistance to clindamycin and erythromycin in *Bacteroides fragilis*. J. Infect. Dis. **139**:83–88.
8. **Young, F. E., and L. Mayer.** 1979. Genetic determinants of microbial resistance to antibiotics. Rev. Infect. Dis. **1**:55–62.

Molecular Cloning of the Oxa-β-Lactamase Gene of Plasmid R46

DIANNE GODWIN* AND JEREMY W. DALE

University of Surrey, Guildford, England

The oxa-2 β-lactamase of the N-group plasmid R46 is one of the few penicillinases which hydrolyze oxacillin more readily than benzylpenicillin. With a molecular weight (45,000) twice that of the majority of β-lactamases and with a structure which is believed to consist of two apparently equal-size subunits, it is an unusual β-lactamase (3). It is further distinguished by its unusual sensitivity to chloride ions and its binding to the dye Cibacron blue (2). By the cloning and eventual nucleotide sequencing of the β-lactamase *bla* gene, we hoped to investigate the evolutionary relationship of this β-lactamase enzyme to other groups of penicillinases.

The plasmid pKM101 (Fig. 1), derived from R46 by a single deletion of 14 kilobases (kb) which left the *bla* gene intact, was used as a source of DNA (6). Langer et al. (4) had localized the *bla* gene to a region surrounding the unique *Eco*RI site of the plasmid (Fig. 1). A preliminary cloning experiment, which involved the double digestion of pKM101 DNA with the restriction endonucleases *Bam*HI and *Sal*I followed by insertion of the 2.59-kb fragment into the plasmid vector pACYC184 (1), resulted in the formation of unstable recombinant plasmids. Recombinant clones were selected for by resistance to ampicillin and chloramphenicol and tested for susceptibility to tetracycline. However, growth in liquid culture of plasmid-carrying cells resulted in a reversion to ampicillin susceptibility that, on investigation by restriction endonuclease analysis and agarose electrophoresis, was found to be caused by the deletion of all or part of the cloned fragment. In some cases insertion of the cloned fragment had initially caused deletions in the plasmid vector which produced a number of recombinants smaller than the plasmid vector. Transformation of the recombinant plasmids into three different host strains indicated that the deletion event was independent of the *recA* nature of the host strains. Similar problems were encountered with the insertion of the *bla*-containing fragment into the plasmid pMB9.

The same standard procedures were used to insert the 2.59-kb fragment containing the *bla* gene into the single-stranded phage vector M13mp7 (5). Cloning into the *Bam*HI and *Sal*I sites of the phage caused insertional inactivation of its β-galactosidase gene, and so phage isolated from colorless plaques were used to infect *Escherichia coli* JM103 to test for β-lactamase pro-

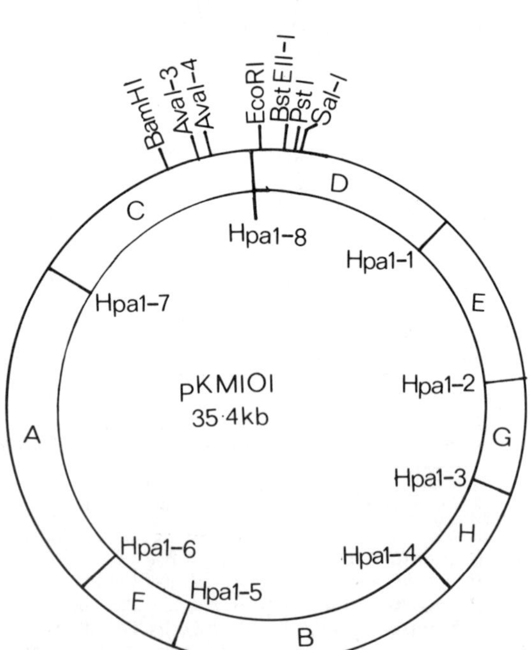

FIG. 1. *Restriction endonuclease map of the plasmid pKM101 (4).*

duction. After growth for 4 h at 37°C to allow for expression of phage genes, the culture was spotted onto L agar plates which were plus and minus ampicillin (10 μg/ml). After incubation at 37°C for 12 h, the colonies infected with phage were scored for ampicillin resistance or susceptibility, and the chromogenic cephalosporin nitrocefin was used to detect β-lactamase production. A number of recombinant phage expressing the oxa-2 β-lactamase were isolated and appeared to maintain the cloned fragment.

In a separate experiment, the insertion of *Hpa*I-generated fragments of pKM101 (Fig. 1) into the plasmid vector pKN80 (7) resulted in the formation of a recombinant clone which carried *Hpa*I fragments B and D. This clone was found to express an oxa-2 β-lactamase as well as the TEM β-lactamase of the plasmid vector. The *bla* gene, therefore, appears to extend from the *Hpa*I-VIII site to the *Sal*I-I site of pKM101 which is a fragment of approximately 1 kb. A current cloning experiment involving the insertion of the length of DNA contained between the *Bam*HI and *Pst*I sites into the phage M13mp7 may reduce the size of the *bla* gene by a further 200 bp. The size of the *bla* gene is therefore estimated to be between 800 to 100 bp, and this indicates that the proposed structure for the enzyme as two equal-sized subunits may be an accurate one.

1. **Chang, A. C. Y., and S. N. Cohen.** 1978. Construction and characterization of amplifiable multicopy DNA cloning vehicles derived from the p15A cryptic miniplasmid. J. Bacteriol. **134:**1141–1156.
2. **Dale, J. W., and J. T. Smith.** 1974. R-factor mediated β-lactamases that hydrolyze oxacillin. Evidence for two distinct groups. J. Bacteriol. **119:**351–356.
3. **Dale, J. W., and J. T. Smith.** 1976. The dimeric nature of an R-factor mediated β-lactamase. Biochem. Biophys. Res. Commun. **68:**1000–1005.
4. **Langer, P. J., W. G. Shannabruch, and G. C. Walker.** 1981. Functional organization of the plasmid pKM101. J. Bacteriol. **143:**1310–1316.
5. **Messing, J. B.** 1979. Certification of the single stranded DNA *Lac*-phage multipurpose cloning system. Recomb. DNA Tech. Bull. **2:**43.
6. **Mortelmans, K. E., and B. A. D. Stocker.** 1976. Ultraviolet light protection, enhancement of ultraviolet mutagenesis, and mutator effect of plasmid *R46* in *Salmonella typhimurium*. J. Bacteriol. **128:**271–282.
7. **Schumann, W.** 1979. Construction of an *Hpa*I and *Hin*dIII plasmid vector allowing direct selection of transformants harbouring recombinant plasmids. Mol. Gen. Genet. **174:**221–224.

Occurrence, Detection, and Characterization of Extrachromosomal DNA Specifying Ampicillin Resistance in Gram-Negative Bacterial Isolates Obtained from Hospitalized Patients

RÜDIGER R. E. FOCK* AND RAINER LAUFS

Institut für Medizinische Mikrobiologie und Immunologie, Universitäts-Krankenhaus Eppendorf, Hamburg, Federal Republic of Germany

From 76 to 95% of *Enterobacter* species, *Klebsiella pneumoniae*, and *Escherichia coli* strains isolated from throat swabs and urine specimens of hospitalized patients were found to harbor plasmid DNA (6), as shown by agarose gel electrophoresis (7). The influence of hospitalization and of antibiotic treatment on the excretion of *E. coli* strains with R-plasmids in the feces of patients was examined (4). About 70% of the *E. coli* strains isolated from rectal swabs taken from hospitalized cardiac and medical patients harbored plasmids. This frequency increased with the length of the stay in hospital. The percentage of drug resistant strains rose from 30% at the time of admission to 70% or more. There was no significant increase in the excretion of drug-resistant *E. coli* strains in the untreated patients, whereas almost all of the patients with antibiotic therapy excreted drug-resistant strains. The excretion of resistant *E. coli* strains increased with the duration of antibiotic treatment, and the ability of the bacteria to transmit their resistance to other bacteria by conjugation rose from about 42% on admission to 100% about 2 weeks after starting chemotherapy. Nurses working in the same wards harbored *E. coli* strains with the same frequency of plasmids and R-factors as the patients at the time of admission (about 70%); the nurses did not excrete more drug-resistant *E. coli* strains than those patients who had not been treated with antibiotics before hospitalization.

E. coli strains were isolated from weekly feces samples from six healthy persons (8). From 1 to 24% of the 2,150 *E. coli* isolates were found to be resistant to ampicillin. In 89% of the examined 410 strains, plasmids were found. The effect of ampicillin on the plasmid population of the intestinal flora of *E. coli* was examined in three healthy individuals. After 1 week of application

(1.0 g/day), all isolated bacteria were resistant to ampicillin. The occurrence of ampicillin resistance seemed to be significantly accompanied by tetracycline resistance.

The biochemical characteristics and the resistance pattern of the *E. coli* strains as well as the molecular size of the plasmids present in these isolates varied, indicating that neither the *E. coli* isolates nor their R-plasmids were of monoclonal origin. All the ampicillin-resistant isolates investigated, however, produced a similar enzyme, a β-lactamase of the TEM-type. The β-lactamase genes in the plasmids can be characterized by molecular DNA-DNA hybridization studies using ^{3}H-labeled plasmid RSF1030 (3) as molecular probe which contains the whole of Tn*A*. The nuclease S1 method as described by Crosa et al. (2) was used in this study for epidemiological survey work. This enzyme specifically degrades about 95% of the single-stranded DNA, whereas only about 5% of the double-stranded DNA is digested. The single-stranded DNA was solubilized under the reported assay conditions (5) within 2 min, and the incubation of the enzyme with the DNA for 20 min did not increase the effect of the S1 enzyme on double-stranded DNA, which could be maintained at the 5% level.

The assay conditions for the determination of DNA relationship using small plasmids (4.2 and 5.5 megadalton [Mdal]) as molecular probe were examined in detail.

(i) Influence of concentration of purified unlabeled plasmid DNA. The actual degree of hybridization was about 75% (Fig. 1). This maximum level was reached when about 8 to 10 μg of unlabeled purified plasmid DNA was added to the reaction mixture. Higher amounts of unlabeled plasmid DNA did not further increase the amount of homoduplex formation. It was shown that 150 μg of unlabeled whole-cell DNA can be used instead of the unlabeled purified plasmid DNA for the assessment of base homologies without changing the reassociation kinetics significantly.

(ii) Influence of the reassociation time. The maximal 71% level of actual homoduplex formation was reached after 60 min of reassociation, and further incubation did not increase the hybridization rate between unlabeled and labeled plasmid DNA. The amount of self-hybridization of the labeled plasmid DNA, however, increased continually with the reassociation time and reached 22% after 180 min.

(iii) Influence of the molecular size of the plasmid. The kinetic of homoduplex formation is dependent on the molecular size of the plasmid (1). Figure 2 demonstrates this fact using three plasmids of different molecular sizes. Complete reassociation (71%) had occurred within h 1, using the small (4.2-Mdal) pMB8::Tn*A* DNA. After 7 h of reassociation, about 60% homoduplex formation of the 34-Mdal plasmid was observed, whereas the large 62-Mdal plasmid showed only 30% homoduplex formation after a reassociation time of 18 h.

(iv) Relationship between RSF1030 and the plasmids of the ampicillin-resistant

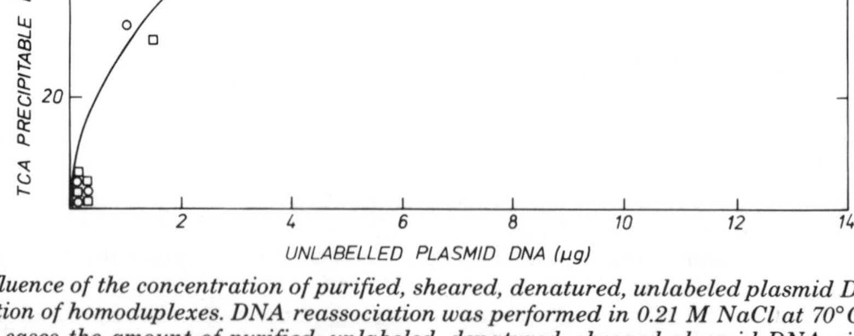

FIG. 1. *Influence of the concentration of purified, sheared, denatured, unlabeled plasmid DNA (4.2 Mdal) on the formation of homoduplexes. DNA reassociation was performed in 0.21 M NaCl at 70°C for 1* (○) *or 2* (□) *h. In all cases the amount of purified, unlabeled, denatured, sheared plasmid DNA given above was incubated with 0.001 to 0.01 µg (about 4,000 cpm) of ^{3}H-labeled, denatured, sheared DNA of the same plasmid. The reassociation is recorded as percentage of trichloroacetic acid-precipitable counts remaining after incubation with S1 nuclease. The self-hybridization was subtracted.*

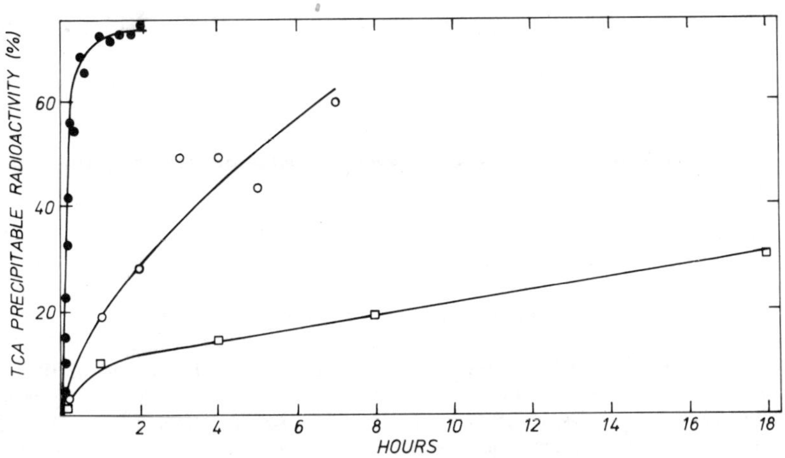

FIG. 2. *Influence of the molecular size of the plasmid DNA on reassociation time. The 4.2-Mdal-size plasmid pMB8::TnA (●), the 34-Mdal-size plasmid RP4 (○), and the 63-Mdal-size plasmid R1 (□) were examined. In all cases 7.5 μg of purified, unlabeled, denatured, sheared plasmid DNA was incubated for reaction with 0.001 to 0.01 μg (about 4,000 cpm) of labeled, denatured, sheared DNA of the same plasmid (see also Fig. 1).*

clinical isolates. The 5.5-Mdal multicopy plasmid RSF1030 contains the whole 3.2-Mdal transposable sequence of DNA (Tn*3*, 58% of the plasmid), which codes for the production of a β-lactamase with a molar substrate profile of a TEM-type β-lactamase (3). Almost all of the investigated ampicillin-resistant isolates showed sequence homology with RSF1030 between 21 and 56% (5, 8). The DNA of the ampicillin-susceptible isolates, which all contained plasmids, and the chromosomal controls as well as two ampicillin-resistant *E. coli* strains, which carried plasmids mediating production of an O-type β-lactamase, did not hybridize significantly with the RSF1030 probe. These findings confirm the observation of others (3) that ^{3}H-labeled RSF1030 forms DNA-DNA duplexes only with plasmids carrying the structural gene for the TEM β-lactamase.

Examining clinical isolates, we were unable to demonstrate gene transfer in vivo. The high incidence of R^+ strains in hospitalized patients is most likely not due to the infectious transfer of R-plasmids throughout the different *E. coli* strains during hospitalization but rather to selection of preexisting resistant clones under the pressure of antibiotic treatment. Analysis of plasmid DNA-DNA duplexes, however, may possibly become a tool in diagnostic work, and the plasmid RSF1030 may be a useful molecular probe for the detection of the TEM β-lactamase specifying DNA sequence Tn*A* (Tn*3*).

1. **Britten, R. J., and D. E. Kohne.** 1966. Nucleotide sequence repetition in DNA. Yearbk. Carnegie Instit. Washington **65:**78–106.
2. **Crosa, J. H., D. J. Brenner, and S. Falkow.** 1973. Use of a single-strand specific nuclease for analysis of bacterial and plasmid deoxyribonucleic acid homo- and heteroduplexes. J. Bacteriol. **115:**904–911.
3. **Heffron, F., R. Sublett, R. W. Hedges, A. Jacob, and S. Falkow.** 1975. Origin of the TEM beta-lactamase gene found on plasmids. J. Bacteriol. **122:**250–256.
4. **Laufs, R., R. Fock, F. B. von Hülst, and R. Ritter.** 1979. Transfer of R-factors during antibiotic treatment in the hospital, p. 74–89. *In* D. van der Waaij, and J. Verhoef (ed.), New criteria for antimicrobial therapy. Proceedings of a Symposium, Utrecht, January 1979. Excerpta Medica, Amsterdam.
5. **Laufs, R., and R. Fock.** 1979. Characterization of genes specifying ampicillin resistance in bacterial isolates using a single-strand specific nuclease for analysis of plasmid DNA-DNA duplexes. J. Gen. Microbiol. **111:**233–237.
6. **Laufs, R., and F. Kleimann.** 1978. Antibiotic resistance factors and other plasmids in bacterial isolates from hospitalized patients. Zentralbl. Bakteriol. Infektionskr. Parasitenkd. Hyg. Abt. 1 Orig. Reihe A **240:**503–516.
7. **Meyers, J. A., D. Sanchez, L. P. Elwell, and S. Falkow.** 1976. Simple agarose gel electrophoretic method for the identification and characterization of plasmid deoxyribonucleic acid. J. Bacteriol. **127:**1529–1537.
8. **Siemens, H. J., G. Gökschu, and R. Laufs.** 1981. Plasmids in intestinal *Escherichia coli* isolates and the influence of ampicillin. Infection **9:**131–136.

Plasmid-Determined Resistance to Aminocyclitols in Enterobacteria

R. GÓMEZ-LUS,* M. C. RUBIO-CALVO, M. NAVARRO, M. A. VITORIA, M. P. CHOCARRO, AND L. LARRAD

Department of Microbiology, School of Medicine, Saragossa, Spain

In previous publications (3–6) we communicated our results concerning the control of plasmids obtained in the University Hospital of Saragossa. Use of gentamicin in our hospital has increased steadily: 887 g in 1976, 1,549 g in 1978, and 2,494 g in 1979. Thus, the gentamicin use in our hospital from 1976 to 1979 shows a threefold increase. At the same time, the incidence of transferable gentamicin resistance increased from 3.08% (from 1 April 1976 to 31 March 1977) to 15.05% (from 1 April 1977 to 22 May 1979), a fivefold increase. From June 1979 to August 1980, gentamicin resistance diminished (11.38%) after restriction of the use of all aminocyclitols in the hospital; the amount of gentamicin used in 1980 was 1,927 g. However, from 1 September 1980 to 31 May 1981, we analyzed 595 resistant gram-negative bacilli, in which the proportion of R^+ gentamicin-resistant isolates increased to 14.95%.

We initially reviewed the data obtained from 468 R^+ strains of enterobacteria isolated in the period from 1 April 1976 to 31 August 1980, regarding those producing aminocyclitol-modifying enzymes. Enzymatic activities against 18 aminoglycoside antibiotics were determined as described by Davies and co-workers (1, 2). We have found the following enzymes: (i) 80 strains were AAC(3)-I (aminoglycoside 3-*N*-acetyltransferase type I) producers, (ii) 152 isolates produced AAC(3)-V, (iii) 3 strains coded for an AAC(6′), (iv) 94 isolates produced APH(3′)-I (aminoglycoside 3′-*O*-phosphotransferase type I), 13 strains coded for an APH(3′)-II, (v) 1 strain produced APH(5″), (vi) 40 strains produced APH(3″), and (vii) 24 isolates produced AAD(3″) (aminoglycoside 3″-*O*-adenyltransferase).

From 1 September 1980 to 31 May 1981, 190 gentamicin-resistant strains of enterobacteria were isolated; of these, we demonstrated the transference of resistance by conjugation in 89 isolates (46.89%). As shown in Table 1, the highest proportion of plasmid-mediated gentamicin resistance was noted in *Citrobacter freundii* (87.5%), *Escherichia coli* (81.48%), *Enterobacter* spp. (65.38%), and *Klebsiella pneumoniae* (57.89%). The smallest proportion was shown by *Proteus* spp. (33.33%) and *Serratia marcescens* (12.12%). Regarding the gentamicin-inactivating enzymes, two susceptibility profiles were obtained when acetylating activity was determined by the radioactive assay method. Eighteen strains (*E. coli*, 8; *Enterobacter* spp., 3; *C. freundii*, 3; *K. pneumoniae*, 2; and *Proteus* species, 2) were capable of producing AAC(3)-I and were resistant to gentamicin and sisomicin. Seventy-one isolates belonging to the species *K. pneumoniae* (31), *E. coli* (14), *Enterobacter* spp. (14), *S. marcescens* (8), and *C. freundii* (4) coded for an AAC(3)-V and were resistant to gentamicin, sisomicin, tobramycin, dibekacin, and netilmicin. From these 89 gentamicin-resistant strains, 55 produced only 3-*N*-acetylating enzymes, but the remaining 34 isolates coded also for other aminoglycoside-modifying enzymes, phosphotransferases and nucleotidyl transferases. In Table 2 are summarized the aminocyclitol resistance patterns and the aminoglycoside-modifying enzymes produced by the 89 R^+ isolates of the enterobacteria studied.

S. marcescens plasmids are known to produce enzymes capable of acetylating gentamicin and other aminocyclitols. In an attempt to analyze the mechanism of aminoglycoside resistance, we studied 65 clinical strains of *S. marcescens* iso-

TABLE 1. *Acetylating enzymes coded by R plasmids from enterobacteria transferred to E. coli K-12*

Donor strains	No. of strains examined	No. of strains carrying R plasmids	AAC(3)-I	AAC(3)-V
S. marcescens	66	8 (12.12%)	0	8
K. pneumoniae	57	33 (57.89%)	2	31
E. coli	27	22 (81.48%)	8	14
Enterobacter species	26	17 (65.38%)	3	14
C. freundii	8	7 (87.5%)	3	4
Proteus species	6	2 (33.33%)	2	0
Total	190	89 (46.84%)	18 (20.22%)	71 (79.77%)

TABLE 2. *Aminocyclitol resistance patterns*[a]

Enzymes	Gm	Tm	Net	Km	Liv	Bt	Sm	Sp	Amk	Tested strains showing pattern
AAC(3)-I	+	−	−	−	−	−	−	−	−	3
AAC(3)-V	+	+	+	−	−	−	−	−	−	52
AAC(3)-I + APH(3′)-I	+	−	−	+	+	−	−	−	−	4
AAC(3)-I + AAD(3″)	+	−	−	−	−	−	+	+	−	7
AAC(3)-I + AAD(3″) + APH(3′)-I	+	−	−	+	+	−	+	+	−	3
AAC(3)-I + AAD(3″) + APH(3′)-II	+	−	−	+	−	+	+	+	−	1
AAC(3)-I + APH(3′)-I + APH(3″)	+	−	−	+	+	−	+	−	−	1
AAC(3)-V + APH(3′)-I	+	+	+	+	+	−	−	−	−	2
AAC(3)-V + APH(3′)-I + AAD(3″)	+	+	+	+	+	−	+	+	−	6
AAC(3)-V + APH(3″)	+	+	+	−	−	−	+	−	−	2
AAC(3)-V + AAD(3″)	+	+	+	−	−	−	+	+	−	6
AAC(3)-V + APH(3′)-II + AAD(3″)	+	+	+	+	−	+	+	+	−	1
AAC(3)-V + APH(3′)-I + AAD(3″) + APH(3″)	+	+	+	+	+	−	+	+	−	1

[a] Gm, Gentamicin; Tm, tobramycin; Net, netilmicin; Km, kanamycin; Liv, lividomycin; Bt, butirosin; Sm, streptomycin; Sp, spectinomycin; Amk, amikacin.

lated in our hospital from 1 January 1977 to 30 May 1980. Among 11 strains harboring conjugative R plasmids (Tra^+), 10 produced AAC(3)-I and 1 coded for an AAC(3)-V. In a second group of 30 isolates bearing nonconjugative R plasmids (Tra^-), 3 strains coded for an AAC(3)-I and 27 strains produced an AAC(3)-V.

Thus, in this collection, transfer-deficient plasmids (Tra^-) are commoner than Tra^+ plasmids, and AAC(3)-V is produced more frequently by Tra^- plasmids.

Twenty-three strains in which plasmids were not detected by conjugation or curing produced the following enzymes: (i) 5 isolates coded for an AAC(3)-I, (ii) 18 strains coded for an AAC(3)-V, and (iii) 1 isolate produced AAC(6′).

Finally, we wish to describe the apparent dissemination of a single plasmid into multiple strains and species of *Enterobacteriaceae* (*K. pneumoniae*, 5; *E. coli*, 4; *E. cloacae*, 2; *E. aerogenes*, 1; and *P. mirabilis*, 1). All these strains harbor conjugative R plasmids, which have in common the following characteristics: not only do they belong to the same incompatibility group (M), possess identical determinants of resistance (ampicillin, tetracycline, gentamicin, tobramycin), and synthesize a β-lactamase type TEM-1, but they also code for an AAC(3)-V with affinity for gentamicin, sisomicin, tobramycin, dibekacin, and netilmicin.

1. **Benveniste, R., and J. Davies.** 1971. Enzymatic acetylation of aminoglycoside antibiotics by Escherichia coli carrying an R factor. Biochemistry **10:**1787–1796.
2. **Brzezinska, M., R. Benveniste, J. Davies, D. J. L. Daniels, and J. Weinstein.** 1972. Gentamicin resistance in strains of Pseudomonas aeruginosa mediated by enzymatic N-acetylation of the deoxystreptamine moiety. Biochemistry **11:**761–766.
3. **Gómez-Lus, R.** 1977. Resistencia bacteriana por plasmidos R, p. 275–283. *In* Symposium de infecciones hospitalarias. Monografias Antibióticos, S. A., Madrid.
4. **Gómez-Lus, R., L. Larrad, M. C. Rubio-Calvo, M. Navarro, and M. P. Lasierra.** 1980. AAC (3) and AAC (6′) enzymes produced by R plasmids isolated in a general hospital, p. 295–303. *In* S. Mitsushashi, L. Rosival, and V. Krčmery (ed.), Antibiotic resistance, transposition and other mechanisms. Avicenum, Prague, and Springer Verlag, Berlin.
5. **Gómez-Lus, R., M. C. Rubio-Calvo, and L. Larrad Mur.** 1977. Aminoglycoside inactivating enzymes produced by R plasmids of Escherichia coli, Citrobacter freundii, Klebsiella pneumoniae, Proteus vulgaris, Providencia stuartii, and Serratia marcescens. J. Antimicrob. Chemother. **3**(Suppl. C)**:**39–41.
6. **Gómez-Lus, R., M. C. Rubio-Calvo, L. Larrad, M. Navarro, P. Lasierra, and M. A. Vitoria.** 1980. 3-N-Aminoglycoside-acetylating enzymes produced by R plasmids-carrying bacteria isolated in a general hospital, p. 708–710. *In* J. D. Nelson and C. Grassi (ed.), Current chemotherapy and infectious disease. American Society for Microbiology, Washington, D.C.

R-Factors and Distribution of Antibiotic Resistance in *Haemophilus influenzae*

P. SOMENZI, G. SERAFINI, M. TONI,* AND G. C. SCHITO

Institutes of Microbiology, Medical Schools, University of Parma, Parma, and University of Genoa, Genoa, Italy*

Strains of *Haemophilus influenzae* resistant to ampicillin have been frequently reported over the past several years (1, 2, 4). Strains resistant to chloramphenicol and other antibiotics have also been detected (1, 3, 5). The occurrence of such resistance is of major clinical consequence since these are the drugs of choice in meningitis caused by *H. influenzae*. Moreover, the existence of plasmid-mediated drug resistance in *H. influenzae* has been demonstrated for ampicillin, chloramphenicol, tetracycline, and kanamycin (3, 5).

Recently, we tested the susceptibility of 145 strains of *H. influenzae* to four antibiotics in clinical use: ampicillin, cefuroxime, chloramphenicol, and tetracycline.

MICs were determined by agar dilution test, using an automated multipoint inoculator. Mueller-Hinton agar medium was supplemented with 5% Fildes blood digest, and each inoculum "spot" contained 10^3 colony-forming units. The results were evaluated after 24 h of incubation at 37°C. The MICs of the four antibiotics for *H. influenzae* strains used in this study are shown in Table 1.

Only against tetracycline was a significant frequency of resistance (9%) observed; ampicillin and chloramphenicol were ineffective against three isolates, and cefuroxime was highly active against all *H. influenzae* strains tested. One isolate was resistant, at the same time, to tetracycline and chloramphenicol, and one was resistant to ampicillin and chloramphenicol as well.

For the demonstration of the presence of plasmids in the resistant strains, agarose gel electrophoresis (0.7%) was done, starting from cleared lysates. Only three strains carried a large plasmid. Strains 37 Tc^r and 55 Tc^r contained a plasmid of approximately 40 megadaltons, and strain 48 Tc^r Cm^r contained a plasmid of 42 megadaltons.

The resistant strains were examined for transfer of ampicillin, chloramphenicol, and tetracycline resistance to an isogenic recipient strain, *H. influenzae* Rif^r Str^r and *E. coli* K-12 J 53 Nal^r. Equal volumes of donor and recipient strain were mixed, filtered through a membrane filter, and placed on plates of Mueller-Hinton agar supplemented with 5% Fildes blood digest (0.1 ml of a culture of 10^9 colony-forming units per ml, with selecting antibiotics).

Only strain 48 Tc^r Cm^r presented a low frequency of transconjugants: 3×10^{-7} for the recipient strain of *H. influenzae* Rif^r Str^r and 2×10^{-8} for *E. coli* K-12 J 53 Nal^r.

This R-factor is similar to that of *H. influenzae* HC 234 reported by Van Klingeren et al. (6). In fact, the plasmid pPR48 Tc^r Cm^r determinant has a molecular weight of 42 megadaltons, and a plasmid of identical size is also found in the transcipient *H. influenzae* Rif^r Str^r, whereas in the transcipient *E. coli* K-12 J 53 Nal^r with phenotype Tc^r Cm^r it was absent. This finding suggests that the resistance determinant of pPR48 is likely to be integrated into the *E. coli* chromosome.

TABLE 1. *Susceptibility patterns of 145 H. influenzae clinical isolates to four antibiotics*

Antibiotic	No. of strains with MICs (μg/ml) of:									
	0.06	0.12	0.25	0.50	1	2	4	8	16	32
Ampicillin	3 (2%)	10 (7%)	46 (32%)	53 (36%)	30 (21%)				3 (2%)	
Cefuroxime	3 (2%)	3 (2%)	25 (17%)	46 (32%)	55 (38%)	13 (9%)				
Chloramphenicol			20 (14%)	55 (38%)	32 (22%)	25 (24%)			3 (2%)	
Tetracycline		4 (3%)	4 (3%)	32 (22%)	80 (55%)	12 (8%)		3 (2%)	6 (4%)	4 (3%)

1. **Center for Disease Control.** 1978. Prevalence of ampicillin and chloramphenicol-resistant strains of *Haemophilus influenzae* causing meningitis and bacteriemia: national survey of hospital laboratories. J. Infect. Dis. **138**:421–424.
2. **Lerman, S. J., J. M. Brunken, and M. Bollinger.** 1980. Prevalence of ampicillin-resistant strains of *Haemophilus influenzae* causing systemic infection. Antimicrob. Agents Chemother. **18**:474–475.

3. **Study, J. H.** 1979. Plasmid transfer in *Haemophilus influenzae*. J. Bacteriol. **139**:520–529.
4. **Thornsberry, C., C. N. Baker, A. Kirven, and J. M. Swenson.** 1976. Susceptibility of ampicillin-resistant *Haemophilus influenzae* to seven penicillins. Antimicrob. Agents Chemother. **9**:70–73.
5. **Van Dang, A., F. Goldstein, J. F. Acar, and D. H. Bouanchaud.** 1975. A transferable kanamycin resistance plasmid isolated from *Haemophilus influenzae*. Ann. Microbiol. (Paris) **126**:397–399.
6. **Van Klingeren, B., J. D. A. Van Embden, and M. Dessens-Kroon.** 1977. Plasmid-mediated chloramphenicol resistance in *Haemophilus influenzae*. Antimicrob. Agents Chemother. **11**:383–387.

Frequency of In Vivo Transfer and Dissemination of Antibiotic Resistance Plasmids Among Gentamicin-Resistant Enterobacteria During Endemic Infection and Colonization

MARK W. CASEWELL[1]* AND SIDONIE KNIGHT

Department of Microbiology, St. Thomas's Hospital Medical School, London, SE1 7EH, England

The intrageneric and intergeneric spread of plasmids conferring resistance to gentamicin and numerous other antibiotics has occasionally been noted in association with hospital outbreaks caused by single strains of multiply resistant coliforms (3, 4). However, little is known about the frequency of plasmid spread and possible in vivo conjugation among hospital bacteria during endemic colonization and infection. We therefore investigated the spread of single plasmids among gentamicin-resistant enterobacteria isolated from patients in one hospital during a non-epidemic period. In view of the frequent association of transferable plasmids to be found in gentamicin-resistant *Klebsiella* spp. (1), we were particularly interested to determine any involvement of this species.

For 13 consecutive months, we identified all inpatients at St. Thomas's Hospital whose bacteriological specimens received by the diagnostic microbiology laboratory yielded more than one strain of gentamicin-resistant enterobacteria. We identified plasmids that were common to multiple strains from individual patients and sought evidence for epidemic plasmids that were common to multiple strains from more than one patient. Standard bacteriological methods were used throughout the study, and *Klebsiella* spp. were K-typed by means of capsular antisera. Gentamicin-resistant enterobacteria from patients with more than one such strain were tested for the presence of plasmids that were transferable to *Escherichia coli* K-12, and the molecular weights of plasmids were determined by agarose-gel electrophoresis of whole-cell lysates (2).

During the 13-month study period, of 184 inpatients with gentamicin-resistant enterobacteria, there were 17 (9.2%) with more than one strain, and the isolates from 14 of these patients possessed plasmids that were transferable to *E. coli* K-12. Eight (4.3%) of the patients with multiple strains of gentamicin-resistant enterobacteria were found to harbor two or more strains with common plasmids that were recognizable by their transferable resistance pattern and indistinguishable electrophoretic mobility, an observation strongly suggestive of in vivo conjugation. The sites of isolation of the 21 strains from these eight patients are shown in Table 1. The resistance patterns and approximate molecular weights of the plasmids identified in the strains from these eight patients are shown in Table 2. *Klebsiella aerogenes* accounted for 52% of the strains, and *E. coli* accounted for 33%. *K. aerogenes* was the first gentamicin-resistant species to be isolated from seven of the eight patients, all but two of whom had at least two distinct strains of *K. aerogenes* in their urine. *K. aerogenes* K21, bearing a transferable plasmid of approximately 110 Mdal which conferred the resistance pattern ApCbCmTcSuTpSmKmNmGmTm, was isolated from four patients (Table 1). This epidemic plasmid was identified in 10 strains belonging to four different genera.

TABLE 1. *Sites of isolation of 21 gentamicin-resistant enterobacteria from eight patients with strains showing indistinguishable plasmids*

Strain	No. of strains isolated from:		
	Urine	Wound	Other
All	13	5	3
Strains with epidemic plasmid	5	5	3
Klebsiella spp.	6	4	1

[1] Present address: Department of Medical Microbiology, The London Hospital Medical College, London E1 2AD, England.

TABLE 2. *Patients harboring several gentamicin-resistant enterobacteria with plasmids common to more than one strain*

Patient no.	Strain	Interval (days)	Plasmid characteristic	
			Resistances transferred	Mol wt
1	*K. aerogenes* K21	0	ApCbCmTcSuTpSmKmNmGmTm	110
	K. aerogenes NT	3	ApCbCmTcSuTpSmKmNmGmTm	110
	E. coli		ApCbCmTcSuTpSmKmNmGmTm	110
2	*K. aerogenes* K21	0	ApCbCmTcSuTpSmKmNmGmTm	110
	E. coli	2	ApCbCmTcSuTpSmKmNmGmTm	110
3	*K. aerogenes* K21	0	ApCbCmTcSuTpSmKmNmGmTm	110
	E. coli	28	ApCbCmTcSuTpSmKmNmGmTm	110
	Enterobacter cloacae	29	ApCbCmTcSuTpSmKmNmGmTm	110
4	*K. aerogenes* K21	0	ApCbCmTcSuTpSmKmNmGmTm	110
	K. aerogenes K3	0	ApCbCmTcSuTpSmKmNmGmTm	110
	Citrobacter freundii	1	ApCbCmTcSuTpSmKmNmGmTm	110
	E. coli	1	ApCbCmTcSuTpSmKmNmGmTm	110
	K. aerogenes K64	24	ApCbCmTcSuTpSmKmNmGmTm	110
5	*K. aerogenes* K21	0	AbCbCmTcTpGmTm	105
	K. aerogenes K60	0	AbCbCmTcTpGmTm	105
6	*E. coli*	0	ApCbCrCmTcSuTpSmKmNmGm	57
	K. aerogenes NT	6	ApCbCrCmTcSuTpSmKmNmGm	57
7	*E. coli*	0	ApCbCmSuTpKmNmGmTm	80
	Serratia marcescens	0	ApCbCmSuTpKmNmGmTm	80
8	*K. aerogenes* K16	0	ApCbCrKfCmTcSuTpSmKmNmGm	62
	E. coli	0	ApCbCrKfCmTcSuTpSmKmNmGm	62

Our finding that as many as 9.2% of the patients with clinical isolates of gentamicin-resistant enterobacteria were infected or colonized by more than one strain and that almost half of these patients (4.3%) harbor several different strains or even different species bearing indistinguishable plasmids indicates that considerable dissemination of plasmids occurs during periods of endemic colonization and infection. The frequency with which we noted urinary and wound isolates (Table 1) and the relative difficulties of achieving in vivo conjugation in the human bowel (5) suggest that the urinary bladder or wound surfaces are more likely anatomical sites for conjugation between enterobacteria. It remains possible that plasmid transfer occurred between several enterobacteria before each patient acquired the strains, but this seems less likely than in vivo conjugation.

Our results show that the 110-Mdal plasmid found in 10 strains of bacteria from four patients is already epidemic at St. Thomas's Hospital. Resistance genes from coliform-derived plasmids have already been implicated in ampicillin-resistant and chloramphenicol-resistant *Haemophilus influenzae*, in penicillinase-producing *Neisseria gonorrhoeae*, and in carbenicillin-resistant *Pseudomonas aeruginosa* (6). Our prediction that *Klebsiella* spp. provide an abundant reservoir of transferable plasmids (1) that will increasingly disseminate among the more pathogenic genera has since been exemplified by the recent description by Datta and colleagues (1a) of the acquisition of plasmid-mediated chloramphenicol and co-trimoxazole resistance in a previously susceptible strain of *Salmonella typhi*, this plasmid almost certainly being derived from *K. aerogenes* isolated previously in the same patient.

In the absence of controlled antibiotic usage and epidemiological containment of these strains, it seems likely that resistance genes derived from gentamicin-resistant, multiply resistant enterobacteria, and *Klebsiella* spp. in particular, will increasingly disseminate to more pathogenic genera.

1. **Casewell, M. W., H. G. Talsania, and S. Knight.** 1981. Gentamicin-resistant *Klebsiella aerogenes* as a clinically significant source of transferable antibiotic resistance. J. Antimicrob. Chemother. **8:**153–160.

1a. **Datta, N., H. Richards, and C. Datta.** 1981. Salmonella typhi in vivo acquires resistance to both chloramphenicol and co-trimoxazole. Lancet **i:**1181–1183.

2. **Eckhardt, T.** 1978. A rapid method for the identification of plasmid deoxyribonucleic acid in bacteria. Plasmid **1:** 584–588.
3. **Markowitz, S. M., J. M. Veazey, Jr., F. L. Macrina, G. Mayhall, and V. A. Lamb.** 1980. Sequential outbreaks of infection due to *Klebsiella pneumoniae* in a neonatal intensive care unit: implication of a conjugative R plasmid. J. Infect. Dis.**142:**106–112.
4. **Tompkins, L. S., J. J. Plorde, and S. Falkow.** 1980. Molecular analysis of R-factors from multiresistant nosocomial isolates. J. Infect. Dis. **141:**625–636.
5. **Wiedemann, B.** 1972. Resistance transfer in vivo and its inhibition, p. 75–90. *In* V. Krcmery, L. Rosival, and T. Wantabe (ed.), Bacterial plasmids and antibiotic resistance. Springer-Verlag, Berlin.
6. **Williams, J. D.** 1978. Spread of R factors outside the Enterobacteriaceae. J. Antimicrob. Chemother. **4:**6–8.

Epidemiology of R-Plasmids in Gentamicin-Resistant *Klebsiella pneumoniae* from Four Associated Hospitals

J. L. BIDWELL,* L. O. WHITE, AND D. S. REEVES

Department of Medical Microbiology, Southmead Hospital, Bristol BS10 5NB, England

Several reports have recently appeared describing resistance plasmids (R-plasmids) in multiresistant strains of *Klebsiella pneumoniae* responsible for outbreaks of hospital-acquired infections in the United Kingdom (3, 6, 8). This report describes the R-plasmids in isolates from four associated Bristol hospitals (Ham Green Hospital [HGH], Southmead Hospital [SMH], Frenchay Hospital [FH], and Bristol Royal Infirmary [BRI]) after the epidemic spread of a single clone of *K. pneumoniae* capsular serotype K2 (2) throughout the region during the period 1976 through 1980.

Isolates at SMH and FH during this period remained sporadic, involving only a few patients. In contrast, outbreaks at BRI and HGH involved the colonization or infection of patients throughout several wards in the hospital concerned. During the period 1978 through 1980, isolates at HGH totaled 147, but differed from isolates at BRI in that 49 (33%) possessed additional resistance to kanamycin. R-plasmids from *K. pneumoniae* K2 isolates at the four Bristol hospitals and from two neighboring centers, Gloucester Royal Hospital (GRH) and Southmead Health Center (SHC), were characterized by genetic and molecular studies and by identification of the R-plasmid-mediated β-lactamases and aminoglycoside-aminocyclitol (AGAC)-modifying enzymes.

Genetic characteristics of R-plasmids were determined by conjugal transfer to *Escherichia coli* K-12 derivatives and by plasmid incompatibility grouping. Preparation of plasmid DNA and molecular weight determination by agarose gel electrophoresis was as described by Eckhardt (5). *E. coli* K-12 transconjugants, derived from matings with *K. pneumoniae* isolates from HGH, SMH, FH, and BRI and containing the isolated nonconjugative plasmid pJB100b (Table 1), were used to prepare purified plasmid DNA for restriction endonuclease analysis. R-plasmid-mediated β-lactamases were prepared by the method of Bidwell and Reeves (1) and identified by analytical isoelectric focusing (7). AGAC-modifying enzymes were prepared and detected as described by Drasar (4).

Kanamycin-susceptible isolates from the four Bristol hospitals transferred the same plasmid complex to *E. coli* K-12 (Table 1). This comprised a conjugative 62-megadalton (Mdal) plasmid designated pJB100a, encoding resistance to trimethoprim and streptomycin (low level) of incompatibility group (Inc) Iα, and a nonconjugative 95-Mdal plasmid designated pJB100b. This plasmid encoded resistance to ampicillin, sulfonamides, gentamicin/sisomicin, tobramycin, tetracycline, streptomycin, and chloramphenicol, was compatible with reference plasmids of IncFI, -FII, -Iα, -Iδ, -C, -D, -H2, -J, -N, -P, and -W, and could not be assigned to an Inc group.

The plasmid pJB100b specified the β-lactamase OXA-1 and the following AGAC-modifying enzymes: AAC (3)-1, responsible for acetylation of gentamicin and sisomicin, APH (3′)-3, responsible for phosphorylation of amikacin (in vitro), and APH (3″), responsible for the phosphorylation of streptomycin. Agarose gel electrophoresis of purified pJB100b DNA preparations, derived from isolates at HGH, SMH, FH, and BRI and digested with restriction endonucleases *Eco*RI and *Bgl*II, showed multiple identical endonucleolytic fragments, strongly inferring epidemiological connection.

Kanamycin-resistant isolates from HGH transferred pJB100a to *E. coli* K-12 and an insertion derivative of pJB100b designated

TABLE 1. *Characterization of R-plasmids from K. pneumoniae K2 serotypes*

Source	No. of isolates examined	Resistance pattern[a]	R-plasmids transferred to *E. coli* K-12: Resistance pattern	Mol size (Mdal)	Inc group[b]	β-Lac[c]	AAC[d]	APH[e]	Plasmid
HGH	4								
SMH	2	ASuGToTpTSC	Tp(S)[f]	62	Iα				pJB100a
FH	1		ASuGToTSC	95	Com	OXA-1	(3)-1	(3′)-3, (3″)	pJB100b
BRI	3								
			Tp(S)	62	Iα				pJB100a
HGH	1	ASuGToTpTKSC	ASuGToTKSC	150	Com	OXA-1	(3)-1	(3′)-3, (3″), (3′)	pJB100b::K
HGH	1	ASuGToTpTKSC	Tp(S)	62	Iα				pJB100a
			ASuGToTSC	95	Com	OXA-1	(3)-1	(3′)-3, (3″)	pJB100b
			ASuGToTC	62	Com	OXA-1	(3)-1	(3′)-3	pJB100bΔS
SMH	1	ASuGToTpTSC	Tp(S)	62	Iα				pJB100a
			ASuGToTSC	95	Com	OXA-1	(3)-1	(3′)-3, (3″)	pJB100b
			ASuGToSC	90	Com	OXA-1	(3)-1	(3′)-3, (3″)	pJB100bΔT
BRI	2	ASuGToTpTKSC	ASuGToTpTKSC	120	ND	OXA-1	(3)-1	(3′), (3″)	pJB101
GRH	1	ASuGToTpTSC	ASuGToTpTSC	86	N	TEM-1	ND	ND	pJB105
SHC	1	ASuGToSC	ASuGToSC	44	P	OXA-1	ND	ND	pJB106

[a] A, Ampicillin; Su, sulfonamides; G, gentamicin/sisomicin; To, tobramycin; Tp, trimethoprim; T, tetracycline; K, kanamycin; S, streptomycin; C, chloramphenicol.
[b] Com, Compatible with all groups tested. ND, Not done.
[c] Type of R-plasmid-mediated β-lactamase.
[d] AGAC-acetylating enzymes.
[e] AGAC-phosphorylating enzymes.
[f] Parentheses indicate low-level resistance.

pJB100b::K (Table 1). This plasmid had a molecular size of 150 Mdal, was unstable, and could revert to the pJB100b type spontaneously on storage of cultures or during transfer to *E. coli* K-12. The 55-Mdal insert encoded the enzyme APH (3′), responsible for phosphorylation of kanamycin. It is probable that pJB100b::K was associated with all of the kanamycin-resistant isolates at HGH. Two deletion derivatives of pJB100b were also characterized. These were designated pJB100bΔT (a tetracycline-susceptible derivative, 90 Mdal) and pJB100bΔS [a streptomycin-susceptible APH (3″)-negative derivative, 62 Mdal].

An unrecorded proportion of isolates at BRI during 1978 were kanamycin resistant. Two representative examples studied transferred a single plasmid (pJB101) to *E. coli* K-12. This plasmid had a molecular size of 120 Mdal and appeared epidemiologically distinct from the pJB100a/b plasmid complex. Similarly, the multiresistant *K. pneumoniae* K2 isolates at GRH and SHC, although phenotypically similar to the isolates from the four Bristol hospitals, contained epidemiologically unrelated plasmids (Table 1).

The results of this and other U.K. studies (3, 6, 8) demonstrate the genetic and molecular diversity of R-plasmids in multiresistant strains of *K. pneumoniae*. It is likely that such diverse plasmids are generated in different centers by the selective action of antibiotics on plasmid gene pools. Since increasing numbers of these genes are known to be transposable, illegitimate recombination between gene complexes in the presence of antibiotic selection pressures would seem to provide an excellent mechanism for generating the observable permutations of genetic material in R-plasmids.

We thank N. Datta, P. M. Bennett, and H. Richards for supplying reference organisms and plasmids and for advice on molecular techniques. The Showering Fund (Southmead Hospital) provided a generous equipment grant.

1. **Bidwell, J. L., and D. S. Reeves.** 1980. Isoelectric focusing of β-lactamases. J. Antimicrob. Chemother **6:**793.
2. **Curie, K., D. C. E. Speller, R. A. Simpson, M. Stephens, and D. I. Cooke.** 1978. A hospital epidemic caused by a gentamicin-resistant *Klebsiella aerogenes*. J. Hyg. **80:**115–123.
3. **Datta, N., S. Dacey, V. Hughes, S. Knight, H. Richards, G. Williams, M. Casewell, and K. P. Shannon.** 1980. Distribution of genes for trimethoprim and gentamicin resistance in bacteria and their plasmids in a general hospital. J. Gen. Microbiol. **118:**495–508.
4. **Drasar, F. A.** 1978. Detection of aminoglycoside degrading enzymes, p. 70–75. *In* D. S. Reeves, I. Phillips, J. D. Williams, and R. Wise (ed.), Laboratory methods in antimicrobial chemotherapy. Churchill-Livingstone, Edinburgh.
5. **Eckhardt, T.** 1978. A rapid method for the identification of plasmid desoxyribonucleic acid in bacteria. Plasmid **1:**584–588.

6. **Hughes, V., N. Datta, and M. C. Faiers.** 1981. Interhospital spread of a multiply resistant klebsiella. Br. Med. J. **282:**696.
7. **Matthew, M., A. M. Harris, M. J. Marshall, and G. W. Ross.** 1975. The use of analytical isoelectric focusing for detection and identification of β-lactamases. J. Gen. Microbiol. **88:**169–178.
8. **Richards, H., V. Hughes, and N. Datta.** 1981. Diversity of plasmids responsible for multiple resistance in klebsiella serotype K2. J. Hyg. **86:**189–194.

Mechanism of Penicillin Resistance in *Streptococcus faecalis*

ROBERTA FONTANA* AND ROBERTO CERINI

Istituto di Microbiologia, Università di Padova, Padova, Italy

Clinical isolates of bacteria that have gained resistance to beta-lactams often arise by the acquisition of a plasmid that carries the genes for beta-lactamase production. However, bacteria can also become resistant to penicillin without producing antibiotic-degrading enzymes (intrinsic resistance). *Streptococcus faecalis* is one of the clinically important species that show the phenomenon of intrinsic resistance. However, the mechanism of such resistance is still unknown.

In this paper, we describe a model system useful in investigating this problem and consisting of the isolation of *S. faecalis* mutants resistant to increasing penicillin concentrations. The analysis of these mutants had led to finding the unique ability of *S. faecalis* penicillin-binding protein (PBP) 5 to bind penicillin with very slow kinetics and to the proposal of a novel hypothesis regarding the mechanism of intrinsic resistance to penicillin in this species. This hypothesis is based on the finding that all resistant strains produced an increased amount of PBP 5 which was proportional to the level of resistance.

S. faecalis ATCC 9790 was used in all the experiments. Cells were grown in SB medium containing, per liter: peptone (Difco Laboratories), 10 g; yeast extract (Difco), 10 g; glucose, 20 g; $NaH_2PO_4 \cdot H_2O$, 16.4 g; and Na_2HPO_4, 26.5 g. For solid medium (SBA), agar (1.5%) was added.

Selection of resistant strains was carried out by serial passages on SBA medium containing increasing amounts of benzylpenicillin. By this procedure, mutants resistant to 5, 20, and 40 μg/ml were obtained and designated R5, R20, and R40, respectively. None of the resistant strains showed beta-lactamase production.

The growth characteristics of the parent and the mutants were similar, although the most resistant strain (R40) showed a growth rate slower than that of the parent (48 and 28 min, respectively).

The acquisition of penicillin resistance was accompanied by increased resistance to other beta-lactamases, but not to other inhibitors of cell wall synthesis or antibiotics with unrelated modes of action (data not shown). The penicillin resistance was very stable, remaining even after 50 transfers in the absence of the antibiotic.

To shed some light on the mechanism of penicillin resistance of these mutants, we evaluated the amount of penicillin bound by cells. We found that the ability of both whole cells and membranes to bind penicillin increased with the increase in the level of resistance. In particular, we found that the amount of radioactivity bound by the parent was nearly 50% lower than that bound by strain R40 (Table 1).

To analyze the characteristics of PBPs, membranes were prepared from the parent and the mutants and treated with [^{14}C]benzylpenicillin for 10 min. The proteins were then fractionated by sodium dodecyl sulfate-polyacrylamide gel electrophoresis, and the PBPs were detected by fluorography as described (1). Under these conditions all mutants showed a PBP pattern identical to that of the parent, but PBP 5 was missing in all of the gels. However, by increasing the time of membrane incubation with radioactive benzylpenicillin, we found that PBP 5 showed a slow penicillin-binding rate. In fact, it bound a detectable amount of radioactivity only after 15 min of incubation and was saturated after 60 min, whereas the other PBPs were saturated after 5 min of incubation with the antibiotic (data not shown). Under these conditions, resistant strains showed an increased amount of PBP 5 which was proportional to the level of penicillin resistance (Fig. 1B).

The evidence that the increase in PBP 5 was due to increased synthesis of this protein came from the fact that in Coomassie-stained gels this protein could be clearly identified as a stained band which had the electrophoretic mobility of PBP 5 and increased in the different strains in amounts equal to the increases seen with PBP 5 (Fig. 1A).

The constitutive synthesis of a protein with

TABLE 1. *Binding of [^{14}C]benzylpenicillin to whole cells and isolated membranes of S. faecalis ATCC 9790 and penicillin-resistant mutants*[a]

Strain	Binding at given penicillin concn (μM)											
	Whole cells (cpm/10^6 cells)					Membranes (cpm/mg of protein)						
	40	100	200	500	1,000	1	2	3	4	5	10	20
ATCC 9790	150	170	450	1,100	1,800	1,520	1,660	1,700	2,080	2,320	2,050	2,140
R5	170	270	480	1,250	1,950	1,510	1,900	2,010	2,200	2,450	2,490	2,410
R20	220	320	550	1,460	2,540	1,780	2,110	2,360	2,570	3,150	3,210	3,260
R40	310	520	970	1,650	3,160	1,920	2,430	2,850	3,230	3,480	3,760	3,970

[a] Two hundred microliters containing 10^9 cells or 1 mg of purified membranes was added to the various dilutions of [^{14}C]benzylpenicillin and incubated for 30 min at 37°C. The binding was stopped with an excess of cold penicillin, and ice-cold trichloroacetic acid (5 ml of a 10% solution) was added. Samples were collected on Whatman filters, washed with trichloroacetic acid, alcohol, and acetone, and radioactivity was counted in a Packard liquid scintillator.

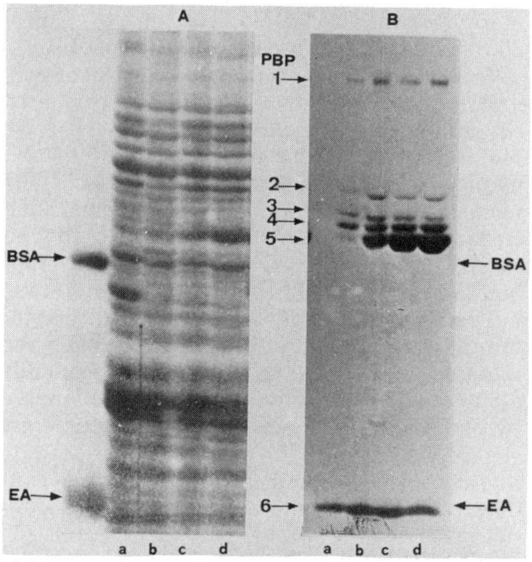

FIG. 1. *PBPs of S. faecalis ATCC 9790 and penicillin-resistant strains. Membrane samples (125 μg of total protein in 20 μl) prepared from cells exponentially growing in SB were treated with 20 μM [^{14}C]-benzylpenicillin (58 Ci/mol) at 37°C for 30 min. After reaction, the samples were supplemented successively with 2 μl of an aqueous solution of 0.01 M nonradioactive benzylpenicillin and 25 μl of denaturing buffer (1). After boiling for 1 min, the samples were subjected to polyacrylamide slab gel electrophoresis in sodium dodecyl sulfate, and PBPs were detected by fluorography as described (1). (A) Coomassie-stained gel; (B) fluorogram; (a) S. faecalis ATCC 9790; (b) S. faecalis R5; (c) S. faecalis R20; (d) S. faecalis R40.*

the characteristics of PBP 5 is probably the cause of the intrinsic penicillin resistance in *S. faecalis.* This possibility is also strongly supported by the properties of some wild resistant strains which we have recently analyzed. A preliminary study showed that such strains synthesized a PBP with the characteristics of PBP 5 which was present in membranes in an amount proportional to the level of the resistance.

PBP 5, because of its low affinity for penicillin (2) and its slow kinetics of penicillin binding, represents the less sensitive target of penicillin. One hypothesis for explaining the role of PBP 5 in resistance is that this protein could take over the function of other PBPs which are essential for cell growth and more sensitive to the antibiotic, such as PBP 3, which has recently been suggested to be the lethal target for penicillin action (3). Since further characterization of PBP 5 could allow a better understanding of its role in the mechanism of penicillin resistance in *S. faecalis,* we are now working on its purification.

1. **Coyette, J., J. M. Ghuysen, and R. Fontana.** 1978. Solubilization and isolation of the membrane-bound DD-carboxypeptidase of *Streptococcus faecalis* ATCC 9790. Eur. J. Biochem. **88:**297–305.
2. **Coyette, J., J. M. Ghuysen, and R. Fontana.** 1980. The penicillin binding proteins in *Streptococcus faecalis* ATCC 9790. Eur. J. Biochem. **110:**445–456.
3. **Fontana, R., P. Canepari, G. Satta, and J. Coyette.** 1980. Identification of the lethal target of benzylpenicillin in *Streptococcus faecalis* by *in vivo* penicillin binding studies. Nature (London) **287:**70–72.

Selection of Unstable Gentamicin-Resistant Variants of *Pseudomonas aeruginosa* in Leukopenic Mice

ANDREAS U. GERBER* AND WILLIAM A. CRAIG

Department of Medicine, William S. Middleton Memorial Veterans Administration Hospital and University of Wisconsin Center for Health Sciences, Madison, Wisconsin 53705, U.S.A.

Gentamicin-susceptible strains of *Pseudomonas aeruginosa* harbor aminoglycoside-resistant subpopulations. This phenomenon was previously demonstrated in our own laboratory by plating high inocula of various strains of *P. aeruginosa* onto agar plates which contained gentamicin in increasing concentrations. The aminoglycoside-resistant subpopulations could easily be selected in vitro by exposing a high inoculum of a gentamicin-susceptible strain of *P. aeruginosa* to two to four times the MIC of an aminoglycoside (Fig. 1). In comparison with the corresponding parental strain, the selected gentamicin-resistant forms exhibited an increased resistance to all current aminoglycosides, including amikacin. Yet, their susceptibility to β-lactam antibiotics was usually retained. These forms were further characterized by slower growth and by formation of smaller colonies on agar plates; they were hence identified as small-colony variants. In a peritonitis model, small-colony variants were less pathogenic for normal mice. Agranulocytic mice, in contrast, were almost as susceptible for small-colony variants as for the parental strain (1).

The present study was designed to evaluate whether aminoglycoside-resistant forms of *P. aeruginosa* could also be selected during gentamicin treatment in vivo and account for aminoglycoside treatment failures and, if so, whether the failures could be prevented by a treatment combining gentamicin with ticarcillin.

Approximately 10^7 colony-forming units (CFU) of gentamicin-susceptible *P. aeruginosa* ATCC 27853 or a clinical isolate, 14974, was injected into the thigh muscle of normal and leukopenic mice. Two hours later, subcutaneous injections of gentamicin up to 30 mg/kg every 3 h were started and continued for 24 h. At various time intervals, three mice were sacrificed, and the thigh muscles were removed and homogenized. The number of CFU per thigh was determined by plating serial 10-fold dilutions of 10% thigh homogenates onto normal and gentamicin-containing agar plates. Gentamicin-resistant organisms could thus be quantitated at the same time as the total population of viable organisms.

A single 30-mg/kg injection of gentamicin resulted in plasma peak levels of 45 μg/ml followed by a half-life time of approximately 20 min. Concentrations in total thigh homogenates peaked after 15 min with 4.6 to 5.1 μg/g and were 0.48 to 1.14 μg/g at 3 h (just before the following injection). Levels in the extracellular fluid (where only *P. aeruginosa* was seen on tissue sections) were estimated to be approximately three to four times higher.

Gentamicin alone easily eradicated *P. aeruginosa* from thighs of normal mice. In leukopenic mice, however, gentamicin resulted in no more than a 1- to 3-log reduction of CFU/thigh (Fig. 2), which was invariably followed by regrowth in all mice despite ongoing treatment. Population analyses of the regrown organisms at 24 h revealed a complete shift to variants resistant to at least 4 μg of gentamicin per ml. Similarly, the subpopulation resistant to 8 μg/ml had grown from less than 10^2 up to 10^5 organisms per thigh. The resistance of these selected subpopulations proved, however, to be unstable and was readily lost. The reversion was observed in vitro (after regrowth of the isolated organisms in drug-free broth) as well as in vivo when the treatment was

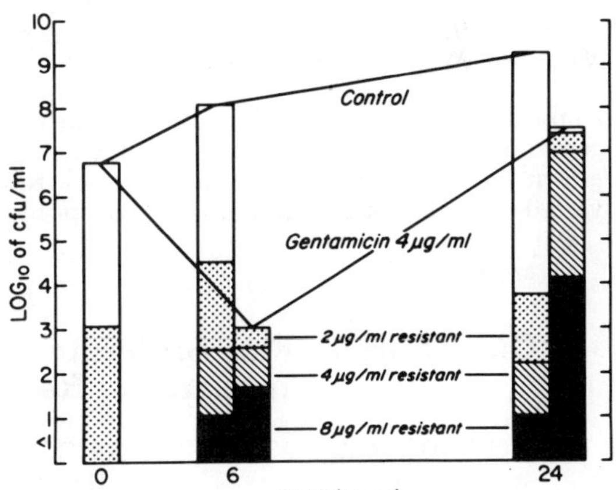

FIG. 1. *Population shift of P. aeruginosa ATCC 27853 exposed to gentamicin (2 × MIC) in vitro. Lines represent the kill-regrowth curve as obtained in the test tube in an extract from Mueller-Hinton agar (Ca^{2+}, 4.8 mg/dl; Mg^{2+}, 1.9 mg/dl). Bars represent the corresponding population analyses obtained by plating on Mueller-Hinton agar containing 0, 2, 4, and 8 µg of gentamicin per ml.*

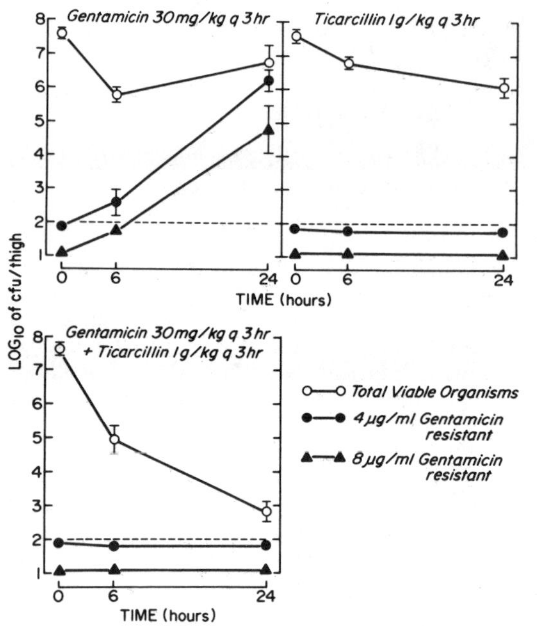

FIG. 2. *Effect of multiple doses of gentamicin and ticarcillin alone and in combination on the number and relative susceptibility of P. aeruginosa ATCC 27853 in infected thighs of leukopenic mice. Gentamicin (30 mg/kg) and ticarcillin (1 g/kg) were administered subcutaneously every 3 h for a total of eight doses. Groups of three mice were killed immediately before and at 6 and 24 h after starting each drug regimen. Total viable organisms (○) and those resistant to 4 (●) and 8 (▲) µg of gentamicin per ml are depicted as geometric means ± 1 SD. The MIC of gentamicin for this strain was 2 µg/ml. The dotted line represents the lower limit for accurate detection of organisms in 10% tissue homogenates.*

stopped after 6 to 12 h. The slowly growing gentamicin-resistant forms were quickly overgrown by the few remaining, or by some reverted, faster-growing gentamicin-susceptible organisms. Hence, we were unable to demonstrate the gentamicin resistance of the selected subpopulations in routine susceptibility testing (Kirby-Bauer).

Ticarcillin (1,000 mg/kg every 3 h) in concomitant or alternate dosing with gentamicin resulted in 99.999% killing of the primary inoculum by 24 h. This combination was very effective in preventing the growth and selection of gentamicin-resistant variants in leukopenic mice.

We draw four major conclusions from our studies. (i) Despite very high dosing and high consequent drug levels in plasma and tissues, *P. aeruginosa* cannot be successfully treated with gentamicin alone in the presence of leukopenia. The same statement was valid in preliminary experiments performed with tobramycin and amikacin. (ii) The therapeutic failures in our model using leukopenic mice are due to a shift of the target organisms to forms which are resistant to gentamicin. (iii) The selected subpopulations of *P. aeruginosa* exhibit a gentamicin resistance which is unstable and which cannot be demonstrated in routine susceptibility test procedures. (iv) The superiority of repeated high doses of the gentamicin-ticarcillin combination in the presence of leukopenia is due to its better coverage of the entire population of the test organisms, including the gentamicin-resistant forms. By 24 h of treatment, ticarcillin proves to be beneficial mainly because of its full suppression of the gentamicin-resistant subpopulations. Our findings could explain, at least in part, the aminoglycoside–β-lactam synergy experienced in the treatment of *P. aeruginosa* infections in leukopenic patients.

1. **Gerber, A. U., and W. A. Craig.** 1980. Small colony variants of *Pseudomonas aeruginosa*: characterization and virulence in normal and leukopenic mice. Clin. Res. **28:**735A.

Outer Surface Fine Structure of Clinical Isolates of *Pseudomonas aeruginosa* Resistant to Antibiotics

THEODORE A. KATSORCHIS, NICHOLAS J. LEGAKIS,* HARRYS PATARYAS, AND JOHN PAPAVASSILIOU

Department of Biology, University of Athens, Panepistimioupolis, Kouponia, and Department of Microbiology, Medical School, University of Athens, Goudi, Athens, Greece*

The importance of the cell envelope of *Pseudomonas aeruginosa* in resistance to antimicrobial drugs by an exclusion mechanism has been demonstrated by EDTA and crypticity studies (14). The outer membrane (OM) of the cell wall, composed of lipopolysaccharides (LPS), proteins, and phospholipids, is mainly involved in this process (1, 11, 12).

In *P. aeruginosa* strains resistant to carbenicillin or polymyxin (3) because of a permeability defect, a correlation between the chemistry of the OM and resistance has been indicated. OM protein alterations have been also reported for *P. aeruginosa* mutants resistant to polymyxin, EDTA, and gentamicin (10). It was also recently shown (8) that trained variants of *P. aeruginosa* resistant to carbenicillin or gentamicin are characterized by increased adherence, evidently due to an altered surface as detected by electron microscopy. In clinical isolates of *P. aeruginosa*, defective permeability contributes greatly to the expression of resistance to β-lactam antibiotics (13, 14), and the same has been reported for resistance to aminoglycosides (2, 7).

In view of these observations, it was considered interesting to study the ultrastructure of the surface of *P. aeruginosa* clinical isolates resistant to carbenicillin or gentamicin to see whether it was different from that of the susceptible stains.

Clinical isolates included in this study were as follows: six susceptible to carbenicillin and gentamicin; four resistant to carbenicillin; three resistant to gentamicin; and four resistant to carbenicillin and gentamicin. All strains studied were resistant to chloramphenicol, tetracycline, and nalidixic acid but susceptible to polymyxin. Organisms were grown at 37°C in Mueller-Hinton broth inoculated from an 18-h broth culture. The cultures in the exponential phase were harvested by refrigerated centrifugation (4°C, 10,000 × *g* for 20 min). The pellets were prefixed in 0.1 M sodium cacodylate containing glutaraldehyde (3%, wt/vol) and formaldehyde (2%, vol/vol). Postfixation was for 20 min at 4°C in $KMnO_4$ (2%, wt/vol). Thin sections (MI-2 ultramicrotome) were double stained with uranyl acetate and lead citrate and then examined with a Philips EM 200 operating at 80 kV.

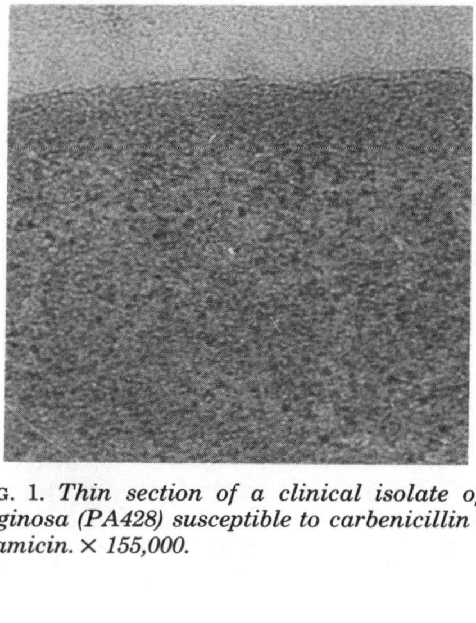

FIG. 1. *Thin section of a clinical isolate of P. aeruginosa (PA428) susceptible to carbenicillin and gentamicin.* × *155,000.*

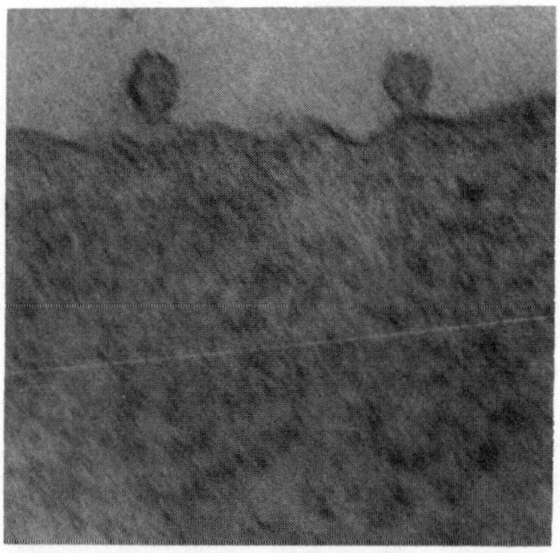

FIG. 2. *Thin section of a clinical isolate of P. aeruginosa (PA388) resistant to carbenicillin and gentamicin.* × *155,000.*

Thin sections of susceptible strains (Fig. 1) showed the typical unit membrane appearance of gram-negative bacteria, with fairly smooth surfaces. Strains resistant to carbenicillin and gentamicin (Fig. 2) were characterized by the presence of bulges in connection with distortion of the tripartite nature of the OM. Furthermore, the OM appeared wavy with cloudy formations. The latter findings in connection with altered stratification of the OM also characterized the strains resistant to carbenicillin or gentamicin. Other experiments not shown here revealed that surface changes were accompanied, in some of the resistant strains, with OM protein alterations (polyacrylamide gel electrophoresis).

In *Enterobacteriaceae*, several lines of evidence support the view that LPS are located only in the outer half and most phospholipid molecules are located in the inner half of the OM (11). Evidence also has been produced that LPS linked with proteins in a protein-LPS complex occupies the outer half of the OM in *P. aeruginosa* (4). The supramolecular organization of these molecules results in the formation of transmembrane pores for the entrance of hydrophilic substances, including polar antibiotics, into the cells (11). This structure appears to be disturbed in LPS-defective mutants of *P. aeruginosa* lacking polymerized O-antigenic side chains, in that membrane components are redistributed so that more hydrophobic molecules (phospholipids) are exposed to the surface of the membrane (9, 11). It is interesting to note that surface changes were recently reported in these mutants (9) that were similar to those observed in our clinical resistant isolates and to those found upon treatment with polymyxin (6).

The bulges observed in carbenicillin- or gentamicin-resistant isolates, as is the case with LPS-deficient mutants (9), may have been fragments of the OM, as is the case in *Escherichia coli* (5), which were extruded from the bacterial surface and which, because of their lipophilicity, were attached to the hydrophobic surface of the OM.

At the moment, it is difficult to assign any role to OM surface alterations in the expression of resistance. However, it might be speculated that OM surface changes reflect impaired penetrability of hydrophilic substances in the sense that essential changes in the OM structure constitute the underlying mechanism for OM surface alterations. The fact that susceptibility to antibiotics was not differentiated in LPS-deficient mutants of *P. aeruginosa* where OM surface alterations were noted (9) apparently contradicts this assumption. However, in some of our resistant isolates, changes in OM proteins were noted which could conform to a decreased permeability. Additionally, in the clinical isolates, other mechanisms of resistance may operate. In these strains, a minor variation of permeability, not detected by the usual tests, could offer an essential increase in the level of the resistant status.

The evidence suggested in this study is in line with previous observations on the role of cellular permeability for the expression of resistance of *P. aeruginosa* to carbenicillin (13) and gentamicin (2, 7) and should initiate interest in the chemistry of the OM. Work is in progress to study further the OM proteins profile and analyze the LPS in these strains.

1. **Costerson, J. W., J. M. Ingram, and K. J. Cheng.** 1974. Structure and function of the cell envelope of gram-negative bacteria. Bacteriol. Rev. **38:**87–110.
2. **Davies, J.** 1979. General mechanisms of antimicrobial resistance. Rev. Infect. Dis. **1:**23–29.
3. **Gilleland, H. E., and R. D. Lyle.** 1979. Chemical alterations in cell envelopes of polymyxin-resistant *Pseudomonas aeruginosa* isolates. J. Bacteriol. **138:**839–845.
4. **Gilleland, H. E., Jr., and R. G. E. Murray.** 1976. Ultrastructural study of polymyxin-resistant isolates of *Pseudomonas aeruginosa.* J. Bacteriol. **125:**267–281.
5. **Hoekstra, D., J. W. Van Der Laan, L. De Leu, and B. Witholt.** 1976. Release of outer membrane fragments from normally growing *Escherichia coli.* Biochim. Biophys. Acta **455:**889–899.
6. **Koike, M., K. Lida, and T. Matsuo.** 1969. Electron microscopic studies on the mode of action of polymyxin. J. Bacteriol. **97:**448–452.
7. **Legakis, N. J., J. Tselentis, E. Courtis, and J. Papavassiliou.** 1979. Cross-resistance of clinical isolates of *Pseudomonas aeruginosa* to five aminoglycosides. J. Antimicrob. Chemother. **5:**487–490.
8. **Lianou, P. E., H. P. Bassaris, G. K. Daikos, T. A. Katsorchis, and N. J. Legakis.** 1980. Increased adherence to human epithelial cells of resistant *Pseudomonas aeruginosa* strains. J. Infect. **2:**354–359.
9. **Meadow, P. M., P. L. Wells, M. Salkinoza-Salonen, and E.-L. Nurmiaho.** 1978. The effect of lipopolysaccharide composition on ultrastructure of *Pseudomonas aeruginosa.* J. Gen. Microbiol. **105:**23–28.
10. **Nicas, T. I., and R. E. W. Hancock.** 1980. Outer membrane protein H1 of *Pseudomonas aeruginosa*: involvement in adaptive and mutational resistance to ethylenediaminetetraacetate, polymyxin B, and gentamicin. J. Bacteriol. **143:**872–878.
11. **Nikaido, H. N., and T. Nakae.** 1979. The outer membrane of Gram-negative bacteria. Adv. Microb. Physiol. **20:**164–220.
12. **Osborn, M. J., and M. C. P. Wu.** 1980. Proteins of the outer membrane of Gram-negative bacteria. Annu. Rev. Microbiol. **34:**369–376.
13. **Richmond, M. H.** 1978. Factors influencing the antibacterial action of β-lactam antibiotics. J. Antimicrob. Chemother. **4**(Suppl. B)**:**1–14.
14. **Sykes, R. B., and A. Morris.** 1975. Resistance of *Pseudomonas aeruginosa* to antimicrobial drugs. Prog. Med. Chem. **12:**333–393.

Transmission Electron Microscopy Investigation of Bacteria with Induced Resistance to Amoxicillin-Fosfomycin Combination

ORNELLA CATTANEO,* GIANFRANCO MARCA, ANNA MARIA CUFFINI, AND NICOLA A. CARLONE

Institute of Microbiology, University of Turin, Turin, and Zambon S.p.A., Laboratory Research, Bresso (Mi), Italy*

Combinations using fosfomycin in conjunction with various other antibiotics have been particularly mentioned among the many associations proposed in the literature. Fosfomycin, in fact, has excellent qualities, such as rapid absorption and establishment of high blood levels (2), as well as bactericidal activity against the majority of pathogenic strains (1). Unfortunately, bacteria frequently become resistant to it (3). For this reason, various workers (5, 6) have suggested that the combination of fosfomycin with amoxicillin is an optimal mixture for the management of infections, since the drugs are synergistic against numerous gram-positive and gram-negative bacteria. Furthermore, the better pharmacological properties of amoxicillin make it preferable to combinations of fosfomycin with other antibiotics (4, 5).

TABLE 1. *MICs of S. aureus and E. coli 12 times subcultured in the presence of amoxicillin, fosfomycin, and their combination*

no culture	amoxycillin MIC mcg/ml		fosfomycin MIC mcg/ml		mixture 1:1 MIC mcg/ml	
	E. coli 0128	S. aureus 6538	E. coli 0128	S. aureus 6538	E. coli 0128	S. aureus 6538
1	4	0 25	2	1	1 · 1	00625·00625
2	8	0 5	32	8	2 · 2	0125·0125
3	16	1	512	16	2 · 2	025·0 25
4	16	1		512	2 · 2	025·0 25
5	16	1			2 · 2	025·0 25
6	16	1			4 · 4	05·05
7	32	1			4 · 4	05·05
8	32	1			4 · 4	05·05
9	32	2			4 · 4	05·05
10	32	2			4 · 4	05·05
11	64	2			8 · 8	05·05
12	64	2			8 · 8	05·05

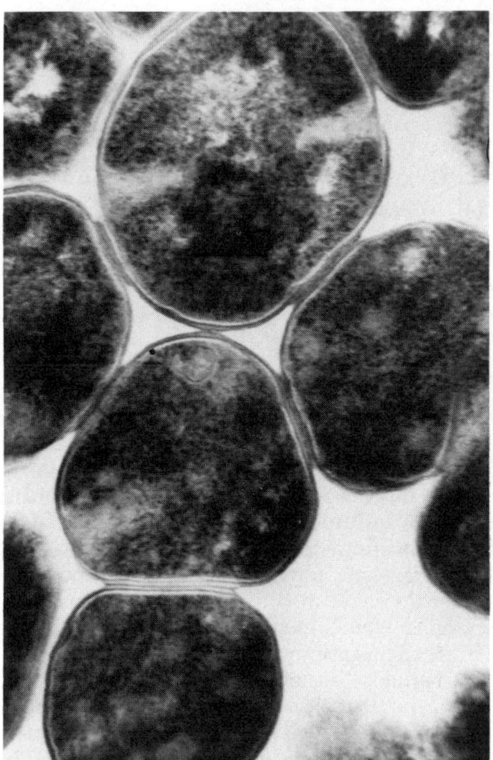

FIG. 1. *Resistant S. aureus after the 12th subculture with the combination. (×55,000).*

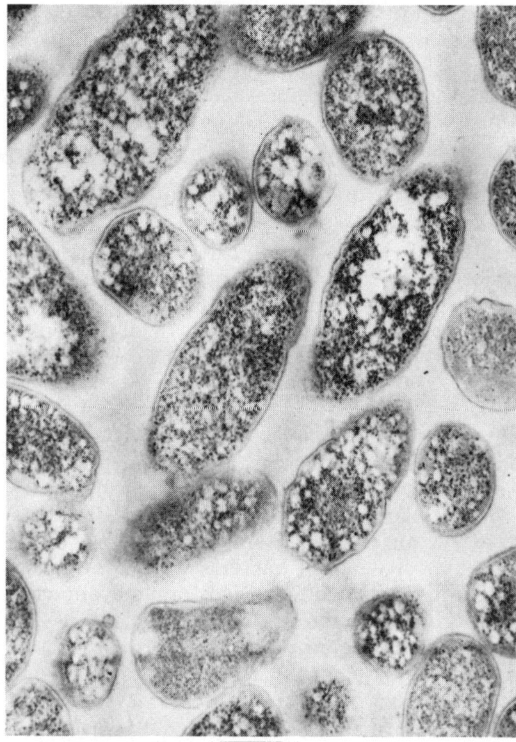

FIG. 2. *Resistant E. coli after the 12th subculture with the combination. (×17,500).*

It was previously reported that 1:1 amoxicillin-fosfomycin combination was effective in reducing natural and induced resistance among bacteria susceptible to both antibiotics (N. A. Carlone et al., in press). In the present study, we investigated changes in antibiotic susceptibility of the same strains (*Staphylococcus aureus* ATCC 6538 and *Escherichia coli* O128) repeatedly subcultured with amoxicillin and fosfomycin, singly and in 1:1 mixture. The studies were performed by use of conventional MIC procedures.

Twelve serial subcultures with amoxicillin resulted in 16- and 8-fold increases in MIC for *E. coli* and *S. aureus*, respectively. In the presence of fosfomycin, a high increase in MIC values was obtained from the third passage for both bacteria. With the combination, bacterial susceptibility decreased throughout the 12 subcultures. These concentrations, however, were lower than those observed with each antibiotic separately (Table 1). In the process of isolating the resistant bacteria, colonies were seen on the isolation plates in the last subculture. The colonies of *S. aureus* obtained through the treatment with amoxicillin and with fosfomycin showed a morphology identical to that of the control. On the other hand, the mixture created colonies with altered edges. In the case of *E. coli*, the control colonies and those treated with fosfomycin manifested smooth and round edges. Treatment with amoxicillin created "fried egg" colonies with frayed edges. This effect was even more pronounced with the combination.

The ultrastructure of the colony-forming organisms was then investigated to elucidate the relationship between their differences to the antibiotic action. We found that *S. aureus* subcultured 12 times with amoxicillin showed abnormally thick and irregular cross walls. In certain bacteria, multiple divisions were noted. Fosfomycin treatment resulted in the formation of chains of damaged and lysed cells; some of them, having irregular shapes, thin septum, and disorganized cytoplasm, presented the beginning of a further septation in a just-divided organism. The low concentrations of the mixture less frequently caused alterations of the cross walls. The majority of the bacteria were even more susceptible to the effect of fosfomycin, showing linked cells with normal cross walls (Fig. 1). Rarely, some bacteria showed abnormal but not hypertrophic septa. On *E. coli*, amoxicillin induced a marked alteration in the cytoplasmic ultrastructure. The cells were aggregated, with rarefied cytoplasm and an indistinguishable DNA region. With fosfomycin, some bacteria were clumped together and showed several vacuoles in their plasmic content. Subcultures treated with the combination had a regular morphology. The cells were separated with well-preserved cell walls. The cytoplasm, on the other hand, showed a more evident vacuolation (Fig. 2). The lower concentrations of amoxicillin and fosfomycin used in the combination (0.5 plus 0.5 μg/ml for *S. aureus* and 8 plus 8 μg/ml for *E. coli*) explain the reduced morphological alterations observed in comparison with those obtained by using each antibiotic separately.

1. **Carlone, N. A., A. M. Cuffini, and O. Cattaneo.** 1977. Fosfomicina I: attività antimicrobica in vitro. G. Batteriol. Virol. Immunol. **70**:100.
2. **Carlone, N. A., A. M. Cuffini, and D. Savoia.** 1977. Fosfomicina II: attività antimicrobica in vivo. G. Batteriol. Virol. Immunol. **70**:215.
3. **Dulaney, E. L., and C. L. Ruby.** 1977. In vitro development of resistance to fosfomycin. J. Antibiot. **30**:252.
4. **Hunter Handsfield, H., H. Clarck, J. F. Wallace, K. K. Holmes, and M. Turck.** 1973. Amoxicillin: a new penicillin antibiotic. Antimicrob. Agents Chemother. **3**: 262.
5. **Neuman, M., and G. Flutaeu.** 1980. The in vitro activity of the association fosfomycin+amoxycillin in the treatment of systemic Salmonella infections in man. Drugs Exp. Clin. Res. **6**:297.
6. **Periti, P.** 1980. Rationale of fixed-dose combinations of fosfomycin with β-lactam antibiotics: co-fosfolactamines. Drugs Exp. Clin. Res. **6**:305.

Microbiological In Vitro and Animal Studies with Combinations of New β-Lactam Antibiotics

A. E. GEHL,* A. DALHOFF, G. DZWILLO, AND H. LODE

Medical Department of Klinikum Steglitz, Freie Universität Berlin, Berlin, and Institute of Chemotherapy, Wuppertal, West Germany

Today, combinations of new cephalosporins with penicillins are increasingly recommended for initial therapy of septicemia without knowledge of the etiological pathogen. A number of studies have demonstrated synergistic as well as antagonistic effects of β-lactam antibiotic combinations (1, 2, 4–6, 9). In this study, we evaluated and compared the in vitro and in vivo antibacterial effects of combinations of ureidopenicillins with new cephalosporins on different randomly selected *Proteus* species and *Pseudomonas aeruginosa.*

MICs were determined by means of a standardized microdilution method (3). An inoculum of 10^6 colony-forming units (CFU)/ml was used. MICs were determined for each drug alone as well as in the presence of a second β-lactam agent. The following definitions were used to characterize the observed effects: antagonism, fourfold or greater increase in the MIC of either antibiotic; indifference, no change in the MIC of either antibiotic or no more than a twofold change in one; partial synergism, twofold or greater decrease in the MIC of each antibiotic; synergism, fourfold or greater decrease in the MIC of each antibiotic.

Bactericidal kinetics were studied by the membrane filtration method (3). The inoculum was approximately 10^6 CFU/ml. Viable counts were determined over a period of 0 to 48 h. The 33 different, randomly selected strains investigated included: 9 of *P. aeruginosa*, 10 of *Proteus*

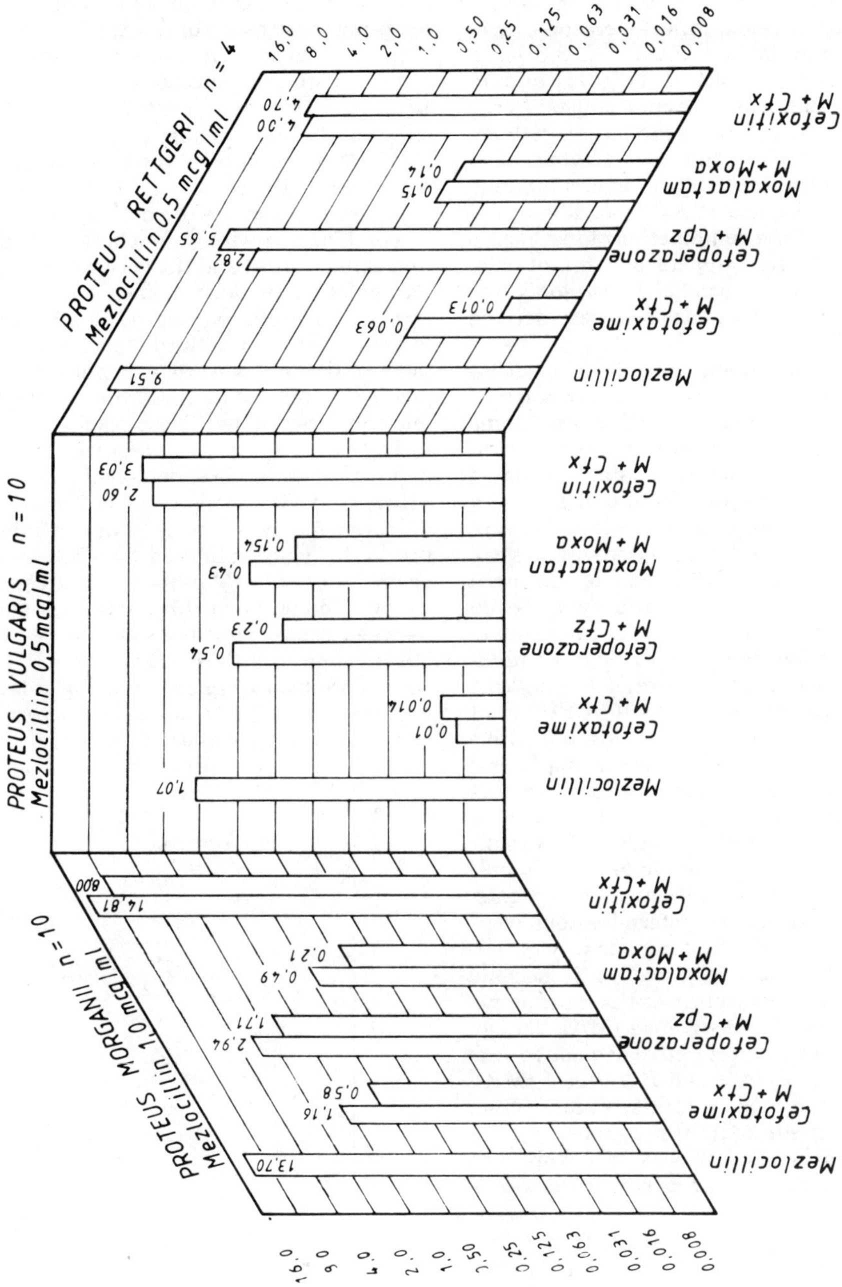

FIG. 1. *In vitro effects of the combination of mezlocillin with cephalosporins against Proteus species.*

vulgaris, 10 of *P. morganii*, and 4 of *P. rettgeri*. Sixteen different combinations of β-lactam antibiotics were tested by microdilution method. Mezlocillin was tested at a constant concentration of 1.0 μg/ml in combination with various concentrations of cefoxitin, cefoperazone, cefotaxime, and moxalactam against *P. morganii* and of 0.5 μg/ml against *P. vulgaris* and *P. rettgeri*. Azlocillin was used at a constant concentration of 2.0 μg/ml in combination with cefoperazone, cefotaxime, and moxalactam against *P. aeruginosa* and of 1.0 μg/ml in combination with cefotaxime against *P. vulgaris*. The bactericidal kinetics of the combination of mezlocillin with cefotaxime and cefoperazone and of azlocillin with cefotaxime against *P. vulgaris* was studied. The concentrations used were derived from the MICs.

The "granuloma pouch" model was used for the in vivo studies (7, 8) as a model of a (sub-) chronic infected inflammation. The granuloma pouch was formed by injecting a given amount of air (20 ml) into the loose subcutaneous tissue of the rat followed by an injection of 1 ml of a solution of 1% croton oil in olive oil. An advantage of this method is that repeated samples can be taken from the same animal on different occasions for a period of several days. Seven days after formation of the pouch, the exudate (6 to 7 ml) was infected with 0.5 ml of an undiluted, washed overnight culture of *P. vulgaris*, so that the final cell count was 10^8 CFU/ml of exudate. The antibiotics were injected alternately intravenously and intramuscularly, respectively, twice daily. The daily doses were as follows: mezlocillin, 200 mg/kg; cefotaxime, 80 mg/kg; and cefoperazone, 80 mg/kg. These substances were injected either alone or in combination. Each regimen was investigated in 20 rats. Samples for viable-count determinations were taken daily prior to the first injection.

Based on the mean MIC values, it became apparent that cefoperazone was the most active antibiotic against *P. aeruginosa* (MIC, 2.0 μg/ml), cefotaxime was most active against *P. vulgaris* (MIC, 0.01 μg/ml) and *P. rettgeri* (MIC, 0.063 μg/ml), and moxalactam was most active against *P. morganii* (MIC, 0.49 μg/ml).

Figure 1 represents the mean MIC values of mezlocillin, cefotaxime, cefoperazone, moxalactam, and cefoxitin and the activity of their combinations against *P. vulgaris*, *P. morganii*, and *P. rettgeri*. As can be deduced from Fig. 1, most of the mezlocillin–cephalosporin combinations produced indifferent effects. Only with strains of *P. rettgeri* did the combination of mezlocillin plus cefotaxime cause a partial synergism (two of four strains). Analogous results were obtained in six of nine *P. aeruginosa* strains with the combination azlocillin plus cefotaxime, which also caused a partial synergism. All the bacterial kinetics experiments exhibited only indifferent effects. In no case could we observe an antagonism between mezlocillin and cephalosporins by adopting these techniques.

In vivo, the combinations were tested against strains exhibiting different β-lactamase production rates and various degrees of inducibility. In spite of the high challenge dose of about 10^8 CFU/ml of exudate, a good therapeutic effect was noted in the course of β-lactam treatment.

Figure 2 illustrates the activity of mezlocillin in combination with cefotaxime as well as an untreated control and the activity of mezlocillin and cefotaxime alone against one *P. vulgaris* strain that produced negligible amounts of β-lactamase. From the third day after commencement of therapy onward, a combined treatment yielded better results than those obtained with one substance alone. These results apply qualitatively for the other *P. vulgaris* strains tested in vivo as well, thus demonstrating that the superior in vitro activity of cefotaxime is not mirrored in vivo. The β-lactam combinations tested in vivo exhibited indifferent activity against those *P. vulgaris* strains with an average to low production of β-lactamase. A synergism between mezlocillin and cefotaxime could be observed only in those cases when *P. vulgaris* strains producing large amounts of β-lactamase were studied. The change in bacterial titers caused by the combinations tested in this study

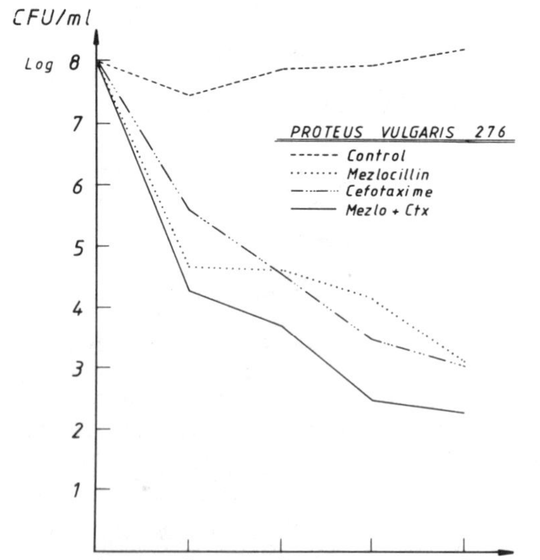

FIG. 2. *Antimicrobial effect of the combination mezlocillin–cefotaxime against P. vulgaris (granuloma pouch).*

was by five $\log_{10}$ titers more effective than a monotherapy with either of these substances.

1. **Andrews, J. M., K. A. Bedford, R. Wise, and A. P. Gillett.** 1980. Azlocillin and ticarcillin in combination with cefoxitin and cefotaxime (HR756); an in vitro study, p. 150–152. *In* J. D. Nelson and C. Grassi (ed.), Current chemotherapy and infectious disease. American Society for Microbiology, Washington, D.C.
2. **Grimm, H.** 1980. Bakteriologische Untersuchungen zum Antagonismus zwischen Acylureidopenicillinen und Cephalosporinen. Arzneim. Forsch. **30:**999–1000.
3. **Klein, P.** 1957. Bakteriologische Grundlagen der chemotherapeutischen Laboratoriumspraxis. Verlag Springer, Berlin.
4. **Knothe, H.** 1980. Sensitivity testing and synergy. J. Antimicrob. Chemother. **6** (Suppl. A):31–35.
5. **Kuck, N. A., R. T. Testa, and M. Forbes.** 1981. In vitro and in vivo antibacterial effects of combinations of beta-lactam antibiotics. Antimicrob. Agents Chemother. **19:** 634–638.
6. **Neuhaus, B., W. Kammer, and D. Förster.** 1981. Resistance to penicillin derivatives inducible by cephalosporins in Enterobacteriaceae and Pseudomonadaceae. Infection **9:**12–17.
7. **Nishida, M., and T. Murakawa.** 1977. Exudate levels and bactericidal activity of cefazolin in a new local infection system using rat granuloma pouches. Antimicrob. Agents Chemother. **11:**1042–1048.
8. **Selye, H.** 1953. Use of "granuloma pouch" technic in the study of antiphlogistic corticoids. Proc. Soc. Exp. Biol. Med. **82:**328–333.
9. **Wise, R., A. P. Gillett, and J. M. Andrews.** 1979. The in vitro activity of mezlocillin when combined with cefoxitin or clavulanic acid. J. Antimicrob. Chemother. **5:**301–306.

Interaction Among Newer Cephalosporins and Azlocillin

CHRISTINA M. J. E. VANDENBROUCKE,* MAJA ROZENBERG-ARSKA, AND JAN VERHOEF

Department of Clinical Bacteriology, University Hospital, Utrecht, The Netherlands

Serious bacterial infections are often treated with the potentially toxic combination of an aminoglycoside and a cephalosporin. The introduction of new cephalosporins with a broad spectrum of activity could possibly help avoid the use of aminoglycosides. A broad-spectrum cephalosporin could be used as a single agent, in combination with another cephalosporin, or in combination with a ureidopenicillin. Antagonism, however, has been shown to exist between certain cephalosporins and between certain cephalosporins and penicillin derivatives. Before combinations of these drugs are to be used clinically, the possibility of antagonism between the drugs should be excluded.

We examined the interaction between azlocillin and cefotaxime, azlocillin and moxalactam, cefsulodin and cefotaxime, and cefsulodin and moxalactam. Cefotaxime and moxalactam are two new cephalosporins with a similar broad spectrum of activity, mainly directed against *Enterobacteriaceae.* Cefsulodin, a cephalosporin, and azlocillin, a ureidopenicillin, both have good activity against *Pseudomonas aeruginosa.*

The four combinations of drugs were tested against clinical isolates of *Staphylococcus aureus* (10 strains), *Pseudomonas aeruginosa* (10 strains), *Escherichia coli* (4 strains), *Klebsiella* species (4 strains), *Enterobacter* species (4 strains), and *Proteus* species (4 strains).

MICs of the different antibiotics and of the combinations of antibiotics were determined by using the broth dilution method. Twofold serial dilutions of each antibiotic were tested alone and in combination with twofold dilutions of the other antibiotics. All tests were performed in duplicate in microtiter plates, with a checkerboard technique. The bacterial inoculum contained 10^5 colony-forming units per ml. The MIC was defined as the lowest concentration of antibiotic that inhibited visible growth. The interaction between the drugs was determined to be synergistic, additive, or antagonistic by means of the fractional inhibitory concentration (FIC) index. The FIC is the ratio between the MIC of a drug in combination and the MIC of the drug alone: FIC = MIC of drug in combination/MIC of drug alone. The FIC index is the sum of the FIC of each of the drugs used in the combination: FIC index = FIC of drug A + FIC of drug B. If the index is less than or equal to 0.5, the combination is considered to be synergistic. If the index is more than 0.5 and less than unity, the interaction is considered to be partially synergistic. In this case, the MIC of one of the drugs in the combination is decreased by only one dilution compared with the MIC of that drug when used alone. If the index is more than unity, the interaction is considered to be antagonistic.

MIC values of azlocillin varied from 2 to more than 256 μg/ml; of cefsulodin, from 1 to more than 256 μg/ml; of cefotaxime, from 0.03 to 32 μg/ml; and of moxalactam, from 0.06 to 32 μg/ml.

The FIC indexes of the MIC values of the antibiotics azlocillin, cefotaxime, and moxalactam used in combination are given in Fig. 1. When the two combinations of azlocillin-cefotaxime and azlocillin-moxalactam were used, no antagonism against any of the 36 strains tested was observed. Both combinations achieved a similar degree of synergy or partial synergy. Synergy between azlocillin and cefotaxime was observed against two strains, and synergy between azlocillin and moxalactam was observed against seven strains. Partial synergy between azlocillin and cefotaxime was observed against 19 strains, and between azlocillin and moxalactam it was observed against 21 strains.

The FIC indexes of the MIC values of the combinations of cefsulodin-cefotaxime and cefsulodin-moxalactam are given in Fig. 2. Antagonism between cefsulodin and cefotaxime was found when they were used against two *Proteus* and two *Enterobacter* strains. The combination cefsulodin-moxalactam showed antagonism when used against the same two *Enterobacter* strains. The antagonism between the drugs increased when increasing amounts of cefsulodin were added to the combination; the more cefsulodin was added, the higher the MIC of cefotaxime and moxalactam. Cefsulodin already had an antagonistic effect when used in amounts of only 2 to 4 μg/ml. Thus, cefsulodin induces resistance against cefotaxime and moxalactam in some strains of *Proteus* and *Enterobacter* species. Fu and Neu (1) found that cephalosporins can induce beta-lactamases in *Enterobacteriaceae.* This mechanism could play an important role in the antagonism observed with some cephalosporin combinations. If this is the case in our experiments, then cefsulodin should induce beta-lactamases directed against cefotaxime and moxalactam. However, Mouton et al.

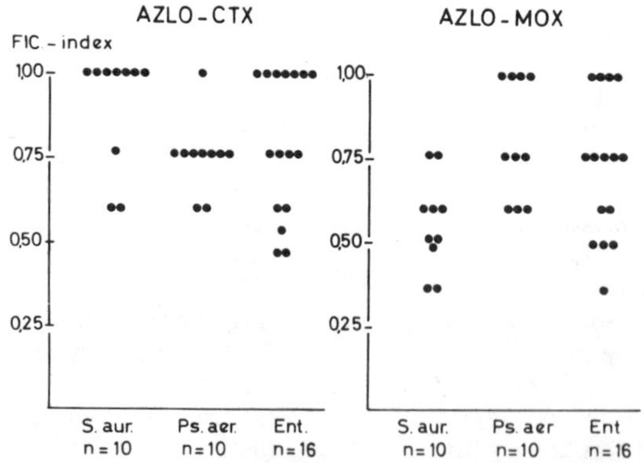

FIG. 1. *FIC indexes of the combinations azlocillin-cefotaxime (AZLO-CTX) and azlocillin-moxalactam (AZLO-MOX). S. aur., S. aureus; Ps. aer., P. aeruginosa; Ent., Enterobacteriaceae.*

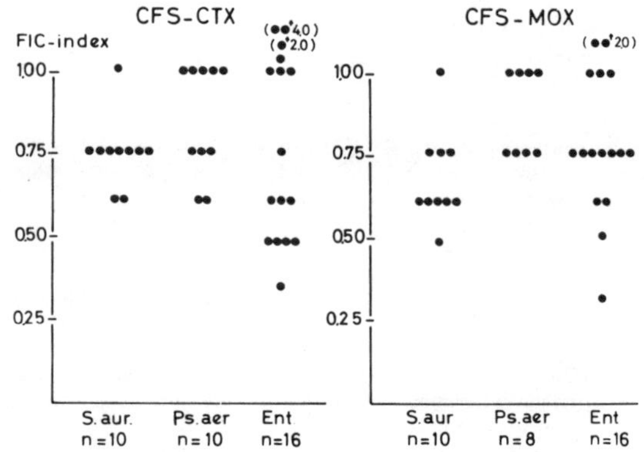

FIG. 2. *FIC indexes of the combinations cefsulodin-cefotaxime (CFS-CTX) and cefsulodin-moxalactam (CFS-MOX).*

(3) showed that cefotaxime is only poorly hydrolyzed by the beta-lactamases of *Proteus* and *Enterobacter* species; according to G. P. A. Bongaerts and R. P. Mouton (personal communication), moxalactam is completely resistant to these beta-lactamases. Mouton et al. (3) also found that there is no correlation between the MIC of some beta-lactam antibiotics for *Enterobacteriaceae* and production of beta-lactamases by *Enterobacteriaceae.* Therefore, it seems likely that mechanisms other than induction of beta-lactamases also play a role in resistance of *Enterobacteriaceae* against beta-lactam antibiotics and in the antagonism observed between cefsulodin and cefotaxime and between cefsulodin and moxalactam. It is possible that factors such as competition for the penicillin-binding proteins of the microorganisms play a role in this antagonism.

Although other investigators (2, 4) observed antagonism between cephalosporins and penicillin derivatives, we were not able to demonstrate any antagonism between azlocillin and cefotaxime or between azlocillin and moxalactam. In some instances, synergism was even observed.

1. **Fu, K. P., and H. C. Neu.** 1981. The role of inducible β-lactamases in the antagonism seen with certain cephalosporin combinations. J. Antimicrob. Chemother. **7:** 104–107.
2. **Graham, W. C., and A. A. Medeiras.** 1980. Antagonism of carbenicillin by cephalosporins in gram-negative bacilli, p. 489–491. *In* J. D. Nelson and C. Grassi (ed.), Current Chemotherapy and Infectious Disease. American Society for Microbiology, Washington, D.C.
3. **Mouton, R. P., G. P. A. Bongaerts, and M. van Gestel.** 1979. Comparison of activity and beta-lactamase stability of cefotaxime with those of six other cephalosporins. J. Antimicrob. Chemother. **16:**757–760.
4. **Neuhaus, B., W. Kammer, and D. Forster.** 1981. Resistance to penicillin derivatives inducible by cephalosporins in Enterobacteriaceae and Pseudomonadaceae. Infection **9:**12–17.

In Vitro Antagonistic Activity of Azlocillin with Cefoxitin Against *Pseudomonas aeruginosa*

H. GIAMARELLOU,* G. L. DAIKOS, K. KANELLAKOPOULOU, AND G. K. DAIKOS

First Department of Propedeutic Medicine, Athens University School of Medicine, King Paul's Hospital, Athens, 609, Greece

The empirical treatment of life-threatening infections, particularly in the neutropenic host, requires a combination of antibiotics to cover most of the probable pathogens. The most common therapeutic regimen includes an antipseudomonal penicillin combined with an aminoglycoside. However, because of the potential hazard of aminoglycoside toxicity, other treatment schedules are under investigation. Azlocillin is a new nontoxic ureidopenicillin with remarkable antipseudomonal activity, including many nosocomial strains resistant to gentamicin or carbenicillin or both (1). On the other hand, cefoxitin has an antibacterial spectrum of activity which includes most of the *Enterobacteriaceae* resistant to first-generation cephalosporins and more than 85% of *Bacteroides fragilis* strains. Cefoxitin, although a very poor substrate for the β-lactamases, is a very effective inducer of the enzymes, as Sanders and Sanders (2) have shown among *Enterobacter* spp., indole-positive *Proteus* spp., and *Serratia* spp.; the same investigators have also described the emergence of resistance to cefamandole in the presence of cefoxitin.

Pseudomonas aeruginosa is the major threat in neutropenic host infections; therefore, the possibility of therapeutic failures on the assumption of cefoxitin β-lactamase induction by *Pseudomonas* strains, which could inactivate azlocillin, should be clarified. Since both antibiotics are nontoxic and inhibit a broad spectrum of microorganisms, the in vitro study of their interaction is justified.

The ability of cefoxitin to antagonize azlocillin was investigated with 20 clinical isolates of *P. aeruginosa* by three methods: (i) the disk approximation test (2) with the use of 75- and 30-μg disks of azlocillin and cefoxitin, respectively; (ii) the broth checkerboard titration procedure; (iii) the bactericidal time-killing curve technique in the presence of 50 μg of cefoxitin per ml and 1× the MBC of azlocillin with an inoculum size of 10^5 colony-forming units/ml.

Antagonism was defined by: (i) a decrease of at least 4 mm in the radius of the azlocillin zone of inhibition between the azlocillin and cefoxitin disks in the disk approximation test, observed in 66% of the strains; (ii) at least a fourfold increase in azlocillin MIC in the checkerboard procedure, as observed in 50% of the strains; (iii) fractional inhibitory concentration determination of $\geq$2, as estimated in 84% of the strains; (iv) a $\geq$2-log difference in the viable counts between azlocillin and azlocillin plus cefoxitin after 6 h of incubation, which occurred in 90% of the *Pseudomonas* strains (Fig. 1).

The observed discrepancies in the results of the applied methods should be explained on the basis of the strictness of the arbitrary criteria used in the definition of antagonism. In the present study, however, whenever a strong antagonism of >2-log difference was observed, all methods were in agreement with the time-killing curve results.

To elucidate the possible mechanism of antagonism, suspensions of cells from eight different *P. aeruginosa* strains were assayed for the production of β-lactamase by the chromogenic cephalosporin procedure (nitrocefin test). Cells were grown overnight on either drug-free (uninduced) or drug-containing (50 μg of cefoxitin per ml, induced) media. The nitrocefin titration assay was thereafter performed with the induced and the uninduced sonicated cell supernatants simultaneously. A strong immediate reaction was observed in five of the eight induced strains but in none of the uninduced strains. After 20 min the remaining three induced strains also exhibited a positive strong reaction, whereas a weak reaction was observed in four and a moderate reaction was observed in another two of the uninduced strains. The possibility that induced β-lactamase production with cefoxitin could decrease azlocillin activity (10 μg/ml) against *P. aeruginosa* was investigated by applying the microbiological assay, recorded on a percentage basis between the induced and uninduced enzymes. Residual azlocillin was assayed by the agar well diffusion method with a very azlocillin-sensitive strain of *P. aeruginosa* used as the assay organism. Results are shown in Table 1. It is obvious that enhanced degradation of azlocillin occurs in the presence of cefoxitin. However, in two of the strains (Table 1, no. 117 and 6394), although an immediate

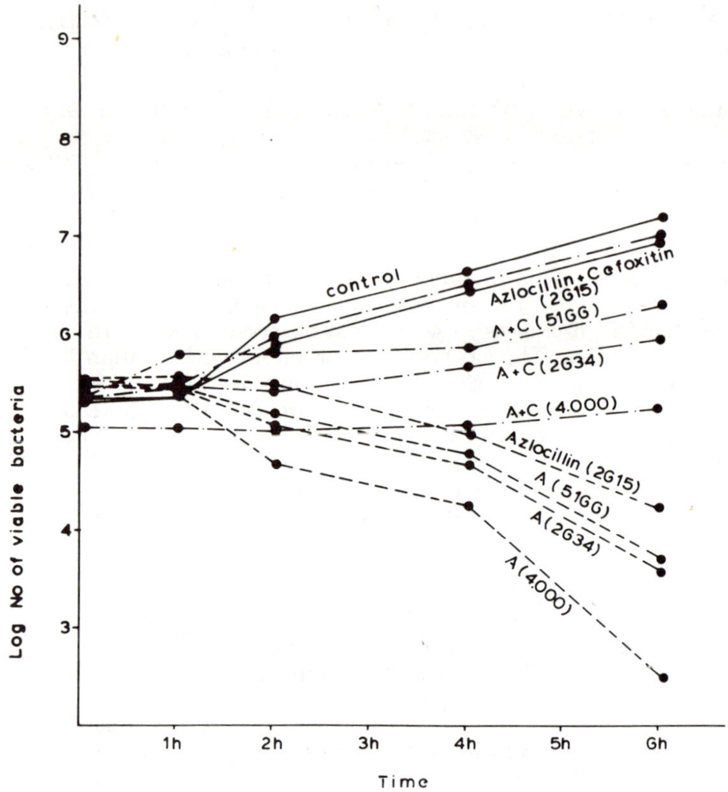

FIG. 1. *Time-killing curves of four P. aeruginosa strains in the presence of azlocillin (A) (1× the MBC) and azlocillin plus cefoxitin (C) (50 μg/ml).*

TABLE 1. *Azlocillin degradation by β-lactamase(s) produced by uninduced and induced cells of P. aeruginosa in the presence of cefoxitin (microbiological assay)*

Strain no.	% Degradation	
	Uninduced (30-min nitrocefin reaction)	Induced (30-min nitrocefin reaction)
2398	10 (L)[a]	100 (S)[b]
2615	12	100 (S)
2707	40 (L)	100 (S)
5116	64 (L)	100 (S)
2634	90 (L)	100 (S)
4028	12 (L)	93 (S)
117	60 (L)	60 (S)
6394	10 (L)	10 (S)

[a] L, Light reaction.
[b] S, Strong reaction.

strong nitrocefin reaction was observed with the induced enzyme and a weak one was observed with the uninduced one, there was no difference in azlocillin degradation between them. Therefore, cefoxitin in the majority of *P. aeruginosa* strains antagonizes azlocillin via the induction of β-lactamase, but also other mechanisms of antagonism within the cell, such as competition for penicillin-binding proteins, should not be excluded. The clinical relevance of the in vitro data reported herein and the relationship between the presence of inducible enzyme(s) and therapy outcome should be further clarified in humans by controlled clinical trials.

1. **Giamarellou, H., K. Hadjipolydorou, K. Kanellakopoulou, D. Bilalis, and G. K. Daikos.** 1978. Clinical efficacy, pharmacokinetics and in vitro evaluation of azlocillin, a new semi-synthetic penicillin, p. 617–622. *In* Proceedings of the First Mediterranean Congress of Chemotherapy, Madrid.
2. **Sanders, C. C., and W. E. Sanders, Jr.** 1979. Emergence of resistance to cefamandole: possible role of cefoxitin-inducible beta-lactamases. Antimicrob. Agents Chemother. **15:**792–797.

Combination Effect of Cefoxitin and Azlocillin in Vitro and in Serum of Volunteers

I. BRAVENY,* K. MACHKA, AND C. GRASSL

Institute of Medical Microbiology, Technical University, Munich, D-8000 Munich 80, Federal Republic of Germany

Combination of two or more antibiotics is necessary, particularly for the initial treatment of serious infections. Aminoglycosides with beta-lactam antibiotics is a widely used combination. Cephalosporins also may be considered, since their activity is similar to that of aminoglycosides. However, not only synergistic effects are seen in beta-lactam combinations: antagonistic effects have also been described, particularly with cefoxitin. Nothing is known of the clinical relevance of this in vitro antagonism. In an attempt to cast more light on this problem, we investigated the activity of cefoxitin combined with azlocillin against 95 clinical isolates, using the checkerboard technique, and compared the results with interactions in the serum of volunteers.

Thirty-one percent of the strains were preselected clinical isolates whereby the cefoxitin disks caused flattening of the zone of inhibition around azlocillin disks. The remaining isolates, belonging to more than 10 different species, were unselected. The fractional inhibitory concentra-

TABLE 1. *Antibacterial effects of cefoxitin plus azlocillin against Serratia marcescens Se8 and Enterobacter cloacae E61 determined by the checkerboard test*

Medium	ϵFIC index	
	Se8	E61
MH[a] broth	5.9	3.0
Urine, pH 6.1	0.8	1.2
Urine, pH 7.5	1.0	1.0
MH broth + 10% serum	3.0	
MH broth + 30% serum	1.5	1.3
Amniotic fluid	1.0	0.8

[a] MH, Mueller-Hinton.

TABLE 2. *Cumulative percentage of serum bactericidal activity (reciprocal) against selected species 1 h after injection of cefoxitin (CEF), azlocillin (AZL), or both*

Organism	Drug	MIC (mg/liter)	% Serum bactericidal activity at given concn (mg/liter)							
			256	128	64	32	16	8	4	2
Escherichia coli (*n* = 11)	CEF	2–128	18	27		36	63	72	82	100
	AZL	4–512	18	36	54			72	100	
	CEF/AZL		18	36	54	72	81		100	
Klebsiella spp. (*n* = 9)	CEF	2–256	11				22	78	100	
	AZL	16–256	11				44	88	100	
	CEF/AZL		11		67	100				
Proteus mirabilis (*n* = 11)	CEF	2–8			18	27	36	63	100	
	AZL	1–4	9	18	82	100				
	CEF/AZL		9	91	100					
Indole-positive *Proteus* spp. (*n* = 12)	CEF	1–32			15	23	31	69	100	
	AZL	4–32				15	45	60		100
	CEF/AZL		8		23	31	100			
Enterobacter spp. (*n* = 12)	CEF	4–256	8	17					25	100
	AZL	4–32	8	17	25	33	83	100		
	CEF/AZL		8	17			34	42	75	100
Serratia spp. (*n* = 6)	CEF	8–32						17	67	100
	AZL	8–16				17	67	84	100	
	CEF/AZL					33	83	100		
Citrobacter spp. (*n* = 6)	CEF	4–256						33	50	100
	AZL	16				50	83	100		
	CEF/AZL				17		34	67	83	100
Pseudomonas aeruginosa (*n* = 12)	CEF	256						8	16	100
	AZL	4–64			8	66	91			100
	CEF/AZL					8	25	50	75	100

tions (FIC) were determined by the checkerboard method in Mueller-Hinton broth and in body fluids. To determine the serum bactericidal activity as described by Klastersky et al. (1) for azlocillin in comparison with the combination, six volunteers received 2 g of cefoxitin on day 1, 5 g of azlocillin on day 2, and cefoxitin combined with azlocillin on day 3. One hour after injection, 100 ml of blood was taken, the sera were pooled and the antibacterial activity against 95 clinical isolates was tested in serial geometric dilutions.

The FIC index ranged from 2.0 to 16.0 in all of the isolates showing antagonism in the agar diffusion test. The FIC indices varied according to the medium used (Table 1). In body fluids such as urine, serum, or amniotic fluid, antagonism was reduced or absent. Table 2 presents the antibacterial activity of sera from volunteers against various species. The combination was considered to be synergistic if the activity against a strain was at least two titer steps higher than that of azlocillin and antagonistic if the combination was two titer steps lower. No antagonism was observed against indole-positive *Proteus* strains, although 10 strains had an FIC index of more than 2.0 in checkerboard titration, nor was antagonism observed against *Serratia* spp. Against seven of the nine *Klebsiella* spp. studied, the combination was clearly synergistic. Of the total of 95 isolates studied, synergism was observed with 24, indifference with 54, and antagonism with 17. The activity of the combination was inadequate against *Pseudomonas aeruginosa* and *Enterobacter* spp.

The interactions between antibiotics are complex and influenced by numerous factors. It can hardly be expected that an in vitro method will create the same conditions for antibiotic interactions as occur in the organism. The terms "antagonism" and "synergism" should therefore be interpreted with caution when applied to clinical situations.

1. **Klastersky, J., D. Dancau, G. Swings, and D. Weerts.** 1974. Antibacterial activity in serum and urine as a therapeutic guide in bacterial infections. J. Infect. Dis. **129:**187–193.

Synergistic Activity of Fortimicin and β-Lactam Antibiotics Against *Pseudomonas aeruginosa* In Vitro and In Vivo

KHOYA SHIBA,* MASAHISA OHMORI, ATSUSHI SAITO, YASUSHI UEDA, KOZO KITAURA, AND KAZUYUKI MINEURA

The Second Department of Internal Medicine, School of Medicine, The Jikei University, Tokyo, and Pharmaceutical Research Laboratory, Kyowa Hakko Kogyo Company, Ltd., Mishima, Japan*

Serious infections due to *Pseudomonas aeruginosa* are often treated with a combination of an aminoglycoside and an antipseudomonal β-lactam antibiotic such as carbenicillin or piperacillin to achieve additive or synergistic antibacterial activity. By lowering antibiotic MICs, synergistic combinations are considered to permit serum levels of an aminoglycoside to exceed the MIC of the infecting *P. aeruginosa* organism and result in therapeutic success.

Fortimicin (KW-1070) is a new broad-spectrum aminoglycoside antibiotic with characteristics of stability to aminoglycoside-inactivating enzymes, except AAC(III)-1 (2), and low-grade oto- and nephrotoxicity (3). This antibiotic exhibits strong activity against gentamicin-resistant bacteria such as *Serratia marcescens*, but its activity against *P. aeruginosa* is low (2, 4). Our previous clinical studies have shown fortimicin to be very effective against various kinds of infection due to gram-negative bacilli, except *P. aeruginosa* (Y. Ueda, A. Saito, and K. Shiba, Program Abstr. Intersci. Conf. Antimicrob. Agents Chemother. 20th, New Orleans, La., abstr. no. 58, 1980).

In the study reported here, the activities of fortimicin and antipseudomonal β-lactam antibiotics, namely, carbenicillin, piperacillin, and cefsulodin, against *P. aeruginosa* were measured in vitro and that of a combination of fortimicin and piperacillin was measured against experimental mouse infections.

Antibacterial activity in vitro. The MICs of the antibiotics alone and in combination were measured by the twofold serial dilution method, using a heart infusion agar plate and an inoculum of 10^4 colony-forming units. Fortimicin inhibited 15 of 27 strains of *P. aeruginosa* at a concentration of 25 μg/ml. It was two to four times more active than carbenicillin and slightly

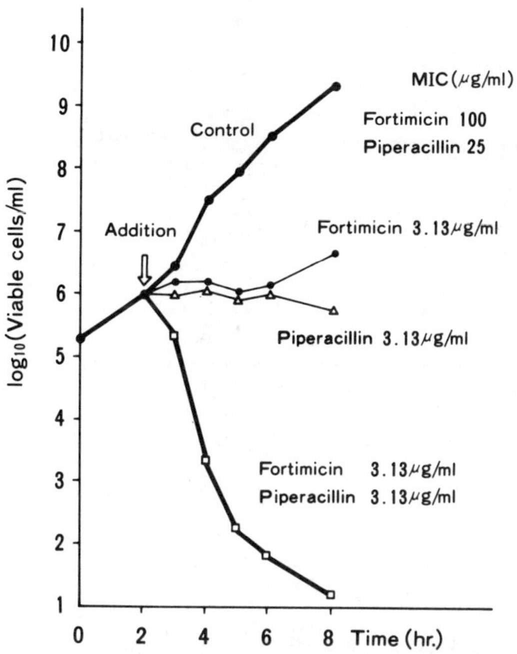

FIG. 1. *Bactericidal activity of fortimicin and piperacillin alone and in combination against P. aeruginosa F-1997.*

less active than piperacillin, but much less active than cefsulodin. Cefsulodin was the most active of the four antibiotics against strains of *P. aeruginosa*, with a MIC_{50} of <6.25 µg/ml.

Synergy in vitro. The inhibitory activities of fortimicin in combination with the β-lactam antibiotics against 27 strains of *P. aeruginosa* were measured by the checkerboard titration method. The effects were considered to be synergistic if the fractional inhibitory concentration index was ≤0.50 and partially synergistic if it was ≤0.75. This index was calculated by dividing the MIC obtained for each of the components in the combination by that for each component alone and adding the two quotients.

Synergy was observed more often when fortimicin was combined with piperacillin (17 strains, 63%) and cefsulodin (15 strains, 56%) than when it was combined with carbenicillin (8 strains, 29.6%). Synergy plus partial synergy were produced against all strains by the fortimicin-piperacillin combination and against 24 (88.9%) and 23 (85.2%) strains by the fortimicin-cefsulodin and fortimicin-carbenicillin combinations, respectively.

Killing curve. Killing curves were performed in heart infusion broth (Difco Laboratories), using a fresh dilution of organisms from an overnight culture in Trypticase soy broth (BBL Microbiology Systems). After incubation for 2 h at 37°C, serial twofold dilutions of fortimicin and piperacillin were added, and samples of culture were taken at selected intervals, immediately diluted in broth, and plated on heart infusion agar. The colony-forming units were counted after overnight incubation.

Figure 1 illustrates the effect of fortimicin-piperacillin when tested against *P. aeruginosa* F1997. When the antibiotics were added alone at a concentration less than the MIC, each antibiotic showed only a bacteriostatic activity. When used in combination, however, a clear bactericidal activity was recognized. The same result was obtained against *P. aeruginosa* E-2.

Synergy in vivo. The efficacy of fortimicin and piperacillin, alone and in combination, was measured against mouse peritoneal infections. Male ddY mice, each weighing 19 ± 1 g, were infected by the intraperitoneal route with suspensions of test organism in 5% hog gastric mucin in a volume of 0.5 ml. The infective inoculum was approximately 10 minimum lethal doses. The antibiotics were administered by the subcutaneous route 2 h after infection. The numbers of animals surviving 7 days after infection were recorded, and the 50% effective dose (in milligrams per kilogram) was determined by the Litchfield-Wilcoxon method. Synergy in vivo was considered to have occurred if the synergistic ratio, which corresponds to the reciprocal of the fractional inhibitory concentration index, was >1 (1).

In Table 1 are summarized the results of in vivo tests performed with three strains of *P. aeruginosa*. Fortimicin-piperacillin in a ratio of 1:5 or 1:10 showed an evident synergistic activity, with synergistic ratios of 2 to 3, against all three strains of *P. aeruginosa*.

Conclusions. The results of experiments reported here show that combination of fortimicin with β-lactam antibiotics exhibited additive or synergistic activity against most strains of *P. aeruginosa* tested. Particularly, fortimicin-piperacillin showed additive or synergistic activity against all strains tested as well as a strong bactericidal activity at a bacteriostatic concentration of each antibiotic alone. The synergy observed in vitro was reproduced against experimental mouse infections, and this combination produced significantly greater protective effects than the individual antibiotics. Therefore, the fortimicin-piperacillin combination is therapeutically promising, although the value of this synergistic combination can be established only by determining its relevance to the therapeutic outcome of clinical infections.

TABLE 1. *Synergistic activity of fortimicin (Fort.) and piperacillin (Pipe.) against intraperitoneal P. aeruginosa infection in mice*

Strain* & Inoculum	Antibiotics (MIC, μg/ml)	Combination Ratio	ED_{50} (mg/kg) Fortimicin / Piperacillin	SR value** (95% C.L.)
F-2043 5.1×10^5 cells/mouse	Fort.		29.3	
	Pipe. (200)		7060	
	Fort. + Pipe.	1 : 5	80.3	2.1 (1.4 3.2)
		1 : 10	95.8	3.2 (2.1 5.0)
F-1997 0.7×10^4 cells/mouse	Fort. (100)		90.3	
	Pipe (25)		639	
	Fort. + Pipe.	1 : 5	143	2.2 (1.5 3.2)
		1 : 10	208	2.0 (1.4 2.8)
E-2 0.8×10^5 cells/mouse	Fort. (25)		208	
	Pipe. (6.25)		2870	
	Fort. + Pipe.	1 : 5	446	2.1 (1.2 3.5)
		1 : 10	740	1.8 (1.0 3.1)

*P. aeruginosa was inoculated with 5% mucin.

Antibiotics were administered subcutaneously 2 hours after infection.

**Confidence limit

1. **Kawakami, M., Y. Nagai, S. Shimizu, and S. Mitsuhashi.** 1971. Anti-microbial effect of combinations of colistin methanesulfonate and chloramphenicol. I. In vitro effect. J. Antibiot. **24:**884–891.
2. **Nara, T., M. Yamamoto, I. Kawamoto, K. Takayama, R. Okachi, S. Takasawa, T. Sato, and S. Sato.** 1977. Fortimicins A and B, new aminoglycoside antibiotics. I. Producing organism, fermentation and biological properties of fortimicins. J. Antibiot. **30:**533–540.
3. **Saito, A., Y. Ueda, and M. Akiyoshi.** 1980. Experimental studies on the ototoxicity and nephrotoxicity of fortimicin A, p. 401–403. *In* J. D. Nelson and C. Grassi (ed.), Current chemotherapy and infectious disease, vol. 1. American Society for Microbiology, Washington, D.C.
4. **Thornsberry, C., A. L. Barry, R. N. Jones, C. N. Baker, R. E. Badal, and R. R. Packer.** 1981. Antibacterial activity of fortimicin A compared with those of five other aminoglycosides, and factors affecting susceptibility tests. Antimicrob. Agents Chemother. **19:** 122–129.

Pharmacokinetic Study of a New Sulfamethopyrazine-Trimethoprim Combination in Children

D. BASSETTI,* I. DE CARNERI, M. FERRECCIO, G. MEINARDI, F. PIAIA, AND V. TAMASSIA

Istituto Malattie Infettive, Genoa, and Farmitalia Carlo Erba, Milan, Italy*

The recently developed combination of trimethoprim (TMP) with the long-acting sulfonamide sulfamethopyrazine (SMPz), in the ratio 5:4 (Kelfiprim), showed antibacterial activity against a large number of gram-positive and gram-negative organisms. Synergism between the two components has been demonstrated with several strains over a wide range of SMPz/TMP ratios (3).

The pharmacokinetic properties of the two

TABLE 1. *Main kinetic parameters of TMP and SMPz in children and adults*

Subjects	Plasma $t_{1/2}$ (h)		Avg vol of distribution (liters/kg)	
	TMP	SMPz	TMP	SMPz
Children	~6	~40	~2	~0.250
Adults	~12	~60	~1.2	~0.190

compounds in adults allow a single daily administration of one capsule (TMP, 250 mg, plus SMPz, 200 mg), with a loading dose of two capsules on the first day (4).

Since literature data suggest that both TMP and SMPz are eliminated faster in children than in adults (1, 4), the simple scaling down of the adult dose, related to the different body weights, could result in suboptimal drug plasma levels in children, particularly for TMP in view of the once a day administration. It seemed important, therefore, to assess the pharmacokinetic properties of Kelfiprim in children to select the pediatric dosage schedule equivalent to the adult dosage schedule in terms of drug plasma levels.

The pharmacokinetic study was carried out in six children, four males and two females aged 5 to 14 years, suffering from various bacterial infections susceptible to the combination TMP-SMPz. The children were given Kelfiprim (oral suspension) at 0.4 ml/kg twice a day, corresponding to 4 mg of TMP plus 3.2 mg of SMPz per kg, every 12 h for 7 days. Blood samples (1.5 ml) were taken at 0, 1, 2, 4, 12, and 24 h on day 1 of treatment and at 0, 1, 2, 4, and 12 h on day 7. Urine excreted on days 1, 2, and 7 of treatment was also collected.

The plasma was separated, and urine samples were kept frozen until analyzed for the determination of TMP by microbiological assay and of SMPz by the colorimetric method of Bratton and Marshall. All children responded favorably to the therapy, and no side effects were observed.

Mean TMP plasma levels ranged between maximum values of about 1.5 to 2 μg/ml and minimum values of about 0.6 to 0.7 μg/ml, and no substantial differences were found between days 1 and 7 of treatment. Mean SMPz plasma levels increased from about 15 to 20 μg/ml in the second part of day 1 up to 55 to 70 μg/ml at day 7 of treatment, with moderate circadian fluctuations.

Fairly high levels of TMP were found in urine, where values were higher than 100 μg/ml from day 1 of treatment. The urine levels of SMPz (free drug) were about 10 to 20 μg/ml over the whole study period.

Table 1 shows the main kinetic parameters of TMP and SMPz calculated, according to conventional methods, from our data for children and from literature data for adults (2). For both drugs, the plasma half-life ($t_{1/2}$) was lower in children than in adults, and the difference was higher (6 versus 12 h) for TMP. There were differences between adults and children also in terms of the apparent volume of distribution, which appears to be 30 and 50% higher in children for SMPz and TMP, respectively.

On the whole, the mean plasma levels observed in children treated with 4 mg of TMP plus 3.2 mg of SMPz per kg twice a day were slightly lower than (for TMP) and similar to (for SMPz) those achieved in adults treated with the standard dosage schedule.

The faster elimination of both drugs in the pediatric age group in comparison with adults suggest that Kelfiprim in children should be given on a twice-daily basis, in contrast to the once a day administration used in adults.

The dose schedule investigated in this study (4 mg of TMP plus 3.2 mg of SMPz per kg every 12 h) appears to be suitable for treating bacterial infections in pediatric patients because it allows achievement of plasma levels of both drugs in the range of those observed in adults treated with the standard doses.

1. **Kremers, P., G. Biertho, J. M. Chantraine, and H. Heusghem.** 1973. Etude pharmacocinétique de l'association sulfaméthoxazole-triméthoprim chez l'enfant. Therapie **28:**1177–1184.
2. **Reeves, D. S., M. J. Bywater, D. W. Bullock, and H. A. Holt.** 1980. Pharmacokinetic study of a Sulphamethopyrazine/Trimethoprim combination (Kelfiprim) in human volunteers. J. Antimicrob. Chemother. **6:**647–656.
3. **Schioppacassi, G., V. Mandelli, R. Mazzoleni, and E. Morvillo.** 1979. Studio dell'interazione sulfametossipirazina-trimethoprim su schizomiceti in vitro. G. Ital. Chemioter. **26:**181–188.
4. **Sereni, F., L. Perletti, E. Marubini, and G. Mars.** 1968. Pharmacokinetic studies with a long-acting sulfonamide in subjects of different ages. Pediatr. Res. **2:**29–37.

Kelfiprim, a Combination of Sulfamethopyrazine and Trimethoprim, in Chronic Prostatitis: Pharmacokinetics and Preliminary Clinical Results

MICHELE PAVONE-MACALUSO,* DANILO DI TRAPANI, F. PAOLO RIZZO, RICCARDO ASCOLI, FRANCESCO CORRADO, ARMANDO MAVER, AND FRANCESCA PIAIA

Institute of Urology, University of Palermo, Palermo; Division of Urology and Division of Andrology, Malpighi Hospital, Bologna; and Farmitalia Carlo Erba, International Division, Medical Department, Milano; Italy*

Chronic prostatitis (CP) is a frequent disease and a common cause of recurrent urinary tract infections in adult males. It may fall under one of the following headings: (i) CP bacteriologically confirmed in the first urine specimen obtained after prostatic massage; (ii) CP with negative bacteriological findings, but leukocytes in the expressed prostatic fluid; (iii) suspicious CP with positive local objective findings but negative bacteriological and microscopical tests (prostatosis), or any condition with suggestive symptoms but negative laboratory tests (prostalgia). Patients falling under headings (ii) and (iii) may still respond to antibacterial treatment.

The treatment of CP is often difficult. Effective antimicrobial agents must be active against the isolated strains and capable of entering the prostatic tissue and fluid. Most aminoglycosides, cephalosporins, nitrofurantoin, and nalidixic acid do not reach prostatic tissue and fluid in therapeutic concentrations. Trimethoprim, sulfamethoxazole, minocycline, tobramycin, indanylcarbenicillin, pipemidic acid, oxolinic acid, and macrolides were reported to reach adequate concentrations in prostatic tissue. Most of such studies were performed only in prostatic adenoma and not in normal or inflamed prostatic tissue or secretion. Since CP requires prolonged treatment, it is not advisable to select parenteral or toxic drugs. Any treatment combining clinical effectiveness with safety and ease of administration can be recommended. Co-trimoxazole (Co-T) is considered the treatment of choice by many urologists. Its effectiveness varies between 30 and 70% in clinical reports.

Kelfiprim (KP) is a combination of trimethoprim (TMP) with a long-acting sulfonamide. It differs from Co-T in that: (i) the sulfa drug is sulfamethopyrazine (SMP) instead of sulfamethoxazole; (ii) the TMP-to-sulfa ratio is 5:4 instead of 1:5; (iii) the presence of a long-acting sulfonamide permits the administration of only one capsule daily after a loading dose of two; (iv) a reduced amount of TMP is given without decrease of efficacy. Preliminary observations by Rotolo et al. (4) suggest that KP is just as active as Co-T in the treatment of urinary tract infections. The pharmacokinetics of KP have been studied by Reeves et al. (2), but no details were given concerning concentrations of both components in prostatic tissue and secretion and in seminal fluid.

In dogs, the TMP concentration in prostatic secretion is two- to threefold higher than in plasma (3). However, the pH of canine prostatic fluid varies between 5.9 and 6.6, whereas in humans the mean value is pH 7.31 ± 0.5 (range, 6.6 to 8.5) and still higher in CP cases: pH 8.34 ± 0.10 (range, 7.0 to 9.0).

Nielsen and Hansen (1) observed that in humans the mean TMP concentration is higher in prostatic fluid (4.76 μg/ml) than in serum (2.81 μg/ml). It is also higher in adenoma (3.42 μg/ml) than in normal prostate (2.98 μg/ml), striated muscle (2.0 μg/ml), and subcutaneous tissue (0.4 μg/ml).

Human normal prostatic tissue is difficult to obtain. Human expressed prostatic secretion is usually scant, and only a few drops are obtained after prostatic massage.

In our studies, the distribution of TMP and SMP was determined in human prostatic tissues, human seminal fluid (40% of which is due to prostatic secretion), and normal rat prostate after oral administration of KP. Seminal fluid was obtained from patients with CP and from healthy volunteers. Human tissue consisted of prostatic adenoma removed by open or transurethral surgery and one normal prostate from a radical cystectomy specimen.

The following methods were employed for determination of TMP and SMP.

(i) TMP. Agar disk plate diffusion was performed, using *Bacillus pumilus* as the susceptible organism. Previous dilution (1:1) of serum was performed to unbind TMP from plasma proteins. The homogenates contained 1 g of fresh tissue in 4 ml of Sörensen solution.

(ii) SMP. Rieder's spectrophotometric method was employed. Homogenates contained 100 mg of fresh tissue in each ml of distilled water.

Two groups of rats were fed 60 mg of TMP per kg and 40 mg of SMP per kg and were sacrificed after 1 and 3 h, respectively. In humans, samples were taken at day 5 of treatment, 1 h after ingestion of a capsule of KP.

Patients with CP were treated with KP in two urological centers in Palermo and Bologna. In Palermo, three different observers recorded their material independently. All patients received two capsules of KP on the first day, followed by a capsule daily for 1 month. The material was not homogeneous: gram-positive strains were more commonly isolated in Bologna than in Palermo, the relative frequency of abacterial CP varied in the different series, and the patients in Bologna presented with infertility problems. The results were similar, however, in the various series. Our pharmacokinetic studies are summarized in Table 1, and our results in bacterial CP are shown in Table 2. The following should be noted. (i) A second month of treatment was successful in 20 of 26 patients who had remained bacteriologically positive. (ii) In 138 patients with nonbacterial CP, leukocytes disappeared from prostatic fluid in 78 (56%); 33 (24%) had symptomatic relief only, and 27 (20%) had no effect. In the series from Bologna disappearance of leukocytes from semen was observed in 12 (48%) of 25 patients with nonbacterial CP. (iii) No significant side effects were observed, and the patients' compliance was excellent.

Although a larger experience is needed, the following conclusions can be drawn. (i) TMP concentrations in prostatic tissues are higher than in serum or plasma after administration of Kelfiprim. Concentrations in prostatic fluid are higher than in spermatic fluid. Semen concentrations in patients with CP were slightly lower than in normal subjects. Such concentrations are above the MIC for most responsible bacterial strains, except *Pseudomonas*. TMP concentrations in adenoma are higher than in normal prostatic tissue. This may bias results based on drug concentrations in adenoma. (ii) SMP concentrations in prostatic tissues and in semen are slightly above the MIC for *Escherichia coli* and below the MICs for *Proteus*, *Pseudomonas*, and *Staphylococcus aureus*. However, as true synergism between SMP and TMP occurs in a wide range of TMP/SMP ratios, even relatively low SMP concentrations are likely to play a synergistic role with TMP. (iii) Clinical results are encouraging. In series from various groups, including different case selections, bacteriological cure was obtained after 1 month of treatment in 69% of cases. In abacterial CP, disappearance of leukocytes from prostatic secretion and semen occurred in about 50% of cases. This compares favorably with Co-T, but patients' compliance was better with KP. Further investigations are needed.

TABLE 1. *Chronic bacterial prostatitis bacteriologically cured after one course of Kelfiprim*

Investigators	No. of cases	No. cured	%
Pavone-Macaluso and Di Trapani	2	2	
Ascoli	7	5	71.4
Rizzo	38	27	71
Maver and Corrado	25	16	64
Total	72	50	69.4

TABLE 2. *Mean TMP and SMP concentrations in biological fluids (μg/ml) or tissues (μg/g) after Kelfiprim administration*

Sample	TMP	SMP
Rat plasma (at 1 h)	0.77	29.5
Rat prostate (at 1 h)	1.42	2.04
Rat prostate (at 3 h)	1.15	0.84
Human normal semen	0.79	0.28
Semen from patients with chronic prostatitis	0.54	0.76
Normal human prostate	1.3	Not determined
Adenoma	4.5	1.14

1. **Nielsen, M. L., and I. Hansen.** 1972. Trimethoprim in human prostatic tissue and prostatic fluid. Scand. J. Urol. Nephrol. **6**:244.

2. **Reeves, D. S., M. J. Byater, D. W. Bullock, and H. A. Holt.** 1980. Pharmacokinetic study of a sulfamethopyrazine/trimethoprim combination (Kelfiprim) in human volunteers. J. Antimicrob. Chemother. **6**:647.

3. **Reeves, D. S., and M. Gilchik.** 1970. Secretion of the antimicrobial substance trimethoprim in the prostatic fluid of dogs. Br. J. Urol. **42**:66.

4. **Rotolo, U., D. Melloni, M. Pavone-Macaluso, D. Natoli, and F. Piaia.** 1979. Ricerca clinica comparativa fra cotrimoxazolo ed una nuova associazione sulfamidico-trimethoprim nelle infezioni dell'apparato urinario. Urologia (Treviso) **46**:873.

In Vitro Bactericidal Activity of Kelfiprim

GIUSEPPE MEINARDI, SILVIO GRASSO, AND IVO DE CARNERI

Farmitalia Carlo Erba, R. & S. Milan, Italy

The interaction between trimethoprim (T) and a long-acting sulfonamide, sulfamethopyrazine (S), the two component drugs in the combination Kelfiprim, was studied to determine its effect on in vitro bactericidal activity. Four gram-negative species of bacteria recently isolated from infected urine were used. The bactericidal activity of Kelfiprim was assessed at low concentrations, below the MIC expected on the basis of the MICs of the two drugs of the combination.

The MICs of T and S were determined in Adams-Roe broth (Biolife) by the twofold dilution method using the microtiter technique (Minidiluter Cooke) and an inoculum of 10^4 colony-forming units per ml. Readings were taken after 18 h of incubation at 37°C. It was not possible to determine the MICs with larger inocula because it became impossible to define the endpoint with precision.

The four strains used were *Escherichia coli* Bs 2, *Klebsiella oxytoca* N 1500, *Proteus morganii* Cr 113, and *Proteus mirabilis* Rho 37113. Bactericidal activity was determined on the same medium but with a larger inoculum: 1×10^5 to 3×10^5 cells per ml. The two folate inhibitors were tested in combination at the following concentrations: ⅛ MIC of S plus ⅛ MIC of T, ⅛ MIC of S plus ¼ MIC of T, ¼ MIC of S plus ⅛ MIC of T, and ¼ MIC of S plus ¼ MIC of T. The drugs were tested singly for comparison at concentrations equal to 1 MIC, ¼ MIC, and ⅛ MIC. At 0, 1, 2, 4, 6, and 8 h, viable cells were counted by streaking 0.1 ml of the cultures or the 1:10 serial dilutions in nutrient agar (Oxoid no. 2) and counting the colonies after 20 h of incubation at 37°C.

Figures 1 and 2 show the course of bactericidal activity of the four combinations of T and S against *K. oxytoca* N 1500 and *P. morganii* Cr 113 compared with the bactericidal activity of the two drugs singly. Kelfiprim's bactericidal activity against the two strains became evident after a short delay, generally around the second hour of contact. With *K. oxytoca* and *P. morganii* the most concentrated drug combination reduced the number of viable cells by 2 to 2.5 log within 8 h. Except for the combination ⅛

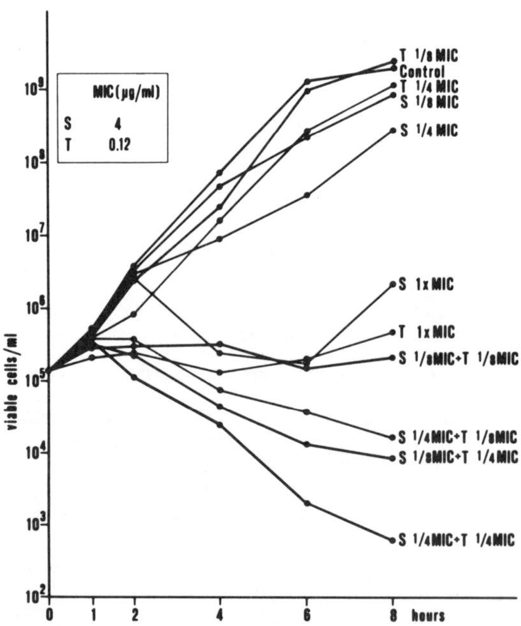

FIG. 1. *In vitro bactericidal activity against K. oxytoca N 1500 of four combinations of S and T in comparison with the two drugs singly.*

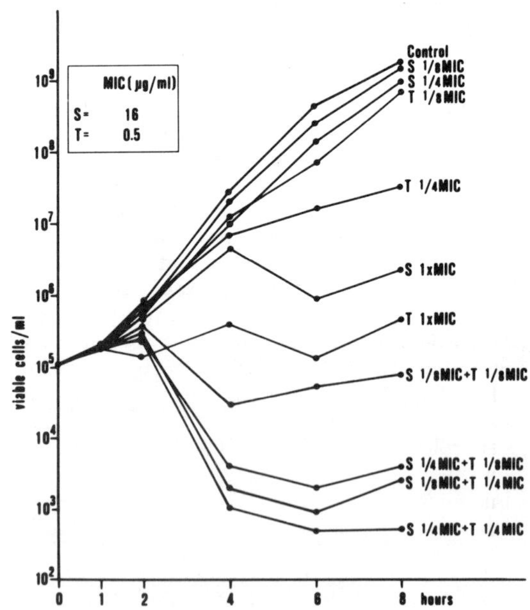

FIG. 2. *In vitro bactericidal activity against P. morganii Cr 113 of four combinations of S and T in comparison with the two drugs singly.*

MIC of S plus 1/8 MIC of T, which was only bacteriostatic, all the other combinations were bactericidal. With *E. coli* Bs 2 the same pattern was observed.

Against these three strains T at the MIC stopped or slowed bacterial growth without killing the organisms; at the MIC, S showed an initial phase of apparent inactivity, then generally transient, slight bactericidal activity which, however, never reduced the bacterial count to base-line values within 8 h. At subinhibitory concentrations T and S only slowed bacterial growth.

With *P. mirabilis* Rho 37113 Kelfiprim showed less bactericidal activity than with the other three strains; the highest concentration of the combination reduced the bacterial count by only just over 1 log. Nevertheless, all four combinations tested were more active than the single components.

The favorable interaction between the combined drugs against four gram-negative bacterial strains isolated from outpatients is in accordance with that observed in bacteriostasis studies by Schioppacassi et al. (1) on collection strains and by Bianchi et al. (2nd Mediterranean Congress of Chemotherapy, Nice, 13–16 October 1980, Abstr. no. 328) on 100 strains isolated from outpatients in northwest Italy.

1. **Schioppacassi, G., V. Mandelli, R. Mazzoleni, and E. Morvillo.** 1979. Studio dell'interazione sulfametossipirazina-trimethoprim su schizomiceti *in vitro*. G. Ital. Chemioter. **26:**181–188.

Experience with Rifampin-Trimethoprim and Rifampin-Erythromycin in the Treatment of Life-Threatening Infection

A. M. EMMERSON,* G. L. RIDGWAY, AND R. N. GRÜNEBERG

Departments of Medical Microbiology, Whittington Hospital, London N19 5NF, and University College Hospital, London WC 1, U.K.*

The treatment of life-threatening infections requires accurate diagnosis and appropriate aggressive therapy. Combination therapy is often used to prevent or delay the emergence of resistance to a single antibiotic or to obtain synergistic interaction against an organism whose initial sensitivity to available antibiotics used separately is too low for complete bactericidal action. Combination therapy is also used to treat infections due to more than one species of bacteria. Clinical experience has shown that debilitated or immunocompromised patients respond poorly to monotherapy, and a combination of antibiotics is recommended (2).

In spite of the numerous antimicrobial agents available for the treatment of life-threatening infections, many regimens are based on the use of the penicillins or cephalosporins, and if the use of these two groups of drugs is contraindicated, then the choice is much restricted. Alternatives such as the aminoglycosides may be inappropriate, and therefore it would seem logical to use rifampin in combination with other antibiotics.

This study reports on the clinical use of rifampin in combination with erythromycin or trimethoprim in five cases with potentially life-threatening illnesses (Table 1).

Case 1. A 24-year-old nurse with extensive cellulitis of the face presented with periorbital swelling and edema of the soft palate, fauces, and larynx. Since she was allergic to penicillin, she was given high-dose parenteral erythromycin. In spite of 36 h of erythromycin and hydrocortisone she failed to respond, and after the isolation of *Staphylococcus aureus* and *Streptococcus pyogenes*, rifampin (300 mg intravenously every 8 h) was added. She made a prompt and uneventful recovery.

Case 2. An 86-year-old lady presented with a right-sided hemiplegia and was found to have a coarse systolic murmur on examination. *S. aureus* was grown from two sets of blood cultures and an infected foot. She was treated with cloxacillin and gentamicin, but in spite of a normal blood urea, gentamicin was not freely excreted and this was stopped after the initial loading dose. Fourteen days after starting cloxacillin she developed a classical penicillin rash, and therapy was changed to rifampin (450 mg daily) plus erythromycin. Within a week her temperature was normal and the systolic murmur was barely audible. Seven days later, her liver function tests became grossly abnormal but returned to their normally high level within 1 week of stopping the rifampin. Her subsequent recovery was remarkable.

Case 3. A 2-month-old girl was admitted from

TABLE 1. *Clinical use of rifampin (RIF) and erythromycin (ERYTH)-trimethoprim (TMP)*

Case	Diagnosis	Organism	Treatment
2-mo-old female	Meningitis	*Flavobacterium meningosepticum*	RIF-ERYTH
86-yr-old female	Endocarditis	*Staphylococcus aureus*	RIF-ERYTH
24-yr-old female	Cellulitis	*Staphylococcus aureus, Streptococcus pyogenes*	RIF-ERYTH
28-yr-old female	Osteomyelitis	*Staphylococcus aureus*, mixed aerobes-anaerobes	RIF-TMP
17-yr-old male	Osteomyelitis	Mixed aerobes-anaerobes	RIF-TMP

TABLE 2. *Treatment regimens of rifampin (RIF) and erythromycin (ERYTH)-trimethoprim (TMP)*

Case	Reason for use	RIF and ERYTH-TMP	Duration
1. Meningitis	Multiple resistance	RIF, 20–46 mg/kg daily; ERYTH, 70 mg/kg every 2 h	28 days
2. Endocarditis	Penicillin allergy	RIF, 300 + 150 mg daily; ERYTH, 500 mg every 12 h	18 days
3. Cellulitis	Penicillin allergy	RIF, 300 mg every 8 h; ERYTH, 500 mg every 6 h	8 days
4. Osteomyelitis	Cloxacillin failure	RIF, 300 mg every 12 h; TMP, 80 mg every 12 h	6 mo
5. Osteomyelitis	Penicillin allergy	RIF, 300 mg every 12 h; TMP, 200 mg every 12 h	3 mo

a hospital in Pakistan having had neonatal meningitis. On admission she was found to have pronounced hydrocephalus and ventriculitis. A heavy growth of *Flavobacterium meningosepticum* was isolated which was resistant to all the available aminoglycosides, cephalosporins, chloramphenicol, trimethoprim, mecillinam, and ticarcillin. It was moderately sensitive to cefoxitin and mezlocillin and sensitive to rifampin (MIC, 1.0 μg/ml) and erythromycin. Intravenous rifampin (20 mg/kg per 24 h) and erythromycin (70 mg/kg every 2 h) was given for 15 days with no effect. At 15 days, rifampin was increased to 46 mg/kg per 24 h and 5 mg was given intraventricularly daily. Four days later, 10 mg of erythromycin was also given intrathecally, but flavobacteria were isolated continuously for 28 days.

Because of the clinical failure and because the bacteria had become resistant to both rifampin and erythromycin, therapy was changed to mezlocillin, 400 mg/kg per 24 h intravenously plus 10 mg intraventricularly, and cefoxitin, 250 mg/kg per 24 h intravenously plus 7.5 intraventricularly per 24 h. Within 24 h of the beginning of this regimen, the cerebrospinal fluid from both ventricles became sterile and remained sterile for the 5 weeks before the patients's discharge.

Case 4. A 17-year-old male patient with spinobifida presented with a large pressure sore on the left side of the buttock which was exposing the sacrum. Surgical exploration revealed an underlying osteomyelitis, and he was treated postoperatively with erythromycin since he was allergic to penicillin and co-trimoxazole. Subsequent addition of metronidazole caused his temperature to settle, but radiographic evidence showed continued bone damage. The erythromycin was stopped and rifampin (300 mg twice daily) and trimethoprim (200 mg twice daily) was added. Nevertheless, further surgery was required; however, after 3 months of rifampin-trimethoprim and metronidazole, a satisfactory outcome was achieved.

Case 5. A 28-year-old female drug addict was admitted with extensive destruction of bone in her left hip after repeated abscesses in her groin. *S. aureus* was isolated from the hip joint, and she was given flucloxacillin postoperatively. This had little effect and radiographs 1 month later showed further damage. Therapy was changed to rifampin (300 mg) and trimethoprim (80 mg twice daily) and continued for 6 months. No adverse effects were recorded, and she was able to walk out of hospital after 3.5 months to continue her oral therapy as an outpatient.

Resistance to rifampin occurs readily when the drug is used alone; thus, other antibiotics have been added to avoid or delay this induced resistance. Because of their essentially similar actions, combinations of trimethoprim and rifampin have been shown to exhibit synergism (3), and others (1) have shown that this combination prevented or delayed resistance developing to either component.

In this study, rifampin in combination with trimethoprim or erythromycin was used in five patients with life-threatening diseases who for various reasons were unable to use or failed treatment with the penicillins (Table 2).

1. **Grüneberg, R. N., and A. M. Emmerson.** 1980. Prevention of emergence of bacterial resistance by combination of two antibiotics: rifampicin and trimethoprim. J. Antimicrob. Chemother. **6**:349–356.
2. **Jensen, K., and H. C. A. Lassen.** 1969. Combined treatment with antibacterial chemotherapeutic agents in staphylococcal infections. Q. J. Med. New Ser. **XXXVIII**(149):91–106.
3. **Kerry, D. W., J. M. T. Hamilton-Miller, and W. Brumfitt.** 1975. Trimethoprim and rifampicin; *in vitro* activities separately and in combination. J. Antimicrob. Chemother. **1**:417–427.

Serum and Prostatic Tissue Levels of Rifampin and Trimethoprim After Administration of a Combination of the Two Drugs

B. ROMEO,* E. FELICI, R. PALLANZA, E. MAPELLI, AND B. GOLDSTEIN

Gruppo Lepetit Research Laboratories, Milan, and Department of Urology, General Hospital, Treviso, Italy*

Chronic prostatitis is an insidious disease because of its tendency to persist asymptomatically and to cause relapsing urinary tract infections. Management of bacterial prostatitis requires that antibacterial agents reach effective levels in tissue and in secretion of the gland. Rifampin (RMP) and trimethoprim (TMP) are broad-spectrum antibacterial agents which are absorbed orally and freely diffuse into body fluids and tissues (2, 6). The combination of RMP with TMP significantly suppresses the in vitro emergence of mutants resistant to both compounds (1, 5). These characteristics suggest that the combination of the two compounds could be suitable for the treatment of bacterial prostatitis.

The aim of the present study was to evaluate the penetration of the RMP-TMP combination into human prostatic tissue (PT). The inflammatory processes in prostatitis apparently take place in prostatic acini as well as in their surrounding tissue, often in the periurethral area, but at times in peripheral PT. Therefore, antibiotic concentrations obtained in the whole PT should be as predictive of therapeutic success as prostatic secretion levels.

Twenty-six patients affected by benign prostatic hypertrophy, in whom excision of the adenoma was required, entered the study. Their age ranged from 52 to 83 years (median, 72). Patients received a single dose of 900 mg of RMP and 240 mg of TMP during the night at about 6, 10, or 14 h before the planned time of surgery.

RMP and TMP concentrations in serum as well as in PT homogenate were determined by microbiological assay, with *Sarcina lutea* ATCC 9341 (RMP) and a rifampin-resistant strain of *Bacillus pumilus* (TMP) as test organisms. A blood sample was obtained at the moment of adenomectomy in order to calculate prostatic tissue/serum (PT/S) concentration ratios for both compounds.

Mean serum and PT concentrations are presented in Fig. 1 (RMP) and 2 (TMP). In all patients RMP levels were higher in serum than in PT at all times. Serum concentrations of RMP in the three groups of patients were 20.0 (6 h), 11.9 (10 h), and 7.4 μg/ml (14 h); PT levels were 8.6, 5.7, and 3.9 μg/g. RMP concentrations decreased more rapidly in serum than in PT. Thus, the PT/S concentration ratio of 0.45 ± 0.08 (mean ± SE of the mean) observed 6 h after the administration increased to 0.51 ± 0.11 and to 0.59 ± 0.13 after 10 and 14 h.

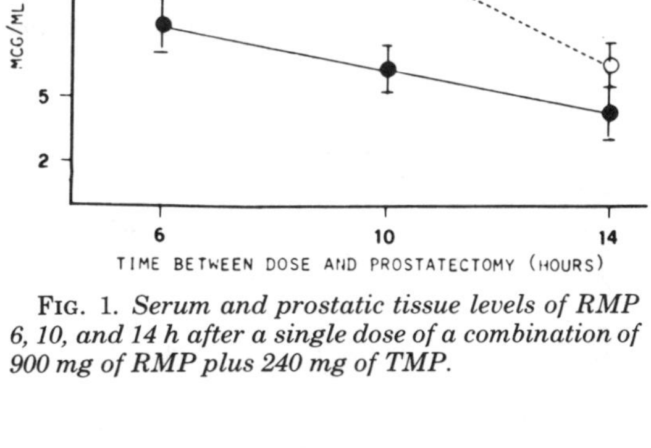

FIG. 1. *Serum and prostatic tissue levels of RMP 6, 10, and 14 h after a single dose of a combination of 900 mg of RMP plus 240 mg of TMP.*

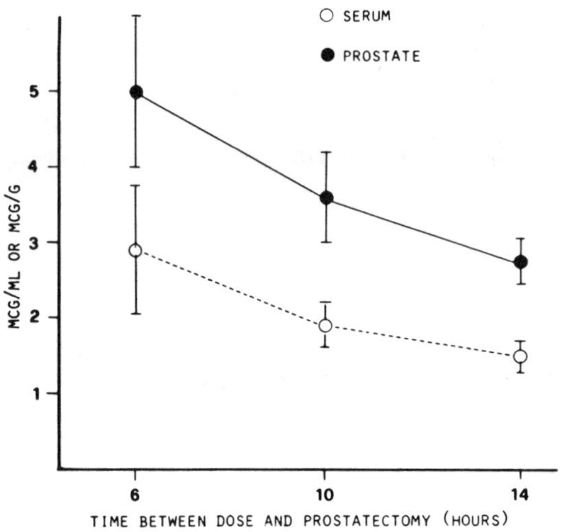

FIG. 2. *Serum and prostatic tissue levels of TMP 6, 10, and 14 h after a single dose of a combination of 900 mg of RMP plus 240 mg of TMP.*

TMP levels were higher in PT than in serum. Mean TMP serum levels were 3.0, 1.8, and 1.3 μg/ml and PT levels were 4.9, 3.6, and 2.7 μg/g at 6, 10, and 14 h. TMP concentrations decreased at comparable rates in both serum and PT; thus, PT/S concentration ratios were 1.8 ± 0.3, 2.3 ± 0.7, and 2.1 ± 0.3.

Because different criteria are used in evaluating comparative bacterial counts in segmented cultures (7), there is some disagreement about which bacterial species are most frequently associated with chronic prostatitis. According to Stamey (7), members of the *Enterobacteriaceae* family are the organisms most frequently isolated from prostatic fluid; *Pseudomonas* and enterococci are less common isolates. In contrast, Drach (3), using the same collection technique, reported a very high proportion of gram-positive bacteria (37% *Staphylococcus epidermidis*, 21% alpha-hemolytic streptococci, 12% diphtheroids, 5% enterococci). In any event, the concentrations of RMP and TMP attained in PT are considerably higher than the MIC for most gram-positive bacteria and are of the order of the MIC for most gram-negative microorganisms involved in chronic prostatitis.

That these tissue levels are satisfactory for therapy was demonstrated by Giamarellou et al. (4); they obtained cure rates of greater than 50% in patients with chronic prostatitis diagnosed by the Meares and Stamey technique.

1. **Arioli, V., M. Berti, G. Carniti, E. Rossi, and L. G. Silvestri.** 1977. Interaction between rifampicin and trimethoprim in vitro and in experimental infections. J. Antimicrob. Chemother. **3:**87–94.
2. **Binda, G., E. Domenichini, A. Gottardi, E. Orlandi, E. Ortelli, B. Pacini, and G. Fowst.** 1971. Rifampicin, a general review. Arzneim. Forsch. **21:**1907–1977.
3. **Drach, G. W.** 1974. Problems in diagnosis of bacterial prostatitis: Gram-negative, Gram-positive and mixed infections. J. Urol. **111:**630–636.
4. **Giamarellou, H., M. Leonidas, M. Papadakis, and G. K. Daikos.** 1978. Rifampicin-trimethoprim efficacy in chronic prostatitis. Proceedings I Mediterranean Congress Chemotherapy, Madrid, 1978, p. 893–895.
5. **Kerry, D. W., J. M. T. Hamilton-Miller, and W. Brumfitt.** 1975. Trimethoprim and rifampicin: in vitro activities separately and in combination. J. Antimicrob. Chemother. **1:**417–427.
6. **Patel, R. B., and P. G. Welling.** 1980. Clinical pharmacokinetics of cotrimoxazole (trimethoprim-sulphamethoxazole). Clin. Pharmacokinet. **5:**405–423.
7. **Stamey, T. A.** 1981. Prostatitis. J. R. Soc. Med. **74:**22–40.

Evidential Support of a Theory of the Bacterial Cause of Secondary Postpartum Hemorrhage with an Analysis of the Results of Treatment, Using Cephradine and Metronidazole

J. VAUGHAN,* D. MACDONALD, AND B. LEEK

National Maternity Hospital, and Veterinary College, Dublin, Ireland*

Secondary postpartum hemorrhage is one of the most urgent and dangerous complications of contemporary obstetrics. At the National Maternity Hospital, Dublin, which currently delivers over 9,000 women annually, there are approximately 40 cases of this type each year, an incidence of 0.5%.

In the past 10 years, 10 hysterectomies were required for this condition as a life-saving procedure; in fact, one woman died (8). Several of the women were primigravidae and the hysterectomy for them was a social tragedy. In all but one of these 10 cases, the bleeding occurred without prior warning.

A detailed study of the 10 cases requiring hysterectomy was made and the following characteristic features emerged. First, the uterine muscle was completely inert and failed to respond to either ergometrine or oxytocin. Second, there was no evidence of retained products of conception. Third, there was no sign of any generalized infection in 9 of the 10 cases. Fourth, there was histological evidence of local infection in every case. Fifth, there was no evidence of generalized coagulopathy (3). Sixth, uterine exploration on admission provoked uncontrollable bleeding.

The organisms most often isolated were anaerobic streptococci, *Bacteroides*, and *Streptococcus faecalis*. In some of the early cases no organisms were found, but this was before the introduction of effective anaerobic cultures. It seems likely now that the failure to identify the causative organism was due to a failure in cultural technique. Immediate plating is imperative when anaerobes are sought.

The following hypothesis was developed. It was suggested that postpartum hemorrhage was possibly due to a localized infection with anaerobic organisms which on the one hand were capable of lysing thrombi in the uterine sinusoids and on the other of paralyzing the uterus and rendering it unresponsive to oxytocin and ergometrine. This theory was tested in the laboratory and verified by the results of therapy at the clinical level. Experiments were devised to test the effects of these organisms, namely anaerobic streptococci, *Bacteroides*, and *S. faecalis*, on human blood clots and on fresh human contracting myometrial strips. Anaerobic streptococci and *S. faecalis* lysed blood clots, whereas *Bacteroides* caused minimal lysis.

Specially prepared strips of fresh uterine muscle obtained either at hysterectomy or caesarean section were suspended in pregassed Krebs solution and their contractions were measured isotonically and isometrically. When cultures of the organisms (30,000 organisms per ml) were added to contracting myometrial strips suspended in pregassed Krebs solution at 37°C, anaerobic streptococci and *Bacteroides* caused uterine paralysis. This paralysis could not be overcome by using ergometrine or oxytocin in concentrations of 30 U/liter. When the muscle preparations so treated were washed out with fresh pregassed Krebs solution, muscle treated with anaerobic streptococci continued to remain unresponsive, whereas that treated with *Bacteroides* tended to recover slowly. *S. faecalis* caused an increase in the frequency of the contractions but a diminution of the muscle tonus. Washing the preparation free of this organism rendered the muscle totally inert and unresponsive to oxytocin and ergometrine. The conditions in an involuting uterus favor the growth of anaerobic organisms because of the diminished blood supply to the myometrium of the upper segment and the anoxic thrombi in the uterine sinusoids.

A policy of treatment based on this theory was evolved. Unless the blood loss was life threatening, immediate exploration of the uterus was abandoned (1, 6). High vaginal swabs were taken immediately and cultured aerobically and anaerobically. Massive antibiotic therapy was started as soon as possible. It was considered that cephradine, a known bactericidal drug active against gram-positive and -negative cocci (*Escherichia coli* and *Proteus mirabilis*), and with minimal plasma albumin binding, together with metronidazole, a drug effective against anaerobes, should be the treatment of choice. The dosage used was 1 g of cephradine parenterally repeated every 6 h. In less serious situations, 500 mg was given orally every 6 h. Metronidazole (400 mg) was given parenterally every 8 h when the condition was grave or 400 mg three times a day in less serious situations (2, 4, 5). Therapy was always continued for 5 days. Since this regime was introduced no hysterectomy has been required and blood loss has been considerably reduced. Curettage was only occasionally required for continuing bleeding but did not provoke the uncontrollable hemorrhage previously seen.

The points of clinical importance are: first, the infection is anaerobic (7) and as such is often missed; second, the infection is localized; third, while local fibrinolysis is intense no fibrin degradation products will be found in the circulation as they are washed out by bleeding. The myometrial paralysis and the failure to respond to either ergometrine or oxytocin are at once the most characteristic and the most dangerous aspects of the condition. With the control of the infection myometrial contractility rapidly returns and involution progresses.

In summary, a theory of origin of secondary postpartum hemorrhage is advanced. It has been tested in the laboratory and clinically.

1. **Berger, E., M. S. Gillieson, and J. H. Waters.** 1981. Puerperal febrile complications and cervical flora following elective manual exploration of the uterus. Am. J. Obstet. Gynecol. **139**:320–323.
2. **Gall, S. A., A. P. Kohan, D. M. Ayers, C. E. Hughes, and W. A. Addison.** 1981. Intravenous metronidazole or clindamycin with tobramycin for therapy of pelvic infections. Obstet. Gynecol. **57**:51–58.
3. **Gilabert, J., J. J. Parrilla, M. Monzonis, et al.** 1979. Changes of haemostasis in severe postpartum infection. Toko-Ginecol. Pract. **38**:285–292.
4. **Koch-Weser, J., and P. Goldman.** 1980. Drug therapy: metronidazole. N. Engl. J. Med. **303**:1212–1218.
5. **Monif, G. R., and R. E. Hempling.** 1981. Antibiotic therapy for the bacteroidacea in post-cesarean section infections. Obstet. Gynecol. **57**:177–181.
6. **Perino, P. L., M. E. Duncan, D. W. Krause and S. A.**

Woke. 1980. Pelvic inflammatory disease and puerperal sepsis in Ethiopia. Am. J. Obstet. Gynecol. **138:**969–973.

7. **Platt, L. D., M. L. Yonekura, and W. J. Ledger.** 1979. The role of anaerobic bacteria in post partum endometritis. Am. J. Obstet. Gynecol. **135:**814–817.

8. **Reports.** 1969–1977. National Maternity Hospital, Dublin.

Combined Effects of Dibekacin and β-Lactams on Gram-Negative Bacterial Infection

KIYOSHI KONNO, KOTARO OIZUMI,* AND SEIICHI AONUMA

Department of Internal Medicine, The Research Institute for Chest Diseases and Cancer, Tohoku University, Sendai 980, Japan

Excellent therapeutic effects of the combination of penicillins and aminoglycosides on pseudomonal infections, as can be anticipated from in vitro synergism, have been demonstrated. Using electron microscopic observations, Nishino and Nakazawa (2) have shown that *Pseudomonas aeruginosa* cells, when exposed to carbenicillin or sulbenicillin (SBPC), became elongated. Usually, treatment with penicillin plus gentamicin causes elongation of bacterial cells and destruction of the cell surface structure.

In the present paper, electron microscopic studies were undertaken to investigate the effects of dibekacin (DKB) on the surface structures of cell walls isolated from mechanically disrupted cells. In addition, morphological changes in bacilli treated with SBPC plus DKB were investigated. Furthermore, the therapeutic efficacy of a β-lactam on respiratory tract infections in patients with lung cancer was compared with that of a β-lactam plus an aminoglycoside.

In the present experiment an in vitro synergism between SBPC and DKB against *P. aeruginosa* IAM 1007 was demonstrated, as evidenced by a fractional inhibitory index of 0.375. Moreover, the bactericidal action of DKB plus SBPC and suppression of the regrowth of the bacilli after treatment with DKB plus SBPC were observed even at subinhibitory concentrations of the two drugs.

To account for the antimicrobial action of aminoglycosides, a theory related to the inhibition of protein synthesis has been proposed, and evidence supporting this theory has accumulated. However, electron microscopic observations of *P. aeruginosa* IAM 1007 cells treated with DKB in the present experiment revealed severe destruction of the cell surface structures, often in association with the leakage of intracellular substances and degenerative changes of ribosomes, which suggested inhibition of protein synthesis. These peculiar destructive changes, caused by aminoglycosides, on the outer membranes of *Pseudomonas* cells have already been reported (1, 2), but the mechanism responsible for these changes has not yet been elucidated.

To find out whether such destructive changes are due to the direct action of aminoglycosides on the cell surface structure or are the consequence of inhibition of protein synthesis, the effects of DKB on cell walls from mechanically disrupted cells were examined. It was found that gradual but progressive release of unidentified substances from the isolated cell walls was followed by complete disappearance of the outer membrane during incubation with DKB. Similar changes of cell surface structures were observed when resting cells in saline were treated with DKB. These findings strongly suggest the direct action of DKB on the outer membrane of *Pseudomonas* cells. On the other hand, SBPC treatment caused elongation of the cells and partial destruction of the peptidoglycan layer, but the outer membrane remained intact.

In contrast, treatment of the bacilli with 1 MIC of SBPC and then with 1 MIC of DKB caused extensive destruction of the membranous structures of the cell walls. These changes were not caused by 1 MIC of DKB alone, unless the bacilli had been pretreated with SBPC. It seems that SBPC, through its action on peptidoglycan layers, enhances the potential destructive effects of DKB on the outer membrane. Moreover, when treated with 1/2 MIC of DKB and then with 1/8 MIC of SBPC, bacilli became much more elongated than when they were exposed to SBPC alone (no DKB pretreatment). Therefore, it is likely that slight damage on the outer membrane caused by subinhibitory concentrations of DKB makes it easier for SBPC to reach its target enzymes. Simultaneous treatment with 1/8 MIC of SBPC and 1/2 MIC of DKB resulted in marked elongation of the bacterial cells and destruction of the cell surface structures. As

TABLE 1. *Comparison of the efficacy on respiratory tract infection in patients with lung cancer between single and combined regimens*[a]

Infectious episodes due to:	Cure rate (no./total episodes) in:					
	Group I			Group II		
	Single regimen	Combined regimen	*P*	Single regimen	Combined regimen	*P*
Gram-positive cocci and *H. influenzae*	14/19 (73.7)[b]	1/3 (33.3)	NS[c]	10/17 (58.8)	12/14 (85.7)	NS
Gram-negative bacilli	2/6 (33.3)	1/2 (50.0)	NS	8/20 (40.0)	19/27 (70.4)	NS
Unknown organisms	6/8 (75.0)	6/7 (85.7)	NS	14/13 (41.2)	12/22 (54.5)	NS
Total %	66.7	66.7	NS	45.1	68.3	0.05

[a] Single, β-lactam; combined, β-lactam plus an aminoglycoside.
[b] Number in parentheses gives percentage.
[c] NS, Not significant.

mentioned above, each of the two drugs caused different changes on the cell surface structures of *Pseudomonas*. When used in combination, SBPC and DKB seem to cause rapid bacteriolysis by mutual enhancement of their actions.

The remarkable decrease in viable counts of the bacilli caused by treatment with SBPC plus DKB was due to destructive changes of the cell surface structures. In addition, the bacilli, which barely escaped the killing effects of SBPC plus DKB, seem to be so profoundly damaged that their regrowth after removal of the drugs is strongly suppressed.

In 89 of 238 patients who were admitted to our hospital due to lung cancer during the last 2 years, a total of 131 infectious episodes occurred. For the precise evaluation of therapeutic efficacy, these infectious episodes were divided into three groups, based on the nature of infections: group I included community-acquired infections which occurred before or within 3 days after admission; the episodes in group II were nosocomial or endogenous infections during hospitalization; and terminal infections fell into group III.

The therapeutic efficacy on infections of a β-lactam alone was compared with that of a β-lactam plus an aminoglycoside. In group III, the cure rate was too low to compare the efficacy between single and combined regimens. Infectious episodes in groups I and II were divided into three categories according to causative organisms (Table 1). In infections due to gram-positive cocci and *Haemophilus influenzae*, no significant difference in cure rate was found between single and combined regimens in either group I or II. In group II, on the other hand, the cure rate of the combined regimens exceeded that of the single regimens in treatment of infectious episodes due to gram-negative bacilli.

1. **Iida, K., and M. Koike.** 1974. Cell wall alterations of gram-negative bacteria by aminoglycoside antibiotics. Antimicrob. Agents Chemother. **5:**95–97.
2. **Nishino, T., and S. Nakazawa.** 1975. Morphological alterations of Pseudomonas aeruginosa by aminoglycoside antibiotics. J. Electron Microsc. **24:**73–86.

Ecological Benefits of Combining Rifamycins with Other Antibiotics

R. N. GRÜNEBERG, A. M. EMMERSON, D. FELMINGHAM,* AND A. W. CREMER

Departments of Microbiology, University College Hospital, London WC1, and Whittington Hospital, London N 19, U.K.*

An experimental model has been developed which is designed to reproduce the characteristics of a treated human infection in vitro. In this experimental procedure, the bacterial growth from an overnight culture of the organism under investigation is separated from the growth medium by centrifugation, washed, resuspended in growth medium containing antibiotic(s), and reincubated in a shaking water bath at 37°C. This procedure is repeated after an incubation period corresponding to half the dose interval for the antibiotic(s) under investigation and repeated thereafter until the experiment is terminated. Total and antibiotic-resistant bacterial counts are performed at each transfer. The concentration of antibiotic(s) in the growth medium is alternated, at each transfer, between concentrations corresponding to the peak and mid-dose pharmacokinetic levels observed in human serum.

Using this experimental procedure, we have investigated a number of antibiotics, used in combination with rifampin, for their ability to suppress the emergence of resistance with either antibiotic used alone.

When a strain of *Escherichia coli* was exposed to rifampin alone, it became rifampin resistant; when exposed to trimethoprim alone, it became trimethoprim resistant. Exposure to a combination of rifampin and trimethoprim resulted in the bacteria being eliminated from the culture without the emergence of bacterial resistance. Similarly, when a strain of *Streptococcus faecalis* was exposed to rifampin alone, it became rifampin resistant, and when exposed to erythromycin alone, it became erythromycin resistant. Exposure to a combination of rifampin and erythromycin resulted in the bacteria being eliminated from the culture without the emergence of bacterial resistance. A strain of *Neisseria gonorrhoeae*, when exposed to rifampin and erythromycin, was eliminated from the culture by either erythromycin alone or in combination with rifampin without the emergence of bacterial resistance. However, when exposed to rifampin alone, the *N. gonorrhoeae* strain became rifampin resistant. Similar results were obtained when the same strain of *N. gonorrhoeae* was exposed to diminishing concentrations of rifampin and erythromycin, either alone or in combination, in an experiment designed to reproduce the characteristics of single-dose therapy in vitro. *N. gonorrhoeae* was also exposed to DL473 (a cyclopentyl rifamycin) and doxycycline either alone or in combination, using the same in vitro single-dose procedure. It became DL473 resistant when exposed to DL473 alone. Exposure to doxycycline alone did not eliminate the organism, although it did not become doxycycline resistant. Exposure to a combination of DL473 and doxycycline resulted in the elimination of the organism without the emergence of bacterial resistance. A strain of *S. faecalis* exposed to rifampin alone became rifampin resistant, but when exposed to tetracycline either alone or in combination with rifampin, it was eliminated from the cultures without the emergence of bacterial resistance. However, when the same strain of *S. faecalis* was exposed to fucidin alone it became fucidin resistant, and when exposed to a combination of rifampin and fucidin, it became doubly resistant to both antibiotics.

Most of the features of the experimental model used in these investigations are intended to reproduce the characteristics of treated human infections in vitro. The exception is the very large bacterial population so arranged that even very rare genetic events may be observed. The predictions arising from experiments conducted in this way are less relevant to the chance of bacterial resistance emerging during a single course of treatment than they are to the likelihood of such events occurring during the course of large numbers of treatments. Experience has shown that the emergence of rifampin resistance during exposure to rifampin alone occurs very readily under the conditions of the experimental procedure but that this can be prevented by a combination of rifampin with some antibiotics. Thus, combinations of rifampin and trimethoprim and rifampin and erythromycin prevented the emergence of bacterial resistance. A combination of rifampin and fucidin failed to prevent the emergence of bacteria doubly resistant to both antibiotics, and a combination of rifampin and tetracycline did not seem preferable to tetracycline alone. In the case of *N. gonorrhoeae*, a combination of either rifampin and erythromycin or DL473 and doxycycline eliminated the organism without the emergence of bacterial resistance.

The experimental procedure described is in principle applicable to any pair of antibiotics and is, in our opinion, a useful technique for predicting the effectiveness of antibiotic combinations in preventing the emergence of bacterial resistance.

Synergistic Effects of Cephalexin with Mecillinam

MASAKO OTSUKI,* NAOMASA GOTOH, TAKESHI NISHINO, AND TERUO TANINO

Department of Microbiology, Kyoto College of Pharmacy, Kyoto, Japan

In vitro and in vivo synergistic effects of cephalexin (CEX) and mecillinam (MPC) against various bacteria were demonstrated, and their action mechanisms are also discussed.

The synergistic effect of CEX and MPC against a total of 21 strains of *Escherichia coli, Klebsiella pneumoniae, Enterobacter* spp., *Serratia marcescens*, and *Proteus* spp. was examined by the checkerboard titration method, using heart infusion agar. Synergistic effects between CEX and MPC were observed against a total of 21 strains. The minimum fractional inhibitory concentration index was less than 0.5 in 16 of 21 strains and had a range of 0.531 to 0.75 in the remaining 5 strains. When the drug was added to log-phase cultures, the lytic activity and bactericidal effects of the combination of both drugs against *E. coli* ST-0198 were determined. When the cells were exposed to the combination of CEX at 3.13 μg/ml and MPC at 0.05 μg/ml, the turbidity and viable counts decreased significantly in the culture media of 10^6 cells per ml, indicating that a synergistic effect occurs between CEX and MPC (Fig. 1). For experimental *E. coli* ST-0198 infection in mice, two drugs were given at the combination ratio of 8:1 (CEX-pivmecillinam). This combination ratio was determined based on the ED_{50} of each antibiotic given alone. The ED_{50} of CEX, pivmecillinam, or the combination of CEX and pivmecillinam was 0.15, 0.017 or 0.039, and 0.0049 mg per mouse, respectively, and the fractional effective dose index was 0.55. The blood concentration ratio of CEX to MPC coincided with the con-

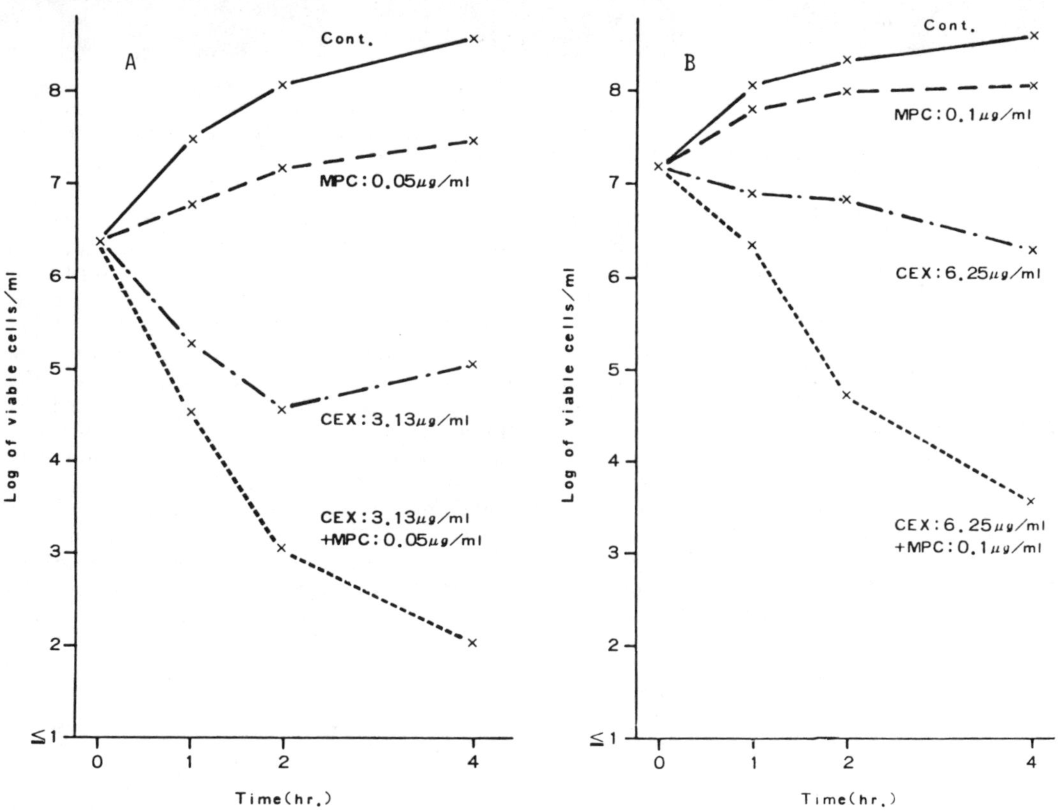

FIG. 1. *Combination effect of CEX and MPC on the viability of E. coli ST-0198. (A) Changes in number of viable cells when drug was added to a culture of 2.5 × 10^6 cells per ml. (B) Changes in number of viable cells when drug was added to a culture of 1.6 × 10^7 cells per ml. Cont., Control.*

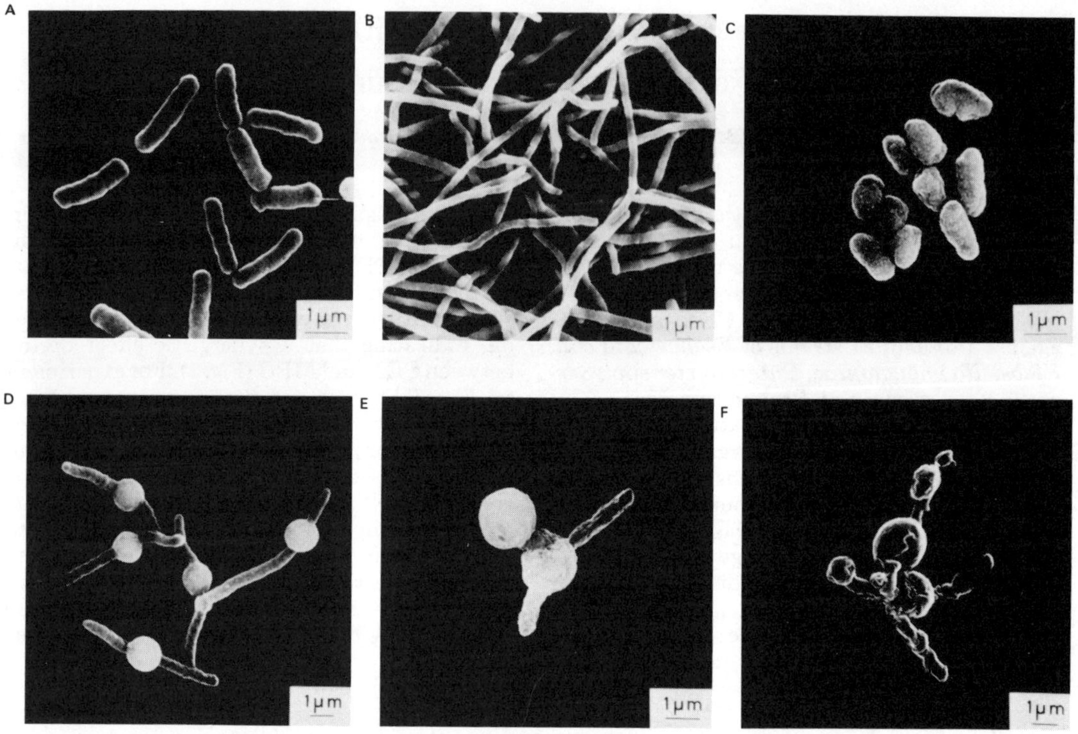

FIG. 2. *Scanning electron micrographs of E. coli ST-0198 exposed to CEX, MPC, and the combination. (A) Normal cells; (B) E. coli cells exposed to CEX at 3.13 μg/ml for 2 h; (C) E. coli cells exposed to MPC at 0.05 μg/ml for 2 h; (D) E. coli cells exposed to the combination for 1 h; (E) E. coli cells exposed to the combination for 2 h; and (F) E. coli cells exposed to the combination for 4 h.*

centration ratio of these antibiotics at which the synergistic effect was observed in vitro. Phase-contrast and scanning electron micrographs of bacterial cells exposed to the combination of CEX at 3.13 μg/ml and MPC at 0.05 μg/ml for 1 h showed somewhat elongated bacteria and formation of spindle cells with swelling in the central part; CEX at 3.13 μg/ml caused formation of filamentous cells, whereas MPC at 0.05 μg/ml caused formation of ovoid cells (Fig. 2). An observation of the internal structure in the swelling part by transmission electron microscope revealed a leakage of the cellular contents from the outermost site expanded by internal pressure. The examination of spheroplast formation proved that the combination of CEX at 3.13 μg/ml and MPC at 0.05 μg/ml caused formation of spheroplasts even when a single antibiotic did not induce formation of spheroplasts. The affinity of the antibiotics for penicillin-binding proteins in *E. coli* K-12 was observed by the competition method with [^{14}C]penicillin G. CEX showed an affinity for penicillin-binding proteins 1a and 3, and MPC showed an affinity for penicillin-binding protein 2. When these antibiotics were used concurrently, they exerted an additive effect to increase the affinity for penicillin-binding proteins. The affinity of [^{14}C]penicillin G was tested by using the cytoplasmic membrane of *E. coli* K-12 cells and observing morphological changes after exposure to each drug for 1 h. When the two drugs were used concomitantly, an affinity similar to one in the presence of a single antibiotic was demonstrated. The *E. coli* ST-0198 cells showed rapid cell lysis 5 min after exposure to both drugs at these concentrations, whereas each drug did not cause lytic activity by itself (CEX at 6.25 μg/ml or MPC at 0.1 μg/ml), and about 60% lytic activity was observed 30 min later.

It would be interesting to study how the inhibition of penicillin-binding proteins 2 and 3 is involved in bacteriolysis.

Clinical and Bacteriological Experiments with Oxolinic Acid in Treatment of Acute Enterocolitis

ANDRÁS SZALKA* AND ÉVA BÁN

Central Hospital for Infectious Diseases, Budapest, Hungary

The term "dysentery" indicates a condition characterized by frequent passage of stools containing blood and mucus and accompanied by straining and painful defecation. There is general agreement that dysentery syndrome is caused by a multiplicity of etiological agents. An acute febrile dysenteric illness in an area where shigellosis is common should be treated with an appropriate absorbable antimicrobial agent. Resistance of *Shigella* strains to ampicillin is currently a worldwide problem. The need for alternative therapy in shigellosis is apparent. Oxolinic acid is a quinoline derivative similar in structure and action to nalidixic acid. The good clinical effectiveness of nalidixic acid as well as the high percentage of in vitro sensitivity of gram-negative rods to this drug led us to investigate the effects of oxolinic acid.

Bacteriological study. The sensitivity of enteric pathogens was tested by a disk diffusion method (Table 1). The oxolinic acid (Chinoin) disk, which contained 30 μg, was made in our laboratory. The MIC estimation was carried out by an agar plate dilution method, using DST (CM 261; Oxoid) agar. The MICs of all *Salmonella*, *Shigella*, and *Escherichia coli* strains varied between 0.38 and 0.19 μg/ml. All isolates that belong to the species *Yersinia enterocolitica* showed a sensitivity lower than 0.19 μg/ml. The nalidixic acid MICs for the corresponding strains were generally four to eight times higher than those of oxolinic acid.

Serum level estimation was carried out on five patients and on two volunteers 0.5 h after oral administration of 500 mg of oxolinic acid three times a day for 3 days and 0.5, 1, 2, 3, and 4 h after the intake of 1,000 mg only for 1 day. To measure the concentration of the microbiologically active oxolinic acid, the cylinder plate technique was used. *E. coli* BE1 (MIC, 0.1 μg/ml) served as the test organism. The sensitivity of the test was 0.2 μg/ml. A detectable concentration of oxolinic acid (0.3 μg/ml) could be seen in the serum of only one patient. These findings conform with those of DiCarlo et al. (2). Fecal excretion of oxolinic acid given 1,500 mg orally per day was also tested in five patients and in five volunteers for 3 days while they were taking the drug as well as for 5 days after discontinuance of therapy. These samples were also examined by the cylinder plate technique (1), using the same *E. coli* test strain. Oxolinic acid could be detected in the feces of every patient in a concentration much higher than the MIC of the enteric pathogens. On the 3rd day after the discontinuance of therapy, all but one sample still contained the drug; by the 5th day the oxolinic acid could not be detected in any fecal sample. The lowest concentration was 5 μg/g; the highest, 180 μg/g.

Bacteriological tests were done every day with every fecal sample of patients receiving oxolinic acid to study the drug's effect on aerobic fecal flora. Some type of alteration could be observed in 28% of the cases, but the normal fecal flora spontaneously regenerated within 2 days.

Clinical study. A total of 118 patients were entered into the clinical study. Each of the patients had had over 15 stools daily, virtually all reported exudate and had observed blood. Most

TABLE 1. *Antibiotic resistance of enteric pathogens isolated in 1980 in the Central Hospital for Infectious Diseases, Budapest*

Organism	% of strains resistant to[a]:					
	AM	CM	PB	TMP + SMZ	NA	OA
Salmonella	8	3.4	0.3	2	0.3	0
Shigella	12	11	6	12	6	0
Y. enterocolitica	100	0	0	5	0	0
Commonest serotypes of enteropathogenic *E. coli*	41	28	1	16	1	0
Campylobacter jejuni[b]	NT	NT	NT	NT	0	0

[a] AM, Ampicillin; CM, chloramphenicol; PB, polymyxin B; TMP + SMZ, cotrimoxazole; NA, nalidixic acid; OA, oxolinic acid; NT, not tested.

[b] Fifteen isolates originated from the National Institute of Health, Budapest.

of the patients had been ill from 1 to 3 days before admission. All patients were young or middle-aged adult males. During the acute phase of the disease, these patients were treated for 3 days with one of the following: (i) oxolinic acid orally, 500 mg three times a day; (ii) nalidixic acid orally, 1 g four times a day; or (iii) supportive therapy consisting of bed rest, fluid and electrolyte replacement, and nutritional supplements.

Stool cultures were made before therapy and on the 5th, 6th, and 7th days after therapy. A sample was regarded as culture negative only when all subsequent examinations failed to isolate the type of *Shigella* or *Salmonella* previously found. Table 2 shows the bacteriological response in these 118 patients. Oxolinic acid was clinically as effective as nalidixic acid. Overall, half of the patients in both groups had no diarrhea beyond the 3rd day. Diarrhea stopped 2 days later in the group treated with supportive therapy. No side effects attributable to oxolinic acid were observed.

In conclusion, we can say that oxolinic acid is a valuable adjunct in the therapy of severe dysenteric illness and may be an effective drug against both ampicillin-susceptible and ampicillin-resistant *Shigella* strains. However, oxolinic acid should not be the drug of choice for eradication of salmonellas, and the consequences of altering the normal bowel flora must be considered when this drug is used.

TABLE 2. *Bacteriological response[a] to oxolinic acid, nalidixic acid, and supportive therapy in 118 patients with severe dysentery syndrome*

Therapy	No. Responding	
	Shigella	Salmonella
Oxolinic acid[b]	14 (1)[c]	10 (5)
Nalidixic acid[d]	3 (1)	12 (11)
Supportive therapy	2 (2)	3 (3)

[a] Stool cultures were performed on the 5th, 6th, and 7th days after therapy.
[b] Three-day treatment (1.5 g orally each day, in divided doses).
[c] Figures in parentheses indicate number of carriers.
[d] Three-day treatment (4.0 g orally each day, in divided doses).

1. **Bognár, S., and L. Binder.** 1967. Post-therapeutic levels of antimicrobial drugs in faeces. Acta Microbiol. **22:** 271–274.
2. **DiCarlo, F. J., M. C. Crew, M. D. Melgar, S. Roemer, S. M. Ringel, L. J. Haynes, and M. Wilson.** 1968. Oxolinic acid metabolism by man. Arch. Int. Pharmacodyn. **174:**413–427.

Infectious Diarrheas: Methodological Aspects and Preliminary Results

P. ALTUCCI,* G. F. ABBATE, L. D'APREA, V. LEONESSA, K. MARCHI, M. RAGANATI, C. DI LENA, V. BUFFA, G. GRANATA, AND G. VISCO

Chair of Medical Therapy (Salmonellosis Service) and Pediatric Clinic, First Faculty of Medicine, Naples University, Naples; SS. Annunziata Pediatric Hospital, Naples; and L. Spallanzani Hospital for Infectious Disease, Rome, Italy*

The infectious diarrheas (ID) are a growing problem today. Despite progress in our knowledge and the discovery of new etiological agents of ID, several problems pertaining to epidemiology, pathogenesis, diagnosis, and therapy are still to be settled.

Our observations in the past years in the Campania area (2) demonstrate the following. First, *Salmonellae* are quantitatively important (about 800 cases for the year evaluated). Since 1975, *Salmonella wien* has been found in large proportions in children and in pediatric institutions (40 to 80% of isolates). A variety of *Salmonella* serotypes other than *S. wien* have been isolated with high frequency from animals and foods. Unlike other *Salmonella* serotypes, *S. wien* spreads, particularly between humans (convalescent or asymptomatic carriers are today the most important reservoir of *S. wien*). A wide spectrum of antibiotic resistance of *S. wien* and its variants has appeared over time and in connection with different environments. As a result, the first and the most frequent (about 65%) pattern of antibiotic resistance was ampicillin, chloramphenicol, cephalosporins, streptomycin, sulfonamides, kanamycin, and tetracyclines, with or without colistin. This pattern is not frequent today because of the loss of one or more previous characters (e.g., CAF or tetracycline resistance) or because other resistances have been gained (e.g., gentamicin, up to 60% of isolates found in pediatric environments; cotrimoxazole, etc.). This phenomenon agrees with the plasmid nature of antibiotic resistance of *S.*

wien (1) as well the different use of antibiotics and the present human parasitism of *S. wien* (4). *Shigellae* are rarely isolated; *S. sonnei* is the most frequent serotype in our area (82% of a total of 124 *Shigella* spp. studied by us), followed by *S. flexneri* (8%). However, the incidence of *Shigellae* is probably underestimated when mucohematic diarrhea is lacking because of both the frequency of mild clinical cases and the poor (or absent) growth in selenite broth and in salmonella-shigella agar of *Shigellae* other than *S. sonnei*. No *Vibrio cholerae* or other enteropathogenic microorganism has been sent to our service for identification and typing. In conclusion, our data indicate that about 70 to 80% of ID appear to lack an identified etiological agent. However, a systematic search has not yet been done in this regard.

On the basis of these observations and our present knowledge, we have started a research program to clarify the incidence in our area of traditional and new etiological agents of ID and to find the eventual clinical-etiological relationships. For microbiological diagnosis, besides the traditional stool culture procedures, both filtration and the Skirrow technique were used for *Campylobacter* spp. isolation (5). The search for *Yersinia enterocolitica* was carried out through enrichment in both potassium-tellurite broth (26°C) and saline buffered at 4°C for 1 month, with weekly subcultures. To screening for enterotoxigenic *E. coli* strains, we preferred, besides serotype identification, the mannose-resistant hemagglutination (HA) test with both group A human erythrocytes and bovine erythrocytes (3).

Our preliminary results (Table 1) show a relatively low incidence of the classical agents of ID, no isolation of *Y. enterocolitica*, and recovery of only one strain of *Campylobacter* spp. The incidence of these agents was low in newborns and in the youngest children (up to 6 months of age; about 90% of our cases). We also found a large circulation of enterotoxigenic serotypes of *E. coli*, which were frequently isolated from asymptomatic patients also (control group). On the other hand, only a few strains displayed a positive mannose-resistant HA. Studies to demonstrate either the invasiveness or the enterotoxin production by the above isolates, through the Serény test, in cellular cultures and in suckling mouse assays, are still in progress. The final results could clarify the reliability of our tests. Finally, in newborns, a non-defined etiology appeared relatively frequently and awaits the virological results.

In the management of all forms of diarrhea, it is necessary to first balance the hydroelectrolyte equilibrium. Chemotherapy in the treatment of

TABLE 1. *Microorganisms isolated from feces of 94 patients (0 to 2 years old)*

Microrganisms		Enteritis (41) No.	Enteritis (41) %	"Control" (53) No.	"Control" (53) %
Salmonella spp		8*	19.5	0	-
Shigella spp		1	2.4	1	1.8
"Enteropathogen." E. coli	A	10	24.4	11	20.7
	B	3	7.3	2**	3.7
Campylobacter spp		1	2.4	0	-
V. cholerae		0	-	0	-
Yersinia spp		0	-	0	-
Viruses		research in progress today			

* 1 patient with both Salmonella and E. coli

**of these patients, one had only one episode of vomiting without dyarrhoea, the other showed dyarrhoea after 10 days

A: on the basis of antigenic classification (the more frequent bioserotypes resulted (O): 44; 78; 86; 125)

B: on the basis of mannose-resistant HA test positivity

Behaviour of tests performed against potentially pathogen E. coli strains

enteritogen serotype	HA* without mannose	HA* with mannose	no. of strains
+	-	-	16
+	+	+	4
-	+	+	1
-	+	-	5

* for detection of Colonizating Factor

ID is controversial due to our poor knowledge about the natural course of the disease.

On the basis of our previous observations in a randomized trial (6), our practice in ID is as follows. (i) In noncomplicated gastroenteritis, we do not use chemoantibiotics because no benefit with regard to clinical picture, course, prognosis, or duration of *Salmonella* excretion is achievable, whereas unwanted effects, such as the selection of multiresistant strains and changing the enteric flora, thereby risking superinfections, can occur. (ii) In high-risk patients or with either suspected or demonstrated bacteremia, we use systemic antibiotics until there is clinical remission, regardless of the persistence of positive stool cultures. In conclusion, chemotherapy is started only to cure or prevent sepsis or metastatic localizations. These latter complications, among 764 salmonellosis cases in a pediatric unit (V. Buffa et al., unpublished data), have been observed in only 20 cases (26%).

TABLE 2. *Clinical and bacteriological course of 66 salmonellosis cases in newborns and children*

CLINICAL PICTURE AND CHEMO. THERAPY	PER CENT OF PATIENTS STERILIZED AT WEEKS 1	2	3	4	>4	COURSE
SUBCLINICAL INFECTIONS, UNTREATED (24 CASES)	54.0	25.0	12.5	4.0	4.0	ALWAYS FAVOURABLE
GASTRO-ENTERITIS, UNTREATED (20 CASES)	40.0	35.0	20.0	5.0	-	ALWAYS FAVOURABLE
GASTRO-ENTERITIS, (COMPLICATED AND/OR IN "HIGH RISK. PATIENTS)*, TREATED (22 CASES)	18.0	13.6	18.0	22.7	18.2	FATAL IN 2 CASES

* = HIGHLY FEBRILE PATIENTS WITH TOXEMIA AND BACTEREMIA SUSPECTED OR DEMONSTRATED. PREMATURE OR PATIENTS WITH SERIOUS UNDERLYING DISEASE.

Our more recent observations (Table 2) confirm our general practice. The untreated infants were not comparable to the treated infants; the latter had an infective complication or symptoms of a more severe and systemic disease. Nevertheless, at least the lack of usefulness of chemoantibiotics in noncomplicated salmonellosis again is evidenced: none of the untreated patients suffered any complication, and the clinical course was always favorable, with spontaneous sterilization in a relatively short time.

1. **Abbate, G. F., I. Alagia, P. Altucci, P. Guarascio, V. Leonessa, P. Narciso, and G. Visco.** 1978. Transfer of resistance in *Salmonella wien*: epidemiological implications, p. 165–166. *In* Current chemotherapy. American Society for Microbiology, Washington, D.C.
2. **Altucci, P., G. F. Abbate, I. Alagia, and V. Leonessa.** 1977. Salmonella e Salmonellosi alla luce dell'esperienza nella Regione Campania. G. Mal. Infett. Parassie. **29:** 553–575.
3. **Evans, D. G., D. J. Evans, Jr., W. S. Tjoa, and H. J. Dupont.** 1978. Detection and characterization of colonization factor of enterotoxigenic *Escherichia coli* isolated from adults with diarrhea. Infect. Immun. **19:**727–738.
4. **Leonessa, V., G. F. Abbate, I. Alagia, L. D'Aprea, and A. P. Pilloni.** 1980. Variations in resistance of *S. wien* and their relationships with use of chemoantibiotics and human transmission mode, p. 124. Proc. 2nd Meditr. Congr. Chemother.
5. **Skirrow, M. B.** 1977. Campylobacter enteritis: a "new" disease. Br. Med. J. **ii:**9–15.
6. **Visco, G., C. Leoni, E. Tornese, C. Carvelli, P. Guarascio, C. Struglia, G. Tocci, G. F. Abbate, V. Leonessa, I. Alagia, and P. Altucci.** 1978. Chemotherapy in salmonellosis, p. 167–169. *In* Current chemotherapy. American Society for Microbiology, Washington, D.C.

Chemotherapy with Bicozamycin in Piglets with Acute Enterotoxigenic *Escherichia coli* Diarrhea

MAX MAURER AND FRIEDRICH KRADOLFER*

Research Department, Pharmaceuticals Division, CIBA-GEIGY Ltd., Basel, Switzerland

Bicozamycin (bicyclomycin; CGP 3543/E) is an antibiotic of unique chemical structure which is active against enterobacterial species commonly implicated in the occurrence of acute diarrhea in humans (2, 3). Its clinical efficacy in patients with acute diarrhea has been reported elsewhere (1). This study on artificially infected piglets was performed to obtain information about the symptomatological and bacteriological responses to treatment with bicozamycin under controlled experimental conditions.

A total of 40 male and female piglets, 18 days old and with a mean weight of 4.6 kg, were infected by gavage, each receiving 1.4×10^{11} cells of an overnight culture of enterotoxigenic *Escherichia coli* O149 K88 *ent*$^+$ *hly*$^+$. The consistency of the feces was estimated visually. Dry and moist samples were considered normal; animals passing loose, watery, and profusely watery feces were considered diarrheic. Ninety-three percent of the animals developed diarrhea within 10 h of infection. Bicozamycin was given 10 h after infection by gavage in doses of 10 mg per kg of body weight and repeated at 6-h intervals for 36 h. Half of the animals were given a sham treatment. The course of the infection and the effect of treatment were assessed by quantitative analysis of *E. coli* excretion in treated and untreated animals. Fresh fecal samples for subsequent viable counts were taken immediately before infection and 2, 4, and 8 days after infection. Appropriate dilutions were plated on MacConkey agar (total fecal coliforms) and brain heart infusion agar supplemented with 5% sheep blood (enumeration of the hemolytic, diarrheagenic strain of *E. coli* used for the infection). Both media were incubated aerobically at 37°C overnight.

In the untreated controls (Fig. 1), high total counts ($10^{8.6}$) of *E. coli* were found 2 days after

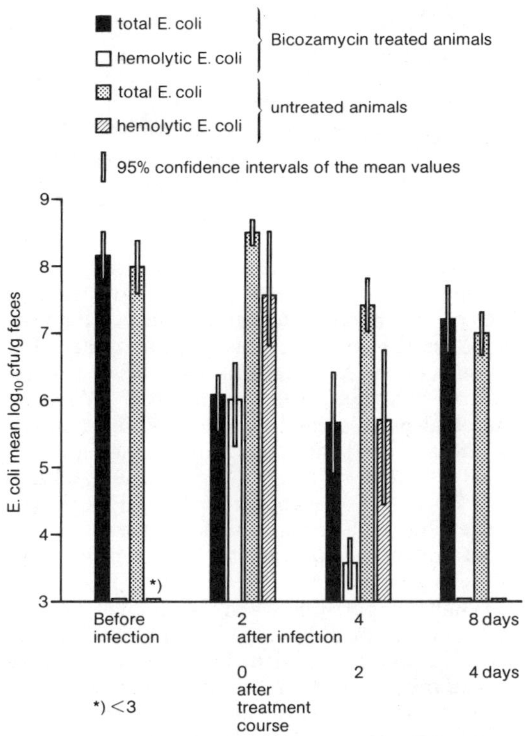

FIG. 1. *Excretion of total and hemolytic (pathogenic) E. coli in treated and untreated animals.*

infection. Thereafter, the total counts decreased, but the differential cultures showed that although the pathogenic hemolytic type was eliminated by the 8th day, the resident *E. coli* did not drop below approximately 1/10 of the number found before the infection. The ratio of the number of infective hemolytic bacilli to the total cultivable *E. coli* population decreased from 1:10 on day 2 to 1:100 on day 4 and to 1:>10,000 on day 8. This indicates the rate of spontaneous elimination of the pathogen from the flora.

In the treated animals, the total *E. coli* population decreased about 500-fold during the treatment period by comparison with the control values. By the 8th day, this difference was no longer demonstrable, reflecting the normalization of the temporarily disturbed colonic flora. On the other hand, the counts of pathogenic *E. coli hly*$^+$ decreased more rapidly in the treated than in the untreated animals. After this period of accelerated elimination during treatment, the pathogenic organisms were excreted at the same rate as in the untreated controls. This observation would seem to indicate that the antibiotic treatment did not impair the microbiocoenotic defense system.

In a separate experiment with 16 piglets infected by the same diarrheagenic strain of *E. coli*, 4 were killed at each of different time intervals after a single oral treatment with bicozamycin. Bacteriological examination in six different intestinal segments revealed a significant reduction of intestinal coliforms for definite time lapses, whereas the bulk of intestinal anaerobes remained numerically unimpaired (M. Maurer, unpublished data).

TABLE 1. *Duration in days of diarrhea after infection (feces of more watery consistency than normal)*

days	treated	untreated	n
0.5	3		3
1	4		4
1.5	4	2	6
2	5	5	10
3	0	4	4
4	0	1	1
>4	1	5	6
Median = 2			34

The duration in days after infection during which the animals continued to pass feces of more watery consistency than normal was different in the two groups (Table 1). Diarrhea of >2 days' duration was observed in only one animal in the bicozamycin group as against 10 in the untreated group; diarrhea of <2 days' duration was seen in 16 treated and 7 untreated animals. The duration of diarrhea in the individual animals was statistically different ($P = 0.001$) in the two groups when tested by the median test (5), and the average value in the treated group was half (ca. 1.5 days) that recorded in the untreated group (>3 days). Treatment with bicozamycin accelerated the process of elimination of the pathogenic *E. coli* and significantly shortened the duration of diarrhea.

1. **Jarumilinta, R., F. Kradolfer, K. Vosbeck, and V. Viranuvatti.** 1980. Effect of bicyclomycin (CGP 3543/E) in acute diarrhoea of various nonparasitic origins, p. 435–437. *In* Current chemotherapy and infectious disease. American Society for Microbiology, Washington, D.C.
2. **Nishida, M., M. Yasuhiro, and T. Matsubara.** 1972. Bicyclomycin, a new antibiotic. III. In vitro and in vivo antimicrobial activity. J. Antibiot. **25:**582–593.
3. **Sackmann, W., R. Jarumilinta, K. Vosbeck, and F. Kradolfer.** 1980. Effect of bicyclomycin (CGP 3543/E) on enterobacterial flora in humans and experimental animals, p. 434–435. *In* Current chemotherapy and infectious disease. American Society for Microbiology, Washington, D.C.
4. **Siegel, S.** 1956. Nonparametric statistics. McGraw-Hill Book Co., New York.

Clinical Efficacy of Bicozamycin in Acute Nonparasitic Nondysenteric Diarrhea: Placebo-Controlled Study

RAWEWAN JARUMILINTA, FRIEDRICH KRADOLFER,* AND P. THANUNGKUL

Research Department, Pharmaceuticals Division, CIBA-GEIGY Ltd., Basel, Switzerland, and Department of Medicine, Bamrasnadura, Infection Disease Hospital, Nonthaburi, Thailand*

Bicozamycin (bicyclomycin; CGP 3543/E), a new antibiotic (2), is distinguished by its activity against enteropathogens belonging to genera *Enterobacteriaceae* and *Vibrionaceae* and to some other species (2, 3). It causes no cross-resistance with other chemotherapeutics, and it is absorbed to only a slight extent after oral administration. This study was undertaken to assess the clinical benefit afforded by short-term treatment with bicozamycin under bacteriologically controlled conditions.

A double-blind placebo-controlled trial was performed in Nonthaburi, Thailand, in 56 hospitalized adult patients suffering from severe nonparasitic (i.e., no *Entamoeba histolytica* or *Giardia lamblia*), nondysenteric (i.e., no blood and mucus) diarrhea of less than 24-h duration. The two groups, with 28 patients each, were comparable before the start of treatment with respect to etiology (Table 1), duration, and severity of diarrhea, fever, abdominal pain, and vomiting. The patients admitted gave their consent to the study.

Bicozamycin or placebo in doses of 500 mg was given orally every 6 h for 36 h. The treatment was allocated at random. All patients received intravenous fluid replacement therapy according to the estimated fluid loss. Patients in whom diarrhea did not stop within 72 h after the start of treatment were given open-label medication.

Stool cultures for enteric bacilli were made on eosin methylene blue, salmonella-shigella, and thiosulfate citrate bile salts sucrose media before and after treatment. The isolates grown on these media were identified according to the API system. The test for enterotoxigenicity was done not later than 2 months after isolation of the organisms by the rabbit jejunal loop method.

Both bicozamycin and placebo were well tolerated. The bacteriological diagnosis and stratification in the two treatment groups are given in Table 1. In approximately three-fifths of the patients, enterotoxigenic pathogens were present; in the remainder, the bacteriological diagnosis was undefined except in one case each of *Salmonella* spp., *Shigella* spp., and *Vibrio parahaemolyticus*.

Fever, abdominal pain, and vomiting ceased rapidly in the patients of both groups. Regardless of the bacteriological diagnosis, the time between the start of the treatment and the passage of the last unformed stool, i.e., the period of diarrhea, was significantly (Wilcoxon matched-pairs, signed-rank test) shorter in the patients treated with bicozamycin: median of 11 to 13 h (range, <1 to 42) as against 49 to 53 h (6 to >72) in the placebo group. Diarrhea lasted longer than 36 h in only one patient treated with bicozamycin, in contrast to 16 patients in the placebo group.

When comparisons are made on an etiological basis, i.e., in the subgroups with enterotoxigenic bacteria and those with diarrhea of unknown origin, the duration of diarrhea after treatment as well as the total duration of diarrhea were significantly shorter in the patients receiving

TABLE 1. *Frequency distribution of strains isolated before and after treatment*

Species[a]	Distribution			
	Bicozamycin		Placebo	
	Before	After	Before	After
E. coli				
Non-ET	41	52	41	48
ET	13	2	10	0
K. pneumoniae				
Non-ET	32	30	34	35
ET	2	0	1	2
Enterobacter spp.				
Non-ET	6	6	4	4
ET	2	0	1	1
Salmonella spp.	0	1	1	1
Shigella spp.	1	0	1	0
V. parahaemolyticus				
Non-ET	1	0	2	0
ET	9	0	8	2
Aeromonas spp.				
Non-ET	13	1	12	7
ET	6	0	3	1
Others				
Non-ET	14	20	8	12
ET	5	1	3	0

[a] Non-ET, Nonenterotoxigenic; ET, enterotoxigenic.

bicozamycin: less than half as long as in placebo-treated patients.

The distribution of the duration of diarrhea in each case in the two treatment groups is shown in Fig. 1. One stool specimen was examined in each patient 1.5 to 4.5 days after the end of treatment. In 16 cases in the bicozamycin group and in 14 in the placebo group in which positive findings for entertoxigenic bacilli were present initially, tests for enterotoxigenicity were also performed after treatment. Two positive cases were found in the bicozamycin group (*E. coli*, *Citrobacter* spp.), and four were found in the placebo group (*Klebsiella*, *Enterobacter*, *Aeromonas*, *V. parahaemolyticus*). Although the enterotoxigenic pathogens evidently tended to disappear from the stools, the concomitant gram-negative flora (*Escherichia*, *Klebsiella*, *Proteus*, *Enterobacter*, *Citrobacter*, *Providencia*) was virtually unchanged.

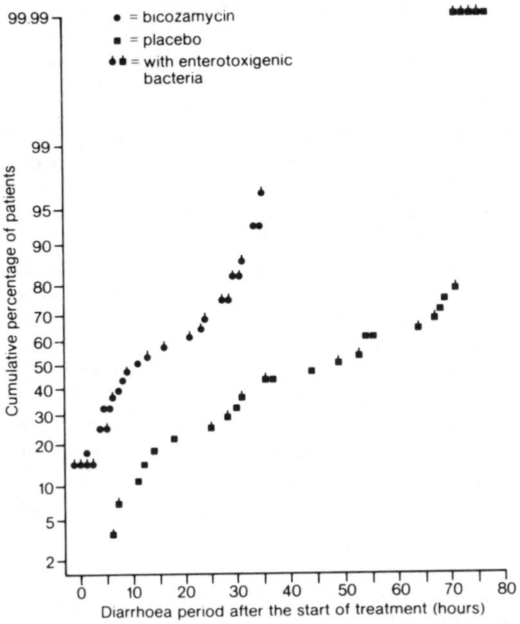

FIG. 1. *Distribution of diarrhea period after treatment in 28 patients treated with bicozamycin and 28 patients given placebo.*

Since similar therapeutic effects and good tolerability of bicozamycin have also been observed elsewhere in diarrhea of various origins, including shigellosis (1), bicozamycin merits further study as a broad-spectrum chemotherapeutic for infectious diarrhea.

1. **Jarumilinta, R., F. Kradolfer, K. Vosbeck, and V. Viranuvatti.** 1980. Effect of bicozamycin (CGP 3543/E) in acute diarrhea of various nonparasitic origins, p. 435–437. *In* Current chemotherapy and infectious disease. American Society for Microbiology, Washington, D.C.
2. **Nishida, M., M. Yasukiro, and T. Matsubava.** 1972. Bicyclomycin, a new antibiotic. III. *In vitro* and *in vivo* antimicrobial activity. J. Antibiot. **25**:582–593.
3. **Sackmann, W., R. Jarumilinta, K. Vosbeck, and F. Kradolfer.** 1980. Effect of bicozamycin (CGP 3543/E) on enterobacterial flora in humans and experimental animals, p. 434–435. *In* Current chemotherapy and infectious disease. American Society for Microbiology, Washington, D.C.

Evidence for the Chromosomal Nature of Bicozamycin Resistance in Enterobacterial Isolates from Humans and Animals

GERHARD LEBEK,* FRIEDRICH KRADOLFER, MAX MAURER, AND KLAUS VOSBECK

Institute of Medical Microbiology, University of Bern, Bern, and Research Department, Pharmaceuticals Division, CIBA-GEIGY Ltd., Basel, Switzerland*

Plasmid-mediated resistance against therapeutic antibiotics is epidemiologically important because of its rapid spread and because it does not impede bacterial growth as chromosomal resistance usually does. The type of resistance of the occasional bicozamycin (bicyclomycin; CGP 3543/E)-resistant enteric bacteria emerging during therapy of acute diarrhea with bicozamycin is therefore important. We examined several such strains for the presence of plasmid-mediated resistance to bicozamycin.

Attempts to transfer bicozamycin resistance with and without using helper plasmids were performed according to Zünd and Lebek (5). Plasmids were isolated as described by Meyers et al. (4) and subjected to gel electrophoresis. Antibiotic resistance patterns were determined with disks on DST agar, using the method of Bauer et al. (1). Attempts to cure *Escherichia coli* strains from conjugative R-plasmids by low cure concentrations (<64 μg/ml) of bicozamycin, using a replica plate technique for detecting a possible loss of resistance, were carried out according to Lebek (3). *E. coli* K-12 921 *lac*$^-$ *leu*$^-$ *thr*$^-$ *met*$^-$ *r*$^-$ *m*$^-$ *rpsL* served as a recipient strain for all tested plasmids.

E. coli O149 K88 E65 (hemolytic, enterotoxigenic, rifampin resistant) with two plasmids (5 and 1 kilobase pairs) was used to infect piglets (Maurer and Kradolfer, this volume).

Nineteen bicozamycin-resistant strains of various bacterial genera were selected from stool specimens of successfully bicozamycin-treated patients in Bangkok (2). Bicozamycin-resistant strains of different enterobacterial species were isolated from feces of infected piglets (Maurer and Kradolfer, this volume). Strains carrying helper plasmids were used for the mobilization of nonconjugative plasmids: *E. coli* K-12 921 *lac*$^-$ *leu*$^-$ *thr*$^-$ *met*$^-$ *r*$^-$ *m*$^-$ *rpsL* pGL (Tc, Sm, Su), 115 kilobase pairs; *E. coli* K-12 921 *lac*$^-$ *leu*$^-$ *thr*$^-$ *met*$^-$ *r*$^-$ *m*$^-$ *rpsL* pGL 231 (Tc, Sm, Su), 115 kilobase pairs; and *E. coli* K-12 921 *lac*$^-$ *leu*$^-$ *thr*$^-$ *met*$^-$ *r*$^-$ *m*$^-$ *rpsL* pGL 231 (Tc, Sm, Cm, Km, Su, Tp), 100 kilobase pairs.

Bicozamycin-resistant strains were isolated on MacConkey or brain heart infusion agar supplemented with 5% sheep blood and bicozamycin, 100 μg/ml. MacConkey agar was used as the selective medium for conjugative R transfer. Antibiotics were added as required at the following final concentrations: streptomycin, 1,000 μg/ml; tetracycline, 20 μg/ml; chloramphenicol, 50 μg/ml; kanamycin, 50 μg/ml; ampicillin, 50 μg/ml; bicozamycin, 100 μg/ml or more if required; and rifampin, 100 μg/ml. For selecting R-plasmids, the following antibiotic disks were added to every selective medium after inoculation with diluted fecal samples: ampicillin, 10 μg/disk; chloramphenicol, 30 μg/disk; streptomycin, 10 μg/disk; trimethoprim/sulfamethoxazole, 25 μg/disk; tetracycline, 30 μg/disk; and kanamycin, 30 μg/disk. Columbia broth was used for conjugative R-transfer experiments.

Enterobacterial strains resistant to 100 μg of bicozamycin per ml isolated from piglets (Table 1) contained no R factors. They did not transfer bicozamycin resistance, even with the use of helper plasmids. Nineteen enterobacterial strains resistant to 100 μg of bicozamycin per ml isolated from stool specimens of patients suffering from diarrhea did not transfer any bicozamycin resistance determinants to receptor strains, regardless of whether they carried conjugative or nonconjugative R factors (Table 2). Three different conjugative R factors were not

TABLE 1. *Enterobacteriaceae from the fecal flora of infected piglets isolated on MacConkey agar containing 100 μg of bicozamycin per ml*[a]

Number of animals	Bicozamycin treatment	Frequency of isolation of enterobacteriaceae at days after infection			
		−1	2	4	8
8	yes	8 animals: 0	5 animals: 0 3 animals: 3×10³*	8 animals: 0	8 animals: 0
8	no	7 animals: 0 1 animal: 5×10²*	7 animals: 0 1 animal: 2×10³*	7 animals: 0 1 animal: 5×10²**	8 animals: 0

[a] Day −1 is 1 day before infection. 0, <5 × 10²/g of feces. *, *Klebsiella* sp.; **, *E. cloacae*.

TABLE 2. *Bicozamycin-resistant enterobacterial strains isolated from feces of bicozamycin-treated diarrhea patients used in plasmid transfer experiments*

Plasmid	Species	Number of strains	Number of patients	Transfer of bicozamycin-resistance to E.coli K12 921
Conjugative R-factor	E.coli	8	8	Ø
Nonconjugative R-factor	E.coli	2	2	Ø
	Proteus mirabilis	2	2	Ø
	Proteus rettgeri	1	1	Ø
	Proteus morganii	1	1	Ø
	Providencia	2	2	Ø
	Enterobacter	1	1	Ø
No plasmid	E.coli	1	1	Ø
	Klebsiella pneumoniae	1	1	Ø

cured by subinhibitory concentrations of bicozamycin. Five hundred to 1,000 clones of each strain were tested.

We conclude that (i) treatment of acute diarrhea with bicozamycin in patients and animals had no influence on the nature and the selection of enterobacterial R factors and (ii) the resistance to 100 μg of bicozamycin per ml in enterobacterial isolates from patients and animals of this study was of chromosomal nature.

1. **Bauer, A. W., W. M. Kirby, J. C. Sherris, and M. Turck.** 1966. Antibiotic susceptibility testing by a standardized single disc method. Ann. J. Clin. Pathol. **45:** 493–496.
2. **Jarumilinta, R., F. Kradolfer, K. Vosbeck, and V. Viranuvatti.** 1980. Effect of bicyclomycin (CGP 3543/E) in acute diarrhea of various nonparasitic origins, p. 435–437. *In* Current chemotherapy and infectious disease. American Society for Microbiology, Washington, D.C.
3. **Lebek, G.** 1969. Die infektiöse bakterielle Antibiotika-Resistenz. Verlag Hans Huber, Bern, Switzerland.
4. **Meyers, J. A., D. Sanchez, L. P. Elwell, and S. Falkow.** 1976. Simple agarose gel electrophoretic method for the identification and characterization of plasmid DNA. J. Bacteriol. **127:**295–309.
5. **Zünd, P., and G. Lebek.** 1980. Generation time prolonging R-plasmids: correlation between increases in the generation time of E. coli caused by R-plasmids and their molecular size. Plasmid **3:**65–69.

Occurrence of *Clostridium difficile* in Antibiotic-Associated Diarrhea in Sweden

BO ARONSSON,* ROLAND MÖLLBY, AND CARL ERIK NORD

Department of Bacteriology, National Bacteriological Laboratory, S-105 21 Stockholm, and Karolinska Institute, S-104 01 Stockholm, Sweden*

Virtually every widely used antimicrobial agent with the exception of vancomycin and parenteral aminoglycosides has been reported to be associated with diarrhea and the intestinal overgrowth of toxin-producing *Clostridium difficile* (2, 6). The mechanism by which this overgrowth takes place cannot solely be explained by resistance among the clostridial strains to offending antibiotics (1). The suppression of normal colon microflora by various antibiotics, thereby enhancing growth of *C. difficile*, seems to play an important role in the pathogenesis of this sometimes deleterious disease (5). In the present study, 1,643 fecal specimens from 1,324 patients suffering from antibiotic-associated diarrhea (AAD) or pseudomembranous colitis were investigated for growth of *C. difficile* and the presence of *C. difficile* toxin.

Collection of specimens. Fecal samples from various Swedish hospitals were sent to the National Bacteriological Laboratory during a 96-week period in 1979 to 1980 with a transportation time of less than 2 days.

Processing of specimens. Stool specimens were diluted 11 times in phosphate-buffered saline. The stool filtrate was diluted in 10-fold serial dilutions; 50 μl of each of these dilutions was added to 100 μl of cell culture medium and incubated for 20 h at 37°C with human embryonic intestinal cells (6). An actinomorphic effect of more than 10% of the cells, which could be neutralized by antiserum from *C. sordelli* (National Institutes of Health, Bethesda, Md., U.S.A.) was regarded as indicative for the presence of *C. difficile* toxin. Isolated strains of *C. difficile* were grown under anaerobic conditions in chopped-meat broth medium, and 50 μl of the culture supernatant was investigated for cytopathogenic activity in a similar manner.

The fecal samples were cultivated anaerobically for 48 h at 37°C on blood agar and CCFA agar (3, 6). Colonies resembling *C. difficile* were identified by colonial and cellular morphology, biochemical tests, and gas-liquid chromatography (4). Isolated strains were tested by the agar dilution method against different antibiotics (Fig. 1).

Isolation and characterization of *Clostridium* strains. Increasing concentrations of *C. difficile* cytotoxin in stool filtrate from patients with AAD were associated with an increased isolation rate of *C. difficile*, from 2.2% when no toxin was detected in the stool to 36% when toxin in the stool filtrate could be demonstrated after dilution more than 10^4 times, and with an increased toxin production by isolated strains in broth medium. Thus, high amounts of *C. difficile* cytotoxin in stool reflected a large number of bacteria and their toxin-producing ability.

Isolated clostridial strains could be divided into three groups: (i) toxin-producing *C. difficile*;

(ii) non-toxin-producing *C. difficile*; and (iii) toxin-producing *Clostridium* sp. These data indicate that not all strains of *C. difficile* produced the cytotoxin and that other clostridial species, as yet unidentified, may produce the toxin.

Antibiotic susceptibility pattern. Most strains required low MICs of metronidazole, benzylpenicillin, and vancomycin. High MICs were seen for the cephalosporins tested. Doxycycline, clindamycin, piperacillin, and thienamycin showed intermediate values (Fig. 1).

Evaluation of AAD risk. The AAD frequency of different antimicrobial agents was compared with the statistics for usage of various antibiotics in Sweden, based upon the defined daily dose statistics (issued by the Nordic Council of Medicine). This enabled us to evaluate the relative risk of achieving AAD for different agents. This risk evaluation (Table 1) found a nearly 100-fold increased frequency of AAD upon usage of lincomycin-clindamycin as compared with that of penicillins and a nearly 200-fold increased frequency of lincomycin-clindamycin-associated diarrhea connected with *C. difficile* toxin in stool samples. After use of cephalosporins, the stool from cases of AAD contained *C. difficile* toxin at a high frequency compared with that of other antibiotics.

The nature of the ecological disturbance associated with the overgrowth of toxin-producing *C. difficile* in AAD is not fully elucidated. The susceptibility of isolated strains from clinical specimens to offending antibiotics seems to be of minor importance in the development of this disease. According to investigations by Larson and others (5) in a hamster model, clindamycin

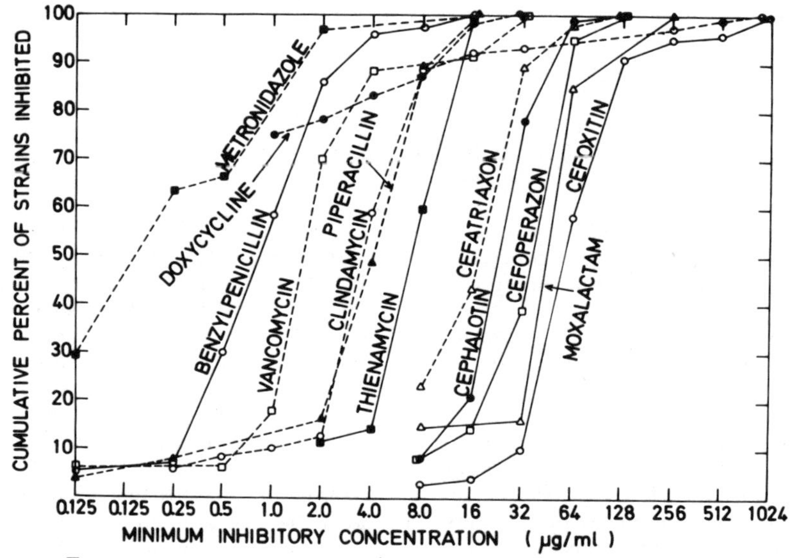

FIG. 1. *Antibiotic susceptibility patterns of 96 clostridial isolates.*

TABLE 1. *Antibiotic sales statistics and evaluation of AAD risk*

Offending antibiotic	A Absolute no. of AAD			B Relative no. of AAD (%)			C Relative sales of antibiotics[a] (%)	D Comparison (B/C × 10)			E Evaluation of AAD risk and narrow-spectrum penicillins ($D_{antibiotic}/D_{penicillin}$)		
	Total	Toxin +	Toxin −	Total	Toxin +	Toxin −		Total	Toxin +	Toxin −	Total	Toxin +	Toxin −
Penicillins													
Narrow spectrum	50	13	37	22	16	26	34	6	5	8	1	1	1
Broad spectrum	23	10	13	10	12	9	19	5	6	5	0.8	1.3	0.6
Cephalosporins	19	15	4	8	18	3	4	21	47	7	3.3	10	1.0
Lincomycin-clindamycin	37	21	16	16	26	11	0.3	543	853	370	84	182	49
Others[b]	46	14	32	20	17	22	42	5	4	5	0.7	0.9	0.7
Multitreatment	51	9	42	23	11	29							
Total	226	82	144	99	100	100	99						

[a] Based on defined daily dose statistics in Sweden, issued by the Nordic Council on Medicine.

[b] Doxycycline, gentamicin, erythromycin, fusidic acid, trimethoprim-sulfa, sulfa, nitrofurantoin, nalidixic acid.

produces a state of susceptibility to intestinal colonization which can be reversed by feeding the animals a suspension of normal hamster feces before challenge with *C. difficile.* Our data support the idea that antibiotics with a pronounced effect on the anaerobic intestinal flora (lincomycin-clindamycin) are more often implicated as causes of AAD in humans, probably due to the disturbance of the normal microecology after the suppression of the anaerobic microorganisms. When antibiotics like cephalosporins are incriminated, the increased resistance among clostridial strains provokes an overgrowth, thus yielding AAD caused by *C. difficile.*

This investigation was supported by the Swedish Medical Research Council (16X-05969).

1. **Bartlett, J. G., N. S. Taylor, T. Chang, and J. Dzink.** 1980. Clinical and laboratory observations in *Clostridium difficile* colitis. Am. J. Clin. Nutr. **33**:2521–2526.
2. **George, W. L., B. D. Kirby, V. L. Sutter, and S. M. Finegold.** 1979. Antimicrobial susceptibility of *Clostridium difficile*, p. 267–271. *In* D. Schlessinger (ed.), Microbiology—1979. American Society for Microbiology, Washington, D.C.
3. **George, W. L., V. L. Sutter, and S. M. Finegold.** 1979. Selective and differential medium for isolation of *Clostridium difficile*. J. Clin. Microbiol. **9**:214–219.
4. **Holdeman, V., E. P. Cato, and W. E. C. Moore (ed.).** 1977. Anaerobe laboratory manual, 4th ed. Virginia Polytechnic Institute and State University, Blacksburg.
5. **Larson, H. E., A. B. Price, and S. P. Borrelio.** 1980. Epidemiology of experimental enterocolitis due to *Clostridium difficile*. J. Infect. Dis. **142**:408–413.
6. **Möllby, R., C. E. Nord, and B. Aronsson.** 1980. Diagnosis of *C. difficile*-associated enterocolitis in Sweden. Laboratory and epidemiological aspects. Scand. J. Infect. Dis. **22**(Suppl.):30–36.

Antibiotic-Associated Pseudomembranous Colitis: Simplified Procedure for Detecting the Causative Organism

PAULINE HONOUR AND SAVERIO P. BORRIELLO*

Clinical Research Centre, Harrow, Middlesex, HA1 3UJ, England

In the past few years, *Clostridium difficile* has been firmly implicated as the etiological agent of both antibiotic- and non-antibiotic-associated pseudomembranous colitis (1). There is also further recent evidence to implicate this microorganism with other intestinal disease states. This has resulted in an increased awareness of, and interest in, analysis of stool samples for the presence of *C. difficile*. Recent investigative procedures have been greatly facilitated by the development of a sensitive selective agar incorporating cycloserine and cefoxitin as selective agents and using long-wave UV light as an aid in detecting *C. difficile* colonies (2). We wanted, however, to evaluate a simplified procedure for the isolation of *C. difficile* from stools that was independent of selective agars and to further modify this procedure so that it was also independent of sophisticated anaerobic facilities.

This study was divided into two parts. The first part was concerned with the evaluation of the use of alcohol to select for clostridial spores (alcohol shock procedure [AP]) compared with a selective antibiotic-containing medium. The second part of the study evaluated a modification of this procedure that used the minimum of anaerobe culture facilities (bench alcohol shock procedure [BAP]). The 266 specimens used in the study were forwarded for investigation from a number of hospitals throughout the United Kingdom. All samples were processed immediately on receipt. Samples were analyzed for the presence of *C. difficile* by use of a selective medium containing cycloserine and cefoxitin at concentrations of 250 and 10 μg/ml, respectively. Stool dilutions were also exposed to an equal volume of absolute ethanol for 1 h at room temperature before seeding onto a blood agar plate. This whole procedure was done under strictly anaerobic conditions (AP) or under atmospheric conditions in the absence of any prereduced media, with the use of a gas kit to generate an anaerobic environment for plate incubation (BAP).

Of the 266 fecal samples, 82 were shown to be positive by a combination of AP and the selective agar procedure (SA). Seventy-seven (94%) of these were detected by SA, and 72 (88%) were detected by AP (Table 1). Ten samples (12%) were positive by SA only, and five samples (6%) were positive by AP only (Table 2). The AP was further modified so that all manipulations before incubation were performed on the open bench. Of 18 positive samples analyzed by BAP, 18 (100%) were detected by SA and 16 (89%) were determined by BAP. (Table 1)

Seven of the ten fecal samples that yielded *C. difficile* by SA only had no demonstrable cytotoxin present, and one of these yielded only noncytotoxigenic *C. difficile* strains. In addition, one of these seven samples came from a patient from whom previous samples were positive for

TABLE 1. *Comparison of methods for recovery of C. difficile from stools*

Method	No. tested	Total no. of *C. difficile*-positive stools[a]	No. of stools yielding *C. difficile* (%)
SA	266	82	77 (94)[b]
AP (anaerobic)	266	82	72 (88)
BAP	55	18	16 (89)

[a] Number of stools shown to harbor *C. difficile* by a combination of all the methods described.

[b] Expressed as a percentage of total *C. difficile*-positive stools.

TABLE 2. *Comparison of AP and cycloserine-cefoxitin selective agar for recovery of C. difficile from 266 stool specimens*

Culture	Response on selective agar	
	Positive	Negative
Alcohol shock positive		
AP	67	5
BAP	16	0
Alcohol shock negative		
AP	10	184
BAP	2	37

stool cytotoxin and for *C. difficile* by both SA and AP. Of the remaining three samples from this set, two were stool cytotoxin positive and one had a cytotoxin that was not neutralized by the cross-reacting *C. sordellii* antitoxin. One of these cytotoxin-positive stools came from a patient from whom previous samples yielded *C. difficile* by both SA and AP.

In two cases, the numbers of *C. difficile* present as determined by SA (100 organisms per g of stool) were below the limit of detection for AP, which is 200 organisms/g, due to the additional 1:2 dilution that this procedure requires. Two of the five specimens that were positive for *C. difficile* by AP only were negative for stool cytotoxin. However, the other three cases were stool cytotoxin positive. Forty-four specimens were analyzed for quantitative recovery of *C. difficile*. Higher counts were obtained by SA than by AP in 31 cases (70%).

The data presented here indicate that the use of alcohol as a selective procedure is an efficient, easily performed method for the detection and isolation of *C. difficile* from stools. In addition, the results show that this method can be successfully performed on the bench with the minimum of anaerobic facilities. An added advantage is that colonies of *C. difficile* isolated by the AP method exhibit a normal cellular morphology, which is not the case for the SA procedure. This cellular morphology can be characteristic and act as an aid in the presumptive identification of *C. difficile*. The AP will also concomitantly isolate other clostridia. Therefore, this sort of screening procedure should increase the likelihood of noting associations between carriage of *C. difficile* and other clostridial species that may enhance its pathogenic effect. Involvement of other clostridia in non-*C. difficile*-associated gastrointestinal tract disease (3) may become apparent by the use of this procedure.

1. **Borriello, S. P., and H. E. Larson.** 1981. Antibiotic and pseudomembranous colitis. J. Antimicrob. Chemother. **7**(Suppl. B):53–62.
2. **George, W. L., V. L. Sutter, D. Citron, and S. M. Finegold.** 1979. Selective and differential medium for isolation of *Clostridium difficile*. J. Clin. Microbiol. **9:** 214–219.
3. **Schwartz, J. N., J. P. Hamilton, R. Fekety, E. G. Green, L. Stamper, D. H. Batts, and J. Silva.** 1980. Ampicillin-induced enterocolitis: implication of toxigenic clostridium perfringens type C. J. Pediatr. **97:** 661–663.

Chlamydial Urethritis in Men: Epidemiology, Diagnosis, and Treatment

WALTER E. STAMM,* LAURA KOUTSKY, BARBARA COLE, ROBERT C. BRUNHAM, AND KING K. HOLMES

Departments of Medicine and Epidemiology, University of Washington, Seattle, Washington 98112, U.S.A.*

Chlamydia trachomatis has been incriminated as a cause of approximately 40% of the cases of nongonococcal urethritis (NGU) in the United States and appears to be an etiological agent in both epididymitis and Reiter's syndrome. However, the epidemiology of *C. trachomatis* urethral infections in unselected men has been less well described, specifically, prevalence, proportion of infections that are asymptomatic, risk factors for infection, and clinical features of these infections. To assess these and other factors, we asked clinicians in our sexually transmitted disease clinic to obtain urethral *C. trachomatis* cultures from all men attending the clinic for a new complaint between 1 February and 1 July 1980. During this period, as well as for 8 additional months, men who presented with NGU were involved in a treatment study in which rosaramicin (250 mg four times a day for 7 days) was compared with tetracycline (500 mg four times a day for 7 days).

Urethral cultures for *Neisserea gonorrhoeae* and *C. trachomatis* were obtained from 1,193 of 1,771 men (or 67%) attending the clinic during this period. Between 1 April and 1 July 1980, the last three months of the study, clinicians were also asked to obtain sera from all men that had cultures taken. Sera were obtained from 654 men and were assayed for antibody to *C. trachomatis* in the microimmunofluorescence assay. After the screening was completed, clinic records of all 654 men who had sera drawn, as well as all *C. trachomatis* and gonococcal infection (GC) cases from the preserology period, were reviewed to obtain demographic and clinical information about men with *C. trachomatis* or GC infection alone, both infections, or neither infection.

Prevalence of both infecting organisms was strongly linked to sexual preference ($P < 0.001$). Of the heterosexual men, 14% had *C. trachomatis* urethritis versus 6% of the homosexual men. In contrast, 25% of the homosexual men had GC versus only 12% of the heterosexual men.

Age was strongly related to the prevalence of urethral chlamydia infection in both heterosexual and homosexual men. Prevalence progressively decreased in both groups during each 5-year period between the ages of 15 and 40.

Discharge and dysuria were seen significantly less frequently in heterosexual and homosexual men with *C. trachomatis* infection than in men with GC. In heterosexual men, 63% with *C. trachomatis* infection had discharge, 62% had dysuria, and 71% had either, versus 93, 78, and 96% for GC. Among homosexual men, 55% with *C. trachomatis* infection had either symptom, versus 99% of the men with GC.

The amount of urethral discharge upon examination was significantly greater in men with GC as compared with men having *C. trachomatis* infection. Only 10% of the heterosexual men with GC had no discharge, but 32% of the men with *C. trachomatis* infection lacked an expressible discharge. Of the men with GC, 77% had moderate or severe discharge, versus 25% of the men with *C. trachomatis* infection. Men with both infections closely resembled men with GC in terms of discharge, and homosexual men closely resembled heterosexual men.

The character of the urethral discharge, like the amount, differed in *C. trachomatis*- and *N. gonorrhoeae*-infected men. Only 5% of the heterosexual men with *C. trachomatis* infection had a purulent discharge, versus 71% of the men with GC and 48% of the men with both GC and *C. trachomatis* infection. Most men with *C. trachomatis* infection (53%) had a clear discharge, versus only 6% of the men with GC and 16% of the men with both.

The number of polymorphonuclear leukocytes per oil immersion field (PMN/OIF) on a Gram stain of urethral secretions has been used in many sexually transmitted disease clinics to define urethritis. In this group of patients, 73% of the heterosexual men and 79% of the homosexual men had ≤5 PMNs/OIF. Only 6% of men with GC and none of men with GC and *C. trachomatis* infection fell in this range, but 33% of the heterosexual and 20% of the homosexual men with *C. trachomatis* infection had ≤5 PMN per high-power field (HPF). The majority of men with *C. trachomatis* infection had 6 to 20 PMN/HPF (54% of the heterosexuals and 73% of the homosexuals), and most men with GC fell into the >20 PMN/OIF category (48% of the heterosexuals and 67% of the homosexuals).

The proportions of patients infected with *N. gonorrhoeae* or *C. trachomatis* who were given an effective therapeutic regimen on their initial clinic visit before the results of cultures were known differed. With *N. gonorrhoeae*-infected patients, 96% were given a regimen that would have been effective. With *C. trachomatis*-infected patients, in contrast, only 61% overall were given effective therapy, 73% of those with *C. trachomatis* infection alone and 15% of those with both *C. trachomatis* infection and GC (most of these patients received intramuscular penicillin or single-dose ampicillin). If NGU was diagnosed, all received effective therapy.

In all, 182 men with NGU (demonstrable urethral discharge, ≥5 PMN/OIF; negative cultures for GC) were randomized to receive rosaramicin (250 mg four times a day for 7 days) or tetracycline (500 mg four times a day for 7 days). All patients completed follow-up visits 2 to 3 and 14 to 16 days posttherapy and had cultures for *N. gonorrhoeae*, *C. trachomatis*, and *Ureaplasma urealyticum* at each visit. The study was double-blinded. The rosaramicin- and tetracycline-treated groups did not differ in age, marital status, sexual preference, race, history of previous NGU, or proportion defaulting.

Of 87 men given rosaramicin, 76 (87%) achieved satisfactory clinical responses, as did 81 (85%) of 95 given tetracycline (Table 1). No significant differences in clinical cure rates were seen in *C. trachomatis*-positive and *C. trachomatis*-negative patients. Three patients given rosaramicin and two given tetracycline had recurrent chlamydial urethritis on their third fol-

TABLE 1. *Comparison of rosaramicin and tetracycline for treatment of NGU*

Drug	Treated	Cure			Gastrointestinal side effects[b]
		Clinical	Bacteriological		
			C. trachomatis	*U. urealyticum*[a]	
Rosaramicin	87	76/87	18/21	29/36	43/87
Tetracycline	95	81/95	34/36	19/31	25/95

[a] $P = 0.07$.
[b] $P < 0.05$.

low-up visit. Persistence or recurrence of *U. urealyticum* occurred more often after tetracycline than after rosaramicin treatment (Table 1). Mild gastrointestinal side effects were seen in both groups but were significantly more frequent in those given rosaramicin.

We conclude that in heterosexual men, the prevalence of *C. trachomatis* urethral infection exceeds the prevalence of GC, whereas in homosexual men the reverse is true. Further, *C. trachomatis* was asymptomatic in one-third of patients, and when symptoms did occur, they were milder than those of gonococcal urethritis. Many patients with *C. trachomatis* urethritis did not have abnormal numbers of PMN/OIF in their urethral smears and would not have been recognized by this criterion alone. Since about 30% of men with *C. trachomatis* urethral infection were recognized as infected only by screening cultures and since only 61% of *C. trachomatis*-infected men were appropriately treated on their initial clinic visit (compared with 96% of the *N. gonorrhoeae*-infected men), a strong need for the availability of *C. trachomatis* cultures in sexually transmitted disease clinics and for other high-risk populations is evident.

Our treatment trial indicated that rosaramicin in the dose and duration given was as effective as tetracycline for the treatment of *C. trachomatis*-positive and -negative NGU. The drug, however, was a cause of frequent, mild gastrointestinal side effects.

High-Performance Liquid Chromatography Analysis of Some Brands of Gentamicin Used Clinically

L. O. WHITE* AND D. S. REEVES

Department of Microbiology, Southmead Hospital, Bristol BS10 5NB, England

The aminoglycoside antibiotic gentamicin is commonly used for antibacterial chemotherapy because of its wide spectrum of activity and its clinical efficacy. Nevertheless, in common with other similar aminoglycosides, gentamicin has a narrow therapeutic range, and serum concentrations should be monitored (3, 4) to avoid toxic levels and to ensure adequate dosage.

Gentamicin as used clinically is a mixture (the gentamicin C complex) of at least three components (gentamicins C1, C1a, and C2) which differ only in the degree of methylation at the 6′ carbon of the amino-hexose which is linked to the 2-deoxystreptamine moiety at the C-4 position.

The various methods used to assay gentamicin in serum may differ in their sensitivity to the different gentamicin C components (4); this is particularly important in the case of the acetyltransferase assay with the enzyme AAC(6′) (1) since AAC(6′) does not acetylate gentamicin C1. There are now numerous brands of gentamicin commercially available, and variations in component ratio are known to occur (5). Because the component ratio of the gentamicin used in a particular hospital might affect the accuracy of clinical gentamicin assays, and because of recent evidence that gentamicin C1 is less toxic than the complex, we have investigated the composition of a number of different brands of gentamicin by a recently described high-pressure liquid chromatographic method (2) which resolves components C1, C1a, C2, and also component C2a, an epimer of C2 which may also be significant.

Samples of gentamicin for clinical usage were collected worldwide and stored at 4°C. They were analyzed in batches as described by Freeman et al. (2) on a Hypersil 5-ODS column except that Waters HPLC equipment was used and the flow rate of the mobile phase was 2 ml/

min. Quantitation was by reference to a standard gentamicin powder of known component ratio, and nonylamine was used as an internal standard. Figure 1 shows typical chromatograms; retention times (minutes) were 2.0 (C1), 6.5 (C1a), 8.75 (C2a), and 10 (C2). Assay precision was good; replicating a single sample six times gave coefficients of variation (percent) of 0.79 (C1), 0.44 (C1a), 1.03 (C2a), and 0.88 (C2). Thirty-four batches of several brands of gentamicin were assayed, and representative results are shown in Table 1. Taking account of all the samples assayed, the mean C1 content was (percent) 34.6 (SD, 4.09), the highest, 45.2, and the lowest, 24.5; mean C1a content was 20.9 (SD, 5.10), the highest, 31.2, and the lowest, 9.0; mean C2 content was 33.4 (SD, 4.31), the highest, 44.8, and the lowest, 26.9; and mean C2a content was 11.03 (SD, 3.39), the highest, 18.1, and the lowest, 6.7. Thus, whereas the major component of most samples was gentamicin C1, over 30% had C2 as the major component, and in one case (Diakarmon batch 81161), the major component was C1a. Gentamicin C1a was the minor component of three samples (Cortolexan 3686, Gentacidon 28G9, Cusi Biogen N2/7), and C2a was the minor component of all of the others, the proportion of C2a ranging from 6 to 18%. In seven samples, the proportion of C2a was similar to that of C1a.

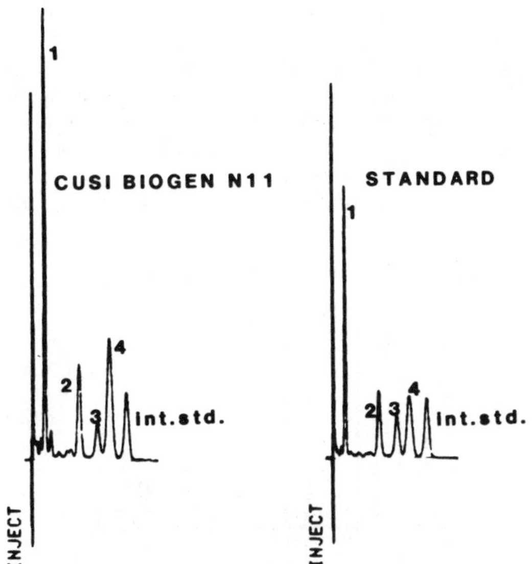

FIG. 1. *Sample chromatograms showing the four gentamicin components. Peak 1 = C1; peak 2 = C1a; peak 3 = C2a; peak 4 = C2. int. std. = Nonylamine internal standard.*

TABLE 1. *Gentamicin component ratios as measured by high-performance liquid chromatography*

Gentamicin brand/batch	% of component			
	C1	C1a	C2a	C2
Gentaroger/N9	34.3	23.1	11.7	30.9
Gentaroger/N11	34.6	28.1	7.5	29.8
Gentamicina/0400279	32.0	16.1	10.2	41.8
Cortolexan/3686	34.7	16.0	16.1	33.3
Garbilocin/30096	37.6	25.7	7.3	29.4
Gentagen/800203	34.0	18.7	16.5	30.8
Diakarmon/2	34.8	20.7	12.5	31.9
Diakarmon/81161	24.9	31.2	16.3	27.6
Garamycin/CA8	33.0	27.2	9.4	30.4
Garamycin/CA9	45.2	21.1	6.7	26.9
Gentacidon/28G9	36.2	9.0	10.0	44.8
Jintamicin/206	29.4	24.3	11.0	35.3
Cusi Biogen/N11	39.7	16.9	7.8	35.6
Cusi Biogen/N5	37.0	11.2	9.8	42.0
Cusi Biogen/N2/7	34.7	14.2	17.1	34.0
Gentapromes/79/2	32.4	25.8	8.2	33.6
Tefoval/792-175	24.4	25.1	18.1	32.4
Garamycin/9AMK48	36.6	23.5	9.4	30.5
Genticin/9124214	35.2	24.0	9.7	31.1

We concluded that there are wide variations in component ratios between different brands of gentamicin and that many batches of gentamicin contain significant amounts of C2a, a newly recognized component about which relatively little is known. The significance of these findings is twofold. When clinical assays are being performed, inaccuracy may result if the gentamicin used to prepare calibrator solutions differs markedly in composition from that used in the patient. The effect would be greatest if the assay methodology were acetyltransferase [AAC(6′)] or high-performance liquid chromatography. Second, if toxicity of the different components varies, then the incidence of toxic side effects may vary with the brand and batch of gentamicin used.

There seems to be a case for manufacturers stating the composition of batches of gentamicin on the package insert. Trials comparing the toxicity of gentamicin with other aminoglycosides should state the component composition of the gentamicin used.

1. **Broughall, J. M., and D. S. Reeves.** 1975. The acetyl transferase method for the assay of serum gentamicin concentrations and a comparison with other methods. J. Clin. Path. **28**:140–145.
2. **Freeman, M., P. A. Hawkey, J. S. Loran, and J. A. Stead.** 1979. The analysis of gentamicin sulphate in pharmaceutical specialties by high performance liquid chromatography. J. Liq. Chrom. **2**:1305–1317.
3. **Reeves, D. S., and L. O. White.** 1981. Antibiotics; clinical aspects, p. 445–456. *In* A. Richens and V. Marks (ed.), Therapeutic drug monitoring. Livingstone, Edinburgh.
4. **White, L. O., and D. S. Reeves.** 1981. Antibiotics; analytic techniques, p. 457–470. *In* A. Richens and V. Marks (ed.), Therapeutic drug monitoring. Livingstone, Edinburgh.
5. **Wilson, W. L., G. Richard, and D. W. Hughes.** 1973. Chemical determination of component ratio and potency of gentamicin complex. J. Pharm. Sci. **62**:282–284.

Microbiological and Therapeutic Evaluation of Twelve Antibiotics in Three Groups of Patients with Urinary Tract Infections

HEDVIG GRABER AND MAGDOLNA ÁRR

Department of Medicine and Clinical Pharmacology, Municipal Hospital Péterfy, H-1441 Budapest, Hungary

The choice of the most effective and safe treatment of urinary tract infection (UTI) is a worldwide problem in clinical practice (1). In a 2-year survey (1979–1980) we have assessed the in vitro susceptibilities of 2,076 UTI pathogens to 12 antibiotics and evaluated the therapeutic results.

Bacteria were isolated from inpatients with acute (or acute exacerbation of) UTI (1,281 isolates), outpatients with chronic UTI (602 isolates), and bacteriuric, mostly asymptomatic pregnant women (193 isolates).

In vitro susceptibilities, determined by the disk method, are presented in Fig. 1. Among the penicillins, mezlocillin inhibited the greatest number of *Escherichia coli*, indole-positive *Proteus*, and *Klebsiella-Enterobacter* strains. The resistance rate of *Pseudomonas* to carbenicillin

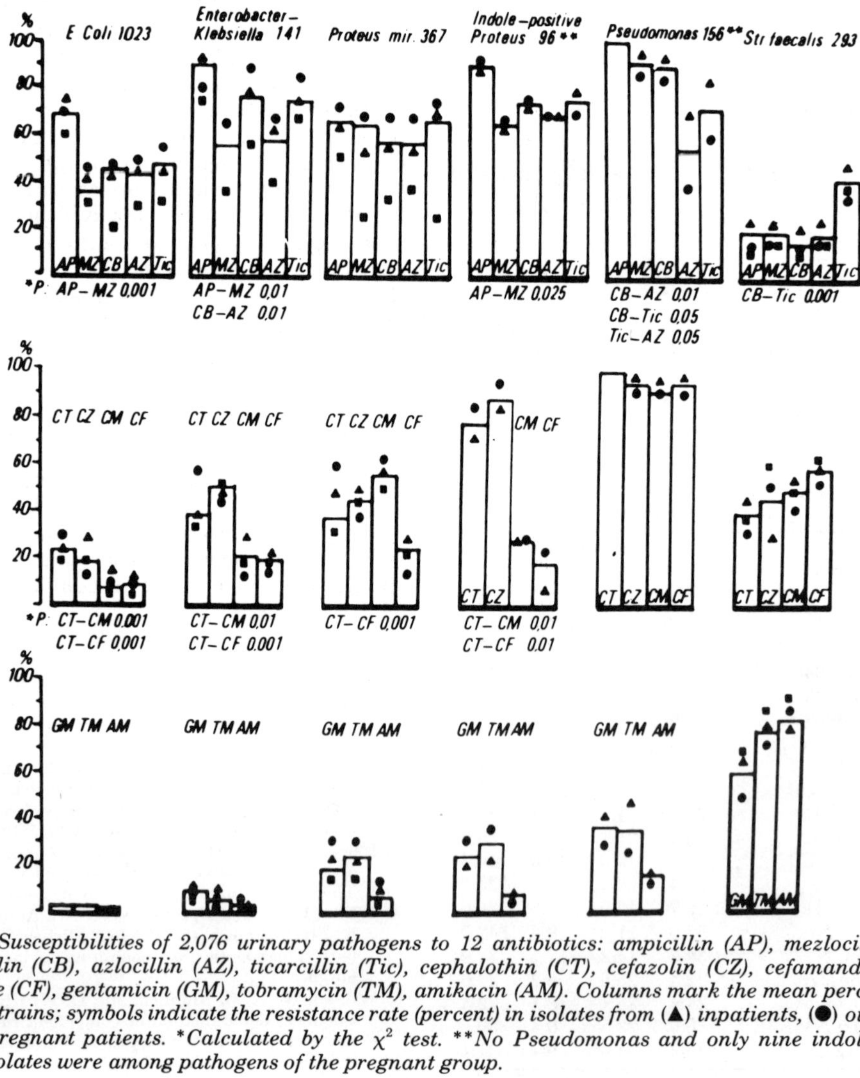

FIG. 1. *Susceptibilities of 2,076 urinary pathogens to 12 antibiotics: ampicillin (AP), mezlocillin (MZ), carbenicillin (CB), azlocillin (AZ), ticarcillin (Tic), cephalothin (CT), cefazolin (CZ), cefamandole (CM), cefuroxime (CF), gentamicin (GM), tobramycin (TM), amikacin (AM). Columns mark the mean percentage of resistant strains; symbols indicate the resistance rate (percent) in isolates from (▲) inpatients, (●) outpatients and (■) pregnant patients. *Calculated by the χ^2 test. **No Pseudomonas and only nine indole-positive Proteus isolates were among pathogens of the pregnant group.*

TABLE 1. *Results of 360 treatments of UTI patients*

Treatment	Daily dose (g)	No. of patients				Cure rate (%)
		Treated		Cured		
Penicillins						
Ampicillin	2–6	29	64	14	36	56.3
Carbenicillin	2–15	35		22		
Mezlocillin	6	21	40	16	31	77.5
Azlocillin	6	13		10		
Ticarcillin	6	6		5		
All penicillins		104		67		64.4
Cephalosporins						
Cephalothin	2–6	69		44		63.7
Cefazolin	2–3	20	50	16	42	84.0
Cefamandole	3–6	12		9		
Cefuroxime	1.5–4.5	18		17		
All cephalosporins		119		86		72.2
Aminoglycosides	(mg/kg)					
Gentamicin	3	87		72		
Tobramycin	3	31		27		
Amikacin	15	19		27		
All aminoglycosides		137		116		86.1
Total		360		269		74.1

was surprisingly high; ticarcillin inhibited about one-quarter and azlocillin one-half of the isolates. Remarkably enough, resistance to penicillins was lower in isolates from the pregnant group than in strains from either hospitalized or chronic patients.

Among cephalosporins, the lactamase-resistant compounds cefamandole and cefuroxime inhibited considerably more strains than cephalothin and cefazolin. The spectrum of cefuroxime approached that of gentamicin; in some cases it was even broader. As expected, none of the cephalosporins studied was active against *Pseudomonas.* According to the literature (2), cephalosporins show minimal activity against *Streptococcus faecalis*; however, 40 to 60% of our strains were inhibited by them.

Aminoglycosides had the broadest spectrum against gram-negative *Enterobacteriaceae* isolates; amikacin inhibited 5 to 10% more isolates than gentamicin or tobramycin. *Streptococcus faecalis* strains were mostly resistant to aminoglycosides.

Our microbiological data indicate a higher resistance rate than that generally described (2, 4).

Therapy was adjusted to in vitro susceptibility. We have evaluated 360 courses, using disappearance of symptoms and eradication of the pathogens as criteria for cure (Table 1). Treatment lasted 8 to 14 days.

Cure rate has been 64% in patients treated with penicillins, 72% with cephalosporins, and 86% after aminoglycoside therapy. The newer β-lactam antibiotics definitely had a better therapeutic effect than their well-known congeners. Whereas the percentage of cured patients has been merely 56 to 60% with ampicillin, carbenicillin, or cephalothin treatment, the cure rate amounted to 77 and 84% with the newer penicillins and cephalosporins, respectively, approaching the efficacy of aminoglycosides. New β-lactam compounds, being potent and atoxic antibiotics, were extremely useful in the treatment of pregnant patients with pyelonephritis and chronic UTI patients with impaired renal function. The good results obtained are ascribed to increased antimicrobial activity (2) and favorable pharmacokinetic properties (3, 4) of the new compounds.

In conclusion it may be stated that new β-lactam compounds represent a significant progress in the therapy of UTI; they are of special value when a powerful antibacterial agent is needed and aminoglycosides are for some reason contraindicated.

1. **Fairley, K. F., and J. A. Whitworth.** 1980. Problems in the treatment of urinary tract infections. Drugs **19:**190–194.
2. **Fass, R.** 1980. In vitro activities of beta-lactam and aminoglycoside antibiotics. Arch. Intern. Med. **140:**763–768.
3. **Graber, H., M. Árr, A. Csiba, E. Ludwig, and T. Magyar.** 1981. Azlocillin and mezlocillin: evaluation of new ureido-penicillins. Int. J. Clin. Pharmacol. Ther. Toxicol. **19**, in press.
4. **O'Callaghan, C. H.** 1979. Description and classification of the newer cephalosporins and their relationships with the established compounds. J. Antimicrob. Chemother. **5:**635–671.

Double-Blind Clinical Trial of Trimethoprim Versus Amoxicillin in Acute Symptomatic Urinary Infection

ROBERT C. SPENCER,*[1] DONALD J. FAIRCLOUGH, AND JOHN COOPER

Department of Microbiology, Barnsley District General Hospital, Barnsley, General Practice, Barnsley, and Wellcome Foundation Limited, Crewe, United Kingdom

Trimethoprim is an antibacterial agent which is active against a wide variety of bacterial species, particularly those commonly considered to cause urinary tract infections. It has been used extensively since 1968 in a fixed (1:5) combination with sulfamethoxazole (as co-trimoxazole). However, synergy in vitro is rare in the urinary tract because of the dominance of trimethoprim (4). Alone, trimethoprim has been studied relatively little in the treatment of acute urinary infections despite its having been available in Finland for 5 to 6 years, where it is used chiefly in low-dose, long-term treatment of chronic urinary infections (6).

This study was undertaken to investigate the efficacy and tolerability of trimethoprim as a single 300-mg dose in acute urinary infections and compare the results with those obtained with amoxicillin, the use of which in urinary infections is well documented (1). It was considered that such a dosage schedule for trimethoprim would appeal to both the physician and patients, who frequently discontinue their treatment once symptoms resolve. The dosage was high enough to ensure sufficient concentrations of trimethoprim in the urine for a period of 36 to 48 h even if the patient forgot to take one dose.

Patients included in this study were those who presented with signs and symptoms which the general practioner considered to be due to an acute urinary infection and who proved subsequently to have significant bacteriuria. Patients were exluded if they were known to be pregnant, were under 16 years of age, had impaired renal function, had known abnormalities of the urinary tract, or were allergic to either drug. On entry personal details were recorded, and patients were given a diary card on which to record their symptoms, adverse drug reactions, etc. (Table 1). Each patient was then randomly allocated to one of two treatment groups. In group A patients were treated with one 300-mg tablet of trimethoprim to be taken at night; those in group B were given 250 mg of amoxicillin three times a day. Both treatments lasted 7 days. Patients were asked to return in 4 days should their symptoms persist; otherwise they were to return on day 14 for a symptomatic assessment and clinical examination.

A urine specimen for laboratory investigation was collected before treatment began and on day 14. The urine specimens were examined as soon as possible in the laboratory, and a semiquantitative count was performed by use of dip slides (Oxoid Ltd.). Isolates were identified by the API biochemical tests, and susceptibility to trimethoprim and amoxicillin was determined by a disk method. Isolates were saved on agar slopes, and strains of *Escherichia coli* found at the second visit were retyped by the method of Davies (3).

Seventy-five patients were included in this study, 37 in group A and 38 in group B (Table 1). There were no statistical differences between the two groups. Generally speaking, there was an even distribution of infecting organisms between the two groups, though there were almost twice as many staphylococcal infections in group B (Table 2). A microbiological cure was taken to be the eradication of the original infecting organism by species or type at follow-up. The microbiological cure rate in group A was 35 of 37 (95%), with two (5%) failures, one relapse (same infecting organism), and one reinfection (new organism). In group B, 34 of 38 (89%)

TABLE 1. *Demographic data of patients in the two treatment groups*

	Group A—Trimethoprim	Group B—Amoxicillin
No. of patients	37	38
Female	35	36
Male	2	2
Age (range) in years	53 (16–82)	42 (17–84)
Past history of urinary infection	17 (46%)	16 (42%)
Presenting symptoms		
Frequency	34 (92%)	36 (95%)
Dysuria	31 (84%)	32 (84%)
Vaginal/vulval symptoms	14 (38%)	10 (26%)
Fever	4 (11%)	10 (26%)
Loin pain	3 (8%)	2 (5%)
Abdominal pain	3 (8%)	4 (11%)
Hematuria	2 (5%)	3 (8%)

[1] Present address: Department of Medical Microbiology, University of Sheffield Medical School, Sheffield S10 2RX, United Kingdom.

TABLE 2. *Distribution of infecting bacteria isolated from patients in the two treatment groups*

Pathogen isolated from urine	Group A—Trimethoprim ($n = 37$)	Group B—Amoxicillin ($n = 38$)	Total ($n = 75$)
Escherichia coli	26 (70% of infections)	22 (58% of infections)	48
Staphylococcus spp. (including *Micrococcus*)	6	11	17
Proteus mirabilis	5	2	7
Streptococcus group D	—	2	2
Klebsiella aerogenes	—	1	1

achieved microbiological cure, with two relapses and two reinfections. However, treatment cure rates with complete resolution of symptoms were 36 of 37 (97%) in group A and 36 of 38 (95%) in group B. There were no statistical differences between the two treatment groups for either microbiological or treatment cure rates.

All adverse drug reactions were recorded, and fewer were found in group A (4 of 37) than in group B (8 of 38). Diarrhea, anorexia, nausea, sore mouth, and headache were the most common complaints. Patient compliance was equally good for both treatment groups.

Acute symptomatic urinary infection is a complaint mostly found in women and is a cause of considerable stress to the patient. In general practice antibiotic treatment is usually started immediately, before the results of the urine culture are known. Therefore, any treatment must possess a high likelihood of being successful against all probable pathogenic bacteria. Also, the treatment regimen must be simple for the patient to use and the drug must have as few side effects as possible. These three factors should ensure as high a patient compliance as possible. In this study comparing trimethoprim with an antibiotic (amoxicillin) whose use in treating urinary tract infections has been well documented, both groups achieved effective cure rates in excess of 90%, and the incidence of side effects with trimethoprim was half that of the amoxicillin group.

Arguments for the use of trimethoprim alone have centered around the lower incidence of associated side effects and the arguments against concern themselves with the possible emergence of resistance. The toxicity of co-trimoxazole is largely attributed to the sulfonamide component. Skin rashes occur in about 5% of cases and gastrointestinal problems in about 10%. Such problems are significantly less common with trimethoprim alone (7). The possibility of the emergence of resistance is the major argument against the widespread use of trimethoprim alone, the mechanism of which is not yet fully understood (2). Trimethoprim resistance is uncommon in general practice amongst urinary pathogens, occurring in 2 to 4% of coliform bacilli (8). Our own figures agree with this. Nevertheless, recent authors have indicated that among some hospital populations it may be higher (around 10%) and on the increase (5). It should be noted that this sort of trend occurred *prior* to the availability of trimethoprim alone. There is presently no firm evidence that the use of trimethoprim alone will have a greater effect on the prevalence of trimethoprim resistance than the use of sulfonamide combinations, and there is no precedent for the routine use of antibiotic combinations to suppress the emergence of resistance in urinary tract infections. The use of trimethoprim alone has been supported (2, 5, 7), but with the qualification that its use in hospitals should be limited and monitored until the questions regarding the risk of development of resistance have received closer study.

We conclude that in general practice the use of trimethoprim alone can be recommended. For acute symptomatic urinary infections the use of a single dose of 300 mg of trimethoprim for 7 days has been very effective, with cure rates in excess of 90%, few side effects, and good patient compliance.

1. **Bailey, R. R., and G. D. Abbott.** 1977. Treatment of urinary tract infection with a single dose of Amoxycillin. Nephron **18:**316–320.
2. **Brumfitt, W., and J. M. T. Hamilton-Miller.** 1980. Trimethoprim. Br. J. Hosp. Med. **24:**281–288.
3. **Davies, B. I.** 1977. Biochemical typing of urinary *E. coli* strains by means of the API 20E enterobacteriaciae system. J. Med. Microbiol. **10:**293–298.
4. **Greenwood, O., and F. O'Grady.** 1976. Activity and interaction of trimethoprim and sulphamethoxazole against *E. coli*. J. Clin. Pathol. **29:**162–166.
5. **Hamilton-Miller, J. M. T., A. Gooding, and W. Brumfitt.** 1981. Resistance to trimethoprim in 1978–79 compared with 1973–75. J. Clin. Pathol. **34:**439–442.
6. **Kasanen, A., M. Anttila, R. Elfuing, P. Kahela, H. Saarimaa, H. Sundquist, R. Tikkanen, and P. Toivanen.** 1978. Trimethoprim: pharmacology, antimicrobial activity and clinical use in urinary tract infections. Ann. Clin. Res. **10** (Supp. 22):5–39.
7. **Lacey, R. W., L. V. Lord, H. K. W. Gunasekera, P. J. Leiberman, and D. E. A. Luxton.** 1980. Comparison of trimethoprim alone with trimethoprim-sulphamethoxazole in the treatment of respiratory and urinary infections with particular reference to selection of trimethoprim resistance. Lancet **i:**1270–1273.
8. **Towner, K. J., N. J. Pearson, P. A. Pinn, and F. O'Grady.** 1980. Increasing importance of plasmid-mediated trimethoprim resistance in enterobacteria: two six-month clinical surveys. Br. Med. J. **i:**517–519.

Co-trimazine Once Daily Versus Co-trimoxazole Twice Daily in Urinary Tract Infection in Children

C. HAGER, P. BAMBERG,* G. DORN, AND D. ADAM*

*University Childrens' Hospital, Munich, Federal Republic of Germany, and Astra Läkemedel AB, Södertälje, Sweden**

Co-trimazine, the combination of sulfadiazine and trimethoprim (TMP), has earlier been used twice daily with good results in the treatment of urinary tract infections (UTI) at half of the established dosage of co-trimoxazole (sulfamethoxazole-TMP). In a double-blind randomized trial a once-daily dose of co-trimazine was compared with the usual twice-daily dose of co-trimoxazole in 49 nonhospitalized children (2 to 12 years) suffering from UTI, i.e., presenting with symptomatic bacteriuria ($>10^5$ bacteria per ml of urine), caused by a sulfadiazine TMP- or sulfamethoxazole TMP-susceptible organism. The patients were controlled once during treatment and then 1 and 2 to 3 weeks after end of treatment. Urine samples were collected either from suprapubic bladder puncture or as clean-catch midstream samples, and the bacteria were identified. MCU and IVP were obtained from all cases with a medial history of anomalies of the urinary tract as well as in the cases in which the therapy failed. The daily dosage of co-trimazine was 5 ml once daily in patients aged 2 to 5 years and 10 ml once daily in those aged 6 to 12 years; dosage of co-trimoxazole was 5 and 10 ml twice daily in the two age groups.

The drugs were given for 10 days as oral suspensions of co-trimazine (TMP, 9 mg/ml; sulfadiazine, 41 mg/ml) or co-trimaxazole (TMP, 8 mg/ml; sulfamethoxazole, 40 mg/ml). After informed consent, patients on co-trimazine received an active dose in the evening and a placebo in the morning. Patients on co-trimoxazole received active drug twice daily.

The mean age for the co-trimazine and co-trimoxazole groups was 6.6 and 6.1 years, respectively. Complicating factors such as obstructions, reflux, or renal anomalies were present in seven patients, five in the co-trimazine and two in the co-trimoxazole group.

Cure, defined as elimination of bacteriuria and symptoms at the last control, was achieved in 20 of 24 of the co-trimazine and in 19 of 25 of the co-trimoxazole patients. Two of the failures in each treatment group could be related to underlying anomalies of the urinary tract. Cure of complicated UTI was achieved in 3 of 5 patients treated with co-trimazine. In the co-trimoxazole group both patients with complicated UTI failed. Sulfonamide-TMP-resistant bacteria were isolated in one of the therapeutic failures in each treatment group. We did not observe any side effects.

The once daily administration of co-trimazine should facilitate the treatment of children, and our results suggest that this regimen, including a comparatively low dose, is an adequate therapy for UTI in childhood.

Co-trimazine Versus Co-trimoxazole as Therapy for Acute Symptomatic Urinary Infection

S. T. CHAPMAN,* D. S. REEVES, R. W. MORRIS, M. R. WATTS, AND R. E. T. REEVES

General Practice, Thornbury, and Department of Medical Microbiology, Southmead Hospital, Bristol, United Kingdom*

Co-trimoxazole has been successfully used extensively for treating urinary infection for 12 years. The sulfonamide component sulfamethoxazole is, however, highly metabolized, only a small amount of the ingested dose appearing as active drug in the urine (3). Co-trimazine (sulfadiazine plus trimethoprim) has a potential advantage in urinary infection because sulfadiazine is much less metabolized than sulfamethoxazole (2), and therefore, dose for dose, the urinary concentration of active sulfonamide will be higher. Thus, a lower dose of co-trimazine than that of co-trimoxazole can be recommended, with potentially fewer side effects.

Patients of both sexes aged 16 years or older presenting to a general practice office with symptoms of acute urinary infection (dysuria/frequency, with or without nocturia, hematuria, or suprapubic pain) were admitted to the study. Clinical details were recorded, a urine specimen was taken, and treatment commenced, allocated by random administration, physician blind, of either co-trimazine (Coptin; Pfizer Inc.), one tablet (90 mg of trimethoprim plus 410 mg of sulfadiazine), or co-trimoxazole (Septrin; Wellcome Research Laboratories), two tablets (160 mg of trimethoprim plus 800 mg of sulfamethoxazole), both given every 12 h for 7 days. Treatment was continued in all patients, whether bacteriuric or not. Clinical follow-up and a urine culture were done 2 weeks after treatment was started. A further urine culture by dip slide was taken at 6 weeks in patients initially infected. Standard semiquantitative urine cultures were made, pathogens being identified by normal laboratory methods and typed when necessary to distinguish reinfection from relapse. Susceptibilities to trimethoprim and sulfonamide were determined by a disk method. Urines were also examined microscopically for pyuria. At follow-up patients were also questioned about drug compliance and possible side effects. They were initially asked a general question about the treatment (volunteered side effects) and in the event of a negative response, about specific side effects of sulfonamide/trimethoprim treatment (questioned-for side effects). Overall, a high rate of follow-up was achieved by having a nurse specifically for pursuing defaulters.

TABLE 1. *Patients entered into trial and infecting organisms*

Item	Co-trimazine	Co-trimoxazole
Patients entered	49	51
Patients assessable	47	50
Female-male ratio	46:2	49:1
Mean (SD) age, years	41.6 (17)	41.5 (12)
Patients not infected	32	26
Patients infected	16 (34%)	23 (46%)
Infecting organisms:		
Escherichia coli (no. sulfonamide resistant)	13 (1)	19 (5)
Enterobacter spp.	0	1
Proteus mirabilis	2	0
Streptococcus faecalis	1	0
Micrococcus spp.	0	3

The results (Table 1) show that 100 patients were entered who were, as might be expected, almost exclusively females of predominantly child-bearing age. Overall, 39% of the patients had significant bacteriuria with typical infecting organisms, mostly *Escherichia coli*. Rather more patients taking co-trimoxazole had significant bacteriuria (46%) than did patients taking co-trimazine (34%), and had sulfonamide-resistant pathogens. At 2-week follow-up, no patient had bacteriuria (Table 2). At 6 weeks, three patients had bacteriuria with organisms indistinguishable from the initial isolate (all fully susceptible *E. coli*) on typing. They were classed as failures, although at that time interval reinfection was a strong possibility. About half the patients in each group had initial pyuria, and this almost invariably disappeared. In all patients symptoms improved, but in a minority they persisted in an abated form.

Twenty-seven percent of patients on co-trimazine and 29% on co-trimoxazole complained of symptoms (one or more of anorexia, nausea, vomiting, diarrhea, rash, headache, dizziness, perineal irritation) which might have been due to the antimicrobials taken. In five patients on co-trimoxazole (none on co-trimazine), these were graded as severe enough to limit the patients' normal activities and in two of these treatment was stopped prematurely.

High rates of cure of bacteriuria have usually been reported in acute urinary infection, and our results compare favorably with other series (ampicillin, 88% [1] and 86% [6]; sulfametopyrazine, 83% [7] and 81% [6]; co-trimoxazole, 91% [1]; trimethoprim, 100% [1]). With such similar rates

TABLE 2. *Results after therapy*

Result	Co-trimazine	Co-trimoxazole
Cure rates		
At 2 weeks	16/16 (100%)	22/22 (100%)
At 6 weeks	13/14 (93%)	20/22 (91%)
Patients with pyuria		
Before therapy	22	25
After therapy	1 (+1 reinfection)	1
Patients with some urinary symptoms after therapy	11	7 (1 severe)
Patients volunteering or stating possible side effects on questioning	13 (27%)	15 (29%)
Patients with serious side effects	0	5
Patients who stopped treatment	0	2

significant differences between treatments would emerge only if enormous numbers of infections were treated. In similar patients attending the same general practice office, a sulfadiazine/nitrofurantoin combination gave a cure rate of 92% (4). It is likely that bacteriuria would have resolved spontaneously, although not so quickly, in some patients without any antimicrobial therapy.

In questioning for possible side effects, no attempt was made to distinguish symptoms which may have been due to non-drug-related causes. There were no differences in the rates of minor side effects during the two treatments, but co-trimoxazole was associated with more severe symptoms and the spontaneous premature cessation of treatment in two patients. This may be an effect of the larger dose of sulfonamide in co-trimoxazole. We have previously reported more side effects from sulfonamide in full doses than from single-dose therapy with sulfametopyrazine (3). We concluded that both co-trimazine and co-trimoxazole are highly effective treatments for acute urinary infections, but that co-trimoxazole is more likely to give more discommoding side effects. This might have been related to its larger dose.

1. **Brumfitt, W., and R. Pursell.** 1972. Double-blind trial to compare ampicillin, cephalexin, co-trimoxazole, and trimethoprim in treatment of urinary infection. Br. Med. J. **2**:673–676.
2. **Ortengren, B., H. Fellner, and T. Bergan.** 1979. Development of sulphonamide-trimethoprim combinations for urinary tract infections. Infection **7** (Suppl. 4):5367–5370.
3. **Reeves, D. S.** 1975. Laboratory and clinical studies with sulfametopyrazine as a treatment for bacteriuria in pregnancy. J. Antimicrob. Chemother. **1**:171–186.
4. **Reeves, D. S., R. W. Morris, M. R. Watts, and K. F. T. Reeves.** 1980. Double-blind clinical trial of a nitrofurantoin/sulphadiazine combination at two dosage levels in acute symptomatic urinary infections. Curr. Med. Res. Opinion **6**:481–487.
5. **Reeves, D. S., and P. J. Wilkinson.** 1979. The pharmacokinetics of trimethoprim and trimethoprim/sulphonamide combinations, including penetration into body tissue. Infection **7** (Suppl. 4):S330–341.
6. **Slade, N., and S. T. Crowther.** 1972. Multicentre survey of urinary tract infections in general practice. Br. J Urol. **44**:105–109.
7. **Windsor, B. P. G., G. A. Langsdale, J. Hill, W. L. Wooper, and H. A. Allen.** 1973. Sulfametopyrazine single dose treatment of urinary tract infections in general practice. Br. J. Clin. Pract. **27**:15–17.

Treatment of Chronic Infections of the Urinary Tract with a Combination of Rifampin and Trimethoprim

VLADIMIR PRÁT AND MILAN HATALA

Institute for Clinical and Experimental Medicine, Prague, Czechoslovakia

In 1975, Kerry et al. (3) demonstrated synergism in the in vitro antibacterial effects of rifampin (RMP) and trimethoprim (TMP) against a large number of bacteria strains. It was also found that TMP decreased the number of mutants resistant to RMP. Further in vitro studies, in which large bacterial populations were exposed to changing concentrations of RMP and TMP simulating urine concentrations of the two drugs (2), demonstrated that RMP and TMP had a reciprocal effect in preventing the resistance to each other.

In this paper we report the results of our own experience when we gave tablets containing 300 mg of RMP and 80 mg of TMP to a selected group of difficult patients with chronic and recurrent urinary tract infections (UTI) who had been previously treated with several other antimicrobials, including co-trimoxazole, β-lactam agents, and aminoglycosides.

In this open, noncomparative trial 23 patients (19 women and 4 men) with a mean age of 55.6 years were treated. The high bacterial counts in urine were most often due to *Escherichia coli* strains (16 times), with other organisms found less frequently (*Proteus mirabilis,* 4 times; *Klebsiella-Enterobacter,* twice; *Pseudomonas aeruginosa,* once). Various kinds of kidney and urinary tract pathologies were found along with the urinary infections (Table 1). Kidney function, evaluated from the plasma creatinine levels, was not markedly decreased in any patient. In 17 patients they were less than 130 μmol/liter and were above that level in only 6, with the highest value found being 151 μmol/liter. The localization tests were performed in all patients but one, for the most part by examination of the antibody-coated bacteria in the urinary sediment but in some cases by bladder lavage, as described by Fairley et al. (1). In 11 patients the infection was in the lower urinary tract, and in 11 it was in the upper urinary tract. All patients had recurrent urinary tract infections, sometimes with acute exacerbation of pye-

TABLE 1. *Clinical forms of the diseases with bacteriuria*

Form	No. of patients
Nephrolithiasis	
Occasional small concretions	4
Many large concretions	4
Recurrent UTI (lower tract)	6
Congenital abnormalities	3
Chronic pyelonephritis without obstruction	2
Prostatitis	2
Phenacetin nephropathy	1
Renal transplant	1
Total	23

TABLE 2. *Short-term results of treatment*

Patient characteristic	No. of patients/total	Percent
Site of infection		
Lower UTI	9/11	81.8
Upper UTI	5/10	50
Infection with *E. coli* strains	13/15	87
Infection with other organisms	2/7	28.6
UTI without obstruction	7/8	87.5
UTI with obstruction	8/14	57.1

lonephritis or cystitis, and all had undergone several previous treatments with antibacterial agents.

The drug was given only to those patients whose urinary pathogens were susceptible in vitro to RMP and TMP. Treatment was given for 7 days. Those patients with upper tract infections took two tablets in the evening and one in the morning; those with lower tract infections took only two capsules in the evening before going to bed.

Bacterial examination of the urine was carried out between the third and seventh days after the end of treatment and in many of the subjects again 3 to 5 weeks later. The urinary levels of RMP and TMP were determined in three patients on the first and last days of treatment. The common biochemical laboratory tests were run before and after treatment to detect possible toxic effects of the drug.

Antibacterial effects of the combination of RMP and TMP in UTI could be evaluated in only 22 of the 23 patients because 1 patient stopped treatment. Among the 22 patients, 14 had sterile urine on the third to seventh days after the end of treatment; in one case there was a reinfection during treatment. From our data short-term therapy caused good effects in 15 of 22 patients (68.2%). In the other 7 cases significant bacteriuria was still present even on the first days after the end of treatment. For 4 of these 7 the urine samples were investigated bacteriologically also during treatment; there had been only a temporary lowering in the microbial counts, and after the end of treatment the bacteriuria returned to the pretreatment level. Of the 15 patients whose urines became bacteria-free, 13 were checked again 3 to 5 weeks later. Ten of them still had sterile urine (45.4% of the initial number of patients), and 3 patients had relapse of infection.

Different aspects of the therapeutic results were analyzed (Table 2). In terms of the site of infection, bacteriuria was overcome by treatment in 9 of 11 patients with lower tract infection (81.8%); from the 10 patients with upper tract infections, positive effects were obtained in 5 (50%). When the results were analyzed according to the type of infecting organisms, treatment was found to have been successful in 13 of the 15 cases with *E. coli* in the urine (87%) and in only 2 of the 7 cases with other bacterial infections (28.6%). Finally, the results were evaluated according to the presence of urinary tract obstructions. In 8 patients without obstruction, there was therapeutic success in 7 cases (87.5%). In 14 patients with obstruction treatment succeeded in 8 (57.1%). Urinary levels of RMP and TMP were measured on the first and last days of treatment. Both drugs were present in the urine at concentrations sufficient for antibacterial activity.

There were no signs or laboratory findings of organ toxicity with the exception of transitory hepatic disturbances in two patients. The first patient had serum glutamic pyruvic and oxalacetic transaminase (SGPT and SGOT) levels elevated on the third day after the end of treatment, but there was no increase in bilirubin and no signs of jaundice. By 12 days after the end of treatment, the SGOT values were normal and the SGPT were still higher than before treatment but had decreased from 44 to 21 U. In the other patient jaundice could be seen on the third day of treatment. Laboratory tests confirmed the increase in total serum bilirubin to 4 mg/100 ml; the SGOT and SGPT values remained normal. The bilirubin level had returned to normal values after 5 days.

In summary, a 7-day treatment with RMP-TMP was found to have a satisfactory efficacy and tolerability in 23 patients with different forms of recurrent urinary tract infections. Shortly after the end of treatment, bacteriuria disappeared in 68% of patients. After 3 to 5 weeks, the urines remained sterile in 45% of patients. As expected, the therapeutic results were considerably better in patients with lower urinary tract infection and in the absence of urinary tract obstruction. However, the results obtained in patients with upper UTI and in the presence of obstruction are encouraging, especially considering that our patients were a selected group of problem cases with a previous history of multiple relapses despite several antibacterial courses. In our experience, one point of relevance is that RMP-TMP is given by the oral route so that these difficult patients could be treated on an ambulatory basis and did not require hospitalization.

1. **Fairley, K. F., A. G. Bond, R. B. Brown, and P. Habersberger.** 1967. Simple test to determine the site of urinary-tract infection. Lancet **ii**:427–428.
2. **Goldstein, B. P., I. F. Ripamonti, G. Bolzoni, G. Carniti, and V. Arioli.** 1979. Rifampin plus trimethoprim: bactericidal activity and suppression of resistance in human urine in vitro. Antimicrob. Agents Chemother. **16**:736–742.
3. **Kerry, D. W., J. M. T. Hamilton-Miller, and W. Brumfitt.** 1975. Trimethoprim and rifampicin: in vitro activities separately and in combination. J. Antimicrob. Chemother. **1**:417–427.

Comparative Study of Rifaprim and Cephalexin in Urinary Tract Infections

M. S. SABBOUR* AND L. M. OSMAN

Departments of Medicine and Clinical Pathology, Ain-Shams University, Cairo, Egypt*

Rifaprim is a combination of rifampin (RMP) and trimethoprim (TMP) in the ratio of 3.75:1. A dosage schedule of 600 mg of RMP and 160 mg of TMP once daily gives maximum serum levels of about 15 μg/ml for RMP and 1.75 μg/ml for TMP; the mean urinary levels are about 200 μg/ml and 100 μg/ml, respectively, during the first 12 h after dosing. These values exceed the MIC for the common urinary pathogens with the exception of *Pseudomonas* (1). These facts led us to investigate the efficacy and tolerability of rifaprim in patients with urinary tract infection (UTI). Cephalexin was chosen as a comparison drug in view of its established value in UTI, its safety, and its excellent tolerability.

One hundred patients of both sexes with chronic or recurrent UTI were subjected to this comparative experimental study. The diagnostic criterion was the presence of significant bacteruria (10^5 bacteria per ml of urine) in a midstream specimen. Urine was cultured on C.L.E.D.; susceptibility of the organisms was determined by disk diffusion by the Kirby-Bauer method. Organisms were considered resistant if the estimated MIC of RMP was above 50 μg/ml and that of TMP was above 25 μg/ml. Only patients in whom the isolated organisms were susceptible to both cephalexin and RMP were included. A random allocation list defined which treatment was to be given to the patient. Rifaprim was administered at bedtime as a single daily dose containing 600 mg of RMP and 160 mg of TMP. Cephalexin was administered as 500-mg capsules four times a day. Treatment was continued for 10 days with both agents.

Table 1 shows the distribution of the organisms isolated from both therapeutic groups; the pattern of organisms was nearly the same. The overall results of the treatment are listed in Table 2. No significant difference was found between the cure rates of the two groups with regard to *Proteus* infections; however, in *Klebsiella* infections, cephalexin was significantly superior to rifaprim, whereas in *Escherichia coli* and staphylococcal infections, rifaprim was significantly superior to cephalexin. Persistence of a sterile urine 6 weeks after treatment was found in 39 of 42 of the rifaprim-treated group and in 35 of 39 of the cephalexin-treated group.

TABLE 1. *Distribution of organisms isolated before treatment*[a]

Organism	Rifaprim group	Cephalexin group
Escherichia coli	33	27
Proteus	5	8
Klebsiella	6	9
Staphylococcus aureus	2	3
Mixed infection	4[b]	3[c]

[a] All isolated strains of *Pseudomonas aeruginosa* were resistant to the three antimicrobials tested. Enterococci were not encountered in the present series.

[b] *E. coli* and *Proteus* in two and *E. coli* and *Klebsiella* in two.

[c] *E. coli* and *Proteus* in one, *E. coli* and *Staphylococcus* in one, and *E. coli* and *Klebsiella* in one.

TABLE 2. *Primary success rate in the two experimental therapeutic groups (percentage in parentheses)*

Organism	Rifaprim group	Cephalexin group
Escherichia coli	31/33 (94)	22/27 (81)
Proteus	4/5 (80)	6/8 (75)
Klebsiella	3/6 (50)	8/9 (89)
Staphylococcus aureus	2/2 (100)	1/3 (33)
Mixed infection	2/4	2/3
All cases	42/50 (84)	39/50 (78)

Rifaprim was tried in a larger dose in seven patients with *Klebsiella* infections; a single dose of 900 mg of RMP plus 240 mg of TMP was administered for 10 days. On the third posttreatment day, the success rate was six of seven (85%); after 6 weeks, one patient had a recurrence, leaving the success rate five of seven (71%). It seems that this larger dose should be utilized from the beginning if the isolate is a *Klebsiella* strain or if there is a mixed infection including a *Klebsiella* strain.

Both therapeutic regimens were well tolerated in most patients. There were no significant changes in any of the hematological parameters measured, and there was no evidence of nephrotoxicity.

The combination of RMP and TMP appears to have two valuable effects: synergism and delay in the emergence of bacterial resistance (2). Successful eradication of bacteria from dense cultures treated by RMP plus TMP is possibly due to the bactericidal action of RMP and the ability of TMP to suppress the emergence of RMP-resistant bacteria. RMP is bactericidal even at high inocula; reduction of the inoculum by RMP allows TMP to express its bactericidal activity, particularly against RMP-resistant cells. Therefore, both components contribute to the sterilization of the urine.

1. **Acocella, G., and R. Scotti.** 1976. J. Antimicrob. Chemother. **2:**271–277.
2. **Kerry, D. W., J.M. T. Hamilton-Miller, and W. Brumfitt.** 1975. J. Antimicrob. Chemother. **1:**417–427.

Comparative Studies of Cefmenoxime (SCE-1365) and Cefazolin in Complicated Urinary Tract Infections

YUKIMICHI KAWADA* AND TSUNEO NISHIURA

Department of Urology, Gifu University School of Medicine, Gifu, Japan

Cefmenoxime is a new semisynthetic cephalosporin antibiotic which is highly active against most gram-negative bacteria (2). The present study was designed to compare the safety and efficacy of cefmenoxime and cefazolin in the treatment of complicated urinary tract infections by a prospective, randomized, double-blind method.

A total of 207 patients in the urology ward were enrolled from 23 institutes in Japan. All of these patients were shown to have underlying urinary tract disease, pyuria of over five leukocytes per high-power field, and bacteriuria of over 10^4 bacteria per ml of urine. The patients were prospectively assigned at random to one of two groups and received either 0.5 g of cefmenoxime or 1 g of cefazolin twice a day, every 12 h, for 5 days by intravenous drip infusion.

Urine culture with colony counting and routine urinalysis were carried out on midstream specimens in male and catheterized specimens in female patients before and after treatment. Routine hematological and biochemical examinations were also carried out before and after treatment for the evaluation of side effects.

The overall clinical efficacy of treatment was evaluated by the criteria proposed by the UTI Committee in Japan as excellent, moderate, or poor (including failure) based on the combination of changes in pyuria and bacteriuria (3). In addition, bacteriological responses to the treatment were determined in relation to the MICs of the drugs for the infecting organisms. Bacteriological response was defined as eradicated if bacteria identical to the original strain were not isolated after treatment and as persistent if bacteria identical to the original strain were isolated after treatment regardless of bacterial count. MICs were determined by the agar plate streak method proposed by the Japan Society of Chemotherapy (1).

Of the 207 patients admitted to the series, 104 received cefmenoxime and 103 received cefazolin. The sex and age distribution, site of infection, severity of pyuria before treatment, incidence of infecting organisms, and the MIC distribution of both cefmenoxime and cefazolin were compared between the two treatment groups. There were no significant differences in the background characteristics. Forty-four patients (42.3%) in the cefmenoxime group and 32 patients (31.1%) in the cefazolin group had indwelling catheters, but the frequency of patients with indwelling catheters showed no significant difference between the two groups. Forty-six patients (44.2%) in the cefmenoxime group and 43 patients (41.7%) in the cefazolin group were infected with two or more organisms, but no significant difference was observed in the incidence of polymicrobial infection.

The overall clinical efficacies of treatment were evaluated in relation to the type of infection, which was classified into four categories depending on whether an indwelling catheter was present and whether the infecting organism was single or multiple. As shown in Table 1, cefmenoxime was significantly more effective than cefazolin in patients with indwelling catheters in both mono- and polymicrobial infections. No significant differences in overall clinical efficacies were observed between the two groups in patients without indwelling catheters. On the whole, significantly higher efficacy of treatment was obtained in the cefmenoxime group.

The bacteriological responses to the treatment are shown in Table 2. Significantly higher eradication of *Serratia* was observed in the cefmenoxime group. The overall eradication rate of bacteria in the cefmenoxime group was also significantly higher than in the cefazolin group. However, the eradication rate of *Pseudomonas aeruginosa* in the cefmenoxime group was rather low in comparison with the other bacterial species in the same group.

When strains for which MICs of cefmenoxime and cefazolin were 6.25 μg/ml or lower were regarded as susceptible, 64 of 144 strains (44.4%) in the cefmenoxime group were susceptible to cefmenoxime and 31 of 134 strains (23.1%) in the cefazolin group were susceptible to cefazolin. Overall eradication rates of bacteria in the cefmenoxime-susceptible and -resistant groups were 89.1% and 65.0%, respectively. This differ-

TABLE 1. *Overall clinical efficacy of the treatment in relation to the type of infection*

Infected with	Indwelling catheter	Treatment group	Responses[a]			Wilcoxon rank sum test
			Excellent	Moderate	Poor	
Single organism	Present	Cefmenoxime (n = 19)	5 (26.3)	6 (31.6)	8 (42.1)	$P < 0.05$
		Cefazolin (n = 13)	0	3 (23.1)	10 (76.9)	
	Not present	Cefmenoxime (n = 39)	14 (35.9)	17 (43.6)	8 (20.5)	NS[b]
		Cefazolin (n = 47)	12 (25.5)	16 (34.0)	19 (40.4)	
Multiple organisms	Present	Cefmenoxime (n = 25)	5 (20.0)	7 (28.0)	13 (52.0)	$P < 0.01$
		Cefazolin (n = 19)	0	2 (10.5)	17 (89.5)	
	Not present	Cefmenoxime (n = 21)	3 (14.3)	9 (42.9)	9 (42.9)	NS
		Cefazolin (n = 24)	2 (8.3)	8 (33.3)	14 (59.3)	
Total		Cefmenoxime (n = 104)	27 (26.0)	39 (37.5)	38 (36.5)	$P < 0.01$
		Cefazolin (n = 103)	14 (13.6)	29 (28.2)	60 (58.3)	

[a] Values in parentheses indicate percentage.
[b] NS, Not significant.

TABLE 2. *Bacteriological response to the treatment*

Organism	Cefmenoxime		Cefazolin		χ^2 test
	Eradicated[a]	Persisted	Eradicated	Persisted	
E. coli	19 (86.4)	3	21 (87.5)	3	NS[b]
Klebsiella	10 (100.0)	0	7 (77.8)	2	NS
Indole-negative *Proteus*	8 (100.0)	0	10 (90.0)	1	NS
Indole-positive *Proteus*	8 (100.0)	0	5 (71.4)	2	NS
Enterobacter	1 (100.0)	0	5 (55.6)	4	NS
Citrobacter	7 (77.8)	2	2 (22.2)	7	NS
Serratia	13 (68.4)	6	3 (18.8)	13	$P < 0.01$
P. aeruginosa	12 (40.0)	18	4 (22.2)	14	NS
Other gram-negative bacilli	14 (77.8)	4	17 (81.0)	4	NS
S. faecalis	24 (82.8)	5	13 (86.7)	2	NS
Other gram-positive cocci	17 (94.4)	1	18 (85.7)	3	NS
Total	133 (77.3)	39	104 (65.0)	56	$P < 0.05$

[a] Values in parentheses indicate percentage.
[b] NS, Not significant.

ence was statistically significant. All of 28 strains of *P. aeruginosa* in the cefmenoxime group were resistant to cefmenoxime. Overall eradication rates of bacteria in the cefazolin-susceptible and resistant groups were 90.1% and 60.2%, respectively. This difference was also statistically significant. When bacteriological responses to the treatment were compared between cefmenoxime and cefazolin, no significant differences were observed in either the susceptible or the resistant group.

Forty-six strains which were not present in the urine before treatment were newly isolated after treatment from 32 patients (30.8%) in the cefmenoxime group. Similarly, 54 new strains were isolated after treatment from 38 patients (36.9%) in the cefazolin group. *P. aeruginosa*, *Streptococcus faecalis*, *Candida*, and yeastlike organisms in the cefmenoxime group and *Serratia* and *P. aeruginosa* in the cefazolin group were predominant.

Side effects were evaluated in 32 patients in the cefmenoxime group and 40 patients in the cefazolin group. There were no significant differences between the two treatment groups regarding the incidence of side effects, and cefmenoxime appeared to be as well tolerated as cefazolin.

From the results obtained, we concluded that cefmenoxime, at the dose employed in this study, was more useful than cefazolin in the treatment of complicated urinary tract infections.

1. **Japan Society of Chemotherapy.** 1981. Standard method for the determination of minimum inhibitory concentrations. Chemotherapy (Tokyo) **29:**76–79.
2. **Tsuchiya, K., M. Kondo, M. Kida, M. Nakao, T. Iwai, T. Nishi, Y. Noji, M. Takeuchi, and Y. Nozaki.** 1981. Cefmenoxime (SCE-1365), a novel broad-spectrum cephalosporin: in vitro and in vivo antibacterial activities. Antimicrob. Agents Chemother. **19:**56–65.
3. **UTI Committee, Japan.** 1980. Criteria for the evaluation of clinical efficacy of antimicrobial agents on urinary tract infections. Chemotherapy (Tokyo) **28:**321–323.

Comparative Clinical Evaluation of Cefmenoxime with Cefotiam in Complicated Urinary Tract Infection by a Randomized Double-Blind Method

J. ISHIGAMI,* T. KURODA, S. MOMOSE, S. NAKAMUTA, AND J. KUMAZAWA

Kobe University, Kobe, Kyushu University, Fukuoka, and Saga Medical College, Saga, Japan*

Cefmenoxime (SCE-1365, CMX), a new injectable cephalosporin synthesized at the Central Research Division of Takeda Chemical Industries Ltd., has as its chemical feature an aminothiazolyl-methoxyiminoacetyl group at the 7 position of the cephalosporin nucleus and a tetrazole ring at the 3 position (Fig. 1). It has been described to have the characteristics of being several times more active against gram-negative rods than the previously introduced injectable cephalosporins and, moreover, to possess a broader antibacterial spectrum, expanded to include *Enterobacter*, *Citrobacter*, indole-positive *Proteus*, and *Serratia* (Symposium on New Drugs, 28th Annual Conference, Japan Society of Chemotherapy, Tokyo, 1980).

Therefore, a double-blind controlled clinical trial of cefmenoxime was conducted to evaluate its efficacy and safety in the treatment of chronic, complicated urinary tract infections by intergroup comparison with cefotiam.

Subjects were over 15 years of age and suffering from underlying urinary tract disease, with pyuria of five or more leukocytes per high-power field and bacteriuria of 10^4 or more viable organisms per ml.

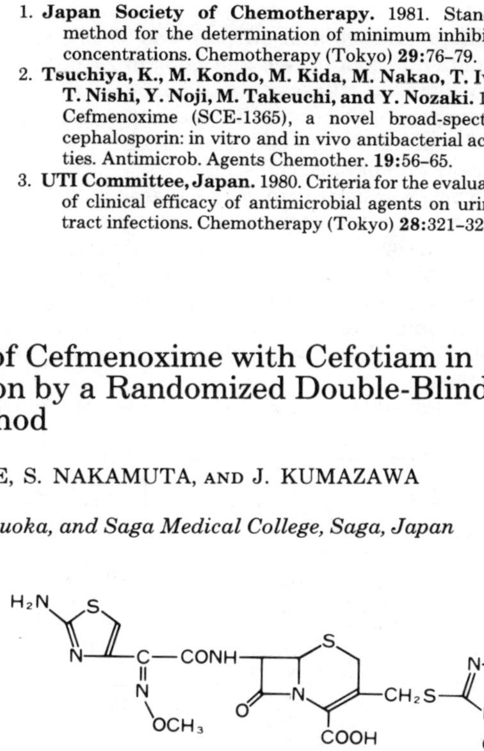

FIG. 1. *Chemical structure of cefmenoxime.*

The two medications were used at 1 g (potency) per vial and supplied as preparations identical in appearance, color, shape, and volume by adding mannitol to cefmenoxime and cefotiam. The daily dosages of cefmenoxime and cefotiam were 2 g. Each dose in a vial was diluted with 300 ml of 5% xylitol solution and administered by intravenous drip infusion over approximately 1 h, twice daily (morning and evening), for 5 consecutive days.

Treatment was carried out on a total of 241 patients, 120 with cefmenoxime and 121 with cefotiam. Of the 241 patients admitted to the trial, 211 (107 on cefmenoxime and 104 on cefotiam) were eligible for efficacy judgment; the remainder were excluded from the judgment because the conditions did not satisfy the criteria of the Committee of Urinary Tract Infections Study, Japan Society of Chemotherapy (1) or because of discontinuation of the treatment. In the safety evaluation, data from 240 patients treated were included; one case was omitted because of concomitant use of other antibiotics and short period of medication.

Background characteristics and patient factors in both treatment groups were fairly equivalent.

The overall clinical efficacy was excellent in 24 patients, good in 49, and poor in 34 on cefmenoxime, an efficacy rate of 68.2%. In the cefotiam group, there were 16 patients with excellent result, 28 with good, and 60 with poor, an efficacy rate of 42.3% ($P < 0.001$).

Pyuria was cleared in 35, decreased in 26, and unchanged in 46 patients in the cefmenoxime group. In the cefotiam group, pyuria was cleared in 24, decreased in 18, and unchanged in 62 patients. The cefmenoxime group showed a higher improvement (cleared plus decreased) rate (57.0%) than the cefotiam group (40.4%) ($P < 0.05$).

Bacteriuria was eliminated in 63 patients, suppressed in 4, replaced with other organisms in 16, and unchanged in 24 in the cefmenoxime group, an improvement (eliminated plus suppressed) rate of 62.6%. The corresponding numbers were 29, 3, 34, and 38 in the cefotiam group, an improvement rate of 30.8%. The microbial replacement rate was 15.0% in the cefmenoxime group and 32.7% in the cefotiam group ($P < 0.001$).

Bacteriological evaluation showed no significant difference in the eradication rate for all species of isolates between the cefmenoxime group (107 of 137 strains, or 78%) and cefotiam group (101 of 145 strains, or 70.0%). The eradication of *Escherichia coli*, *Klebsiella*, *Enterobacter*, indole-positive *Proteus*, and *Serratia* occurred more frequently with cefmenoxime, especially in the case of *E. coli* ($P < 0.10$) and *Serratia* ($P < 0.05$).

The two treatment groups were compared as to overall clinical efficacy and effects on pyuria and bacteriuria in the patients stratified according to group of diseases, indwelling catheter, type of infection, and kinds of organism (Fig. 2). Stratified analyses favored cefmenoxime over cefotiam in most strains. Cefmenoxime especially was significantly superior to cefotiam.

Side effects of cefmenoxime and cefotiam were

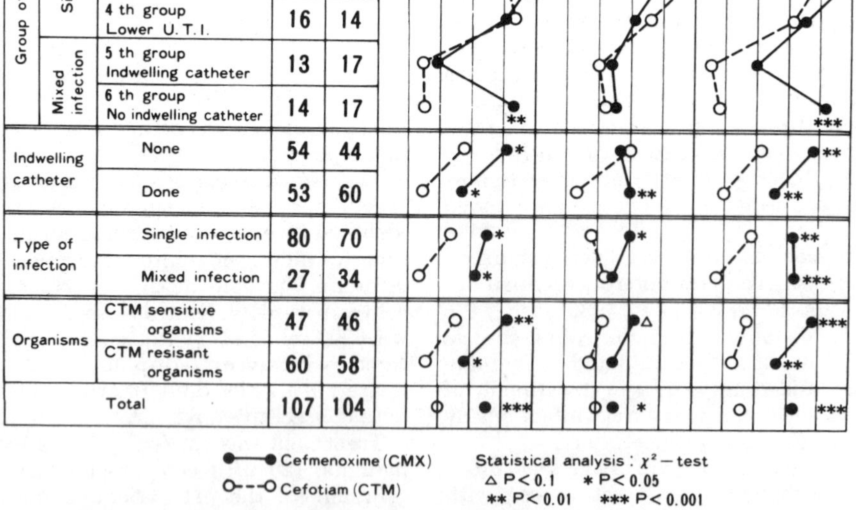

FIG. 2. *Comparison of the efficacy rates of cefmenoxime and cefotiam.*

0.8% (1 of 119) and 0.8% (1 of 121), respectively. One patient receiving cefmenoxime developed a moderate eruption, and administration of the drug was discontinued. In the cefotiam group, one patient recorded a moderate eruption, ache of urethral tract, and malaise, leading to the discontinuation of treatment. All of these findings are, however, commonly observed in the course of cephalosporin treatment.

Abnormal laboratory findings were noted in nine patients on cefmenoxime and eight patients on cefotiam, though all were found to have returned to normal after completion of treatment. In the cefmenoxime group, slight elevation of serum glutamic oxalacetic and pyruvic transaminase, alkaline phosphatase, and bilirubin were noted. In the cefotiam group, elevation of serum glutamic oxalacetic and pyruvic transaminase, alkaline phosphatase, and eosinocytes and decreased platelets were the main abnormal laboratory findings. The safety of cefmenoxime and cefotiam appeared to be essentially comparable.

In summary, the results of the present comparative study with cefotiam showed that cefmenoxime is a more valuable chemotherapeutic agent for treatment of chronic, complicated urinary tract infections. Cefmenoxime showed a higher efficacy rate in the treatment of the aforementioned infections, and safety evaluation did not show any difference between the two drugs.

1. **Ogoshi, M.** 1980. Criteria for drug efficacy evaluation in urinary tract infections. Chemotherapy (Tokyo) **28:** 1351–1358.

Comparison of Lymecycline and Erythromycin in Treatment of Nongonococcal Urethritis

J. M. HUBRECHTS,* B. GORDTS, F. KHODJASTEH, R. J. DENOLF, R. VANHOOF, AND J. P. BUTZLER

St. Pieters Hospital, Brussels, Belgium

The objective of this randomized open study was to assess the clinical efficacy of lymecycline and erythromycin treatment in patients suffering from nongonococcal urethritis (NGU). Patient selection was based on the presence of a clinical history of NGU, dysuria, or urethral discharge. Bacteriological criteria consisted of exclusion of *Neisseria gonorrhoeae*-positive patients, presence of *Chlamydia trachomatis* or *Ureaplasma urealyticum*, and presence of polymorphonuclear leukocytes in the urethral smear.

A total of 221 male NGU patients attending our venereal disease center were included in the study (St. Pieters Hospital, Brussels, Belgium). One hundred twenty-six patients received 300 mg of lymecycline twice a day for 8 days, and 95 received 500 mg of erythromycin stearate twice a day for 8 days. No other simultaneous treatment was allowed.

Randomization consisted of changing the antibiotic every 4 weeks for the new NGU patients taken into the study. Patients were to report to the clinic 8 days after the end of the treatment for cultures and clinical evaluation (i.e., clearing of discharge and dysuria). After treatment, 174 NGU patients returned for follow-up and could be classified into three groups. (i) A first group of 78 NGU patients with positive cultures for *C. trachomatis* (Table 1) showed 95.5% cure (44 of 46) with lymecycline and 87.5% cure (28 of 32) with erythromycin. (ii) A second group of 51 patients with positive cultures for *U. urealyticum* showed 88.5% cure (23 of 26) with lymecy-

TABLE 1. *Treatment of Chlamydia-positive but Ureaplasma-negative patients with lymecycline and erythromycin*

Total no. of patients	No. of dropouts	No. of complete cases	Drug	No. (%) of patients: Bacteriologically and clinically cured	Bacteriologically cured only	Not cured
55	9	46	Lymecycline	44 (95.5)[a]	1 (2.2%)	1 (2.2)
36	4	32	Erythromycin	28 (87.5)[a]	4 (12.5)	

[a] No statistically significant difference between the drugs: $0.5 > P > 0.3$.

TABLE 2. *Treatment of Chlamydia-negative but Ureaplasma-positive patients with lymecycline and erythromycin*

Total no. of patients	No. of dropouts	No. of complete cases	Drug	No. (%) of patients:		
				Bacteriologically and clinically cured	Bacteriologically cured only	Not cured
32	6	26	Lymecycline	23 (88.5)[a]	2 (7.7)	1 (3.8)
29	4	25	Erythromycin	18 (72)[a]	7 (28)	

[a] No statistically significant difference between the drugs: $0.3 > P > 0.2$.

cline and 72% cure (18 of 25) with erythromycin (Table 2). (iii) The last group of 45 nonspecific urethritis patients showed 81.8% cure (18 of 22) with lymecycline and 82.6% cure (19 of 23) with erythromycin.

The analysis of these results showed no statistically significant difference in the effectiveness of either drug in the three groups, nor was there a statistical difference between the results obtained in the *Chlamydia*-positive and *Chlamydia*-negative groups. Lymecycline and erythromycin must be regarded as excellent drugs for the treatment of nongonococcal urethritis.

The interest of this study was twofold: first, to try out the efficacy of a relatively short tetracyline treatment (lymecycline) of 8 days for NGU; second, to study the efficacy of an 8-day treatment with erythromycin (especially of interest in cases of tetracycline intolerance and pregnancy). Both drugs were clinically and bacteriologically very effective, and considering the given dose, the tolerance was excellent.

Chemotherapeutic Design Against Superinfections in Severe Chronic Respiratory Infections

YOSHIO UZUKA,* KEIZO MATSUMOTO, TSUYOSHI NAGATAKE, HARUMI SHISHIDO, AND NAOTO RIKITOMI

Department of Internal Medicine, Institute for Tropical Medicine, Nagasaki University, Nagasaki, Japan

Superinfection is considered to be a serious problem during antibiotic treatment of patients with severe chronic respiratory infections because it results in a poor prognosis. Very little is known of the incidence and clinical course of such superinfection. Therefore, this clinical study was performed by utilizing our quantitative sputum culture method (1), cytological examination, and titration of serum antibodies. This study revealed the difference between "colonization" and "superinfection" and made it clear that a chemotherapeutic design against these superinfections can improve the prognosis of the patients with severe chronic respiratory infections.

All sputum specimens were homogenized with *N*-acetylcysteine, and the number of bacteria was measured by the quantitative culture method; potential bacterial pathogens detected at $\geqq 10^7$/ml were considered "significant" organisms. From 1971 to 1979, 89 episodes (58 patients) of changes of significant bacteria in sputum (i.e., the appearance of other potential pathogens at $\geqq 10^7$/ml in sputum after the disappearance of primary pathogens) were observed during antibiotic treatment of 1,442 respiratory infections. Almost none of the newly observed pathogens seemed to endanger the patients at first, but some of them clearly showed pathogenicity later. Thus, we defined "colonization" to mean a change of significant bacteria in sputum during antibiotic treatment without clinical manifestation and "superinfection" to mean a true infection by newly observed bacteria. This definition is almost the same as that described by Tillotson and Finland (2).

A total of 89 episodes in 58 patients (chronic bronchitis, 31; chronic bronchiolitis, 13; bronchiectasis, 6; chronic pulmonary emphysema, 8) were examined and divided into two periods: 1971 to 1974 and 1975 to 1979. From 1971 to 1974, 30 episodes (22 patients) of colonization were observed (Table 1). The primary pathogens were mainly *Haemophilus influenzae* (25 isolates) or *Streptococcus pneumoniae* (5 isolates) or both, eight species of bacteria colonized, and 17 of 30 colonizations (57%) were by *Pseudomonas aeruginosa*. Fourteen patients were administered antipseudomonal antibiotics, but seven of them developed severe superinfections

TABLE 1. *Relationship between incidence of superinfection and antibiotic treatment after colonization*

Period	Antibiotic treatment after colonization (no. of cases)	Potential pathogenic bacteria	No. of cases				
			Primary pathogens	Colonization	Significant bacteria in sputum after change of chemotherapy	True infection developed	Death resulted
1971–1974	+, 22	None	0	0	1	0	0
		H. influenzae	17 (2)[a]	0	2	2	0
		P. aeruginosa	0	14 (2)	16 (1)	7[b]	4
		Others (4 species)	7	10	4	0	0
	−, 8	None	0	0	1	0	0
		H. influenzae	8	0	7	7	0
		P. aeruginosa	0	3	0	0	0
		Others (3 species)	0	5	0	0	0
1975–1979	+, 3	None	0	0	0	0	0
		H. influenzae	2	0	0	0	0
		P. aeruginosa	0	2 (1)	3 (2)	2 (1)[b]	0
		Others (2 species)	1	2	2	1[b]	0
	−, 56	None	0	0	8	0	0
		H. influenzae	46 (3)	2	46	46	0
		P. aeruginosa	2	19 (3)	1	1[b]	0
		Others (10 species)	11	38	0	0	0

[a] Number of cases in which other bacteria were present is given in parentheses.
[b] Superinfection.

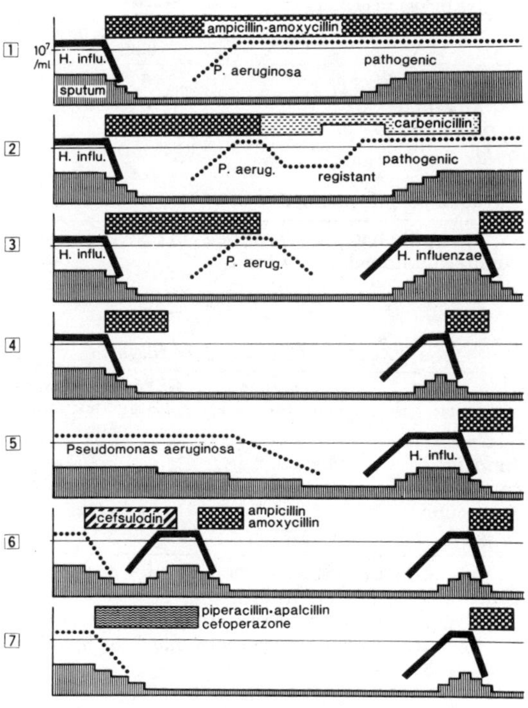

FIG. 1. *Chemotherapeutic design against superinfection. (1 & 2) Clinical course from colonization to superinfection. (3) Colonized bacteria disappear after cessation of antibiotic treatment. (4) Colonization prevented by short-term antibiotic treatment. (5–7) Retrograde superinfection—from P. aeruginosa infection to the stage of recurrent infection by H. influenzae.*

by *P. aeruginosa* and four of them died of respiratory failure. However, in three patients who received no antibiotic treatment after colonization, *P. aeruginosa* disappeared spontaneously; later two of these patients developed a recurrent *H. influenzae* infection.

Therefore, from 1975 to 1979, antibiotic treatment was stopped in 56 of 59 episodes (36 patients) of colonization. Two of the patients were colonized by *H. influenzae*, and both developed clinical superinfection after cessation of antibiotic treatment. In 52 of the other 54 colonizations (including 21 by *P. aeruginosa*), colonized bacteria disappeared spontaneously, and later, 44 of them developed *H. influenzae* infection. Severe clinical superinfections were not observed during this period.

Another study on serum antibody titers in 51 patients revealed that *H. influenzae* infections preceded *P. aeruginosa* infections.

These studies revealed that superinfection by *P. aeruginosa* is most harmful to patients with severe chronic respiratory infections, because the destruction of pulmonary tissues may be accelerated by proteolytic enzymes of *P. aeruginosa*. The chemotherapeutic schedule shown in Fig. 1 was thus designed to prevent superinfection by *P. aeruginosa* and revealed that short-term antibiotic treatment of *H. influenzae* infection can prevent not only superinfection by *P.*

aeruginosa, but also colonization. Retrograde superinfection, i.e., the change from *P. aeruginosa* to *H. influenzae*, can be actively induced by cefsulodin, and this may mean a good prognosis for patients.

From these results, it is concluded that a chemotherapeutic design to prevent superinfections by *P. aeruginosa* and to keep patients in the stage of chronic and recurrent infections by *H. influenzae* can improve the long-term prognosis of patients with severe chronic respiratory infections.

1. **Matsumoto, K., Y. Uzuka, T. Nagatake, Y. Nogushi, and H. Suzuki.** 1978. A quantitative sputum culture method—the significance of the quantity $\geqq 10^7$/ml of isolated organisms. Jpn. J. Thorac. Dis. **16:**77–89. (In Japanese.)
2. **Tillotson, J. R., and M. Finland.** 1969. Bacterial colonization and clinical superinfections of the respiratory tract complicating antibiotic treatment of pneumonia. J. Infect. Dis. **119:**597–624.

Randomized Comparative Study of Amoxicillin and Ampicillin During the Onset of Bacterial Meningitis in Children

ERIC MALLET,* ANNIE LEROY, CATHERINE DESNEIGES, AND CLAUDE HELLOUIN DE MENIBUS

Service de Pédiatrie and Laboratoire d'Antibiothérapie, Centre Hospitalo-Universitaire, Hôpital Charles Nicolle, 76031 Rouen Cédex, France*

Recently, a parenteral form of amoxicillin has become available (Beecham Sévigné Laboratories). The present study was designed to evaluate the therapeutic value of amoxicillin with respect to bacterial eradication from cerebrospinal fluid (CSF) and CSF diffusion of the drug during the onset of bacterial meningitis in children.

At the present time, 37 children (aged 2 months to 13 years) with bacterial meningitis have already been treated intravenously (i.v.) with amoxicillin and ampicillin in a randomized comparative study. The infecting organisms were: meningococcus (n = 15), *Haemophilus influenzae* (n = 4), *Streptococcus pneumoniae* (n = 4), and *Salmonella* (n = 1). All organisms were ampicillin or amoxicillin susceptible. There were eight cases of purulent aseptic meningitis. Antibiotics were administered i.v. in a daily dose of 200 mg/kg, which was equally divided among six 1-min bolus i.v. administrations on day 1 and four on each following day.

The CSF antibiotic concentration, determined by a microbiological method, was evaluated 1 h after dose administration (50 mg/kg i.v.) on day 2 (24 to 30 h). There was almost no difference in the number and nature of bacterial meningitis cases treated by each antibiotic (Table 1).

There was no significant difference between data on CSF antibiotic concentration and CSF bacterial eradication on day 2 (Table 2). There were two cases of ampicillin-treated bacterial meningitis (one *Salmonella* and one *S. pneumoniae*) with positive CSF culture on day 2 in spite of antibiotic CSF concentrations of 6 and 2.7 µg/ml, respectively.

TABLE 1. *Bacterial meningitis repartition*

Etiological organism	No. of children treated with: Amoxicillin	Ampicillin
N. meningitidis	8	7
H. influenzae	5	3
S. pneumoniae	2	3[a]
Salmonella		1
Purulent aseptic meningitis	4	4

[a] One child had positive antigen in CSF detected by counterimmunoelectrophoresis.

TABLE 2. *CSF day 2 findings*

Drug	CSF antibiotic concn after 1 h (µg/ml)[a]	CSF bacterial eradication (no./total cases)[b]
Amoxicillin (n = 19)	5.4 ± 4.4 (2.1–18)	7/16
Ampicillin (n = 18)	5.5 ± 3.3 (1.2–12.2)	4/12[c]

[a] 50-mg/kg i.v. bolus injection. Mean ± SD is given. Range is given in parentheses.

[b] Negative in CSF by Gram stain and culture.

[c] Includes two positive cultures, one *S. pneumoniae* and one *Salmonella*.

The results of this study suggest that amoxicillin is at least as effective as ampicillin in the treatment of bacterial meningitis in children. It would be useful to continue this study on a larger scale.

Comparative Clinical Study of Apalcillin and Sulbenicillin Against Postoperative Infections

K. SAKAI,* T. TANAKA, K. ISHIBIKI, I. NAKAYAMA, K. SHIBATA, J. YURA, N. SHINAGAWA, AND N. KAWABATA

The Second Department of Surgery, Osaka City University Medical School, Osaka; Department of Health Administration, School of Health Sciences Faculty of Medicine, University of Tokyo, Tokyo; Department of Surgery, School of Medicine, Keio University, Tokyo; The Third Department of Surgery, Nihon University, School of Medicine, Tokyo; and The First Department of Surgery, Nagoya City University School of Medicine, Nagoya, Japan*

Apalcillin, sodium (2*S*,5*R*,6*R*)-6-[(R)-2-(4-hydroxy-1,5-naphthyridine- 3-carboxamido)-2-phenylacetamido]-3,3- dimethyl-7-oxo-4-thia-1-azabicyclo[3.2.0]heptane-2-carboxylate (PC-904), is a semisynthetic penicillin having a broad antibacterial spectrum which has been newly developed at the Laboratory of Sumitomo Chemical Co., Ltd., Japan. It has a particularly strong antibacterial effect upon *Pseudomonas aeruginosa* and other gram-negative bacteria (1, 2).

To ascertain the therapeutic effects and clinical usefulness of apalcillin (APPC) objectively, a well-controlled, comparative study was performed at 99 medical institutions in Japan, using sulbenicillin (SBPC) as the control drug in the patients of postoperative wound infections in trial A and postoperative localized peritonitis and dead-space infections or both in trial B.

Either 1 g of APPC or 5 g of SBPC was administered to patients by intravenous drip infusion twice a day for 7 days in trial A and 10 days in trial B.

In this comparative study, the total number of patients was 270 cases; 136 cases in the APPC-administered group and 134 cases in the SBPC-administered group. They were all inpatients in the period from April 1979 to June 1980. The subcommittee compared the safety between APPC and SBPC on all of the cases. However, excluding 49 cases by predetermined criteria, a comparison of the background factors of patients and the efficacy between the drugs was made for 221 cases. APPC was administered in 112 cases, and SBPC was administered in 109 cases.

Overall clinical improvement rates judged by committee members were 91.5% in the APPC group and 66.7% in the SBPC group in trial A (Table 1) and 88.7% in the APPC group and 47.3% in the SBPC group in trial B (Table 2). In both trials, APPC was significantly superior to SBPC.

Overall clinical improvement rates of both drugs were compared in subgroups divided by the depth of infections classified into superficial wall and deep wall in trial A and divided by the site of infections such as abdominal cavity, perineo-pelvic dead space, and pleural cavity in trial B. In trial A, the improvement rates were 100% in the APPC group and 69.6% in the SBPC group in cases of superficial wall infections and 88.4% in the APPC group and 64.5% in the SBPC group in cases of deep-wall infections. In trial B, the improvement rates were 87.9% in the APPC group and 48.5% in the SBPC group in infections of the abdominal cavity and 89.5% in the APPC group and 47.6% in the SBPC group in infections of perineo-pelvic dead space. Therefore, APPC was significantly superior to SBPC in all subgroups in both trial A and trial B. In pleural infections, each drug was administered to only one case. The case in which APPC was administered was assessed as improved and the case in which SBPC was administered was assessed as not changed.

As to bacteriological effects, eradication rates of clinical isolates were 90% in the APPC group and 50% in the SBPC group in trial A and 99% in the APPC group and 51.4% in the SBPC group in trial B. Thus, APPC was significantly superior to SBPC in both trials A and trial B.

As to the frequency of eradication of each clinical isolate, 17 of the 20 strains of *P. aeruginosa* in the APPC group and 5 of the 11 strains in the SBPC group were eradicated, indicating a higher rate of eradication in the APPC group. Higher eradication rates were also noted for gram-positive coccal bacteria and gram-negative rod bacteria, especially *Escherichia coli* and *Klebsiella pneumoniae*, as well as for anaerobic bacteria, such as *Bacteroides fragilis*, by the administration of APPC, although the differences between the drugs were not statistically significant.

As to usefulness as judged by the surgeons for each patient, APPC was significantly superior to SBPC in both trial A and trial B.

Regarding the elimination or improvement of clinical symptoms and findings such as redness, swelling, induration, pain, local heat, discharge, and body temperature in trial A, and pain, abdominal distension, tenderness, muscular de-

TABLE 1. *Overall clinical improvement judged by committee members (trial A)*

Drug	No. of cases	Overall clinical improvement[a]					Improvement rate (%)		Statistical analysis[a]	
		M	I	F	Unchanged	Undecided	M + I	M + I + F	U	χ^2
APPC	59	20	34	3	1	1	91.5	96.6	***	* (M) ** (M + I) * (M + I + F)
SBPC	54	7	29	7	11	0	66.7	79.6		

[a] M, Markedly improved; I, improved; F, fairly improved. * $P < 0.05$; ** $P < 0.01$; *** $P < 0.001$.

TABLE 2. *Overall clinical improvement judged by committee members (trial B)*

Drug	No. of cases	Overall clinical improvement[a]					Improvement rate (%)		Statistical analysis[a]	
		M	I	F	Unchanged	Undecided	M + I	M + I + F	U	χ^2
APPC	53	18	29	2	3	1	88.7	92.5	***	+ (M) *** (M + I) ** (M + I + F)
SBPC	55	10	16	10	18	1	47.3	65.5		

[a] M, Markedly improved; I, improved; F, fairly improved. + $P < 0.1$; ** $P < 0.01$; *** $P < 0.001$.

fense, discharge, and body temperature in trial B, APPC was significantly superior to SBPC in most of the areas.

Side effects and abnormalities of laboratory findings were more frequently observed in the SBPC group than in the APPC group. A total of 3 of the 136 cases in the APPC group and 18 of the 134 cases in the SBPC group were evaluated as having side effects. Thus, a significant difference was found between the two drug groups. However, each incidence of side effects or laboratory abnormalities was not significantly different between the two drug groups, except that elevated GPT was found significantly more frequently in the SBPC group.

From the results, it is concluded that APPC is more useful against postoperative infections than SBPC at a dosage of one-fifth of that of SBPC.

1. **Noguchi, H., Y. Eda, H. Tobiki, T. Nakagome, and T. Komatsu.** 1976. PC-904, a novel broad-spectrum semisynthetic penicillin with marked antipseudomonal activity: microbiological evaluation. Antimicrob. Agents Chemother. **9:**262–273.
2. **Komatsu, T.** 1975. PC-904, a new semi-synthetic penicillin: *in vitro* and *in vivo* activities. Abstr. no. 257, 15th Interscience Conference on Antimicrobial Agents and Chemotherapy. American Society for Microbiology, Washington, D.C.

Septicemia After Gastroenterological Surgery

KYUYA ISHIBIKI,* NAOKI AIKAWA, TETSURO KUBOTA, MUNEHIKO NAKADA, HIROSHI TAKAMI, AND OSAHIKO ABE

Department of Surgery, School of Medicine, Keio University, Tokyo, Japan

Septicemia is still one of the most fatal complications after gastroenterological surgery. In this study, 50 cases of postoperative septicemia with clinical signs and symptoms were studied to analyze causative organisms and their antibiotic susceptibility patterns and to evaluate the clinical effect of chemotherapy.

Fifty cases of septicemia with positive blood culture after gastroenterological surgery consisted of 12 cases of esophageal, 21 cases of gastroduodenal, 5 cases of small and large intestinal, 10 cases of hepatobiliary, and 2 cases of other surgeries. Their ages ranged from 40 to 79 years, there were 40 males and 10 females, and surgery occurred from August 1975 to December 1979.

The total number of isolates from postoperative septicemias was 87 strains. They mainly consisted of *Klebsiella* (24.1%), *Pseudomonas* (12.6%), *Bacteroides* (12.6%), *Enterobacter*

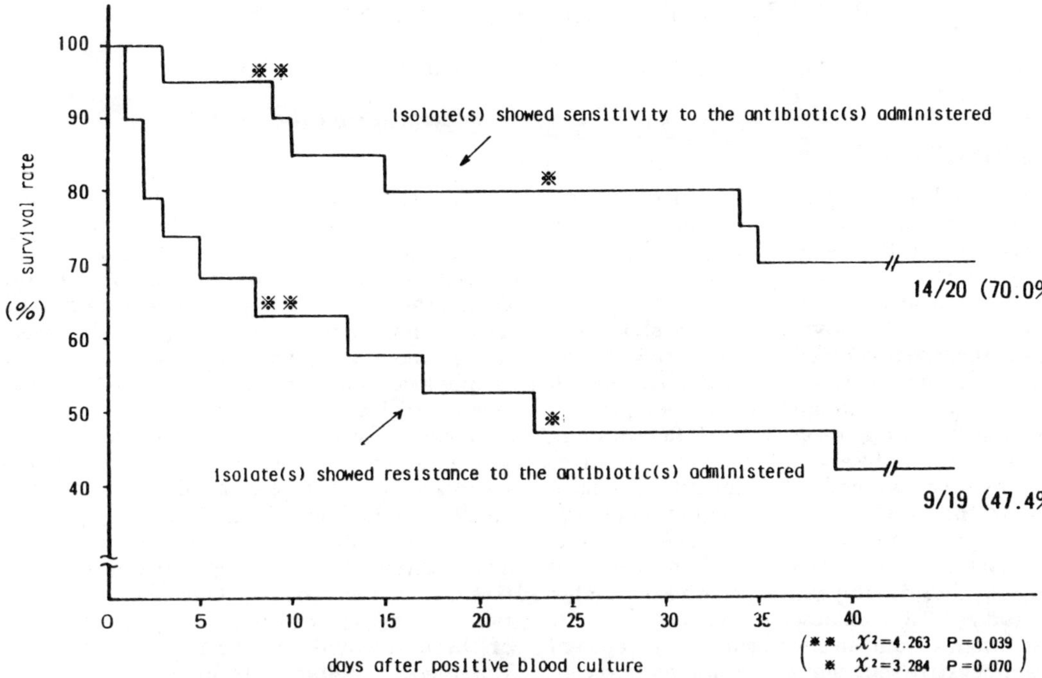

FIG. 1. *Survival curves of septicemia after gastroenterological surgery.*

(9.2%), *Serratia* (9.2%), *Candida* (6.9%), and *Staphylococcus aureus* (5.7%). Staphylococci and streptococci were found most frequently in upper gastrointestinal tract surgery. *Klebsiella* was isolated most often in biliary tract surgery. *Bacteroides* was revealed in surgery of both the lower and upper gastrointestinal tract. These data showed the close relationship between the causative organism and the bacterial population in the resident flora of each digestive organ. *Candida* was found in cases of long-term indwelling intravenous catheter for intravenous hyperalimentation.

Out of 50 cases, 29 (58%) developed septic shock and 20 died. The mortality rate of 69% in septic shock was significantly higher than that of 29% in nonshock patients ($P < 0.005$). The overall mortality rate was 52%. *Klebsiella, Enterobacter, Escherichia coli, Serratia,* and *Bacteroides* were isolated in patients who developed septic shock within 30 postoperative days, whereas *Pseudomonas aeruginosa, S. aureus,* and *Candida* were distributed widely throughout the postoperative period in patients with positive blood culture and septic shock. From the clinical standpoint, it should be noticed that stomal leakage and failure of drainage may contribute to the development of postoperative septicemia, in addition to the characteristic pathogenicity of the causative organism.

The susceptibility to antibiotics of isolates from the septicemias was lower than that of strains from other surgical infections. Susceptibility of causative organism, except for *Candida*, to given antibiotic(s) during 3 days after positive blood culture influenced significantly the prognosis of septicemia after gastoenterological surgery. Thirty-nine cases in which the isolate was tested for susceptibility to given antibiotic(s) by the one-disk method were found susceptible; whereas 3 cases of *Candida* and 11 cases of unknown disk susceptibility, because of new antibiotics, were divided into two groups of susceptible and resistant organisms. Survival curve of the resistant group showed a steep decrease within 5 days after positive blood culture. On day 8, the survival rate of 95% in the susceptible group was significantly higher than that of 63% found in the resistant group. Final survival rates in the susceptible and resistant groups were 70.0 and 47.4%, respectively (Fig. 1). It was concluded from these results that antibiotic chemotherapy should be effective in controlling postoperative septicemia when the antibiotic(s) is selected according to the susceptibility of the causative organism(s).

Septicemias 1979: A Prospective One-Year Study of 220 Patients

C.-M. WARNS,* B. FANGMANN, J. WAGNER, AND H. LODE

Klinikum Steglitz, Medical Department, Free University of Berlin, Berlin, Federal Republic of Germany

The etiology and pathogenesis of septicemia have undergone a clear change since the introduction of antibiotics. Streptococci of group A and pneumococci of the preantibiotic era are now increasingly replaced by gram-negative pathogens and staphylococci. This shifting of the pathogen spectrum is related to the advancing age of our patients as well as to the greater number of risk patients with severe primary diseases. More aggressive types of therapy offer, even to primarily apathogenic germs such as *Staphylococcus epidermidis*, an entrance pathway to the cardiovascular system by implantation of foreign bodies. Further, frequent nonspecific application of antibiotics in clinics leads to the selection of highly resistant germs. A number of studies (2, 3) conducted in the past few years have pointed out an increasing significance of gram-negative septicemias. Several more recent investigations (1, 4), however, emphasize the importance of gram-positive pathogens, especially in connection with nosocomial infections. The present study was done to clarify to what extent this development is applicable to our clinic, a university clinic with 2,200 beds and 13 different departments.

We defined septicemia as a general infection with cultural germ detection in blood cultures. In addition, we applied clinical criteria for a septicemia, such as temperatures above 38.5°C, chills, somnolence, renal failure, shock, embolism phenomena, consumption coagulopathy, predisposing primary diseases, or an initial focus with identical germ detection.

In the year 1979 we registered 220 patients with septicemias, some prospectively and some retrospectively. Gram-positive (n = 103) and gram-negative (n = 99) organisms were found with equal frequency in the positive blood cultures. There was a polymicrobial infection in 14 cases and a fungus infection in 4. In the gram-positive cultures, *Staphylococcus aureus* predominated (over 50%), followed by enterococci in 16% (Table 1). The greatest fraction of the gram-negative cultures consisted of *Escherichia coli* with 50% and *Klebsiella* with 15% (Table 2). Staphylococci, enterococci, and *E. coli* were mainly involved in the 14 polymicrobial infections.

In our group of patients, 73 patients did not have a severe primary disease. The others had malignomas, hematological primary diseases, hepatic cirrhosis, or diabetes mellitus. Twenty-three patients were under cytostatic or immunosuppressive therapy. The most frequent initial focus of a sepsis was the urogenital tract (57 cases), the predominant organism being *E. coli*. Twenty-four postoperative septicemias were mainly induced by enterococci and *S. aureus*. Staphylococci were primarily involved in septicemias originating from foreign bodies, such as pacemakers, venous catheters, bladder catheters, or synthetic prostheses: we found staphylococci in 25 of the 33 clinically confirmed foreign-body infections. The majority of all patients (119) came from the Medical Department. Only 30% of these developed a septicemia during hospitalization (nosocomial). One-third of all patients were from the Surgical Department; 95% of these acquired the sepsis in the hospital. Enterococci predominated in nosocomial septicemias in the Surgical Department. Striking was the fact that, of the total of 21 patients with clinically confirmed enterococci in the blood—including the enterococci in polymicrobial infections—13 of the 14 surgical and 2 of the 7 internal patients had been treated with cefazolin or cefamandole before the septicemia started. It must remain open to what extent a role is played here by a selection mechanism through the enterococcus gap of the cephalosporins. Streptococci, pneumococci, *E. coli*, and *Klebsiella* were most frequently isolated among septicemias acquired outside the hospital.

The total lethality of the septicemias amounted to 74 of 220 patients (33%). The lethality was highest for the gram-positive and polymicrobial infections. The high lethality in the gram-positive septicemias was connected

TABLE 1. *Occurrence of organisms in gram-positive septicemias (n = 103)*

Pathogen	No. of isolates
Staphylococcus aureus	50
Staphylococcus epidermidis	18
Streptococci	25
Group A	2
Group B	3
Group viridans	3
Group anhemolyticus	1
Enterococci	16
Streptococcus pneumoniae	6
Anaerobic *Corynebacterium*	4

TABLE 2. *Occurrence of various organisms in gram-negative septicemias (n = 99)*

Pathogen	No. of isolates
Escherichia coli	50
Klebsiella pneumoniae	15
Proteus mirabilis	6
Proteus morganii	3
Salmonella B	7
Salmonella typhi	1
Bacteroides spp.	3
Bacteroides fragilis	3
Pseudomonas aeruginosa	4
Enterobacter cloacae	2
Enterobacter hafniae	1
Enterobacter agglomerans	1
Citrobacter	1
Acitrobacter	1
Haemophilus influenzae	1

with the high staphylococcus lethality of 40% and that of the pneumococci of 84%. In this connection, it should be taken into consideration that 32 of the 50 patients with a staphylococcus septicemia had a severe primary disease and 5 of the 6 patients with a pneumococcus septicemia were over 80 years of age.

The results of this 1-year study in 220 patients with septicemias show an increased predominance of gram-positive germs, particularly *S. aureus* and *S. epidermidis* as well as enterococci, which particularly occur as nosocomial pathogens. The dominance of gram-positive germs in hospital infections should definitely be taken into consideration in the initial treatment of septicemias when the pathogen has not yet been isolated.

1. **Daschner, F.** 1981. Krankenhausinfektionen in einem Universitätsklinikum. Dtsch. Med. Wschr. **106**:101–105.
2. **Finland, M., and M. W. Barnes.** 1978. Bacteriemic superinfections of patients with bacteriemia: occurrence, bacteriology, mortality, and duration of hospitalization at Boston City Hospital during 12 selected years between 1935 and 1972. J. Infect. Dis. **138**:829–836.
3. **McGowan, J. E., M. W. Barnes, and M. Finland.** 1975. Bacteriemia at Boston City Hospital: occurrence and mortality during 12 selected years (1935–1972), with special reference to hospital-acquired cases. J. Infect. Dis. **132**:316–335.
4. **Spengler, R. F., W. B. Greenough III, and P. D. Stolley.** 1978. A descriptive study of nosocomial bacteriemias at the Johns Hopkins Hospital, 1968–1974. Johns Hopkins Med. J. **142**:77–84.

Combined Initial Treatment with Amikacin and Cephalothin or Ampicillin for Febrile Neutropenic Patients with Hematological Malignancies

JAN PALMBLAD* AND BERIT LÖNNQVIST

Department of Medicine, Karolinska Institutet at Södersjukhuset, and Huddinge Hospital, Section of Clinical Haematology and Oncology, Stockholm, Sweden*

Antimicrobial therapy for infections in neutropenic cancer patients must be instituted promptly, since these infections are associated with a high initial mortality. Hence, a prospective, randomized trial protocol was adopted to study (i) present types of infections occurring in neutropenic patients with hematological malignancy in Stockholm, Sweden, and (ii) the comparative efficacy and toxicity of amikacin plus ampicillin or cephalothin in these patients. Between 1977 and 1979, all patients with a malignant hematological disease, granulocytopenia ($<10^9$ neutrophils per liter), and fever (temperature $> 38°C$) were included in the study. After cultures from blood, urine, and clinically relevant sites, serum for antibody assessments, and chest X-ray and audiograms were obtained, patients were randomly given either amikacin (0.5 g twice daily) plus ampicillin (2 g four times daily) or amikacin (as above) plus cephalothin (2 g four times daily). This initial therapy was continued for at least 7 days. If no or susceptible organisms had been isolated but the patient had not improved after therapy for 72 h or 7 days, respectively, optional drugs could be added. Drugs were administered until the patient had been afebrile for 5 days.

Each febrile episode and the response to therapy were classified according to the EORTC (1) as a microbiologically documented infection, a clinically documented infection, or fever of unknown origin. Antibiotic response was classified as improvement, temporary improvement, failure, or not evaluable.

Statistical analyses were performed with Fisher's exact test.

During 43 episodes of fever, 33 patients were randomized, and 39 of these febrile episodes

TABLE 1. *Pathogens isolated from microbiologically documented infections*

Organism	No. of isolates from episodes treated with:				Total
	Amikacin + ampicillin		Amikacin + cephalothin		
	With bacteremia	Without bacteremia	With bacteremia	Without bacteremia	
Staphylococcus aureus	1 (1)[a]	3[b]	1 (1)	4 (2)[c,d]	9
Escherichia coli	2 (1)[a]			1	3
Pseudomonas aeruginosa	1 (1)			2 (2)	3
Proteus sp.		1		1 (1)[c]	2
Haemophilus parainfluenzae				1	1
Klebsiella sp.			1		1
β-Hemolytic streptococci group A		1		1[d]	2
γ-Hemolytic streptococci			1 (1)		1
Bacillus cereus	1				1
Candida albicans		1 (1)[b]			1

[a] Combined *S. aureus* and *E. coli* bacteremia. Number in parentheses denotes cases in which therapy failed.
[b] Combined *S. aureus* and *C. albicans* infection.
[c] Combined *S. aureus* and *Proteus* infection.
[d] Combined *S. aureus* and β-hemolytic streptococcal infection.

could be evaluated for response to therapy. Patients were equally distributed between the two antibiotic regimen groups with regard to degree of neutropenia, age, sex, and hematological disease. Of the fever episodes, 18% were due to a bacteremia, 36% were otherwise microbiologically documented, 41% were clinically documented, and only 5% were fevers of unknown origin.

The microorganisms isolated are listed in Table 1. The majority of infections were localized to the lungs (43%), the skin (36%), or the oral cavity (33%). No bacteremia with unknown primary site was noted, and no perianal infections were noted either. Two sites were infected simultaneously in 11 episodes. In 24% of the pneumonias, this primary site served as the source for a bacteremia. Similarly, bacteremia occurred in 14% of the skin infections and in 38% of the oral cavity infections.

The results of the response to antibiotic treatment are given in Table 2, where it will be seen that the combination of amikacin plus ampicillin was associated with a nonsignificantly ($P > 0.05$) higher rate of successful responses than the combination of amikacin plus cephalothin. The efficacy of the therapy was similar (65%) whether or not B-neutrophil counts changed (which occurred for a similar proportion of patients in both regimen groups), and the two antibiotic combinations did not differ in this respect.

Serial audiograms were normal in all but two patients, who showed slight high-frequency hearing loss.

The incidences of hypokalemia were 15%, of renal dysfunction (serum creatinine > 110 μmol/liter or a rise >50% of the initial value), 17%, and of thrombophlebitis, 10%, and results were similar for both antibiotic regimens.

TABLE 2. *Response to treatment: number of episodes*

Response	No. of patients with response		Total (%)
	Amikacin + ampicillin	Amikacin + cephalothin	
Improvement	14	11	64
Failure	4	9	33
Not evaluable	1		3
Total	19[a]	20[b]	100

[a] Two patients died from their infections during therapy, and three more died after discontinuation of therapy because of a second infection, a hepatic failure, and a hemorrhage.
[b] Two patients died from cerebral hemorrhage during therapy, and three more patients after discontinuation of antibiotic therapy for the same reason, with no signs of persistent infection.

No bacterial strain was resistant to both antibiotics in the combination, and in 10 strains, resistance to one of the actual antibiotics was noted. Failure of therapy was equally frequent whether both or only one antibiotic in the actual combination was appropriate, according to this susceptibility testing.

Serum levels of amikacin were measured on 49 occasions. The peak levels were above the recommended level (35 μg/ml) in six cases and below that level (10 μg/ml) in one case. The 12-h value, i.e., prior to administration, was higher than recommended (10 μg/ml) in none. Changes of the amikacin dosage were undertaken in two episodes.

In this study, *Staphylococcus aureus* was the most common single bacteria among patients with hematological malignancies in Stockholm. The incidence of *Pseudomonas* infections was low in comparison with figures from many other countries. In accordance with previous studies, we found no infections caused by anaerobic bacteria and a low frequency of *Pneumocystis carinii* and *Candida* infections. It was possible to document infections as the cause of fever in the great majority of the patients. The initial antibiotic therapy was effective in most fever episodes. There was no significant difference between the two combinations. Amikacin has been found in this study to represent an easily administered aminoglycoside, since the standard dosage gave appropriate serum levels in most cases and the dosage seldom required alteration.

1. **EORTC International Antimicrobial Therapy Project Group.** 1978. Three antibiotic regimens in the treatment of infection in febrile granulocytopenic patients with cancer. J. Infect. Dis. **137:**14–29.

Infections Complicating Leukemia and Malignant Lymphoma

Y. UEDA,* H. OKUBO, Y. OKAMOTO, AND K. MAEHARA

First Department of Internal Medicine, Kansai Medical University, Osaka, Japan

In step with the recent progress made in the therapy of leukemia and malignant lymphoma, including such improved measures against bleeding as platelet transfusion, the incidence of complicating infections in these diseases has increased, and the opportunistic pathogens of these infections have become quite diverse (3). We have examined the features of complicating infections occurring in all of the patients with acute leukemia, malignant lymphoma, and adult T cell malignancy treated in our Department of Internal Medicine from 1975 to 1980.

We listed 96 cases of hematological malignancies, including lymphomas: 26 cases of acute myelocytic leukemia, 9 cases of acute lymphocytic leukemia, 13 cases of acute monocytic leukemia, 7 cases of acute promyelocytic leukemia, 1 case of acute erythroblastic leukemia, 6 cases of blast crisis of chronic myelocytic leukemia, 24 cases of malignant lymphoma, and 10 cases of adult T cell leukemia-lymphoma.

The disease represented here as adult T cell leukemia-lymphoma is a peculiar subtype of chronic lymphocytic leukemia with lymphoma of the T cell type in Japan (4).

If mild infections of the skin, the soft tissues, and the oral cavity were included, the presence of infections of some sort could be observed in almost every case. However, summed up here are febrile episodes over 38°C and with durations of over 48 h, exclusive of fevers alleviated by steroid therapy or fevers induced by blood transfusion or by therapeutic drugs. The febrile episodes in question were found in 76% of the acute leukemia cases, 58% of the malignant lymphoma cases, and 70% of the adult T cell leukemia-lymphoma cases.

The most frequent infectious disease in the fever episodes was pneumonia, i.e., 39.2% in acute leukemia, 38.6% in malignant lymphoma, and 70% in adult T cell leukemia-lymphoma. In the acute leukemia cases, the frequencies of septicemia and abscess followed that of pneumonia: septicemia, 15.2%; abscess, 8%. On the other hand, fever of unknown origin was also frequently observed, totaling about 30% of the fever episodes, most of which should be attributed to septicemia, despite the fact that repeated blood cultures failed to detect the presence of pathogens.

In almost all of the septicemia cases complicating acute leukemia, granulocytopenia of less than 500 neutrophils per mm^3 was found on day 1 of the febrile episodes (1). The neutrophil count recovered in concomitance with cure of the septicemia. Similar tendencies, although less significant, were also seen in pneumonia and fever of unknown origin in cases of acute leukemia.

In contrast, in the abscess cases complicating acute leukemia, and in infections complicating malignant lymphoma or adult T cell leukemia-lymphoma, granulocytopenia was mostly not significant on day 1 of the fever. Therefore, triggers for these infections other than granulocytopenia should be considered, such as oppression by lymphoma or soft tissue damage by bleeding.

The isolated organisms were mostly gram-negative rods, 76.6% of the total. Among them, the most frequent species isolated were *Pseudomonas aeruginosa, Klebsiella* sp., and *Escherichia coli*, totaling 64.8%. However, infections by fungi, *Pneumocystis carinii*, or *Cytomegalo-*

virus sp. have recently been increasing (2). Infections by *P. carinii* and by *Cytomegalovirus* sp. were found in T cell malignancy cases among those examined and were found to be related to lymphocytopenia rather than to granulocytopenia.

Direct causes of death were examined. In the acute leukemia cases, the percentage of bleeding was about 21%, that of infection was about 34%, and that of bleeding with infection was about 39%; i.e., over 70% of the fatal causes in those patients were related to the complicating infections. In the malignant lymphoma cases, about 33% of the fatalities were attributed to infections, and in the adult T cell leukemia-lymphoma cases, about 63% were attributed to infections.

When the numbers of cases and the numbers of fatalities were itemized according to kind of infection, 40% died of septicemia, and 21% died of pneumonia. Pneumonia followed by septicemia proved to be about 90% fatal. The fatality rate of pneumonia in adult T cell leukemia-lymphoma was as high as 70%.

When infectious foci or organisms were plural, the fatality rate became remarkably elevated. If the number of infectious foci or the number of organisms were more than three, the fatality rate was 100%.

As mentioned above, infectious diseases were very often found in the leukemia and lymphoma cases. In these cases, infections may occur during any stage of the disease, but those occurring in the patients who show no response to the therapy for their underlying diseases have the most bitter prognosis. As for these cases, the early detection of infectious foci and organisms is imperative for successful treatment.

This means that primary efforts must be made in detecting foci and organisms. After obtaining specimens for appropriate cultures, broad-spectrum combined antibiotic therapy should be immediately commenced. In our own department, for example, frequent use is made of penicillins with aminoglycosides or cephalosporins with aminoglycosides.

During these treatments, care should be taken regarding the substitution of pathogens: in other research, we found that the pathogens are often replaced by *Klebsiella* sp. after failure of penicillin administration combined with aminoglycosides and by *P. aeruginosa* after failure of cephalosporin administration combined with aminoglycosides.

On the other hand, such supportive therapeutic measures as isolation in a bio-clean room and regimens for improving the general condition of patients to prevent anemia, bleeding tendency, hypoproteinemia, dehydration, etc., are also important in the treatment of those patients with opportunistic infections.

1. **Bodey, G. P., et al.** 1978. Fever and infection in leukemia patients—a study of 494 consecutive patients. Cancer **41:**1610–1622.
2. **Fujii, H., Y. Yoshida, T. Ikai, K. Ogino, S. Takeuchi, and M. Yamada.** 1979. A study of 14 cases with Pneumocystis carinii infection accompanied with hematopoietic disorders. Jpn. J. Clin. Hematol. **20:**15–24.
3. **Takenaka, T., M. Shimoyama, K. Minato, T. Kitahara, T. Sakano, C. Konda, and K. Kimura.** 1979. Clinical study of septicemia in patients with leukemia and its antibiotic therapy. Jpn. J. Clin. Hematol. **20:** 261–267.
4. **Uchiyama, T., K. Takatsuki, J. Yodoi, K. Sagawa, and H. Uchino.** 1977. Adult T cell leukemia: clinical and hematological features of 16 cases. Blood **50:**481–492.

Febrile Episodes in Neutropenic Hosts: Comparative Efficacy of Carbenicillin/Gentamicin Versus Azlocillin/Cefoxitin

H. GIAMARELLOU,* P. TAPRATZI, A. SAHIN, B. SEITANIDES, A. KATRAHOURA, AND G. K. DAIKOS

*Metaxas Memorial Hospital of Piraeus, Piraeus 30, and First Department of Propedeutic Medicine, Athens University School of Medicine, King Paul's Hospital, Athens 609, Greece**

Today it has become a rule to treat febrile granulocytopenic episodes in compromised hosts empirically with a combination of broad-spectrum antibiotics while waiting for the results of cultures. No one combination has yet been acknowledged to be the most efficacious, although it is believed that carbenicillin should always be part of any such antibiotic regimen (1).

This study reports preliminary results of response to therapy in 52 granulocytopenic patients allocated on a random basis to two separate antibiotic regimens: carbenicillin plus gentamicin or azlocillin plus cefoxitin. The study has been scheduled to finally include 80 patients, 40 in each group; therefore, it is still in progress.

Granulocytopenia was defined as less than

1,000 circulating granulocytes per mm^3. Material from blood, throat, tracheal secretions, and sputum in the presence of pulmonary infiltrates, urine, stool, and rectal swabs were routinely cultured by conventional methods before antibiotics were started. Before treatment was started and during and on the last day of treatment, hematology, liver, and renal toxicity tests as well as a complete investigation for bleeding disorders were performed.

A total of 23 patients, 13 male and 10 female, with a mean age of 54 ± 15.8 years, were given carbenicillin (5 g, 0.5-h infusion, every 4 h) plus gentamicin (1.5 mg/kg every 8 h, intravenously), and 29 patients, 17 male and 12 female, with a mean age of 51.2 ± 20.3 years, were given azlocillin (5 g, 0.5-h infusion, every 6 h) plus cefoxitin (2 g, 0.5-h infusion, every 6 h) at separate time intervals. Underlying diseases included the following in the respective groups: acute non-lymphocytic leukemia in 9 versus 11 patients, acute lymphocytic leukemia in 4 versus 5, non-Hodgkin lymphoma in 7 versus 5, Hodgkin lymphoma in 1 versus 3, chronic myelocytic leukemia in 1 versus 2, and preleukemia in 2 patients of the second group.

The distribution of infections is shown in Table 1. Clinical presentation of infection was rather poor, with physical findings of exudate, fluctuation, ulceration, local heat, swelling, dysuria and frequency, cough, sputum production and purulence, as well as rales and signs of pulmonary consolidation being encountered in only a minority of patients, as has also been pointed out by Sickles et al. (5).

TABLE 1. *Distribution of infection in 52 neutropenic patients treated either with gentamicin plus carbenicillin (23) or azlocillin plus cefoxitin (29).*

Type of infection	No. of infections	
	Gentamicin + carbenicillin	Azlocillin + cefoxitin
Pneumonia	12 (3)[a]	12 (5)[a]
Urinary	7 (6)[a]	8 (7)[a]
Pharyngitis	5 (2)[a]	5 (5)[a]
Soft tissue	1	3
Anorectal	1	3
Septicemia	2 (2)[a]	
Total	28[b] (13)[a]	31[b] (17)[a]

[a] Bacteriological confirmation.
[b] Double infections in seven patients.

Predominant isolates in cultures included *Escherichia coli* (9), *Klebsiella pneumoniae* (9), *Pseudomonas aeruginosa* (5), *Streptococcus pneumoniae* (4), *Staphylococcus aureus* (1), *Enterococcus* sp. (1), and indole-positive *Proteus* (1). Therefore, a total of 30 microorganisms were isolated from 13 and 17 patients in each group, respectively, and another 15 and 14 infections in each group (10 of which were in the first group and 4 of which were in the second) constituted double coexisting infections in five and two patients, respectively. Treatment would be discontinued if patients did not respond after at least 96 h of treatment, whereas if they responded, antibiotics were stopped at least 48 h after the granulocytes were considered adequate (≥1,000/mm^3).

Clinical response data are shown in Table 2. Statistical analysis by the χ^2 test of the results obtained did not prove any statistically significant difference in the cure rate or number of failures between the two groups. Also, considering the promptness of therapeutic response, no difference was observed in favor of one of the two therapeutic regimens. However, it should be pointed out that a successful response to antibiotics was closely correlated with an increase in the absolute number of granulocytes, since about 75% of the observed treatment failures occurred when the granulocyte number was <100/mm^3, whereas only 3 patients out of the 38 who responded successfully had such a low number of granulocytes. This critical point has also been stressed by several investigators (3, 4), also indicating the need for granulocyte transfusions in the nonresponders.

Among patients who ultimately failed to respond, in five of the gentamicin group and two of the azlocillin group anaerobes, which had not been initially isolated in cultures, should have been implicated, since all seven cases responded successfully thereafter to the administration of

TABLE 2. *Clinical response in 52 neutropenic patients treated with either gentamicin plus carbenicillin (23) or azlocillin plus cefoxitin (20)*

Combination	Clinical response				
	Cure		Improvement (no.)	Failure	
	No.	%		No.	%
Gentamicin + carbenicillin	11 (5)[a]	47.8 (45.5)[a]	2	10 (6)[a]	43.4 (54.5)[a]
Azlocillin + cefoxitin	15 (7)[a]	51.1 (63.6)[a]	3 (1)[a]	11 (3)[a]	37.9 (27.3)[a]

[a] Bacteriological confirmation.

clindamycin. The remaining seven failures finally responded to different antibiotic regimens which included amikacin. On the other hand, the successful response excluded the possibility of viral diseases while confirming the existence of bacterial infections in all 14 patients in whom treatment failed regardless of the administered antibiotic combination.

Considering side effects, six patients in the first group, versus one in the second, developed severe hypokalemia, in one patient in the gentamicin group serum creatinine increased to abnormal levels, and twice in the azlocillin group diffuse maculopapular rash forced the discontinuation of the combination.

Although from the results reported herein it is clear that the response rate for the antibiotic regimens was similar, the less frequent occurrence of hypokalemia in the second group, as well as the probability of covering more anaerobes by cefoxitin administration while escaping the possibility of gentamicin nephrotoxicity, should be in favor of the combination of azlocillin plus cefoxitin. On the other hand, since treatment in febrile granulocytopenic patients should always be started empirically, the high percentage of resistance among *P. aeruginosa* strains (2) to both gentamicin and carbenicillin (50 and 80%, respectively) constitutes a strong indication in favor of the combination of azlocillin plus cefoxitin. However, the in vitro observation that cefoxitin, by β-lactamase induction in *P. aeruginosa* strains, could antagonize azlocillin should be kept in mind, although such an effect has not been confirmed in the present series (Giamarellou et al., this volume).

1. **Bodey, G. P., M. Buckley, Y. S. Sathe, and E. J. Freireich.** 1966. Quantitative relationships between circulating leukocytes and infection in patients with acute leukemia. Ann. Intern. Med. **64:**328–340.
2. **Daikos, G. K., H. Giamarellou, R. Hadjipolydorou, and K. Kanellakopoulou.** 1980. In vitro and in vivo activity of azlocillin against *Pseudomonas aeruginosa*, p. 626–628. *In.* W. Siegenthaler and R. Lüthy (ed.), Current chemotherapy, vol. 1. American Society for Microbiology, Washington, D.C.
3. **Lank, B., A. R. Ronald, G. K. M. Harding, and D. W. Mecullough.** 1978. Granulocytopenia in hospitalized patients. Part II. Am. J. Med. **64:**127–132.
4. **Schimpff, S. C.** 1977. Therapy of infection in patients with granulocytopenia. Med. Clin. N. Am. **61:**1101–1118.
5. **Sickles, E. A., W. H. Greene, and P. H. Wiernik.** 1975. Clinical presentation of infection in granulocytopenic patients. Arch. Intern. Med. **135:**715–719.

Moxalactam Therapy of Anaerobic Infections in Cancer Patients

HJALMAR LAGAST, PHILIPPE VAN DER AUWERA, FRANÇOISE MEUNIER-CARPENTIER, MARIO CRUCIANI, AND JEAN KLASTERSKY*

Department of Medicine, Institut Jules Bordet, Université Libre de Bruxelles, Bruxelles, Belgium

We report here our experience with moxalactam therapy of anaerobic infections in cancer patients. This compound has a broad spectrum of activity which includes aerobic gram-negative bacilli and anaerobes, including *Bacteroides fragilis* spp. It is less active on gram-positive cocci and is inactive on enterococci (2).

Anaerobic infections in cancer patients are frequently mixed aerobic and anaerobic infections, as shown by Klastersky et al. (1), with aerobic gram-negative bacilli being the most frequently isolated pathogens. Moxalactam, with its broad spectrum, seemed to us an appropriate therapy for these infections.

Twenty-three patients with cancer entered this open study. There were 15 men and 8 women with a median age of 58 years. Head and neck cancer (eight patients) along with colorectal cancer (four patients) accounted for half of the underlying cancers.

Clinical sites of infection were divided into four main types: ulcerated tumor, 10 patients; abscess, 5 patients; laryngotracheitis, 4 patients; and pulmonary infection, 3 patients.

Fever was of rather low grade; only 7 of 23 patients had fever above 38.5°C before therapy. All of the patients presented foul smell of the infected focus. Only 9 of 23 patients had leukocytosis above 12,000/μl. Two patients were neutropenic (acute leukemia), and 2 were leukopenic (chemotherapy).

The initial bacteriological specimens allowed the isolation of 62 pathogens. Forty-two could be tested for susceptibility to moxalactam, and seven of these were resistant by either disk sensitivity or minimal inhibitory concentration. Aerobic pathogens were associated with the offending anaerobes in 12 of the 23 infections. Aerobic gram-negative bacilli were present in 9 of the 12 cases.

TABLE 1. *Outcome of anaerobic infections treated with moxalactam*

Infection	Success[a]	Recurrence	Failure
Pure anaerobic	9	1	1
Mixed	9	1	2

[a] A 78% total success rate.

Table 1 shows the outcome of the anaerobic infections treated with moxalactam. There was no difference in outcome between pure anaerobic and mixed infections. The overall cure rate was 78%.

The pathogen of both recurrences was *Bacteroides melaninogenicus*, and relapse occurred rapidly after withdrawal of moxalactam.

The three failures had each a different cause. One was due to superinfection with *B. fragilis*, *Clostridium* sp., and aerobic gram-negative bacilli resistant to moxalactam. Another patient died from massive hemoptysis due, probably, to involvement of a major artery by a mediastinal abscess. The last one developed a pure anaerobic cerebral abscess from an otitis media. He died, with sterile cerebrospinal fluid after 16 days of moxalactam therapy. At the autopsy, pus remained at the floor of the temporal lobe and inadequate surgical drainage was likely responsible for the failure.

At the end of the moxalactam therapy, bacteriological specimens showed the presence of aerobic pathogens at the infected focus in six patients. One of these patients failed, and another one had a recurrence. Reversible side effects of moxalactam without its withdrawal included a rash in one patient, one episode of diarrhea, and two patients with elevation of alkaline phosphatase levels. One patient developed an important elevation of alkaline phosphatase (eight times the upper limit of normal values), gamma glutamyltransferase, and bilirubin levels. Moxalactam was withdrawn, and abnormal values returned to normal within 3 weeks.

Moxalactam, with its broad spectrum, proved to be very effective therapy against anaerobic and mixed infections in cancer patients. Aerobic superinfection was scarce. Comparative studies are needed to investigate whether antiaerobic therapy is essential in mixed infections.

1. **Klastersky, J., J. Coppens, and G. Mombelli.** 1979. Anaerobic infections in cancer patients: comparative evaluation of clindamycin and cefoxitin. Antimicrob. Agents Chemother. **16:**366–371.
2. **Reimer, L. G., S. Minett, and L. B. Reller.** 1980. Comparison of in vitro activity of moxalactam with cefazolin, amikacin, tobramycin, carbenicillin, piperacillin, and ticarcillin against 420 blood culture isolates. Antimicrob. Agents Chemother. **17:**412–416.

Moxalactam Therapy of Serious Nosocomial *Serratia* Infections in Patients with Neoplastic Disease

ARTHUR E. BROWN,* OFELIA QUESADA, AND DONALD ARMSTRONG

Memorial Sloan-Kettering Cancer Center, New York, New York 10021, U.S.A.

Hospital-related infections are often caused by resistant bacteria and cause significant morbidity and mortality in patients with neoplastic diseases. We recently reported a gradual increase in the recovery of aminoglycoside-resistant gram-negative bacilli, all capable of multiplying and surviving in water and appearing most frequently on a 42-bed pediatric unit at Memorial Sloan-Kettering Cancer Center. (A. Blevins, T. Kiehn, G. Bell, A. Brown, and D. Armstrong, Abstr. Annu. Meet. Am. Soc. Microbiol. 1981, L18, p. 81). From June 1978 through June 1981, aminoglycoside-resistant *Serratia* species were isolated from one or more sites in 64 pediatric patients.

Moxalactam, a semisynthetic beta-lactam antibiotic, has an extended antibacterial spectrum which includes *Serratia* species (3, 4, 6, 7). In March 1980, an investigational protocol to study the efficacy and safety of moxalactam was begun at Memorial Sloan-Kettering Cancer Center. This is a report of the results of moxalactam therapy of patients with serious nosocomial *Serratia* infections from March 1980 through June 1981.

Patients were chosen for moxalactam therapy if they had a positive culture for *Serratia* species. Moxalactam was given at doses of 200 mg/kg per day intravenously every 8 h (maximum: 12 g/day). Aminoglycoside antibiotics were continued when patients were already receiving them. Aminoglycoside doses were adjusted according to aminoglycoside serum concentrations determined by radioimmunoassay. Cultures and laboratory parameters were obtained before, during, and after moxalactam therapy. Antimicrobial susceptibility of bacterial isolates was determined initially by standardized disk-diffusion methods (1), and MICs were subsequently determined by broth dilution with microtiter techniques (2, 5). Patient outcome was evaluated as either a success or a failure. The outcome was a success if the patient became afebrile, signs of infection cleared, and follow-up cultures demonstrated eradication of *Serratia* species. The outcome was regarded as a failure if the signs of infection persisted and/or follow-up cultures remained positive for *Serratia* species.

MICs (Table 1) of 23 *Serratia marcescens* isolates and one *Serratia liquifaciens* isolate revealed that all were susceptible to moxalactam. Four of 24 *Serratia* isolates were susceptible to gentamicin, 5 of 24 to tobramycin, and 11 of 24 to amikacin. In addition, 10 of 24 *Serratia* isolates were moderately susceptible to amikacin.

Twenty-three patients had 24 *Serratia* infections. There were 18 males and 5 females; 20 were children and 3 were adults. Underlying diseases were: nine with leukemia; two with aplastic anemia; three with lymphoma; and nine with solid tumors. Two-thirds of the patients had an absolute granulocyte count <1,000/mm^3 when moxalactam was started. The median duration of moxalactam therapy was 14 days.

Nineteen of 24 (79.2%) infections due to *Serratia* species were successfully treated. Six of seven (85.7%) urinary tract infections were successfully treated with moxalactam alone. Of 12 *S. marcescens* septicemias, 10 (83.3%) were successfully treated with moxalactam and an aminoglycoside. Three of five (60.0%) *S. marcescens* infections involving cultures of two respiratory sites, two wounds, and one stool were successfully treated with moxalactam with or without an aminoglycoside. Whereas the *S. marcescens* isolated from stool in pure culture while the patient was on other antibiotics after gut sterilization may have represented recolonization after bone marrow transplantation, the child's clinical response after eradication of *Serratia* bacteria from the stool cultures suggested that he had been infected.

TABLE 1. *MICs*

Antibiotic	MICs (μg/ml)		
	MIC$_{50}$[a]	MIC$_{90}$[a]	Range
Moxalactam	8	16	0.125–16
Gentamicin	>16	>16	0.5–>16
Tobramycin	>16	>16	1.0–>16
Amikacin	16	32	2.0–64

[a] Concentrations at which 50 and 90% of the *Serratia* isolates were inhibited, respectively.

There were five failures. Moxalactam-susceptible *S. marcescens* was recovered from the urine from a 12-year-old boy with acute myelogenous leukemia and neutropenia after receiving moxalactam alone for 3 days. Moxalactam was discontinued, amikacin was started, and the organism was eradicated.

S. marcescens (moxalactam MIC = 0.25 μg/ml) was isolated from the endotracheal aspirate of a 67-year-old man with adenocarcinoma of the stomach and pneumonitis while on amikacin. Moxalactam was added, and he died 12 days later. A moxalactam-resistant *S. marcescens* (MIC = 128 μg/ml) was recovered from the postmortem blood culture.

A 1-year-old boy with neuroblastoma and severe combined immunodeficiency disease had pharyngitis due to *S. marcescens*. Although the *Serratia* infection was cleared after 8 days of moxalactam therapy, *S. marcescens* recurred in the respiratory site and a wound site 7 days after moxalactam was stopped. He was successfully retreated with moxalactam and amikacin. Whether this was indeed a failure of treatment or a reinfection cannot be determined with certainty.

S. marcescens sepsis and meningitis occurred in a 12-year-old boy with acute lymphoblastic leukemia and neutropenia while he was receiving ampicillin and gentamicin. The antibiotics were changed to moxalactam alone. *S. marcescens* was recovered 24 h later from cerebrospinal fluid. Amikacin was added. Cerebrospinal fluid cultures were persistently positive for *S. marcescens*, and he died.

A 9-year-old boy with aplastic anemia and neutropenia had positive blood cultures for *S. marcescens* while on antibiotics. All antibiotics were stopped except for amikacin, and moxalactam was added. He initially responded, but subsequently died due to *Aspergillus* pneumonitis. While the initial blood culture isolate of *S. marcescens* was susceptible to 8 μg of moxalactam per ml, a highly resistant *S. marcescens* strain (moxalactam MIC > 1,024 μg/ml) was isolated from the blood at autopsy.

Toxicity and side effects were limited to a prolonged prothrombin time in 6 of 24 cases. All six cases had clinical evidence of bleeding. Although there were seven episodes of bleeding, in no cases could hemorrhage be attributed to moxalactam alone, as all seven were thrombocytopenic due to their underlying disease or their chemotherapy or both. Six of those with bleed-

TABLE 2. *Superinfections*

Case no.	Site(s)	Organism(s)	Moxalactam resistance	Outcome
17	Blood	*S. sanguis* II	Yes	Died with fungemia
	Blood	*T. glabrata*		
24	Urine	*P. putida*	Yes	Cleared spontaneously without treatment
83	Blood (autopsy)	*S. faecium*	Yes	Died with fungemia
		C. difficile	Yes	
		C. tropicalis		
106	Blood	*Corynebacterium* species CDC group JK	Yes	Died of fungal pneumonitis
	Lung (autopsy)	*Aspergillus* species		

ing had evidence of partial or complete disseminated intravascular coagulopathy.

Superinfections occurred in four patients (Table 2). Among bacterial isolates, moxalactam-resistant *Streptococcus sanguis* II, *Streptococcus faecium*, *Clostridium difficile*, and *Corynebacterium* species CDC group JK were isolated from the blood cultures of three different patients while they were receiving moxalactam or from autopsy blood specimens. Moxalactam-resistant *Pseudomonas putida* was isolated from the urine culture of a patient on day 12 of moxalactam therapy. This isolate cleared spontaneously without specific antimicrobial therapy. *Torulopsis glabrata* and *Candida tropicalis* fungemia occurred in two patients.

Moxalactam alone or in combination with an aminoglycoside appears to be safe and effective in the treatment of serious nosocomial *Serratia* infections in patients with neoplastic diseases and deserves further investigation. Resistant *S. marcescens* developed during therapy in two cases.

1. **Bauer, A. W., W. M. M. Kirby, J. C. Sherris, and M. Turck.** 1966. Antibiotic susceptibility testing by a standardized single disc method. Am. J. Clin. Pathol. **45:** 493–496.
2. **Ericcson, H. M., and J. C. Sherris.** 1971. Antibiotic sensitivity testing: report of an international collaborative study. Acta Path. Microbiol. Scand. Suppl. Sect. B. **217:**1–90.
3. **Fass, R. J.** 1979. In vitro activity of LY127935. Antimicrob. Agents Chemother. **16:**503–509.
4. **Flournoy, D. J., and F. A. Perryman.** 1979. LY127935, a new beta-lactam antibiotic, versus *Proteus, Klebsiella, Serratia*, and *Pseudomonas*. Antimicrob. Agents Chemother. **16:**641–643.
5. **Harwick, H. S., P. Weiss, and F. R. Fekety, Jr.** 1968. Application of microtitration techniques to bacteriostatic and bactericidal antibiotic susceptibility testing. J. Lab. Clin. Med. **72:**511–516.
6. **Jones, R. N., P. C. Fuchs, H. M. Sommers, T. L. Gavan, A. L. Barry, and E. H. Gerlach.** 1980. Moxalactam (LY127935), a new semisynthetic 1-oxabetalactam antibiotic with remarkable antimicrobial activity: in vitro comparison with cefamandole and tobramycin. Antimicrob. Agents Chemother. **17:**750–756.
7. **Jorgensen, J. H., S. A. Crawford, and G. A. Alexander.** 1980. In vitro activities of moxalactam and cefotaxime against aerobic gram-negative bacilli. Antimicrob. Agents Chemother. **17:**937–942.

Clinical Trials of Antibiotic Prophylaxis in Colorectal Surgery

M. R. SERTOLI,* F. CAFIERO, E. CAMPORA, E. PARODI, R. ROSSO, AND E. BERTI-RIBOLI

Istituto di Oncologia, Università di Genova, Istituto Scientifico per lo Studio e la Cura dei Tumori, and I Clinica Chirurgica, Università di Genova, Genova, Italy*

A high incidence of postoperative infections complicates colorectal surgery. Infections specifically related to this kind of surgery are principally of endogenous origin and are frequently caused by either direct contamination of the surgical field or dissemination from a postoperative anastomotic dehiscence. Both anaerobic and aerobic bacteria are responsible, and the most frequent wound isolates are *Bacteroides fragilis* and *Escherichia coli*, respectively. Various attempts have been made to decrease postoperative infections by reducing the endoluminal bacterial pool. The basic approach, mechanical bowel preparation, eliminating gross feces, reduces the total amount of bacteria but does not decrease endoluminal bacterial concentration. Antibiotic prophylaxis with drugs effective against both aerobic and anaerobic flora is therefore indispensable, as previous controlled studies have demonstrated.

Three successive randomized studies of prophylactic antibiotic treatment for elective colon surgery have been carried out. The first trial compared erythromycin and neomycin (E-N) given orally with the same preparation plus lincomycin to assess the eventual benefit of a systemic additive. Since the oral preparation was poorly tolerated, a second trial was started comparing E-N to cefoxitin given intravenously (i.v.). The two treatment regimens were found to be equally effective; therefore, a third trial was designed to identify the best short-term schedule for cefoxitin.

Only clinical evidence was used to classify patients as infected. Appropriate specimens were always collected when infection was clinically evident. The same mechanical bowel preparation was common to the three studies: preoperative days 5 and 4, residue-free diet; preoperative days 3 and 1, clear liquid diet; preoperative days 2 and 1, sennoside A and B calcium salts (150 mg orally at 8:00 a.m.), magnesium sulfate (15 g orally at 4:00 p.m.), hydration for the following 2 h (1 liter orally).

The E-N association was chosen for the first study since previous studies have proven it to be a successful prophylactic oral preparation able to reduce the intestinal bacterial pool, and consequently infections of an endogenous source (1). The aim of the study was to determine whether a systemic preoperative treatment given with lincomycin, whose MIC is active against 90% of anaerobic flora, was able to give added protection against eventual *B. fragilis* bacteremia. According to Clarke et al. (1), the E-N schedule was as follows: preoperative day 1, 1 g of E plus 1 g of N at 1:00, 2:00, and 11:00 p.m. Lincomycin, 1 g i.v., was added at random with premedication. Thirty successive, fairly comparable patients undergoing elective colon surgery were entered in the study over a 4-month period. The rates of complications directly related to surgery were comparable in the two groups (Table 1). Lincomycin was therefore not used further to avoid eventual aminoglycoside-linked complications such as pseudomembranous colitis.

Nausea and vomiting were frequent during E-N oral treatment, hampering drug absorption. Therefore, a second trial was started to evaluate whether cefoxitin administered i.v. exhibits a comparable effect. Cefoxitin, a cephamycin derivative, was chosen since its wider spectrum of activity includes both aerobic and anaerobic bacteria (3). Systemic treatment with cefoxitin was not meant to reduce the endogenous bacterial pool as with E-N but rather to create a plasmatic drug barrier against endoluminal spread. The aim of the study was to exclude any major therapeutic difference between the two. Over a 10-month period, 80 successive, fairly comparable patients undergoing elective surgery were entered in a randomized trial. The treatment plan was as follows: group A—oral E-N preparation according to the previous schedule; group B—cefoxitin, 2 g i.v., 1 h before surgery, at the end of surgery, and 10 h from the first dose. With the above cefoxitin schedule an active plasmatic peak is reached at surgery and maintained in the postoperative period. Septic complications directly related to colorectal surgery were not statistically different in the two groups: 12% in group A and 7.5% in group B. Overall, severe septic complications were only 3.75% (Table 2). It appears that perioperative systemic cefoxitin is as effective as preoperative oral E-N treatment, as other studies also suggest (2). On the other hand, cefoxitin has no appreciable side effects and it can be precisely administered. In addition, in emergency surgery, when oral treat-

TABLE 1. *Septic complications directly related to colorectal surgery*

Type of surgery	Treatment group	No. of patients	Wound infections	Intraperitoneal abscess and/or peritonitis	Septicemia	Death	Total septic patients
Extraperitoneal	E-N	3	0	0	0	0	0
	E-N-L[a]	2	0	0	0	0	0
Intraperitoneal	E-N	9	1	2	0	1	4
	E-N-L	9	0	0	1	0	1
A-P resections[b]	E-N	3	0	0	0	0	0
	E-N-L	4	0	0	0	0	0
Total	E-N	15	1	2	1	0	4
	E-N-L	15	0	0	1	0	1

[a] L, Lincomycin.
[b] A-P, Abdominal-perineal.

TABLE 2. *Septic complications directly related to colorectal operations*[a]

Type of surgery	Treatment group	No. of patients	Wound infection	Intraperitoneal abscess and/or peritonitis	Total septic patients (%)
Extraperitoneal	A	0	0	0	0
	B	2	0	0	0
Intraperitoneal	A	33	3	1	4 (12.1)
	B	32	1	2	3 (9.3)
A-P resections	A	7	1	0	1 (14.3)
	B	6	0	0	0
Total	A	40	4	1	5 (12)
	B	40	1	2	3 (7.5)[b]

[a] No septicemia or deaths were recorded.
[b] $P = 0.125$, chi-square test.

ment is impossible, i.v. cefoxitin could represent a valid alternative treatment.

At this point, the effectiveness of cefoxitin having been proven, a third study was undertaken to establish the most appropriate perioperative schedule. Seventy successive, comparable patients were given cefoxitin, either 2 g i.v. at 1 h before surgery, at the end of surgery, and at 10 h from the first administration or 2 g i.v. at 1 h before surgery, at the end of surgery, and then every 6 h for 24 h. Again, no statistically significant difference in sepsis rate was demonstrated in the two groups, 11.4 versus 8.5%, respectively. Since the two schedules gave similar results, either can be recommended as prophylactic treatment in elective colon surgery, even if pharmacokinetics suggest that the second schedule is preferable.

1. **Clark, J. S., R. E. Condon, J. G. Bartlett, S. L. Gorbach, R. L. Nichols, and S. Ochi.** 1977. Preoperative oral antibiotics reduce septic complications of colon operations: results of prospective, randomized, double-blind clinical study. Ann. Surg. **186:**251–259.
2. **Hoffmann, C. E. J., M. Reznikov, P. H. Hakendorf, P. J. McDonald, and J. M. Watts.** 1980. Short-course prophylaxis with cefoxitin in colorectal surgery, p. 1217–1218. *In* J. D. Nelson and C. Grassi (ed.), Current chemotherapy and infectious disease. American Society for Microbiology, Washington, D.C.
3. **Stapley, E. O., J. Birnbaum, A. K. Miller, H. Wallick, D. Hendlin, and H. B. Woodruff.** 1979. Cefoxitin and cephamycins: microbiological studies. Rev. Infect. Dis. **1:**73–87.

Comparative Evaluation of Antibiotic Prophylaxis and Surgical Techniques in Gunshot and Knife Wounds of the Colon

ASHIS K. MANDAL,* SISTER MARY ANN LOU, AND HARAGOPAL THADEPALLI

Departments of Surgery and Internal Medicine, Charles R. Drew Postgraduate Medical School, Martin Luther King, Jr. General Hospital, and the University of California at Los Angeles School of Medicine, Los Angeles, California 90059, U.S.A.*

Homicidal injuries usually are caused by knives and low-velocity handguns. Infection is the major threat to patients with colonic trauma. During the last decade, the mortality of patients with colon wounds ranged from 3 to 7%, compared to 60% during World War I and 37% during World War II (1). This retrospective study evaluates and compares the risks of infection in relation to the anatomical location of the colon injuries, the surgical techniques used to repair the perforation of the colon to prevent fecal contamination, and the groups of antibiotics administered.

Seventy consecutive patients with penetrating colon injuries were treated from March 1972 to June 1978 at Martin Luther King, Jr. General Hospital. Fifty-three of these patients suffered gunshot wounds, and the other 17 patients had stab wounds. Since no septic complications occurred in any of the 17 knifed victims, they have been excluded from this study. The other 53 patients were analyzed in detail. Of the 53 patients, 15 had injuries in the ascending colon, 16 had injuries in the transverse colon, and 22 had injuries in the descending colon. There were three types of surgical procedures used in the management of these colon injuries: primary repairs in 17 patients, primary repairs with loop exteriorizations in 21 patients, and colostomies in 15 patients.

All 53 gunshot victims received preoperative and postoperative antibiotics. Twenty-seven of these patients received 600 mg of intravenous clindamycin every 6 h and 80 mg of gentamicin every 8 h. Ten patients received a single drug, carbenicillin, 6 g intravenously every 6 h. Also, 16 patients received 3 g of intravenous cephalothin every 6 h and 500 mg of intramuscular kanamycin every 12 h. Aerobic and anaerobic cultures were obtained from the purulent exudates. The cultures for aerobes were processed by routine methods. The Virginia Polytechnic Institute method was used for the processing of anaerobic cultures (2).

The clinical outcome of these patients is shown in Fig. 1 and Table 1. Fourteen patients (26.4%) developed 16 serious infections. Six patients had gram-negative septicemia, and one (2%) died because of this infection. Two (13.3%) of the 15 patients with injuries in the ascending colon had infections. Two (12.5%) of the 16 injured in the transverse colon had infections. Furthermore, 10 (45.5%) of the 22 patients who suffered injuries in the descending colon developed septic complications. The difference between the right colon and the left colon was significant, $P < 0.01$.

Since the frequency of the infections was high in the descending colon, the 22 patients with

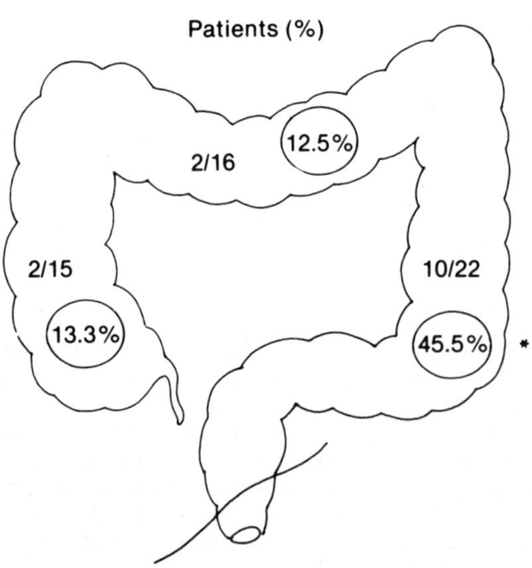

* P < 0.01

FIG. 1. *Gunshot wounds of colon: postoperative infections analyzed by site of injury.*

TABLE 1. *Large-bowel injuries: comparison of three antibiotic regimens*[a]

MECHANISM OF INJURY	ANTIBIOTIC THERAPY	Number Of Patients	DEEP INFECTIONS	
			Number of Patients	Percent Infected
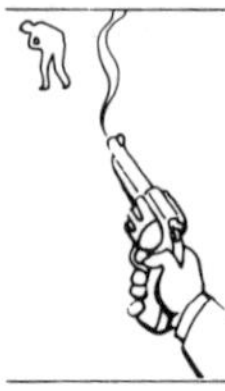	CLINDAMYCIN & GENTAMICIN	27	4	14.8
	CARBENICILLIN	10	2	20
	CEPHALOTHIN & KANAMYCIN	16	8	50 *

[a] *$P < 0.01$.

descending colon injuries were analyzed further by surgical procedures. Three (75%) of 4 patients with primary repairs, 4 (36.4%) of 11 patients with primary repairs and loop exteriorizations, and 3 (42.9%) of 7 patients with colostomies had septic complications. These differences were not statistically significant. When the three surgical procedures were used for the management of all 53 patients, it was found that infections occurred in seven (41%) primary repair patients, four (19%) primary repair and loop exteriorization patients, and three (20%) colostomy patients. Although there was a higher number of infections in patients who only had primary repairs, there were no statistical differences noted among the three surgical methods. The infections associated with clindamycin and gentamicin therapy, as well as with carbenicillin therapy, did not reveal any significant difference; however, patients under cephalothin and kanamycin therapy had a statistically significant difference, $P < 0.01$.

Twenty percent of fecal mass is composed of bacteria which are predominantly anaerobic microorganisms (3). The perforated colon immediately will contaminate the peritoneal cavity with its own microflora content and produce significant abdominal and distant metastatic infections with generalized sepsis. Hence, the risk of developing infectious complications from secondary colonic perforations is very high. To prevent such infections, antibiotics effective against anaerobes should be given preoperatively. Although no statistically significant difference was noted among the three types of surgical procedures, there seem to be appreciable numerical and clinical differences among these methods of repair. Primary repairs may be adequate for knife wounds. However, either primary repairs with loop exteriorizations or colostomies are preferred for gunshot wounds.

We thank Aloke Mandal for editing and preparation of this manuscript.

1. **Chilimidris, C., D. R. Boyd, L. E. Carlson, F. A. Folk, R. J. Baker, and R. J. Freeark.** 1971. A critical review of management of right colon injuries. J. Trauma **11:** 651–660.
2. **Holdeman, L. V., and W. E. C. Moore.** 1975. Anaerobic laboratory manual, 3rd ed., pp. 1–128. Virginia Polytechnic Institute and State University, Blacksburg.
3. **Thadepalli, H.** 1979. Principles and practice of antibiotic therapy for post traumatic abdominal injuries. Surg. Gynecol. Obstet. **148:**937–951.

Bacteriological Evaluation of Three Methods of Bowel Preparation for Elective Colorectal Surgery

A.E.J.M. VAN DEN BOGAARD,* W. J. WEIDEMA, M. J. HAZEN, AND R. I. C. WESDORP

Department of Medical Microbiology and Department of Surgery, State University of Limburg, 6200 MD Maastricht, The Netherlands*

The preparation of the gastrointestinal tract for elective colorectal surgery is still a controversial issue (2). The conventional preparation consists of dietary restriction, mechanical cleansing with cathartics and enemas, and often administration of antibiotics. In 1973 Cox et al. (1) described whole-gut irrigation (WGI) as an economic, rapid, and more efficient alternative method for mechanical cleansing of the bowel. With this method a nasogastric tube is passed into the stomach and an isotonic irrigation fluid is introduced through the tube (50 to 75 ml/min) while the patient is seated on a special toilet. WGI continues until the rectal fluid becomes clear. This takes about 10 to 20 liters of irrigation fluid over a period of 2 to 4 h.

To compare this new method with the conventional bowel preparation, a prospective randomized study was performed in three groups of patients. All patients eligible for elective colorectal surgery were included and divided randomly into three groups. The first group was prepared for 3 days by the conventional method and received 3 × 1 g of neomycin and 3 × 0.5 g of metronidazole on day 3. Group 2 was prepared by WGI, and group 3 was prepared by WGI with antibiotics (1 g of neomycin and 0.5 g of metronidazole per liter) added to the irrigation fluid. Only patients with a complete obstruction of the bowel and patients who had received antibiotics within 10 days before surgery were excluded from the trial.

Aerobic and anaerobic bacterial counts were performed by a decimal dilution method from fecal samples taken just before and immediately after bowel preparation and from bowel biopsies of the resected part of the colon. Bacteriological procedures and anaerobic incubation were performed in an anaerobic glovebox. The wounds were inspected for infection on days 3, 7, and 10 by the same surgeon, and other septic complications were monitored.

The reduction of the bacterial flora (Fig. 1) in the feces was significantly higher after WGI plus antibiotics than after conventional cleansing. WGI caused a higher reduction than conventional cleansing, but this was only significant for the aerobic flora. In four conventionally cleansed patients the total bacterial count per gram of feces was higher after preparation than before. The contaminating mass encountered during surgery was considerably lower in both irrigated groups. The bacterial anaerobic counts per gram of gut wall were significantly higher in group 2 (WGI) than in the two other groups of patients who had received antibiotics.

In group 1 ($n = 21$) there was only one patient with a rectum extirpation (Fig. 2). The three wound infections (14%) in this group were due to aerobic bacteria (coliforms). In group 2 ($n =$

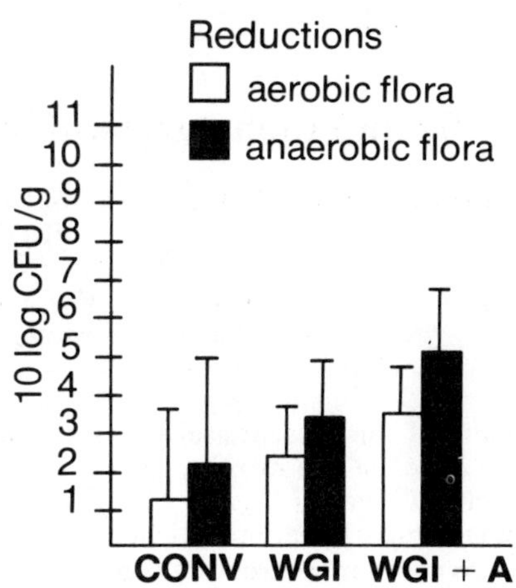

FIG. 1. *Reduction in colony counts in fecal samples taken before and after bowel preparation. Aerobic: WGI + antibiotics (A) > conventional (CONV), P = 0.04. Anaerobic: WGI + A > conventional, P = 0.0003; WGI + A > WGI, P = 0.03. CFU, Colony-forming units.*

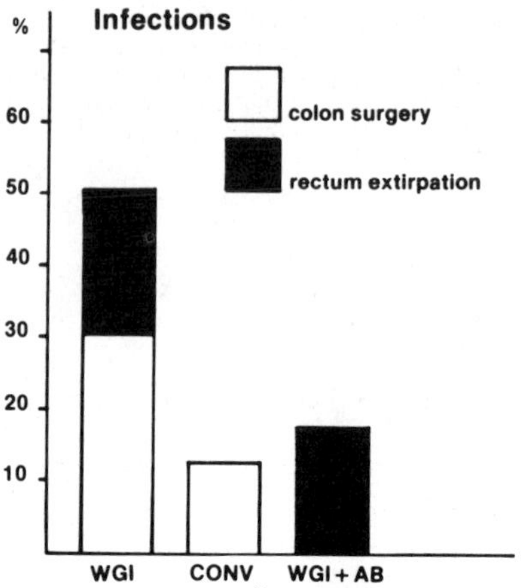

FIG. 2. *Infection rate with preparation by WGI, conventional, and WGI + antibiotics (WGI + AB). The infection rate in group 3 was negatively influenced by the high percentage of patients with a rectum extirpation compared with the conventionally prepared group (25 versus 5%).*

20) ten patients (50%) developed a wound infection, and anaerobic bacteria (*Bacteroides fragilis*) as well as aerobic microorganisms were isolated from all wounds. In group 3 ($n = 19$) no wound infections or other septic complications were observed in patients with colon surgery. Three of five patients with a rectum extirpation developed an infection of the perineal wound. Cultures of these wounds yielded only aerobic bacteria (coliforms, enterococci, and *Staphylococcus aureus*). The infection rate in this group was 16%.

The mortality which occurred in the three groups was, respectively, 0 (WGI + antibiotics), 4 (conventional), and 6 (WGI) patients. The hospital stay after surgery was also considerably shorter for the groups of patients who had received antibiotic prophylaxis (mean, 21 days) than for the WGI group (mean, 29 days).

WGI with or without antibiotics gave a significantly higher reduction of the bacterial flora than did conventional cleansing of the bowel. However, the reduction did not correlate with the wound infection rate. A low bacterial count per gram of gut wall (groups 1 and 3) seems to correlate better with the postoperative septic complication rate. The low bacterial counts in the biopsies were probably due to the administration of antibiotics. The mean serum levels of metronidazole during surgery, measured by high-performance liquid chromatography, had mean concentrations of 13.5 mg (group 1) and 18.7 mg (group 2) per liter. The concentrations were adequate to protect against anaerobic infections.

In conclusion, WGI is an excellent method for mechanical cleansing of the intestinal tract. If it is used to prepare patients for elective colorectal surgery, the preoperative administration of antibiotics is necessary.

1. **Cox, A. G., J. Hewitt, J. Rigby, and J. Reeve.** 1973. Whole gut irrigation in preparation for large bowel surgery. Lancet **ii:**337–340.
2. **Hirschmann, J. V., and T. S. Inui.** 1980. Antimicrobial prophylaxis: a critique of recent trials. Rev. Infect. Dis. **2:**1–23.

Short-Term Prophylaxis with Ornidazole in Elective Colorectal Surgery

ROAR HOEL,* AUD SALVESON, SVERRE REINERTSEN, CHRISTIAN NEESS, AND INGRID MATHESON

Department of Surgery, Central Hospital of Rogaland, and Microbiology Laboratory, 4000 Stavanger, and Department of Clinical Research, F. Hoffman-La Roche, Lilleaker, Oslo 2, Norway*

The aim of the present study was to investigate the effect of the nitroimidazole derivative ornidazole (Tiberal) used prophylactically against anaerobic infections in colonic and rectal surgery. We also measured the concentration of ornidazole in serum and bowel tissue in 10 patients.

The control group was given doxycycline according to the previous routine at the hospital and with the awareness of this drug's effect on both aerobic and anaerobic bacteria. One hundred consecutive patients requiring colonic or rectal surgery were admitted to the trial and randomly allocated into two groups receiving either ornidazole or doxycycline.

Ornidazole was given as an oral dose 24 h preoperatively and intravenously for the 3 following days, corresponding to 25 mg/kg of body weight daily. The doxycycline group received 200 mg perorally 24 h preoperatively and intravenously for the 3 following days.

Preoperative preparations, with bowel irrigation and dietary restrictions for 2 days, and the surgical technique were standardized, and a restricted number of surgeons participated.

All patients were evaluated daily during the hospital stay and finally after 1 month. All infectious complications were registered, and specimens for bacteriological examination were taken and forwarded to the laboratory under anaerobic conditions.

The concentrations of ornidazole in serum, bowel tissue, and subcutanous fat were assayed microbiologically in 10 patients 24 h after the first dose and in serum only after a further 2 days of medication.

No anaerobic infections were observed in the ornidazole group compared with five infections involving anaerobic bacteria in the doxycycline group (Table 1). The difference was statistically significant ($P < 0.05$, Fischer exact test). In the ornidazole group two strains of *Staphylococcus aureus* were isolated; the rest of the pathogens in this group consisted of various aerobic intestinal microbes. The pathogens in the doxycycline group included seven anaerobic strains, chiefly *Bacteroides*.

The majority of the infectious complications were uncomplicated wound infections not requiring additional antibiotics. With the exception of one anastomotic leakage, no serious complication occurred.

The serum and tissue concentrations measured in 10 patients after an ornidazole dose of 21.8 ± 2.7 mg/kg were as follows (mean ± SD): serum, 7.4 ± 1.4 μg/ml; subcutaneous fat, 4.7 ± 3.1 μg/ml; intestinal wall, 5.6 ± 3.7 μg/ml. The minimum steady-state plasma concentration was 12.6 ± 2.8 μg/ml. In vitro studies have shown ornidazole to be effective against anaerobic bacteria, with an MIC of 3.1 μg/ml (4, 7, 8). The serum levels in our patients exceeded the MIC 24 h after administration of the drug. Four patients had an inadequate drug level in subcutaneous fat, and three of these also had inadequate levels in the intestinal wall. However, the calculated mean values, as well as the median values, of tissue concentrations showed levels exceeding 3.1 μg/ml.

The mean half-life of ornidazole is 13.8 ± 1.8 h (3), and the drug level calculated from the second postoperative day should therefore indicate the minimum steady-state plasma concentration. All minimum steady-state plasma concentrations were above the accepted MIC for ornidazole.

No idiosyncratic reactions or side effects attributable to the drugs administered were seen during the observation period, and all laboratory tests were within the normal range.

TABLE 1. *Incidence of anaerobic and aerobic infections*

Type of infection	No. of infections	
	Ornidazole group ($n = 44$)	Doxycycline group ($n = 48$)
Anaerobic	0	3
Combined anaerobic-aerobic	0	2
Aerobic	11	4

This study demonstrates that ornidazole is effective in preventing anaerobic infections postoperatively, but does not prevent complications with aerobic pathogens. Other studies have pointed out that prophylaxis against anaerobes prevents the more severe postoperative complications, and our study confirms this observation (1, 6).

The serum concentrations measured at 24 h are in the same range as those found by Palmu et al. (4); however, they found a higher tissue concentration than we did. This indicates that the drug rapidly reaches the peripheral bowel compartment but may have attained its maximum level before the samples were taken. Ornidazole should therefore be administered at a time closer to the time of the operation. A dosage interval of 12 h seems satisfactory.

The complete absence of side effects is in contrast to other studies (2, 5), but may be explained partly by the patients' condition after the operation and partly by the effect of analgesics and sedatives given at the same time.

1. **Fiddian, R. V.** 1978. Prophylaxis in colonic surgery. J. Antimicrob. Chemother. **4**(Suppl. C):39–47.
2. **Goldring, J., A. Scott, W. McNaught, and G. Gillespie.** 1975. Prophylactic oral antimicrobial agents in elective colonic surgery. Lancet **ii**:997–999.
3. **Matheson, I., K. Hernborg Johannessen, and B. Bjørkvoll.** 1977. Plasma levels after a single oral dose of 1.5g ornidazole. Br. J. Vener. Dis. **53**:236–239.
4. **Palmu, A., O. V. Renkonen, and U. Aromaa.** 1979. Ornidazole and anaerobic bacteria: in vitro sensitivity and effects on wound infections after appendectomy. J. Infect. Dis. **139**:586–589.
5. **Tally, F. P., V. L. Sutter, and S. M. Finegold.** 1975. Treatment of anaerobic infections with metronidazole. Antimicrob. Agents Chemother. **7**:672–675.
6. **Willis, A. T., I. R. Ferguson, et al.** 1977. Metronidazole in prevention and treatment of Bacteroides infections in elective colonic surgery. Br. Med. J. **1**:607–610.
7. **Wise, R., J. M. Andrews, and K. A. Bedford.** 1977. The activity of four agents including three nitroimidazole compounds against Bacteroides sp. Chemotherapy (Basel) **23**:19–24.
8. **Wüst, J.** 1977. Susceptibility of anaerobic bacteria to metronidazole, ornidazole, and tinidazole and routine susceptibility testing by standardized methods. Antimicrob. Agents Chemother. **11**:631–637.

Infective Endocarditis: Ten Years of Experience in a German University Hospital

H. LODE,* C. M. WARNS, J. WAGNER, AND R. SCHRÖDER

Medical and Microbiological Departments, Klinikum Steglitz, Freie Universität Berlin, 1000 Berlin 45, Federal Republic of Germany*

Bouillaud (1) was the first to define, in 1841, the term endocarditis as "an exudative and proliferative phlogistic lesion of the valvular endothelium, in rare cases also of the parietal endocardium." Up to 1945, bacterial endocarditis practically always took a lethal course; this was fundamentally different after antibiotics had been introduced, which significantly improved the prognosis. Today, the frequently vague symptoms, the increased shifting of the bacterial spectrum from the gram-positive to the gram-negative range, the more frequently occurring connections with cardiosurgical interventions, dialysis treatment, drug abuse, and hospital infections, as well as the possibilities of the illness taking a severe course, are all reasons why infective endocarditis is still considered to be a disease with numerous diagnostic and therapeutic problems.

In a prospective study over 10 years (March 1971 to May 1981), the data of 92 patients (38 females, 54 males) between 19 and 79 years of age with 97 manifestations of endocarditis were collected uniformly on standardized investigation forms and then analyzed. All patients were observed for at least 8 weeks after conclusion of the therapy. Two negative blood cultures were considered to be a successful treatment up to this stage.

The most frequent general symptoms of the patients were: 86 occurrences (89%) of temperature of more than 38°C, 39 with simultaneous shivering attacks; 39 complaints of an increased tendency to sweat; 38 cases of weight loss; 38 mentions of decrease ~~in~~ vitality, tiredness, and fatigue; and 22 patients with nausea, loss of appetite, and arthritic complaints.

As clinical findings, we detected temperatures increasing to more than 38°C in 86 cases of illness (89%), signs of manifest cardiac insufficiency in 64 (66%), and cardiac murmurs in 95 (98%). Embolic phenomena and splenomegaly were also observed in 22 (23%) and 20 (21%) cases, respectively. The aortic valve was involved in 39 cases (24 insufficiencies, 1 stenosis, 8 combinations, 6 prostheses); the mitral valve, in 26 cases (10 insufficiencies, 6 stenoses, 7 combinations, 1 prosthesis); and both the aortic and mitral valves, in 15 cases. Ten cases were congenital vitia, 7 of which were ventrical septum defects, 1 tricuspidal atresia, and 1 cor triloculare monoventriculare.

The laboratory findings showed anemia (hemoglobin less than 12 g/100 ml) in 42 (44%) of the patients. A total of 80% of the patients had an accelerated blood sedimentation rate of more than 30 mmHg (ca. 2 kPa) in the first hour. We registered an increase of gamma globulin of more than 20% (relative) in 41% and a decrease of albumin concentration (<50% [relative]) in 34% of the patients. It was striking that an increase of leukocytes (>10,000/ml) or a deviation to the left (more than four stabs) occurred only in 44% of the patients. No patient with proof of gram-negative bacteria showed increased granulocytes.

Before therapy was initiated, three to six venous blood cultures were taken from our patients and prepared over a period of 8 to 10 days by aerobic and anaerobic culture procedures. In 75 (77%) cases, it was possible to secure bacteriologically at least two positive identical blood cultures. In 15 (16%) cases without positive bacteriology, a definite pathological-anatomical confirmation of infective endocarditis was achieved. The remaining 7 (8%) patients had the typical clinical symptoms, but, even after 12 blood cultures, it was not possible to isolate any germs. Five of these patients had been pretreated with antibiotics for several days by their family doctors.

A total of 82 different strains were isolated, 68 gram-positive germs with 39 hemolytic streptococci versus 14 gram-negative strains, as follows: 39 streptococci, 12 *Staphylococcus aureus*, 5 *S. epidermidis*, 11 enterococci, 6 *Escherichia coli*, 4 *Pseudomonas aeruginosa*, 3 *Klebsiella pneumoniae*, and 1 each *Alcaligenes faecalis* and *Erysipelothrix*, the latter two being rather unusual. When comparing our bacteriological findings with earlier information on bacterial distribution, the remarkable change of bacterial endocarditis becomes obvious. From 1946 to 1957 (4, 5, 7), only viridans streptococci and *Streptococcus faecalis* were detected, whereas between 1958 and 1967 Cherubin and Neu (3) in New

York isolated only 50% viridans streptococci. Of the 97 illnesses in 92 patients, 74 cases of endocarditis (all viridans streptococcal infections) could be treated successfully.

A total of 23 patients died; a postmortem examination was performed on all of them. Of the deaths, there were two early and one late endocarditis case with gram-negative bacteria after prosthetic replacement of the aortic valve, six staphylococcal endocarditis, and two *Pseudomonas* infections. The most frequent cause of death was irreversible cardiac insufficiency in 17 patients, which in 5 cases was not repairable even with acute replacement of the valve. The high death rate of 25% (23 of 92 patients) correlates exactly with numerical data from Zürich, New York, and Boston (3, 4, 7, 9) pertaining to the last 15 years. To increase the favorable outcome of endocarditis, some authors (2, 6, 8) recommend relatively early replacement of the infected aortic valve if a cardiac insufficiency develops, if arterial embolisms are manifest, and if the chemotherapeutic success is not sufficient.

1. **Bouillaud, B.** 1936. *In* C. B. Perry (ed.), Bacterial endocarditis, p. 3. Wright, Bristol.
2. **Buchbinder, N. H., and W. C. Roberts.** 1972. Left-sided valvular active infective endocarditis. Am. J. Med. **53:** 20–35.
3. **Cherubin, C. E., and H. C. Neu.** 1971. Infective endocarditis at the Presbyterian Hospital in New York City from 1938–1967. Am. J. Med. **51:**83–96.
4. **Finland, M., and M. W. Barnes.** 1970. Changing etiology of bacterial endocarditis in the antibacterial era. Ann. Intern. Med. **72:**341–348.
5. **Germer, W. D.** 1951. Endocarditis lenta. Ergeb. Inn. Med. Kinderheilkd. **2:**296–341.
6. **Lode, H., B. Behn, H. Langmaack, and R. Schröder.** 1977. Bakterielle Endokarditis. Dtsch. Med. Wochenschr. **102:**599–606.
7. **Nager, F., F. Urthaler, and M. Rothlin.** 1971. Der Wandel der infektiösen Endokarditis. Schweiz. Med. Wochenschr. **101:**105–109.
8. **Richardson, J. V., R. B. Karp, J. W. Kirklin, and W. E. Dismukes.** 1978. Treatment of infective endocarditis: a 10-year comparative analysis. Circulation **58:**589–597.
9. **von Reyn, C. F., B. S. Levy, R. D. Arbeit, G. F. Friedland, and C. S. Crumpacher.** 1981. Infective endocarditis: an analysis based on strict case definitions. Ann. Intern. Med. **94:**505–518.

Streptococcal Endocarditis: Single Versus Combination Therapy and Role of Various Species

CARMELITA U. TUAZON,* VEE GILL, AND FRED GILL

Division of Infectious Diseases, George Washington University Medical Center, Washington, D.C. 20037, and Department of Microbiology, National Institutes of Health, Bethesda, Maryland 20205, U.S.A.*

Streptococci are the most common cause of infective endocarditis, and those of the viridans group are the predominant isolates. Most recently, certain features of the disease have been emphasized, e.g., subgrouping of group D into enterococcal and non-enterococcal groups and its therapeutic implications, association of *Streptococcus bovis* with colonic carcinoma, significance of *S. mutans*, role of vitamin B_6-dependent strains, incubation period, and recommendations for prophylaxis. However, few studies have looked at the microbial characteristics and differences among infections caused by various species of the viridans streptococci. In addition, treatment of streptococcal endocarditis has remained controversial, with some groups favoring single therapy with penicillin and others preferring penicillin plus aminoglycoside.

Over the last 5 years (1975–1980), we accumulated 48 patients with 51 episodes of streptococcal endocarditis seen at the George Washington University Medical Center, Washington, D.C., and Suburban Hospital, Bethesda, Md. The hospital records of all of these patients were reviewed. Included in this group were 33 patients from George Washington University and 15 from Suburban Hospital.

Criteria for the diagnosis of endocarditis included the isolation of the same streptococcus from two or more blood cultures in patients either with or without underlying valvular disease and no obvious focus of infection elsewhere. In addition, patients with clinical illnesses consistent with endocarditis with no extracardiac focus of infection and isolation of streptococcus from a single blood culture and two or more peripheral signs of endocarditis and patients in whom diagnosis was confirmed at surgery or autopsy were also included.

Strains of streptococci isolated from blood cultures were identified by standard methods and serologically grouped. Hemolysis was determined by using sheep blood agar incubated anaerobically at 37°C. Beta-hemolytic streptococci were identified by precipitin grouping on isolates prior to 1978; thereafter, by latex agglutination.

Group D streptococci were identified to species by the following reactions: bile-esculin, arginine hydrolysis, growth at 45°C, growth in 6.5% NaCl, production of extracellular polysaccharide on 5% sucrose agar (mitis-salivarius agar), starch hydrolysis, and acid production from glucose, mannitol, lactose, sucrose, salicin, arabinose, glycerol, raffinose, sorbitol, and trehalose. Identification to species of non-group D alpha- and nonhemolytic streptococci was performed by using the above reactions in addition to acid production from inulin and also hydrolysis of esculin. Identification criteria of Facklam (Centers for Disease Control) were used for the group D streptococci. The MIC and MBC were determined in vitro by the microtiter broth dilution, using Trypticase soy broth (BBL Microbiology Systems) and an inoculum of 10^5 organisms. The maximum serum bactericidal titer in serum specimens obtained at or near the expected nadir of antibiotic concentration was determined by a serum dilution technique.

There was a male predominance, with 33 of 48 (69%) being males. The racial distribution of this group of patients was 35 whites and 13 blacks of 48 patients. The patients in this study ranged in age from 19 to 85 years (mean, 50 years).

Seven of 48 (15%) patients had definite history of rheumatic valvular disease. Fourteen of 48 (29%) patients were diagnosed as having valvular disease of nonrheumatic etiology: 7 with mitral regurgitation secondary to papillary muscle dysfunction or chorda tendinae rupture, 2 with bicuspid aortic valves, 2 with mitral valve prolapse, 1 with aortic insufficiency post-pneumococcal endocarditis, 1 with patent ductus arteriosus, and 1 with combined ventricular septal defect and aortic insufficiency. Three patients had murmurs with undefined anatomic abnormality. There were five drug users. Nineteen of 48 (40%) did not have any underlying disease.

Of the 24 patients with underlying valvular lesions or murmurs or both, only 6 had antecedent procedures which could be temporally related to the development of endocarditis. Two of six received penicillin prophylaxis before the procedures. One other patient received penicillin prophylaxis for a dental procedure after his initial episode of endocarditis.

Eighteen of the 48 patients received antibiotics before admission. Two patients received penicillin for rheumatic fever prophylaxis, and another two received it for dental procedures. The other patients received antibiotics for symptoms related to the endocarditis, and one patient received prophylaxis for a coronary bypass procedure. A wide variety of antibiotics were prescribed: penicillin (5), tetracycline (5), erythromycin (3), cephalosporins (3), and ampicillin (2). The MIC for isolates from four patients who received tetracycline was 8 μg/ml, that for one isolate from a patient treated with erythromycin was 8 μg/ml, and that for one isolate from a patient who received ampicillin was 2 μg/ml.

A total of 20 patients had had procedures, dental, endoscopic, or surgical, ranging from 1 week to 6 months before their hospitalization for infective endocarditis. Onset of symptoms in this group of patients varied from 10 days to 2 months. Fifteen patients had some type of dental procedure, e.g., dental capping, cleaning, filling, tooth extraction, cavity filling, dental work for bleeding, or root canal. Nondental procedures included two sigmoidoscopies, one barium enema, one coronary bypass procedure, and 1 surgery for a sex change.

Microbiological studies to look at the species and antibiotic susceptibilities were performed. There were a total of 52 isolates from 48 patients: 1 patient had 2 relapses, 1 patient had a reinfection, and another patient had 2 organisms isolated. Identification of the streptococcal isolates and susceptibility to penicillin are shown in Table 1. The majority of isolates, 35 of 48, were

TABLE 1. *Penicillin suscepticility of streptococcal isolates*

Streptococci	No. of isolates	MIC (μg/ml)
Oral		
S. sanguis II	11	≤0.05 (10) 1(1)
S. sanguis I	9	≤0.05 (7) 0.08 (2)
S. mitis	3	≤0.05
S. mutans	3	>6(1) <0.05 (2)
S. intermedius	2	0.06 <0.05
S. morbillorium	2	≤0.05
S. anginosus constellatus	1	0.05
α *Streptococcus* (not identified)	3	NA[a]
γ *Streptococcus* (not identified)	1	NA
Group D		
S. bovis	6	≤0.05
S. fecalis	2	0.8–1.0
S. faecium	1	<3≥60
Beta-hemolytic		
Group B	5	0.03–0.12
Group G	2	0.01–0.05
S. pneumoniae	1	ND[b]

[a] NA, Not available.
[b] ND, Not done.

alpha-hemolytic or nonhemolytic streptococci (oral streptococci), which were the most common in this group. Nine of the 52 isolates were group D streptococci, 3 enterococci and 6 were *S. bovis*; of the remaining isolates, 7 were beta-hemolytic streptococci of groups B and G. One case of *S. pneumoniae* endocarditis was encountered. Twenty-six of 31 isolates of oral streptococci had penicillin MICs of ≤0.05 μg/ml. Two *S. sanguis* biotype I isolates had penicillin MICs of 0.08 μg/ml. Only one isolate, an *S. mutans*, had an original penicillin MIC relatively resistant at >6 μg/ml. This result was obtained twice upon repeated testing of the isolate, but upon continued subculture of the organism this resistance was lost.

The three enterococcal group D steptococci had penicillin MICs of >0.5 μg/ml, as would be expected. Streptomycin susceptibilities of the enterococci showed a high level of resistance, >2,000 μg/ml. Six isolates of *S. bovis* were all susceptible to penicillin at <0.05 μg/ml.

Five group B streptococci had susceptibilities to penicillin of between 0.03 and 0.12 μg/ml, whereas two group G streptococci were extremely susceptible (MIC <0.05 μg/ml). One of the group B strains was resistant to erythromycin at 8 μg/ml.

Serum bactericidal levels were performed in 34 of 48 (71%) patients. A total of 88% of patients had levels of ≥1:8, and in 35% of patients the level was ≥1:128. There was no correlation between serum bactericidal concentration level and clinical course.

We looked at the efficacy of single versus combination therapy in 46 patients with 48 episodes of endocarditis. In the analyses of the treatment regimens, two patients were excluded (one patient with an *S. pneumoniae* isolate and another patient with an *S. fecalis* isolate since standard therapeutic regimens are recommended for these diseases). The other two enterococcal endocarditis cases were included since diagnosis was made retrospectively. Twenty-two episodes were treated with a single antibiotic and 26 episodes were treated with combination therapy for at least 1 week with an aminoglycoside. The two patient groups were comparable as to age, race, sex, mean duration of symptoms, and mean duration of fever after antibiotic therapy. Of the patients who received single antibiotic therapy, one had two episodes of relapse which subsequently responded to combination therapy. There was no statistical difference in the clinical course, toxicity, and mortality rate among patients on single and those on combination therapy.

There were six deaths in this series of patients. Two died of ruptured mycotic aneurysms, and two died after valvular replacements (one due to arrhythmia and the other to progressive congestive heart failure and severe coronary artery disease), and one died from severe congestive heart failure. The other death was due to gastrointestinal bleeding unrelated to endocarditis. Other complications seen were two mycotic aneurysms, two renal infarcts, and two multiple emboli. Eight patients had drug reactions in the form of eosinophilia, skin rash, and hemolytic anemia.

Viridans Streptococci with Reduced Bactericidal Susceptibility to Penicillin from Patients with Endocarditis: Susceptibilities to Erythromycin, Rifampin, Vancomycin, and Aminoglycosides

DAVID SHANSON* AND SIMON NAMNYAK

Department of Clinical Microbiology, St. Stephen's Hospital, Chelsea, London S.W. 10 9th, England

The use of bactericidal antibiotics is essential for the effective treatment of bacterial endocarditis. The majority of viridans streptococcus strains isolated from patients with endocarditis are susceptible to penicillin with an MIC of ≤0.1 mg/liter, and most strains are killed completely by 1.0 mg of penicillin per liter. However, an important minority of strains of viridans streptococci isolated from some patients with endocarditis are not killed by 1.0 mg of penicillin per liter (1, 3), and then an appropriate antibiotic combination is frequently required to obtain a complete bactericidal effect (2). Bactericidal synergy between penicillin and streptomycin against penicillin-susceptible strains of viridans streptococci has been previously reported (4), but there is a lack of published data about the effects of antibiotic combinations on relatively penicillin-resistant strains of viridans streptococci. The purpose of the present study was to test the susceptibilities of a selected group of viridans streptococcal strains, with a penicillin

MBC of >1.0 mg/liter, to penicillin, erythromycin, rifampin, vancomycin, streptomycin, and gentamicin by using each drug alone and in combination with another agent.

A total of 14 strains of viridans streptococci, isolated from the blood cultures of 14 patients with bacterial endocarditis, were selected for this study; these included 7 strains of *Streptococcus mitior*, 4 strains of *Streptococcus sanguis*, 2 strains of *Streptococcus salivarius*, and 1 strain of *Streptococcus mutans*. The MIC and MBC of each antibiotic for each strain were determined by the tube serum broth dilution technique, using an inoculum of approximately 10^6 colony-forming units per ml and Iso-Sensitest broth (Oxoid Ltd.) containing 25% serum. The broths were subcultured after overnight incubation onto blood agar, using a standard 10-μl loop. The endpoint for the MBC determinations and for the tests of the bactericidal effects of antibiotics in combination was taken as less than five colonies on the subculture plate. All of the antibiotic combination tests were carried out in serum Iso-Sensitest broth, using an inoculum similar to that described above.

The MICs of benzylpenicillin for 11 strains were ≤0.12 mg/liter, but the MBCs of penicillin were between 3.1 and >12.5 mg/liter for these strains. The MICs of penicillin for three other strains were 0.2 to 1.5 mg/liter, and the MBCs for these strains were >12.5 mg/liter. A reduced susceptibility to ampicillin and amoxicillin was also noted for all 14 strains; the MBCs of ampicillin and amoxicillin were 6.2 to >12.5 mg/liter and 1.6 to >12.5 mg/liter, respectively. As the ratio of MBC to MIC of a penicillin drug was always >26:1, these viridans streptococci behaved as "penicillin-tolerant" strains.

The MICs of streptomycin and gentamicin for the 14 streptococcal strains were 16 to >256 mg/liter and 4 to 64 mg/liter, respectively. At a concentration of 32 mg/liter, only 7% of the strains were killed by streptomycin, as compared with 57% killed by gentamicin. However, a bactericidal effect of gentamicin was demonstrable only in therapeutic concentrations when it was combined with another antibiotic.

A comparison of the MICs and MBCs of erythromycin, rifampin, and vancomycin for the 14 streptococcal strains is shown in Table 1. Erythromycin was the most active single bactericidal drug, with 50% of the strains killed by a concentration of 1.6 mg/liter, followed by rifampin, which killed only 14% of the strains at this concentration.

The results of antibiotic combination tests are shown in Table 2. Marked bactericidal synergy was demonstrated between benzylpenicillin and gentamicin for all 14 streptococcal strains. Erythromycin plus gentamicin was also effective in killing all 14 strains at concentrations which could easily be achieved in the serum after therapeutic doses. Bactericidal synergy was marked between erythromycin and rifampin for 13 of the strains tested, but one strain of *S. sanguis* grew after subculture even when concentrations of up to 3.0 mg of each drug per liter were combined in a full chessboard titration. Erythromycin plus rifampin was more frequently bactericidal than a combination of rifampin plus gentamicin. However, synergy was often demonstrable between rifampin and gentamicin or vancomycin. Four streptococcal strains that were not killed by a combination of rifampin and vancomycin were killed when the concentration of the antibiotics was increased to 10 mg of vancomycin per liter plus 2 mg of rifampin per liter. Bactericidal synergy was demonstrated between vancomycin plus gentamicin for just over half the strains when a low concentration of vancomycin was tested. Four streptococcal strains which survived this combination were tested again, using

TABLE 1. *Susceptibilities of 14 penicillin-tolerant strains of viridans streptococci to erythromycin, rifampin, and vancomycin*

Antibiotic	No. of strains susceptible to antibiotic at following concn (mg/liter):											
	<0.02	0.02	0.05	0.1	0.2	0.4	0.8	1.6	3.2	6.4	12.8	>12.8
Erythromycin												
MIC	6	1	3	—	1	1	1	—	—	—	—	1
MBC	—[a]	—	—	1	—	1	2	3	1	1	3	2
Rifampin												
MIC	1	—	1	1	5	6	—	—	—	—	—	—
MBC	—	—	—	—	—	1	—	1	1	2	7	2
Vancomycin												
MIC	—	—	—	—	—	5	6	3	—	—	—	—
MBC	—	—	—	—	—	—	—	—	—	—	2	12

[a] —, No strains.

TABLE 2. *Effects of antibiotic combinations on 14 penicillin-tolerant strains of S. viridans*

Antibiotic combination[a]	MBCs (mg/liter) each drug alone	Concn (mg/liter) of drugs tested in combination	No. of strains tested	No. (%) of strains killed by combination
P + G	P: 3.1 to >12.5 G: 8.0 to 250	P: 0.005 to 0.1 G: 1.0 to 2.0	14	14 (100)
E + G	E: 0.1 to >12.5 G: 8.0 to 250	E: 0.01 to 1.6 G: 2.0	14	14 (100)
E + R	E: 0.1 to >12.5 R: 0.4 to >12.5	E: 0.01 to 1.6 R: 0.05 to 0.4	14	13 (93)
R + G	R: 0.4 to >12.5 G: 8.0 to 250	R: 0.05 to 0.4 G: 2.0	14	10 (71)
R + V	R: 0.4 to >12.5 V: ≥12.5	R: 0.05 to 0.4 V: 0.8	14	10 (71)
E + V	E: 0.1 to >12.5 V: ≥12.5	E: 0.02 to 1.6 V: 0.8 to 3.1	14	8 (56)
V + G	V: ≥12.5 G: 8.0 to 250	V: 0.8 G: 2.0	14	8 (56)
V + S	V: ≥12.5 S: 32 to >250	V: 0.8 S: 2.0	14	4 (29)

[a] P, Penicillin; G, gentamicin; E, erythromycin; R, rifampin; V, vancomycin.

vancomycin at 10 mg/liter combined with gentamicin at 2.0 mg/liter, and all four strains were then completely killed. Vancomycin plus gentamicin was more frequently bactericidal than vancomycin plus streptomycin when equivalent concentrations were compared.

These results suggest that most viridans streptococcal strains with a reduced bactericidal susceptibility to penicillin, isolated from patients with endocarditis, are likely to be completely killed by therapeutic concentrations of antibiotics included in one of the following combinations: penicillin plus gentamicin, erythromycin plus gentamicin, erythromycin plus rifampin, or vancomycin plus gentamicin. Other combinations with rifampin plus vancomycin or rifampin plus gentamicin may also be effective, but it is important to carry out combination tests on each isolate. Erythromycin combined with gentamicin or rifampin should be especially considered when penicillin-tolerant strains of viridans streptococci are isolated from endocarditis patients with penicillin allergies.

1. **David, S.** 1979. Penicillin resistant streptococci. N. Engl. J. Med. **300**:500–501.
2. **Parrillo, J., G. C. Borst, M. H. Mazur, M. S. Klempner, R. C. Moellering, and S. E. Anderson.** 1979. Endocarditis due to resistant viridans streptococci during oral penicillin chemoprophylaxis. N. Engl. J. Med. **300**: 296–300.
3. **Pulliam, L., S. Inukuchi, W. K. Hadley, and J. Mills.** 1979. Penicillin tolerance in experimental streptococcal endocarditis. Lancet **ii**:957.
4. **Wolfe, J. C., and W. D. Johnson.** 1974. Penicillin sensitive streptococcal endocarditis. In vitro and clinical observation on penicillin-streptomycin therapy. Ann. Intern. Med. **81**:178–181.

Long-Term, Low-Dose, Thrice Weekly Prophylaxis with Trimethoprim-Sulfamethoxazole for Recurrent Urinary Infection in Females

GODFREY K. M. HARDING,* ALLAN R. RONALD, MARGARET J. THOMSON, AND GLORIA J. GRAY

Departments of Medicine and Medical Microbiology, University of Manitoba, and Infectious Diseases Section, Health Sciences Centre, Winnipeg, Manitoba, Canada R3E OW3

Reinfection by organisms from outside the urinary tract is the common reason for recurrence in females after a course of therapy. Antimicrobial prophylaxis has been shown to prevent these recurrences (2, 3, 5). In a previous controlled prospective study, we have shown that trimethoprim (TMP)-sulfamethoxazole in a dose of one-half tablet (40 mg of TMP and 200 mg of sulfamethoxazole) daily at bedtime is more effective than 500 mg of sulfamethoxazole daily at bedtime or 500 mg of methenamine mandelate four times daily together with 500 mg of ascorbic acid four times daily (3).

In subsequent studies, we determined that the minimum effective dose of TMP-sulfamethoxazole for prophylaxis in women is one-half regular-strength tablet thrice weekly (Sundays, Wednesdays, and Fridays) at bedtime (2). This regimen was more effective than one tablet of TMP-sulfamethoxazole once weekly or one-half tablet twice weekly (5). These studies demonstrated that prophylaxis for 3 to 6 months prevented recurrences throughout the course of therapy. Except for that by Pearson et al. (4), other studies of systemic antimicrobial prophylaxis in women have been for 6 months or less. In the present study, we continued prophylaxis for 2 years and carefully followed the periurethral and rectal flora as well as urine cultures of women treated prophylactically with TMP-sulfamethoxazole, one-half tablet three times weekly.

Thirteen adult females who had previously been treated for 6 months with one-half regular-strength tablet of TMP-sulfamethoxazole (TMP, 40 mg, and sulfamethoxazole, 200 mg) and whose infections had recurred within 6 months (2) were entered in the present study. Two preadolescent females who had received half the adult dosage were also enrolled in this study.

After the existing urinary tract infection was eradicated, the women received TMP (40 mg) in combination with sulfamethoxazole (200 mg) (one-half regular-strength tablet) thrice weekly (Sundays, Wednesdays, and Fridays) at bedtime. The two preadolescent females received one-quarter regular-strength tablet. Once started, the prophylactic regimen was to be continued for 24 months.

Patients were seen initially and at 3-month intervals during prophylaxis. On discontinuation of prophylaxis they were seen at 2, 4, 8, and 16 weeks and at 8-week intervals thereafter until recurrence or for 1 year. In addition, patients were interviewed and examined whenever they were symptomatic.

At each clinic visit, a periurethral swab, an anal canal swab, and a clean-voided midstream urine specimen were obtained as previously described (3, 5). At the initial visit and at the visits during prophylaxis, blood specimens were also obtained to monitor complete blood cell count, platelet count, and levels of serum glutamic oxaloacetic acid, serum alkaline phosphatase, serum bilirubin, blood urea nitrogen, and serum creatinine. Patients were also questioned regarding any urinary symptoms as well as compliance with and tolerance to the drug regimen during the preceding 3 months. Quantitative cultures were carried out on all isolates from periurethral and anal canal swabs and from urine specimens as previously described (3, 5). In this study no attempt was made to routinely distinguish *Staphylococcus epidermidis* from *Staphylococcus saprophyticus*.

All *Escherichia coli* isolated from urine specimens and the periurethral and anal canal cultures were biotyped with a nine-test system to aid in differentiating reinfection from relapse (1). A urinary tract infection was defined as bacteriuria of 10^5 or more organisms per ml when patients were symptomatic. Asymptomatic patients were required to have two separate urine specimens containing 10^5 or more of the same organism per ml.

Agar dilution MICs of TMP and sulfamethoxazole were obtained for all aerobic gram-negative bacilli isolated before and during prophylaxis from periurethral and anal canal cultures and on all urinary pathogens in significant counts isolated from urine specimens obtained before, during, and at the first recurrence after discontinuation of prophylaxis.

Fifteen female patients, including 13 women ranging in age from 20 to 73 years (mean, 49 years; median, 50 years) and two girls of ages 11 and 12, were entered in the study of 24-month prophylaxis. Of 15 intravenous urograms obtained, 12 were normal. In three, there was radiographic evidence of chronic pyelonephritis. The mean number of urinary tract infections occurring in these 15 patients during the year preceding entry into the initial 6-month prophylaxis study was 3.6. These 15 patients recurred within 6 months after discontinuation of the low-dose, thrice weekly, 6-month course of prophylaxis. The mean time to recurrence was 3.3 months after discontinuation of prophylaxis.

Potential aerobic gram-negative pathogens isolated from periurethral and anal canal cultures during prophylaxis are shown in Table 1. Of 116 periurethral cultures, 106 did not yield any aerobic gram-negative rods. The 10 positive cultures were obtained from five patients.

During prophylaxis, 66 of the 97 anal canal cultures failed to yeild aerobic gram-negative bacilli. In one patient the anal canal was simultaneously colonized with a *Klebsiella* sp. (MIC, 0.25 μg of TMP per ml) and a *Citrobacter* sp. (MIC, 8 μg of TMP per ml). The three strains of *Pseudomonas aeruginosa* were all from the same patient.

TABLE 1. *Antimicrobial susceptibility to TMP and sulfamethoxazole of potential aerobic gram-negative pathogens isolated from 116 periurethral and 97 anal canal cultures during prophylaxis*

Organism/susceptibility	No. of pathogens from: Periurethral cultures (n = 116)	Anal canal cultures (n = 97)
Escherichia coli	7	27
TMP susceptible	3	24
TMP resistant[a]	4	3
Sulfamethoxazole susceptible	0	0
Sulfamethoxazole resistant[b]	7	27
Other *Enterobacteriaceae*		2
TMP susceptible		1
TMP resistant[c]		1
Sulfamethoxazole susceptible		0
Sulfamethoxazole resistant[d]		2
Pseudomonas aeruginosa	3	3
TMP resistant[e]	3	3
Sulfamethoxazole resistant[b]	3	3

[a] MIC ⩾ 2 μg/ml (six strains from three patients, MIC of 2 μg/ml; one, MIC of 4 μg/ml).
[b] MIC > 512 μg/ml.
[c] MIC = 8 μg/ml.
[d] MIC ⩾ 32 μg/ml (one strain, MIC of 32 μg/ml; one, MIC of 128 μg/ml).
[e] MIC = 256 (all strains from the same patient).

TABLE 2. *Infecting pathogens isolated from urine cultures during prophylaxis and at the first recurrence after prophylaxis with thrice weekly TMP-sulfamethoxazole for 2 years and their antimicrobial susceptibility to TMP*

Organism[a]	No. isolated: During prophylaxis (n = 4)	At first recurrence (n = 8)
Escherichia coli	2[b]	5
Pseudomonas aeruginosa		1[c]
Streptococcus faecalis	1	
Streptococcus agalactiae		1
Staphylococcus epidermidis	1	
Staphylococcus aureus		1[d]

[a] MICs for *S. faecalis*, *S. agalactiae*, and *S. epidermidis* were ⩽1 μg of TMP per ml.
[b] One *E. coli* isolate had a TMP MIC of 2 μg/ml. All other *E. coli* isolates had TMP MICs of ⩽1.0 μg/ml.
[c] MIC of TMP = 256 μg/ml.
[d] MIC of TMP = 2 μg/ml.

The infecting urinary pathogens and their susceptibility to TMP isolated during prophylaxis and at the first recurrence of infection after prophylaxis are listed in Table 2. Four infections occurred during 29.1 cumulative patient years of prophylaxis, for a frequency of infection of 0.14 infection per patient year. The number of breakthrough infections was similar in both the first and second years of prophylaxis, suggesting that long-term prophylaxis will not increase the frequency or predispose patients to more resistant reinfections.

We have followed 13 patients until recurrence or for up to 1 year if they have remained infection-free after discontinuation of prophylaxis. Five patients have not recurred within 1 year of follow-up. These five patients also did not have any breakthrough infections during the 2 years of prophylaxis. Recurrences occurred in eight patients. The mean time to recurrence in these eight patients was 1.5 months. One patient became infected with a *P. aeruginosa* strain (MIC, 256 μg of TMP per ml). The other infecting strains had TMP MICs of ⩽1 μg/ml with the exception of one strain of *Staphylococcus aureus*, which had a TMP MIC of 2 μg/ml.

None of the 15 patients experienced any side effects during the thrice weekly period of prophylaxis. Hematological and biochemical parameters were not altered appreciably in any patient.

We concluded that prophylaxis with 40 mg of TMP and 200 mg of sulfamethoxazole, thrice weekly at bedtime, is an effective well-tolerated regimen which is able to maintain an infection-free state in women who have a history of multiple closely spaced episodes of infection. Until the biological defect that permits these recurrences is delineated or until other regimens are proven to be equally effective without predisposing to colonization or infection with resistant organisms, TMP-sulfamethoxazole in a low dose remains our prophylactic agent of choice.

1. **Buckwold, F. J., A. R. Ronald, G. K. M. Harding, T. J. Marrie, L. Fox, and C. Cates.** 1979. Biotyping of *Escherichia coli* by a simple multiple-inoculation agar plate technique. J. Clin. Microbiol. **10:**275–278.
2. **Harding, G. K. M., F. J. Buckwold, T. J. Marrie, L. Thompson, R. B. Light, and A. R. Ronald.** 1979. Prophylaxis of recurrent urinary tract infection in female patients. Efficacy of low-dose, thrice-weekly therapy with trimethoprim/sulfamethoxazole. J. Am. Med. Assoc. **242:**1975–1977.
3. **Harding, G. K. M., and A. R. Ronald.** 1974. A controlled study of antimicrobial prophylaxis of recurrent urinary infection in women. N. Engl. J. Med. **291:**597–601.
4. **Pearson, N. J., A. M. McSherry, K. J. Towner, and W. R. Cattell.** 1979. Emergence of trimethoprim-resistant enterobacteria in patients receiving long-term co-trimoxazole for the control of intractable urinary-tract infection. Lancet. **ii:**1205–1208.
5. **Ronald, A. R., G. K. M. Harding, R. Mathias, C. K. Wong, and P. Muir.** 1975. Prophylaxis of recurring urinary tract infection in females: a comparison of nitrofurantoin with trimethoprim-sulfamethoxazole. Can. Med. Assoc. J. **112** (Suppl.)**:**13–16.

Bacampicillin Twice a Day in Acute Exacerbations of Chronic Bronchitis

RUDOLF FERLINZ,* WOLFGANG MÜLLER, JOACHIM SCHÖNEN, AND KARL BARTMANN

Department of Pneumology, University of Mainz, and Laboratory-Department Clinic Aprath, Wülfrath, Federal Republic of Germany

Aminopenicillins have been used in dosage regimens of three to four times daily in the treatment of acute exacerbations of chronic bronchitis. Animal studies and clinical results indicate that a twice daily (b.i.d.) dosage regimen for bacampicillin can be recommended as an appropriate treatment (2, 4, 5). A decrease in the number of daily intakes might reduce dose-dependent side effects and result in better patient compliance.

In a randomized double-blind trial during 10 to 14 days, bacampicillin, 800 mg b.i.d., was compared with the established therapy of doxycycline in a starting dose of 200 mg on the 1st day followed by 100 mg once daily. Forty hospitalized patients suffering from acute exacerbations of chronic bronchitis caused by a bacterial infection were included. The bacterial etiology was judged by sputum purulence, bacteria in the sputum, or both. For bacterial and cytological determination (1), sputum was sent in special cooled boxes to the laboratory and analyzed by the method of Mulder (3). The progress of the therapy was judged daily according to sputum quantity and color, purulence, dyspnea, and wheezing. The final therapeutic effect was assessed on the 14th day after the start of therapy.

Before the antibiotic treatment was started, a probable causative pathogenic bacterium was isolated in 23 of the 40 patients. Nineteen (83%) patients carried *Haemophilus influenzae*; in two of these patients, *Staphylococcus aureus* also was found. Two patients carried only *S. aureus*, one carried *Branhamella catarrhalis*, and one likely had a *Pseudomonas aeruginosa* infection. Two patients were not included in the evaluation: one patient with *P. aeruginosa* treated with doxycyline and one patient without bacteriological findings treated with bacampicillin. According to clinical and bacteriological criteria, 18 of 19 patients on bacampicillin and 19 of 19 on doxycycline were cured. In the patient who failed under bacampicillin treatment. *S. aureus* and *H. influenzae* were isolated before treatment. At the end of the therapy, *P. aeruginosa*, which is not susceptible to ampicillin, was found.

TABLE 1. *Average patient score obtained in evaluation of sputum purulence, sputum color, dyspnea, and wheezing*

Drug	Score (% of initial)		
	Day 4	Day 7	Day 10
Bacampicillin	76.8	57.7	42.0
Doxycycline	79.4	53.1	40.7

Among the culture-proven infections with only *H. influenzae*, 10 of 10 patients on bacampicillin and 7 of 7 patients on doxycycline were cured. No drug-related side effects were observed. It was noteworthy that the initial pathogens were eliminated in all cases treated with the b.i.d. dosage of bacampicillin.

The symptoms were followed by a score system (Table 1) and showed that an improvement could still be observed between days 7 and 10. Both therapeutic courses worked well in our hands and gave comparable results.

1. **Bartmann, K.** 1978. Sputumuntersuchung zur Diagnose von Infektionen des Atemtraktes. Med. Klin. **73:**1074–1079
2. **Ekström, B., L.-P. Jalar, and L. Magni.** 1979. Comparative in vivo activity of bacampicillin and amoxycillin.
3. **Mulder, J.** 1938. Haemophilus influenzae (Pfeiffer) as an ubiquitous cause of acute and chronical purulent bronchitis. Acta Med. Scand. **94:**98.
4. **Pauwels, R., and J. J. Detiege.** 1980. Deux prises quotidiennes de bacampicilline dans le traitment des infections des voies respiratoires en pratique de médicine générale. An. Med. **35:**529–543
5. **Sjövall, J.** 1977. Lower respiratory tract infections treated with bacampicillin: a dose comparison. J. Intern. Med. Res. **5:**313–321

Pathogens in Quinsy and Its Chemotherapy

RINYA SUGITA,* SHOZO KAWAMURA, GINICHIRO ICHIKAWA, YUTAKA FUJIMAKI, MIYAKO OHTANI, AND MASAHIRO FUKUDA

Juntendo University School of Medicine, 2-1-1, Hongo Bunkyo-ku, Tokyo, Japan

Peritonsillar abscess (quinsy) occurs when a bacterial infection of the tonsils spreads to the potential peritonsillar space deep behind the tonsil between the tonsillar capsule and the superior constrictor pharyngeal muscle. Treatment of this condition consists of first confirming the presence of an abscess formation by puncture, followed by incision, drainage, and chemotherapy.

Most textbooks of otorhinolaryngology describe the causative organisms as aerobes. However, the fact that the site of the infection is near the oral mucosa and away from open air strongly suggests that anaerobes may play an etiological role. Nevertheless, there are few reports of attempted investigations into both aerobic and anaerobic organisms as possible causative agents. Under such circumstances, it is not uncommon for us to be at a loss as to the choice of antibiotic for treatment of quinsy.

The present study represents our attempt to reevaluate the bacteriology of quinsy with due emphasis placed on both aerobic and anaerobic organisms as possible invaders. The purpose of this paper is to report mainly on the antibiotic susceptibility of microorganisms detected from quinsy.

Thirty patients with quinsy who were seen at the outpatient service of the Department of Otorhinolaryngology of Juntendo University Hospital between January 1978 and February 1980 were involved in the study. This series of patients had the following age distribution: 2 people from 10 to 20 years, 10 from 20 to 30 years, 9 from 30 to 40 years, 6 from 40 to 50 years, 2 from 40 to 50 years, 2 from 50 to 60 years, and 1 from 60 to 70 years.

At the time of the first examination, pus was collected by puncture of the most severely affected portion of the soft palate with a syringe and 18-gauge needle. The specimens were studied at the Bacteriological Division of the Clinical Laboratories of Juntendo University Hospital. Anaerobic cultivation was carried out with the GasPak anaerobic system (BBL Microbiology Systems).

From the 30 cases, 9 species and 46 strains of microorganisms were isolated and identified (Table 1). There were 18 strains of aerobes, of which group A streptococci (26.1%), *Streptococcus pneumoniae* (4.3%), and *Haemophilus influenzae* (2.2%) were most frequent. Twenty-eight strains of anaerobes were also detected, the most common of which were *Peptostreptococcus* sp.

TABLE 1. *Results of bacterial analysis in 30 cases of peritonsillar abscess*

Type of organism	Organism	Frequency of isolation	%
Aerobe	Group A streptococci	12	26.1
	H. influenzae	1	2.2
	S. pneumoniae	2	4.3
	Alpha-hemolytic streptococci	3	6.5
	Total	18	39.1
Anaerobe	*Peptostreptococcus* sp.	13	28.3
	Peptococcus sp.	7	15.2
	Fusobacterium sp.	4	8.7
	B. fragilis	1	2.2
	Propionibacterium sp.	1	2.2
	Microaerophilic streptococci	2	4.3
	Total	28	60.9
Total		46	100.0

TABLE 2. *EEI according to antibiotic in cases of peritonsillar abscess*

Organism	Antibiotic[a]								
	ABPC	SBPC	CEZ	GM	CP	TC	EM	JM	LCM
Group A streptococci	26.1	26.1	26.1	9.7	18.0	15.8	19.0	18.0	17.8
Peptostreptococcus sp.	28.3	28.3	28.3	0	24.6	21.5	28.3	28.3	28.3
Peptococcus sp.	15.2	15.2	15.2	2.8	12.6	11.4	11.1	15.2	15.2
Fusobacterium sp.	8.7	8.7	8.7	1.3	8.7	8.7	2.1	3.9	5.5
Total expected EEI	78.3	78.3	78.3	13.8	63.9	57.4	60.5	65.4	66.8

[a] Abbreviations not given in text: TC, ticarcillin; EM, erythromycin; JM, josamicin.

(28.3%), *Peptococcus* sp. (15.2%), and *Fusobacterium* sp. (8.7%).

Antibiotic susceptibility ratios of four kinds of microorganisms found were as follows: for ampicillin (ABPC), sulbenicillin (SBPC), and cefazolin (CEZ), *Peptostreptococcus*, *Peptococcus*, *Fusobacterium*, and group A streptococci (100%); for chloramphenicol (CP), group A streptococci (68.9%), *Peptostreptococcus* (86.9%) *Peptococcus* (82.9%), and *Fusobacterium* (100%); for lincomycin (LCM), group A streptococci (68.0%), *Peptostreptococcus* (100%), *Peptococcus* (100%), and *Fusobacterium* (63.2%); for gentamicin (GM), group A streptococci (37.0%), *Peptostreptococcus* (0%), *Peptococcus* (5.4%), and *Fusobacterium* (6.7%).

There are a few studies on anaerobes in quinsy, and those concerning anaerobes and aerobes simultaneously are also rare. Hansen (2) isolated 151 strains of anaerobes from 153 cases. Gram-positive cocci accounted for 32%, and 62% were gram-negative rods, among which *Bacteroides* and fusiform bacilli were predominant. Hallander et al. (1) recovered anaerobes from 26 of 30 cases, stating that *Bacteroides*, *Fusobacterium*, *Peptostreptococcus*, and *Peptococcus* were the dominant pathogens. Our results show anaerobes to be predominant over aerobes, especially gram-positive cocci.

Almost all cases of quinsy occur after several days of acute tonsillitis, and the pathogen of most acute tonsillitis is group A streptococci. The site of peritonsillar infection is a closed space away from the atmosphere and adjacent to the oral mucosa; aerobic culture of pus from quinsy frequently proves to be negative. Moreover, in occasional cases incision of the abscess yields pus with an offending odor. Our results indicated that the main causative pathogens are *Peptostreptococcus* sp. and *Peptococcus* sp. (anaerobes) and group A streptococci (aerobes).

From the detection ratio of pathogens in cases of quinsy and the antibiotic susceptibility ratios of these pathogens, the EEI, or expected efficacy index (tentative term), was determined for each antibiotic by the following formula, which can be used as a reliable guide for treatment: EEI of ABPC = (detection ratio of *Peptostreptococcus* × ABPC susceptibility ratio of *Peptostreptococcus*) + (detection ratio of *Peptococcus* × ABPC susceptibility ratio of *Peptococcus*) + (detection ratio of *Fusobacterium* × ABPC susceptibility ratio of *Fusobacterium*) + (detection ratio of group A streptococci × ABPC susceptibility ratio of group A streptococci). EEI values so determined for various antibiotics against quinsy were: SBPC, 78.3; ABPC, 78.3; CEZ, 78.3, and LCM, 66.8. The antibiotics of first choice are penicillins or cephalosporins, and those of second choice are LCM or CP.

1. **Hallander, H. O., A. Flodstrom, and K. Holmberg.** 1975. Influence of the collection and transport of specimens on the recovery of bacteria from peritonsillar abscess. J. Clin. Microbiol. **2**:504–509.
2. **Hansen, A.** 1950. Nogle undersogelsen over gramnegative anaerobe ikkesporendannende bacterier, isolerede fra peritonsilloere abscesser bos monnesker. Munksgaard, Copenhagen.

Role of Newer Antibiotics in Tropical Developing Countries

DAVID MONTEFIORE, ADE OJENIYI,* NATHANIEL ROTOWA, AND FOLORUSO ADEYEMI-DORO

Department of Medical Microbiology and Department of Preventive and Social Medicine, University of Ibadan and University College Hospital, Ibadan, Nigeria*

Infectious diseases, especially those due to bacteria, remain an important cause of morbidity and death in developing countries. The most recent report from the Nigerian Federal Ministry of Health refers to the year 1977 and shows that infections accounted for 32% of all hospital admissions, 42.6% of hospital attendances, and 46.4% of total deaths. Malaria was the most frequent diagnosis, followed by enteritis and other diarrheal diseases. Although these data may not be accurate, they do illustrate the great difference between disease patterns experienced in the developing tropical countries and those found in other parts of the world.

Antibiotics are extensively used both in hospitals and by the general public (1), to whom they are readily available despite formal regulations requiring their sale by prescription only. Their use may not always be suitable, since even in hospitals it is only the larger centers that have laboratory facilities to identify infecting organisms and determine their antibiotic susceptibility. In most cases the physician chooses his treatment by clinical judgment, aided to some extent by knowledge from other centers of the most likely infecting bacteria and the likely susceptibility pattern.

The consequences have been much as one would expect. In centers where studies have been possible over a number of years, a steady increase has been found in the proportion of common bacterial isolates which are resistant to many of the older antibiotics. Probably because these same agents are widely used for self-treatment by the general population, at least in urban areas, there is often little difference in susceptibility patterns between strains isolated from inpatients and those obtained from outpatients.

Two examples from our hospital (University College Hospital, Ibadan) will illustrate the increase in the proportion of resistant strains over the years. In 1963, 28% of 170 strains of *Staphylococcus aureus* isolated from infected wounds or blood cultures among inpatients were susceptible to benzylpenicillin. By 1981 the proportion of susceptible strains from similar cases had fallen to 15% of 92 isolates. Corresponding figures for *Escherichia coli* show that, in 1974, 40% of 158 strains were susceptible to ampicillin, but by 1979 this had fallen to 20% of 138 strains. The proportion of susceptible strains has remained virtually unchanged since then. Other organisms have responded similarly (K. O. Alausa and D. Montefiore, in press), and the complete findings can be briefly summarized by saying that plasmid-determined, multiple, transmissible resistance is extremely common among bacterial strains isolated in Ibadan (A. Ojeniyi, Ph.D. thesis, 1980).

There is little doubt, therefore, that in the coming years newer agents will be required in the tropics, as elsewhere, to treat a proportion of patients with severe bacterial infections.

Three of these newer agents, cefuroxime, amikacin, and cefotaxime, have been introduced to the Nigerian market during the last year or so. Although not all of them are new in other parts of the world, it was worthwhile to examine the in vitro susceptibility patterns of common bacterial isolates from hospital inpatients during 1980.

Preliminary findings for the older penicillins were obtained from disk diffusion tests, using benzylpenicillin (2 U), ampicillin (10 μg), and methicillin (10 μg). Beta-lactamase production was determined by the nitrocefin and iodometric methods. All of 70 *S. aureus* isolates were penicillinase producers, and 12 strains (17%) were also resistant to methicillin. Of 61 strains of *E. coli*, 87% were beta-lactamase producers and resistant to ampicillin. As expected, 96% of 70 *Klebsiella* strains were resistant to ampicillin, as were 51% of 51 strains of *Proteus mirabilis*. It was clear that these two older antibiotics would be of very limited value in treating infections due to these common organisms.

MICs were then determined, using the agar dilution method, for 336 strains of commonly isolated bacteria, including most of those already tested by the disk method. The results are given in Table 1.

The findings were very similar to those originally reported from other parts of the world when the three newer agents, cefuroxime, amikacin, and cefotaxime, were first introduced. All strains of *S. aureus*, except those that were methicillin resistant, were susceptible to the two cephalosporins. Resistance to the cephalosporins among the *Enterobacteriaceae* was rare but did occasionally occur, whereas amikacin was

TABLE 1. *MICs for a cumulative percentage of isolates with inocula of 10^4 colony-forming units*

Organism (no. of strains)	Antibiotic	MIC (μg/ml)		
		MIC_{50}	Range	MIC_{90}
Staphylococcus aureus (patients; 70)	Kanamycin	0.5	0.25–>64.0	1.0
	Gentamicin	0.125	0.125–>16.0	0.5
	Cefotaxime			
	Methicillin susceptible	1.0	0.5–2.0	2.0
	Methicillin resistant	>16.0	4.0–>16.0	>16.0
	Cefuroxime			
	Methicillin susceptible	1.0	0.25–2.0	1.0
	Methicillin resistant	>64.0	2.0–>64.0	>64.0
S. aureus (carriers; 25)	Kanamycin	0.5	0.125–1.0	1.0
	Gentamicin	0.125	0.015–0.5	0.25
	Cefotaxime	1.0	1.0–2.0	2.0
	Cefuroxime	0.5	0.5–2.0	1.0
Escherichia coli (61)	Kanamycin	0.5	0.25–>16.0	>16.0
	Gentamicin	0.5	0.25–>15.0	1.0
	Amikacin	1.0	0.25–4.0	2.0
	Cefotaxime	0.06	≤0.015–1.0	0.25
	Cefuroxime	4.0	2.0–>64.0	8.0
Klebsiella sp. (70)	Kanamycin	0.25	0.125–>16.0	>16.0
	Gentamicin	0.125	0.06–>16.0	>16.0
	Amikacin	0.5	0.25–1.0	1.0
	Cefotaxime	0.06	0.03–>16.0	0.25
	Cefuroxime	4.0	1.0–>64.0	16.0
Proteus mirabilis (38)	Kanamycin	2.0	1.0–>16.0	>16.0
	Gentamicin	1.0	0.125–>16.0	4.0
	Amikacin	2.0	0.5–8.0	4.0
	Cefotaxime	≤0.015	≤0.015–1.0	0.03
	Cefuroxime	2.0	1.0–64.0	8.0
Indole-positive *Proteus* spp. (6)	Kanamycin	2.0	0.5–16.0	16.0
	Gentamicin	0.5	0.25–16.0	16.0
	Amikacin	0.5	0.5–1.0	1.0
	Cefotaxime	0.03	≤0.015–0.03	0.03
	Cefuroxime	64.0	4.0–>64.0	>64.0
Pseudomonas aeruginosa (83)	Carbenicillin	128.0	64.0–>256.0	>256.0
	Gentamicin	0.5	≤0.06–>64.0	2.0
	Amikacin	2.0	0.25–64.0	4.0
	Cefotaxime	32.0	8.0–>64.0	>64.0
Pseudomonas sp. (8)	Carbenicillin	>256.0	>256.0	>256.0
	Gentamicin	0.06	0.06–0.125	0.125
	Amikacin	0.25	0.06–2.0	2.0
	Cefotaxime	32.0	4.0–64.0	64.0

active against the rare strain which proved resistant to gentamicin. Occasional strains of *Pseudomonas aeruginosa* were resistant to gentamicin and amikacin, whereas approximately 50% were susceptible to attainable serum levels of cefotaxime.

What, then, is the place of the newer antibiotics in the context of Nigeria, as representative of a tropical developing country?

It has been seen that the high prevalence of resistance to the older antibiotics means that newer agents are required and that demand for them is likely to increase as time goes on. But new antibiotics are expensive. It is difficult to give a precise figure for the annual per capita expenditure on health services in Nigeria, as funding comes from different sources and varies to some extent in different parts of the country. In general, however, it probably totals rather less than the present cost of one-half of a single adult dose of any of the three newer antibiotics. With increasing emphasis being rightly placed on preventive rather than curative medical services in the tropics, this inevitably means that the new antibiotics will be used only in exceptional circumstances, which may be very difficult for the physician to define in the absence of adequate laboratory facilities.

It is therefore likely that the older and cheaper agents will remain the mainstay of treatment in the tropics, even though their effective use may be difficult because of bacterial resistance and lack of facilities in most hospitals to determine susceptibility patterns. The need for antibiotic policies and control which may help to prolong the useful life of the older agents is obvious. But even if supplies were available, unrestricted use of the newer agents could be highly undesirable, as the prevalence of resistant strains would no doubt increase, just as it has with the older agents.

There is no easy answer to the problem, but it is one which may have far-reaching implications. Antibiotic-resistant bacteria can travel, as evidenced by the epidemiology of penicillinase-producing strains of *Neisseria gonorrhoeae*. Problems and their solutions in the tropics must therefore be of concern to countries in other parts of the world.

1. **Alausa, K. O., and D. Montefiore.** 1978. Bacterial infections, sensitivity patterns and chemotherapy among hospital patients in the tropics. Scand. J. Infect. Dis. **10:**295–302.

Stability of BRL 17421, a Novel β-Lactam Antibiotic, to a Wide Range of β-Lactamases

R. A. EDMONDSON,* B. SLOCOMBE, AND M. COLE

Beecham Pharmaceuticals, Research Division, Betchworth, Surrey RH3 7AJ, England

BRL 17421 is a new semisynthetic β-lactam antibiotic with a methoxy substituent in the 6α-position and an α-carboxy-3-thienylacetamido side chain in the 6β-position (Fig. 1). The combination of these two substituents confers a remarkably high stability to a very wide range of bacterial β-lactamases.

The stability of BRL 17421 to a large number of cell-free β-lactamase preparations has been determined in comparison with cefuroxime, cefotaxime, and cefoxitin. The enzyme preparations were made by growing the bacteria in Nutrient Broth No. 2 (Oxoid) for 7 h with shaking at 37°C. *Bacteroides fragilis* was grown anaerobically (GasPak) for 48 h in brain heart infusion medium (Oxoid). For those bacteria which produce inducible β-lactamases, for example strains of *Enterobacter*, indole-positive *Proteus*, *Citrobacter*, and *Serratia*, benzylpenicillin was added after 2.5 h of growth to give a concentration of 500 μg/ml in the culture, except for *Staphylococcus aureus* where the inducer was methicillin at 1 μg/ml in the culture. Bacterial cells were collected by centrifugation and resuspended in a 1/50 volume of water. After disruption of the cells by ultrasonication in the cold the debris was removed by high-speed centrifugation, and the supernatants were retained as concentrated stock enzyme preparations.

The reaction mixtures consisted of 200 μg of β-lactam antibiotic per ml in 0.05 M, pH 7, potassium phosphate buffer and a 1/10 dilution of the concentrated stock enzyme preparation. The reaction mixtures were maintained at 37°C, and residual antibiotic was determined after 0, 30, and 60 min using a paper tape bioassay procedure based on a method first described for penicillin acylase (1). In this assay procedure, samples taken from the reaction mixtures were spotted onto strips of chromatography paper and dried in a stream of warm air to stop any further reaction. The residual antibiotic was then assayed by placing the paper strips on agar seeded with an appropriate indicator organism. After 10 min contact, the strips were peeled from the agar, thus removing the β-lactamase firmly bound to the paper. This method avoids interference from continuing β-lactamase action which would occur during a conventional hole-in-plate bioassay procedure. Antibiotic standards, free of β-lactamase, were also spotted onto

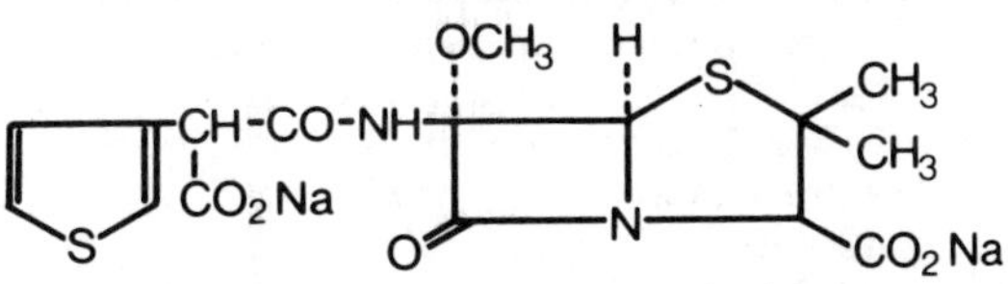

FIG. 1. *Structure of BRL 17421, disodium 6, β-(2-carboxy-2-thien-3-ylacetamido) 6,α-methoxy-penicillanate.*

TABLE 1. *Stability of BRL 17421 to a range of β-lactamases compared with cefuroxime, cefotaxime, and cefoxitin*

Source of β-lactamase	Substrate remaining after 1 h (%)[a]			
	Cefoxitin	Cefuroxime	Cefotaxime	BRL 17421
Plasmid mediated:				
TEM 1	100	22	0	100
TEM 2	100	0	0	100
PSE 4(pMG19)	100	60	47	100
OXA 1(pGN238)	100	0	0	100
OXA 3(p57b)	85	100	17	100
SHV 1(pR1010)	100	34	0	100
HMS 1(pR997)	100	65	34	100
Chromosomally mediated:				
Escherichia coli (5)[b]	47–100[c]	0–100	0–70	100
Enterobacter spp. (10)	0–100	0–75	0–85	100
Citrobacter spp. (5)	100	100	18–100	100
Serratia marcescens (3)	100	0–32	0–17	100
Pseudomonas aeruginosa (5)	32–100	24–100	32–100	100
Providencia spp. (10)	90–100	0–100	0–100	0–100
Proteus spp. (6)	80–100	0–100	0–100	100
Klebsiella pneumoniae (4)	100	0–100	0–8	100
Miscellaneous:				
Acinetobacter calcoaceticus (5)	100	75–100	30–100	100
Bacteroides fragilis (3)	100	0	0	100
Staphylococcus aureus (2)	100	100	100	100

[a] Substrate concentration, 200 μg/ml, temperature 37°C, pH 7.0, same enzyme concentration for all substrates (see text).
[b] Number of strains tested.
[c] Range of results for strains tested.

paper strips and treated in an identical way. *Staphylococcus aureus* (Oxford) NCTC 6571 was used for the assay of cefuroxime and cefotaxime, *Sarcina lutea* NCTC 8340 for cefoxitin, and *Neisseria catarrhalis* NCTC 3622 for BRL 17421.

Representative results for various types of plasmid-mediated, chromosomally mediated, and miscellaneous β-lactamases are shown in Table 1. Against all of the plasmid-mediated β-lactamases, BRL 17421 was completely stable, whereas cefuroxime and/or cefotaxime were inactivated by all of the preparations, and cefoxitin was slowly inactivated by OXA 3-type β-lactamase. Of the chromosomally mediated β-lactamases tested, BRL 17421 was stable to all, except for the preparations from 2 out of 10 strains of *Providencia* species. These two were isolates of *Providencia alcalifaciens*, and both had been grown in the presence of benzylpenicillin to induce β-lactamase. In the absence of inducer no loss of BRL 17421 was observed. Both strains of *P. alcalifaciens* were susceptible to BRL 17421, being inhibited by concentrations of 2.5 μg/ml. BRL 17421 was stable to the β-lactamase preparations from *Acinetobacter calcoaceticus*, *B. fragilis*, and *S. aureus*.

BRL 17421 is a poor inhibitor of many β-lactamases, for example those produced by *Enterobacter* spp., and induces production of β-lactamase in organisms such as *Serratia marcescens*, *Enterobacter cloacae*, and *S. aureus*, but not *Pseudomonas aeruginosa*. However, it is stable to the induced enzymes produced by these bacteria.

In summary, the β-lactamase stability of BRL 17421 to 69 β-lactamase preparations has been tested in comparison with cefuroxime, cefotaxime, and cefoxitin. Of these 69 preparations, 67 had no measurable effect on BRL 17421 under the conditions of the test. Even at high substrate concentration (5 mg/ml), the TEM 1 β-lactamase preparation used caused no detectable loss of BRL 17421 over a 4-h period. The stability of BRL 17421 to β-lactamases appears to be due to a combination of low affinity for the enzymes and low rate of hydrolysis of any enzyme-substrate complex which is formed.

1. **Cole, M.** 1969. Factors affecting the synthesis of ampicillin and hydroxypenicillins by the cell-bound penicillin acylase of *Escherichia coli*. Biochem. J. **15**:757–764.

BRL 17421, a Novel β-Lactam Antibiotic: In Vitro and In Vivo Properties

RONALD A. DIXON, DAVID J. MERRIKIN, LINDA W. MIZEN, AND BRIAN SLOCOMBE*

Beecham Pharmaceuticals Research Division, Brockham Park, Betchworth, Surrey RH3 7AJ, England

BRL 17421, 6β-(2-carboxy-2-thien-3-ylacetamido)-6α-methoxy-penicillanic acid, disodium salt, is a new semisynthetic β-lactam antibiotic combining potent antibacterial activity with exceptional stability to a wide range of bacterial β-lactamases (R. A. Edmonson, B. Slocombe, and M. Cole, this volume).

BRL 17421 exhibits good antibacterial activity against members of the *Enterobacteriaceae*, including *Escherichia coli, Klebsiella pneumoniae, Enterobacter* spp., *Citrobacter* spp., *Serratia* spp., *Providencia* spp., *Proteus* spp. (indole positive and negative), *Salmonella, Shigella*, and *Yersinia enterocolitica*, including strains highly resistant to many of the penicillins and cephalosporins currently available. The majority of *Enterobacteriaceae* were inhibited by a concentration of 5 μg/ml or less. Strains of *Serratia marcescens* were generally twofold less susceptible to BRL 17421 and required 10 μg/ml for inhibition. The compound was highly active against *Haemophilus influenzae* and *Neisseria gonorrhoeae*, including strains producing plasmid-mediated β-lactamase, as well as strains of *Branamella catarrhalis, Brucella*, and *Pasteurella*. The antibacterial activity of BRL 17421 was markedly less against *Pseudomonas aeruginosa* and *Bacteroides fragilis* subspecies than against members of the *Enterobacteriaceae*. The majority of *P. aeruginosa* and *B. fragilis* tested at an inoculum of 10^6 colony-forming units (CFU) required concentrations of 250 μg/ml for inhibition. A reduction in inoculum size to 10^4 CFU resulted in a 5- to 10-fold increase in susceptibilities, with MIC values of 25 to 50 μg/ml being observed. Against aerobic gram-positive organisms such as *Staphylococcus aureus, Streptococcus pyogenes, Streptococcus pneumoniae*, and *Streptococcus faecalis*, as well as the anaerobic gram-positive bacteria, BRL 17421 exhibited a very low level of antibacterial activity.

When tested against 260 recent clinical isolates of *Enterobacteriaceae* (Table 1), the majority were inhibited at 5 μg/ml or less, with remarkably few strains resistant to the compound. BRL 17421 inhibited 75% of 60 isolates of *E. coli* (40 isolates highly resistant to ampicillin) at 2.5 μg/ml or less, and all were inhibited by 5 μg/ml. The compound showed good activity against *K. pneumoniae* with all strains inhibited by 5 μg/ml or less, including two strains highly resistant to cefuroxime. BRL 17421 was active against isolates producing chromosomally mediated cephalosporinases, such as *Enterobacter, Citrobacter, Providencia*, and *Proteus* (indole-positive and -negative strains). All were inhibited in a range of 1.0 to 10 μg/ml, including a number of isolates highly resistant to both cefuroxime and cefotaxime. The majority of *S. marcescens* isolates were inhibited by 10 μg/ml, and BRL 17421 was considerably more active than cefuroxime.

The antibacterial activity of BRL 17421 against *Enterobacteriaceae*, including strains producing large amounts of β-lactamase, was little affected by inoculum sizes ranging from 10^3 to 10^7 CFU when tested in agar or from 10^3 to 10^6 CFU/ml in a nutrient liquid medium. BRL 17421 was bactericidal as determined by viable count measurements at concentrations close to the MIC, with MBC values generally the same, or twofold greater when tested with an inoculum of 10^5 CFU/ml in a variety of different media. The rate of in vitro selection of resistant variants from BRL 17421-susceptible bacteria, by repeated subculture in the presence of increasing concentrations of the compound, was slow and stepwise in character.

BRL 17421 was found to be approximately 85% bound to human serum proteins, as determined by the Centriflo membrane cone (CF50A) filtration method (Amicon Ltd., Woking, England), and highly stable in human serum at 37°C ($t_{1/2} > 150$ h). The antibacterial activity was generally reduced twofold or, in a few instances, fourfold in the presence of 50% human serum. The presence of 50% human serum in nutrient broth had little adverse effect on the rate of kill achieved with BRL 17421 against the majority of bacteria tested.

Serum concentrations achieved in different animal species after parenteral administration of 100 mg/kg (monkey, 10 mg/kg) were high, mean peak serum concentrations occurring between 5 to 30 min after dosing: mice, 194 μg/ml; rats, 117 μg/ml; rabbits, 57 μg/ml; dogs, 271 μg/ml; and squirrel monkeys, 38 μg/ml. The corresponding serum elimination half-lives were 18, 16, 35, 63, and 126 min, respectively. BRL 17421 was ex-

TABLE 1. *Comparative antibacterial activities of BRL 17421, cefuroxime, and cefotaxime against clinical isolates of Enterobacteriaceae*

Organism (no. of isolates)	Antibiotic	MIC[a] (μg/ml) against: (cumulative % of isolates)		
		Range	75	90
E. coli (ampicillin-susceptible) (20)	BRL 17421	1.0–5.0	2.5	5.0
	Cefuroxime	0.5–2.5	2.5	2.5
	Cefotaxime	0.005–0.05	0.02	0.02
E. coli (ampicillin-resistant) (40)	BRL 17421	1.0–5.0	2.5	5.0
	Cefuroxime	1.2–2.5	5.0	10
	Cefotaxime	0.01–2.5	0.5	1.0
K. pneumoniae (40)	BRL 17421	1.0–5.0	2.5	5.0
	Cefuroxime	0.5–>500	2.5	2.5
	Cefotaxime	0.01–0.5	0.05	0.5
P. mirabilis (27)	BRL 17421	1.0–5.0	5.0	5.0
	Cefuroxime	0.5–>500	10	50
	Cefotaxime	0.01–2.5	0.01	0.01
Indole-positive *Proteus* (20)	BRL 17421	1.0–10	5.0	5.0
	Cefuroxime	0.2–>500	250	>500
	Cefotaxime	0.01–50	0.01	2.5
Providencia spp. (13)	BRL 17421	1.0–5.0	2.5	5.0
	Cefuroxime	0.2–>500	10	50
	Cefotaxime	0.01–2.5	0.1	1.0
Enterobacter spp. (40)	BRL 17421	1.0–10	5.0	10
	Cefuroxime	2.5–250	5.0	50
	Cefotaxime	0.02–50	5.0	50
Citrobacter spp. (20)	BRL 17421	1.0–10	2.5	5.0
	Cefuroxime	1.0–50	10	50
	Cefotaxime	0.02–50	0.1	25
Serratia spp. (40)	BRL 17421	2.5–500	10	10
	Cefuroxime	25–>500	>500	>500
	Cefotaxime	0.05–500	0.5	1.0

[a] MIC determined by serial dilution into nutrient agar, inoculated with 0.001 ml of approximately 10^9 CFU/ml (to give 10^6 CFU per spot).

TABLE 2. *In vivo efficacy of BRL 17421 in systemic infections in mice*

Organism	ED_{50} (mg/kg)[a] of:			
	BRL 17421	Cefazolin	Cefuroxime	Cefoxitin
E. coli 96 (R^-)	19	9	12	21
E. coli 96 (R^+)	18	7	5	13
K. pneumoniae T767	16	12	16	40
K. pneumoniae D192 (R^+)	60	>1,200	465	26
E. cloacae T626	22	>1,200	60	840
S. marcescens US 39	53	>1,200	171	48

[a] Mice dosed 1, 3, and 5 h post-intraperitoneal infection.

creted unchanged in high concentrations in the urines of the different species with the percentage of the dose recovered after parenteral dosing ranging from 42% in rabbits to 67% in dogs. There was no significant absorption after oral administration of the compound.

The chemotherapeutic efficacy of BRL 17421, cefazolin, cefuroxime, and cefoxitin was compared in mice infected with different strains of *Enterobacteriaceae* (Table 2). The mice were challenged by the intraperitoneal route with an infective inoculum of 10 to 100 LD_{50}. Groups of 10 mice were treated subcutaneously with a total of 4 dose levels for each antibiotic 1, 3, and 5 h postinfection. The numbers of animals surviving on day 4 after infection were recorded and the

ED_{50} values (milligram per killigram per total dose) were calculated by probit transformation.

BRL 17421 showed a broad spectrum of in vivo activity and exhibited good protection against lethal infections caused by bacteria producing large quantities of chromosomal or plasmid-mediated β-lactamases. BRL 17421 was equally effective in protecting mice infected with an ampicillin-susceptible strain of *E. coli* and an ampicillin-resistant strain, producing plasmid-mediated β-lactamase. Against a cefazolin-susceptible strain of *K. pneumoniae* T767, BRL 17421, cefazolin, and cefuroxime exhibited a similar degree of protection, whereas against an infection induced by a cefazolin-resistant strain, *K. pneumoniae* D192, BRL 17421 was more effective than either cefuroxime or cefazolin. The compound showed good protection against infections of cefazolin-resistant strains of *E. cloacae*, *C. freundii*, *S. marcescens*, and *P. alcalifaciens*.

Pharmacokinetics of BRL 17421, a Novel Semisynthetic Beta-Lactam Antibiotic

JILL D. GURNEY* AND DERRICK JACKSON

Beecham Pharmaceuticals, Brockham Park, Betchworth, Surrey, England

BRL 17421, disodium 6α-(2-carboxy-2-thien-3-ylacetamido)-6α-methoxypenicillanate, is a novel, semisynthetic β-lactam antibiotic with a broad spectrum of stability to β-lactamases. It has good antibacterial activity against most *Enterobacteriaceae* and *Neisseria gonorrhoea*. Its spectrum includes those strains which are highly resistant because of their production of plasmid-mediated β-lactamases. The pharmacokinetics of BRL 17421 were studied in 15 normal, healthy, fasting volunteers. The antibiotic was administered both intramuscularly and intravenously at mean total doses of 750, 1,000, and 1,250 mg, the precise dosages being calculated according to the surface area of each individual.

For intramuscular administration all three doses were dissolved in a solution containing 1% lignocaine and, in addition, the lowest dose was given in plain water. For intramuscular dosing each gram of BRL 17421 was given in a total volume of 2.9 ml. In the case of intravenous administration each dose was dissolved in 10 ml of water for injection. Pain was recorded by volunteers on visual analog scores at 0, 30, 60, 90, and 120 min after each of the four intramuscular injections. The study was of a random crossover design, and the volunteers were not told which injection they were receiving. Blood was taken immediately before each dose for estimation of clinical chemistry and hematology. The hematological investigations were also undertaken 24 h after each dose, and the serum chemistry was taken 10 days after the final dose.

Comparison of the effects of 750 mg intramuscularly with and without lignocaine showed several differences. The volunteers who had experienced previous intramuscular injections of antibacterials did not consider the discomfort following BRL 17421 to be worse than would be expected after any intramuscular injection. Nonetheless the visual analog scores did show that the inclusion of lignocaine in the solution significantly reduced the degree of discomfort both at rest and on movement immediately after and 30 min after the injection. The injection with lignocaine gave significantly higher serum levels (70 compared to 64 μg/ml) and a slightly shorter time (1.42 h) to reach peak levels. The injection with lignocaine gave significantly higher serum levels at all time points up to 2 h. From 4 to 12 h the levels achieved were slightly lower with lignocaine than without, but these differences were not statistically significant. The area under the curve and percentage of urinary recovery were slightly, but not significantly, greater after the injections containing lignocaine.

Attempts were made to fit an appropriate compartment model to the data for each volunteer at each dose. The model best fitting the curves following intravenous administration was a two-compartment model following the equation $C = Ae^{-\alpha t} + Be^{-\beta t}$. For intramuscular dosing the curve fitted a one-compartment model with absorption according to the equation $C = Ae^{-\alpha t} - Be^{-\beta t}$. On the basis of the intravenous model, it may have been expected that a two compartment model would fit the intramuscular data satisfactorily, but it is difficult to distinguish between the phases of absorption and redistribution into the extra compartment. From the intravenous results it can be seen that the con-

TABLE 1. *BRL 17421: pharmacokinetic parameters after intramuscular administration*

Dose (mg)	Parameters[a]						
	AUC (μg.h/ml)	Peak (μg/ml)	Time to peak (h)	Half-life absorption (h)	Half-life elimination (h)	UR (mg)	UR (%)
750 (water)	449	58	1.7	0.51	3.5	584	80
750	451	68	1.4	0.40	3.4	595	80
1,000	595	84	1.7	0.47	3.5	794	81
1,250	697	104	1.7	0.43	3.3	1,002	81

[a] AUC, Area under the curve; UR, urinary recovery.

TABLE 2. *BRL 17421: pharmacokinetic parameters after intravenous administration*

Dose (mg)	Parameter[a]										
	AUC (μg.h/ml)	Peak (μg/ml)	α-half-life (min)	β-half-life (h)	K_{12} (h^{-1})	K_{21} (h^{-1})	V_D central (1)	V_D tissue (1)	V_DSS (2)	UR (mg)	UR (%)
750	468	158	10	3.6	1.7	2.3	4.5	3.3	7.8	635	86
1,000	589	196	10	3.6	1.8	2.3	4.7	3.5	8.3	846	85
1,250	711	244	8.6	3.4	2.0	2.6	4.7	3.6	8.3	982	80

[a] UR, Urinary recovery; AUC, area under the curve.

tribution of the first term $Ae^{-\alpha t}$ is minimal by 1 h after injection. The means of the pharmacokinetic parameters calculated from the curve-fitting program by using the appropriate model were very similar to the means of the parameters calculated directly from the raw data. Tables 1 and 2 show the pharmacokinetic parameters calculated from the curve-fitting model.

At each dose level the area under the curve was very similar after each route of administration, implying total absorption after intramuscular dosing. A graphic plot against dose for each individual at each dose level suggested a linear dose response, though this was difficult to assess accurately for three dose levels over a relatively small range. The serum elimination half-life for all six dosage levels varied from 3.3 to 3.6 h.

After the three intravenous dosages, the steady-state volume of distribution was 7.8 to 8.3 liters, comprised of a central compartment of 4.5 to 4.7 liters and a tissue compartment of 3.3 to 3.6 liters.

From the above data, administration of BRL 17421, 1 g every 12 h for 4 days, would be expected to give minimum serum concentrations of about 10% greater in the steady state than after a single dose.

Total urinary recovery after 48 h was 79 to 81% for all intramuscular doses and for the highest intravenous dose. Urinary recovery after intravenous 750- and 1,000-mg doses was 86 and 85%, respectively. Most was excreted shortly after dosing, between 67 and 78% of the total dose administered having been recovered within 12 h of injection.

No adverse events were reported that were considered attributable to BRL 17421, nor were there any relevant changes in the wide range of biochemical and hematological parameters that were measured on approximately 10 occasions before, during, and after treatment.

Clinical, Bacteriological, and Kinetic Studies with BRL 17421, A Novel Semisynthetic β-Lactam Antibiotic

JOHN KOSMIDIS,* ARIS POLYZOS, HELEN GIAMARELLOU, AND GEORGE K. DAIKOS

First Department of Propedeutic Medicine, Athens University School of Medicine, King Paul's Hospital, Athens 609, Greece

BRL 17421 is 6β-(2-carboxy-2-thien-3-ylacetamido)-6α-methoxypenicillanate disodium. This novel semisynthetic β-lactam antibiotic is active against most clinically important gram-negative bacteria, including all genera of *Enterobacteriaceae, Haemophilus influenzae, Neisseria gonorrhoeae, Pasteurella* spp., and *Brucella* spp., with an extremely low incidence of resistant strains. It is not active against *Pseudomonas aeruginosa, Bacteroides fragilis*, or gram-positive bacteria. It is remarkably stable to β-lactamases of all Richmond types produced by gram-positive or gram-negative organisms, chromosomal or plasmid mediated, and its action is bactericidal. BRL 17421 has a rather long half-life and administration every 12 and even 24 h may be sufficient.

BRL 17421 was used in the treatment of urinary tract infection in 17 patients, 12 females and 5 males, aged 25 to 73 years. Infecting organisms included *Escherichia coli* (13), *Proteus mirabilis* (2), indole-positive *Proteus* spp. (1), and indole-positive *Proteus* spp. plus *Providencia stuartii* (1). Of the above 18 organisms, 11 were resistant to ampicillin, 13 to tetracycline, 3 to cephalothin, 1 to nalidixic acid, 4 to nitrofurantoin, and 8 were resistant to cotrimoxazole. Dosage was 500 mg intramuscularly once daily for 10 days. The usual clinical parameters were tested before, during, and after treatment. Urine cultures were performed at −2, 0, 2, 4, 7, 11, 31, and 59 days, and the usual laboratory tests to detect toxicity on the liver, kidney, and hematopoietic system were performed before and after therapy.

In vitro activity of BRL 17421 was tested against 120 consecutive clinical isolates of *Enterobacteriaceae*. MIC was determined by the standard microtiter tube dilution method in tryptose phosphate broth (Difco) with an inoculum size of 10^5 colony-forming units/ml, after diluting an overnight culture. The MIC was defined as the concentration of the antibiotic giving no visible growth after 24 h of incubation.

A full profile of measurements of serum and urine concentrations of BRL 17421 was performed in six patients after the first intramuscular dose of 500 mg. A conventional agar-well plate assay technique was used with *P. aeruginosa* 10701 as assay organism and a concentration of 10 mM of calcium chloride in the assay medium.

Results of treatment are presented in Table 1. In patients with uncomplicated infection, a cure rate of 83% was achieved in spite of such a small dosage given once daily. In contrast, infections in the presence of stone or anatomical abnormality could not be cured with this dosage. No side effect or toxicity was observed in any of the patients treated.

Results of our in vitro studies are presented in Table 2. It can be seen that the majority of strains had an MIC of 1 to 8 mg/liter, whereas 96% of the *E. coli* strains and 87% of the total population studied were susceptible to 16 mg/liter or less.

TABLE 1. *Results of treatment with BRL 17421 at an intramuscular dosage of 500 mg once daily for 10 days*

Diagnosis	No. of Cases	Result[a]					
		Clinical			Bacteriological		
		Cure	Fail	NA	Erad	Part erad	Pers/rel
Cystitis/uncomplicated	11	9	2		9		2
Cystitis-orcheoepididymitis	1	1			1		
Cystitis/stone-anatomical abnormality	2		2				2
Pyelonephritis/stone	1		1				1
Asymptomatic bacteriuria/stone	2			2		1	1

[a] Fail, Failure; NA, not assessable (asymptomatic); Erad, eradication; Part erad, partial eradication; and Pers/rel, persistence or relapse.

TABLE 2. *In vitro activity of BRL 17421 against 120 consecutive clinical isolates of Enterobacteriaceae*

Organism	Total no. of strains	No. of strains inhibited by indicated MIC (mg/liter)										
		0.125	0.25	0.5	1	2	4	8	16	32	64	≥128
E. coli	32	2	1	1	4	4	11	7	1	1		
K. pneumoniae	28	4	4	1	5	5	3		1		1	4
Enterobacter spp.	22	2	1		1	3	7	2	1	1	1	3
P. mirabilis	19		1	5	3	4	1	2				3
Proteus spp. (indole positive)	19	1	1	1	6	1	2	4	1	1	1	

Mean serum levels after 500 mg intramuscularly were as follows: at 1 h, 39 mg/liter; at 2 h, 44 mg/liter; at 4 h, 36 mg/liter; at 6 h, 26 mg/liter; at 8 h, 21 mg/liter; at 12 h, 12 mg/liter, and at 24 h, 2.1 mg/liter. Half-life averaged 5.1 h. Mean urine concentrations were 421 mg/liter at 0 to 2 h, 512 at 2 to 4 h, 297 at 4 to 8 h, 122 at 8 to 12 h, and 81 mg/liter at 12 to 24 h. Mean 24-h urinary recovery was 78% of dose.

Our studies confirmed the excellent in vitro activity of BRL 17421 against *Enterobacteriaceae* and the advantageous pharmacokinetics. A serum concentration above 12 mg/liter was sustained for 12 h due to a long serum half-life, whereas 83% of *Enterobacteriaceae* had an MIC of 8 mg/liter or less. Urine concentrations exceeded 80 mg/liter for 24 h. Further, our therapeutic results with the small dosage of 500 mg intramuscularly were very encouraging: an 83% cure rate in uncomplicated urinary infections was observed. Complicated infections could not be cured, but a higher dosage may be more successful.

In conclusion, BRL 17421 seems a very promising antibiotic because of its excellent in vitro activity against *Enterobacteriaceae* and other gram-negative organisms, its favorable pharmacokinetics, and lack of side effects or toxicity. In our hands it had excellent activity against uncomplicated urinary tract infections given at an intramuscular dosage of 500 mg once daily.

EM5210 (SQ 26,445), a Novel Monobactam

WEN-CHIH LIU, WILLIAM L. PARKER,* JERRY SCOTT WELLS, PACIFICO A. PRINCIPE, WILLIAM H. TREJO, DANIEL P. BONNER, AND RICHARD B. SYKES

The Squibb Institute for Medical Research, Princeton, New Jersey 08540, U.S.A.

We have recently isolated from bacterial fermentation seven members of a new class of β-lactam antibiotics called monobactams (5). One of these, SQ 26,445, is produced by strains of *Gluconobacter* and *Acetobacter* species that have been isolated from many sources. The antibiotic, shown to be acidic by electrophoresis, was isolated by absorption on Dowex 1 resin, elution with aqueous NaCl, desalting with charcoal, chromatography on Bio-Rad AG 1×2 resin eluting with a gradient of NaCl in 0.01 M NaH_2PO_4, and chromatography on Diaion HP20AG. SQ 26,445 thus obtained as the amorphous sodium salt is most stable at pH 3 to 5 and has an R_f of 0.25 on silica gel eluting with 2-butanol–HOAc–water, 3:1:1. The specific rotation of the free acid in water (pH 2.7, c = 0.15) is +73° at 589 nm. Absorption at δ3.49 and 3.94 ppm in the ${}^1H$-nuclear magnetic spectrum (D_2O) indicated that SQ 26,445 might be closely related to SQ 26,180 **1** (Fig. 1), which has resonances at these positions for the methoxyl group (δ3.50) and position 4 (3.98 ppm) of the azetidinone. The ${}^{13}C$-NMR spectrum supported this relationship with absorption at δ162.9, 91.8, and 55.1 ppm corresponding to positions 2, 3, and 4 (δ160.5, 89.5, and 53.1 ppm) in **1**. The infrared spectrum of SQ 26,445 has peaks at 1,770 (β-lactam carbonyl), 1,242, 1,051 (—SO_3^-), 1,384 (—CO_2^-), 1,640, and 1,530 cm^{-1} (amide I and II), the latter two peaks indicating, in conjunction with the NMR spectra, that SQ 26,445 is a peptide. Hydrolysis of the antibiotic in 6 N HCl (115°C, 16 h) gave D-glutamic acid, D-alanine, and ammonia in a ratio of 2:1:2. Another hydrolysis product was observed by electrophoresis (ninhydrin and Pauly reagent) but was not isolated. This may be the imidazole **2** in analogy to the imidazole **3** that is formed from **1** under these conditions. Glutamic acid was shown to be N-terminal by the Sanger method. Failure to undergo Edman degradation indicated that the glutamic acid was connected to the γ-carboxyl group, and this was confirmed by ${}^1H$-NMR spec-

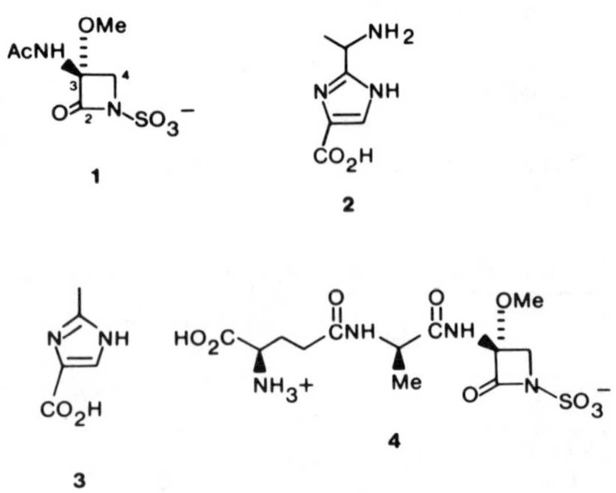

FIG. 1. *Structure of* **1**, **2**, **3**, *and* **4**.

TABLE 1. *Antibacterial activity of SQ 26,445 (EM5210)*[a]

Organism	SC#	MIC (μg/ml)
Staphylococcus aureus	1276	>100
Staphylococcus aureus	2399	>100
Staphylococcus aureus	2400	>100
Staphylococcus aureus	10165	>100
Streptococcus faecalis	9011	>100
Streptococcus agalactiae	9287	50
Micrococcus luteus	2495	50
Escherichia coli	8294	50
Escherichia coli	10857	100
Escherichia coli	10896	25
Klebsiella aerogenes	10440	50
Klebsiella pneumoniae	9527	50
Proteus mirabilis	3855	12.5
Proteus rettgeri	8479	6.3
Proteus vulgaris	9416	25
Salmonella typhosa	1195	25
Shigella sonnei	8449	50
Enterobacter cloacae	8236	25
Enterobacter aerogenes	10078	50
Citrobacter freundii	9518	25
Serratia marcescens	9783	25
Pseudomonas aeruginosa	9545	50
Pseudomonas aeruginosa	8329	>100
Acinetobacter calcoaceticus	8333	25

[a] Medium: DST agar (Oxoid Ltd.). Inoculum: 10^4 colony-forming units. SC#: Squibb collection number.

troscopy of SQ 26,445 at pH 1 to 6 (3, 4). The full structure of SQ 26,445 was therefore deduced to be **4**, in which the configuration at position 3 of the azetidinone is assumed to be the same as that in **1** (determined by synthesis). An antibiotic of this structure was isolated independently by workers at Takeda Chemical Industries, Ltd. (1, 2).

SQ 26,445 has moderate antibacterial activity (Table 1).

1. **Asai, M., K. Haibara, M. Muroi, K. Kintaka, and T. Kishi.** 1981. Sulfazecin, a novel β-lactam antibiotic of bacterial origin. Isolation and chemical characterization. J. Antibiot. **34**:621–627.
2. **Imada, A., K. Kitano, K. Kintaka, M. Muroi, and M. Asai.** 1981. Sulfazecin and isosulfazecin, novel β-lactam antibiotics of bacterial origin. Nature (London) **289**: 590–591.
3. **Kasai, T., and S. Sakamura.** 1973. NMR spectra of glutamic acid-containing dipeptides in relation to sequence determination. Agric. Biol. Chem. **37**:2155–2157.
4. **Kristensen, I., and P. O. Larsen.** 1973. Differentiation between α-glutamyl peptides, γ-glutamyl peptides, and α-aminoacyl glutamic acids by PMR spectroscopy. Acta Chem. Scand. **27**:3123–3125.
5. **Sykes, R. B., C. M. Cimarusti, D. P. Bonner, K. Bush, D. M. Floyd, N. H. Georgopapadakou, W. H. Koster, W. C. Liu, W. L. Parker, P. A. Principe, M. L. Rathnum, W. A. Slusarchyk, W. H. Trejo, and J. S. Wells.** 1981. Monocyclic β-lactam antibiotics produced by bacteria. Nature (London) **291**:489–491.

Phase I Clinical Study of TA-058

HARUMI SHISHIDO,* KEIZO MATSUMOTO, YOSHIO UZUKA, TAKESHI NAGATAKE, MASASHI YAMAMOTO, YOSHIMITSU SAKUMA, AND TOTARO YAMAGUCHI

Department of Internal Medicine, Institute for Tropical Medicine, Nagasaki University, Nagasaki, and Microbiological Research Laboratory, Tanabe Seiyaku Co., Ltd., Saitama, Japan*

TA-058, 6-[D-2-(D-2-amino-3-*N*-methylcarbamoylpropionamido)-2-*P*-hydroxyphenylacetamido] penicillanic acid trihydrate, is a new semisynthetic penicillin for parenteral use, and is superior to some other penicillins in its in vitro and in vivo antibacterial activity as well as for its lack of toxicity (1).

In this study, the clinical safety of TA-058 was examined in a phase I trial with healthy volunteers, and pharmacokinetic data with these subjects were analyzed and compared with those of piperacillin.

Clinical safety study. Eight healthy adult male volunteers were equally divided into two groups. Those in group A were administered intravenously (i.v.) 1 g of TA-058 per man once a day at 9:00 a.m. for the first 2 days and twice a day at 9:00 a.m. and 7:00 p.m. for the following 3 days, and those in group B were administered the same dose twice a day at 9:00 a.m. and 7:00 p.m. for 5 consecutive days. All of the volunteers were hospitalized for 6 days and were subjected to physical examinations and laboratory tests. Some of the laboratory tests were repeated 2 and 4 weeks after their discharge.

Abnormalities attributable to TA-058 were not observed in any of the physical examinations (blood pressure, pulse rate, electrocardiogram, and respiratory rate) or the laboratory tests (hematological examination, blood chemistry, and urinalysis).

Serum concentration and urinary excretion. Serum and urinary concentrations of TA-058 were determined by the agar diffusion method, using *Bacillus subtilis* ATCC 6633.

TA-058 gave its peak serum concentration 5

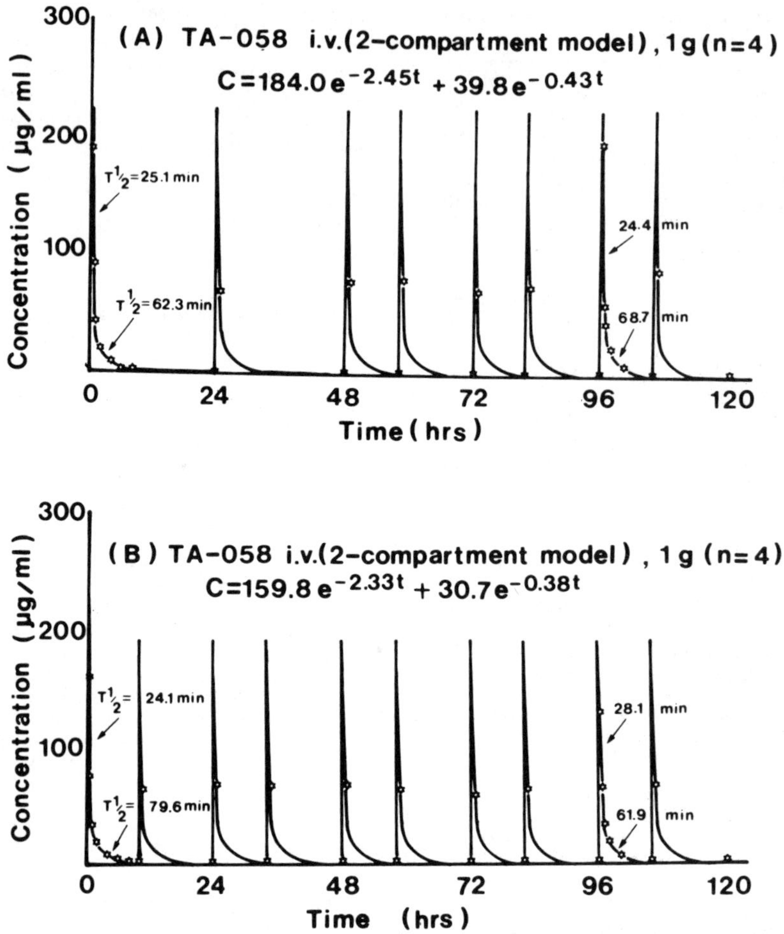

FIG. 1. *Serum concentration curves in healthy volunteers administered i.v. injections of TA-058 8 (A) and 10 (B) times.*

TABLE 1. *Pharmacokinetic parameters of TA-058 and piperacillin in eight volunteers given single 1.0-g i.v. and d.i. doses (crossover)*[a]

Drug	Route[b]	n[c]	A (µg/ml)	B (µg/ml)	α (h^{-1})	β (h^{-1})	$T_{1/2}$ (β) (h)	K_{12} (h^{-1})	K_{21} (h^{-1})	K_{el} (h^{-1})	Vc (liters)	V_T (liters)	Vc + V_T (liters)	$AUC_{0-\infty}$ (µg.h/ml)
TA-058	i.v.	4	106.4	18.0	1.81	0.42	1.7	0.38	0.62	1.23	8.05	4.92	12.97	101.7
PIPC	i.v.	4	93.0	14.0	2.55	0.65	1.1	0.46	0.90	1.84	9.31	4.79	14.10	58.0
TA-058	d.i.	4	127.5	18.3	1.89	0.43	1.6	0.38	0.61	1.33	6.86	4.27	11.13	110.0
PIPC	d.i.	4	72.7	4.8	1.83	0.51	1.4	0.17	0.59	1.58	12.90	3.72	16.62	49.1

[a] PIPC, Piperacillin; n, number of volunteers (crossover); A and B, drug concentration at time zero in α and β phase; α and β, hybrid rate constant for distribution and elimination phase; T/2 (β), biological half-life (β phase), K_{12} and K_{21}, transfer rate constant; K_{el}, elimination rate constant; Vc, volume of distribution in central compartment; V_T, volume of distribution in tissue compartment; AUC, area under the curve. Calculation: least square method using NONLIN; i.v. and d.i., two-compartment model, i.m., one-compartment model.

[b] The drugs were dissolved in 20 ml of distilled water for i.v., 250 ml of physiological saline for d.i. (over 1 h), and 3 ml of 0.5% lidocaine solution for i.m. administration.

[c] All volunteers were fasted overnight before administration. There was a 2-week washout period between the crossover experiments.

TABLE 2. *Pharmacokinetic parameters of TA-058 and piperacillin in five volunteers given single 1.0-g i.m. doses (crossover)*[a]

Drug	Route[b]	n[c]	V/F (liters)	K_a (h^{-1})	K_{el} (h^{-1})	$T_{1/2}$ (K_{el}) (h)	C_{max} (μg/ml)	t_{max} (h)	$AUC_{0-\infty}$ (μg.h/ml)
TA-058	i.m.	5	31.1	3.15	0.40	1.7	23.8	0.75	80.4
PIPC	i.m.	5	45.2	4.66	0.55	1.3	16.6	0.52	40.0

[a] V, Volume of distribution; F, fraction of dose absorbed; K_a, absorption rate constant; C_{max}, maximum serum concentration; t_{max}, time of maximum concentration. For other abbreviations and description of calculation, see Table 1, footnote *a*.

[b] See Table 1, footnote *b*.

[c] See Table 1, footnote *c*.

min after the i.v. administration. The mean peak concentration on days 1 and 5 (5 min after the first injection) in group A were 188.5 and 194.0 μg/ml, respectively, and those in group B were 161.0 and 131.0 μg/ml. The half-lives of the serum concentration in the α-phase ($T_{1/2}\alpha$) and β-phase($T_{1/2}\beta$) were calculated to be 24.1 to 25.1 and 62.3 to 79.6 min, respectively. The mean serum concentration data were fitted to a two-compartment open model (Fig. 1). Within 4 h after administration, 75% of the dose was excreted as TA-058 into the urine. Examination by thin-layer chromatographic bioautography revealed that there was no active metabolite in serum, though a trace amount of amoxicillin was in the one urine sample collected 10 h after the administration on the first day. No evidence of accumulation was obtained after 5 consecutive days of administration.

Absorption and excretion of TA-058 were compared with those of piperacillin in 13 healthy adult male volunteers after i.v. injection, intramuscular (i.m.) injection, or intravenous drip infusion (d.i.). The administration schedule and the model parameter studies are shown in Tables 1 and 2. The serum and urinary curves for i.v. and d.i. administration were shown to be well fitted to a two-compartment open model, whereas the curves for i.m. injection were best represented by a one-compartment model. The serum half-life of TA-058 in the β-phase ($T_{1/2}\beta$) was longer than that of piperacillin and the area under the curve of TA-058 was two- to threefold greater than that of piperacillin by any route of administration. The peak serum concentrations of TA-058 were always higher than those of piperacillin, regardless of the administration route.

The 8-h urinary recovery rates of TA-058 after d.i., i.v., and i.m. administration were 87.9, 75.1, and 74.9%, respectively. In contrast, the urinary recovery of piperacillin up to 8 h ranged from 70 to 75%.

In a separate experiment, three groups of volunteers consisting of four healthy male adults each were administered (d.i.) 0.5, 1.0, and 2.0 g of TA-058 per man, respectively. The mean area under the curve values were 47.5, 100.0, and 219.5 μg.h/ml, respectively, and thus were in proportion to the dose.

In view of the in vitro and in vivo antibacterial activities of TA-058, superior to those of piperacillin and other established semisynthetic penicillins, and also the clinical safety and the excellent pharmacokinetic properties compared with those of piperacillin, as described in this study, further extensive phase II studies of TA-058 are warranted.

1. **Nishino, T., N. Ishii, T. Tanino, S. Ohshima, and T. Yamaguchi.** 1980. In vitro and in vivo antibacterial activity of TA-058, a new broad-spectrum semisynthetic penicillin, p. 362–363. *In* J. D. Nelson and C. Grassi (ed.), Current chemotherapy and infectious diseases. American Society for Microbiology, Washington, D.C.

Pharmacokinetic Studies of TA-058 in Laboratory Animals

TOTARŌ YAMAGUCHI,* ISAO MAEZAWA, YOSHIMITSU SAKUMA, KATO TANI, HIROTSUGU YOSHIDA, AND SATOSHI OHSHIMA

Microbiological Research Laboratory, Tanabe Seiyaku Co., Ltd., Saitama, Japan

The in vitro and in vivo antibacterial activities of TA-058, 6-[D-2-(D-2-amino-3-*N*-methylcarbamoylpropionamido)-2-*P*-hydroxyphenyl-acetamido] penicillanic acid trihydrate, a new semisynthetic penicillin derivative for parenteral use, were reported previously (1).

In this study, the pharmacokinetics and metabolism of TA-058 in laboratory animals and its serum protein binding were investigated and compared with those of piperacillin and carbenicillin.

A single dose of 20 or 100 mg of TA-058 per kg was administered intravenously or intramuscularly into mice, rats, rabbits, and dogs, and its serum levels were determined (Fig. 1). All of the species attained comparable serum concentrations after intramuscular administration, but the decay of TA-058 concentrations in serum differed from species to species; i.e., it was fastest in rats and mice and slowest in dogs. The increase in the dose of TA-058 from 20 to 100 mg/kg resulted in a proportionate increase in the serum level.

After intravenous injection in rats, TA-058 tissue levels in the body were in the descending order of kidney, serum, liver, and lung (Table 1). The kidney concentrations in the rats were found to be higher than those in the mice, whereas the liver concentrations were lower in the rats than in the mice. In comparison with piperacillin and carbenicillin, TA-058 gave higher concentrations in the serum, lung, and kidney of rats than did the other two semisynthetic penicillins. Intramuscular administration of TA-058 in rats gave its peak tissue concentrations at 15 min, and the order of the tissue levels was the same as that after the intravenous administration. The tissue levels of TA-058 in the serum, kidney, and lung were higher than those of piperacillin and carbenicillin and persisted much longer than those of the latter compounds.

The 24-h urinary and biliary recovery rates of TA-058 in rats after intramuscular injection of 20 mg/kg were 63 and 19%, respectively (Table 1). The urinary and biliary excretion were almost complete within the first 2 and 4 h, respectively. On the other hand, the 24-h urinary and biliary recovery rates of piperacillin under the same conditions were 50 and 20%, respectively.

The 24-h urinary and biliary recovery rates of TA-058 in rabbits after intravenous injection of 20 mg/kg were 86 and 13%, respectively, and those of piperacillin were 52 and 43%, respectively.

To compare the serum levels of TA-058 and piperacillin, four beagle dogs were administered each drug by an intravenous drip-infusion method in a crossover study. The serum level of TA-058 just after the completion of the administration was two times higher than that of piperacillin, and the former persisted much longer than the latter (Table 1). In this crossover study, the urinary excretion rates of TA-058 were 47% of the dose during the drip-infusion period (1 h) and 23% in the following 4 h. Piperacillin was excreted into the urine with a pattern similar to that of TA-058.

In the rats and rabbits given probenecid, the peak serum concentrations of TA-058 were about two times higher than those in control animals without probenecid. This result would be expected if TA-058 is excreted into the urine through the uriniferous tubules of the kidney.

When 100 mg of TA-058 per kg was intravenously injected into rats, practically no amoxicillin was detected in samples of serum, lung,

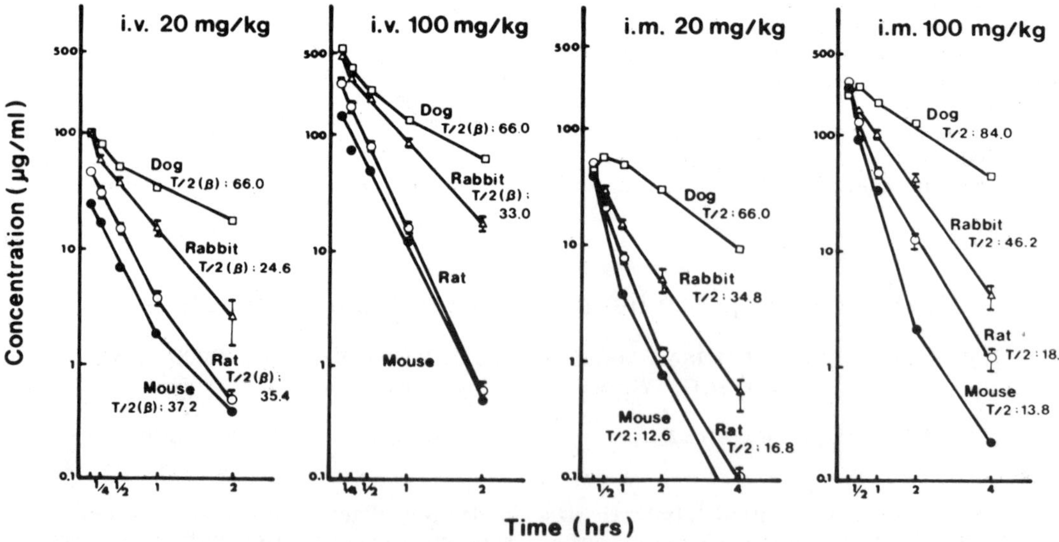

FIG. 1. *Serum levels of TA-058. i.v., Intravenous; i.m., intramuscular.*

TABLE 1. *Tissue distribution levels and other pharmacokinetic parameters of TA-058 and piperacillin after parenteral administration in various laboratory animals*[a]

Animal	Drug	Route	Dose (mg/kg)	Serum or tissue	Concn (μg/ml)						$AUC_{0-\infty}$ (μg.h/ml)	$T_{1/2}$ (min)[c]	Recovery (%)			
					7.5 min[b]	15 min	30 min	1 h	2 h	4 h			Urinary 0–5 h	Urinary 5–24 h	Biliary 0–4 h	Biliary 4–24 h
Rat	TA-058	i.v.	20	Serum	46.6	31.3	14.8	3.7	0.5	NT[d]	23.2	35.4	NT	NT	NT	NT
				Lung	19.7	13.1	6.3	1.9	0.3	NT						
				Liver	35.7	31.4	17.2	6.2	1.6	NT						
				Kidney	148.1	104.3	62.9	31.5	5.8	NT						
	PIPC	i.v.	20	Serum	13.2	6.5	0.1	—	—	NT			NT	NT	NT	NT
				Lung	8.4	2.3	0.6	—	—	NT						
				Liver	115.0	32.1	10.0	3.7	1.6	NT						
				Kidney	115.0	34.8	5.1	—	—	NT						
	TA-058	i.m.	20	Serum	NT	48.5	21.2	7.5	1.1	0.1	32.7	16.8	61.9	2.0	15.8	2.9
				Lung	NT	14.3	8.5	3.1	0.4	—						
				Liver	NT	30.3	24.8	9.3	1.8	0.2						
				Kidney	NT	163.1	113.4	49.3	14.5	2.0						
	PIPC	i.m.	20	Serum	NT	11.8	4.1	0.3	—	—			21.7	0.5	53.4	1.6
				Lung	NT	6.1	2.8	0.3	—	—						
				Liver	NT	52.1	26.5	3.5	—	—						
				Kidney	NT	81.5	30.9	3.5	0.5	—						
Rabbit	TA-058	i.v.	20	Serum	102.0	57.0	36.5	14.7	2.6	1.2	65.1	24.6	66.2[e]	21.3[e]	12.8	0.3
	PIPC	i.v.	20		NT	NT	NT	NT	NT	NT			54.0[e]	0.25[e]	41.7	2.0
	TA-058	i.m.	20	Serum	NT	NT	30.0	15.3	5.2	—	42.8	34.8	NT	NT	NT	NT
Dog	TA-058	i.v.	20	Serum	96.3	79.7	49.0	35.0	17.2	5.1	114.5	66.0				
	TA-058	i.m.	20	Serum	24.0	43.7	58.0	49.7	29.7	9.0	134.7	66.0	NT	NT	NT	NT
	TA-058	d.i.	20	Serum	17.9	30.2	52.4	77.2					70.6			
					58.5	48.8	34.4	20.6	6.6	1.3					NT	NT
	PIPC	d.i.	20	Serum	11.8	20.5	27.5	36.4								
					28.2	21.4	12.6	5.4	1.3	0.09			64.6		NT	NT

[a] PIPC, Piperacillin; AUC, area under the curve; i.v., intravenous; i.m., intramuscular; d.i., intravenous drip-infusion. Intravenous drip-infusion was given over 1 h. —, None detected.

[b] Time after injection.

[c] Half-life: intravenous, β-phase of two-compartment model; intramuscular, one-compartment model.

[d] NT, Not tested.

[e] At 0 to 4 and 4 to 24 h after injection.

liver, kidney, urine, and bile collected at 2 to 6 h after administration. Incubation of TA-058 with the serum, urine, bile, or any of the above tissues yielded no amoxicillin in the 4-h incubation period, whereas a trace amount of amoxicillin was detected in each incubation mixture after the succeeding 20 h of incubation.

The rate of human serum protein binding of TA-058 was 24%, which was lower than those of carbenicillin (69%) and piperacillin (35%). With rat and dog sera, the protein-binding rates (22% in rats and 18% in dogs) of TA-058 were also lower than those of carbenicillin and piperacillin.

The results obtained may be summarized as follows: TA-058 is well absorbed from the site of injection (intramuscular), distributed to most tissues in high concentrations, resistant to metabolic inactivation, and excreted into urine efficiently through the uriniferous tubules of the kidney, and, especially, it gives higher serum concentrations compared with the other semisynthetic penicillins.

1. **Nishino, T., N. Ishii, T. Tanino, S. Ohshima, and T. Yamaguchi.** 1980. In vitro and in vivo antibacterial activity of TA-058, a new broad-spectrum semisynthetic penicillin, p. 362–363. *In* J. D. Nelson and C. Grassi (ed.), Current chemotherapy and infectious disease. American Society for Microbiology, Washington, D.C.

Carboxamides of Ampicillin with Anti-*Pseudomonas* Activity

A. GUERRATO, L. MORELLI, P. ORSOLINI, D. PIERACCIOLI, B. TAMBURINI,* L. XERRI, AND G. COPPI

Glaxo Research Laboratories, Inc., Verona, Italy

During recent years, pyridone carboxamides of ampicillin or amoxicillin have attracted the attention of medicinal chemists on account of their activity against *Pseudomonas* spp., responsible for very serious infections in hospitals.

A synthetic program at Glaxo Research Laboratories in Verona, Italy, undertaken to come up with penicillins capable of combatting these infections, has led to a series of pyrimidinone derivatives of ampicillin which are characterized by significant activity against *Pseudomonas* spp.

Table 1 shows the generic structure of these ampicillin derivatives (compounds 7 through 15) and their in vitro activity against a number of gram-positive and gram-positive bacteria, including *Pseudomonas* spp. Included for purposes of comparison are the activities of ampicillin, carbenicillin, and mezlocillin.

A preliminary study of ampicillin amides with cycloalcane carboxilic acids (see Table 1, compounds 1 through 6) yielded interesting information with regard to the correlation between certain physicochemical characteristics of the molecules and their activity.

Even though their spectra are not very broad and they prove less active than the reference standards, it is interesting to note that the activity against *Pseudomonas* spp. is correlated to the increase in the size of the ring, i.e., to the increase in the steric hindrance and in the lipophilic character of the side chain substituents. This information was then applied to a few derivatives of a thiazole-pyrimidinone carboxamide of ampicillin (compound 7), which revealed a broad spectrum of activity against gram-positive and gram-negative strains, in particular, of *Pseudomonas* spp.

The substitution of methyl or phenyl (compounds 8 and 9) for one hydrogen atom in the thiazole ring led to a reduction in activity against *Pseudomonas* spp. (Table 1); moreover, the thiazolidine derivative (compound 10), although more lipophilic, is less active than the thiazole derivative. Compound 11 possesses a structure which is correlated to that of compound 9, except in the case of the former compound the phenyl ring is coplanar with the thiazole-pyrimidine ring, yet is similar to compound 7 in terms of its activity against *Pseudomonas*, and there is an appreciable increase in its activity against gram-negative strains with consequent broadening of the spectrum of this penicillin.

Substitutions in the phenyl ring of benzothiazole derivative 11 led to less active compounds, and the isosteric substitution of a benzoxazole ring (compound 14) for the benzothiazole ring also failed to yield better results.

Attempts to make compound 7 more hydrophilic by substituting a triazole ring (compound 15) for the thiazole ring again yielded a less active compound.

In conclusion, of the molecules thus far synthesized, the most active appears to be the parent compound 7. Further syntheses of penicillins of this type are under way to verify the correlation, if any, between the cycloalcane and the pyrimidinone series.

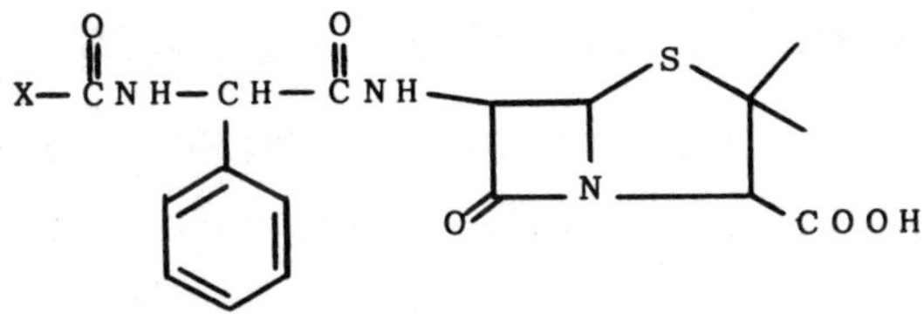

TABLE 1. *In vitro activity (MIC in μg/ml) of carboxamides of ampicillin*

No.	Compound	*Staphylococcus aureus* 663	*Staphylococcus aureus* 1612	*Streptococcus faecalis* 850	*E. coli* 851	*Proteus mirabilis* 431	*Proteus vulgaris* 1356	*Pseudomonas aeruginosa* 150
1	Cyclopropyl	3.9	125	15.6	62.5	31.2	>250	250
2	Cyclobutyl	<1.9	125	15.6	62.5	31.2	>250	250
3	Cyclopentyl	3.9	125	15.6	62.5	31.2	>250	250
4	Cyclohexyl	<1.9	125	31.2	62.5	31.2	>250	125
5	Cycloheptyl	<1.9	125	31.2	62.5	31.2	>250	62.5
6	Cyclooctyl	<1.9	125	31.2	31.2	31.2	250	62.5
7	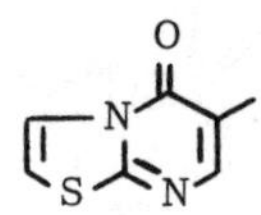	<1.9	>250	15.6	62.5	15.6	>250	7.8
8	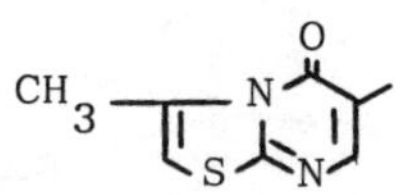	<1.9	250	31.2	31.2	31.2	250	62.5
9	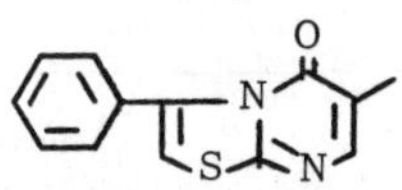	<1.9	250	125	7.8	15.6	62.5	125
10	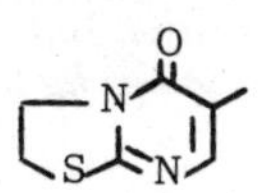	<1.9	250	250	125	62.5	>250	250
11	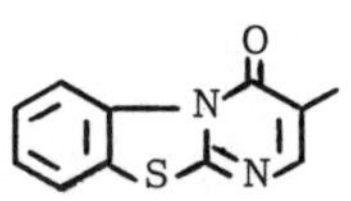	<1.9	250	15.6	7.8	3.9	62.5	31.2
12	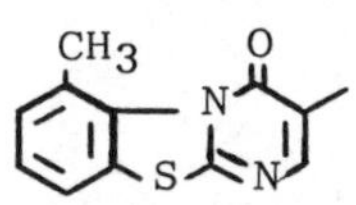	<1.9	125	>250	7.8	15.6	31.2	125
13	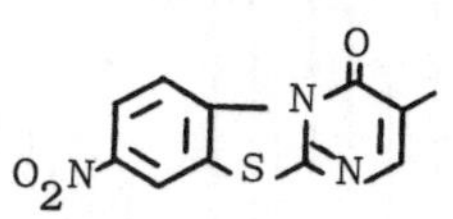	<1.9	250	125	62.5	31.2	>250	250
14	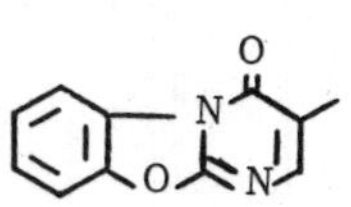	<1.9	250	250	31.2	3.9	>250	62.5
15	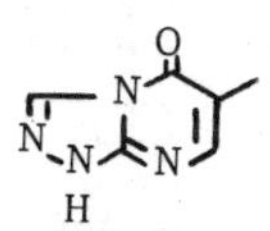	<1.9	250	62.5	31.2	15.6	>250	62.5
	Ampicillin	<1.9	>250	<1.9	7.8	<1.9	>250	250
	Carbenicillin	<1.9	125	62.5	7.8	<1.9	250	31.2
	Mezlocillin	<1.9	250	31.2	3.9	<1.9	62.5	15.6

Comparative Pharmacokinetic Study of KB1585 and Talampicillin

C. L. AFFOO,* F. MOOSDEEN, J. D. WILLIAMS, AND S. YAMABE

Department of Medical Microbiology, The London Hospital Medical College, London E1 2AD, U.K.

KB1585 is a dioxolene ester of ampicillin. Studies in experimental animals have shown that after oral administration the drug is readily absorbed and hydrolyzed to ampicillin. We therefore thought it of interest to compare the pharmacokinetics of KB1585 with those of the closely related antibiotics talampicillin and ampicillin.

We studied six healthy, fasting, adult subjects and administered single oral doses of the three drugs at 1-week intervals in a dosage of 4 mg/kg (of ampicillin equivalent) in a randomized, blind crossover pattern. Hematological and biochemical parameters were monitored before and after the administration of KB1585 and talampicillin. Venous blood samples were taken at 5, 10, 15, 20, 25, 30, 40, 50, 60, 90, 120, 180, and 240 min. Samples of urine were collected at intervals of 0 to 2, 2 to 4, 4 to 6, and 6 to 12 h, the volumes were recorded, and each sample was stored at −20°C.

Serum samples, within 24 h of collection, and urine samples were assayed for ampicillin by the agar-diffusion technique, using nutrient agar. *Staphylococcus aureus* (NCTC 6571) was incorporated in the agar as the indicator organism. Standard and test samples, in duplicate, were applied in a randomized fashion to wells in large plates (23 cm^2). Standard curves were obtained for the range of 0.25 to 8 mg/liter, ampicillin was dissolved in sterile water, and dilutions were made in serum and 0.1 M phosphate buffer, pH 7.4, for serum and urine assays, respectively.

The linear regression coefficient

$$r = \frac{\Sigma XY - \dfrac{\Sigma X \Sigma Y}{n}}{\sqrt{\left(\Sigma X^2 - \dfrac{(\Sigma X)^2}{n}\right)\left(\Sigma Y^2 - \dfrac{(\Sigma Y)^2}{n}\right)}}$$

was calculated for each standard curve and, using the regression equation ($Y_{est} = mx + b$), free ampicillin levels in serum and urine samples were computed.

Both KB1585 and talampicillin gave peak levels (of free ampicillin) 30 min after administration which ranged from 4.5 to 7.3 mg/liter; doses of ampicillin gave peak levels of between 1.5 and 2.7 mg/liter at 60 min (Fig. 1). At 4 h after administration of each drug, the concentration of ampicillin was less than 0.5 mg/liter. High serum levels correlated with high recovery of ampicillin from the urine. Figure 2 shows the urinary excretion for each drug. Of the free ampicillin, 71% was recovered in the urine 4 h after talampicillin administration, and 59% was

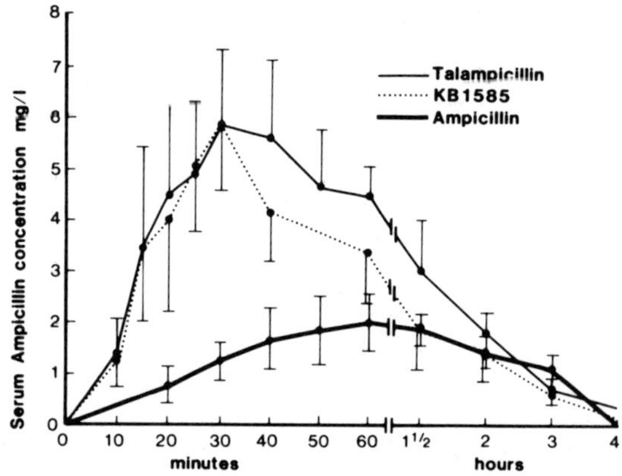

FIG. 1. *Serum levels of ampicillin after single oral doses of KB1585, talampicillin, and ampicillin equivalent to 4 mg of ampicillin per kg (mean values for six normal volunteers).*

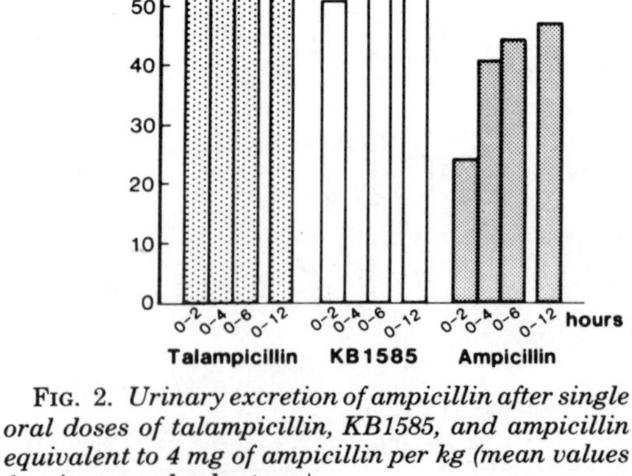

FIG. 2. *Urinary excretion of ampicillin after single oral doses of talampicillin, KB1585, and ampicillin equivalent to 4 mg of ampicillin per kg (mean values for six normal volunteers).*

recovered 4 h after the dose of KB1585. After the dose of ampicillin, 47% was recovered in the urine by 12 h.

No hematological or biochemical abnormalities were noted before or after the administration of KB1585 or after talampicillin. There were no side effects in any of the six subjects.

The serum levels for KB1585 and talampicillin at various time intervals were compatible with a single-compartment open model. KB1585 and talampicillin had similar half-lives, namely, 0.75 ± 0.04 and 0.75 ± 0.06 h, respectively. Their elimination constants were both 0.92 h^{-1}. The mean area under the curve for KB1585 and talampicillin was 58.7 ± 8.0 and 80.5 ± 12.8 mg.h/liter, respectively.

The results of this study suggest that the absorption of talampicillin is more complete than that of KB1585 and that both esters are better absorbed than ampicillin. KB1585 and talampicillin have similar peak levels that are higher, and occur much earlier, than those of ampicillin. KB1585 and talampicillin are otherwise similar in terms of their half-lives and elimination constants. None of the three drugs produced side effects.

Cellular and Molecular Action of Clofoctol on Bacteria

F. YABLONSKY, J. COMBE, F. SIMONNET, AND G. SIMONNET

C.E.N. Saclay, Institut National des Sciences et Techniques Nucleaires, Laboratoire de Radiobiologie, 91191 Gif sur Yvette Cedex, France

Clofoctol, (tetramethyl-1,1,3,3-butyl)-4-(dichloro-2,4-benzyl)-2-hydroxy-1-benzene, is a new synthetic antibacterial agent active against gram-positive bacteria. This compound is used in human medicine for the treatment of upper respiratory tract infections. The mechanism of action of this antibacterial agent is at present unknown. However, clofoctol is not a specific inhibitor of one of the nucleic acid syntheses (DNA, RNA) or proteins (4).

In this report, we determined an interaction of clofoctol with the cell envelope, either or morphology, on cell wall synthesis, or on biochemical properties associated with the envelope: membrane permeability and energetic me tabolism.

Action of clofoctol on the structure of the cellular envelope and cell wall synthesis. Whole cells of *Bacillus subtilis* were incubated in a synthetic medium and treated with a bacteriostatic concentration of clofoctol for 30 min. Sectioned and stained cells were examined by electron microscopy. Among the nonlysed cells, we observed physical damage to the cell wall and the cytoplasmic membrane. These holes in the bacterial envelope seemed to be located always at the septum or the potential septum of the bacteria.

Clofoctol is active only against gram-positive bacteria. However, this antibacterial agent lyses gram-negative bacteria when they are treated with lysozyme and EDTA (spheroplasts). The lack of activity of clofoctol, which is a very hydrophobic drug, against gram-negative bacteria is certainly due to its inability to penetrate the lipopolysaccharide layer. Gram-positive bacteria bind clofoctol (10^6 to 10^7 molecules per cell), whereas gram-negative bacteria do not (2). Both protoplasts and spheroplasts bind clofoctol.

Like many antibiotics, such as penicillins, cycloserine, and vancomycin, clofoctol (4 μg/ml) has been observed to cause an accumulation of UDP-*N*-acetylmuramyl pentapeptide in *B. cereus*. Peptidoglycan synthesis was measured by the incorporation of *N*-acetyl[^{14}C]glucosamine into glucosamine and muramic acid residues of the peptidoglycan (5). Clofoctol at 4 μg/ml inhibited the incorporation of *N*-acetylglucosamine into peptidoglycan after 30 min of incubation and caused a concomitant intracellular accumulation of UDP-*N*-acetylmuramyl pentapeptide.

However, in vitro incorporation of [^{14}C]UDP-*N*-acetylmuramyl pentapeptide into peptidoglycan is not inhibited by clofoctol when a particulate enzymatic preparation from *Escherichia coli* JE5605 is used (3). Under these conditions, the overall course of peptidoglycan synthesis is considered. These results indicate that clofoctol acts differently from penicillin or vancomycin, even though it causes an accumulation of mucopeptide within the cells. It is conceivable that this drug affects the synthesis of various membrane components and that the observed inhibition of cell wall synthesis is a consequence of this action.

Action of clofoctol on the biochemical

properties associated with the envelope. The membrane is the site of many enzymes which control the active transport of amino acids and sugars into the cell. It may also be the site of cell wall synthesis and electron transport. The action of clofoctol on *B. subtilis* is characterized by a rapid leakage of intracellular materials that absorb light at 260 nm. Treatment of whole cells, protoplasts, or vesicles from *B. subtilis*, and of spheroplasts or vesicles from *E. coli* with clofoctol after loading with [^{14}C]glutamate, resulted in a very rapid leakage of radioactivity (Fig. 1).

In the same way, the uptake of [^{14}C]glutamate was inhibited by clofoctol in the same cellular structures. This leakage upon exposure of susceptible bacteria to clofoctol is thought to be evidence of membrane-damaging action. The disorganization of this structure would be lethal for the cell. As a consequence, membrane-localized enzymes or carriers would be affected. We tried to evaluate the relationship between the effects of clofoctol on bacterial metabolism and the effects on the viability of the cells.

Clofoctol does not inhibit the oxygen consumption of *B. subtilis* even at very high concentrations (50 μg/ml). Since all macromolecular syntheses are stopped after treatment with clofoctol, the effect of the drug on intracellular ATP concentration was studied (1). A culture of *B. subtilis* was treated with 4 μg of clofoctol per ml, and we observed a very rapid decrease in the intracellular ATP pool (Fig. 2) but an increase in the intracellular ADP pool. This observation may be explained by a disruption of the cytoplasmic membrane. Consequent loss of small molecules, ions, and ATP may cause the inhibition of the incorporation of labeled precursors into macromolecules. We have observed also that clofoctol alters both membrane potential and pH gradient.

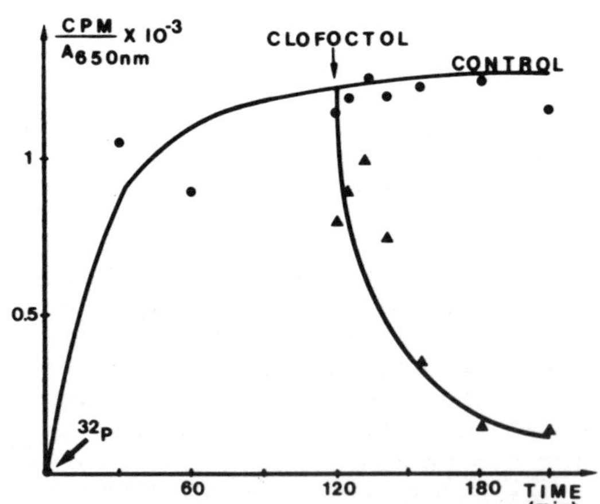

FIG. 1. *Efflux of glutamate from preloaded B. subtilis cells. The cells were allowed to accumulate [^{14}C]glutamate for 30 min at 37°C (10^{-4} M; 0.025 μCi/ml). At zero time, clofoctol was added (·—·, control; △, 3.3 μg/ml), and equal portions were filtered at various times to measure the amount of radioactivity remaining in the cells.*

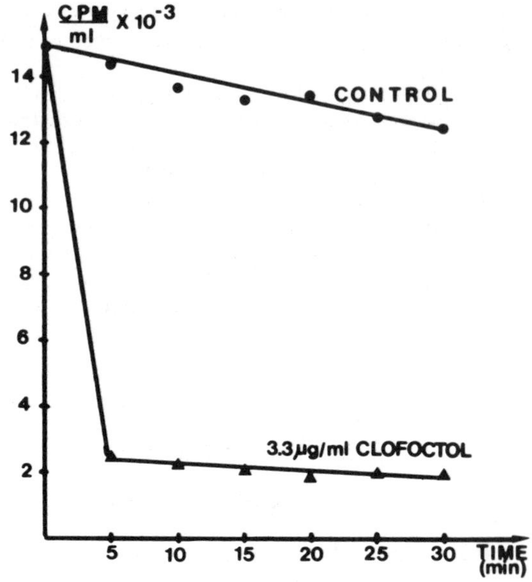

FIG. 2. *Intracellular pool of ATP in B. subtilis cells. Incorporation of $H_3{}^{32}PO_4$ (5.10^{-4} M; 100 μCi/ml) into the intracellular pool of ATP was measured after extraction of the cells with 2 M formic acid and chromatography. Clofoctol was added after 2 h at the steady state. Symbols: ·—·, control; △, 4 μg of clofoctol per ml.*

Conclusions. The morphological alterations observed in the surface structure of clofoctol-treated *B. subtilis*, as well as the inhibition of cell wall synthesis, can explain the modifications of cell permeability properties. These modifications result in a release of 260-nm-absorbing materials. These alterations do not lead to any inhibition of oxygen uptake, but lead to a rapid decrease in the intracellular pool of ATP and to variations of pH gradient and membrane potential, which can explain the lethal action of clofoctol.

1. **Cashel, M.** 1969. The control of ribonucleic acid synthesis in *Escherichia coli.* J. Biol. Chem. **244:**3133–3141.
2. **Combe, J., F. Simonnet, F. Yablonsky, and G. Simonnet.** 1980. Clofoctol binding by the bacteria. J. Pharmacol. **11:**411–426.
3. **Isaki, K., M. Matsuhashi, and J. L. Strominger.** 1968. Biosynthesis of peptidoglycan of bacterial cell walls. J. Biol. Chem. **243:**3180–3192.
4. **Simonnet, F., G. Simonnet, and J. Combe.** 1979. Action of clofoctol on Gram positive bacteria. J. Pharmacol. **10:**303–314.
5. **Tynecka, Z., and J. B. Ward.** 1975. Peptidoglycan synthesis in *Bacillus licheniformis.* Biochem. J. **146:**253–267.

Target Binding Sites for Various Chemotherapeutic Agents Containing γ-Pyridone-β-Carboxylic Acid

TOSHIHIKO ARAI

Department of Microbiology, Keio University School of Medicine, Tokyo, Japan

Compounds containing a γ-pyridone-β-carboxylic acid structure represent an important group of antibacterial agents. It is well known that these drugs inhibit DNA replication by blocking the elongation of DNA chains and that their γ-pyridone-β-carboxylic acid structure is essential for their antibacterial function (2–4). Thus, these drugs are expected to have the same target. But we found that the combined use of nalidixic acid (NA) and pipemidic acid (PPA) had synergic action against bacteria (1). This could only be explained by the idea that these drugs have different binding sites on the target protein. In this paper, we discuss the relation among binding site specificities and chemical structures of these compounds by their antibacterial functions in combinational uses.

Compounds used for this study are shown in Fig. 1. NA, MPNA, MONA, and TQA were kindly supplied by R. Domori of Daiichi Seiyaku Co.; PPA, PA, AT, and ATO were supplied by M. Shimizu of Dainippon Pharmaceutical Co.; and OA and AM were supplied by Tanabe Seiyaku Co. and Kyorin Pharmaceutical Co., respectively. These drugs were dissolved in 0.1 N NaOH to 10 mg/ml and diluted stepwise with sterile distilled water. Combinations of 0.5 ml each of two different drug solutions with various concentrations and 14 ml of molten sensitivity disk agar (modified Mueller-Hinton agar; Nissui Seiyaku Co.) were mixed and solidified in petri dishes. *Escherichia coli* NIHJ JC2 was cultured in Trypticase soy broth (BBL Microbiology Systems) to mid-exponential growth phase and diluted with sterile physiological saline solution to about 10^4 cells/ml. Then 0.1 ml of this suspension was plated on the petri plates. Colonies grown on the plates were counted after 18 h of incubation at 37°C, and antibacterial effects of combinations of these drugs were estimated.

MPNA, AT, and ATO, which have a methyl (MM) residue at their terminal structure at the 7 position, and OA, which has a methylene (MM) residue at the 7 position, were all found to have an additive effect with NA and a synergistic effect with PPA. AM, which has a piperazinyl (PP) residue at the 7 position, was found to have an additive effect with PPA and a synergistic effect with NA. PA, which has a pyrrolidinyl (PR) residue at the 7 position, was found to have a synergistic effect with both NA and PPA. MONA, which has a morpholinoyl (MP) residue at the 7 position, was found to have only an additive effect with both NA and PPA, whereas TQA, which has a methylthiazol (MT) residue at the 5 and 6 positions, was found to have an independent or antagonistic effect with NA and PPA. It was also found that PA had a synergistic effect with MONA but an additive effect with TQA, and that MONA and TQA had additive effects. These results (Fig. 2) indicated that NA, MPNA, AT, ATO, and OA had the same function, that PPA and AM had also the same function, and that the functions of PA, MONA, TQA, and these two groups were different from one another. That is, these drugs could be classified into five groups by their synergistic, additive, or antagonistic relations in combinational uses.

If the major target of these compounds is common, as documented, since each group always has the common structure at the terminal 7 position, a direct relationship between chemi-

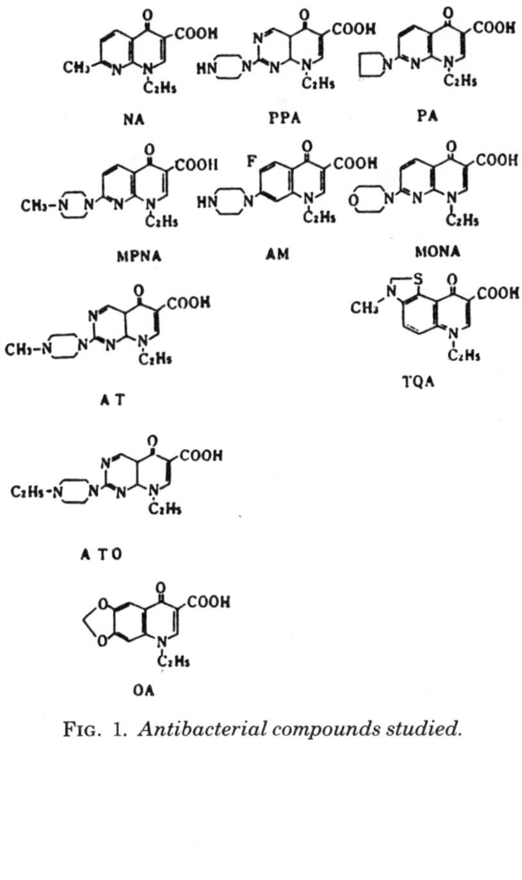

FIG. 1. *Antibacterial compounds studied.*

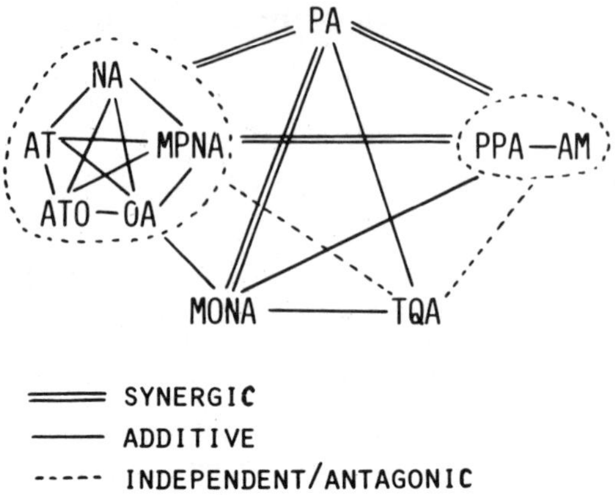

FIG. 2. *Antibacterial relationships among the compounds tested.*

cal structure and target binding specificity of these compounds is strongly suggested. The active structure to block DNA chain elongation could be due to the common 1-ethyl-4-oxoquinoline-3-carboxylic acid structure, as has been well documented, but the binding sites of the target enzyme for these compounds might be different by their terminal structure at the 7 position. That is, MM, PP, PR, and MP residues at the 7 position and the MT residue at the 5 and 6 positions took different binding sites. Sites for MM, PP, and PR accepted the corresponding compounds independently, but the binding of the MR compound to the site interfered with the binding of MM and PP for their sites. This could be explained by the idea that the MR site is located close to both MM and PP sites and that the binding of MR interferes with the binding of both MM and PP. The binding of the MT compound was found to actively remove already bound MM and PP compounds. This could also be explained by the idea that the binding of MT can cause an allosteric change of the target protein and that this change can close MM and PP sites.

1. **Arai, T.** 1980. Screening of drugs effective for combinational applications with pipemidic acid. Chemotherapy **28:**1060–1063. (In Japanese.)
2. **Bourguignon, G. J., M. Levitt, and R. Sternglanz.** 1973. Studies on the mechanism of action of nalidixic acid. Antimicrob. Agents Chemother. **4:**479–486.
3. **Darvas, F., Z. Mészáros, L. Kováca, I. Hermerz, M. Balogh, and J. Kardos.** 1979. Investigation of the common mechanism of action of antibacterial compounds containing γ-pyridone-β-carboxylic acid structure by principal component. Arzneim. Forsch. **29:** 1334–1339.
4. **Gellert, M., K. Mizzuuchi, M. H. O'Dea, T. Itoh, and J. Tomizawa.** 1977. Nalidixic acid resistance: a second genetic character involved in DNA gyrase activity. Proc. Natl. Acad. Sci. U.S.A. **74:**4772–4776.

Activity of Alafosfalin Against Bacterial Pathogens of the Gastrointestinal Tract In Vitro and In Vivo

DONALD WESTMACOTT,* MICHAEL J. HALL, CEDRIC H. HASSALL, LORNA J. LEES, BERNARD ROWE, AND LINDA R. WARD

Roche Products Limited, Welwyn Garden City, and Central Public Health Laboratories, Colindale, London, England*

Phosphonopeptides are novel peptide mimetics with acid-terminal residues simulating natural amino acids (5). The potent antibacterial activity of phosphonopeptides depends on three distinct stages: (i) transport into bacteria via peptide permeases, (ii) intracellular hydrolysis by aminopeptidases, and (iii) in the case of peptides derived from L-1-aminoethylphosphonic acid, inhibition of peptidoglycan biosynthesis essentially as a result of inactivation of alanine racemase by the released alanine mimetic (4).

Several properties of alafosfalin (L-alanyl-L-1-aminoethylphosphonic acid) suggested that this phosphonopeptide might be of use in gastrointestinal (GI) infections. The activity of alafosfalin is known to be especially potent against gram-negative bacteria and is not subject to cross-resistance with other commonly used antibacterial agents (7). Alafosfalin has also been shown to be effective against *Escherichia coli* infections in the mouse septicemia model both by oral and subcutaneous routes (1). In addition, high levels of agents are present in the small intestine of rats after dosing with [^{14}C]alafosfalin (2). Alafosfalin also offers a low order of toxicity to animals by all routes of administration (2) and is well tolerated in humans (3). In this paper we report a detailed examination of susceptibility of bacterial isolates from clinical cases of GI infections to alafosfalin and present data on the performance of alafosfalin in veterinary and preliminary human clinical trials in *E. coli* enterocolitis and shigellosis.

In vitro activity. The susceptibility to alafosfalin of 2,519 GI infection clinical isolates from wide-ranging geographical origins was determined by an agar dilution method using a defined, antagonist-free, susceptibility testing medium (1). *Shigella* spp. isolated from United Kingdom cases between June 1980 and February 1981 (mainly *S. flexneri*) were by far the most susceptible organisms to alafosfalin (Table 1). Only 2 out of 410 strains were not inhibited by 0.5 μg/ml. The few *S. sonnei* tested (n=8) were especially susceptible, all isolates being inhibited by 0.12 μg/ml. These results were comparable to the activity of mecillinam and trimethoprim against *Shigella* (6), but unlike these two agents no resistance to alafosfalin was observed in any of the 410 isolates.

A uniform pattern of susceptibility of *E. coli* to alafosfalin was observed in three United Kingdom centers and one Swedish center. A majority of isolates were highly susceptible (Table 1), with 97% of organisms being inhibited by 4 μg/ml. It would appear that the background level of resistance to alafosfalin in clinical isolates is very low.

TABLE 1. *Activity of alafosfalin against clinical isolates of bacteria from GI tract infections*

Organism	No. of isolates	MIC (μg/ml) Range	For 50% of isolates	For 90% of isolates
Shigella spp.	410	0.06–1	0.25	0.5
E. coli	318	0.03–64	0.5	2
V. cholerae	300	<1–>32	2	32
Salmonella spp. (not *S. paratyphi* A)	1521	0.25–>32	8	8
S. paratyphi A	70	>32	>32	>32

Isolates of *Vibrio cholerae* from 13 countries were generally inhibited by 2 μg of alafosfalin per ml (Table 1). The relatively high MIC_{90} value reflects the unexpectedly localized resistance to alafosfalin in Indonesia where 87% of isolates were inhibited only by 64 or 128 μg of alafosfalin per ml.

The majority of *Salmonella* isolates examined were susceptible to 8 μg of alafosfalin or less per ml (Table 1), although *S. typhi* was consistently more susceptible. *S. paratyphi* A strains isolated in Britain in 1978 from patients mainly infected in Southeast Asia were exceptional in being uniformly resistant to alafosfalin. The mechanism of this resistance is currently being investigated.

Piglet studies. Pharmacokinetics of alafosfalin in newborn swine indicated that this agent may be useful in treatment of scours of piglets. Alafosfalin was rapidly absorbed after intramuscular administration (500 mg/kg or 100 mg/kg) and cleared relatively slowly from the general circulation with a half-life of about 100 min. A trial of alafosfalin activity in an experimental infection of neonatal swine with the enterotoxigenic *E. coli* NADC 987 was initiated. Piglets were infected with 2×10^8 to 9×10^8 cells, and 1 h after onset of scouring were treated orally with water (placebo) or alafosfalin at 125 to 1,000 mg/kg. Doses were repeated after a further 4, 12, 24, 36, 48, 72, 96, and 120 h. A dose-dependent response to treatment was apparent at 500 and 1,000 mg/kg. With the highest dose, survival was increased from 29% (placebo) to 53%, weight

TABLE 2. *Summary of clinical and bacteriological responses to treatment of E. coli enterocolitis and shigellosis*

Bacterial diagnosis	Treatment[a]	No. of patients	Clinical response: Excellent/good	Clinical response: Moderate	Clinical response: Poor	Bacteriological response: Clearance	Bacteriological response: Failure	Bacteriological response: No record
E. coli[b] positive	Alafosfalin, 10 to 20 mg/kg/day (i.m.)	51	35 (69%)		16	38 (75%)	13	
	Bactrim, 20 mg/kg/day (i.m.)	20	12 (60%)		8	15 (75%)	5	
	Gentamicin, 5 mg/kg/day (i.m.)	15	8 (53%)		7	10 (66%)	5	
Shigella[c] positive	Alafosfalin, 250 mg q.d.s. (p.o.)	44	44 (100%)	0	0	42 (95%)	0	2
	Bactrim, 480 mg b.d. or q.d.s. (p.o.)	40	38 (95%)	2	0	37 (92.5%)	0	3

[a] i.m., Intramuscular; p.o., per oral; b.d., twice a day; q.d.s., four times a day.
[b] One noncomparative and two randomized comparative 6-day trials.
[c] Three randomized comparative 6-day trials.

gain per pig increased from 136 g to 413 g, and general appearance and autopsy scores improved significantly.

Clinical trials. An open pilot study of alafosfalin in the treatment of infantile enterocolitis (14 infants) was followed by a further two open, randomized trials comparing alafosfalin (51 infants) with co-trimoxazole (Bactrim) (20 infants) or gentamicin (15 infants), all administered intramuscularly. Table 2 summarizes results for bacteriologically confirmed *E. coli* cases. Alafosfalin was at least as effective as the standard agents, especially in terms of clinical response. When isolates at day 5 were tested for susceptibility to alafosfalin, no development of resistance to the agent was detected. No side effects of alafosfalin were reported in any of these trials.

A further three randomized trials were set up comparing orally administered alafosfalin with Bactrim in treatment of shigellosis in children and adults (total of 46 patients in each treatment group). All bacteriologically confirmed shigellosis cases which were treated with alafosfalin showed complete clinical and bacteriological recovery, this agent being at least as effective as Bactrim (Table 2). Side effects of alafosfalin were minimal, with nausea equivalent to that after Bactrim being reported in one trial and headache in two children in a second trial.

In conclusion, the consistent, marked in vitro activity of alafosfalin against *Shigella* spp. and *E. coli* was also expressed in GI infections caused by these organisms in adults and children. Efficacy in natural infections of humans appeared to be greater than in the experimental infection of piglets with an especially virulent enterotoxigenic *E. coli* strain. These results indicate that alafosfalin offers significant potential for chemotherapy of bacterial GI infections in adults and children.

1. **Allen, J. G., F. R. Atherton, M. J. Hall, C. H. Hassall, S. W. Holmes, R. W. Lambert, L. J. Nisbet, and P. S. Ringrose.** 1979. Phosphonopeptides as antibacterial agents: alaphosphin and related phosphonopeptides. Antimicrob. Agents Chemother. **15**:684–695.
2. **Allen, J. G., L. Havas, E. Leicht, I. Lenox-Smith, and L. J. Nisbet.** 1979. Phosphonopeptides as antibacterial agents: metabolism and pharmacokinetics of alafosfalin in animals and humans. Antimicrob. Agents Chemother. **16**:306–313.
3. **Allen, J. G., and L. J. Lees.** 1980. Pharmacokinetics of alafosfalin, alone and in combination with cephalexin, in humans. Antimicrob. Agents Chemother. **17**:973–979.
4. **Atherton, F. R., M. J. Hall, C. H. Hassall, R. W. Lambert, W. J. Lloyd, and P. S. Ringrose.** 1979. Phosphonopeptides as antibacterial agents: mechanism of action of alaphosphin. Antimicrob. Agents Chemother. **15**:696–705.
5. **Atherton, F. R., M. J. Hall, C. H. Hassall, R. W. Lambert, and P. S. Ringrose.** 1979. Phosphonopeptides as antibacterial agents: rationale, chemistry, and structure-activity relationships. Antimicrob. Agents Chemother. **15**:677–683.
6. **Hansson, H. B., M. Walder, and I. Juhlin.** 1981. Susceptibility of shigellae to mecillinam, nalidixic acid, trimethoprim, and five other antimicrobial agents. Antimicrob. Agents Chemother. **19**:271–273.
7. **Maruyama, H. B., M. Arisawa, and T. Sawada.** 1979. Alafosfalin, a new inhibitor of cell wall biosynthesis: in vitro activity against urinary isolates in Japan and potentiation with β-lactams. Antimicrob. Agents Chemother. **16**:444–451.

Teichomycin A_2, a New Antibiotic from *Actinoplanes*: Activity In Vitro and In Vivo

MARISA BERTI,* ROSA PALLANZA, BETH P. GOLDSTEIN, AND VITTORIO ARIOLI

Research Laboratories, Gruppo Lepetit S.p.A., Milan, Italy

Teichomycin A_2 is a new glycopeptide antibiotic of molecular weight 2,000 obtained from fermentation of *Actinoplanes teichomyceticus* (1). It inhibits bacterial cell-wall synthesis. Teichomycin A_2 is chemically related to the vancomycin-ristocetin group of antibiotics. It is active on gram-positive aerobic and anaerobic bacteria; MIC values on the various species in comparison with those of vancomycin, cephaloridine, and erythromycin are reported in Table 1. Teichomycin A_2 was the most active of the antibacterials against *Streptococcus faecalis*, *Streptococcus faecium*, *Clostridium perfringens*, and *Clostridium difficile*. Against the other species, it was somewhat less active than cephaloridine and erythromycin but more active than vancomycin. The in vitro activity of teichomycin A_2 was not significantly affected by pH, presence of serum, or increasing inoculum size; only a fourfold increase in the MIC value was observed when serum content was increased from 2 to 70%. Teichomycin A_2 was bactericidal for growing cells but not for resting cells. After 5 h of contact with a concentration five times the MIC, 99.9% of *Staphylococcus epidermidis* were killed, while for *Staphylococcus aureus* and

TABLE 1. *In vitro activity against gram-positive aerobic and anaerobic bacteria*

Species	No. of strains	Median MIC (μg/ml)[a]			
		A_2	VN	CE	ER
Staphylococcus aureus	7	0.4	0.8	0.2	0.4
S. epidermidis	8	0.8	1.6	0.05	0.2
Streptococcus pneumoniae	8	0.08	0.47	0.2	0.06
S. pyogenes	9	0.08	0.62	0.02	0.04
S. faecalis/S. faecium	8	0.31	1.6	25	1.25
Other streptococci	5	0.1	0.8	0.02	0.02
Clostridium diphtheriae	1	0.2	0.8	0.05	0.02
C. perfringens	1	0.1	1.6	0.8	6.2
C. difficile	2	0.4	1.6	2.3	2.3
Propionibacterium acnes	2	0.4	0.8	0.1	0.1

[a] A_2, Teichomycin A_2; VN, vancomycin; CE, cephaloridine; ER, erythromycin.

TABLE 2. *Efficacy in experimental infections*[a]

Organism	Subcutaneous ED_{50} (mg/kg/day)[b]			
	A_2	VN	CE	ER
Staphylococcus aureus L 165	0.72	7.2	2.8	28
Streptococcus pyogenes L 143	0.1	1.1	0.62	3.8
S. pyogenes L 49	0.11	0.58	0.03	0.44
S. pneumoniae L 44	0.41	1.9	0.93	26

[a] Treatment schedule: once daily for 3 days starting soon after infection.

[b] A_2, Teichomycin A_2; VN, vancomycin; CE, cephaloridine; ER, erythromycin.

Streptococcus pyogenes killing was about 99%; by 24 h, killing was more than 99.9% for all three strains. On *S. faecalis* killing was somewhat more than 90% by 24 h. The mutation rate toward resistance is $<10^{-10}$/cell per generation. No cross-resistance was observed with clinically used antibiotics; cross-resistance to vancomycin could not be studied because of inability to isolate bacteria resistant to either antibiotic.

In experimental infection in mice (Table 2), teichomycin A_2 administered subcutaneously was 5 to 10 times more effective than vancomycin, 4 to >20 times more effective than erythromycin, and somewhat better than cephaloridine except for the infection caused by *S. pyogenes* L 49 where cephaloridine was more effective. The apparent half-life of teichomycin A_2 in mice was 2.5 h. Teichomycin A_2 gave higher and more prolonged blood levels than an equivalent dose of vancomycin (at 50 mg/kg, peak concentrations were ~5 for vancomycin and ~100 for teichomycin A_2). The subcutaneous LD_{50} of teichomycin A_2 in mice is 2,860 mg/kg.

1. **Parenti, F., G. Beretta, M. Berti, and V. Arioli.** 1978. Teichomycins, new antibiotics from *Actinoplanes teichomyceticus* nov. sp. I. Description of the producer strain, fermentation studies, and biological properties. J. Antibiot. **31**:276–283.

Mechanism of Action of Teichomycin A_2, A New Antibiotic

SERGIO SOMMA* AND LUCIANO GASTALDO

Research Laboratories, Gruppo Lepetit S.p.A, Milan, Italy

Teichomycin A_2 (TA_2) is a new antibiotic produced by *Actinoplanes teichomyceticus*, and having an outstanding bactericidal activity against several species of gram-positive microorganisms (3). TA_2 is a glycopeptide of 2,000 molecular weight, belonging to the vancomycin-like group of antibiotics. The molecule includes a bis-diphenyl-ether moiety with two chlorine atoms, which appears to be identical with a corresponding structure in vancomycin; TA_2, however, differs from the other members of the family in the sugar moieties containing D-mannose and D-glucosamine (1).

TA_2 inhibits specifically the biosynthesis of

the cell wall in susceptible organisms. The data supporting this assumption are based on the following experiments: TA_2 added to a growing culture of *Bacillus subtilis* blocks immediately the uptake of *N*-acetyl-glucosamine, a peptidoglycan precursor, without affecting, for at least 10 min, the incorporation of the precursors of other macromolecular syntheses such as DNA, RNA, and protein. Furthermore, the treated organisms show an intracellular accumulation of *N*-acetylaminosugar-nucleotides, mainly represented by a product identified as a uridine-5′-diphosphate-*N*-acetylmuramyl-pentapeptide; this fact indicates that the polymerization process of the peptidoglycan, by either transglycosilation or transpeptidation, was inhibited, rather than the synthesis of some of the precursors. The antibiotic was active in a particulate enzyme preparation from *Bacillus stearothermophilus* capable of carrying out the synthesis of cross-linked peptidoglycan (3); the transglycosilation reaction is blocked by addition of TA_2, with a concomitant accumulation of the peptidosaccharide-phospholipid intermediate (Fig. 1).

TA_2, at a concentration of 200 μg/ml, partially prevents the lysis of whole cells of *Micrococcus lysodeikticus* by lysozyme treatment; the same effect was observed with vancomycin and ristocetin. The growth inhibition activities of TA_2, vancomycin, and ristocetin are reversed in an agar plate bioassay when purified cell wall fragments are incorporated in the nutrient medium. The action of TA_2 undergoes reversion after the addition of wall fragments also in a cell-free extract carrying out peptidoglycan synthesis; the cell membranes added to the reaction mixture contain all the enzymes necessary for peptidoglycan polymerization, but are free from cell wall fragments. In contrast, gardimycin (current name, actagardin), a peptide antibiotic inhibitor of transglycosilation (4), exerts a suppressive effect which is not affected by the walls but is completely reversed by the addition of membranes (Fig. 2).

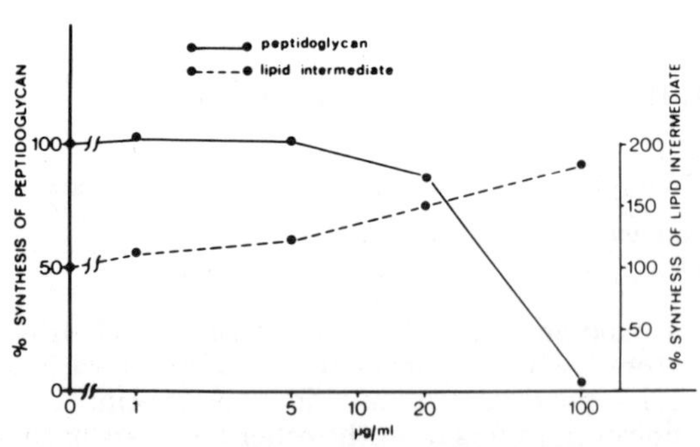

FIG. 1. *Effect of Teichomycin A_2 on the in vitro synthesis of peptidoglycan and lipid intermediate. The abscissa shows the concentration of the antibiotic.*

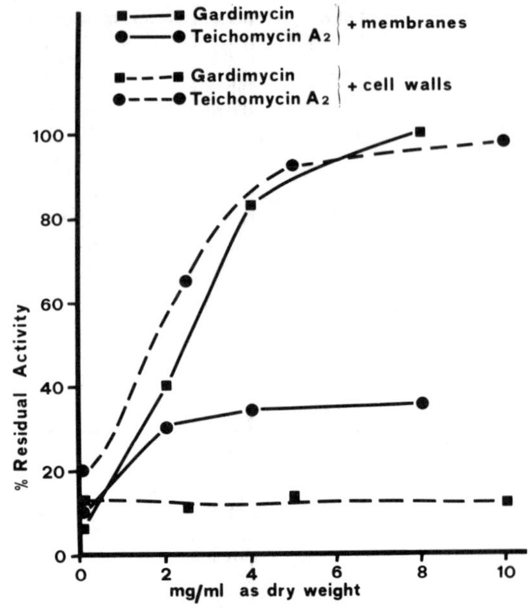

FIG. 2. *Suppression of the inhibitory effect of Teichomycin A_2 and gardimycin on peptidoglycan synthesis in a cell-free system after addition of cell wall fragments or cell membranes. The concentration of the antibiotics was 100 μg/ml. The abscissa shows the concentration of the cell membranes or walls.*

TA_2 and vancomycin were also tested in an assay of D-alanyl-D-alanine carboxypeptidase from cell membranes of *Escherichia coli*; inhibition of the enzyme is detectable with both products only when the molar ratio of the antibiotic versus the substrate (uridine-5′-diphosphate-*N*-acetylmuramyl-pentapeptide) approaches 1 or more; in contrast, the carboxypeptidase is inhibited by a low amount of ampicillin, regardless of the substrate concentration.

All of the data presented here indicate that TA_2 has a mode of action very similar to that of vancomycin (2), the characteristic features being: the selective action of the cell wall biosynthesis, the inhibition of the polymerization of the peptidoglycan, and the stronger affinity for the cell wall or for some of its precursors, such as uridine-5′-diphosphate-*N*-acetylmuramyl-pentapeptide, rather than for specific enzymes involved in the peptidoglycan synthesis. The latter fact is demonstrated by the reversion of antibiotic inhibition exerted by cell walls or nucleotide precursors, but not by cell membrane preparations, as in the case of enzyme inhibitors such as gardimycin and ampicillin. It has not yet been ascertained whether TA_2 prevents only the transglycosilation or also the transpeptidation reaction.

1. **Bardone, M. R., G. Tuan, and C. Coronelli.** 1978. Preliminary structural studies on Teichomycin A_2, a new antibiotic. Abstr. 239, 11th Int. Symp. on Chemistry of Natural Products, Sofia, Bulgaria.
2. **Jordan, D. C., and P. E. Reynolds.** 1975. Vancomycin, p. 704–718. *In* J. W. Corcoran and F. E. Hahn (ed.), Antibiotics, vol. 3. Springer-Verlag, Inc., Heidelberg, Germany.
3. **Parenti, F., G. Beretta, M. Berti, and V. Arioli.** 1978. Teichomycin, new antibiotics from *Actinoplanes teichomyceticus* nov. sp. I. Description of the producer strain, fermentation studies and biological properties. J. Antibiot. **31:**276–281.
4. **Somma, S., W. Merati, and F. Parenti.** 1977. Gardimycin, a new antibiotic inhibiting peptidoglycan synthesis. Antimicrob. Agents Chemother. **11:**396–401.

Synthesis of the Antibiotic SA 85.530 and its Conversion to Ring-Substituted and Ring-Transformed Derivatives

H. BERNER,* G. FISCHER, J. HILDEBRANDT, G. LABER, AND H. VYPLEL

Sandoz Forschungsinstitut, A-1235 Vienna, Austria

Nucleophilic substitution of the activated side-chain of the tricyclic diterpene pleuromutilin (structure 1) afforded SA 85.530 (4a) in good yield. The diazoketone (6) and the Mannich-Base (15) were shown to be the most versatile key intermediates for the syntheses of ring-substituted derivatives as well as for the transformation to the cyclobutanone analog (14). See Fig. 1 for chemical structures.

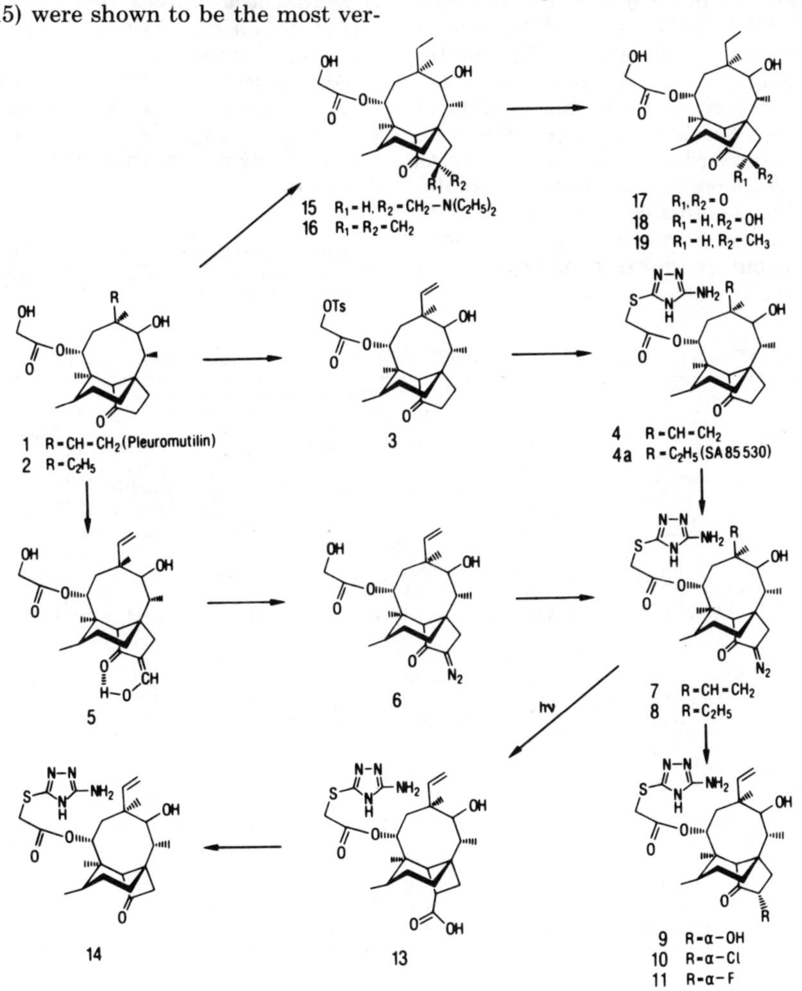

FIG. 1. *Chemical structures.*

SA 85.530 b, a New Semisynthetic Pleuromutilin Derivative with Antibacterial Activity: In Vitro Evaluation

JOHANNES F. HILDEBRANDT,* HANS BERNER, GEORG LABER, FRIEDERIKE TURNOWSKY, AND EBERHARD SCHÜTZE

Sandoz Research Institute, Vienna, Austria

SA 86.530 b, 19,20-dihydro-14-o[(3 amino-1,2,4-triazol-5yl)-thioacetyl]mutilin, is a new semisynthetic antibiotic. It is a derivative of pleuromutilin, a fermentation product from basidiomycetes species which was described by Knauseder et al. (1) and H. Berner et al. (this volume).

The antibacterial activity of SA 85.530 b was determined by standard bacteriological procedures after dissolving the water-insoluble substance in dimethyl sulfoxide or suspending it in 0.15% agarose. The in vitro activity, 50% MIC (MIC_{50}), 90% MIC (MIC_{90}) and MIC ranges of 85.530 in comparison with doxycycline, erythromycin, clindamycin, and rosaramicin are shown in Tables 1 and 2. From this data, it can be seen that SA 85.530 b is comparable in its activity to all standards against *Staphylococcus aureus*, *Staphylococcus epidermidis*, streptococci, and *Haemophilus* spp. It is superior to doxycycline and erythromycin against *Bacteroides fragilis* but inferior to clindamycin by a factor of 10 to 20.

With respect to sexually transmitted bacterial infections, SA 85.530 b was shown to be a very potent substance against *Chlamydia trachomatis*, *Ureaplasma urealyticum*, *Mycoplasma* species, and *Neisseria gonorrhoeae*; its activity against this latter organism was superior to those of all substances with which it was compared. Since it is a new antibiotic, no cross-resistance was observed in tetracycline-, penicillin-, and erythromycin-resistant strains. Under laboratory conditions, resistance development by *Staphylococcus aureus*, *Streptococcus faecalis*, and *Bacteroides fragilis* followed the multistep mutation pattern.

MIC values for *Staphylococcus aureus*, *Streptococcus faecalis*, and *Klebsiella pneumoniae* were not or only slightly (by a factor of 2) influenced by varying the pH of tryptic soy broth from 6 to 8.

1. **Knauseder, F., and E. Brandl.** 1976. Pleuromutilins. Fermentation, structure and biosynthesis. J. Antibiot. **29:**125–131.

TABLE 1. *Antibacterial activity of SA 85.530 compared with those of other antimicrobial agents*

Antimicrobial agent	MIC (μg/ml) against following organism							
	Staphylococcus aureus (*n* = 105)	*Staphylococcus epidermidis* (*n* = 9)	*Streptococcus* spp. (*n* = 19)	*Haemophilus* spp. (*n* = 14)	*Neisseria gonorrhoeae* (*n* = 56)	*Bacteroides fragilis* (*n* = 19)	*Ureaplasma urealyticum* (*n* = 12)	*Mycoplasma* spp. (*n* = 12)
SA 85.530								
MIC_{50}	0.4	0.06	0.10	0.78	0.25	2.0	1	0.03
MIC_{90}	0.63	0.5	0.25	3.95	1.0	4.0	16	0.11
MIC range	0.156–5 (>10)	0.039–0.625	0.015–10	0.16–5	0.06–2	0.25–4	0.13–16	0.015–0.125
Doxycycline								
MIC_{50}	0.16	0.5	0.13	0.31	0.13	4.0	0.18	5.0
MIC_{90}	6.25	2.5	0.16	0.62	8.0	8.0	16	5.0
MIC range	0.039–10 (>10)	0.019–5	0.031–10	0.16–1.25	0.06–8	0.12–8.0	0.03–16	0.125–5.0
Erythromycin[a]								
MIC_{50}	0.16	0.05	0.02	1.97	0.25	8.0	2.83	>50
MIC_{90}	>10	0.09	0.16	2.79	3.03	8.0	16	>50
MIC range	0.078–>10	0.039–0.156	0.015–>10	0.63–3.12	0.06–8	1–16	0.5–16	>50
Clindamycin								
MIC_{50}	0.06	0.007	0.02	2.5		0.12	2.8	0.25
MIC_{90}	0.125	0.16	0.10	5.59	NT[b]	0.12	16	0.50
MIC range	0.039–>10	0.005–0.312	0.015–>10	0.39–5		0.12	0.5–16	0.06–0.5

[a] Erycinum.
[b] NT, Not tested.

TABLE 2. *In vitro activity of SA 85.530 compared with those of other antimicrobial agents against Chlamydia trachomatis in McCoy cell cultures*[a]

Antimicrobial agent	Activity (μg/ml) against following *Chlamydia* strain											
	SA_2F	UW-3	UW-4	UW-55	UW-57	L404	L434	TW-3	TW-5	G-17	AP-2	MOPN
SA 85.530												
MLC[b]	0.05	0.05	0.05	0.005	0.05	0.05	0.5	0.05	0.5	0.05	0.05	0.05
MIC	0.05	0.05	0.05	0.005	0.05	0.05	0.05	0.05	0.05	0.05	0.005	0.005
Doxycycline												
MLC	0.05	0.5	0.05	0.005	0.5	0.05	0.5	0.5	0.5	0.5	0.5	0.005
MIC	0.05	0.5	0.005	0.005	0.005	0.005	0.05	0.5	0.05	0.5	0.05	0.005
Erythromycin[c]												
MLC	>5	0.5	>5	>5	0.5	>5	>5	0.5	5	0.5	0.5	0.5
MIC	5.0	0.05	0.5	0.5	0.5	5.0	0.5	0.5	0.5	0.5	0.05	0.05
Clindamycin												
MLC	0.5	0.5	5.0	0.5	7.5	5.0	7.5	0.5	5.0	0.5	0.5	7.5
MIC	0.5	0.5	5.0	0.5	5.0	5.0	5.0	0.5	5.0	0.5	0.5	5.0
Rosaramicin												
MLC	5.0	0.5	0.5	0.5	0.5	5.0	0.5	0.05	0.5	0.05	0.05	0.5
MIC	5.0	0.05	0.05	0.5	0.05	0.05	0.05	0.05	0.05	0.05	0.005	0.005

[a] Strains were kindly provided by San Pin Wang, Seattle, Wash., and P. Reeve.

[b] MLC, Minimum lethal (bactericidal) concentration, determined after three passages of monolayers which showed no inclusions at MIC or higher drug concentrations.

[c] Lactobionat.

SA 85.530 b, a New Semisynthetic Pleuromutilin Derivative with Antibacterial Activity: Chemotherapeutic, Toxicological, and Pharmacokinetic Properties in Laboratory Animals

AXEL F. WENZEL,* ROBERT BAUMGARTNER, APOSTOLOS GEORGOPOULOS, JOHANNES HILDEBRANDT, GEORG LABER, EBERHARD SCHÜTZE, AND HUBERT WALZL

Sandoz Research Institute, Vienna, Austria

SA 85.530 is a representative of a new class of semisynthetic antibiotics derived from a fermentation product of *Pleurotus mutilis* (and other basidiomycetes) named Pleuromutilin (H. Berner et al., this volume). The compound is active in vitro against bacteria causing sexually transmitted diseases, such as *Chlamydia trachomatis*, *Ureaplasma*, and *Mycoplasma* species and *Neisseria gonorrhoeae*. In addition, the spectrum comprises obligate anaerobic organisms, *Haemophilus* spp., and the gram-positive bacteria, including tetracycline-, erythromycin-, and penicillin-resistant organisms (J. Hildebrandt et al., this volume).

In vivo antimicrobial efficacy. Septic infections in mice were produced by intraperitoneal inoculation of overnight cultures of *Streptococcus pyogenes*, *Streptococcus aronson*, *Staphylococcus aureus*, and also *Sphaerophorus necrophorus* (A. Wenzel, unpublished data). The antibacterial activity against *Chlamydia trachomatis* was evaluated in experimental mouse pneumonia. Animals were intratracheally inoculated, and 8 days after infection and therapy, the therapeutic effect was calculated by macroscopically scoring the lung lesions. Polyarthritis was produced in rats by intraperitoneal infection with *Mycoplasma arthritidis*. The criteria for effective antimicrobial therapy was the prevention of death or arthritis and paralysis.

In mice infected intraperitoneally with *Sphaerophorus necrophorus*, liver and abdominal abscess formation occurs at about 3 days postinfection. Prevention of these lesions was the basis for evaluation of chemotherapeutic efficacy.

Comparative 50% effective dose (ED_{50}) values of SA 85.530 and four commercially available drugs are presented in Table 1. The statistical significance of differences was calculated by Student's *t* test.

In the systemic infections with gram-positive

bacteria, SA 85.530 exhibits an in vivo activity which is significantly superior to those of erythromycin and tetracycline and similar to that of clindamycin. The therapy of the *Sphaerophorus necrophorus* septicemia with SA 85.530 was more effective than that with clindamycin and metronidazole. The superiority over metronidazole is also demonstrated in the abscess formation model by *Sphaerophorus necrophorus*. Against chlamydial lung infection, the therapeutic activity of SA 85.530 is significantly better than that of tetracycline and erythromycin. The 50% effective dose values of 85.530 in the rat-mycoplasma-polyarthritis model are inferior to clindamycin and superior to tetracycline.

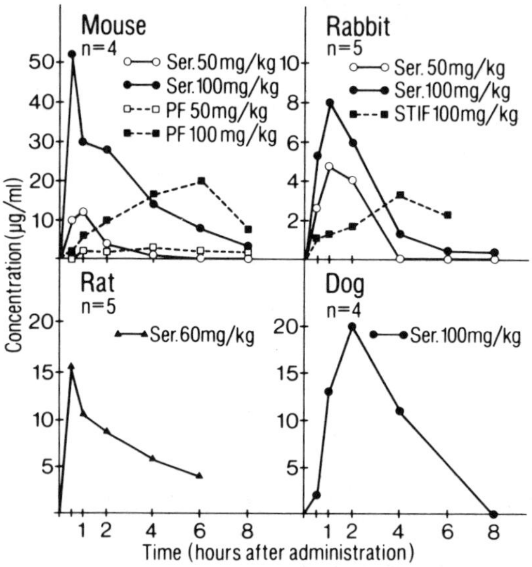

FIG. 1. *Levels of SA 85.530 b in serum and body fluids of four animal species after a single oral dose. Abbreviations: Ser., serum; PF, peritoneal fluid; STIF, soft-tissue interstitial fluid; n, number of animals (rabbits, rats, dogs) investigated; in mice, number of animals per time point.*

In summary, SA 85.530 proved to be a very potent antibacterial agent in the treatment of experimental infections. Compared wtih relevant commercially available drugs, its activity is superior in most of the model infections tested.

Pharmacokinetics. Concentrations of SA 85.530 in the serum of fasted mice, rats, rabbits, and dogs, in the peritoneal fluid of mice, and in soft-tissue interstitial fluid of rabbits after oral administration were determined by the microagar diffusion method described by Georgopoulos (1). Body fluids were collected, using diffusion chambers with permeable membranes which were implanted intraperitoneally or subcutaneously 3 days before the experiments. Details of implantation and collection techniques were described by Laber et al. (3), and the composition and definition of the fluids was described by Laber et al. (2) and Schmook et al. (4). Concentration-versus-timecurves are shown in Fig. 1. In mice given a single oral dose of 50 or 100 mg of SA 85.530 per kg, the average peak serum levels were 12 and 53 µg/ml after 1 and 0.5 h, respectively, with an elimination half-life of 0.6 and 2 h, respectively. Peak concentrations in peritoneal fluid which occurred after 4 h were 3 and 17 µg/ml. A maximum serum level of 16 µg/ml was measured 0.5 h after application of 60 mg/kg to rats, with a half-life of 3.1 h. Rabbits

TABLE 1. *Efficacy of SA 85.530 b and other antibiotics in systemic and nonsystemic infections after oral application*

Microorganism	Infection model	Challenge dose (CFU per animal)	No of doses (h postinfection)	ED_{50} values (mg/kg) b.w. per dose: SA 85.530 b	Erythromycin	Tetracycline	Clindamycin	Metronidazole
Streptococcus pyogenes (A)	Mouse septicemia	1×10^1	2 (1, 4)	15.5	34	23.5	13	ND[a]
Streptococcus aronson (B)	Mouse septicemia	5×10^1	2 (1, 4)	16	34	39	17.5	ND
Staphylococcus aureus	Mouse septicemia	2×10^8	2 (1, 4)	11	70.5	4.5	3	ND
Sphaerophorus necrophorus	Mouse septicemia	1×10^7	2 (0, 1)	16	ND	16.5	>500	>500
Chlamydia trachomatis	Mouse pneumonia	2×10^{2b}	10[c]	10	36	14	ND	ND
Mycoplasma arthritidis	Rat polyarthritis	1×10^9	5 (1, 6, 24, 30, 48)	4.4	ND	14.4	0.8	ND
Sphaerophorus necrophorus	Mouse intraperitoneal abscess formation	1×10^6	3 (1, 3, 5)	131	ND	ND	ND	144

[a] ND, Not done.
[b] Inclusion bodies.
[c] Twice daily over 5 days.

were given 50 or 100 mg of SA 85.530 per kg orally. After 1 h, serum peaks of 5 and 8 μg/ml were observed, and the half-lives were 1.1 and 1.5 h, respectively. In soft-tissue interstitial fluid of rabbits, 3 μg/ml was measured as the maximal concentration after 4 h (dose, 100 mg/kg). A peak serum level of 20 μg/ml was attained in dogs 2 h after oral application of capsules. The half-life was determined to be 2.7 h. These results demonstrate an oral absorption in different animal species which is dose dependent. At 4 h after administration, the drug concentrations in the body fluids (soft-tissue interstitial fluid, peritoneal fluid) exceeded the declining serum level curves, indicating a useful penetration of SA 85.530 into possible infection sites.

Toxicology. The 50% lethal dose of SA 85.530 after a single oral administration to mice was more than 1,000 mg/kg. No significant abnormalities were observed in rats and dogs given up to 500 and 120 mg/kg, respectively, of SA 85.530 once daily over 4 weeks.

Conclusion. SA 85.530 proved to be an effective antibacterial agent against experimental infections caused by chlamydiae, obligate anaerobes, streptococci, and staphylococci. This in vivo efficacy was, in most cases, significantly superior to those of relevant commercially available drugs, such as erythromycin, tetracycline, clindamycin, and metronidazole. Preliminary pharmacokinetic studies demonstrated oral absorption in mice, rats, rabbits, and dogs and penetration into peritoneal and soft-tissue interstitial fluids in mice and rabbits, respectively. Acute and subchronic toxicological studies revealed no side effects in mice, rats, or dogs.

1. **Georgopoulos, A.** 1978. A simple micro agar diffusion method for the determination of antibiotic concentrations in blood and other body fluids. Zentralbl. Bakteriol. Parasitenk. D. Infektionskr. Hyg. Abt. I. Orig. A **242**:387–393.
2. **Laber, G., H. Obenaus, and H. Walzl.** 1980. Pressure measurements and histological investigations after subcutaneous implantation of diffusion chambers in rabbits. Infection **8**(5):187–189.
3. **Laber, G., E. Schütze, R. Leskova, R. Kolb, and A. Georgopoulos.** 1980. A diffusion chamber technique for measuring concentrations of antibiotics in interstitial fluids. Infection **8**(2):58–62.
4. **Schmook, F. P., M. Nefzger, G. Laber, A. Georgopoulos, R. Czok, and E. Schütze.** 1980. Composition of fluids from diffusion chambers implanted in the soft tissue and kidneys of rabbits. Infection **8**(4):156–161.

Siderochelin: A New Ferrous-Ion Chelating Agent Produced by *Nocardia*

J. SCOTT WELLS,* CAROL M. RICCA, WEN-CHIH LIU, SUSAN M. FISHER, WILLIAM H. TREJO, DANIEL P. BONNER, AND RICHARD B. SYKES

The Squibb Institute for Medical Research, Princeton, New Jersey 08540, U.S.A.

During a screening program designed to detect inhibitors of lipopolysaccharide biosynthesis, we detected a novel compound with ion-chelating properties. The compound was produced by *Nocardia* sp. SC 11,430 and has been named siderochelin. The structure is shown in Fig. 1.

Cultures of aerobic actinomycetes were isolated from soil samples by stamping air-dried soils onto an agar medium containing (g/liter): glucose, 5; KNO_3, 1; K_2HPO_4, 0.5; $MgSO_4 \cdot 7H_2O$, 0.5; NaCl, 0.5; $FeSO_4 \cdot 7H_2O$, 0.01; and agar, 20 (pH 7.0). After incubation at 28°C for 10 to 14 days, isolated colonies were picked for testing in the screen.

Nocardia sp. SC 11,430 was isolated from a soil sample collected in Virginia. Vegetative mycelium of the culture fragmented into rod and coccal forms within 5 days. The cells were nonacid fast and gram positive. Colonies growing on agar were smooth to doughy in consistency. No aerial mycelium was formed.

Acid hydrolysates of whole-cell walls analyzed by the method of Becker et al. (1) revealed the presence of *meso*-diaminopimelic acid, with galactose and arabinose as the major sugar components.

The culture produced acid from adonitol, glucose, glycerol, inositol, maltose, and sucrose. Casein and hypoxanthine were decomposed, but not tyrosine, xanthine, and guanine. There was hydrolysis of gelatin, but not of starch.

Fermentations were done in a 380-liter, stainless-steel fermentor containing 250 liters of fermentation medium consisting of (g/liter): yeast extract, 4; malt extract, 10; and glucose, 4. Samples of fermentation broth were tested by a paper disk assay on agar plates (3.5% seed agar [BBL Microbiology Systems] and 0.5% NaCl)

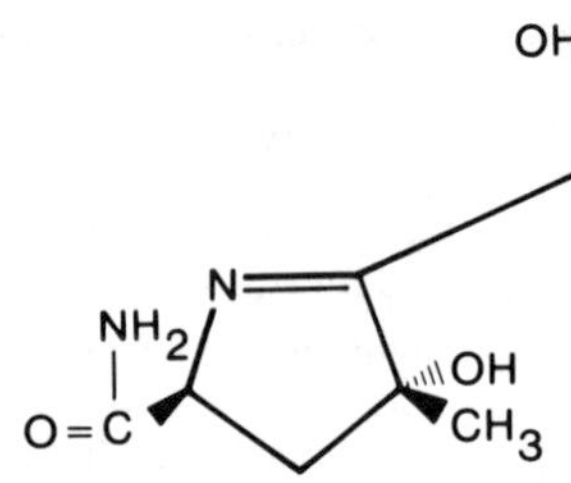

FIG. 1. *Structure of siderochelin A.*

containing 10 μg of diumycin per ml (2) and seeded with *Escherichia coli* SC 10,888. Zones of inhibition were recorded after overnight incubation at 37°C.

Siderochelin was isolated from fermentations of *Nocardia* sp. SC 11,430 by first concentrating the broth filtrate (60×). The concentrate was extracted with methanol, which was then reconcentrated and extracted sequentially with hexane, toluene, and three extractions with methanol-chloroform (1:9). Concentrates of the combined methanol-chloroform extracts yielded 4.1 g of crude crystalline siderochelin. The crystals contained two diastereoisomers that were separated on the basis of shape into platelets (A) and needles (B). Separation of the isomers was carried out by fractional crystallization from acetonitrile. Both siderochelin A and B were soluble in methanol, ethanol, ethylacetate, acetone, and chloroform, but insoluble in hexane and water. Their physical and chemical properties are listed in Table 1.

Siderochelin A was weakly active against a range of aerobic and anaerobic bacteria. The compound had a spectrum of activity similar to that of apoferrosamine, a ferrous-ion chelating agent produced by a strain of *Pseudomonas fluorescens* (3). The compound appeared to be less active than apoferrosamine against dermatophytic fungi but had similar activity against *Trichomonas vaginalis*. Both compounds were inactive against *Candida albicans*.

The mode of action of siderochelin has been attributed to its ability to chelate metal ions.

TABLE 1. *Physical and chemical properties of siderochelins A and B*

Property	Siderochelin A	Siderochelin B
Crystalline form	Platelets	Needles
Melting point (°C)	165–168	200–201
UV (MeOH): λ_{max} ($E^{1\%}$)	315 (220)	315 (220)
Mass spectrometry, molecular ion	235	235
Empirical formula	$C_{11}H_{13}N_3O_3$	$C_{11}H_{13}N_3O_3$
Elemental analysis calculated for $C_{11}H_{13}N_3O_3$ (%)	Found	
C = 56.22	56.14	56.38
H = 5.58	5.44	5.60
N = 17.88	17.66	17.78
Optical rotation (nm)	(c, 0.30, MeOH)	(c, 0.21, MeOH)
λ	$[\alpha]^{22}$	$[\alpha]^{22}$
598	+1.7°	−1.9°
578	+2.3°	+2.4°
546	+2.3°	+1.4°
436	+43.9°	−23.0°
Thin-layer chromatography (silica gel MeOH/ $CHCl_3$, 1:19)	R_f = 0.40	R_f = 0.40

Iron uptake studies with *E. coli* showed a 75% inhibition of uptake of $^{55}Fe^{2+}$ by siderochelin A at the MIC. In addition, the activity of siderochelin A was antagonized in the presence of Fe^{2+}, Fe^{3+}, Co^{2+}, and Zn^{2+} ions.

1. **Becker, B., M. P. Lechevalier, R. E. Gordon, and H. A. Lechevalier.** 1964. Rapid differentiation between *Nocardia* and *Streptomyces* by paper chromatography of whole-cell hydrolysates. Appl. Microbiol. **12:**421–423.
2. **Meyers, E., D. S. Slusarchyk, F. E. Pansy, H. I. Basch, W. H. Trejo, and P. J. DeBaecke.** 1972. Biological characterization of diumycin, a phosphorus-containing glycolipid antibiotic. J. Antibiot. **25:**163–170.
3. **Pouteau-Thourenot, M., A. Gaudemer, and M. Barbier.** 1965. Sur la ferrosamine, pigment de *Bacillus roseus fluorescens*. Bull. Soc. Chim. Biol. **47:**2085–2091.

Norfloxacin (MK-0366, AM-715), a New Orally Absorbed Synthetic Compound for the Treatment of Bacterial Infections

HANS H. GADEBUSCH,* LAWRENCE R. KOUPAL, EVEMARIE CELOZZI, DANIEL L. SHUNGU, JUDITH BLAND, BARBARA WEISSBERGER, BARBARA A. PELAK, ELLEN FISCH, SALLY K. CHUNG, AND JOANN HUBER

Merck Institute for Therapeutic Research, Rahway, New Jersey 07065, U.S.A.

Norfloxacin (MK-0366, AM-715), 1-ethyl-6-fluoro-1,4-dihydro-4-oxo-7-(1-piperazinyl)-3-quinoline carboxylic acid, is a new bactericidal agent whose safety exceeds that of every known compound of this type yet reported. Unlike earlier compounds, MK-0366 exhibits a very broad spectrum of antibacterial activity against both gram-positive and gram-negative organisms, and potency that exceeds that of nalidixic acid, pipemidic acid, and miloxacin (1), as well as that of oxolinic acid, cinoxacin, and rosoxacin (Table 1).

The present study further compares the antibacterial activity in vitro of the title compound with that of nalidixic acid, cinoxacin, amoxicillin, cefaclor, tetracycline, trimethoprim, and the combination sulfamethoxazole/trimethoprim, compounds that are presently marketed as active oral agents for the treatment of bacterial infections. The MICs in this instance were determined with a multipoint inoculator (10^5 colony-forming units per spot) in agar dilution tests on Mueller-Hinton agar. For tests with trimethoprim and sulfamethoxazole/trimethoprim, Mueller-Hinton agar was supplemented with 5% lysed horse blood; GC agar base supplemented with hemoglobin and IsoVitaleX (BBL Microbiology Systems) was used when testing *Haemophilus* and *Neisseria*. All organisms were incubated at 35 to 37°C for 16 to 24 h. The potential for development of resistance was studied by comparing the mutational frequency of MK-0366 with that of oxolinic acid, by means of direct selection of mutants on Trypticase soy agar (BBL) (2).

Experimental chemotherapeutic studies in mice were conducted by infecting animals intraperitoneally with challenge doses of pathogens sufficient to cause death within 48 h. All compounds were given by gavage at 0 and 6 h postinfection.

Blood levels and urinary concentrations of

TABLE 1. *Comparison of the antibacterial activity in vitro of MK-0366 with four other organic acids[a] against gram-positive and gram-negative organisms*

Organism	MIC (μg/ml)[b]				
	MK-0366	NAL	OA	CIN	RSX
Staphylococcus aureus MB 2865	0.5	128	4	128	2
S. epidermidis CLC 874	0.03	2	0.125	8	0.125
Streptococcus pyogenes MB 1114	4	>128	>128	>128	32
S. faecalis MB 2864	4	>128	32	128	8
S. pneumoniae MB 4336	4	>128	64	>128	16
Acinetobacter lwoffi MB 3579	0.5	8	1	32	1
Citrobacter freundii MB 2478	0.03	8	1	8	1
Enterobacter cloacae MB 2646	0.06	16	1	8	1
Escherichia coli MB 4392	0.25	>128	8	128	16
Klebsiella rhinoscleromatis MB 4467	0.25	32	8	16	8
Morganella morganii MB 2833	0.03	4	0.25	4	0.5
Proteus mirabilis MB 2829	0.015	4	0.125	4	0.25
Providencia rettgeri MB 3722	0.125	>128	8	>128	32
Proteus stuartii MB 2850	1	>128	8	>128	>128
Pseudomonas aeruginosa MB 2835	0.5	>128	16	>128	16
Serratia marcescens MB 2840	2	64	8	>128	16
Shigella sonnei MB 3261	0.03	4	1	8	1
Salmonella typhi CLC 1202	0.03	8	0.25	8	0.5
Yersinia enterocolitica CLC 865	0.03	2	0.25	2	0.5

[a] Nalidixic acid (NAL), oxolinic acid (OA), cinoxacin (CIN), and rosoxacin (RSX).
[b] Agar dilution test, multipoint inoculator, inoculum 10^5 colony-forming units per spot, Trypticase soy agar (BBL Microbiology Systems), incubation at 35°C for 20 h.

MK-0366 in pharmacokinetic experiments were measured by bioassay as a function of time after oral doses of the drug to mice, rats, and rhesus monkeys. Preliminary interpretive standards for disk susceptibility tests were determined from MICs and zone diameters from 127 bacterial species using the error rate-bounded method.

Before proceeding with studies in vitro, the effect of various factors on antibacterial activity of MK-0366 was determined. From these studies, it was concluded that the antibacterial activity of MK-0366 was not affected adversely by changes in culture medium composition (Trypticase soy, Mueller-Hinton, nutrient, or brain heart infusion agar), pH of culture medium (pH 6.0 to 9.0), inoculum size (10^3 to 10^6 colony-forming units per spot), or the presence of 50% inactivated human plasma in nutrient agar. A survey of more than 350 fresh clinical isolates clearly showed MK-0366 also to be more potent in vitro than any of the structurally unrelated antibiotics tested against 13 genera of *Enterobacteriaceae*, as well as *N. gonorrhoeae*, *H. influenzae*, and *Pseudomonas aeruginosa*. Ninety percent of the isolates in these four groups of bacteria were inhibited by MK-0366 at less than 1 μg/ml, 0.6 μg/ml, 0.25 μg/ml, and 8 μg/ml, respectively. MK-0366 was not cross-resistant with any of the antibiotics tested. Spontaneous mutation rates of representatives from four genera of bacteria (*Escherichia*, *Klebsiella*, *Proteus*, *Staphylococcus*), strains that were susceptible to both MK-0366 and oxolinic acid in media containing drug concentrations of 10 μg/ml, were consistently lower for MK-0366 (ca. 10^{-12}) than for the comparison drug (range, 10^{-6} to 10^{-10}). The spontaneous mutation rate of a strain of *P. aeruginosa* to MK-0366 was ca. 10^{-12}.

MK-0366, like related organic acids, inhibits bacterial DNA synthesis. At the molecular level three specific events were attributed to this new compound: (i) inhibition of the ATP-dependent DNA supercoiling reaction by *E. coli* DNA gyrase, (ii) inhibition of the relaxation of supercoiled DNA, an activity that is induced by DNA gyrase in the absence of ATP, and (iii) promotion of double-stranded DNA breakage in *E. coli* cells (M. Gellert, personal communication).

The potent antibacterial activity of MK-0366 demonstrated earlier in vitro was translated into high cure rates in experimentally infected animals (Table 2). In every instance MK-0366 was significantly more effective than nalidixic acid and most of the other agents tested. Included among these were several β-lactamase–producing isolates (*E. coli* 2891, *Morganella morganii* 2833, *P. vulgaris* 2829), a tetracycline-resistant

TABLE 2. *Comparison of the therapeutic efficacy of MK-0366, nalidixic acid (NAL), amoxicillin (AMOX), cefaclor (CEF), tetracycline (TET), and cotrimoxazole (SXT/TMP) in experimental septicemia in mice*[a]

Pathogens	MK-0366		NAL		AMOX		CEF		TET		SXT/TMP	
	MIC[b]	ED_{50}[c]	MIC	ED_{50}	MIC	ED_{50}	MIC	ED_{50}	MIC	ED_{50}	MIC	ED_{50}
Escherichia coli MB 289	0.03	0.7	2	6.3	>128	>200	>128	>200	>128	>200	0.24/0.01	1.2/0.2
Klebsiella pneumoniae MB 4005	0.06	1.6	2	41.4	32	6.3	0.5	11.8	0.5	50	>122/>6.4	>200/>40
Salmonella schottmuelleri MB 2837	0.5	0.8	64	25	2	1.6	0.25	1.2	1	53	1.9/0.1	3.0/0.6
Proteus mirabilis MB 3125	0.06	0.9	4	15.1	4	3	64	1.6	64	>200	1.9/0.1	1.2/0.2
Morganella morganii MB 2833	0.03	1.3	4	4.2	>128	>200	>128	NT[d]	8	NT	3.8/0.2	6.7/1.3
Proteus vulgaris MB 2829	0.02	3.3	8	16.4	>128	>200	>128	60.5	8	200	3.8/0.2	1.6/0.3
P. mirabilis CL 794	0.06	5.2	>128	>200	>128	>200	32	15.1	128	>200	>128	>200/>40
Klebsiella pneumoniae CL 15	2	13.3	>128	143	>128	>200	0.5	1.17	4	>200	64	18.7/3.74

[a] Infection induced by intraperitoneal injection of pathogen with challenge doses ranging from 9 to 562 LD_{50}s.
[b] MIC in micrograms per milliliter at 10^5 colony-forming units, agar dilution test, Mueller-Hinton agar.
[c] Median effective dose in milligrams per kilogram per dose calculated after oral administration to mice in divided doses at 0 and 6 h postinfection.
[d] Not tested.

E. coli (MB 2891), and a trimethoprim/sulfamethoxazole-resistant *Klebsiella* (MB 4005). Lastly, MK-0366 was as effective orally as gentamicin given parenterally (ED_{50}, ca. 15 mg/kg) in controlling infections due to two strains of *P. aeruginosa*, organisms that were resistant in vitro to carbenicillin. These excellent therapeutic results were made possible by the rapid absorption of MK-0366 from the gastrointestinal tract in mice and efficient distribution from the vascular compartment to various extravascular tissues. Absorption and elimination kinetics were similar for mice, rats, and rhesus monkeys. The combination of potent activity against a broad spectrum of bacteria, oral absorption in mammals, and high cure rates in experimentally infected mice have focused attention on MK-0366 as a superior developmental candidate for the treatment of a wide variety of infections in humans.

1. **Ito, A., K. Hirai, M. Inoue, H. Koga, S. Susue, T. Irikura, and S. Mitsuhashi.** 1980. *In vitro* antibacterial activity of AM-715, a new nalidixic acid analog. Antimicrob. Agents Chemother. **17**:103–108.
2. **Stanier, R. Y., E. A. Adelberg, and J. Ingraham.** 1976. The microbial world, 4th ed. Prentice Hall, Englewood Cliffs, N.J.

Antibacterial Activity of HR-221, a New Oxim-Cephalosporin

W. STILLE,* S. SPIELER, AND P. M. SHAH

Zentrum der Inneren Medizin, J. W. Goethe Universität, Frankfurt, Federal Republic of Germany

HR-221 is a new thiazol derivative of cefotaxime, developed by Hoechst-Roussel (Fig. 1). The MICs (50 and 90%) of HR-221 are shown in Table 1.

HR-221 is slightly less active than cefotaxime. Cefotaxime-resistant strains are also resistant to HR-221. HR-221 has good bactericidal activity. The 99% kill rate times in minutes are as follows: *Escherichia coli*, 105, 130, 135, 140, and 195; *Klebsiella pneumoniae*, 60, 60, 75, 85, and 156; *Enterobacter* sp., 45, 70, 75, 80, and 90; *Citrobacter freundii*, 50, 90, and 135; *Serratia marcescens* 55, 90, 135, and 195; and *Staphylococcus aureus*, 65, 135, 165, 195, and 525. The bactericidal activity of HR-221 was determined at two times the MIC. Kill rate times were determined with Mueller-Hinton medium and membrane filtration, using an inoculum of 10^6 organisms per ml.

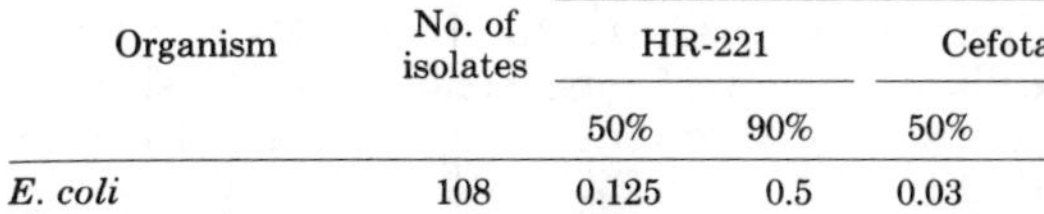

FIG. 1. *Structure of HR-221.*

HR-221 is highly active against enterobacteria and moderately active against *S. aureus* and *Pseudomonas*. It fulfills the basic requirements of a potential agent for the treatment of urinary tract infections.

TABLE 1. *MICs of HR-221*[a]

Organism	No. of isolates	MIC (μg/ml)									
		HR-221		Cefotaxime		Cefazolin		Cefoxitin		Piperacillin	
		50%	90%	50%	90%	50%	90%	50%	90%	50%	90%
E. coli	108	0.125	0.5	0.03	0.06	1	4	2	8	1	32
K. pneumoniae	87	0.25	4	0.125	0.5	4	≥128	4	64	4	≥128
Enterobacter sp.	71	2	512	1	128	≥512		256	≥512	16	128
Proteus mirabilis	54	0.015	0.25	0.015	0.125	2	16	1	8	0.25	16
Proteus (indole positive)	21	0.015	1	0.015	0.25	4	128	2	8	0.5	8
Salmonella sp.	40	0.25	0.5	0.03	0.06	2	4	4	8	4	32
Citrobacter	20	8	64	2	16	256	≥512	128	≥512	8	64
Staphylococcus aureus											
Penicillinase negative	48	4	8	1	2	0.25	1	2	8	2	8
Penicillinase positive	38	4	16	1	4	0.5	2	2	8	1	4

[a] Determined by agar dilution in Mueller-Hinton agar.

Comparative Studies of SM-1652 and Other Recently Developed Cephalosporins

MASUHIRO KATO,* MASATOMO FUKASAWA, HIROSHI NOGUCHI, TAKAO OKUDA, TOSHIAKI KOMATSU, KUNIICHIRO YANO, AND SUSUMU MITSUHASHI

School of Medicine, Gunma University, Maebashi, Sumitomo Chemical Co., Pharmaceuticals Division, Osaka, and Yamanouchi Pharmaceutical Co., Tokyo, Japan*

SM-1652 (Fig. 1) had potent antipseudomonal activity coupled with a broad antibacterial spectrum, high bactericidal activity, and long-acting effects (2, 3). The antibacterial activities were determined by the agar dilution method. For *Pseudomonas aeruginosa* strains IFO3445, NCTC 10490, and PAO1, the MICs of SM-1652, cefsulodin (CFS), cefoperazone (T-1551; CPZ), and cefotaxime (CTX) were as follows: IFO3445, 0.78, 0.39, 6.25, and 12.5; NCTC 10490, 1.56, 0.78, 3.13, and 12.5; PAO1, 3.13, 3.13, 6.25, and 6.25 μg/ml, respectively. Against clinically isolated *P. aeruginosa* (200 strains), SM-1652 was almost as active as CFS, two times as active as CPZ, and 8 to 16 times as active as CTX, cefmenoxime, and moxalactam. It was concluded that SM-1652 has the highest anti-*P. aeruginosa* activity among new generation β-lactams.

Activity against clinical isolates of species other than *P. aeruginosa* was measured (Table 1). SM-1652 exhibited broad-spectrum antibacterial activity. The features of the spectrum were as follows. (i) On glucose-nonfermentative gram-negative bacteria such as *P. cepacia*, *P. maltophilia*, and *Acinetobacter*, the concentrations of SM-1652 which inhibited 50% of clinical isolates (MIC_{50}) were in the range of 1.38 to 6.77 μg/ml, being the lowest, whereas MIC_{50} values of CPZ and CTX were 5.51 to 26.63 and 4.48 to 7.47 μg/ml, respectively. (ii) Against gram-positive cocci, SM-1652 was comparable to CPZ and CTX. (iii) SM-1652 inhibited most *Enterobacteriaceae* at concentrations lower than 3 μg/ml except for *Proteus* sp. (4 to 9 μg/ml) and *Serratia marcescens* (18.4 μg/ml). Some differences between MIC_{50} and MIC_{75} of SM-1652 were found in *S. marcescens*, *Escherichia coli*, *Klebsiella pneumoniae*, and *Enterobacter cloacae*.

It was observed that SM-1652 exhibited long-acting activity (3). For example, the plasma (SM-1652) or serum levels 4 h after bolus intravenous injection of 1 g in humans were 70.7, 22.0, 3.1, and 15.4 μg/ml for SM-1652, CPZ, CTX, and cefazolin (CEZ), respectively (3–6). As one of the ways to estimate clinical usefulness, we calculated the inhibition percentage of clinical isolates at the concentration described above. As shown in Table 1, SM-1652 inhibited all the strains tested not less than 90%, except for *E. cloacae* (88.5%) and *S. marcescens* (68.54%). It should be noted that in gram-positive cocci and in glucose-nonfermentative gram-negative bacteria, SM-1652 showed very high inhibition percentages: *Staphylococcus aureus* (100%); *S. epidermidis* (100%); *Streptococcus pyogenes* (100%); *P. aeruginosa* (99.25%); *P. cepacia* (98.18%); *P. maltophilia* (97.06%); and *Acinetobacter* (100%). On the contrary, CPZ and CTX inhibited only 41.87 to 97.95% and 11.85 to 28.53%, respectively, of glucose-nonfermentative gram-negative bacteria.

The MBCs were determined with a loop transfer method. In *E. coli* and *Proteus*, the MBCs were almost the same or only twofold higher than the MICs of SM-1652. In CPZ, the differences between MBCs and MICs were almost the same as for SM-1652 in *E. coli*; however, in indole-positive *Proteus* the MBCs were higher than the MICs by two to eight times. The more potent bactericidal activity of SM-1652 than CPZ in *E. coli* ML4707 was also confirmed by a growth inhibition experiment. In *P. aeruginosa* GN3315, SM-1652 exhibited almost the same bactericidal activity as CPZ and CFS, which was somewhat less cidal than the effect observed in *E. coli*.

Additionally, morphological changes were performed by the film-agar method for SM-1652, CPZ, CEZ, CBPC, and piperacillin (PIPC) in *E. coli* NIHJ JC-2. SM-1652, CPZ, and PIPC made the test organism filamentous in a wide range of drug concentrations. However, SM-1652 lysed cells at the lowest concentration. The lysis concentrations were reduced in the order PIPC > CBPC > CPZ ≧ CEZ = SM-1652.

The affinity to the penicillin-binding proteins (PBPs) was measured by preincubation method

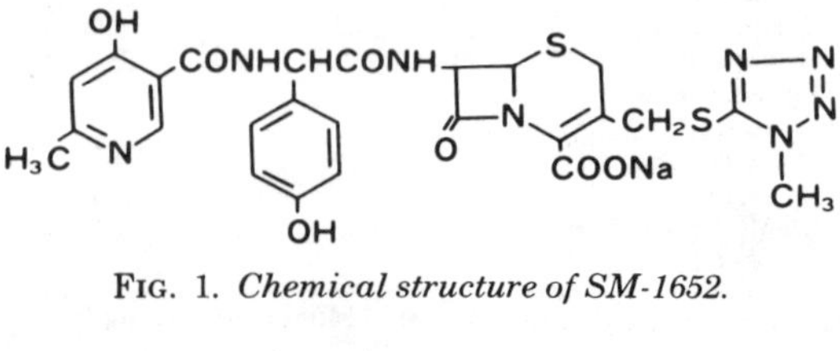

FIG. 1. *Chemical structure of SM-1652.*

TABLE 1. *Antimicrobial susceptibility of clinical isolates to SM-1652 and other cephalosporins*

Organism	No. of strains	SM-1652			CPZ			CTX			CEZ		
		MIC_{50}	MIC_{75}	Inhibition (%)[a]	MIC_{50}	MIC_{75}	Inhibition (%)	MIC_{50}	MIC_{75}	Inhibition (%)	MIC_{50}	MIC_{75}	Inhibition (%)
S. aureus	100	1.02	1.38	100	1.06	1.41	99.00	0.84	1.19	98.90	0.23	0.32	99.0
S. epidermidis	53	0.65	1.15	100	0.67	1.18	99.31	0.40	0.77	95.94	1.09	1.51	96.23
S. pyogenes	92	0.05	0.08	100	0.06	0.08	100	≦0.03	≦0.03	100	0.07	0.08	100
E. coli	200	1.44	13.87	94.75	0.22	1.26	97.91	≦0.20	≦0.20	98.97	1.42	2.79	95.45
K. pneumoniae	200	1.56	10.88	91.00	0.23	1.71	94.18	≦0.20	≦0.20	100	1.22	2.38	92.91
P. vulgaris	40	6.73	12.60	97.96	1.30	2.44	97.59	≦0.20	≦0.20	95.92	21.6	>100	30.61
P. rettgeri	35	5.26	11.61	98.57	1.43	3.88	98.95	≦0.20	≦0.20	97.14	62.1	>100	18.87
P. morganii	50	8.84	12.33	92.00	0.98	1.66	99.27	≦0.20	≦0.20	95.95	>100	>100	13.16
P. inconstans	32	7.08	11.74	96.88	1.37	2.41	96.88	≦0.20	≦0.20	96.79	57.4	>100	15.05
P. mirabilis	100	4.88	7.32	99.50	0.73	1.31	100	≦0.20	≦0.20	98.00	3.19	5.23	89.00
E. cloacae	110	2.85	12.14	88.55	0.25	1.02	99.33	≦0.20	0.88	79.04	>100	>100	26.83
E. aerogenes	24	1.86	2.63	100	≦0.20	0.28	100	≦0.20	≦0.20	100	>100	>100	26.26
C. freundii	26	2.21	5.73	94.23	0.28	0.66	98.59	≦0.20	≦0.20	88.36	28.7	>100	43.47
S. marcescens	205	18.4	>100	68.54	1.55	15.83	78.04	≦0.20	0.66	88.11	>100	>100	1.12
P. aeruginosa	200	1.32	2.17	99.25	2.28	3.13	97.95	6.31	10.86	15.46	1.11[b]	1.49[b]	96.91[b]
P. cepacia	55	1.38	5.26	98.18	5.51	22.53	74.70	4.48	9.10	28.53	>100	>100	0
P. maltophilia	34	4.96	7.97	97.06	11.02	17.68	87.12	6.25	17.68	17.50	>100	>100	0
Acinetobacter	100	6.77	11.10	100	26.63	45.02	41.87	7.47	13.21	11.85	ND[c]	ND	ND

[a] Inhibition percentage of clinical isolates at the plasma or serum level 4 h after a 1-g intravenous bolus injection in humans.
[b] Data for cefsulodin.
[c] ND, Not determined.

TABLE 2. *Protective effect against systemic infection in mice*

Organism	Challenge dose[a]	Drug[b]	MIC (μg/ml)	ED_{50} (mg/kg)[c]
E. coli ML4707	25 LD_{50} (2.5×10^6 CFU/mouse)	SM-1652	0.39	7.30 (4.08–13.1)
		CPZ	0.05	4.10 (2.46–6.85)
		CTX	0.05	1.65 (0.91–2.48)
		CZX	0.05	1.13 (0.78–1.64)
		CFX	3.13	37.0 (24.3–56.2)
		CEZ	1.56	34.0 (21.5–53.7)
K. pneumoniae GN6445	5 LD_{50} (7.3×10^6 CFU/mouse)	SM-1652	0.39	4.60 (2.36–8.97)
		CPZ	0.10	0.88 (0.42–1.85)
		CTX	0.05	0.36 (0.20–0.66)
		CZX	0.05	0.34 (0.19–0.61)
		CFX	3.13	62.5 (39.1–100.0)
		CEZ	1.56	6.10 (3.89–10.98)
P. aeruginosa GN3315	15 LD_{50} (1.2×10^5 CFU/mouse) + mucin	SM-1652	1.56	31.0 (22.1–43.3)
		CPZ	6.25	102.0 (61.8–168.3)
		CFS	0.78	17.0 (11.1–26.0)
		CTX	ND[d]	>200
		CZX	ND	>200
		CBPC	ND	>200

[a] Mice (male ICR, weighing 19.0 to 21.0 g) were intraperitoneally infected. CFU, Colony-forming units.
[b] Medication, 1 and 4 h after infection. Abbreviations not given in text: CZX, ceftizoxime; CFX, cefoxitin.
[c] Numbers in parentheses, 95% confidential limits.
[d] ND; Not determined.

with *E. coli* JE1011 membrane fraction. The finding that SM-1652 had high affinity for PBP-3, -1A, -1Bs, and -2 supported the above-mentioned antibacterial activities and morphological changes. That is, the concentrations of SM-1652 to prevent [^{14}C]benzylpenicillin binding by 50% were: 1A, 0.12; 1Bs, 0.65; 2, 0.35; 3, 0.04; 4, 100; and 5/6, 100 μg/ml. These values are nearly equal to those found with CPZ.

The stability to various β-lactamases was measured with purified enzymes by the UV method. To most cephalosporinases tested, SM-1652 was very stable. But it was hydrolyzed by 8% with cephalosporinase from *S. marcescens* GN10857 (with cephaloridine [CER] normalized to 100%). Cefuroxime-hydrolyzing β-lactamases (1) from *P. vulgaris* GN7919, *P. cepacia* GN11164, and *B. fragilis* GN11478 hydrolyzed SM-1652, CPZ, CTX, CEZ, CER, and penicillin G. But V_{max} values of SM-1652 and CPZ were 1/10 to 1/5 of those of CTX. SM-1652 and CPZ were hydrolyzed by penicillinase type I (V_{max} ratios were 52.6 and 26.0 for SM-1652 and CPZ, with penicillin G normalized to 100) but were very stable to penicillinase from *S. aureus*.

Protective effects of SM-1652 against experimental systemic infections in mice are illustrated in Table 2. SM-1652 showed protective effects comparable to those of CPZ in *E. coli* ML4707 in spite of the difference in MIC. Against *P. aeruginosa* GN3315, SM-1652 exhibited potent antipseudomonal activity in vivo as well as in vitro compared with other β-lactams.

In conclusion, SM-1652 has high antipseudomonal activity with a broad antibacterial spectrum, potent bactericidal activity, and high in vivo efficacy. This antibiotic is now under phase III clinical evaluation.

1. **Hirai, K., S. Iyobe, M. Inoue, and S. Mitsuhashi.** 1980. Purification and properties of a new β-lactamase from *Pseudomonas cepacia*. Antimicrob. Agents Chemother. **17**:355–358.
2. **Komatsu, T., T. Okuda, H. Noguchi, M. Fukasawa, K. Yano, M. Kato, and S. Mitsuhashi.** 1980. SM-1652, a new parenterally active cephalosporin: microbial studies, p. 275–278. *In* Current chemotherapy and infectious disease. American Society for Microbiology, Washington, D.C.
3. **Koyama, M., N. Nakatsuru, K. Yoshinaga, H. Matsui, C. Ikeda, K. Yano, and T. Noguchi.** 1980. Human pharmacokinetics of SM-1652, p. 149. Proc. 20th Intersci. Conf. Antimicrob. Agents Chemother.
4. **Nakayama, I., Y. Akieda, H. Mizuashi, K. Sakao, A. Nishimoto, H. Sawaguchi, and S. Ishiyama.** 1980. Studies on cefoperazone (T-1551) in surgery—antibacterial activity, absorption, excretion, metabolism, tissue distribution and its clinical application. Chemotherapy **28**:595–608.
5. **Shimzau, R., N. Kato, Y. Ban, Y. Kawada, and T. Nishiura.** 1980. Antimicrobial activity in urine and clinical efficacy of Ceftizoxime. Chemotherapy **28**:696–705.
6. **Shimizu, K., T. Kumada, and K. Okuzumi.** 1980. Basic and clinical studies on Cefotaxime. Chemotherapy **28**: 228–236.

In Vitro Antibacterial Activity of Cephalosporins and Moxalactam Compared with That of Aminoglycosides and Ureidopenicillins

FRANK G. C. HEILMANN,* MAJA ROZENBERG-ARSKA, AND JAN VERHOEF

Department of Clinical Bacteriology, University Hospital, Utrecht, The Netherlands

Recently a new generation of cephalosporins with a very broad antibacterial spectrum has been developed. Now the possibility arises of treating patients with serious infections with these less toxic drugs. However, before these drugs become the drug of choice in treating serious infections, the susceptibility of microorganisms to these drugs must be known in a hospital setting. Therefore, we compared the in vitro antibacterial activity of cefaclor (COR), cefamandole (CML), cefoperazone (T-1551; CPZ), cefotaxime (CTX), cefotiam (CAM), cefsulodin (CFS), ceftazidime (CTZ), cefuroxime (CUR), and cephalothin (CPT) with that of moxalactam (MOX), amikacin (AMK), gentamicin (GEN), netilmicin (NET), tobramycin (TOB), ampicillin (AMP), azlocillin (AZL), and piperacillin (PIP) against clinical isolates from patients of the University Hospital of Utrecht.

The antibiotic susceptibility of *Acinetobacter* spp. (8 strains), *Pseudomonas* spp. (30 strains), *Klebsiella* spp. (25 strains), *Proteus* spp. (33 strains), *Escherichia coli* (65 strains), *Enterobacter* spp. (30 strains), *Enterococcus* spp. (20 strains), *Staphylococcus aureus* (43 strains), and *S. epidermidis* (7 strains) was tested by standard agar diffusion and agar dilution methods.

Table 1 shows the cumulative results of MICs of bacterial strains as the concentrations of the drugs which inhibited growth of 50% (MIC_{50}) and 90% (MIC_{90}) of the microorganisms.

These results indicate that cephalothin remains the cephalosporin of choice against staphylococci. None of the new cephalosporins are effective against enterococci. MOX, CTX, CTZ, and CAM have similar antibacterial activities against *Enterobacteriaceae* and are at least as potent as the aminoglycosides. CFS and CTZ are the most effective cephalosporins against *Pseudomonas* and *Acinetobacter* but less potent than aminoglycosides.

TABLE 1. *Cumulative MIC_{50} and MIC_{90} values.*

	COR	CML	CPZ	CTX	CAM	CFS	CTZ	CUR	CPT	MOX	AMK	GEN	NET	TOB	AMP	AZL	PIP
STAPHYLOCOCCUS																	
MIC 50	1.5	1.5	6	0.8	0.8	0.8	3	0.4	0.4	1.5	0.4	0.1	0.2	0.1	-	12	6
MIC 90	6	6	12	1.5	3	3	6	1.5	0.8	6	1.5	0.8	0.8	0.8	-	25	12
PSEUDOMONAS / ACINETOBACTER																	
MIC 50	>100	>100	3	6	>100	0.8	1.5	>100	-	3	0.4	0.4	1.5	0.1	-	1.5	0.4
MIC 90	>100	>100	25	50	>100	25	6	>100	-	25	3	100	50	6	-	25	12
ENTEROBACTERIACEAE																	
MIC 50	0.8	1.5	0.8	0.1	0.4	50	0.4	1.5	-	0.1	1.5	0.4	0.8	0.8	-	12	1.5
MIC 90	6	6	12	0.4	1.5	>100	0.8	6	-	0.4	3	1.5	3	3	-	>100	50
ENTEROCOCCUS																	
MIC 50	25	25	25	6	>100	>100	>100	12	-	>100	>100	25	50	50	0.8	0.8	0.8
MIC 90	50	50	100	>100	>100	>100	>100	>100	-	>100	>100	>100	100	100	1.5	3	3

Cefmenoxime Concentration in Infected Tissues from Patients After Intramuscular or Intravenous Administration and Clinical Effect on Patients with Cholecystitis and Peritonitis

IKUO HASHIMOTO,* YASUO SAWADA, TAKASHI NAKAMURA, JIROH MIKAMI, EIICHI BEKKI, HIDEO FUJITA, MICHIKO SAITOH, HIROYUKI NISHINDAI, MASAMI NAKANISHI, AND YOICHI KASAI

Departments of Surgery and Internal Medicine, St. Franciscan Tenshi Hospital, and First Surgical Department, School of Medicine, Hokkaido University, Sapporo, Japan*

Only a few of the studies on pharmacokinetics in patients treated with antibiotics have reported data on antibiotic concentration in the tissues (2). These studies have showed the concentrations at a single time point after drug administration (3, 4). A previous study was done to determine the concentration of cefmetazole (CMZ) in the infected tissue, plasma, and bile of patients as a function of time (5). However, it is doubtful whether the effective concentration in the infected tissue can be obtained by changing the drug or the route of administration. Therefore, the present study was undertaken to investigate the concentration of cefmenoxime (SCE-1365; CMX) tissue after intramuscular (i.m.) and intravenous (i.v.) administration.

TABLE 1. *Clinical effect of CMX after i.m. injection or i.v. drip infusion for preoperative patients with cholecystitis and cholangitis (patients 1 to 10) and for postoperative patients with acute peritonitis (patients 11 to 24)[a]*

Patient no.	Age (yr)	Sex	Wt (kg)	Daily dose	Method	Duration (days)	Organism	MIC, 10^6 cells/ml (μg/ml)	Clinical effect
1	67	F	44.5	1 g, 0.5 × 2	i.m.	6	No growth		Good
2	33	F	59	1 g, 0.5 × 2	i.m.	20	*E. coli*	0.05	Good
3	68	F	51	1 g, 0.5 × 2	i.m.	7	*K. pneumoniae*	0.025	Good
4	36	F	64	1 g, 0.5 × 2	i.m.	7	No growth		Good
5	57	M	54	1 g, 0.5 × 2	i.m.	5	No growth		Excellent
6	53	F	61	2 g, 1 × 2	i.v.	6	No growth		Good
7	60	F	62.5	2 g, 1 × 2	i.v.	6	No growth		Good
8	50	F	57	2 g, 1 × 2	i.v.	6	No growth		Good
					i.v.				
9	65	F	64.5	1 g, 1 × 1	i.v.	10	No growth		Good
10	46	F	64	2 g, 1 × 2	i.v.	8	No growth		Excellent
11	15	M	63	1 g, 0.5 × 2	i.m.	4	*E. coli*	0.025	Excellent
12	42	F	43.5	1 g, 0.5 × 2	i.m.	5	*E. coli*	0.05	Excellent
13	16	F	54.4	1 g, 0.5 × 2	i.m.	4	*E. coli*	0.05	Good
14	11	F	36	1 g, 0.5 × 2	i.m.	7	*E. coli*	0.05	Good
15	19	F	55	1 g, 0.5 × 2	i.m.	4	*E. coli*	0.05	Excellent
16	24	M	45.5	1 g, 0.5 × 2	i.m.	8	*E. coli*	0.0125	Good
17	35	M	71	1 g, 0.5 × 2	i.m.	3	No growth		Good
18	6	M	28	1 g, 0.5 × 2	i.m.	4	*E. coli*	0.025	Excellent
19	56	M	58	1 g, 0.5 × 2	i.m.	4	*E. coli*	0.0125	Excellent
20	49	M	64	1 g, 0.5 × 2	i.m.	5	*E. coli*	0.05	Excellent
21	9	F	35	1 g, 0.5 × 2	i.v.	4	*E. coli*	0.05	Excellent
22	71	F	54.5	2 g, 1 × 2		10	*E. coli*	0.05	Excellent
							K. pneumoniae	0.05	
23	45	M	46	2 g, 1 × 2	i.v.	10	*Enterobacter aerogenes*	1.56	Excellent
24	8	M	23	2 g, 1 × 2	i.v.	4	*E. coli*	0.05	Excellent

[a] Patient 1 was diagnosed as having choledocho-duodenal fistula. In patients 3 through 6, 9, and 10, the cystic duct was obstructed. Patients 2, 3, 5, 6, and 10 were diagnosed as having acute cholecystitis, and patients 1, 4, and 7 through 9 had subacute cholecystitis. Patients 11 to 14, 18, 20 to 22, and 24 were diagnosed as having acute peritonitis with perforate appendicitis. Patients 15 to 17 were diagnosed as having localized peritonitis with phlegmous empyemic appendicitis. Patient 19 was diagnosed as having diffuse peritonitis with intestinal obstruction. Patient 23 was diagnosed as having panperitonitis with intestinal perforation. No adverse effects of the drug treatment were observed in any of the 24 patients.

CMX is a new semisynthetic cephalosporin with marked resistance to β-lactamase, having a low MIC for gram-negative bacilli and a broad spectrum of antibacterial activity against various pathogenic bacterial species, including *Haemophilus influenzae*, indole-positive *Proteus*, *Serratia marcescens, Citrobacter freundii*, and *Enterobacter cloacae* (1). The patients were hospitalized between November 1979 and September 1980 in the Surgical Department of Tenshi Hospital. They included 13 females and 9 males, and their ages ranged from 6 to 71 years. The patients included 14 with acute peritonitis (12 due to acute appendicitis and 2 others) and 10 with acute or subacute cholecystitis. In 14 cases, CMX (Takeda Chemicals Co. Ltd.) in a dose of 500 mg was given i.m. before the operation. In the other eight cases, CMX in a dose of

TABLE 2. *CMX concentration in various body fluids and tissues during operation after i.m. administration of 500 mg to patients 1 to 5 and 11 to 19 and i.v. administration of 1,000 mg to patients 6 to 10, 20, and 22 to 24*[a]

Patient no.	Cefmenoxime concn at indicated time after injection			
	Plasma (μg/ml)	A-bile in cases 1–10; ascites with pus in cases 11–24 (μg/ml)	B-bile in cases 1–10; pus in appendix in cases 11–24 (μg/ml)	Gall bladder wall in cases 1–10; appendix wall, others in cases 11–24 (μg/g)
1	5.1 at 110 min	402.0 at 104 min		0.9 at 85 min (++)[b]
		387.0 at 120 min		7.0 at 110 min
2		34.0 at 164 min	3.9 at 120 min[c]	55.7 at 210 min (++)
		24.4 at 177 min	10.2 at 210 min	
3	4.8 at 133 min	216.0 at 132 min	1.8 at 160 min	1.6 at 150 min (++)
		213.0 at 135 min		
4		302.5 at 160 min	18.5 at 138 min	7.2 at 138 min (++)
5	3.8 at 165 min	213.7 at 164 min		2.0 at 142 min (+++)
				7.7 at 150 min
				7.4 at 160 min
6		1,454.0 at 50 min	1.6 at 20 min[c]	48.8 at 40 min (+++)
		575.0 at 56 min[d]	72.3 at 40 min	
7		66.1 at 20 min	2.5 at 20 min[c]	13.4 at 40 min (+)
		203.7 at 23 min	3.5 at 40 min	
		1,157.0 at 40 min		
8	33.9 at 60 min		4.3 at 52 min[c]	10.2 at 60 min (+)
			14.8 at 60 min	
9	18.5 at 59 min	1,030.0 at 64 min	3.0 at 94 min	16.5 at 94 min (+++)
		886.0 at 67 min		
		411.5 at 84 min		
10		777.0 at 76 min	11.9 at 100 min	16.8 at 100 min (+++)
		826.5 at 85 min		
		1,409.0 at 90 min		
11	5.1 at 72 min	3.4 at 73 min	2.8 at 85 min	4.1 at 85 min
12	1.6 at 247 min	1.3 at 225 min		1.4 at 240 min
13	3.5 at 155 min			2.8 at 148 min
14	5.6 at 156 min			
15	2.1 at 188 min		3.4 at 215 min	2.7 at 215 min
16	2.0 at 40 min		0.2 at 30 min	3.3 at 30 min
17	0.5 at 255 min		0.2 at 240 min	0.8 at 240 min
18	12.9 at 70 min		0.8 at 60 min	9.2 at 60 min
19	7.1 at 135 min			3.9 at 111 min
20	32.6 at 80 min	35.3 at 75 min		16.5 at 80 min
21	28.6 at 27 min		0.5 at 18 min	12.9 at 18 min
22		42.3 at 18 min	52.5 at 20 min	45.5 at 20 min
23		2.2 at 30 s		32.9 at 90 min
		10.6 at 5 min		(mesenterial
		39.5 at 41 min		lymph node)
		29.9 at 65 min		
		26.1 at 95 min		
		71 min	0.4 at 75 min	0.8 at 75 min

[a] Patient 21 was given 500 mg i.v. and patient 24 was given 1 g i.v. for 2 h.
[b] Inflammatory degree of gall bladder wall.
[c] Punctured bile in gall bladder.
[d] Diluted with Biligrafin solution.

1 g was given i.v. during the operation. In one case, 500 mg of CMX was given i.v. during the operation, and in one case 1 g was given by i.v. drip infusion for 2 h before the operation. During the operation, plasma, bile, and tissue specimens were taken and sent to Takeda Chemicals Co. (Osaka, Japan) for determination of CMX concentration. This determination was carried out by microbioassay, with *Proteus mirabilis* ATCC 21100 as the test organism.

Since it is very important in chemotherapy to know the distribution of drugs in the infected tissues and the MIC of the drug for the pathogenic bacteria, this study was performed to determine the CMX concentrations in infected target organs or tissues of the patients. Our findings (Tables 1 and 2) are as follows. (i) When given in a dose of 500 mg i.m. before operation, the CMX concentration in A-bile (bile in the common duct) increased gradually up to 2 h, reaching maximal levels of 300 to 402 μg/ml, and then declined slowly. (ii) When given in a dose of 1 g i.v., the concentration reached a peak of 1,030 to 1,454 μg/ml at 1 h and then declined slowly. (iii) CMX was observed in B-bile (bile in the gall bladder) through the gall bladder wall in the cases of obstructed cystic ducts and reached a high level comparatively quickly after injection. (iv) CMX levels in the gall bladder wall after i.v. administration were four to five times higher than those after i.m. administration. (v) Concentrations of CMX in the gall bladder wall and appendixes were directly proportional to the degree of the pathological changes of inflammation. (vi) In a case of acute panperitonitis due to intestinal perforation, the CMX concentration in the purulent ascites was 10.6 μg/ml at 5 min after i.v. administration. In this case, the CMX concentration in purulent ascites was 26.1 μg/ml at 95 min after i.v. administration. (vii) The CMX concentrations in plasma, purulent ascites, A-bile, B-bile, appendix, pus in the appendix, gall bladder wall, and other infected tissues were higher than the MIC of CMX for *Escherichia coli* and *Klebsiella pneumoniae* after 500 mg to 1 g of CMX by parenteral administration.

For therapeutic purposes, CMX was given in a daily dose of 1 g (0.5 g twice) by i.m. administration in 16 cases (5 cholecystitis and 11 peritonitis) for 3 to 20 days; in the other 8 cases (5 cholecystitis and 3 peritonitis), CMX was given in a dose of 1 g by drip infusion twice a day for 4 to 10 days. Clinical responses were rated excellent in 12 cases, good in 12 cases, fair in none, and poor in none. No clinical adverse effect was observed. Therefore, CMX appears to be a very useful drug when used for chemotherapy of acute peritonitis and cholecystitis.

1. **Goto, S., et al.** 1980. SCE-1365, a new cephalosporin: in vitro antibacterial activities, p. 264–266. *In* J. D. Nelson and C. Grassi (ed.), Current chemotherapy and infectious disease. American Society for Microbiology, Washington, D.C.
2. **Kiss, I. J., et al.** 1978. Pharmacokinetic study of rifampicin in biliary surgery. Int. J. Clin. Pharmacol. **16:**105–109.
3. **Nakamura, T., et al.** 1978. Dibekacin concentration in various tissues of patients. Chemotherapy (Tokyo) **27:** 377–378.
4. **Nakamura, T., et al.** 1979. Bacampicillin concentration in various tissues of patients. Chemotherapy (Tokyo) **27:**202–205.
5. **Nakamura, T., et al.** 1980. Cefmetazole concentration in infected tissues from patients after intravenous administration and clinical effect for patients with cholecystitis and peritonitis, p. 236–238. *In* J. D. Nelson and C. Grassi (ed.), Current chemotherapy and infectious disease. American Society for Microbiology, Washington, D.C.

Clinical Usefulness of Cefmetazole in Newborn and Premature Infants

RYOCHI FUJII

Department of Pediatrics, Teikyo University School of Medicine, Tokyo, Japan

We investigated the usefulness of cefmetazole (CMZ) in newborn and premature infants. Blood level was measured after intravenous injection of 20 mg/kg to 16 newborn and 8 premature infants.

The biological half-life ($t_{1/2}$) in full-term infants up to 3 days old was, on average, 4.18 h and became shorter with age. A similar tendency was observed in premature infants. With a dose of 25 mg/kg, comparable results were obtained in 14 full-term newborns and seven premature infants. Five cases given CMZ by drip infusion revealed changes in blood level similar to those seen in infants who had received a single intravenous injection.

The following three points were confirmed. First, the $t_{1/2}$ was extremely long the first few days after birth, shortening markedly thereafter

(Fig. 1). In 2-week-old newborns, $t_{1/2}$ declined to about the same level as in infants more than 1 month old. Second, in premature infants, individual differences were greatest on the day of birth, and $t_{1/2}$ was longer than in full-term infants. In both full-term and premature infants, particular care should be taken with regard to CMZ administration during the first 3 days after birth. This is still true, but to a lesser degree, for the succeeding 2 days. After infants reached 5 days of age, $t_{1/2}$ showed a trend toward rapid normalization. Third, the longer $t_{1/2}$ and greater individual differences in premature infants correlated with their lower body weights. Even in full-term infants, great individual differences were observed at the age of 3 days or less.

Urinary excretion was investigated in 10 cases who were less than 7 days old. Urinary volume had a very high correlation with urinary antibiotic recovery. It was suggested that, in general, ultimate urinary recovery is hard to estimate from urinary excretion during the first 6 h after administration in newborn infants.

In 51 cases (37 newborns and 14 infants), clinical efficacy was 94.1% and administration was generally good at a total daily dosage of 60 to 100 mg/kg, given three to four times a day. Dose response was not clearly observed. Clinical effect classified by diagnosis (Table 1) was 100% (excellent in 2 and good in 2) in 4 cases of purulent meningitis, the severest infection in infants (isolated bacteria: *Escherichia coli* in 2 cases, *E. coli* and *Serratia* in 1, and group B *Streptococcus* in 1), 100% (excellent in 4 and good in 3) in 7 cases of sepsis (isolated bacteria: *E. coli* in 5 cases and *Staphylococcus aureus* in 2), 100% (excellent in 6 and good in 11) in 17 cases of respiratory tract infection (mainly pneumonia), 100% (excellent in 1 and good in 2) in 3 cases of SSS syndrome, and 91.7% (excellent in 9 and good in 2) in 12 cases of urinary tract infection. Clinical efficacy on the whole was 94.1% (excellent in 23, good in 25, and poor in 3) among 51 cases, even though many very severe infections were included.

Bacteriological effect (rate of eradication of bacteria) was 100% in 10 cases of gram-positive bacteria, including *Staphylococcus aureus*, and 95.7% in 23 cases of gram-negative bacilli, including *E. coli* and *Serratia marcescens*. Overall bacteriological effect was 97.0% in 35 cases with gram-positive and gram-negative organisms, excluding two cases on which the bacteriological follow-up was not carried out; also, instead of a decrease in the number of causative agents, complete eradication of bacteria was always observed. No particular side effects (except for an increase in serum glutamic oxalacetic and serum glutamic pyruvic transaminases and eosinophils, eruption, etc., in a few cases) were observed.

Thus, CMZ is believed to be a safe and effective antibiotic for the treatment of severe bacterial infections during the neonatal period. This will continue to be true in the future, as the number of β-lactamase-producing bacteria increases. The recommended dosage of CMZ is 20 mg/kg twice a day for infants younger than 3 days old and three times a day for those 4 to 7 days old. In infants 8 days old or more, the dosage should be 60 to 100 mg/kg daily administered three to four times a day. The method of administration must be intravenous injection (one shot), intermittent intravenous infusion, or drip infusion. In cases of serious infection, the dosage may be proportionately increased in accordance with the symptoms. Very small premature infants must be injected with care, since $t_{1/2}$ in the serum may be prolonged.

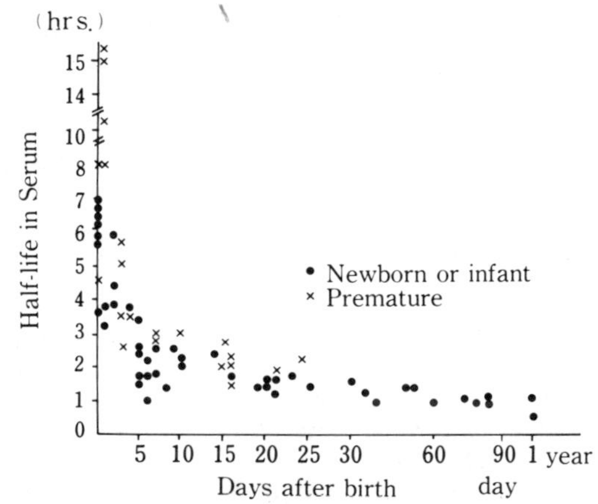

FIG. 1. *Correlation between half-lives of CMZ in serum and days of age.*

TABLE 1. *Clinical results classified by diagnosis*

Diagnosis	Excellent	Good	Poor	Unknown	Total	Efficacy(%)*
Respiratory tract infection	6	11			17	100
Purulent meningitis	2	2			4	100
Sepsis	4	3			7	100
Urinary tract infection	9	2	1		12	91.7
SSS syndrome	1	2			3	100
FUO		2			2	100
Other infection*	1	3	2		6	66.7
Total	23	25	3		51	94.1

* Fibrosis of the lung, Group B Streptococcosis.peritonitis. Salmonella enteritis. purulent cephalohematoma. pyoderma.

* Percent efficacy = (excellent + good)/(total number of patients − unknown) ×100

Pharmacokinetics of YM 09330 (Cefotetan) in Normal Subjects and Patients with Renal Insufficiency

SHOJI HIRANO,* MITSUO OHKAWA, SHUJI TOKUNAGA, ISAMU MOTOI, RYOCHU SHODA, AKIYOSHI IKEDA, TOSHIAKI SUGATA, MASARU SAWAKI, MASAYOSHI SHIMAMURA, AKIRA OKASHO, EINOSUKE NAKASHITA, AND KYOICHI KURODA

Department of Urology, School of Medicine, Kanazawa University, Kanazawa 920, Japan

YM 09330 (cefotetan) is a new 7-methoxy cephalosporin derivative demonstrated to have high and prolonged blood levels and high urinary recovery after intramuscular or intravenous injection (1). The pharmacokinetics of YM 09330 was studied after a single 500-mg intravenous injection in 8 healthy volunteers and 41 patients with impaired renal function (38 males and 11 females; age, 27 to 88 years; body weight, 39.0 to 80.0 kg). The subjects were divided into five groups according to endogenous creatinine clearance (Ccr) corrected for 1.73 m^2 of body surface area: group 1, 8 healthy volunteers with Ccr of 110 to 167 ml/min; group 2, 8 patients with Ccr of 68.6 to 93.9 ml/min; group 3, 16 patients with Ccr of 30.9 to 57.7 ml/min; group 4, 10 patients with Ccr of 8.1 to 28.2 ml/min; and group 5, 7 patients with Ccr of 0 to 7.8 ml/min. All seven patients in group 5 periodically underwent hemodialysis. Blood samples were obtained just before injection and 5, 15, and 30 min and 1, 2, 5, 8, 12, and 24 h after injection. Urine samples were collected from 0 to 2, 2 to 4, 4 to 6, 6 to 8, and 8 to 24 h. Serum and urinary concentrations of YM 09330 were determined by the thin-layer paper disk method, using *Escherichia coli* NIHJ as the titration strain and sensitive test agar as the culture medium. A standard dilution series was prepared by using pooled human serum obtained from normal subjects and 0.1 M phosphate buffer (pH 7.0). The assay range for both serum and urine samples was 0.78 to 100 μg/ml. Urinary concentration of YM 09330 and its tautomer were additionally determined by high-pressure liquid chromatography, using a model ALC 202 chromatograph (Waters Co., Ltd.). The detection limit was 1 μg/ml for both compounds. Pharmacokinetic parameters were estimated according to a two-compartment open model, using a NONLIN program.

Mean serum concentrations and mean cumulative urinary recoveries in each group after a single 500-mg intravenous injection of YM 09330 are shown in Table 1; pharmacokinetic parameters are summarized in Table 2. Serum concentrations during the β-phase increased in parallel with the degree of renal impairment. The mean serum half-life (β) and mean serum concentration of YM 09330 8 h after dosing were 3.0 h and 8.3 μg/ml in normal subjects as compared with 13.1 h and 45.7 μg/ml in hemodialysis patients. There was a significant correlation between Ccr and cumulative urinary recovery ($P < 0.001$). Mean cumulative urinary recovery at 24 h was 83.3% in the normal subjects as compared with 4.7% in group 5. Statistical analysis demonstrated a significant correlation between Ccr and the elimination rate constant ($P < 0.001$) and Ccr and β ($P < 0.001$). A hyperbolic relationship was observed between Ccr and the serum half-life (β). The apparent volume of distribution of YM 09330 was not influenced by the degree of renal impairment. The results demonstrated significant correlations between body clearance and Ccr ($P < 0.001$), renal clearance and Ccr ($P < 0.001$), and body clearance and renal clearance

TABLE 1. *Mean serum concentration of YM 09330 and mean cumulative urinary recovery*

Determination	Time (h)	Group 1	Group 2	Group 3	Group 4	Group 5
Serum concn (μg/ml ± SD)	1	45.6 ± 2.1	47.0 ± 8.7	56.2 ± 8.2	71.2 ± 16.9	77.1 ± 16.5
	2	31.9 ± 1.4	37.5 ± 6.8	45.3 ± 5.4	64.2 ± 16.8	67.0 ± 12.6
	5	15.9 ± 0.6	21.5 ± 5.2	26.7 ± 4.8	48.9 ± 12.5	54.4 ± 14.2
	8	8.3 ± 0.5	13.1 ± 3.6	18.4 ± 4.3	39.7 ± 12.1	45.7 ± 10.4
	24	0.2 ± 0.1	1.4 ± 1.3	3.5 ± 3.4	17.3 ± 7.9	24.5 ± 11.5
Urinary recovery (% ± SD)	0–2	39.3 ± 6.1	23.6 ± 6.0	16.2 ± 7.4	4.3 ± 7.6	1.0 ± 0.9
	0–4	54.7 ± 8.7	37.8 ± 4.7	28.5 ± 8.6	7.3 ± 10.8	1.7 ± 1.5
	0–6	65.0 ± 7.7	45.4 ± 11.2	36.3 ± 35.5	10.2 ± 13.3	2.5 ± 2.2
	0–8	71.9 ± 5.6	51.9 ± 11.4	44.1 ± 13.4	13.3 ± 15.9	3.2 ± 2.7
	0–24	83.3 ± 3.8	66.2 ± 12.6	61.1 ± 13.2	21.2 ± 20.6	4.7 ± 4.2

TABLE 2. *Pharmacokinetic parameters of YM 09330 after a single 500-mg intravenous injection in 8 normal subjects and 41 patients with impaired renal function*[a]

Patient group	Ccr (ml/min per 1.73 m^2)	β (h^{-1})	Elimination rate constant (h^{-1})	Half-life (β) (h)	AUC[b] (μg.h/ml)	V_d (liters)[c]	Body clearance (ml/min per 1.73 m^2)	Renal clearance (ml/min per 1.73 m^2)
1	133.1 ± 17.9	0.234 ± 0.031	0.612 ± 0.113	3.00 ± 0.37	254.0 ± 25.0	8.04 ± 1.60	38.7 ± 3.9	32.3 ± 3.6
2	79.5 ± 9.3	0.193 ± 0.037	0.557 ± 0.170	3.72 ± 0.79	323.8 ± 75.0	6.72 ± 2.81	31.5 ± 6.9	20.2 ± 7.9
3	47.2 ± 8.3	0.164 ± 0.042	0.438 ± 0.157	4.59 ± 1.62	427.8 ± 91.8	7.34 ± 1.21	23.9 ± 5.1	13.6 ± 5.0
4	16.0 ± 7.6	0.075 ± 0.039	0.184 ± 0.114	11.09 ± 4.38	1,171.0 ± 486.9	7.06 ± 1.63	10.1 ± 5.9	3.3 ± 4.9
5	5.0 ± 2.9	0.062 ± 0.024	0.147 ± 0.062	13.11 ± 6.60	1,452.9 ± 767.7	6.59 ± 0.98	8.3 ± 3.6	0.5 ± 0.5

[a] Results are given as the mean ± SD.
[b] Area under the serum concentration curve (zero to infinity).
[c] Apparent volume of distribution at steady state.

($P < 0.001$). There was a hyperbolic relationship between Ccr and the area under the serum concentration curve. The ratio of the 24-h cumulative urinary recovery of the tautomer to that of YM 09330 was 3.5 to 9.9% in each group; there was no correlation with renal function. To investigate potential differences in pharmacokinetics between periods out of hemodialysis and during hemodialysis, serum concentrations were measured for 5 h in five hemodialysis patients of group 5 by a crossover design. The mean serum concentrations of YM 09330 during hemodialysis were higher than those out of hemodialysis until 1 h after administration, but this relationship was reversed from 2 h after administration onwards. Mean serum concentrations at 5 h after administration were 49.8 μg/ml out of hemodialysis and 38.7 μg/ml during hemodialysis. The serum half-life (β) during hemodialysis was 5.7 h as compared with 9.4 h out of hemodialysis, showing that the mean half-life (β) was shortened an average of 3.7 h by dialysis. The serum half-life (β) of YM 09330 in hemodialysis patients was 13.1 h, 4.4-fold longer than that in normal subjects. This prolongation was, however, milder than the 30 h reported for ceftizoxime or the more than 30 h reported for cefazolin.

Our pharmacokinetic study confirmed that YM 09330 was excreted chiefly via the kidneys. There was only a slight difference between patients with moderate renal impairment and normal subjects, so that modification of the dosage is probably unnecessary in patients with Ccr of more than 30 ml/min. Although YM 09330 is a substance with good therapeutic tolerance, dose reduction or prolongation of dosage interval may be appropriate in patients with severe renal dysfunction to avoid excessive serum concentrations of the drug. For hemodialysis patients, treatment should be administered at the end of each hemodialysis session.

1. **Tachibana, A., M. Komiya, Y. Kikuchi, K. Yano, and K. Mashimo.** 1980. Pharmacological studies on YM 09330, a new parenteral cephamycin derivative, p. 273–275. *In* J. D. Nelson and C. Grassi (ed.), Current chemotherapy and infectious disease. American Society for Microbiology, Washington, D.C.

Intramuscular Ceforanide Therapy of *Staphylococcus aureus* Endocarditis in Parenteral Drug Abusers

RICHARD GREENMAN,* RICHARD ZWEIG, GORDON DICKINSON, AND THOMAS HOFFMAN

Division of Infectious Diseases, University of Miami School of Medicine, and Miami Veterans Administration Medical Center, Miami, Florida 33101, U.S.A.*

Infectious endocarditis is a common complication of parenteral drug abuse. In drug addicts, endocarditis is most frequently caused by *Staphylococcus aureus* and usually involves the valves of the right side of the heart (4). Single-drug intravenous β-lactam antibiotic therapy for 4 weeks has been shown to result in low mortality rates, and no advantage of combination antimicrobial therapy has been demonstrated in this setting (1). A frequent problem with intravenous therapy has been the difficulty in continuing intravascular access for 4 weeks in patients with already traumatized veins. This has frequently led to the necessity for central catheters or surgical cut-down placement, or in patients leaving the hospital after incomplete therapy because they would not tolerate such procedures.

Ceforanide (BL-S786R) is an investigational cephalosporin antibiotic that is well tolerated intramuscularly in doses up to 1 to 2 g. The pharmacokinetics of the agent are such that peak and trough (12 h) plasma levels of approximately 50 μg/ml and 3 μg/ml are demonstrable after 1 g administered intramuscularly (BL-S786R, Basic data brochure, Bristol Laboratories, Syracuse, N.Y.). Mean MICs of ceforanide for *S. aureus* have been shown to be approximately 1 μg/ml, with all strains susceptible to 4 μg/ml (3). Cooper et al. (2) treated nine patients with endocarditis caused by a variety of susceptible organisms with ceforanide and found generally favorable results.

The purpose of this study was to compare the efficacy of ceforanide therapy with that of a standard intravenous regimen in the treatment of staphylococcal endocarditis in parenteral drug abusers. Intravenous drug-abusing patients admitted to Jackson Memorial Hospital or the Miami Veterans Administration Medical Center with signs and symptoms suggestive of endocarditis were eligible for the study. Patients were excluded if they had a creatinine level greater than 3 mg/100 ml, were pregnant, or had a history of penicillin or cephalosporin allergy. After informed consent was obtained, patients were randomly assigned to therapy with 1 g of ceforanide intravenously (if an intravenous catheter was in place for other reasons) or intramuscularly every 12 h or 2 g of cephapirin intravenously every 4 h. If *S. aureus* was isolated from at least three blood cultures, the patient was continued on the protocol. Susceptibility of the infecting organisms was determined by both a modified Bauer-Kirby-Sherris method and by broth dilution studies. Bactericidal titers were determined on sera obtained at times corresponding to peak (30 min after either drug) and trough (11.5 h after ceforanide and 3.5 h after cephapirin) antibiotic concentrations.

Twenty-one patients with *S. aureus* endocarditis were begun on one of the regimens, 10 on ceforanide and 11 on cephapirin. Four patients did not complete therapy. Two were switched by their primary physicians to "standard therapy," and two left the hospital after less than 2 weeks of therapy. Patients ranged in age from 22 to 50 years (mean, 31). There were 11 female and 10 male patients. Eighteen patients were black. Valve involvement included 17 patients with right-sided disease only, 2 with mitral and tricuspid, and 2 with aortic valve disease. There were no differences between the two groups in the above-mentioned parameters or any other parameters studied.

Mean MICs and MBCs for the infecting organisms were 0.69 ± 0.46 μg/ml and 1.88 ± 1.73 μg/ml, respectively, for ceforanide and 0.10 ± 0.17 μg/ml and 0.19 ± 0.22 μg/ml, respectively, for cephapirin (Fig. 1). Geometric mean peak and trough serum killing levels were 1:7.5 and 1:1.8, respectively, for ceforanide and 1:75 and 1:3.1, respectively, for cephapirin (Fig. 2).

Seventeen patients were treated long enough

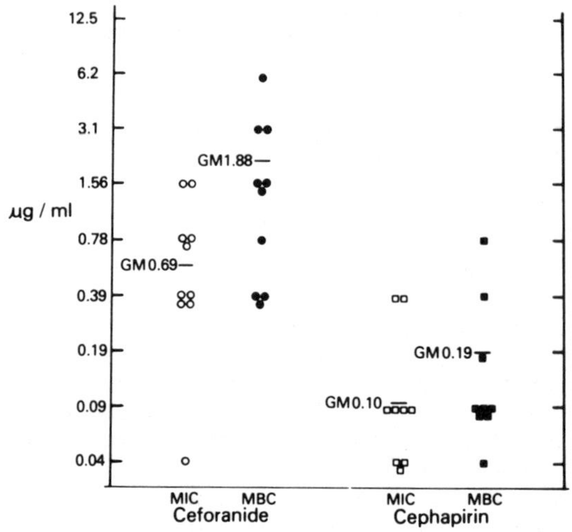

FIG. 1. *MIC and MBC of ceforanide and cephapirin for clinical isolates of S. aureus. GM, Geometric mean.*

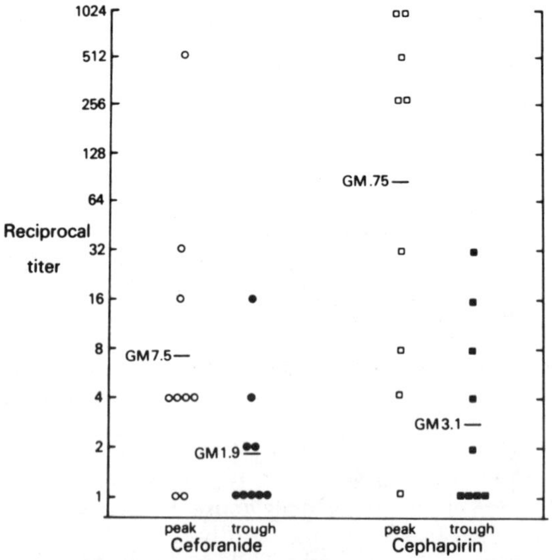

FIG. 2. *Serum killing levels of peak and trough samples of patients receiving ceforanide and cephapirin. GM, Geometric mean.*

to be considered evaluable. Of these patients, there was one immediate relapse among eight ceforanide-treated patients. There was one primary drug failure among nine patients treated with cephapirin. Both of these patients were subsequently cured with retreatment with other antibiotic regimens. In two patients treated with cephapirin, parenchymal brain abscess became apparent while on therapy. They were subsequently cured with surgical extirpation and continued antibiotics. Of the 15 patients apparently cured, 13 returned for follow-up at 1 to 3 months. None of these patients had evidence of relapse. Mean numbers of days to defervescence were identical in the two groups (ceforanide, 6.5 days; cephapirin, 6.3 days). No patients developed congestive heart failure or required placement of a prosthetic heart valve. There was no mortality in either group.

Ceforanide therapy was well tolerated by all patients. Four cephapirin patients developed significant phlebitis at the injection site, and one patient each had neutropenia or elevation of serum transaminase seemingly related to drug therapy. Two cephapirin patients left the hospital against medical advice, refusing further intravenous therapy.

Previous studies at our institution (1, 4) have included 71 patients treated with oxacillin alone or in combination with an aminoglycoside drug. In these patients there were no primary drug failures and no relapses noted, though follow-up was not necessarily as good as in the present study. Also, no brain abscesses were noted in these previous patients though such complications have been well described by others. Two of the 11 cephapirin-treated patients in this study had brain abscesses. Two unanswered questions can be posed by this study. First, do cephalosporins lead to a higher rate of failure or relapse than semisynthetic penicillins, and second, might cephalosporin therapy lead to a higher incidence of clinically apparent brain abscesses?

In conclusion, ceforanide appears to be a useful antimicrobial in the treatment of *S. aureus* endocarditis in parenteral drug abusers. Despite higher MIC and MBC values and lower serum killing levels, no significant differences in outcome were noted between patients treated with ceforanide versus cephapirin. Intramuscular ceforanide was better tolerated by patients than was intravenous cephapirin.

1. **Abrams, B., A. Sklaver, T. Hoffman, and R. Greenman.** 1979. Single or combination therapy of staphylococcal endocarditis in intravenous drug abusers. Ann. Intern. Med. **90**:789–791.
2. **Cooper, R., J. Mills, and P. Joseph.** 1980. Ceforanide therapy of endocarditis, p. 902–904. *In* J. D. Nelson and C. Grassi (ed.), Current Chemotherapy and infectious disease. American Society of Microbiology, Washington, D.C.
3. **Leitner, F., M. Misiek, T. Pursiano, R. Buck, D. Chisholm, R. DeRegis, Y. Tsai, and K. Price.** 1976. Laboratory evaluation of BL-S786, a cephalosporin with broad spectrum antibacterial activity. Antimicrob. Agents Chemother. **10**:426–435.
4. **Sklaver, A., T. Hoffman, and R. Greenman.** 1978. Staphylococcal endocarditis in addicts. South. Med. J. **71**:638–643.

Bacteriological, Clinical, and Pharmacokinetic Evaluation of Cefonicid (SK&F 75073) in Urinary Tract Infections

G. MASCART,* L. MARCELIS, R. VANHOOF, P. MASCART, M. VANHAERVERBEECK, M. MARCHETTI, AND J. P. BUTZLER

I.M.C. Anderlecht, Edith Cavell Clinic, St. Pierre University Hospital, Brussels, Belgium

Cefonicid is a new broad-spectrum cephalosporin with special activity against *Enterobacter*, indole-positive *Proteus*, *Proteus mirabilis*, some strains of *Serratia*, and *Haemophilus influenzae* (1). This work presents the first clinical, bacteriological, and pharmacokinetic evaluation in patients with urinary tract infections.

Twenty-one patients were divided into two groups. One group (10 patients) received 0.5 g/day for 10 days, and the other group (11 patients) received 1.0 g/day for 7 days. In all cases the drug was given as a single daily intramuscular (i.m.) injection. Patients were not included in the study if there was: serum creatinine of >2 mg/100 ml, known allergy to beta-lactam antibiotics, simultaneous treatment with furosemide or ethacrinic acid, urinary tract catheter, or antibiotic therapy during the 3 days before starting cefonicid. There were 19 women and 2 men; their age range was from 53 to 91 years.

Diagnosis of urinary tract infection was made when two urine cultures were positive for the same strain (10^5 colony-forming units/ml). The susceptibility of the infecting pathogen to cefonicid was determined by the Kirby-Bauer method and by MIC, using the broth dilution method with Mueller-Hinton medium. Inoculum size for MIC was 10^5 colony-forming units/ml.

Safety tests were performed on days 0, 4, 7, and also on day 10 in those who received the drug for 10 days. Tests consisted of erythrocyte, leukocyte, and platelet counts, hemoglobin, PVC, urea, creatinine, transaminases, and urine microscopy. Urine culture was performed before, during, and at the end of treatment.

On the first and last days of treatment, serum levels were determined at 1, 2, 8, 12, and 24 h after the i.m. injection. Serum concentrations were determined by an agar well method, using *Bacillus subtilis* as the test organism. All samples were assayed at least in triplicate, and drug concentrations were calculated from the dose-response curve constructed from the standard solutions. The sensitivity of the assay was limited to 1 μg/ml, and its accuracy was in the range of ±5% as for any microbiological assay.

On day 1 of treatment, the mean peak blood levels were 61.6 μg/ml after 0.5 g and 94.7 μg/ml after 1 g. These concentrations were attained at 1.9 h after 0.5 g and at 2.2 h after 1 g. The mean peak serum levels on the last day was 73.7 and 135.6 μg/ml, respectively, after 0.5 and 1 g. These values were reached at 1.6 h after 0.5 g and at 1.8 h after 1 g.

Twenty-four hours after cefonicid injection, the mean serum concentration on the first day was 7.3 μg/ml after 0.5 g and 15.2 μg/ml after 1 g. On the last study day, the values after 24 h were 6.6 and 12.6 μg/ml, respectively, for 0.5 and 1 g.

A comparison of the results obtained by Pitkin et al. (2) in healthy volunteers receiving 1 g i.m. showed a mean peak serum level of 98.6 μg/ml in their volunteers versus 94.7 μg/ml in our patients. However, 24-h serum concentrations were higher in our patients (15.2 μg/ml versus 4.5 μg/ml), probably because of diminished excretory ability in this series of elderly patients. The mean elimination half-life was 4.5 h in volunteers versus 7.2 h in our patients. No important accumulation of the drug can therefore be expected in patients receiving cefonicid according to a once-daily dosing regimen.

Clinical and bacteriological data are summarized in Tables 1 and 2. The infecting pathogen was *Escherichia coli* in 19 cases and *Providencia* and *Klebsiella* in the remaining 2 cases.

The MIC measured in 20 cases was 1 μg or less 14 times, 2 to 4 μg in 5 cases, and 16 μg in 1 instance. Therapeutic success was obtained in 100% of the patients at the end of the treatment period; long-term follow-up was not available in this group of patients. Neither clinical nor laboratory side effects were noted in any of the patients. Ten patients complained on occasion of moderate local pain after the injection.

The results obtained in this limited series of patients indicate that cefonicid given at either

TABLE 1. *Results in patients receiving 0.5 g for 10 days*

No.	Sex	Age (yr)	Pathogen	Disk test (mm)	MIC (μg/ml)	Tolerance	Underlying condition
1	M	72	*Providencia*	36 (S)[a]	<0.5		Cerebrovascular accident, ischemic cardiopathy
2	F	76	*E. coli*	26 (S)	0.5		Latent diabetes, Parkinson's disease
3	F	91	*E. coli*	30 (S)	<0.5		Cancer of breast, Vaquez's disease
4	F	84	*E. coli*	—	<0.5	Pain at injection	Anemia, diverticulosis, Paget's disease
5	F	79	*E. coli*	35 (S)	0.5		Coronary insufficiency, chronic bronchitis
6	F	76	*E. coli*	20 (S)	2	Pain at injection	Diabetes, arthrosis, cardiac insufficiency, liver cirrhosis, hypothyroidism
7	F	74	*E. coli*	25 (S)	4		Cerebral sclerosis
8	F	87	*E. coli*	26 (S)	1	Pain at injection on day 7	Cerebral sclerosis, cataract
9	F	75	*E. coli*	21 (S)	4		Hypertension, cerebrovascular accident
10	F	76	*E. coli*	S	—	Pain at injection on day 7	Diabetes, polyneuritis

[a] S, Susceptible.

TABLE 2. *Results in patients receiving 1 g for 7 days*

No.	Sex	Age (yr)	Pathogen	AB (mm)	MIC (μg/ml)	Clinical response	Tolerance	Underlying condition
1	F	87	*E. coli*	25 (S)[a]	2			Diabetes, cerebrovascular accident
2	F	80	*E. coli*	19 (S)	0.5		Pain at injection day 2	Ischemic cardiopathy, liver stasis, Hbs carrier
3	F	77	*E. coli*	21 (S)	4			Chronic pyelonephritis, diabetes
4[b]	F	60	*E. coli*	22 (S)	16		Pain at injection	Cirrhosis
5	F	72	*E. coli*	33 (S)	<0.5	Dysuria on days 1–3	Pain at injection on day 6	Hypertension, arteritis, hypoparathyroidism, goiter, macrocytic anemia
6	F	63	*E. coli*	25 (S)	0.5		Pain at injection	Hypertension, angina pectoris, gastric ulcer, diabetes
7	F	74	*E. coli*	26 (S)	<0.5			Obesity
8	M	53	*E. coli*	38 (S)	<0.5			Pulmonary tuberculosis Gastritis
9	F	82	*E. coli*	32 (S)	<0.5			Ischemic cardiopathy, hypertension, diabetes
10	F	81	*Klebsiella*	27 (S)	<0.5		Pain at injection	Right mastectomy
11	F	72	*E. coli*	26 (S)	<0.5	Temp of 38.9°C on day 1	Pain at injection on days 3–7	Cerebrovascular accident, myocardial infarction

[a] S, Susceptible.
[b] Not included for calculation of the mean.

0.5 or 1 g once daily for up to 10 days achieves satisfactory microbiological and clinical results in uncomplicated urinary tract infections.

1. **Actor, P., J. V. Uri, I. Zajac, J. R. Guarini, C. S. Sachs, L. Phillips, D. A. Berges, G. L. Dunn, J. Hoover, and J. A. Weisbach.** 1976. Laboratory studies with SK&F 75073, a new parenteral cephalosporin with high serum levels. Program Abst. 16th Intersci. Conf. Antimicrob. Agents Chemother., Chicago, 27–29 October, abstr. no. 86.
2. **Pitkin, D. H., P. Actor, F. Alexander, J. Dubb, R. Stote, and J. A. Weisbach.** 1980. Cefonicid (SK&F 75073) serum levels and urinary recovery after intramuscular and intravenous administration, p. 252–254. *In* J. D. Nelson and C. Grassi (ed.), Current chemotherapy and infectious disease. American Society for microbiology, Washington, D.C.

Activity of Nine Cephalosporins Against *Nocardia asteroides*

F. MARTIN-LUENGO,* F. LOPEZ-AZORIN, AND M. BERNAL

Department of Microbiology, Faculty of Medicine, University of Murcia, Murcia, Spain

Nocardia asteroides is the species within the genus *Nocardia* that most frequently causes nocardiosis. Infections due to *Nocardia* are not uncommon; 500 to 1,000 new cases occur every year in the United States (2). Nocardiosis appears more frequently in patients receiving immunosuppressive therapy. The lung is the preferred site of infection, but any organ may be involved. Sulfonamides and streptomycin are the accepted drugs as chemotherapy for nocardiosis; nevertheless, an alternative therapy must be established when sulfonamide treatment fails or because of side effects with such a therapy.

Twenty-five strains of *Nocardia asteroides*

isolated from clinical samples that had been maintained by subculture in brain heart infusion agar were used in our study. All strains were identified as *Nocardia* by studying the nocardiomicolic acids and menaquinones by thin-layer chromatography. The identification of the species was made biochemically.

Nine drugs of the cephalosporin family (cefoperazone, cefotaxime, cefoxitin, cephaloridine, cephacetrile, cephalothin, cephradine, cefazolin, and moxalactam) were tested for their activity against *N. asteroides* strains. Appropriate dilutions of the drugs were added to melted diagnostic sensitivity test agar (Oxoid Ltd.) to give final concentrations ranging from 0.3 to 100 μg/ml.

The strains were inoculated in brain heart infusion broth medium, and the cultures were maintained with agitation for five days at 35°C. The cultures were then adjusted to a turbidity of 1 on the McFarland scale. This concentration was used as inoculum, and the inoculation was performed with a Steers replicator. The plates were incubated at 35°C for 7 days. The MIC of a drug was considered the lowest concentration that inhibited the growth of a strain. The appearance of few colonies, i.e., fewer than three, was considered as no growth.

Table 1 shows the cumulative percentage of strains inhibited at the different concentrations tested. Among the drugs studied, cefotaxime was the most active, inhibiting 65.3% of the strains at 25 μg/ml. At the same concentration, the other drugs showed less activity. Cephaloridine and moxalactam followed cefotaxime in activity, inhibiting 47.8 and 32% of the strains, respectively, at 25 μg/ml. Several papers have reported good in vitro activity of other drugs against *Nocardia;* i.e., minocycline and erythromicin (1), doxycycline, minocycline, and lincomycin (4), and amikacin (3).

TABLE 1. *Activity of nine cephalosporins against N. asteroides*[a]

Drugs	Concn (μg/ml)					
	3.1	6.2	12.5	25	50	100
Cefoperazone				4.5	13.6	36.3
Cephacetrile				11.5	26.9	38.4
Cefazolin		8	20	24	52	80
Moxalactam		8	24	32	64	92
Cephalothin	4	8	12	12	36	56
Cephradine	4.3	4.3	8.6	17.2	17.2	21.7
Cefoxitin	5.2	5.2	10.4	15.7	36.8	42.1
Cephaloridine	8.6	17.3	39.1	47.8	65.2	78.2
Cefotaxime	19.2	42.3	46.1	65.3	80.7	84.6

[a] Results are given as the cumulative percentage of strains inhibited. Lower concentrations tested (0.75 and 1.5 μg/ml) did not cause any inhibition.

Some authors have reported contradictory results on the in vitro susceptibility of *Nocardia* spp. to different drugs (1); however, the in vitro studies are necessary before chemotherapy can be started.

In vivo studies using an experimental model, as developed by Wallace et al. (5), may be helpful in establishing the drugs and combination chemotherapy most useful in treating infections caused by *Nocardia* spp.

1. **Bach, M. C., L. D. Sabath, and M. Finland.** 1973. Susceptibility of *Nocardia asteroides* to 45 antimicrobial agents in vitro. Antimicrob. Agents Chemother. **3:**1–8.
2. **Beaman, B. L., J. Burnside, and B. Edwards.** 1976. Nocardial infections in the United States 1972–1974. J. Infect. Dis. **134:**286–289.
3. **Dalovisio, J. R., and G. A. Pankey.** 1978. In vitro susceptibility of *Nocardia asteroides* to amikacin. Antimicrob. Agents Chemother. **13:**128–129.
4. **Lerner, P. I., and G. L. Baum.** Antimicrobial susceptibility of *Nocardia* species. Antimicrob. Agents Chemother. **4:**85–93.
5. **Wallace, R. J., E. J. Septimus, D. M. Musher, M. B. Berger, and R. R. Martin.** 1980. Treatment of experimental nocardiosis in mice: comparison of amikacin and sulfonamide. J. Infect. Dis. **140:**244–248.

Influence of In Vitro Methods on Phenotypic Expression of Bacterial Susceptibility to Cephalosporins

F. H. KAYSER,* FRANÇOISE HOMBERGER, AND GIOVANNA MORENZONI

Institute of Medical Microbiology of the University of Zürich, Zürich, Switzerland

Examination of the activity of cefoperazone against various ampicillin-resistant, gram-negative bacteria in agar dilution (3) and simultaneously in microbroth dilution tests (3) revealed that strains could be divided into three classes. Class I strains were organisms which were susceptible in agar as well as in microbroth dilution tests (MICs, ≤16 mg/liter). Class II strains were susceptible in agar dilution, but resistant in microbroth dilution procedures (MICs, ≥32mg/liter). Class III strains showed resistance in both test systems.

Among 100 randomly selected, Amp[r] *E. coli* strains freshly isolated from hospitalized patients, 51 belonged to class I, 48 belonged to class II, and 1 belonged to class III. Class III cultures were very rarely observed, not only in *Escherichia coli,* but also in other bacterial species (1).

The geometric means of the MICs of cephalosporins against 100 *E. coli* strains (Amp[r]) of classes I, II, and III are summarized in Table 1. It can be seen that cultures susceptible to cefoperazone in agar dilution but resistant in microbroth dilution (class II strains) showed a similar behavior also against cefamandole and cephalothin. The other cephalosporins, as well as moxalactam, were highly active against all of the strains examined.

Various strains containing R-plasmids which code for the production of TEM–beta-lactamase, cured derivatives of these strains, and transconjugants were examined for resistance to cefoperazone, cefamandole, and cephalothin. The results indicated that the resistance of strains to these drugs was plasmid mediated due to the production of TEM-beta-lactamase. Cefoperzone, cefamandole, and cephalothin are known to be rather unstable against this type of beta-lactamase (2). Figure 1 shows the events which occurred in a cefoperazone-containing culture of a class II strain. After a short lag phase, the number of viable cells of the culture decreased by 2 to 3 logs in 4 to 5 h of incubation. Thereafter, regrowth occurred and, after 24 h, the density of the culture equalled that of the control. Determination of cefoperazone during growth showed complete inactivation of the drug in the first 4 h.

To explain the differences in the phenotypic response to cefoperazone in strains of classes I, II, and III, the amount of beta-lactamase produced was measured in representative organisms. Cells were grown and harvested at the end of logarithmic growth and adjusted to an optical density equivalent to approximately 10^{10} colony-forming units per ml. Ten milliliters of the suspensions were exposed to short, controlled ultrasonic treatment. Samples were centrifuged, and supernatants were used as crude enzyme preparations. Enzymatic activity was measured with benzylpenicillin as a substrate at pH 5.9 and 30°C. Enzyme preparations of class I *E. coli* strains contained 38 to 40 nanocatals (ncat) and class II cultures 250 to 1,000 ncat of beta-lactamase activity in 10 ml of the suspensions. Two class III strains were examined. One, *Salmonella dublin* HK246, was found to contain 530 ncat, and the other, *Klebsiella pneumoniae* HK212, had 620 ncat of enzymatic activity.

TABLE 1. *MICs of ampicillin and cephalosporins against 100 Amp[r] E. coli strains*[a]

Antibiotic	Geometric mean of MICs (mg/liter) in class:					
	I		II		III	
	Agar	Broth	Agar	Broth	Agar	Broth
Ampicillin	229	308	501	572	>256	>256
Cefoperazone	0.48	1.5	0.9	182	32	>256
Cefamandole	2.0	3.4	2.2	54	64	>256
Cephalothin	16	29	9.6	40	64	>256
Cefoxitin	4.4	2.8	2.7	1.4	1	2
Cefuroxime	5.7	1.5	3.5	0.8	4	4
Cefotaxime	0.1	0.08	0.06	0.06	<0.1	<0.1
Ceftazidime	0.2	0.1	0.08	0.06	<0.1	<0.1
Ceftriaxone	0.09	0.08	0.06	0.06	<0.1	<0.1
Moxalactam	0.1	0.06	0.07	0.06	<0.1	<0.1

[a] MICs of antibiotics were determined in Mueller-Hinton agar or Mueller-Hinton broth (BBL Microbiology Systems) according to the procedure proposed by the National Committee for Clinical Laboratory Standards (NCCLS). In agar dilution tests, an inoculum of 10^4 cells per spot was used. In microbroth dilution, the inoculum was 5×10^5 cells per ml.

Transfer of R-plasmids from HK246 and HK212 to *E. coli* K-12 resulted in transconjugants which phenotypically were now class II strains. The transconjugants produced 430 and 960 ncat of beta-lactamase, respectively. Thus, the amount of beta-lactamase produced seems to be the cause of the different responses to cefoperazone in class I and class II cultures. The difference in phenotype between class II and III strains, however, is probably due to the different architecture of these organisms (beta-lactam binding sites and barrier function of the outer membrane), since cultures of both classes produced similar amounts of beta-lactamase.

Several class I, II, and III strains examined showed a significant inoculum effect. MICs of cefoperazone against *E. coli* K-12 (RP4), for instance, in microbroth dilution were >256, 32, and 2 mg/liter, using an inoculum of about 5×10^5, 5×10^4, or 5×10^3 cells per ml. In agar dilution, MICs were >256, 4, and 2 with an inoculum of 10^5, 10^4, or 10^3 cells per spot. Addition of the enzyme inhibitor CP 45899 in concentrations from 1 to 10 mg/liter reduced MICs of cefoperazone considerably (10 to 20 times against class III strains, 100 times and more against class II and class I cultures).

The results of this work indicate that about half of the Amp[r] *E. coli* strains were resistant to cefoperazone, cefamandole, and cephalothin in microbroth dilution, using an inoculum of about 5×10^5 cells per ml as proposed by the National Committee for Clinical Laboratory Standards (3). In some representative strains examined,

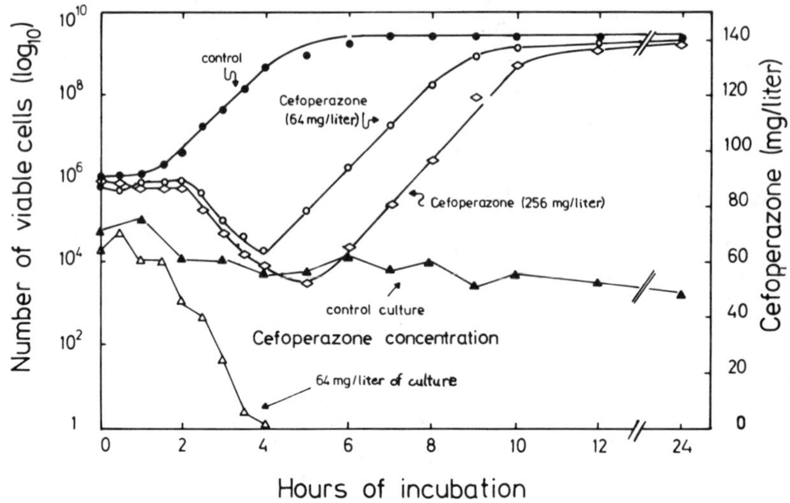

FIG. 1. *Growth of E. coli K-12 (RP4) in broth with and without cefoperazone and concentration of cefoperazone in cultures.*

resistance to cefoperazone was due to enzymatic destruction of the drug. By using an inoculum of $<10^5$ cells per ml in microbroth dilution or by using the standard agar dilution procedure, strains were susceptible. Rarely, strains were observed to be resistant in broth dilution with inocula of $<10^5$ cells per ml or in agar dilution. These strains probably owed their high-level resistance to production of beta-lactamase in concurrence with their cell envelope architecture. Addition of an enzyme inhibitor (CP 45899) to strains that produced TEM-beta-lactamase reduced the MICs of cefoperazone by about 10 to more than 100 times.

1. **Kayser, F. H.** 1980. Microbiological studies on cefoperazone. Clin. Therapeut. **3**:24–33.
2. **Mitsuhashi, S., S. Minami, N. Matsubara, A. Yotsuji, S. Kurashige, and I. Saikawa.** 1980. In vitro and in vivo antibacterial activity of cefoperazone. Clin. Therapeut. **3**:1–13.
3. **National Committee for Clinical Laboratory Standards.** 1980. Standard methods for dilution antimicrobial susceptibility tests for bacteria which grow aerobically. National Committee for Clinical Laboratory Standards proposed standard, PSM-7.

Antibacterial Effects of Cephalothin, Cefazolin, Cefuroxime, and Cefotaxime on Gentamicin-Resistant Bacteria

W. FEGELER* AND W. RITZERFELD

Hygiene-Institut der Westfälischen Wilhelms-Universität, Münster/W., Federal Republic of Germany

Gentamicin is one of the efficacious standard antibiotics, but nevertheless 2,444 bacterial strains were found to be gentamicin resistant by the agar diffusion method. This represents 13% of the 18,032 bacterial strains which were isolated from clinical specimens and tested in 1980. More than a quarter (27%) of the pathogens from the intensive care units were gentamicin resistant.

Among the gentamicin-resistant bacteria, 13% were gram-negative rods ($n = 316$) and 85% were gram-positive cocci ($n = 2,109$). The group of gram-negative rods consisted mainly of *Escherichia coli* (29%, $n = 91$), the *Klebsiella* group (16%, $n = 55$), the *Enterobacter* group (10%, $n = 31$), the *Pseudomonas* group (18%, $n = 58$), and *P. aeruginosa* (18%, $n = 56$). The main components of the gram-positive cocci were *Staphylococcus aureus* (39%, $n = 825$) and *Streptococcus faecalis* (37%, $n = 782$).

This report concerns investigations of the efficacies of cephalothin (CEP), cefazolin (CEZ), cefuroxime (CXM), and cefotaxime (CTX) against the gentamicin-resistant strains and a comparison of the efficacies of CTX, CEP, CEZ, and CXM against this group as well as all of the gentamicin-susceptible bacterial strains tested in 1980.

When the gentamicin-resistant gram-negative rods were tested with the individual cephalosporin antibiotics, an increase in activity of the latest cephalosporin groups was clearly seen. For example, the percentage of *E. coli* strains susceptible was 41% with CEZ, 68% with CXM, and 91% with CTX; for the *Klebsiella-Enterobacter* group susceptibility was 9% with CEZ, 43% with CXM, and 71% with CTX, and for the genus *Pseudomonas* it was 1% with CEZ, 21% with CXM, and 49% with CTX.

Against *S. aureus,* exactly the opposite result was found. CEP was most efficacious; 79% of the isolates were susceptible to CEP and 63% were susceptible to CTX. The susceptibility of the enterococci was 60% with CEP and 41% with CTX.

Even with these percentages in hand, a comparison of the cephalosporins is not possible. This becomes clear when the following facts are considered. In testing for resistance, between 16 and 24 different antibiotics were used in one and the same test. The results showed a specific "resistance pattern." A comparison between antibiotics can be made only inside this resistance pattern because only here are conditions exactly the same.

In 1980 CEZ was tested against only 78 enterococci, the result being that 29 (37%) were susceptible, whereas the test of CTX showed 1,242 susceptible enterococci in 2,408 strains investigated, i.e., 51%. The comparison between CEZ and CTX was limited to only 78 strains of enterococci. The result was that CEZ, as well as CTX, was active in 5 of 78 cases (6%), when the antibiotic of comparison was inactive.

We next compared CEP, CEZ, and CXM with CTX because the antibacterial activity of CTX comes closest to that of gentamicin. When comparing the efficacies of two antibiotics, there will be a combination in which the bacteria are resistant to one of the antibiotics whereas they are susceptible to the other and vice versa.

Table 1 shows the comparison between CTX and CEP. Against *S. aureus*, CEP was active on 13% (n = 105) of the CTX-resistant organisms of the gentamicin-resistant group. In this group only a 1% CTX susceptibility of the CEP-resistant bacteria could be found. Against the enterococci CEP had a 20% activity, whereas that of CTX was only 2%. Against the group of gentamicin-susceptible strains, the activities of both cephalosporins, CEP and CTX, were very similar. The 13% of the gentamicin-resistant group can be explained by the higher activity of CEP against primary susceptible staphylococci.

Though the classification of the gentamicin-resistant gram-negative rods showed that the largest group was that of *E. coli* with a frequency of 91 strains and the smallest was that of the *Enterobacter* group with 31 strains, an attempt will be made to offer the data in percentages to make a better comparison possible (Table 2).

TABLE 1. *Comparison of CTX with CEP*

Susceptibility[a]		Percentage of strains			
		S. aureus		*S. faecalis*	
		G-R[b] (818)	G-S (4,360)	G-R (777)	G-S (1,619)
CTX	CEP				
ϕ	+	13	1	20	18
+	ϕ	1	1	2	2

[a] ϕ, Resistant; +, susceptible.
[b] G-R, Gentamicin resistant; G-S, gentamicin susceptible. The number of strains tested is shown in parentheses.

TABLE 2. *Comparison of CTX with CEZ and CXM*

Susceptibility[a]		Percentage of strains									
		E. coli		*Klebsiella* group		*Enterobacter* group		*Pseudomonas* group		*P. aeruginosa*	
		G-R (89)	G-S (4,814)	G-R (51)	G-S (615)	G-R (31)	G-S (410)	G-R (58)	G-S (332)	G-R (56)	G-S (1,480)
CTX	CEZ										
ϕ	+	2	<1	0	<1	0	1	0	1	2	<1
+	ϕ	39	13	55	19	48	38	40	51	54	65
CTX	CXM										
ϕ	+	2	<1	0	<1	0	<1	2	<1	4	<1
+	ϕ	19	7	14	8	19	17	10	48	46	64

[a] ϕ, Resistant; +, susceptible.
[b] G-R, Gentamicin resistant; G-S, gentamicin susceptible. The number of strains tested is shown in parentheses.

In the CTX/CEZ comparison the different antibacterial activity is made clear by the increase of the susceptible proportion in the gentamicin-susceptible strains. The susceptibility of *E. coli* was 13% and that of *P. aeruginosa* was 65%. In the gentamicin-resistant group the superiority of CTX was made evident by the high percentages of susceptible strains among CEZ-resistant bacteria. The lowest susceptibility was that of *E. coli* (40%) and the highest was that of the *Klebsiella* group (55%). Only twice in *E. coli* and once in *P. aeruginosa* was a CTX-resistant strain susceptible to CEZ.

The proportions of CXM-susceptible strains were small in the CTX-resistant bacteria of the gentamicin-resistant group. The highest percentage was 4% in *P. aeruginosa*. If there was CXM resistance, there was the following percentage of CTX susceptibility for the individual species; 19% for *E. coli*, 14% for the *Klebsiella* group, 19% for the *Enterobacter* group, 10% for the *Pseudomonas* group, and 46% for *P. aeruginosa*. The distribution of the CTX activity in gentamicin-resistant strains was very similar to that with susceptible strains except that 48% of the *Pseudomonas* group were susceptible. This can be explained as a specific part of the antibacterial activity of CTX.

Summing up, we found that *S. aureus* and enterococci were most susceptible to CEP. For gram-negative rods CTX proved to be the most efficacious cephalosporin. Furthermore, the above results show that the new antibiotics cannot be considered a substitute for the other antibiotics but rather as an enrichment of the therapeutic possibilities.

Method for Assessing Timed Bacteriostatic and Bactericidal Activities of Cephalothin

GOHTA MASUDA,* MASAYOSHI NEGISHI, HAJIME YAMAGATA, MIEKO KASEDA, AND SHIGENORI TAMAGAWA

Department of Infectious Diseases and Clinical Laboratory Department, Tokyo Metropolitan Komagome Hospital, 3-18-22 Honkomagome, Bunkyo-ku, Tokyo 113, Japan*

The in vitro activity of antimicrobial agents is often expressed today in terms of MIC or minimum lethal concentration (MLC). To determine these concentrations, prolonged exposure (usually 18 to 24 h) of microbes to drug(s) is required. Such prolonged exposure is, however, not usual in clinical medicine. If antimicrobial drugs are administered parenterally as in many clinical situations, they will produce in serum or at the focus of infection antimicrobic concentrations exceeding the MIC or MLC for several hours at the most. Variation of exposure time will give apparently discrepant results when one attempts to analyze the correlation between in vitro antimicrobial susceptibility data and clinical results. On the basis of this, a method for assessing timed bacteriostatic and bactericidal activities of an antibiotic, cephalothin, has been developed.

Figure 1 gives the schematic presentation of, potentially, the maximum number of colony-forming units (CFU) surviving after exposure to various antimicrobial activities of a drug. The theoretical bacteriostatic concentration is also illustrated. As the MIC is currently defined as the lowest drug concentration producing no turbidity of broth after overnight incubation of microbes with antimicrobial agents, there remains the possibility that the CFU could, in some instances, slowly multiply in the presence of the drug with concentrations lower than its bacteriostatic concentration. Such a minimal increase of CFU would often fail to produce visible turbidity, and the drug concentration is therefore apt to be interpreted as "inhibitory." Minimally reducing concentration (MRC) is, on the other hand, defined as the minimum concentration producing minimal reduction of CFU—another approximation to the theoretical bacteriostatic concentration as well as the MIC.

To assess the MRC, we prepared small test tube series containing 1 ml of heart infusion broth (Difco Laboratories) and twofold dilutions of cephalothin. Each tube was inoculated with CFU adjusted to contain $n \times 10^6$ (n = a few to 30 at most) per ml of broth (referred to as "standardized suspension") (4). After incubation of these tubes at 35°C for a certain number of hours, a 0.001-ml sample was removed from each tube and placed in 1 ml of phosphate buffer solution. After blending on a Vortex mixer to obtain uniform suspension of CFU, a 0.001-ml sample from the phosphate buffer suspension was transferred onto agar plates (numbers of

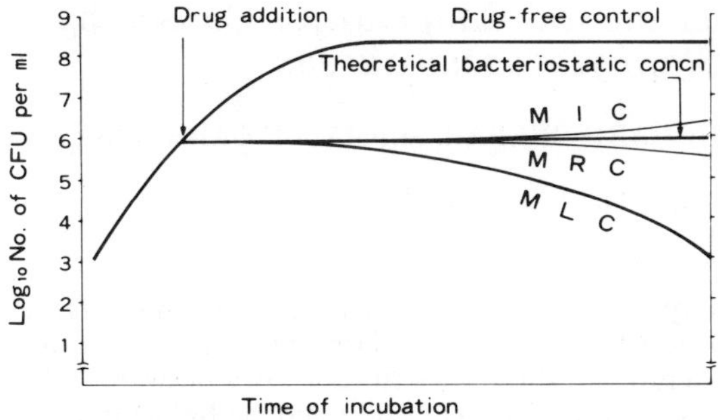

FIG. 1. *Schematic presentation of the potentially maximal number of CFU surviving after exposure to indicated antimicrobial activities (MIC, MRC, and MLC) of a drug. Theoretical bacteriostatic concentration is also illustrated.*

CFU should be n per inoculation spot if no change in numbers occurred during incubation of the standardized suspension). These plates were incubated at 35°C overnight. The minimum drug concentration yielding $n/2$ colonies on the plates, indicating the concentration producing minimal reduction of CFU numbers, was designated as the MRC. Determinations were made on the test tubes at time intervals of 6, 18, and 42 h of exposure to cephalothin and designated as 6-h, 18-h and 42-h MRCs, respectively. The MLC, defined as the lowest concentration producing a 99.9% reduction of CFU numbers (1), was also determined at time intervals of 6, 18, and 42 h of exposure and designated as 6-h, 18-h, and 42-h MLCs, respectively.

The timed bacteriostatic concentration with brief exposure (6-h MRC) to cephalothin for *Escherichia coli* and *Klebsiella* spp. was generally two to four times lower than the MIC. These results are in accord with the data on *Staphylococcus aureus* reported by Lindberg et al. (3). We failed to obtain, however, such a low 6-h MRC value for our strains of *S. aureus* and *Enterococcus*. Table 1 shows the comparative ratios of bacteriostatic to bactericidal concentrations with various times of exposure of bacteria to cephalothin. If the mode of action of this drug is categorized as bactericidal when the ratio is low (4 or less) and bacteriostatic when high (8 or more) (2), then cephalothin is bactericidal to 33 and bacteriostatic to 3 of the 36 strains of *E. coli* with the ratio of 6-h MLC/6-h MRC used as the measure. The drug appeared to be bactericidal to all these strains when the ratio was made up of longer (18-h MLC/18-h MRC, 42-h MLC/42-h MRC, and 18-h MLC/MIC) exposure times. The result with 27 strains of *Klebsiella* spp. was similar to that with *E. coli*. Cephalothin was bacteriostatic to a large number of strains of *S. aureus* and *Enterococcus*, especially when organisms were exposed to the drug over a brief period of time. The study of *Enterococcus* with an exposure time of 6 h revealed, in particular, that the drug is bacteriostatic to all the strains except for those two showing 6-h MLC and 6-h MRC exceeding 12,800 μg/ml of cephalothin.

TABLE 1. *Comparison of bacteriostatic with bactericidal concentrations of cephalothin for E. coli, Klebsiella spp., S. aureus, and Enterococcus*

Bacteria (no. of strains)	Type of comparison	Ratio			
		1	2	4	8≦
E. coli (36)	6-h MLC/ 6-h MRC	13	12	8	3
	18-h MLC/18-h MRC	33	3		
	42-h MLC/42-h MRC	33	3		
	18-h MLC/MIC	27	8	1	
Klebsiella spp. (27)	6-h MLC/ 6-h MRC	3	5	11	8
	18-h MLC/18-h MRC	22	5		
	42-h MLC/42-h MRC	22	5		
	18-h MLC/MIC	21	4	2	
S. aureus (27)	6-h MLC/ 6-h MRC	2	6	3	16
	18-h MLC/18-h MRC	14	11	1	1
	42-h MLC/42-h MRC	20	6	1	
	18-h MLC/MIC	11	11	3	2
Enterococcus (54)	6-h MLC/ 6-h MRC				52[a]
	18-h MLC/18-h MRC	9	6	10	29
	42-h MLC/42-h MRC	21	19	4	10
	18-h MLC/MIC	2	12	8	32

[a] Of 54 strains of *Enterococcus* tested, two strains with 6-h MRC and 6-h MLC values exceeding 12,800 μg of cephalothin per ml were excluded from the tally.

As presented, the mode of activity in vitro varies significantly with the time of exposure to cephalothin and the bacteria tested. These data would be of significance in the deductive analysis of in vitro antimicrobial susceptibility data and effectiveness in clinical medicine.

1. **Anhalt, J. P., L. D. Sabath, and A. L. Barry.** 1980. Special tests: bactericidal activity, activity of antimicrobics in combination, and detection of β-lactamase production, p. 478–484. In E. H. Lennette, A. Balows, W. J. Hausler, and J. P. Truant (ed.), Manual of clinical microbiology, 3rd ed. American Society for Microbiology, Washington, D.C.
2. **Fuchs, P. C., C. Thornsberry, A. L. Barry, T. L. Gavan, E. H. Gerlach, and R. N. Jones.** 1977. Ticarcillin, carbenicillin and BL-P1908: in vitro comparison of three anti-pseudomonal semisynthetic penicillins. J. Antibiot. **30:**1098–1106.
3. **Lindberg, D. A. B., and G. T. Stewart.** 1966. Exercises in the logistics of chemotherapy, p. 168–176. Antimicrob. Agents Chemother. 1965.
4. **Masuda, G., T. Yajima, K. Nakamura, T. Yanagishita, and H. Hayashi.** 1979. Comparative bactericidal activities of beta-lactam antibiotics determined in agar and broth media. J. Antibiot. **32:**1168–1173.

Cefazolin Versus Cephalothin in Experimental Endocarditis Caused by β-Lactamase–Producing *Staphylococcus aureus*

KENNETH M. KAYE,* WILLIAM D. KOBASA, RICHARD SNEPAR, AND JAIME CARRIZOSA

The Medical College of Pennsylvania, Philadelphia, Pennsylvania 19129, U.S.A.

The effectiveness of cefazolin and cephalothin was compared in endocarditis in rabbits produced by two strains of β-lactamase–producing *Staphylococcus aureus*. The MICs for both strains were 0.8 μg/ml of cefazolin and 0.4 μg/ml of cephalothin. In vitro inactivation studies indicated that strain 1 inactivated 50% of the cefazolin present in 2 h and strain 2 inactivated 50% in 3 h at 37°C. In contrast, over 50% of cephalothin remained even after 24 h.

Rabbits were anesthetized, and the right carotid artery was cannulated. One day later, each rabbit was inoculated by ear vein with 10^7 *S. aureus* strain 1 or 2 organisms. Inoculated control animals were left untreated. In treatment groups, antibiotic therapy was begun 24 h after infection; the regimens were cefazolin, 15 mg/kg, and cephalothin, 70 mg/kg, given every 6 h intramuscularly.

After 4 days of therapy, following a period of 12 h without treatment, the surviving rabbits were killed. All aortic valve vegetations from each rabbit were excised and pooled, and the number of *S. aureus* cells per gram was determined. The catheter was left in place throughout the experiment.

Serum bactericidal activity was determined by diluting serum in twofold steps in tubes containing normal rabbit serum. The maximal bactericidal dilution was the highest dilution of serum in normal rabbit serum that resulted in a 10,000-fold decrease or 99.99% kill in 48 h of incubation.

Rabbits were inoculated with *S. aureus* strain 1. After 24 h, 10% had died. The remaining rabbits were divided into three groups of 18 to 20, one untreated, one cefazolin treated, and one cephalothin treated. The subsequent mortality of untreated controls was 50% at 1 day, 83% at 2 days, 89% at 3 days, and 94% at 4 days. The mortality in cefazolin-treated rabbits was 15% at 1 day and 20% at 2, 3, and 4 days of treatment. The mortality in the cephalothin-treated rabbits was 22, 44, 44, and 55%. All rabbits that died had infected vegetations.

Cefazolin and cephalothin protected against mortality. P values for cefazolin versus controls were $P < 0.05$ on day 1 and $P < 0.01$ on days 2, 3, and 4 after initiation of therapy. P values for cephalothin versus controls were $P > 0.05$ on day 1 and $P < 0.05$ on days 2, 3, and 4 after initiation of therapy. However, there was no significant difference in mortality between rabbits treated with cefazolin and cephalothin.

Similar results were observed with strain 2. Rabbits were inoculated with *S. aureus* strain 2. After 24 h, 15% had died. The remaining rabbits were divided into three groups of 20 to 24: one untreated, one cefazolin treated, and one cephalothin treated. The subsequent mortality of untreated controls was 40% at 1 day, 75% at 2 days, and 95% at 3 and 4 days. The mortality in cefazolin-treated rabbits was 19% at 1 day, 29% at 2 days, and 43% at 3 and 4 days of treatment. The mortality in the cephalothin-treated rabbits was 38, 41, 50, and 50%. All rabbits that died had infected vegetations.

Cefazolin and cephalothin protected against mortality ($P > 0.05$ for cefazolin versus controls on day 1 and $P < 0.01$ on days 2, 3, and 4 after initiation of therapy; $P > 0.05$ for cephalothin versus controls on days 1 and 2 and $P < 0.01$ on days 3 and 4 after initiation of therapy). However, there was no significant difference in mortality between rabbits treated with cefazolin and cephalothin.

The mean $\log_{10}$ of *S. aureus* strain 1 per gram of vegetation in surviving rabbits was 5.2 for rabbits treated with cefazolin, with 25% sterile, and 3.3 for rabbits treated with cephalothin, with 38% sterile. The mean log colony-forming units of *S. aureus* strain 2 was 8.4 for rabbits treated with cefazolin, with 9% sterile, and 6.9 for rabbits treated with cephalothin, with none sterile. The results for cefazolin versus cephalothin were not significantly different.

After the first injection of antibiotic, mean cefazolin levels were about 93, 81, 58, and 7 μg/ml at 15, 30, 60, and 120 min. Mean cephalothin levels were about 130, 103, 39 and 14 μg/ml. The serum half-life was 0.45 and 0.53 h for cefazolin and cephalothin, respectively.

The median maximal bactericidal dilutions for cefazolin in rabbits infected with strain 1 were 1:64, 1:16 to 1:32, 1:16, and 1:4 to 1:8 at 15, 30, 60, and 120 min. The median maximal bactericidal dilutions for cephalothin were >1:64, >1:64, 1:32, and 1:16. The median maximal bactericidal dilutions for cefazolin in rabbits infected with strain 2 were 1:32, 1:16 to 1:32, 1:16, and 1:8. In those treated with cephalothin the median maximal bactericidal dilutions were 1:16 to 1:32, 1: 64, 1:32, and 1:16.

Although with both of these β-lactamase–producing strains the mortality rate was higher in animals treated with cephalothin than in those treated with cefazolin, these differences were not significant. In a previous study from our laboratory, similar results were reported with strain 1 (1). In contrast, Goldman and Petersdorf (2) reported that cefazolin was significantly less effective than cephalothin in preventing deaths from strain 2. They attributed the lesser effectiveness of cefazolin to its β-lactamase sensitivity. They explained the difference between the two studies by the fact that in our studies the serum levels of cefazolin were much higher than those of cephalothin. To test this hypothesis, in the present study the same doses were used as in Goldman and Petersdorf's study, in which equivalent levels were achieved with cefazolin and cephalothin. However, in contrast to their study, no significant differences were found in mortality rate with either strain. In fact, although not significant, the mortality rate was higher in cephalothin-treated rabbits with both strains.

In the present study the titers of *S. aureus* in vegetations of rabbits sacrified after 4 days of treatment were higher in cefazolin-treated animals than in cephalothin-treated rabbits for both strains, but the differences were not significant. The serum half-life of cefazolin in rabbits is about 30 min, and the half-life of cefazolin mixed with β-lactamase in vitro is 2 to 3 h. Considering that the rate of excretion of cefazolin is much more rapid than the rate of inactivation, it is not surprising that the slow rate of inactivation does not interfere with the effectiveness of cefazolin in *S. aureus* endocarditis.

1. **Carrizosa, J., J. Santoro, and D. Kaye.** 1978. Treatment of experimental *Staphylococcus aureus* endocarditis: comparison of cephalothin, cefazolin, and methicillin. Antimicrob. Agents Chemother. **13**:74–77.
2. **Goldman, P. L., and R. G. Petersdorf.** 1980. Importance of β-lactamase inactivation in treatment of experimental endocarditis caused by *Staphylococcus aureus*. J. Infect. Dis. **141**:331–337.

Comparative Evaluation of Cefamandole and Carbenicillin in Gunshot and Stab Wounds of the Abdomen

SISTER MARY ANN LOU,* HUM DAC BUI, ASHIS K. MANDAL, THEODORE L. SCHLATER, AND HARAGOPAL THADEPALLI

Divisions of General Surgery and Infectious Disease, Martin Luther King Jr. General Hospital and Charles R. Drew Postgraduate Medical School, Los Angeles, California 90059, U.S.A.*

In our previous studies of penetrating abdominal injuries, we reported the efficacy of preoperative administration of intravenous antibiotics in lowering the incidence of intraabdominal sepsis and wound infections (2, 3). In search of a single antibiotic that will be effective in controlling aerobic and anaerobic contaminants from the gastrointestinal tract, we have found carbenicillin to be equally as effective as the combination of clindamycin and gentamicin (1). A newer cephalosporin, cefamandole nafate, has shown superior in vitro activity against a wide range of gram-negative and gram-positive aerobes as well as anaerobes, and in high doses it can even inhibit 75% of *Bacteroides fragilis* isolates (1), although not *Pseudomonas*. This prospective, randomized, open-label study was undertaken to evaluate the in vitro activity of cefamandole and compare its effectiveness with that of carbenicillin as control in preventing infectious complications following gunshot and stab wounds of the abdomen.

Forty-one patients admitted with gunshot or stab wound to the abdomen were randomized into group I and group II (Table 1). Group I received carbenicillin, 6 g every 6 h. Group II received cefamandole, 2 g intravenously every 6 h. All received antibiotics as soon as possible in the emergency room, approximately 0.5 to 4 h before laparotomy. If gastrointestinal injury was found, the antibiotic was continued for a minimum of 5 days. If no gastrointestinal injury was found, it was discontinued after 72 h. No other antibiotic was added unless clinical course and culture report indicated the need for change.

Aerobic and anaerobic cultures were taken from peritoneal fluid upon entering the colonic cavity and from fascia and subcutaneous tissue upon closing. Follow-up cultures of blood and fluid from surgical drains were taken on the third postoperative day. Additional cultures were done as indicated.

The two groups were well matched in sex, age, race, and extent of injury. None of the 41 pa-

TABLE 1. *Patient characteristics*

Characteristic	Carbenicillin	Cefamandole
No. of patients	20	21
Age (avg)	18–37 (26.7) yr	18–39 (26.9) yr
Sex	19 male, 1 female	19 male, 2 female
Race	14 black, 6 hispanic	18 black, 2 hispanic, 1 white
Gunshot	18	13
Stab	2	8
Colon injury	6	6
Upper gastrointestinal	10	12
Solid organ injury	10	10

tients died. Only 1 patient in the cefamandole group developed a subhepatic abscess. This was attributed to faulty surgical technique of using too many large hemostatic metal clips, causing focal necrosis of the liver and secondary infection. One patient in the carbenicillin group developed septic shock following cervical laminectomy, unrelated to his recovery from laparotomy.

Four patients had negative laparotomies, two had gunshot wounds (one carbenicillin, one cefamandole), two had stab wounds (one carbenicillin, one cefamandole). The most common solid organ injury was the liver, and the most common hollow viscus injured was the small bowel. The average number of organs injured was 1.6 per patient in group I and 1.5 in group II.

Bacteriological study of the peritoneal fluid and surgical incision at laparotomy grew a variety of organisms, mostly gram-negative aerobes with a few anaerobes (Table 2). None of these patients developed clinical infection. Among the 24 of 41 patients (58%) who had negative cultures, 11 of 20 patients (55%) were in the carbenicillin group and 14 of 21 (67%) were in the cefamandole group, indicating the effectiveness of the preoperative antibiotic therapy.

Each group had six patients with colon injuries comparatively managed according to a separate colon injury protocol. Neither group had septic complications. The total number of febrile days over 101°F (38.3°C) was 12 days in group I and 13 days in group II. The average hospital stay was 11.4 days for group I and 9.2 days for group II.

TABLE 2. *Bacteriology at laparotomy*

Organism	Group	
	Carbenicillin	Cefamandole
Peritoneal		
Peptostreptococcus		1
Ruminicola		1
Bacteroides		2
Staphylococcus epidermidis	2	3
Alpha- and beta-hemolytic streptococci	3	
Enterococcus	*1*	
Escherichia coli	4	1
Proteus spp.	2	
Enterobacter		1
Klebsiella		1
Citrobacter	1	
Fascia		
Alpha-hemolytic *Streptococcus*	1	
E. coli	2	
S. epidermidis		3
S. aureus		1
Pseudomonas		1

Although we intend to extend this study to a larger group of patients, the initial data indicated that a single drug, cefamandole or carbenicillin, can effectively prevent postoperative infections associated with abdominal trauma. Routine addition of aminoglycoside therapy is not necessary. Antibiotic therapy should begin before surgery and should cover the endogenous aerobes and anaerobes of the gastrointestinal tract. Sound surgical technique is equally important.

1. **Bach, V., and H. Thadepalli.** 1980. Susceptibility of anaerobic bacteria in vitro to 23 antimicrobial agents. Chemotherapy (Basel) **26:**344–353.
2. **O'Donnell, V., M. A. Lou, J. L. Alexander, and A. K. Mandal.** 1978. Role of antibiotics in penetrating abdominal trauma. Am. Surg. **44:**574–577.
3. **O'Donnell, V., A. K. Mandal, M. A. Lou, and H. Thadepalli.** 1978. Evaluation of carbenicillin as a single antibiotic in the prevention of infections following abdominal trauma, p. ii. *In* W. Siegenthaler and R. Lathy (ed.), Current chemotherapy. American Society for Microbiology, Washington, D.C.
4. **O'Donnell, V., A. K. Mandal, M. A. Lou, and H. Thadepalli.** 1979. Evaluation of carbenicillin and a comparison of clindamycin and gentamycin combined therapy in penetrating abdominal trauma. Surg. Obstet. Gynecol **147:**525–528.

Cephalexin: Twice-Daily Dosage in Children

ANDREW K. BROWNING

Glaxo Group Research Ltd., Greenford, Middlesex, U.K.

The total daily dose of cephalexin is usually taken in three or four divided doses. Frequency of administration is known to be a factor contributing to noncompliance with drug regimens, and reducing the number of doses per day is one way in which compliance may be improved. The aim of the study reported here was to compare the efficacy and tolerance of cephalexin (Ceporex) in two groups of children randomly allocated to receive their total daily dose in two or four divided doses. The multicenter study involved 14 general practitioners in the United Kingdom. The patients were all aged 16 years or under and had a respiratory or soft tissue infection. Depending on their age and the severity of infection, the children were given a total daily dose of 500 mg, 1 g, or 2 g of cephalexin, as a syrup, in two or four divided doses according to a randomization code. The study was single blind; the physicians selected the appropriate total daily dose but were unaware of the dosage regimen for each patient. Treatment was for 5 days initially, with clinical assessments after 48 h (day 3) and at the end of the 5-day course (day 6). The physicians had the option of continuing therapy for a further 5 days (total of 10 days) if considered necessary at the second assessment. Patients who received 10 days' treatment were reassessed at the end of the therapeutic course (day 11). All patients with a beta-hemolytic streptococcal throat infection were treated for 10 days, even if clinically well at the second assessment, for consistency with medical recommendations.

A total of 533 patients were included in the study, 262 given two doses per day (group A) and 271 given four doses per day (group B). The patients were well matched for sex, severity of infection, and clinical history. Twenty-four patients had been treated unsuccessfully with other antibacterial therapy (mainly penicillin V, ampicillin, or erythromycin) during the week before entering this trial. The groups were again well matched for age with median ages as follows: 500 mg/day, 3.0 years (group A) and 3.0 years (group B); 1 g/day, 6.5 years (group A) and 6.0 years (group B); 2 g/day, 13.0 years (group A) and 12.5 years (group B). The majority of patients (158 in group A and 183 in group B) had upper respiratory infections, mainly tonsillitis (50%) and otitis media (30%). One hundred and fifty-four (84 in group A and 70 in group B) had lower respiratory infections, mainly acute bronchitis (76%), and there were 38 soft tissue infections (20 in group A and 18 in group B).

The clinical response after 48 h of treatment (Table 1) indicated 50% (group A) and 52% (group B) much improved at this stage (i.e., marked improvement in symptoms and signs compared with the pretreatment assessment). There was no statistically significant difference between the two groups at this assessment (chi squared = 3.953 with 2 df). Sixteen patients were withdrawn at this assessment, seven due to inadequate response, seven due to side effects, and two for other reasons. The remainder continued therapy and were assessed again on day 6. The clinical response at this second assessment (Table 2) indicated 89% of the patients in each group cured or improved considerably (i.e., complete remission or considerable improvement in symptoms and signs). Another four patients were withdrawn at this assessment due to side effects, and four were withdrawn for other reasons. The largest group of patients comprised the upper respiratory infections. In this group, twice-daily dosage was as effective as four doses per day, with 140 of 154 (91%) in group A cured or improved considerably compared with 163 of 177 (92%) in group B. Similarly, the success rate on day 6 in the lower respiratory tract infections was 91% in both groups. The number of patients with soft tissue infections was much lower, but all were cured or considerably improved after 5

TABLE 1. *Clinical response after 48 h of treatment*

Response	Two doses/day (group A)	Four doses/day (group B)
Much better	130 (50%)	141 (52%)
Slightly better	98	109
No better or worse	34	21

TABLE 2. *Clinical response after 5 days of treatment*

Response	Two doses/day (group A)	Four doses/day (group B)
Success or considerable improvement	233 (89%)	240 (89%)
Slight improvement	19	18
Failure	4	10
Withdrawn for reason other than inadequate response	6	3

days of treatment except two, in group B, who had improved slightly. A total of 110 patients (56 in group A and 54 in group B) continued for a further 5 days, but this included 35 with a beta-hemolytic streptococcal throat infection given 10 days of therapy in accordance with the protocol. Of the 110 patients, only 3 were not cured or considerably improved at the end of treatment.

There was a total of 32 (6%) side effects, considered by the physicians to be drug related, reported at one or other of the assessments. They were mainly gastrointestinal disturbances, and most were transient. Only 9 of the 24 side effects present on day 3 were also present on day 6, and none reported at the first or second assessment was present on day 11. In the 18 patients who were hypersensitive to penicillin, a rash occured in only 1 patient during therapy.

The results show that the daily dose of cephalexin is effective when given in two divided doses, with results equivalent to those obtained with four doses a day with the same total daily dose. Twice-daily dosage is more convenient to the patient and should aid patient compliance.

Pharmacokinetics of Cefoxitin Given by Intravenous Infusion in Patients with Pleural Effusion

A. DOMINGUEZ-GIL, M. J. GARCIA, M. BARRUECO, AND M. J. OTERO*

Practical Pharmacy Department and Medical Pathology Department, University of Salamanca, Salamanca, Spain*

The serum levels reached by antibiotics during treatment are of great use in clinical practice with respect to their efficiency and safety. Various studies have shown the organism to be a multicompartmental system where the incorporation and presence of drugs in different organs and tissues follows individualized kinetic processes which are frequently different from those taking place in the systemic circulation (3, 4). The penetration of antibiotics and chemotherapeutic agents into various tissues should therefore become a criterion for selection in antiinfective therapy. The levels reached by antibiotics in the pleural fluid are of great interest in the treament of infectious processes localized in this place.

The pharmacokinetics of cefoxitin were studied in six healthy volunteers (63 to 74 years old) and five patients with pleural effusion (54 to 69 years old). The dose administered was 30 mg/kg by intravenous (i.v.) perfusion lasting 2 h. Samples of blood and pleural fluid were withdrawn at previously programmed times, the latter being obtained through a permanently fixed catheter. Serum and pleural fluid levels of cefoxitin were determined by a microbiological plate diffusion method, using *Bacillus subtilis* (ATCC 6633) as the test organism. Standard curves of pooled human serum and pleural fluid were prepared with a concentration range of 100 to 5 μg/ml. Repeated analyses of the reference standards showed the variation coefficient of the technique to be less than 5%, and the lowest limit of susceptibility was shown to be 2 μg/ml.

The antibiotic followed a two-compartment open kinetic model, according to the MAICE test (5). The pharmacokinetic parameters corresponding to the model were established from the concentration reached by the antibiotic in both fluids, using a programmable Hewlett-Packard 97 calculator (2).

In healthy volunteers, the antibiotic reached a maximum serum concentration of 102.54 μg/ml, falling to 4 μg/ml 6 h after administration. Figure 1 shows the average concentration curves of cefoxitin in serum and pleural fluid after i.v. perfusion. At the end of the perfusion, the serum cefoxitin level had an average value of 90.44 μg/ml, which fell to 7 μg/ml 6 h after beginning administration. The antibiotic was incorporated into the pleural fluid, where it reached a maximum concentration of 17.01 μg/ml, similar to that established when the same dose of cefoxitin is given by bolus administration (C_{max} = 19.73 μg/ml) (1). The amount of cefoxitin which reached the pleural fluid represented an average value of 2.42% of the dose administered and was conditioned in each case by the volume of pleural fluid obtained by needle aspiration.

Table 1 shows the pharmacokinetic parameters of cefoxitin established in the group of patients. The half-life of the slow disposition phase had an average value of 1.54 h. This value, greater than that described in the literature, is attributable to the slight degree of renal impairment which some of the patients in the survey were suffering from. The incorporation of cefoxitin into the pleural fluid followed first-order

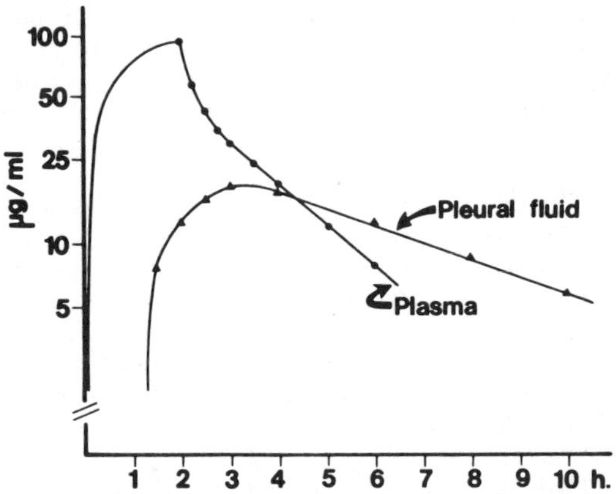

FIG. 1. *Average plasma (●) and pleural fluid (▲) levels of the antibiotic established in the five patients included in the survey.*

kinetics defined by the constant K_i, which had an average value of 1.37 h^{-1}. The incorporation rate into the pleural fluid was conditioned by the administration route used, the bolus i.v. type being faster than i.v. perfusion. The disappearance of the antibiotic from the pleural fluid was defined by the constant K_d, whose average value was 0.18 h^{-1}, corresponding to a half-life ($t_{1/2d}$) of 3.85 h. As a consequence, the elimination rate of cefoxitin from the pleural fluid was less ($P < 0.005$) than the elimination rate from serum.

On establishing a multiple-dosage regimen, the antibiotic concentrations in the pleural fluid will be maintained higher as a consequence of the difference between the two kinetic processes.

TABLE 1. *Pharmacokinetic parameters obtained from the average plasma and pleural fluid levels of cefoxitin in the five patients included in the survey*

$\alpha = 4.44\ h^{-1}$	$K_0 = 878.00$ mg/h	$V_c = 3.78$ l
$t_{1/2\alpha} = 0.16$ h	$K_{12} = 1.94\ h^{-1}$	$V_t = 6.97$ l
$\beta = 0.45\ h^{-1}$	$K_{21} = 1.05\ h^{-1}$	$V_{dss} = 10.85$ l
$t_{1/2\beta} = 1.54$ h	$K_{13} = 1.90\ h^{-1}$	$Cl_p = 119.70$ ml/min
		$AUC_0^{\infty a} = 242.31$ µg.ml/h
$K_d = 0.18\ h^{-1}$	$t_0 = 1.32$ h	$\%D = 2.42$
$t_{1/2d} = 3.85$ h	$t_{max} = 3.02$ h	$Cl_{pl} = 4.02$ ml/min
$K_i = 1.37\ h^{-1}$	$C_{max} = 17.01$ µg/ml	$AUC_0^{\infty} = 143.19$ µg.ml/h
$t_{1/2i} = 0.50$ h		

[a] AUC, Area under the serum concentration curve.

The administration of 30 mg of cefoxitin per kg by i.v. perfusion every 8 h ensures antibiotic levels greater than the MICs reported for many cefoxitin-susceptible organisms.

1. **Barrueco, M., M. J. Garcia, M. J. Otero, A. Dominguez-Gil, and J. Martinez L. de Letona.** 1981. Disposition of cefoxitin in patients with pleural effusion. Clin. Ther. **3**:425–435.
2. **Foster, T. S., and D. W. A. Bourne.** 1977. Use of a programmable hand-held calculator for clinical pharmacokinetics. Am. J. Hosp. Pharm. **34**:70–75.
3. **Lanao, J. M., A. Dominguez-Gil, J. G. Macias, J. L. Diez, and M. J. Nieto.** 1980. The influence of ascites on the pharmacokinetic of amikacin. Int. J. Clin. Pharmacol. **17**:171–175.
4. **Vicente, M. V., T. Olay, M. C. R. Quecedo, and A. Rodriguez.** 1979. Diffusion of beta-lactam antibiotics and Fosfomicin to interstitial tissue fluid in rabbits. Chemotherapy **25**:329–335.
5. **Yamakoa, K., T. Nakagawa, and T. Uno.** 1978. Application of Akaike's information criterion in the evaluation of linear pharmacokinetics equations. J. Pharmacokin. Biopharm. **6**:165–175.

Effects of Cefoxitin in Patients with Diseases of the Hematopoietic System with Complicating Severe Infections

ATSUSHI HORIUCHI,* HIROFUMI HASEGAWA, TORU MASAOKA, AND KIYOYASU NAGAI

Kinki University School of Medicine and Center for Adult Diseases, Osaka, and Hyogo College of Medicine, Hyogo, Japan*

Patients with hematopoietic disease such as acute or chronic myelocytic leukemia are liable to develop complications of severe infections because of a markedly reduced neutrophil count and immunological incompetence. Cefoxitin (CFX) was administered to patients with such severe complicating infections at a daily dose of 3 to 12 g for a period of 4 days or longer by intravenous drip infusion. The underlying diseases of these 64 patients were acute leukemia (44 patients), blastic crisis of chronic myelocytic leukemia (10), erythroleukemia (2), malignant lymphoma (2), aplastic anemia (2), and others. Of the complicating infections in these patients (Table 1), suspected septicemia was the largest in number (47), followed by respiratory tract infection (including pleurisy) (7), septicemia (3), oral infection (3), and urinary tract infection (2).

The efficacy rate of CFX was 66.7% for septicemia, 66.0% for suspected septicemia, 42.9% for respiratory tract infection, and 66.7% for oral infection, with an overall efficacy rate of 60.9%. Therapeutic effects were excellent in 13 patients and good in 26.

TABLE 1. *Infections associated with hematopoietic diseases and clinical effects of CFX*

Infection[a]	No. of cases	Efficacy rate[b] (%)
Septicemia	3	66.7
Septicemia (probable)	47	66.0
Oral infection	3	66.7
RTI (including pleurisy)	7	42.9
UTI	2	50.0
Others	2	0
Total	64	60.9

[a] RTI, respiratory tract infection; UTI, urinary tract infection.
[b] Defined as [(excellent + good)/total] × 100.

TABLE 2. *Clinical effects classified by daily dose of CFX*

Daily dose (g)	Judgment (no. of cases)					Efficacy rate[a] (%)
	Excel-lent	Good	Fair	Poor	Total	
3		1			1	100.0
4	1	3	1	1	6	66.7
6	3	12	4	7	26	57.7
8	6	8	1	7	22	63.6
≧9	3	2		4	9	55.6
Total	13	26	6	19	64	60.9

[a] Defined as in Table 1.

The relationship between efficacy rate and daily dose is shown in Table 2. There was no appreciable difference in the efficacy rate among the groups of patients who received daily doses of 4, 6, 8, or ≧9 g, and the efficacy rate ranged from 55.6 to 66.7%. Moreover, there was no appreciable difference in the efficacy rate between the patients who had failed to respond to prior antibiotic therapy and those treated with CFX from the beginning. The efficacy rates were 56.5% (13 of 23) for the former and 63.4% (26 of 41) for the latter.

The efficacy rate of CFX was also classified on the basis of the change in neutrophil count during treatment. CFX was effective in 20 (57.1%) of the 35 patients with an initial neutrophil count less than 500/μl. Generally, the response to treatment was better in patients whose neutrophil count increased during treatment than in those whose neutrophil count decreased or was unchanged.

Causative microorganisms were identified in 10 patients, and a good or excellent therapeutic response was observed in 6 patients. The efficacy rate was 61% (33 of 54) for the remaining 54 patients whose causative microorganisms were not identified.

Side effects were observed in three patients: skin eruptions in two and transient abnormality of hepatic function in another. These patients, however, had also received antileukemic agents or blood transfusions. Consequently, it is difficult to say that these adverse effects were attributable to CFX treatment.

These findings are especially impressive since they come from patients with reduced neutrophil count and immunological incompetence. Thus, CFX is considered an appropriate broad-spectrum antibiotic for the treatment of patients with hematopoietic diseases complicated by severe infections in which identification of the causative microorganisms may be very difficult.

Penetration of Cefoxitin into Peritoneal Fluid

R. WISE, I. A. DONOVAN, N. S. AMBROSE, AND J. E. ALLCOCK

Departments of Microbiology and Surgery, Dudley Road Hospital, Birmingham B18 7QH, U.K.

Cefoxitin is a broad-spectrum cephamycin active against the majority of clinically important enterobacteria and *Bacteroides fragilis*. This range gives cefoxitin a role in the treatment and prevention of abdominal sepsis. Cefoxitin is highly bound, which may lead to poor tissue penetration and thus to a diminution in its activity. We have devised a simple method of measuring the peritoneal penetration of antibiotics and comparing this to serum levels; we have evaluated the method with cefoxitin.

Twenty-five patients (mean age, 57 years; range, 22 to 78 years) undergoing abdominal surgery have been studied. Two patients had peritonitis at the time of surgery. Each received 2 g of cefoxitin as an intravenous bolus injection at between 10 min and 3 h before surgery and at the time noted. After the peritoneal cavity was opened and good hemostasis was ensured, a preweighed, sterile, 13-mm-diameter filter paper disk was placed behind the transverse mesocolon on the posterior abdominal wall. A serum sample was taken and the time was noted. After a period of 5 min, the paper disk was removed. At the

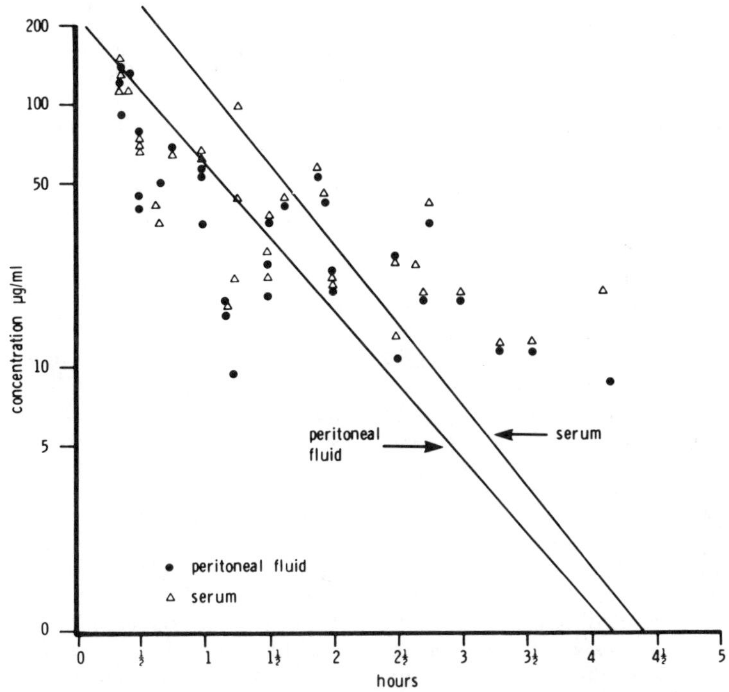

FIG. 1. *Serum and peritoneal fluid levels after 2 g of cefoxitin was given intravenously.*

end of the procedure, if contamination with blood was not too excessive, another disk was placed in the peritoneal cavity and another serum sample was taken. The time was again noted. Assay of the serum and paper disk samples was carried out within 2 h.

At the laboratory, disks were compared with standard disks prepared in 5, 10, and 20% human blood and isotonic saline solution. Any disk found to be contaminated with more than 10% blood was discarded.

An agar diffusion assay was employed, using *Bacillus subtilis* NCTC 8236 as the indicator organism. Serum samples were assayed in triplicate against standards prepared in pooled human serum. The peritoneal fluid disk samples were reweighed to measure the amount of fluid absorbed (mean weight of fluid absorbed, 108 ± 37 mg). The disks were then assayed by using standard disks prepared with 20% human serum in the same volume as the test disk. The 95% confidence limit of the serum assay was ±14.5%.

Of the 47 peritoneal fluid samples obtained from 25 patients, 9 had to be discarded because of blood contamination. Standard regression line analysis for both serum and peritoneal fluid samples is shown in Fig. 1. Serum and peritoneal fluid levels declined almost in parallel. Using only paired data between 10 and 20 min (n = 34), the mean peritoneal fluid level was 86% (SD, 27%) that of the simultaneous serum level. At between 10 and 20 min, the mean serum and peritoneal fluid levels were 132 and 110 µg/ml, respectively.

The study shows that cefoxitin, although highly protein bound, penetrates rapidly into peritoneal fluid, achieving 80 to 90% of the simultaneous serum levels. Since both levels decline in an almost parallel fashion, equilibrium between the peritoneal and vascular compartment must be rapid. This suggests a more rapid and complete equilibration than previous blister studies (1) have shown.

Although only two patients with peritonitis have been studied, there is no suggestion that peritonitis improved or hindered the penetration of cefoxitin into peritoneal fluid.

Since the peritoneal fluid levels fall below the level of 16 µg/ml (the 90% mean inhibitory concentration for *B. fragilis*) after 2 h, it is suggested that a further 2-g intravenous dose be given to maintain effective levels during the surgical procedure.

1. **Wise, R., B. Cadge, A. P. Gillet, A. Bhamjee, and D. P. Thornhill.** 1979. The pharmacology of cefoxitin and the comparison of two human blister models. J. Infect. **1**(Suppl.):49–56.

Concentration of Cefoxitin in Oral Tissues and Serum

KENICHI SAITO,* KENICHI MICHI, AND KENJI HASHIMOTO

School of Dentistry, Showa University, and Faculty of Dentistry, Tokyo Medical and Dental University, Tokyo, Japan*

Cefoxitin (CFX), a new semisynthetic cephamycin derivative, has a broad antibacterial spectrum which includes anaerobes. After intravenous administration, it appears in high concentrations in serum. However, no report has been published on CFX concentrations in oral tissues. In the present study, therefore, with an intention of evaluating the therapeutic effects of CFX in the treatment of oral tissue infections, we measured the serum and tissue concentrations of CFX in laboratory animals and in patients, using a bioassay method.

Wistar rats weighing 150 to 200 g received a single subcutaneous injection of CFX at a dose of 100 mg/kg. CFX concentrations in the submaxillary gland, masseter muscle, tongue, gum and buccal mucosa, lower jaw bone, and serum were determined at 15, 30, 60, 120, and 180 min after injection, using a thin double-layer disk method. *Escherichia coli* MB3804 was used as the test microorganism.

Mean peak concentrations observed were 91.5 μg/ml in the serum, 34.7 μg/g in the gum and buccal mucosa, 23.5 μg/g in the tongue, 16.6 μg/g in the submaxillary gland, 12.5 μg/g in the lower jaw bone, and 11.8 μg/g in the masseter muscle (Fig. 1).

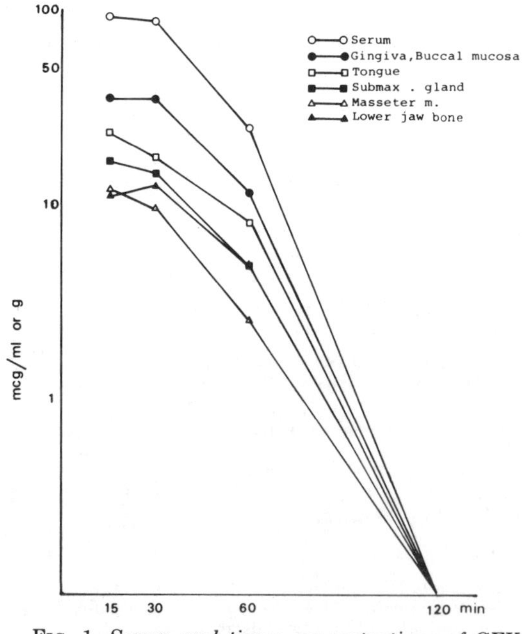

FIG. 1. *Serum and tissue concentrations of CFX after subcutaneous administration to rats (100 mg/kg; n = 4).*

The mean peak concentration in the lower jaw bone was observed at 30 min; in the gum and buccal mucosa, at 15 and 30 min; and in other tissues, at 15 min after injection. The gum and buccal mucosa-versus-serum ratio was approximately 1:3. Only trace amounts were observed in all tissues at 120 min after injection.

Using the 18 patients who had undergone surgical operations, we determined CFX concentrations in the oral mucosa, muscle, sinus mucosa, salivary gland, and serum at 30, 60, 90, 120, 150, and 180 min after starting a 1-h intravenous drip infusion of CFX in a dose of 2 g, using a thin double-layer disk method. Tissues were taken from sites where blood flow had not been disturbed by the surgical procedure. *E. coli* MB3804 was used as the test microorganism. The 18 patients (13 males and 5 females) had normal renal function. Their ages ranged from 20 to 72 (mean, 44.2) years. The mean body weight was 57.8 kg, and the mean dose was 35.9 mg/kg.

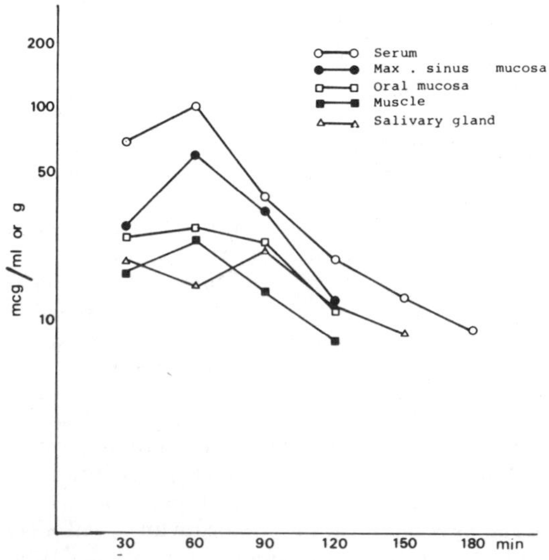

FIG. 2. *Serum and tissue concentrations of CFX after intravenous infusion in patients (2 g/60 min, drip infusion).*

The mean peak concentration in the serum was 101.7 μg/ml. Other mean peak concentrations were 59.4 μg/g in the maxillary sinus mucosa, 27.0 μg/g in the oral mucosa, 23.7 μg/g in the muscle, and 21.2 μg/g in the salivary gland (Fig. 2).

Peak serum concentrations were observed at 60 min, followed by a rapid decrease to 1/10 of the peak value by the end of 180 min after infusion was started. The peak concentration in the salivary gland was observed at 90 min and in other tissues it was observed at 60 min after the infusion was started. The highest peak tissue concentration was observed in the sinus mucosa, and its ratio versus the serum concentration was approximately 2:3. These tissue concentrations of CFX decreased in the same manner as did the serum concentration, except in the salivary gland.

The serum CFX concentration-time curve was obtained by the least-squares method of fitting serum concentrations to an open two-compartment model. The elimination half-life calculated from the β-slope was 0.915 h.

We studied CFX concentrations in oral tissues in animals and in patients by means of a bioassay method. In laboratory animals, the highest peak concentrations were observed in the gum and buccal mucosa, followed by the tongue, submaxillary gland, lower jaw bone, and the masseter muscle in that order. These findings are consistent with those for the cephalosporins.

In patients, the highest peak concentrations were observed in the sinus mucosa, and peak concentrations in oral tissues were from 1/4 to 2/3 of the corresponding serum concentrations. Further study is needed to elucidate the reason for the high-peak CFX concentration in the sinus mucosa and the apparent delayed peak concentration in the salivary gland.

The data presented furnish evidence to support the clinical efficacy of CFX in the treatment of oral infections.

Comparative Study of Concentrations of Four Cephalosporins in Dog Lymph

JOHN KOSMIDIS,* GEORGE KOUKOULIDIS, ARIS POLYZOS, AND ANASTASSIOS RIGAS

First Department of Propedeutic Medicine and Second Department of Propedeutic Surgery, Athens University School of Medicine, King Paul's Hospital, Athens 609, Greece*

The concentration of antibiotics in interstitial fluid is very important for the success of chemotherapy, probably more so than blood levels.

Several techniques have been used for sampling material that is considered to correspond to interstitial fluid: skin abrasion, skin blister formation, tissue cage implantation, fibrin clot implantation, and tissue homogenization. Various problems, such as protein concentration in the collected fluid differing from that in the interstitial fluid, contamination with blood, proliferation of cells possibly binding antibiotics, and the formation mechanism of collected fluid differing from that of normal interstitial fluid, reduce the reliability of results obtained by these techniques and make confirmation necessary (1).

Thoracic duct lymph is, on the other hand, considered to accurately represent the extracellular fluid of many tissues of the body and was chosen for a comparative study of four cephalosporins.

Sixteen dogs were used for the experiments, four for each drug. A single dose of 15 mg/kg of one of the following antibiotics was given: cephaloridine (CRD), cephalothin (CFT), cefotaxime (CTX), or cefoxitin (CFX). CRD was given intramuscularly, and the others were given intravenously.

After induction of general anesthesia, thoracotomy was performed and the major thoracic duct was intubated. Injection of the antibiotic was performed, and serial specimens of lymph (every 15 min) and blood (every hour) were taken for 4 h. Blood pressure and other life parameters were closely monitored to ensure adequate kidney and liver function throughout the experiment. After collection of the last specimen, the animals were sacrificed.

Concentrations of antibiotics in lymph and serum were measured by conventional microbiological well plate techniques, with a strain of *Staphylococcus aureus* as the indicator organism for CRD, *Sarcina lutea* for CFT, and *Bacillus subtilis* for CTX and CFX.

Mean levels of the four cephalosporins in lymph and serum throughout the 4-h study period are given in Table 1. CRD levels in lymph reached a peak of 91 mg/liter after 1.25 h and

TABLE 1. *Concentration of four cephalosporins in dog lymph after a dose of 15 mg/kg*

Drug	Fluid	Mean concn (mg/liter) at indicated times after dose															
		15 min	30 min	45 min	60 min	1.25 h	1.5 h	1.75 h	2 h	2.25 h	2.5 h	2.75 h	3 h	3.25 h	3.5 h	3.75 h	4 h
CRD	Lymph	11.8	15.3	48	79	91	72	77	74	64	64	52	39	30	22	23	20
	Serum				86				51				31				14
CFT	Lymph	78	70	133	138	138	116	120	104	102	88	87	88	76	60	54	52
	Serum				28.5				16.5				15.8				14.2
CTX	Lymph	3.3	3.9	5.2	14	17	26	28	28	35	41	47	46	36	38	36	31
	Serum				125				92				74				40
CFX	Lymph	10.8	19.4	27	27	49	43	62	72	67	70	68	72	72	71	70	68
	Serum				110				92				75				64

declined to 20 mg/liter at 4 h, with a half-life of 60 min. Serum levels were slightly higher than those in lymph at 1 h but were lower thereafter, exhibiting a decay curve almost parallel to that of lymph levels. CFT gave a much higher lymph peak of 138 mg/liter at 1 h, when blood levels had already fallen to 28.5 mg/liter. Lymph levels declined slowly, with a half-life of 112.5 min, and remained much higher than the corresponding serum levels. CTX was very slow to pass into lymph, reaching a peak of 47 mg/liter only after 2.75 h. A decline ensued, giving a curve running parallel to the always higher serum levels. CFX was also slow to reach a peak in lymph, 72 mg/liter at 2 h, and then reached a plateau until the end of the experiment. Blood levels declined slowly, and at 4 h they were just lower than those in lymph.

All four cephalosporins studied were adequately concentrated in lymph. They have all been successfully used in the treatment of various infections where tissue levels are important. Some differences, however, were observed, and are worth comment. CRD reached an early and high lymph peak, although it was administered intramuscularly, and then had a quick decline. It seems that it can move freely and quickly from blood to interstitial fluid and vice versa. CFT seems to move more easily from blood to interstitial fluid than vice versa, since its lymph levels were always much higher than those in serum. CTX moves slowly from blood to lymph, but it seems to have no difficulty in disappearing from the latter. Removal from lymph has taken place in spite of higher blood levels. This can only be explained by some kind of inactivation of CTX in the tissues. Finally, CFX moves slowly in both directions. It reached a peak after 2 h and then exhibited a plateau until the end of the experiment.

1. **Chisholm, G. D., P. M. Waterworth, J. S. Calnan, and L. P. Garrod.** 1973. Concentration of antibacterial agents in interstitial tissue fluid. Br. Med. J. **1:**569–573.

Pharmacokinetic and Clinical Studies with Cefuroxime Sodium in Total Joint Replacement

CLIVE H. DASH,* SEAN P. F. HUGHES,[1] MARGARET R. K. KENNEDY, SUSAN WANT, AND JOHN H. DARRELL

Glaxo Group Research Ltd., Greenford, Middlesex, UB6 OHE, and Royal Postgraduate Medical School (and Hammersmith Hospital), London, United Kingdom*

In orthopedic operations, many dosage schedules advocated for prophylaxis against infection have involved several days of antibiotics. Resistance of bacteria is less likely to occur with shorter regimens. This report summarizes the prophylactic effect of short dosage regimens of cefuroxime in total joint replacement and details the concentrations in bone, synovial capsule, and serum.

A total of 95 patients (29 males, 66 females), aged 25 to 84 (median, 61) years, underwent 106 operations (69 hips, 37 knees). They have been

[1] Present address: University Department of Orthopaedic Surgery, Princess Margaret Rose Orthopaedic Hospital, Fairmilehead, Edinburgh, EH10 7ED, Scotland.

followed for 1.25 to 3.5 years. Concentrations of cefuroxime were assayed in bone, capsule, and serum from 77 operations. In 42 operations (25 hips, 17 knees) cefuroxime was given as 1 g intravenously (i.v.) with induction of anesthesia; then 1 g was given intramuscularly (i.m.) about 6 and 12 h later. In 62 operations (42 hips, 20 knees) 1.5 g i.v. was given with induction of anesthesia, and 750 mg was given i.m. about 6 and 12 h later. For two separate operations a patient with chronic renal failure was given single i.v. doses of 500 or 750 mg. In all knee operations a tourniquet was applied to the thigh a few minutes after injection.

At operation samples of excised capsule and bone (femoral head or from around the knee) were collected together with blood at similar times. In addition, blood samples were collected postoperatively every half hour for about 6 h. Serum was separated and, together with capsule and bone, was stored at −20°C pending assay. Bone and synovial capsule samples were broken or cut into small pieces and agitated for 4 h in buffer to achieve equilibrium. Concentrations of cefuroxime in the supernatant were measured in two separate laboratories (Royal Postgraduate Medical School and Glaxo Group Research) by similar large-plate bioassays, with *Bacillus subtilis* 1904E as test organism. The hemoglobin concentration was also measured in the supernatant to allow calculation of the degree of blood contaminating the tissue specimens.

There was a good correlation between the assay results in the two laboratories, although the results from Royal Postgraduate Medical School tended to be about 10 to 15% lower than those from Glaxo Group Research. Slight differences in technique could account for this variation. Serum concentrations were often in excess of 100 mg/liter at 30 min after 1.5 g i.v. and were about 40 mg/liter at 2 h, with a half-life of 80 min. After 1.0 g the concentrations were about two-thirds and the half-life was 74 min. Most of the bone and capsule samples were taken within 1 h of injection, so the results were divided into two groups: those taken up to 30 min after injection and those taken between 30 and 60 min. After 1 g, a clear pattern seemed to emerge. The mean concentration in the femoral head up to 30 min was higher than in the later group. In the bone from the knee, the higher mean levels occurred between 30 and 60 min. In the synovial capsule, the mean concentrations followed the same pattern (Table 1). This pattern was less clear after 1.5 g, but there was a suggestion that the higher concentrations around the knee occurred in the 30- to 60-min period (Fig. 1).

The ratio of the tissue concentration to the simultaneous serum concentration was calculated for each sample. The mean values are given in Table 1. The capsule consistently gave a higher ratio than the bone. Likewise, the hip tissues gave a higher ratio than those from the knee. However, when the ratio of the results of bone to capsule was calculated, the two joints produced almost identical values (Table 1). This suggests that the lower concentrations around the knee are a result of the tourniquet present during the operation, but that the penetrability of the tissues is of a similar degree. It would be of interest in the future to assay blood distal to the tourniquet in knee operations and relate the levels to the excised tissues.

TABLE 1. *Mean concentrations of cefuroxime in two timed periods (≤30 min, >30 min) after injection of 1 g and 1.5 g and the mean ratios of tissue concentrations to blood and to capsule concentrations*

Dose (g)	Time (min)	Joint	Bone	Capsule
1	≤30	Hip	13.2	23.4
	>30		8.8	19.3
1	≤30	Knee	11.1	16.6
	>30		17.8	40.1
1.5	≤30	Hip	17.6	26.2
	>30		16.8	34.9
1.5	≤30	Knee	14.8	11.8
	>30		37.1	50.8
Ratio: tissue/blood (%)		Hip	19.0	33.7
		Knee	14.4	23.7
Ratio: bone/capsule (%)		Hip	56.4	
		Knee	60.8	

The amount of contaminating blood did not appear to differ between bone and capsule, but there was a large difference between hip and knee tissues. The assayed levels in the hip tissues were on average about 40% higher than those quoted in Table 1 and Fig. 1 as a result of contamination, whereas the knee tissues were assayed about 10% higher. Again, these differences between hips and knees are explicable by the presence of the tourniquet.

Two patients developed deep infections. Both patients had had total knee replacements. One patient was on steroids for rheumatoid arthritis and developed a *Staphylococcus aureus* infection 6 months after operation. The other patient had had a previous operation on the knee for osteoarthritis and developed an anaerobic streptococcal infection 1 year postoperatively. It may be that the perioperative management of patients undergoing knee replacement or other operations distal to a tourniquet should be modified so that the injection is given some time before operation, for example, with the premedication. However, i.v. injection is preferable to

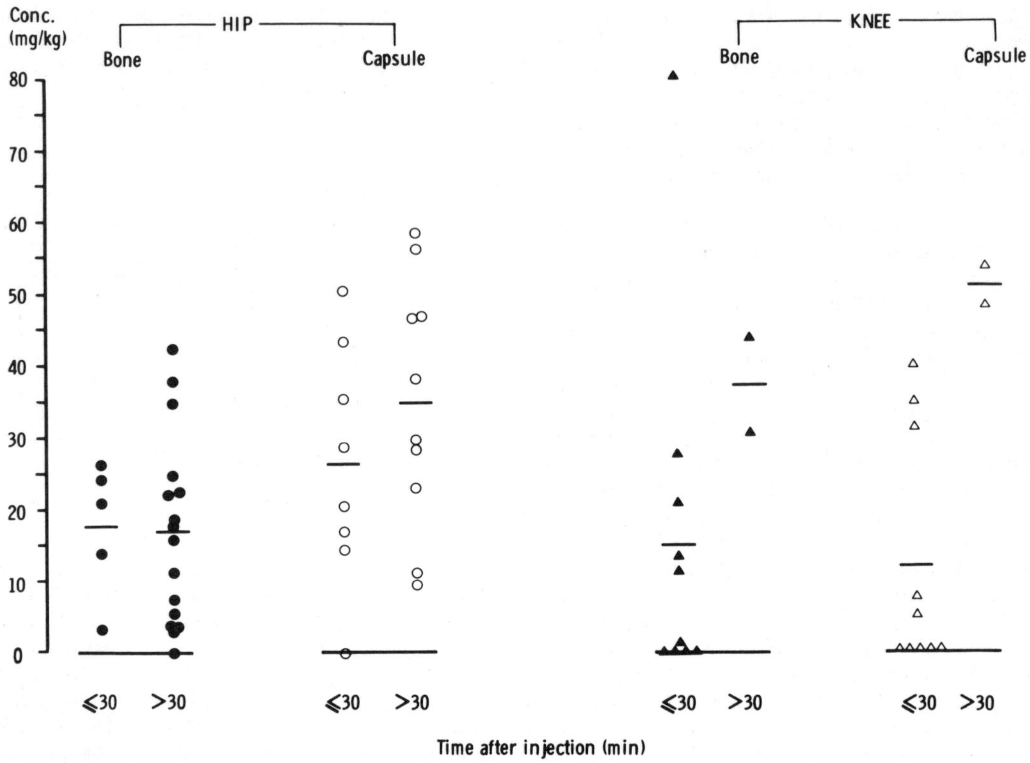

FIG. 1. *Concentrations of cefuroxime in bone (solid symbols: hip, ●; knee, ▲) and capsule (open symbols: hip, ○; knee, △) during two timed intervals after i.v. injection of 1.5 g. The horizontal bars represent mean values.*

i.m. because of the higher concentrations achieved.

Overall, the deep infection rate in this series of patients compares satisfactorily with the best results quoted in the literature. This is encouraging considering the low dose, short-term regimen that was used in a group of patients containing unusually large numbers with rheumatoid arthritis who were on corticosteroids.

Cefuroxime Penetration into Cerebrospinal Fluid in Patients with Purulent Meningitis

JACQUES MODAI, ALAIN MEULEMANS, JACQUES LEBAS, MICHEL WOLFF, AND BERNARD REGNIER

Claude-Bernard Hospital, Paris, France

Cefuroxime has a broad antibacterial spectrum and a high resistance to degradation by β-lactamases (5). Although the use of cephalosporins in purulent meningitis has so far been controversial because of their poor penetration into the cerebrospinal fluid (CSF), preliminary studies of CSF penetration (6; J. Modai, J. Pierre, E. Bergogne-Berezin, and M. F. Avril, Program Abstr. Intersci. Conf. Antimicrob. Agents Chemother. 18th, Atlanta, 1978, abstr. 323) suggest that cefuroxime may achieve therapeutic concentrations in CSF against most of the pathogens associated with meningitis including *Haemophilus influenzae* (both ampicillin susceptible and ampicillin resistant), *Neisseria meningitidis,* and *Streptococcus pneumoniae.*

The results of these studies prompted us to evaluate the CSF penetration of cefuroxime in nine patients hospitalized with bacterial meningitis and treated with other antibiotics. In all patients CSF was macroscopically purulent, with leukocyte counts varying between 550 and 17,400 cells per mm^3. There was a dominance of polymorphonuclear leukocytes (63 to 100%). There were increased concentrations of protein in CSF (120 to 650 mg/100 ml), and the ratio between CSF and blood glucose was decreased in all patients. The causative pathogens were isolated in eight patients: *N. meningitidis* in two; *S. pneumoniae,* two; *S. pyogenes,* one; *Staphylococcus aureus,* one; *Serratia marcescens,* one; *Listeria monocytogenes,* one. The remaining patient had a negative CSF culture.

Six of the patients received antibiotic treatment with ampicillin in daily doses varying between 12 and 16 g; two patients received a combination of either methicillin or ampicillin and amikacin. In addition to the above antibiotics, all patients received cefuroxime administered intravenously as four 1.5-g doses at 6-h intervals. These doses were administered on days 2 to 20 of treatment with the appropriate antibiotic.

Cefuroxime concentrations in serum and CSF were studied in samples drawn 60, 120, or 180 min after the fourth cefuroxime dose. In all cases lumbar puncture was performed only when clinically indicated and in no case purely for the purpose of this study. Cefuroxime levels in serum and CSF samples were determined by high-performance liquid chromatography using a modification of the procedure described by Nilsson-Ehle and Nilsson-Ehle (3).

The serum and CSF concentrations of cefuroxime are given in Table 1. When the patients within each of the three sampling groups (i.e., 60, 120, and 180 min after cefuroxime administration) were compared, some variations were found in both serum and CSF concentrations. These variations were probably due to differences in age, weight, renal function, and the degree of meningeal inflammation. In all patients, cefuroxime gave detectable CSF concentrations that varied with the sampling time and with the time elapsed since the onset of the disease. As a result of pronounced individual variations, it was difficult to compare the concentrations obtained 60, 120, and 180 min after administration of cefuroxime. However, although not statistically significant, a tendency toward higher concentrations at about 120 min after intravenous administration of the drug was noted. All patients were followed for adverse reactions to cefuroxime, and none was reported. Since cefuroxime was not used therapeutically, no evaluation was made of the outcome of the treatment.

The CSF concentrations of cefuroxime achieved in all patients were by far higher than the MICs for meningococci (0.06 μg/ml) and pneumococci (0.06 μg/ml), the organisms most frequently responsible for bacterial meningitis in adults. There is no question that cefuroxime supersedes ampicillin or penicillin therapy for infections with these organisms although these agents have been used effectively for more than a decade. What is needed is a better therapy than ampicillin or penicillin for meningitis due to *H. influenzae,* considering the increasing frequency of ampicillin-resistant strains, and for other gram-negative bacilli, mainly *Escherichia coli, Klebsiella, Proteus* spp., and, as the result of neurosurgical procedure, *Pseudomonas*

TABLE 1. *Concentrations in serum and CSF of cefuroxime after administration of four 1.5-g doses intravenously at 6-h intervals*

Patient no. (age, sex)	Sampling time (min)	Time elapsed since the onset of disease (day)	Cefuroxime concn (μg/ml)		
			Serum	CSF	CSF/serum concn ratio
1 (26, M)	60	2	26	2.5	0.09
2 (53, M)	60	3	55	2	0.03
3 (37, F)	60	2	52	8.4	0.16
4 (47, M)	120	7	19	9	0.47
		20	34	7.5	0.22
5 (48, M)	120	3	13	9.5	0.73
		9	13.5	9	0.69
6 (26, M)	120	3	7.7	4.5	0.33
		12	12.5	3.5	0.28
7 (25, F)	180	3	12	2	0.16
8 (54, M)	180	2	7	3.4	0.48
9 (30, M)	180	3	10	1.5	0.15

TABLE 2. *Range of cefuroxime MICs with gram-negative bacilli*

Pathogen	MICs (μg/ml), minimum-maximum and (mode)
Haemophilus influenzae (including ampicillin resistant)	0.25–0.5 (0.5)
Escherichia coli	1.0–16 (4.0)
Klebsiella pneumoniae	1.0–16 (2.0)
Proteus mirabilis	0.5–2.0 (0.75)
Proteus spp., indole positive	0.12–>32 (>32)
Enterobacter spp.	2.0–>32 (4.0)
Serratia marcescens	16–>32 (>32)
Pseudomonas spp.	16–>32 (>32)

aeruginosa. The MICs of cefuroxime for these pathogens (1) are shown in Table 2. Most of the CSF concentrations of cefuroxime observed in our patients would be in a therapeutic range. However, the MIC for indole-positive *Proteus* spp., *S. marcescens,* and *P. aeruginosa* would be beyond the cefuroxime levels attainable in the CSF. The penetration of cefuroxime into the CSF has not been widely studied in humans. In a previous study, we investigated the penetration of cefuroxime into CSF by measuring the cefuroxime concentrations of simultaneous CSF and serum specimens from 12 patients hospitalized for viral meningitis (Modai et al., 18th ICAAC, abstr. 323). Mean serum levels at 30, 90, and 180 min after administration of 1 g of cefuroxime intravenously were 22, 8.7, and 2.5 μg/ml, respectively, but only 0.17, 0.45, and 0.58 μg/ml in corresponding CSF samples. Norrby et al. (4) tried cefuroxime in two cases of severe bacterial meningitis, one caused by *Klebsiella* and one caused by *S. pneumoniae.* In both patients higher cefuroxime concentrations than ours were assayed in CSF, as a result of the degree of meningeal inflammation, which is higher in bacterial meningitis than in viral meningitis. The ability of cefuroxime to penetrate the blood-CSF barrier when the meninges are inflamed was also demonstrated by Muller et al. (2) in a recent study. The concentrations of cefuroxime in CSF and serum after a single 2.5-g intravenous bolus injection were measured in patients with varying degrees of meningeal inflammation, and cefuroxime was found to pass into the CSF of those patients with inflamed meninges, the amount being dependent on the degree of inflammation.

Our results, in combination with those of others, indicate that cefuroxime has a good penetrability into the CSF when the meninges are inflamed and that it might be considered in selected cases of purulent meningitis when the susceptibility pattern indicates its usefulness.

1. **Barry, A. L., C. Thornsberry, R. N. Jones, P. Fuchs, T. L. Gavan, and E. M. Gerlach.** 1977. Cefuroxime, an in vitro comparison with six other cephalosporins. J. R. Soc. Med. **70**(Suppl. 9):63–70.
2. **Muller, C., A. Netland, A. F. Dawson, and E. Andrew.** 1980. The penetration of cefuroxime into the cerebrospinal fluid through inflamed and non-inflamed meninges. J. Antimicrob. Chemother. **6**:279–283.
3. **Nilsson-Ehle, I., and P. Nilsson-Ehle.** 1978. Liquid chromatographic assay of cefuroxime in serum. Clin. Chem. **24**:365.
4. **Norrby, R., R. D. Foord, J. D. Price, and P. Hedlung.** 1977. Pharmakokinetic and clinical studies of cefuroxime. J. R. Soc. Med. **70**(Suppl. 9):25–33.
5. **O'Callaghan, C. H., K. B. Sykes, A. Griffiths, and J. E. Thornton.** 1976. Cefuroxime, a new cephalosporin antibiotic : activity in vitro. Antimicrob. Agents Chemother. **9**:511–519.
6. **Renlund, M., and O. Pettay.** 1977. Pharmacokinetics and clinical efficacy of cefuroxime in the newborn period. Proc. R. Soc. Med. **70**(Suppl. 9):179–182.

Prevention of Wound Infection and Abdominal Wound Disruption with Prophylactic Cefuroxime

THOMAS T. IRVIN,* JOHN B. F. GRANT, NEIL J. McC. MORTENSEN, AND CLIVE H. DASH

Department of Surgery, Royal Devon and Exeter Hospital (Wonford), and Medical Division, Glaxo Group Research Limited, Middlesex, England*

Infection has adverse effects on wound repair and, in the case of abdominal wounds, may result in the complications of burst abdomen and incisional hernia (1). These complications might be avoided by the use of an alternative method of wound closure such as the mass suture technique (2) or by the use of antibiotics to prevent wound infection. These factors were examined in a randomized prospective clinical trial in 300 patients undergoing elective laparotomy.

The 300 patients were randomly allocated to three treatment groups; 8 patients were subsequently withdrawn from the trial either because the treatment protocol was incorrectly administered or because they died before an assessment of wound healing could be made. In group 1 (97 patients) the abdominal wound was closed with monofilament nylon and a mass suture technique. In group 2 (98 patients) the wound was closed with polypropylene suture material and a conventional layered suture technique supported by retention sutures. In group 3 (97 patients) the wound suture technique was identical to that used in group 2, but the patients also received two doses of the antibiotic cefuroxime: an intravenous dose of 1.5 g was given after induction of anaesthesia, and a second dose of 0.75 g was given intramuscularly 8 h later. The incidence of wound infection, burst abdomen, and incisional hernia was recorded, and the patients were followed for 6 months after surgery. A diagnosis of wound infection was made only when there was discharge of frank pus from the abdominal incision.

Eighty percent of the operations were of the clean-contaminated type involving surgical procedures on the biliary or gastrointestinal tracts, and the three groups of patients were well matched for age, sex, and multiple clinical variables including the nature of the operative procedure and the surgical pathology. Nine patients in group 1, 11 patients in group 2, and 4 patients in group 3 died in hospital, but the differences in postoperative mortality in the three groups are not statistically significant. Most deaths resulted from cardiopulmonary complications. The incidence of overt postoperative wound infection in the three groups is shown in Table 1. There were no wound infections in the group treated with cefuroxime (group 3), whereas 10 to 13% of the wounds in the other two groups became infected, a difference which is statistically significant (Fisher's exact test, $P = 0.0001$). There was no significant difference in the incidence of wound sepsis in groups 1 and 2, and the different methods of wound closure had no significant effect on the incidence of wound infection. The incidence of burst abdomen and incisional hernia in the three groups of patients is shown in Table 2. No patient in group 3 (the cefuroxime group) developed these complications, but they occurred in four patients in group 1 and in two patients in group 2. In each case, a wound infection preceded the onset of these complications. In four patients coliform organisms were responsible for the wound disruption, one patient developed an incisional hernia after a staphylococcal infection, and one patient developed a burst abdomen in the presence of a mixed infection of coliform organisms and staphylococci.

TABLE 1. *Incidence of wound infection in the three groups of patients*

Group	No. of patients	No. with wound infection
1	97	13 (13.4%)
2	98	10 (10.2%)
3	97	0

TABLE 2. *Incidence of wound disruption (burst abdomen or incisional hernia) in the three groups of patients*

Group	No. of patients	No. with burst abdomen	No. with incisional hernia	Total (wound failure)
1	97	2	2	4 (4.1%)
2	98	0	2	2 (2.0%)
3	97	0	0	0

The study has shown that attention to the mechanical aspects of abdominal wound closure does not prevent wound disruption in the presence of infection, and earlier claims that the mass suture technique of abdominal wound closure prevented the disruption of infected wounds were not substantiated in this controlled clinical trial. On the other hand, two systemic doses of the broad-spectrum antibiotic cefuroxime before and after the surgical operation prevented wound infection in elective abdominal surgery, and the complications of burst abdomen and incisional hernia were also abolished.

We conclude that wound infection is a significant factor in the pathogenesis of abdominal wound disruption, but it appears that disruption can be prevented by the prophylactic use of an antibiotic such as cefuroxime in abdominal surgery.

1. **Irvin, T. T., C. J. Stoddard, M. G. Greaney, and H. L. Duthie.** 1977. Abdominal wound healing: a prospective clinical study. Br. Med. J. **2**:351–352.
2. **Jenkins, T. P. N.** 1977. Burst abdomen—a preventable condition. Br. Med. J. **1**:771–772.

Prophylactic Antibiotics in Chest Surgery: Comparison Between Cefuroxime and Magnapen

KEYVAN MOGHISSI,* IAN LEIGHTON, FRANCOISE STRUGNELL, MARY DENCH, AND CLIVE H. DASH

Humberside Cardio-Thoracic Surgical Centre, Castle Hill Hospital, Hull, England

In spite of the wealth of information which exists in the literature concerned with antibiotics, relatively few publications are available in regard to prophylactic use of antibiotics in the specific situations of chest surgery.

Over the past few years, a series of studies were set up in our department with the object of evaluating the necessity of using prophylactic antibiotics in chest surgery and determining the optimal duration of the treatment.

The present communication is concerned with the results of one such study, a clinical trial comparing cefuroxime and Magnapen (flucloxicillin plus ampicillin; Beecham Research Laboratories, U.K.) in pulmonary and esophageal surgery.

A total of 171 patients, comprising 105 pulmonary and 66 esophageal surgery patients, were admitted to and completed the trial. Pulmonary surgery patients were allocated at random to group A (cefuroxime), group B (Magnapen), and group C (no antibiotics). Esophageal surgery patients were randomized to group A (cefuroxime) and group B (Magnapen).

Group A patients were given cefuroxime, 1.5 g intravenously, at the start of the operation followed by cefuroxime, 750 mg intramuscularly, twice daily for 2 days. Group B patients were given Magnapen, 2 g intravenously, at the start of the operation followed by Magnapen, 1 g intramuscularly, twice daily for 2 days. Group C patients were given no antibiotics prophylactically. All patients were given appropriate antibiotics postoperatively if there was an infective complication requiring antibiotic therapy.

During the operation, serum, lung, and muscle tissue samples were obtained for estimation of their antibiotic concentration. Serum and sputum samples were also obtained on the second postoperative day for estimation of antibiotic levels. Patients were monitored postoperatively: clinically for signs of infective complications and microbiologically by repeated sampling of sputum or infective materials for identification of microorganisms and their antibiotic susceptibility.

In pulmonary surgery there were 34, 35, and 36 patients in groups A, B, and C, respectively. In esophageal surgery there were 31 and 35 patients in groups A and B, respectively. There was no significant difference of age or sex in different groups.

The incidence and the type of infective complications for each group and for the pulmonary

TABLE 1. *Incidence of infection by treatment group and type of surgery*

Group	No. of patients				
	Wound sepsis	Pleuropulmonary infection	General infection	Total	
Pulmonary surgery[a]					
A Resection (20)[b]	0	2	1	3	3 (8.8%)
No resection (14)	0	0	0	0	
B Resection (14)	1	8	0	8	8 (22.8%)
No resection (21)	0	0	0	0	
C Resection (19)	3	6	1	7	15 (41.6%)
No resection (17)	1	7	2	8	
Esophageal surgery					
A Resection (21)	2	3	1	4	5 (16.0%)
No resection (10)	0	1	0	1	
B Resection (19)	0	4	2	6	4 (11.4%)
No resection (16)	0	0	0	0	

[a] The difference between group A and group C was statistically significant ($P < 0.05$).
[b] Number of patients treated.

TABLE 2. *Mean antibiotic concentrations during pulmonary and esophageal operations*

Antibiotic	Specimen	Concn (μg/liter)[a]			
		0–30 min	31–60 min	61–90 min	>90 min
Cefuroxime	Blood	63.2 (12)	28.4 (22)	21.1 (13)	8.8 (13)
	Lung	9.2 (12)	3.0 (18)	5.3 (7)	0.8 (15)
	Muscle	3.2 (4)	4.8 (11)	2.6 (17)	1.4 (27)
Ampicillin	Blood	48.5 (16)	28.9 (36)	21.4 (9)	15.5 (7)
	Lung	5.3 (6)	5.9 (20)	2.6 (9)	2.4 (23)
	Muscle	4.3 (5)	4.4 (14)	4.6 (13)	3.4 (41)
Flucloxacillin	Blood	53.0 (16)	32.4 (36)	25.5 (9)	16.3 (7)
	Lung	6.1 (6)	6.1 (20)	3.2 (9)	3.7 (23)
	Muscle	6.2 (5)	5.4 (14)	4.3 (13)	3.8 (41)

[a] The figures in parentheses indicate number of samples in mean.

and esophageal surgery are shown in Table 1. In pulmonary surgery the incidence of infective complication was 8.8, 22, and 41.6% for groups A, B, and C, respectively. Fifteen of the 36 patients in group C (i.e., with no prophylactic antibiotics) had postoperative infective complications requiring therapeutic antibiotics, of whom 13 had pleuropulmonary infections, as opposed to 11 of the total of 69 patients in the combined groups A and B (i.e., groups treated with prophylactic antibiotics). The difference between groups A and C was statistically significant ($P < 0.05$).

In esophageal surgery patients, the incidence of postoperative infective complication was 16 and 11.4% for groups A and B, respectively. The difference was not statistically significant.

A detailed study of infected patients indicates that the postoperative infection was not dependent on the preoperative recovery of pathogenic microorganisms. However, in some patients in group C the offending microorganisms recovered from infected materials were identical to those which were present preoperatively in the sputum. The levels of antibiotic in serum and tissues (Table 2) were as expected with respect to the time elapsed between the administration and sampling for each antibiotic. Antibiotics were also present in the tissue samples which were examined. Detailed analysis of our patients shows, however, that there was no relationship between the blood or tissue concentration of antibiotic and the development or lack of postoperative infection. All except one of the infected patients had antibiotic concentrations in blood and tissues that were higher than the mean.

Ceftizoxime: In Vitro and In Vivo Microbiological Properties

IVO DE CARNERI,* GIUSEPPE MEINARDI, SILVIO GRASSO, GISELLA MONTI, AND ALBERTA BIANCHI

Farmitalia Carlo Erba R. & S., Milan, Italy

Over the last few years, great qualitative leaps forward have been made in the development of new cephalosporins. One of them of the latest generation, ceftizoxime (FK 749), has attracted much attention, mainly because of its in vivo stability and excellent activity against gram-negative microorganisms, producers or not of β-lactamases, together with a good activity against streptococci and other gram-positive bacteria (1, 2).

We studied the activity of this drug in vitro and in vivo on collection bacterial strains and on strains isolated in hospital or in out-patient clinics. In vitro activity was studied by MIC determination on diagnostic sensitivity test agar with an inoculum of 2×10^5 to 5×10^5 viable cells.

The spectrum of activity of ceftizoxime was compared with those of cefuroxime, cefoxitin, and cefotaxime on collection strains, most of them susceptible to traditional cephalosporins. The drug was slightly more active (twice) than cefotaxime against enterobacteria and about 100 times more active than the other two reference drugs.

A study was also performed on β-lactamase-producing strains. Seven of these were *Escherichia coli* strains producing different plasmid-mediated β-lactamases, and two were *Klebsiella aerogenes* 1082E and *Enterobacter cloacae* P99, producing chromosomally mediated β-lactamases. On *E. coli* strains, ceftizoxime was basically as active as cefotaxime; cefoxitin and cefuroxime were about 100 times less active. It is worth noting that against *K. aerogenes* 1082E, which produces Richmond's class IVc β-lactamases, ceftizoxime was 23 times more active than cefotaxime and 32 times more active than cefoxitin or cefuroxime. The *Enterobacter* P99 strain tested showed resistance to all four antibiotics.

The activity against six strains of *Haemophilus influenzae* was studied in Bordet Gengou agar with 12% defibrinated rabbit blood added; ceftizoxime (MIC, 0.004 to 0.015 μg/ml) was about twice as active as cefotaxime and 50 times more active than cefuroxime. Cefoxitin was definitely less active.

The distribution of susceptibility among 180 bacterial strains, 116 isolated in 1979 from outpatients at 17 laboratories in Lombardy, Piedmont, and Liguria and 64 isolated in 1975 to 1976 in the three sections of the Milan Ospedale Maggiore, was studied with the method described for the collection strains.

Against *E. coli* (30 strains), ceftizoxime and cefotaxime showed the same activity. This was also true against 30 strains of *Klebsiella* spp. Against *Proteus mirabilis* (30 strains), ceftizoxime was more active than cefotaxime. Against indole-positive *Proteus* spp. (40 strains), the difference in activity of ceftizoxime compared with the reference drugs was even more marked.

It is worth stressing that seven strains of *Proteus* spp. resistant or poorly susceptible to cefotaxime showed susceptibility to ceftizoxime (Table 1).

Even against 20 opportunistic strains (14 strains of *Enterobacter* spp., 2 strains of *Citrobacter* spp., and 4 strains of *Serratia* spp.), ceftizoxime was somewhat more active than cefotaxime. Against all of these gram-negative bacterial species, cefuroxime and cefoxitin were much less active.

In *Staphylococcus* spp., the activity differed only slightly between the various cephalosporins, except for cefoxitin, which showed the least activity of all.

In vivo activity of ceftizoxime and cefotaxime was compared in acute systemic infection of mice, using eight collection strains. Against these strains the two drugs showed equivalent activity, with cefotaxime slightly more active on *Staphylococcus aureus* Smith and ceftizoxime more active on *Salmonella typhi* Watson. The seven strains of *Proteus* spp. resistant or slightly susceptible to cefotaxime in vitro proved equally resistant or slightly susceptible to this drug in vivo, but responded to ceftizoxime (Table 2).

In local subcutaneous infection by *K. aerogenes* 1082E, a producer of β-lactamase, ceftizoxime was only slightly more active than cefoxitin, but definitely more effective than cefotaxime.

The findings reported show that ceftizoxime is a stable cephalosporin antibiotic offering considerable intrinsic activity and a broad spectrum. It may thus have some advantages over cefotaxime.

TABLE 1. *In vitro activity of ceftizoxime against seven strains of Proteus spp. resistant or poorly susceptible cefotaxime*

Organisms	MIC (μg/ml)	
	Ceftizoxime	Cefotaxime
P. mirabilis 119L	2	128
P. mirabilis 1S	1	>128
P. mirabilis 14S	0.12	128
P. rettgeri 10C	0.5	8
P. vulgaris 126G	0.06	64
P. vulgaris 127G	0.12	16
P. vulgaris 128G	0.5	128

TABLE 2. *Therapeutic activity of ceftizoxime and cefotaxime in acute systemic infection in mice with seven strains of Proteus spp. in vitro resistant or poorly susceptible to cefotaxime*

Organisms	ED_{50} (mg/kg)[a]	
	Ceftizoxime	Cefotaxime
P. mirabilis 119L	9	120
P. mirabilis 1S	0.9	35
P. mirabilis 14S	12	>400
P. rettgeri 10C	3.5	94
P. vulgaris 126G	0.3	7.5
P. vulgaris 127G	1.7	9
P. vulgaris 128G	0.13	5.8

[a] Graphically estimated.

1. **Kamimura, T., Y. Matsumoto, N. Okada, Y. Mine, M. Nishida, S. Goto, and S. Kuwahara.** 1979. Ceftizoxime (FK 749), a new parenteral cephalosporin: in vitro and in vivo antibacterial activities. Antimicrob. Agents Chemother. **16:**540–548.

2. **Kojo, H., M. Nishida, S. Goto, and S. Kuwahara.** 1979. Antibacterial activity of ceftizoxime (FK 749), a new cephalosporin, against cephalosporin-resistant bacteria, and its stability to β-lactamase. Antimicrob. Agents Chemother. **16:**549–553.

Pharmacokinetics of Ceftizoxime (Single Dose) in Adult Volunteers and Patients with Renal Dysfunction

FUSANOSUKE YAMASAKU,* YASUTOSHI SUZUKI, HAJIMU TAKEDA, OSAMU SEKINE, AND YOSHIMARU USUDA

Department of Internal Medicine, Suibarago Hospital; The Second Department of Internal Medicine, Niigata University School of Medicine; and Department of Internal Medicine, Shinrakuen Hospital, Niigata, Japan*

Ceftizoxime (CZX) is a new broad-spectrum cephalosporin antibiotic which has especially potent antibacterial activity against a wide variety of gram-negative bacilli.

A study was made to determine the recommended dosage schedule for CZX in patients with varying degrees of renal impairment.

Serum and urinary concentrations of CZX were determined by bioassay in 5 healthy adult volunteers and 14 patients with varying degrees of renal impairment.

Bioassay of CZX was made by a disk-agar diffusion method, using *Bacillus subtilis* ATCC 6633 as the test organism in the test medium of sodium citrate agar (1.0% sodium citrate, 0.5% polypeptone, 0.3% beef extract, and 1.0% agar). The paper disk used was 8 mm in diameter. The standard solutions were prepared with human serum (Consera) for serum samples, and with 0.067 M phosphate buffer for urine samples.

Volunteers consisted of five males varying in age from 22 to 24 years whose average body surface was 1.68 m^2 and whose creatinine clearance (C_{cr}) was from 104 to 120 ml/min.

Pharmacokinetic parameters of CZX were calculated from serum concentrations in three of the five volunteers after a 0.5-g intravenous bolus injection of CZX on the basis of a two-compartment open model by a FACOM 230-38 computer. The pharmacokinetic parameters are shown in Table 1.

Eleven of the 14 patients were classified into four grades. Serum concentrations were measured four or five times during 1 to 6 h in the volunteers and the patients with C_{cr} values of more than 30 ml/min and five times during 2 to 24 h in patients with C_{cr} values of less than 30 ml/min after a 0.5-g intravenous bolus injection of CZX. In each group, pharmacokinetic parameters of CZX were calculated from serum concentrations on the basis of a one-compartment open model by a FACOM 230-38 computer, and the pharmacokinetic parameters are shown in Table 2.

Distribution volumes (V_d) of CZX remained unchanged although renal function decreased, and the elimination rate constant (K_{el}) decreased with a decrease in renal function. As a result, biological half-lives prolonged markedly. The linear correlation between C_{cr} and K_{el} was found, and the following first-order equation was derived:

$$K_{el} = 0.0285 + 0.00478 \cdot C_{cr} \qquad (1)$$

where $r = 0.948$ and $P < 0.01$.

In three patients undergoing hemodialysis during 3 to 8 h after the 0.5-g intravenous bolus injection of CZX, pharmacokinetic parameters of CZX were calculated from average serum concentrations at 4, 6, and 8 h on the basis of a one-compartment open model by a FACOM 230-38 computer. The average V_d, K_{el}, and serum half-life ($T_{1/2}$) were 11.5 liters, 0.218 h^{-1}, and 3.18 h, respectively. The average serum concentration at 8 h after injection was 7.7 μg/ml, which was about one-third of the average serum concentration of 24.8 μg/ml in the anuric group.

Average cumulative urinary recovery rates in the first 6 h were 95% in group I, 78% in group II, 71% in group III, and 21% in group IV.

The dosage schedule in patients with impaired renal function may be adjusted according to the degrees of renal failure, that is, the dosage is reduced or dose intervals are prolonged. When a single dose is the same as that in patients with normal renal function regardless of renal failure, the dose intervals are estimated as follows. In general, repetition of the single dose every third

TABLE 1. *Pharmacokinetic parameters of CZX in healthy volunteers*[a]

Case	A (μg/ml)	B (μg/ml)	α (h^{-1})	β (h^{-1})	$T_{1/2}\beta$ (h)	V_c (liters)	$V_{d\beta}$ (liters)	Cl_β (ml/min)	AUC (μg. h/ml)	C_{max} (μg/ml)
1	27.6	26.5	4.16	0.473	1.47	9.24	16.9	132.8	62.8	54.2
2	40.7	36.2	4.19	0.442	1.57	6.50	12.4	91.0	91.6	76.8
3	48.3	24.7	5.45	0.517	1.34	6.85	17.1	147.2	56.6	73.0
Average	38.7	28.9	4.55	0.467	1.48	7.40	15.2	118.4	70.4	67.6

[a] Blood samples were collected at 5, 15, and 30 min and at 1, 2, 3, 4, and 6 h after a 0.5-g intravenous bolus injection of CZX. AUC, Area under the curve.

TABLE 2. *Pharmacokinetic parameters of CZX in patients with renal dysfunction*

Group	V_d (liters)	K_{el} (h^{-1})	$T_{1/2}$ (h)
I. Healthy volunteers (C_{cr}: 120, 117, 115, 112, 105; $n = 5$)	15.8	0.522	1.33
II. Normal and slightly impaired ($C_{cr} > 60$: 116, 60.3; $n = 2$)	12.4	0.480	1.44
III. Moderately impaired ($60 \geqq C_{cr} > 30$: 53, 49, 46, 39; $n = 4$)	13.3	0.282	2.46
IV. Severely impaired ($30 \geqq C_{cr} > 10$: 29, 12; $n = 2$)	15.5	0.086	8.07
V. Anuric (C_{cr}: 0, 0, 0; $n = 3$)	15.6	0.026	26.56

half-life will result in therapeutic and nontoxic serum levels in patients with impaired renal function (1); the appropriate intervals between doses of CZX, in varying degrees, depending on the stage of renal failure, were calculated by using equation 1.

In the case of treatment with CZX, the dose intervals were 8 h in patients with C_{cr} values of more than 60 ml/min, 8 to 12 h in patients with C_{cr} values of 30 to 60 ml/min, 12 to 24 h in patients with C_{cr} values of 10 to 30 ml/min, and 24 to 48 h in patients with C_{cr} values of 10 ml/min or less.

On the other hand, another therapeutic regimen is also used: the dose interval in patients with impaired renal function is the same as that in patients with normal renal function, and a single dose is reduced relative to the severity of renal impairment. In the case of administration of highly safe drugs like CZX, the maintenance dose is determined to make the maximum serum levels of both groups equal in steady state. The maintenance dose in patients with renal dysfunction can by derived from the following equation. Maintenance dose:

$$\hat{D} = D \cdot \left(\frac{1 - e^{-\hat{K}_{el} \cdot T}}{1 - e^{-K_{el} \cdot T}}\right) \tag{2}$$

Since in patients with impaired renal function it may take a long time to reach the steady state in comparison with patients with normal renal function, an initial dose is determined to make the serum level at T hours, the dose interval time after first dosing, equal to the minimum serum level in steady state. Initial dose:

$$\hat{D}^* = \hat{D} \cdot \left(\frac{1}{1 - e^{-\hat{K}_{el} \cdot T}}\right) = D \cdot \left(\frac{1}{1 - e^{-K_{el} \cdot T}}\right)$$

An initial dose can be calculated from the above equation. When a dose interval of 8 or 12 h and K_{el} values obtained from equation 1 are substituted in the above equation, the initial dose in patients with impaired renal function ($\hat{D}^*$) is almost equal to that in patients with normal renal function, since $\hat{D}^*$ is equal to D, regardless of renal function.

For example, when patients with a C_{cr} value of 10 ml/min acquire serious infections, which in patients with normal renal function are treated in a dose of 0.5 g of CZX every 8 h, they must be administered 0.5 g of CZX as an initial dose. The maintenance dose (0.24 g) is calculated from equations 1 and 2.

1. **Cutler, R. E., and B. M. Orne.** 1969. Correlation of serum creatinine concentration and Kanamycin half life. J. Am. Med. Assoc. **209:**539–542.

Ceftizoxime: Pharmacokinetics and Clinical Evaluation in Respiratory Tract Infection

AKIRA SAITO, EIONOSUKE ODAGAKI,* AND MASUMI TOMIZAWA

The Second Department of Internal Medicine, Hokkaido University School of Medicine, Sapporo, Japan

Ceftizoxime (CZX) is a new cephalosporin antibiotic developed in the Research Laboratories of Fujisawa Pharmaceutical Co., Ltd., Osaka, Japan. Having a unique chemical structure in that it lacks a side chain at the 3-position, this antibiotic is active against various clinically important pathogens that have defied conventional cephalosporin antibiotics. The organisms that are suppressed clinically by this new substance include *Haemophilus influenzae*, indole-positive *Proteus* spp., *Citrobacter*, *Enterobacter*, and *Serratia* spp., the latter three holding an important position as opportunistic pathogens, and *Bacteroides fragilis* and other anaerobic organisms, as well as *Escherichia coli*, *Klebsiella pneumoniae*, and *Proteus mirabilis* (1, 2). This paper is concerned with a study of the pharmacokinetics and clinical efficacy of this agent.

The subjects were six healthy male volunteers without abnormal laboratory findings or a history of allergy to penicillins or cephalosporins. They had taken no medication for 1 month preceding this study. They ranged from 21 to 28 years of age (mean: 22.8 years), from 57 to 80 kg (mean: 64.8 kg) in body weight, from 163 to 177 cm (mean: 167.8 cm) in height, and from 99.3 to 115.8 ml/min (mean: 105.5 ml/min) in creatinine clearance. They were divided into two groups and given 1 g of CZX by an intravenous drip infusion either in 250 ml of physiological saline given over a period of 1 h or in 500 ml of the fluid given over 2 h. The same procedure was conducted at an interval of 1 week to complete a crossover study. Blood and urine specimens were also tested for CZX concentration by a paper disk method using *Bacillus subtilis* ATCC 6633 as the test organism and sodium citrate medium as the test medium. In the assay of concentration in serum, the appropriate standard curve was made by using human serum. For the urine sample, 1/15 M phosphate buffer solution (pH 7.0) was used as the diluent. The blood specimens were examined for changes in biochemical findings.

The mean serum levels, serum half lives ($T_{1/2}$), and urinary concentrations are summarized in Fig. 1. When infusion was over a period of 1 h, the serum levels were 27.5 to 45.0 μg/ml (mean: 34.7 μg/ml) 30 min after the beginning of infusion and at the end of infusion attained a peak of 64.0 to 76.0 μg/ml (mean: 69.0 μg/ml). The levels tapered off after termination of the infusion, with mean levels of 50.8 μg/ml at 15 min, 29.8 μg/ml at 30 min, 19.8 μg/ml at 1 h, 9.8 μg/ml at 2 h, and 3.4 μg/ml at 4 h and with a $T_{1/2}$ of 1.33 h and an area under the serum level curve (AUC) of 103.5 μg.hr/ml. When the drug was injected over 2 h, the serum levels were 14.5 to 18.5 μg/ml (mean: 16.8 μg/ml) 1 h after the beginning of infusion, and levels peaked at 26.0 to 37.0 μg/ml (mean: 30.6 μg/ml) at the end of the infusion. The serum levels after the end of infusion were 21.3 μg/ml at 15 min, 16.5 μg/ml at 39 min, 12.2 μg/ml at 1 h, 5.7 μg/ml at 2 h, and 1.6 μg/ml at 4 h, with a $T_{1/2}$ of 1.06 h and an AUC of 69.0 μg.hr/ml.

The urinary excretion was as follows. The mean recovery in the first 2-h urine sample was 562 (= 315 + 247) mg (56.2%) for the 1-h infusion and 510 mg (51.0%) for the 2-h infusion. The 6-h urinary recovery was 824.8 mg (82.5%) and 860.9 mg (86.1%), respectively. The mean highest urinary level, which may vary with urinary volumes taken, was 4,125 μg/ml (1- to 2-h urine samples) for the 1-h infusion and 6,233 μg/ml (0- to 2-h urine samples) for the 2-h infusion. No contributory abnormalities were detected in GOT, GPT, alkaline phosphatase, BUN, or serum creatinine of the blood specimens collected during these periods.

The subjects were 16 patients with moderate to severe respiratory tract infection (9 with pneumonia, 5 with chronic bronchitis, and 2 with purulent infection of the lung) who were admitted between August 1978 and February 1979 to the Second Department of Internal Medicine, Hokkaido University Hospital, Sapporo, Japan, and affiliated hospitals. They were without a history of drug allergy, and their skin tests were negative for CZX. They were 10 males and 6 females, ranging in age from 26 to 81 (mean: 51.8). The daily dose was 2 to 4 g, which was given by intravenous drip infusion in two divided doses. The period of administration was essentially 14 days.

The assessment of therapeutic effectiveness was ensured by biological follow-up of the sputum for cure, cure associated with relapse, and superinfection. The cessation of expectoration

TABLE 1. *Effectiveness of CZX*

Organisms isolated	No. of strains	Bacteriological effectiveness: Cure	Persisted	MIC_{80}[a] (μg/ml)
S. aureus	1	1	0	3.13[1)]
S. pneumoniae	4	4	0	0.05[1)]
H. influenzae	4	4	0	≦0.025[1)]
K. pneumoniae	3	3	0	≦0.025[1)]
S. marcescens	1	1	0	1.56[1)]

Diagnosis	No. of Patients	Clinical effectiveness: Excellent	Good	Fair	Poor
Pneumonia	9	3	3	2	1
Chronic bronchitis	5	2	2	1	0
Purulent infection of the lung	2	2	0	0	0

[a] MIC of CZX; inoculum size, 10^6 cells per ml. 1), Reference 1.

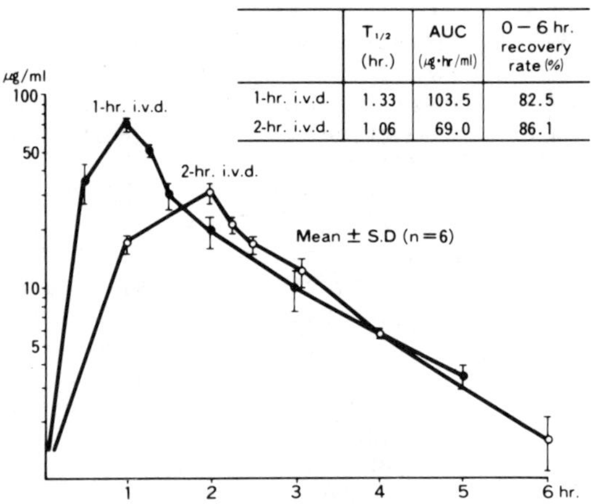

FIG. 1. *Serum levels of CZX after an intravenous dose (i.v.d.) of 1 g.*

was regarded as cure. Some clinical isolates were tested for MIC of CZX. Therapeutic effectiveness, with this understanding, is hereafter defined as "overall clinical efficacy," which was classified by doctors in charge into four groups, including "excellent," "good," "fair," and "poor."

The results are summarized in Table 1. The ratio of effectiveness by diagnosis was 78% for pneumonia, 80% for chronic bronchitis, and 100% for purulent infection of the lung. The overall effectiveness rate was as high as 81.3% (13 of 16). Bacteriologically, CZX proved to be highly active, affording 100% eradication and low MIC values against *Streptococcus pneumoniae*, *H. influenzae*, and *K. pneumoniae*, as exemplified by the MIC of 1.56 μg/ml against *Serratia marcescens*. Side effects, which developed 7 days after the beginning of treatment and consisted of rash and itching in one patient each, were not so severe as to necessitate discontinuation of treatment.

CZX is among the so-called new-era cephalosporins. It has structural resemblance to cefotaxime but differs in that it lacks an alkyl chain at the 3-position. This characteristic makes CZX stable to deacetylation, which is seen with cefotaxime.

The mean serum levels at the end of 1- and 2-h intravenous infusions of 1 g were as high as 69.0 and 30.6 μg/ml, respectively, which are comparable to those obtained by other investigators (1). The $T_{1/2}$ of CZX appeared to be intermediate among the new cephalosporins. The satisfactory urinary recovery, which was as high as 80% in the form of unchanged compound in 6-h urine samples, may give this substance another use in the treatment of urinary tract infections.

The rate of overall clinical efficacy as high as 81.3% agreed well with satisfactory biological activities against the causative organisms. Side effects, rash and itching seen in only one patient each, were not so severe as to require withdrawal of the drug, but require the clinician's attention before its use.

1. **Hara, K.** 1980. FK 749. Chemotherapy (Tokyo) **28:**639–647.
2. **Kamimura, T., Y. Matsumoto, N. Okada, Y. Mine, M. Nishida, S. Goto, and S. Kuwahara.** 1979. Ceftizoxime (FK 749), a new parenteral cephalosporin: in vitro and in vivo antibacterial activities. Antimicrob. Agents Chemother. **16:**540–548.

Pharmacokinetics and Clinical Evaluation of Ceftizoxime in Obstetrics and Gynecology

N. CHO* AND Z. TAKASE

Showa University School of Medicine, Tokyo, and Kawasaki Medical School, Okayama, Japan*

With the aim of assessing the usefulness of ceftizoxime (CZX) in obstetric and gynecological fields, an attempt was made in 18 institutions in different districts of Japan to investigate the antibacterial activity of the antibiotic and its transfer to uterine tissues and retroperitoneal space exudates and also to evaluate the clinical benefit of its use in obstetric and gynecological infections.

The concentration of CZX at which it can inhibit the growth of 80% of the bacterial strains isolated as causative organisms for obstetric and gynecological infections was determined on 226 strains of aerobic and 18 strains of anaerobic organisms. The concentration was 0.1 μg/ml or below for most gram-negative rods, 6.25 μg/ml for *Staphylococcus aureus*, 3.13 μg/ml for *Bacteroides* spp., and 0.78 μg/ml for *Peptococcus* spp.

Determination was made of the concentration of CZX in uterine and adnexal tissues after intravenous bolus injection of 1 g in 42 patients undergoing total hysterectomy. The values of serum and uterine tissue concentrations were analyzed by first-order kinetics, using the NONLIN program to give pharmacokinetic parameters. These data were well described by first-order kinetics. The coefficient of correlation between the concentration in tissues and its regression line was 0.696 to 0.901. The half-life of the antibiotic was 0.9 h in venous blood serum, 2.6 h in the endometrium, 1.1 h in the myometrium, 1.3 h in the cervix, 0.99 h in the fallopian tube, and 1.4 h in the ovary. The estimated concentrations of the antibiotic in uterine tissues and the concentrations at which it inhibited the growth of 80% of clinically isolated strains are shown in Fig. 1. The latter concentration for *S.*

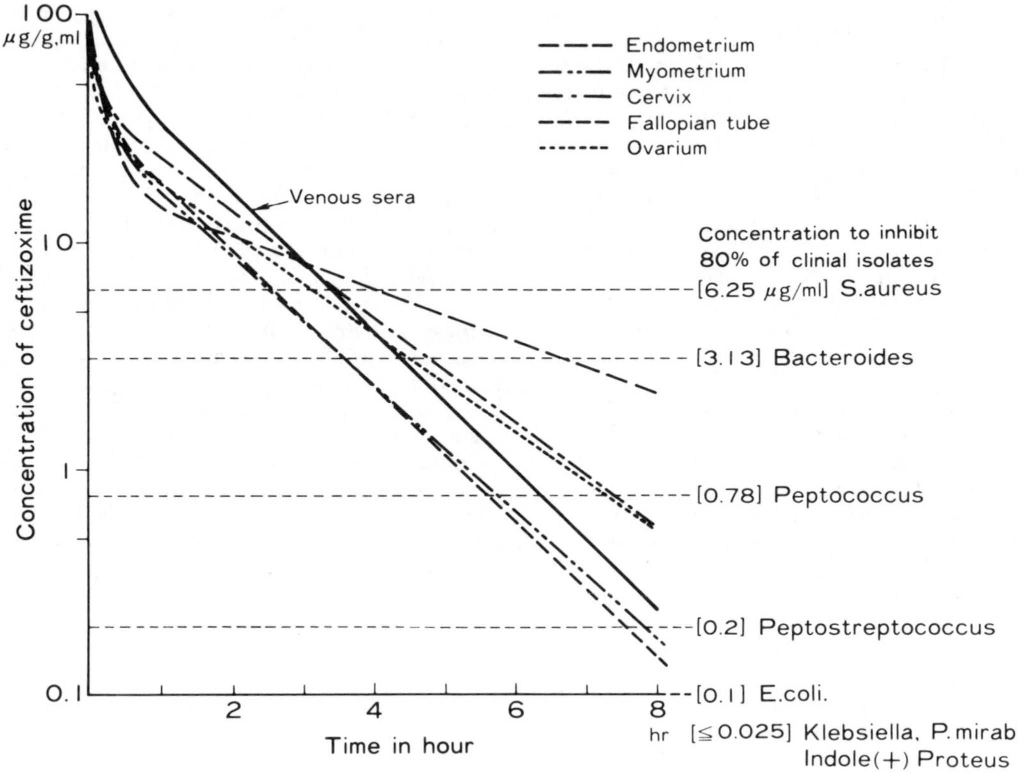

FIG. 1. *Concentrations of CZX in uterine tissues after a 1-g intravenous bolus injection.*

TABLE 1. *Bacteriological response to CZX*

Organism	No. of strain	Eradicated (%)	Persisted
Gram (+) cocci			
S. aureus	15	15 (100 %)	
S. epidermidis	12	10 (83.3%)	2
S. faecalis	12	8 (66.7%)	4
Others	5	5	
sub-total	44	38 (86.4%)	6
Gram (−) rods			
E. coli	44	39 (88.6%)	5
Klebsiella	14	13 (92.9%)	1
P. mirabilis	2	1	1
Indole (+) Proteus	5	4	1
Enterobacter	9	9 (100 %)	
Others	5	5	
sub-total	79	71 (89.9%)	8
Anaerobes			
Peptococcus	14	14 (100 %)	
Peptostreptococcus	4	2	2
B. fragilis	10	6 (60 %)	4
Bacteroides sp.	6	6	
Others	6	6	
sub-total	40	34 (85.0%)	6
Total	163	143 (87.7%)	20

aureus and *Bacteroides* spp. was maintained for 2.5 and 3.5 h, respectively, and that for aerobic gram-negative rods was maintained for over 8 h. Similarly, a study was made of the concentration of CZX in uterine and adnexal tissues after intravenous drip infusion of 1 g in 1 h in 152 patients. The concentration of the antibiotic attained in tissues immediately after drip infusion (at 1 h) and the antibiotic half-life were 71.7 μg/ml and 1.8 h in serum, 19.5 μg/g and 1.1 h in the endometrium, 21.0 μg/g and 1.0 h in the myometrium, 25.4 μg/g and 1.2 h in the cervix, 20.7 μg/g and 1.5 h in the ovary, and 20.1 μg/g and 1.3 h in the fallopian tube. The duration of the concentration at which the antibiotic inhibited the growth of 80% of the organisms of different species was similar to that found with intravenous injection.

In 15 postoperative patients undergoing total hysterectomy, retroperitoneal space exudates were collected through a drain after intravenous drip infusion of 1 g of CZX in 1 h. The concentration of the antibiotic in the exudate was 1.05 to 39.7 μg/ml (mean, 14.8 μg/ml) at 1 h (at end of infusion), reaching a peak 2 h after administration of 12.5 to 55.0 μg/ml (mean, 25.5 μg/ml) and remaining as high as 1.62 to 18.0 μg/ml (mean, 6.81 μg/ml) even at 8 h. Theoretically, the peak concentration was 25.5 μg/ml, which was to have been attained at 2.2 h, and the half-life was 1.8 h.

The clinical benefit of the antibiotic was examined in 151 patients with obstetric or gynecological infections treated with 1 to 4 g of the antibiotic daily. The antibiotic proved useful in 47 of 48 patients with uterine infection, 51 of 57 patients with adnexal infection, 29 of 32 patients with intrapelvic infection, and 11 of 14 patients with infection of the external genitalia, that is, in 138 (90.2%) of 151 patients in all. The bacteriological effect of the antibiotic is shown in Table 1. Treatment with the antibiotic resulted in elimination of 143 (87.7%) of 163 strains of causative organisms.

Adverse reactions observed included facial redness and itching in 2, diarrhea in 2, facial redness or flush in 1, and a mild increase in GOT and GPT in 3 patients.

In summary, CZX was transferred to genital tissue and postoperative retroperitoneal space exudates in concentrations higher than the MIC for the majority of clinically isolated organisms. The antibiotic also was useful in eliminating a large proportion of causative organisms. It may be concluded that CZX is of value in the treatment of obstetric and gynecological infections and in the prevention of postoperative infection.

Pharmacokinetics of Ceftizoxime and Its Clinical Applications in Patients Undergoing Hemodialysis

MASAHIDE TAKII,* OSAMU RIKITAKE, TAKATOSHI OTONARI, YOSHIRO SAWAE, AND KAORU OKADA

Second Department of Internal Medicine, Fukuoka University School of Medicine, and First Department of Internal Medicine, Faculty of Medicine, Kyushu University, Fukuoka, Japan*

Ceftizoxime (CZX), a new cephalosporin, has exhibited an activity greater than that of previously introduced cephalosporins against gram-negative rods, particularly indole-positive *Proteus*, *Enterobacter*, and *Serratia* spp. (1, 2), and is effective in the treatment of infections caused by these susceptible organisms. It is excreted unchanged mainly by the kidney, and toxicity may be increased in patients with impaired renal function.

We have made an attempt to establish its pharmacokinetics in patients on maintenance hemodialysis, in search of recommendable dosage schedules for these patients.

The subjects were 11 patients on maintenance hemodialysis (6 males and 5 females whose creatinine clearances were less than 5 ml/min). Their ages ranged from 39 to 65 years, and body surface areas ranged from 1.17 to 1.68 m^2 (mean: 1.47 m^2). The efficiency of a 6-h hemodialysis session, as determined by creatinine clearance, ranged from 63.4 to 130 ml/min (mean: 100.5 ml/min).

The study was in a crossover design and allowed three or more hemodialysis sessions to elapse between the paired tests.

Nine patients were given 500 mg of CZX intravenously over a 5-min period at the beginning of a hemodialysis session. Four of them participated in the crossover study with this dose. Three patients received one-half that dose of 250 mg during hemodialysis and between the dialysis sessions. Blood specimens were collected at selected time intervals up to 6 h (during dialysis) or up to 24 h (between dialysis sessions) after CZX administration and assayed for serum concentration by the agar diffusion method, using *Escherichia coli* NIHJ JC-2 as the test organism.

Table 1 lists the pharmacokinetic parameters calculated from the mean values of A, B, α, and β of the patients.

The theoretical C_{max} values between dialysis sessions for 500 and 250 mg of CZX were 48.9 and 28.1 μg/ml, respectively, and $T_{1/2\beta}$ values were 28.8 and 46.8 h. In patients on maintenance hemodialysis, C_{max} was reduced and $T_{1/2\beta}$ was prolonged markedly compared with those of normal subjects (3, 4).

During dialysis, C_{max} rose to the normal values and $T_{1/2\beta}$ was markedly shortened to 4.47 and 3.15 h, though still about three times as long as the normal values.

Computer-derived serum CZX levels, together with the mean actual levels, are shown in Fig. 1. Excellent agreement ($r > 0.98$) was obtained between the computer-derived and actual serum levels.

Using these parameters, we devised the following three different dosage schedules for the clinical study: mode 1, 500 mg of CZX at the end of each hemodialysis; mode 2, 250 mg of CZX at the same time as described for mode 1; and mode 3, 250 mg at the end of each dialysis and an additional 100 mg every 24 h between sessions. The predicted trough serum concentrations after

TABLE 1. *Pharmacokinetic parameters of CZX*[a]

CZX given intravenously	C_{max}	K_{12} (h^{-1})	K_{21} (h^{-1})	K_{el} (h^{-1})	$T_{1/2\alpha}$ (h)	$T_{1/2\beta}$ (h)	Vd_β (liters per body)	Cl (ml/min)	AUC (μg.h/ml)
Between dialyses									
500 mg ($n = 4$)	48.9	0.880	2.900	0.0313	0.18	28.8	13.3	5.3	1,560
250 mg ($n = 3$)	28.1	0.288	0.647	0.0215	0.73	46.8	12.9	6.6	1,309
During dialysis									
500 mg ($n = 9$)	71.8	1.621	1.172	0.401	0.22	4.47	18.1	46.8	178
250 mg ($n = 3$)	51.5	1.403	1.857	0.408	0.20	3.15	8.9	32.9	126

[a] Figures in each parameter show the mean values of all patients. The number of patients studied in each experiment is shown within parentheses. AUC, Area under the curve.

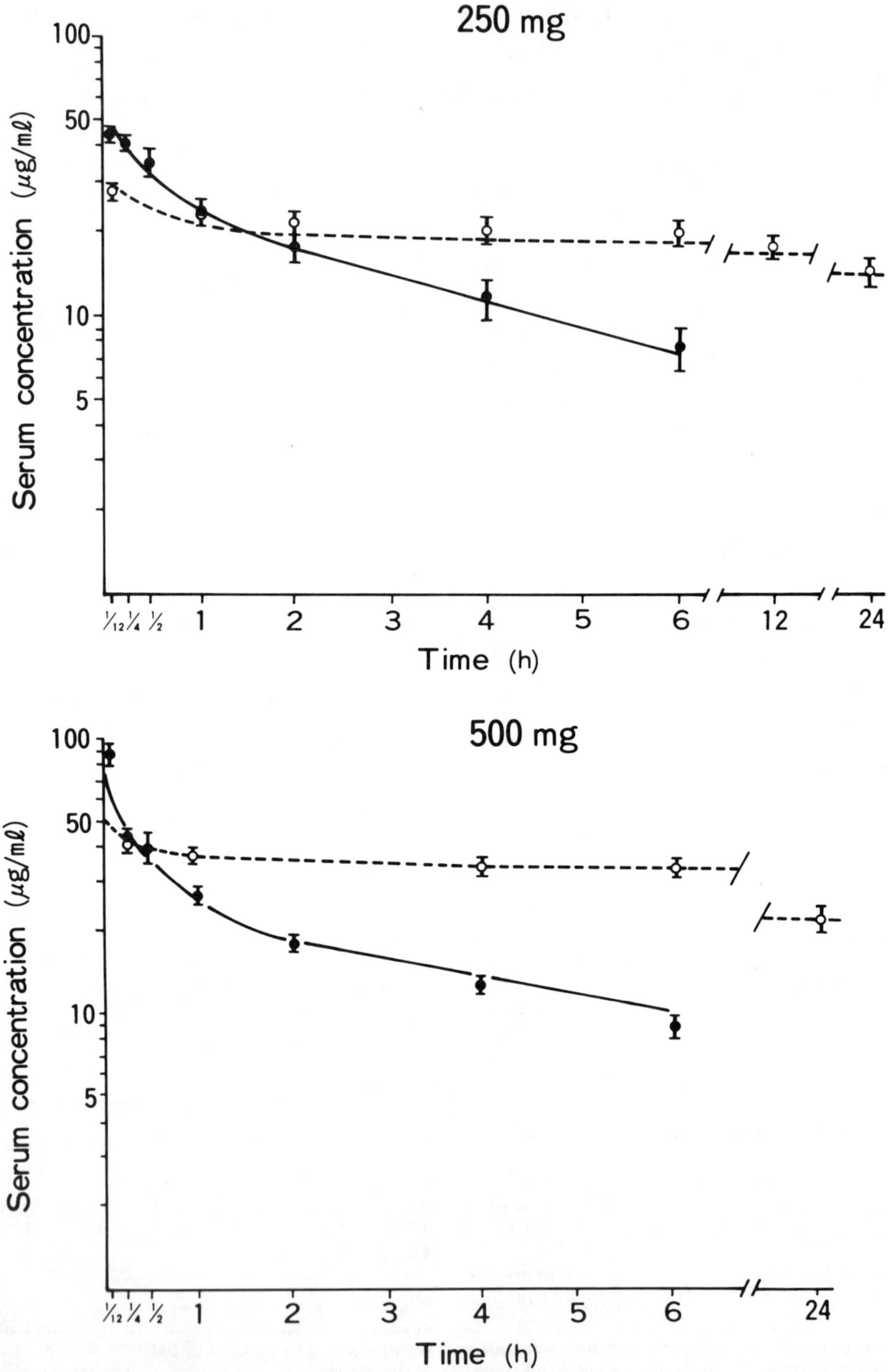

FIG. 1. *Simulated serum concentration of CZX after intravenous bolus injection. ——, During hemodialysis; ----, at interdialysis period; ●, mean serum CZX concentration with standard error during hemodialysis; ○, mean serum CZX concentration with standard error at interdialysis period.*

these three schedules were 2.74, 2.65, and 5.11 μg/ml, respectively, and are considered to be high enough to suppress infections caused by most gram-negative rods.

Four patients, described below, were treated by these dosage schedules.

A 44-year-old woman was cured of upper urinary tract infection due to *E. coli* by mode 3 for 11 days.

A 52-year-old man with spiking fever after thrombectomy was treated by mode 1. Blood cultures grew *Staphylococcus aureus*. The MIC of CZX against this organism was 25 μg/ml. Lincomycin in substitution for CZX led to a salutary response.

A 42-year-old man had suffered from chronic cellulitis on his left leg associated with intermittent fever. Culture of a specimen taken from the affected area grew *Pseudomonas aeruginosa*. Piperacillin, cefsulodin, and aminoglycosides were without effect. Treatment by mode 2 for 19 days alleviated his fever.

A 17-year-old woman developed thrombophlebitis on a site of a cutaneous arteriovenous fistula. No organism was recovered from the blood. Treatment by mode 1 for 12 days resolved her inflammation.

CZX was effective in three of the four patients. No side effect was detected in any of the four patients.

The actual serum CZX concentrations in these patients correlated well with those predicted.

We believe that CZX is clinically useful in the treatment of infections in patients on maintenance hemodialysis, especially when used in conformity with our proposed dosage schedules.

1. **Kamimura, T., Y. Matsumoto, N. Okada, Y. Mine, M. Nishida, S. Goto, and S. Kuwahara.** 1979. Ceftizoxime (FK 749), a new parenteral cephalosporin: in vitro and in vivo antibacterial activities. Antimicrob. Agents Chemother. **16**:540–548.
2. **Nishida, M., T. Kamimura, N. Okada, Y. Matsumoto, Y. Mine, T. Murakawa, S. Goto, and S. Kuwahara.** 1979. Comparison of antibacterial activity of a new cephalosporin, ceftizoxime (FK749), with other cephalosporin antibiotics. J. Antibiot. **32**:1319–1327.
3. **Ohkawa, M., T. Sugata, A. Okasho, K. Kuroda, T. Miyagi, and T. Sato.** 1980. Pharmacokinetics of ceftizoxime (CZX) in patients with impaired renal function. Chemotherapy **28**(Suppl. 5):706–714. (Abstract in English.)
4. **Yamasaku, F., Y. Suzuki, H. Takeda, O. Sekine, and Y. Usuda.** 1980. Pharmacokinetics of ceftizoxime in adult volunteers and patients with impaired renal function. Chemotherapy **28**(Suppl. 5):338–344. (Abstract in English.)

Pharmacokinetics of Ceftizoxime in Aged Patients

T. INAMATSU,* K. SHIMADA, AND K. URAYAMA

Tokyo Metropolitan Geriatric Hospital, Tokyo, Japan

Ceftizoxime is a recently introduced cephalosporin antibiotic for parenteral use, characterized by a broader spectrum of antibacterial action compared with cephalosporins in conventional use, with profound activity against gram-negative bacilli and with notable stability to enzymatic inactivation by β-lactamases (3).

Pharmacodynamic studies in healthy volunteers demonstrated the biological half-life of the compound to be approximately 1.4 h with respect to serum antibiotic level and the 24-h urinary recovery rate to be approximately 85% of the dose given, after an intravenous bolus injection of 1 g (2).

It would be rational to assume, nevertheless, that the pharmacokinetic character of the antibiotic in elderly individuals differs from that observed in younger subjects, which eventually may indicate that dosage of the compound needs to be modified for patients of advanced age.

With a view to exploring the appropriate dosage of ceftizoxime for the treatment of infections in aged patients, we conducted a pharmacodynamic study of the compound in hospitalized aged patients with normal serum creatinine levels.

The subjects studied were 13 Japanese patients, 6 male and 7 female, with a mean age of 79 ± 8 years (mean ± SE; range, 68 to 97 years) and a mean body weight of 43 ± 9 kg (range: 24 to 57 kg). These patients had some depression of renal function associated with aging; their average creatinine clearance was 40 ml/min per 1.48 m^2 of body surface.

For comparative assessments, five younger adult volunteers were also studied. Their average age was 34 ± 4 years, and their mean body weight was 53 ± 7 kg.

Blood samples were obtained at 0.25, 0.5, 1, 2, 4, and 6 h after an intravenous dose of 1 g of ceftizoxime injected slowly over 5 min. Consecutive 2-h urine samples (0 to 2, 2 to 4, and 4 to 6 h) were collected after the injection.

Both serum and urine levels of antibiotic were determined microbiologically by the disk assay.

Figure 1 illustrates the mean serum antibiotic concentrations and excretion in the urine after an intravenous dose. The group of aged patients displayed a mean serum level of 80.1 μg/ml at 15 min after injection, which was a little higher than that in the younger adult group. At 6 h after injection, however, the serum antibiotic level in the aged patient group was still as high as 16.8 μg/ml, approximately eight times as high as that in the younger adult group.

The aged patient group showed a lower average urinary recovery rate of 66.5% during the first 6 h after injection, compared with 83.0% in the younger adult group.

The pharmacokinetic parameters were calculated with the application of a two-compartment open model and nonlinear least-squares regression analysis from the data obtained (Table 1).

As seen from the data, there was a delay in elimination of administered ceftizoxime in the aged patients, with prolongation of the biologic half-life to about 2.5 times that in the younger adult group. Elimination constants of individual aged patients showed a significant correlation with respective creatinine clearance values (r = 0.787). In view of the established fact that ceftizoxime is excreted largely by the kidneys, it seems reasonable to assume that the prolonged biological half-life of this antibiotic observed in the elderly patients after intravenous administration is attributable mainly to subclinical impairment of renal function.

In the aged patient group, the central compartment had a greater distribution volume, whereas the distribution volume at β-phase was comparable to that in the younger adult group.

An attempt was made to estimate the serum levels of ceftizoxime in aged patients after an intravenous injection by simulation with values determined for pharmacokinetic parameters in the aged patient group. The estimated serum

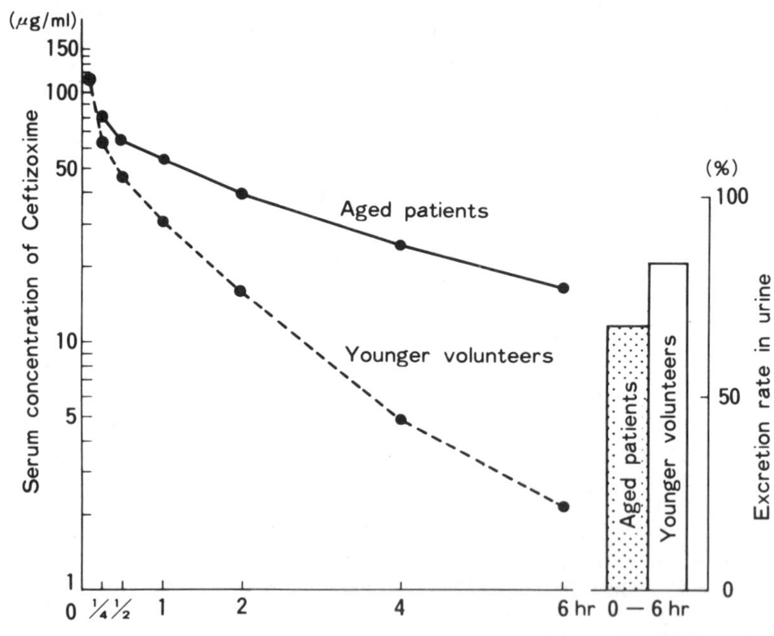

Mean (μg/ml)

	Serum concentration ¼	½	1	2	4	6hr	Urinary recovery (0 – 6 hr)
Aged patients (n = 13)	80.1	65.2	54.5	39.5	24.7	16.8	66.5%
	±4.0	3.6	3.5	2.6	1.9	1.6	± 5.1
Younger volunteers (n = 5)	64.3	46.0	31.0	16.4	4.9	2.2	83.0%
	±3.6	3.0	1.1	0.3	0.1	0.0	± 2.3

FIG. 1. *Serum concentration and urinary excretion of ceftizoxime in aged patients.*

TABLE 1. *Pharmacokinetic parameters of ceftizoxime in aged patients*

Mean ±SE

	A μg/ml	α /hr	B μg/ml	β /hr	K_{12} /hr	K_{21} /hr	Ke /hr	Co μg/ml	$T_{1/2}(\beta)$ hr	Vd l	Vc l	AUC μg·hr/ml
Aged patients	54.7 ±5.6	3.23 0.66	58.2 4.7	0.216 0.02	1.70 0.43	1.79 0.37	0.386 0.046	112.8 8.1	3.20 0.31	17.1 1.7	9.53 0.83	312 23
Younger volunteers	97.4 ±15.9	4.88 2.33	41.2 9.6	0.496 0.064	2.25 1.35	1.84 0.80	1.26 0.25	139.0 24.5	1.42 0.22	18.55 1.23	7.45 1.38	108 6

level was 112.8 μg/ml at time zero and 5.3 μg/ml at 12 h after an intravenous bolus injection of 1 g. By intravenous drip infusion with the same dose over a period of 2 h, a peak concentration of 59.4 μg/ml was estimated to occur at 2 h, followed by a decline to 6.3 μg/ml in the ensuing 10 h. These data indicate that administration yields serum antibiotic concentrations which exceed the MICs of the antibiotic against the principal pathogenic species of clinical bacterial isolates except *Pseudomonas aeruginosa*.

It would be reasonable to conclude from the results that sufficient serum antibiotic concentrations to treat severe gram-negative infections can be maintained in aged patients by intravenous administration of ceftizoxime in doses of 1 g every 12 h.

The results of the present study suggest, as already pointed out by Cockcroft (1), that renal function is impaired with advancing age in aged patients even though the serum creatinine is maintained within normal limits. It would follow, accordingly, that patients of advanced age, when treated with drugs, should be regarded as having a slight to moderate degree of impairment of renal function even though the serum creatinine level shows a normal value.

1. **Cockcroft, D. W., and M. H. Gault.** 1976. Prediction of creatinine clearance from serum creatinine. Nephron **16:**31–41.
2. **Nakashima, M., et al.** Phase I study of ceftizoxime a new cephalosporin—single dosing study. J. Clin. Pharmacol., in press.
3. **Nishida, M., T. Kamimura, N. Okada, Y. Matsumoto, Y. Miwa, T. Murakawa, S. Goto, and S. Kuwabara.** 1979. Comparison of antibacterial activity of a new cephalosporin, ceftizoxime (FK 749), with other cephalosporin antibiotics. J. Antibiot. **32:**1319–1327.

A Comparative Clinical Study of Ceftizoxime and Cefazolin in Patients with Purulent Peritonitis by the Double-Blind Method

HIROSHI TANIMURA,* NOBUAKI KOBAYASHI, AND YORINORI HIKASA

Second Department of Surgery, Kyoto University School of Medicine, Kyoto, Japan

In the chemotherapy of peritonitis, semisynthetic penicillins and cephalosporins with low toxicity are drugs of choice since the more severe the disease, the more frequently it is accompanied with renal dysfunction (1). In addition, appropriate drugs with a broad spectrum of antibacterial activity against not only gram-negative bacilli but also anaerobic bacteria must be selected for the effective treatment of peritonitis because most cases are caused by mixed pathogens.

We conducted a multicenter, double-blind comparative study of ceftizoxime and cefazolin to evaluate therapeutic effectiveness and safety against purulent peritonitis. Ceftizoxime, a new cephalosporin antibiotic, is very stable against β-lactamases and has a broad spectrum and very potent antibacterial activity, especially against gram-negative bacilli and anaerobic bacteria.

Treatment was carried out on a total of 115 patients, 56 receiving ceftizoxime and 59 receiving cefazolin. The daily dosages of ceftizoxime and cefazolin were 2 and 4 g, respectively. Each dose in a vial was diluted with 100 ml of physi-

TABLE 1. *Overall clinical efficacy*[a]

Cases	Drug	Total	No. (%) of patients with response				Effectiveness rate (%)[b]	Statistical test
			Marked	Moderate	Slight	Poor		
Total	CZX	47	13 (27.7)	25 (53.2)	8 (17.0)	1 (2.1)	80.9	NS
	CEZ	53	13 (24.5)	28 (52.8)	10 (18.9)	2 (3.8)	77.4	
Severe	CZX	25	8 (32.0)	13 (52.0)	4 (16.0)		84.0	$P < 0.10$
	CEZ	30	5 (16.7)	14 (46.7)	9 (30.0)	2 (6.7)	63.3	
Caused by perforation of stomach or duodenum	CZX	10	3 (30.0)	5 (50.0)	2 (20.0)		80.0	NS
	CEZ	14	3 (21.4)	6 (42.9)	5 (35.7)		64.3	

[a] CZX, Ceftizoxime; CEZ, cefazolin. NS, Not significant.
[b] Marked + moderate/judged cases.

ological saline and administered by intravenous drip infusion over approximately 1 h, twice daily, for 7 consecutive days.

Of the 115 patients admitted to the trial, 100 (47 on ceftizoxime and 53 on cefazolin) were eligible for efficacy evaluation, and the remainder were excluded from the evaluation because of violation of protocol. Causal diseases were perforated appendix in 55, perforated small or large intestine in 14, perforated stomach or duodenum in 24, and other perforated organs in 7 cases.

There were no significant differences between the two drug groups in the background characteristics of patients such as sex, age, body weight, type and severity of disease, and symptoms before treatment.

Table 1 shows the overall clinical efficacy of the drugs. The response to ceftizoxime was marked in 13 of the 47 patients, moderate in 25, slight in 8, and poor in 1, the effectiveness rate (marked + moderate) being 80.9%. In contrast, the response to cefazolin was marked in 13 of the 53 patients, moderate in 28, slight in 10, and poor in 2, with an effectiveness rate of 77.4%. There was no statistically significant difference between the two drug groups, although ceftizoxime was given at half the dose of cefazolin.

As shown in Table 1, however, the effectiveness rate of ceftizoxime in patients with severe peritonitis was 84.0% (21 of 25 cases) and that of cefazolin was 63.3% (19 of 30 cases), showing the greater effectiveness of ceftizoxime compared with cefazolin ($P < 0.10$). The excellent result of ceftizoxime is also supported by the following facts.

First, the effectiveness rate of ceftizoxime for peritonitis due to perforation of the stomach or duodenum, the general condition of which patients was not good, was 84.0%, and that of cefazolin was only 64.3%. Second, the reason the drug was withdrawn before 7 days of treatment was that ceftizoxime was effective in all four patients, whereas cefazolin was ineffective in one of two patients. Third, the effect of cefazolin was marked in 35.3% of the patients with localized peritonitis and 19.4% of those with diffuse peritonitis. In contrast, the effect of ceftizoxime was marked in 30.8 and 26.5%, respectively.

The usefulness rate (very satisfactory + satisfactory), as judged by each doctor, was 76.6% for ceftizoxime and 60.4% for cefazolin.

With regard to bacteriological effectiveness, the eradication rate of organisms was 91% with ceftizoxime and 87% with cefazolin, with no significant difference between the two groups.

In the safety evaluation, the data from 113 and 112 patients were included in side effects and laboratory findings, respectively. Two patients receiving ceftizoxime showed skin rash, and in one of them, skin rash was accompanied by nausea and vomiting. In the cefazolin group, transient phlebalgia and diarrhea were observed in one case each. All of these findings are, however, commonly observed in the course of cephalosporin treatment. Abnormal laboratory findings were noted in two patients on ceftizoxime (eosinophilia and mild elevation of transaminase) and two patients on cefazolin (elevation of GPT and alkaline phosphatase). The safety of ceftizoxime and cefazolin appeared to be the same.

This study showed that ceftizoxime is a more valuable chemotherapeutic agent than cefazolin for treatment of purulent peritonitis.

1. **Tanimura, H., N. Kobayashi, M. Setoyama, K. Maruyama, Y. Hikasa, et al.** 1978. Chemotherapy of peritonitis with particular reference to concentrations of sulbenicillin in human ascitic fluid. Jpn. J. Antibiot. **31:** 133–144.

Clinical Studies with Ceftizoxime (FK 749)

GEORGE W. COUNTS,* CARTER D. HILL, AND MARVIN TURCK

University of Washington, Seattle, Washington 98104, U.S.A.

Ceftizoxime (FK 749), which is the desacetoxymethyl derivative of cefotaxime, is a new semisynthetic beta-lactamase–resistant cephalosporin. Initial in vitro studies indicated that ceftizoxime extended the microbial spectrum of commercially available cephalosporin antibiotics (1, 2). The current study evaluated the in vitro activity of ceftizoxime and clinical efficacy, safety, and tolerance in the treatment of bacterial infections in hospitalized patients.

Results of testing in Mueller-Hinton agar with an inoculum of 10^5 colony-forming units are shown in Table 1. For the majority of the gram-negative bacilli tested, the MIC_{90} was less than 1.0 μg/ml. The drug exhibited good activity against isolates of *Enterobacter* species and *Serratia marcescens*. The latter strains were highly resistant to most antibiotics, including aminoglycosides, carbenicillin, and commercially available cephalosporins. The drug had little activity against isolates of *Pseudomonas aeruginosa* or enterococcus. MICs and MBCs in broth were somewhat higher than those found in agar. However, the MIC_{90} and MBC_{90} were ≦10 μg/ml for all tested isolates of *Enterobacteriaceae*, including *Serratia* and *Enterobacter* species, and of *Staphylococcus aureus*.

Of 126 adult patients who entered a study of the efficacy, safety, and tolerance of ceftizoxime, 105 were considered evaluable. This group consisted of patients with pneumonia (67), skin and soft tissue infections (33), and miscellaneous other infections (5). The usual dose employed was 0.5 to 1.0 g every 12 h, with a maximum daily dose of 6 g. Patients were excluded from analysis on the basis of insufficient drug therapy (13), absence of confirmatory diagnosis of infection (6), concomitant effective antibiotic (1), and termination of treatment because of development of rash (1).

The overall summary of the study is shown in Table 2. Satisfactory clinical and bacteriological response occurred in 94% of the patients treated (99/105).

Of the patients with pneumonia, 48 infections (78%) were caused by *Streptococcus pneumoniae* and 12 were caused by *Haemophilus influenzae*. Pneumococcal pneumonia was accompanied by bacteremia in 23% of patients. Clinical response was good in 64 of 67 patients with pneumonia (96%). Infiltrates seen on X-rays completely cleared in 33 patients and were substantially improved upon completion of therapy in an additional 29 patients. Follow-up chest radiographs were not obtained in five patients. Within 6 weeks, four patients exhibited a recurrent episode of pneumonitis, in two instances associated with a different bacterium and in two episodes associated with what appeared to be relapse infection caused by the original pathogen.

A microbial etiology was established for 20 of 33 patients with cellulitis and other skin and soft tissue infections. Practically all proved cases were associated with recovery of *S. aureus* or *Streptococcus pyogenes*. No etiology was found for 13 patients with clinically evident cellulitis (cultures were negative in eight instances and were not obtained in five others). No difference was seen in response rate for those with and without established bacterial etiology. Of these patients, 91% were cured. Five patients with *Escherichia coli* pyelonephritis, *Serratia* bacteremia, and *S. pyogenes* conjunctivitis and sinusitis were also cured with ceftizoxime. The drug was well tolerated. One patient developed a pruritic rash, necessitating discontinuation of the drug. Of 48 patients receiving intramuscular injections, one patient complained of moderate to severe injection pain. No phlebitis was seen in the 103 patients who were given intravenous infusions of ceftizoxime. Reversible elevation of liver function tests were noted in 19 of 93 patients tested (20%). Thrombocytosis occurred in approximately one-third of the patients treated

TABLE 1. *Minimal concentrations of ceftizoxime (FK 749) required to inhibit 50% and 90% of 256 isolates tested in Mueller-Hinton agar*

Isolate	No. of isolates	MIC (μg/ml)		
		Range	50%	90%
Staphylococcus aureus	29	1.0–7.5	5.0	7.5
Klebsiella sp.	30	0.015–0.06	0.015	0.03
Escherichia coli	30	0.03–0.125	0.06	0.06
Proteus mirabilis	27	0.007–0.03	0.007	0.015
Proteus sp.	28	0.007–12.5	0.06	5.0
Serratia marcescens	26	0.06–>100	0.25	2.5
Enterobacter sp.	28	0.25–50.0	0.5	2.5
Pseudomonas aeruginosa	30	12.5–>100	50	>100
Enterococci	28	1.0–>100	>100	>100

TABLE 2. *Results of treatment and adverse reactions in 105 patients treated with ceftizoxime*

Type of infection	Outcome (no. cured[a]/no. treated)	Bacteremia (no. positive/no. tested)	Thrombocytosis (no. with increase/no. tested)[b]
Pneumonia	64/67		13/34
S. pneumoniae (48)		7/30	
H. influenzae (12)		0/6	
Other (7)		1/4	
Soft tissue	30/33	1/20	4/15
Pyelonephritis	3/3	0/3	0/4
Other	2/2	1/2	

[a] Clinical and bacteriological response with adequate posttherapy evaluation. Total cured, 94%.

[b] Includes only patients with actual numerical platelet counts recorded before and after treatment. Total with increase, 32%.

(Table 2). For those patients, elevated platelet counts ranged from 406,000 to 913,000/mm^3, with a mean of 617,000/mm^3.

Ceftizoxime appears to be a promising new cephalosporin antibiotic. In addition to good antibacterial activity seen in in vitro tests, ceftizoxime given every 12 h was highly effective therapy for common bacterial infections in hospitalized patients. Three patients with serious *Serratia* infections, two of whom had bacteremia, were also successfully treated with ceftizoxime.

The exact mechanism responsible for the thrombocytosis is not certain. Possible contributing factors in our patient population were alcohol abuse, correction of vitamin or folate deficiencies, stress, and sepsis. No patient had a thrombotic episode and platelet counts returned to normal after cessation of therapy. Thrombocytosis has been previously noted in 30 to 50% of patients receiving penicillin G or cefamandole (3) and ceforanide (4). An exact causal relationship and any possible clinical significance have not been established.

1. **Greenwood, D., N. Pearson, A. Eley, and F. O'Grady.** 1980. Comparative in vitro activities of cefotaxime and ceftizoxime: new cephalosporins with exceptional potency. Antimicrob. Agents Chemother. **17:**397–401.
2. **Kamimura, T., Y. Matsumoto, N. Okada, Y. Mine, M. Nishida, S. Goto, and S. Kuwahara.** 1979. Ceftizoxime (FK 749), a new parenteral cephalosporin: in vitro and in vivo antibacterial activities. Antimicrob. Agents Chemother. **16:**549–553.
3. **Petty, B. G., C. R. Smith, J. C. Wade, G. L. Conrad, J. J. Lipsky, J. J. Ellner, and P. S. Lietman.** 1978. Double-blind comparison of cefamandole and penicillin in pneumococcal pneumonia. Antimicrob. Agents Chemother. **14:**13–18.
4. **Wallace, R. J., R. R. Martin, and S. B. Greenberg.** 1979. Ceforanide (BL-S786) in the treatment of community-acquired bacterial pneumonia. Infection **7:**176–179.

In Vitro Activity, Serum and Sputum Levels, and Clinical Effectiveness of Ceftizoxime, a New Parenteral Cephalosporin

MASAO NAKATOMI,* ATSUSHI SAITO, MASARU NASU, KEIZO YAMAGUCHI, YOSHITERU SHIGENO, AND KOHEI HARA

The Second Department of Internal Medicine, Nagasaki University School of Medicine, Nagasaki City, Japan

This paper is concerned with a laboratory and clinical study of ceftizoxime, a newly developed cephalosporin derivative.

Ceftizoxime was compared with a series of commercially available antimicrobial substances, comprised of cefazolin, cefotiam, cefamandole, cefmetazole, ampicillin, and piperacillin, for in vitro activity against 22 standard strains and 763 routine clinical isolates of gram-positive cocci, *Enterobacteriaceae*, glucose nonfermentative gram-negative bacilli, and *Haemophilus* species by the agar plate method recommended by the Japanese Society of Chemotherapy.

A suspension containing 10^6 cells of bacteria per ml was inoculated onto agar plates containing serial concentrations of the test antibiotics.

Ceftizoxime, though somewhat less active than cefotiam and cefamandole against *Staphylococcus aureus* and *Staphylococcus epidermidis*, was found to be the most active of all of the test substances against a host of test organisms, including *Escherichia coli*, *Klebsiella aerogenes*, *Enterobacter cloacae*, *Enterobacter aerogenes*, *Citrobacter freundii*, *Proteus mirabilis*, *Proteus vulgaris*, *Proteus morganii*, *Proteus rettgeri*, *Proteus inconstans*, *Serratia marcescens*, *Haemophilus parainfluenzae*, and *Haemophilus influenzae* (Fig. 1).

The mean peak serum levels of ceftizoxime

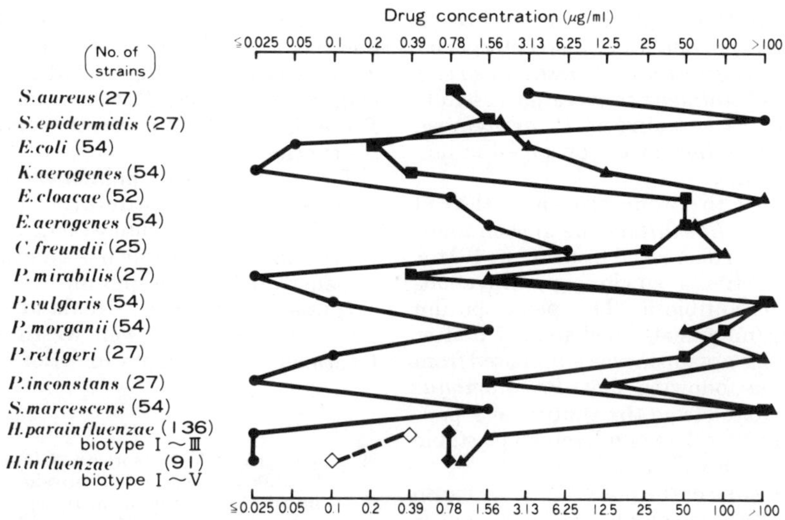

FIG. 1. *Drug concentration required to inhibit 80% of clinical isolates. Inoculum size, 10^6 cells per ml. Symbols: ●, ceftizoxime; ■, cefotiam; ▲, cefamandole; ◆, ampicillin; ◇, piperacillin.*

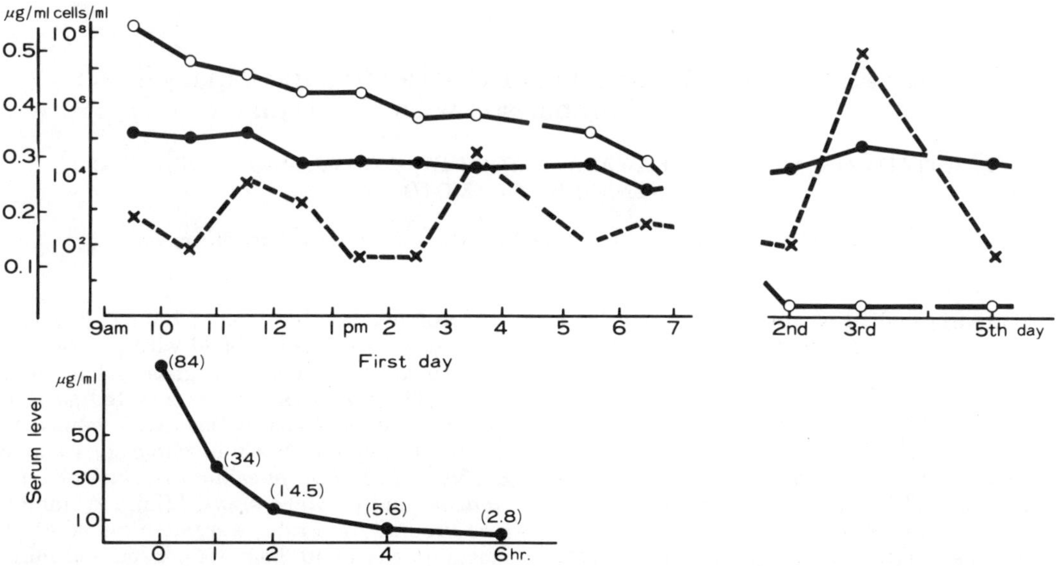

FIG. 2. *Viable count of bacteria in sputum of 46-year-old, 45-kg female with chronic bronchitis. Ceftizoxime was given twice daily by drip infusion over 1 h. Symbols: ○, viable counts of H. influenzae; ●, viable counts of Pseudomonas aeruginosa; ×, sputum levels of ceftizoxime.*

after single intravenous doses of 250 and 500 mg, given to 10 healthy adult volunteers in a crossover design, were 14.3 and 27.0 μg/ml, respectively. The recovery rate of these doses in the 6-h urine was about 80%.

The peak serum levels in 6 patients with chronic bronchitis or lung abscess who received ceftizoxime by intravenous drip infusion were 84 to 101 μg/ml when 1 g was infused over a period of 1 h and 91 to 210 μg/ml when 2 g was infused over 1 to 2 h. The urine recovery amounted to 68.3 and 95.6% in two patients.

The peak sputum levels of ceftizoxime in 6 patients with chronic bronchitis or lung abscess after intravenous drip infusion of 1 to 2 g were 0.29 to 1.8 μg/ml.

The rate of effectiveness of ceftizoxime in 23 patients with pulmonary or pleural infections who were treated with intravenous drip infusion of 2 to 4 g of this antibiotic for 7 to 16 days was as high as 78%. Bacteriologically, one strain each of *Streptococcus pneumoniae*, β-streptococcus, *Enterobacter aerogenes*, and *P. aeruginosa* and six strains of *H. influenzae* were successfully eradicated, but two strains of *P. aeruginosa* persisted. No side effects were observed in any of these 23 patients.

In one patient with chronic bronchitis, the cell count of *Haemophilus influenzae* in each milliliter of the sputum decreased from 10^8 to 10^4 for the first 10 h after a single 1-g intravenous infusion of this antibiotic. The peak sputum level of 0.29 μg/ml was attained about 7 h after the infusion. This organism was eliminated from the sputum the following day. *Pseudomonas aeruginosa*, isolated from the sputum at a population of about 10^5 cells per ml, remained stable throughout the study (Fig. 2).

Ceftizoxime is one of the potent cephalosporin antibiotics recently developed in Japan and is characterized by its strong antimicrobial activity, especially against gram-negative bacilli (1).

Our laboratory study revealed that ceftizoxime has a potent antibacterial activity against gram-negative bacilli, including *Escherichia coli, K. aerogenes, Enterobacter, Citrobacter, Proteus, Serratia marcescens*, and *Haemophilus* species.

The patients with pulmonary infections responded satisfactorily to this cephalosporin antibiotic with a high clinical efficacy rate, which proved that ceftizoxime has an excellent ability to penetrate into the sputum.

It was concluded from this study that ceftizoxime is an antibiotic well worth a try in the treatment of pulmonary infections.

1. **Kamimura, T., Y. Matsumoto, N. Okada, Y. Mine, M. Nishida, S. Goto, and S. Kuwahara.** 1979. Ceftizoxime (FK 749), a new parenteral cephalosporin: in vitro and in vivo antibacterial activities. Antimicrob. Agents Chemother. **16:**540–548.

In Vitro and Clinical Evaluation of Ceftizoxime in Urinary Tract Infection: A Comparison with Cefotiam

YOSHITADA OHI,* TAKASHI KAWABATA, TOSHIHIRO GOTO, MICHIO OBATA, AND KENICHIRO OKAMOTO

Department of Urology, Faculty of Medicine, Kagoshima University, Kagoshima, Japan

The purpose of this study was to develop a better in vitro test method for the prediction of clinical efficacy of antimicrobial agents against urinary tract infection (UTI). The test drugs chosen for this study were ceftizoxime (CZX) and cefotiam (CTM).

Minimum inhibitory concentrations (MICs) of CZX and CTM were determined against 165 strains of gram-negative rods from UTI patients. The concentration of CZX required to inhibit 80% of clinically isolated *Escherichia coli* was 0.2 μg/ml, whereas that of CTM was 0.78 μg/ml. The concentrations of CZX required for inhibition of 80% of clinically isolated strains, i.e., *Klebsiella pneumoniae, Proteus mirabilis, Proteus vulgaris, Enterobacter cloacae, Serratia marcescens*, and *Pseudomonas aeruginosa*, were less than those of CTM.

The urinary antimicrobial activities after an intravenous injection of 500 mg of CZX and 1,000 mg of CTM were determined by diluting the urine samples with Minuth's synthesized urine (1). Urine samples were collected from six healthy adult volunteers receiving the two drugs by a crossover method every 2 h for 12 h. These samples were diluted twofold with the synthesized urine, to which 0.1% glucose had been added. The test strains were selected so that they had similar sensitivities (MIC values) to the most frequent MICs of clinically isolated *Escherichia coli, K. pneumoniae, Enterobacter cloacae*, and *S. marcescens*. Minimum inhibitory tube dilution rates were determined at an inoculum size of 10^5 bacteria per ml, and minimum bactericidal dilution rates were determined by the method of Silverblatt and Turck (2).

Simultaneously obtained pharmacokinetic data of the intravenously injected drugs are listed in Table 1. Although 1,000 mg of CTM is seemingly superior to 500 mg of CZX, the latter excelled the former in the length of serum half-lives.

The recovery rate in the 12-h urine was 92.1% for CZX and 68.8% for CTM.

The rates of minimum bactericidal tube dilution, which refers to the largest serial number of dilution of the urine found to retain bactericidal activity against *Escherichia coli*, are shown in

TABLE 1. *Pharmacokinetic studies of CZX and CTM after intravenous administration*

Drug and dose (mg)	Case no.	Ke[a] (h)	Half-life (h)	V_d[b] (liter per body)	Body clearance (liter/h)	AUC[c] (μg.h/ml)	Cp (t = 0)[d] (μg/ml)
CZX (500)	1	1.048	1.27	18.46	10.11	49.45	51.82
	2	1.194	1.41	19.76	9.74	51.34	61.28
	3	1.366	1.18	18.01	10.55	47.41	64.78
	4	1.448	1.24	13.28	7.43	67.28	97.38
	5	1.440	1.21	14.49	8.30	60.27	86.76
	6	1.102	1.15	12.34	7.47	66.90	73.72
Mean		1.266	1.24	16.06	8.93	57.11	72.62
CTM (1,000)	1	2.506	0.77	15.11	13.61	73.50	184.1
	2	1.707	0.92	16.66	12.55	79.69	136.0
	3	1.978	0.90	20.12	15.53	64.38	127.3
	4	2.254	1.14	27.66	16.89	59.22	133.5
	5	2.098	1.38	37.11	18.62	53.71	112.7
	6	1.794	1.22	28.68	16.31	61.30	110.0
Mean		2.056	1.06	24.22	15.59	65.30	133.9

[a] Ke, Elimination rate constant.
[b] V_d, Distribution volume.
[c] AUC, Area under the curve of concentration.
[d] Cp (t = 0), Peak serum concentration given by extrapolating the curve to the time t = 0.

Fig. 1. Minimum bactericidal tube dilutions were obtained by 315.2, 64, 52, 22.6, 6.5, and 1.6 times the dilution of the urine samples collected at 2, 4, 6, 8, 10, and 12 h, respectively, after CZX injection in an average of six volunteers. As a result, higher concentrations and smaller dilution rates were necessary to obtain the minimum bactericidal concentration values of CTM. No bactericidal activities were demonstrated in the urine collected 12 h after CTM injection. A similar tendency was observed against *K. pneumoniae*. When CZX was given, bactericidal activities against *Enterobacter cloacae* were evident in the urine of up to 10 h. When CTM was given, the urine was active for up to only 4 h.

Furthermore, no urine was bactericidal against *S. marcescens* when CTM was given, whereas when CZX was given, the urine was bactericidal against this organism for up to 4 h.

Consequently, the urine after an intravenous administration of CZX seems to be more active than the urine after the administration of 1,000 mg of CTM against usual urinary isolates.

CZX was given to 30 patients with chronic complicated urinary tract infections in daily doses of 1 or 2 g for 5 days. The overall effectiveness rate was 70% by the criterion proposed by the Japanese UTI Committee. The rate of eradication of urinary bacteria was 72.2%. Persisting bacteria were five strains of *Pseudomonas aeruginosa*, two strains of *Staphylococcus epidermidis*, and one strain each of *Escherichia coli*, *K. pneumoniae*, and *Serratia marcescens*.

It is well known that β-lactam antibiotics are inactivated by β-lactamases in urine (3). In the discussion of chemotherapy of UTI with β-lactam antibiotics, one should preferably take into account the overall effect, which consists of urinary drug levels, inactivation by β-lactamases, permeability of drugs to outer bacterial membranes, intrinsic antibacterial activity, and antibacterial spectra. Evaluation of antimicrobial activities of test antibiotic-containing urines may be useful in the prediction of their in vivo effectiveness.

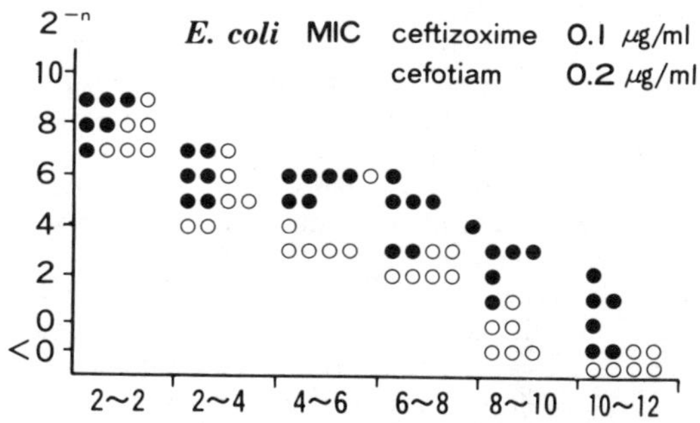

FIG. 1. *The minimum bactericidal dilution rates of urine excreted after injection of drugs for Escherichia coli. This strain was selected as the one which has similar sensitivity (MIC values) to the most frequent MICs of clinical isolates of Escherichia coli. Urine collected after the injection was diluted with synthesized urine. MICs were determined at an inoculum size of 10^6 cells per ml. Dilution rate of urine expressed as 2^{-n} is shown on the vertical line, and time (h) after injection is shown on the horizontal base line. Symbols: ●, CZX; ○, CTM.*

We determined the minimum bactericidal dilution rates of test antibiotic-containing urine against typical urinary isolates. The results of these in vitro tests may possibly reflect the clinical effectiveness of CZX on chronic, complicated UTI.

1. **Minuth, J. N., D. M. Musher, and S. B. Thorsteinsson.** 1976. Inhibition of the antibacterial activity of gentamicin by urine. J. Infect. Dis. **133**:14–21.
2. **Silverblatt, F., and M. Turck.** 1968. Laboratory and clinical evaluation of carbenicillin (carboxybenzyl penicillin). Antimicrob. Agents Chemother. **1968**:279–285.
3. **Ohi, Y., K. Okamoto, T. Kawabata, S. Momose, J. Kumazawa, S. Nakamuta, K. Eto, and N. Miyoshi.** 1979. Laboratory and clinical studies on β-lactamase in urinary tract infection. Nishinihon J. Urol. **41**:1055–1068.

Antimicrobial Activity in Urine and Clinical Efficacy of Ceftizoxime

RYOICHI SHIMAZU,* NAOKI KATO, TATSUO DOI, YUKIMICHI KAWADA, TSUNEO NISHIURA, AKIRA NISHIO, AND YOSHIAKI KUMAMOTO

Gifu University School of Medicine, Gifu, and Sapporo Medical College, Sapporo, Japan*

In vitro antimicrobial activity against urinary isolates, pharmacokinetics, antimicrobial activity in the urine, and clinical efficacy on complicated urinary tract infections of ceftizoxime, a new semisynthetic cephalosporin antibiotic, were studied.

MICs of ceftizoxime for urinary isolates of *Escherichia coli* (97 strains), *Klebsiella* (50 strains), and *Serratia marcescens* (26 strains) were compared with those of cefazolin. MICs were determined by the agar plate streak method proposed by the Japan Society of Chemotherapy (1). The MIC of ceftizoxime for *E. coli* ranged from ≦0.2 to 12.5 μg/ml, and the MIC for 70% of strains (MIC_{70}) was 0.2 μg/ml. The MIC of cefazolin for *E. coli* ranged from 1.56 to >100 μg/ml, and the MIC_{70} was 12.5 μg/ml. The MIC of ceftizoxime for *Klebsiella* ranged from ≦0.2 to 6.25 μg/ml, and the MIC_{70} was 0.2 μg/ml. On the other hand, the MIC of cefazolin for *Klebsiella* ranged from 3.13 to >100 μg/ml, and the MIC_{70} was 12.5 μg/ml. The MIC of ceftizoxime for *S. marcescens* ranged from 0.78 to >3200 μg/ml, and the MIC_{70} was 200 μg/ml. However, the MIC of cefazolin for *S. marcescens* was over 3,200 μg/ml in all of the strains tested.

Serum and urine concentrations after intravenous bolus injection of 0.25-, 0.5- and 1-g single doses of ceftizoxime and a 1-g single dose of cefazolin were determined by a crossover method in six healthy volunteers. The concentrations of ceftizoxime and cefazolin were assayed by a disk diffusion method with *Bacillus subtilis* ATCC 6633 as the test organism.

Average peak serum levels achieved 5 min after intravenous bolus injection of 0.25-, 0.5-, and 1-g single doses of ceftizoxime were 25.9 ± 2.7, 63.9 ± 4.5, and 127.3 ± 11.6 μg/ml, respectively, and were found to be related to the dosage. The half-lives were 1.44, 1.21, and 1.32 h, respectively. An average peak serum level achieved 5 min after the intravenous bolus injection of a 1-g single dose of cefazolin was 143.8 ± 11.4 μg/ml, and the half-life was 1.67 h.

Average peak urine levels achieved within 2 h of administration of 0.25-, 0.5-, and 1-g single doses of ceftizoxime were 585 ± 65, 1,424 ± 398, and 4,630 ± 1,947 μg/ml, respectively, and the urinary recovery within 8 h ranged from 89 to 93%. Urinary excretion of ceftizoxime after a 1-g single dose was quicker and urinary concentration was higher than those achieved after the administration of an identical dose of cefazolin.

Antimicrobial activities in the urine obtained after intravenous injection of various doses of ceftizoxime were compared with those of cefazolin. Urine samples collected for the determination of the urinary concentration of ceftizoxime or cefazolin were filtrated with a Seitz filter and diluted up to 2^{16}-fold with the urine of each volunteer, which was collected before the administration of antibiotics. *E. coli* GMUA-4, *Klebsiella* GMU52-2, and *S. marcescens* GMU51-6 were used as the test organisms. The MICs of ceftizoxime and cefazolin were ≦0.2 and 12.5 μg/ml for *E. coli* and *Klebsiella* and 200 and >3,200 μg/ml for *S. marcescens*, respectively. The MIC values for each test organism agreed with the MIC_{70} values for each bacterial species. The test organism was incubated in urine at 37°C for 24 h, and the urine with the maximum dilution rate in which bacterial growth was inhibited was determined. Then, all the urine specimens in which bacterial growth was inhibited were incubated on the agar plate at 37°C for 24 h, and the urine with the maximum dilution rate in which bacterial growth was completely inhibited was determined.

Antimicrobial activities in the urine obtained

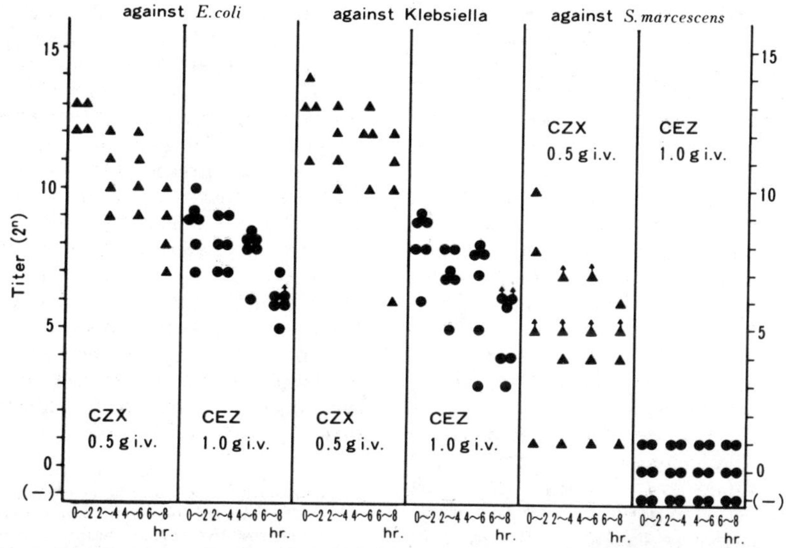

FIG. 1. *Antimicrobial activity of ceftizoxime (CZX [▲]) and cefazolin (CEZ [●]) in urine. The test organisms used and their MICs were: E. coli GMUA-4 and Klebsiella GMU 52-2, ≤0.2 and 12.5 μg/ml for ceftizoxime and cefazolin, respectively, and S. marcescens GMU 51-6, 200 and >3,200 μg/ml for ceftizoxime and cefazolin, respectively. i.v., Intravenous.*

TABLE 1. *Overall clinical efficacy of ceftizoxime in complicated urinary tract infections*

Bacteriuria \ Pyuria	Cleared	Decreased	Unchanged	Effect on bacteriuria
Eliminated	6		5	11 (55%)
Decreased			2	2 (10%)
Replaced		1	4	5 (25%)
Unchanged			2	2 (10%)
Effect on pyuria	6 (30%)	1 (5%)	13 (65%)	Case total 20

		Overall effectiveness rate
Excellent	6 (30%)	14/20 (70%)
Moderate	8 (40%)	
Poor (including Failure)	6 (30%)	

after the administration of a 0.5-g single dose of ceftizoxime were higher than those obtained after the administration of a 1-g single dose of cefazolin against each test strain (Fig. 1). Antimicrobial activities in the urine obtained after the administration of 0.25- and 1-g single doses of ceftizoxime were also higher than those obtained after the administration of cefazolin.

The clinical efficacy of ceftizoxime was evaluated in 14 male and 6 female patients with complicated urinary tract infections. Of these 20 patients, 11 had indwelling catheters. All patients were shown to have underlying urinary tract disease, pyuria of over 5 leukocytes per high-power field, and bacteriuria of over 10^4 bacteria per ml of urine. Daily doses of 0.5, 1, or 2 g of ceftizoxime were injected intravenously in two divided doses every 12 h for 5 days, and the clinical efficacy of treatment was evaluated on day 6. The overall clinical efficacy of treatment was assessed as excellent, moderate, or poor (including failure), based on the combination of changes in pyuria and bacteriuria by the criteria proposed by the Urinary Tract Infection Committee in Japan (2).

The bacteriological response to the treatment, also evaluated in each species, was defined as eradicated if bacteria identical to the original strain were not isolated after treatment and as persistent if bacteria identical to the original strain were isolated after treatment, regardless of bacterial counts.

The overall clinical efficacy of the treatment was excellent in six patients (30%), moderate in eight patients (40%), and poor in six patients (30%) (Table 1). Clinical efficacy was not related to the dosage. When overall clinical efficacies were compared between patients with and without indwelling catheters, excellent plus moderate responses were obtained in 8 (72.7%) of 11 patients with indwelling catheters and in 8 (89%) of 9 patients without indwelling catheters.

Of 25 strains isolated from the urine of 20 patients, 20 (80%) were eradicated after treatment, and only 5 strains (3 strains of *Pseudomonas aeruginosa*, 1 strain of glucose nonfermentative, gram-negative bacteria, and *Streptococcus faecalis*) were persistent. Nine strains which were not present in the urine before treatment were newly isolated from five patients (25%) after treatment. Of the nine new strains, *Streptococcus faecalis* (four strains) were predominant.

Neither side effects nor abnormal findings in laboratory tests were observed.

From the results obtained, we concluded that ceftizoxime was effective and less toxic in the treatment of complicated urinary tract infections.

1. **The Japan Society of Chemotherapy.** 1981. Standard method for the determination of minimum inhibitory concentrations. Chemotherapy (Tokyo) **29:**76–79.
2. **The Urinary Tract Infection Committee, Japan.** 1980. Criteria for the evaluation of clinical efficacy of antimicrobial agents on urinary tract infections. Chemotherapy (Tokyo) **28:**321–323.

Clinical and Laboratory Evaluation of Ceftizoxime for the Treatment of Respiratory Infections

KEIZO MATSUMOTO, HARUMI SHISHIDO,* TSUYOSHI NAGATAKE, YOSHIO UZUKA, MIKIO TAGUCHI, MASASHI YAMAMOTO, AND KIWAO WATANABE

Department of Internal Medicine, Institute for Tropical Medicine, Nagasaki University, Nagasaki, Japan

Ceftizoxime is a new semisynthetic cephalosporin antibiotic, and has an aminothiazolylacetyl group bearing a *syn* methoxyimino function at the 7-position of the cephem nucleus without the 3-substituent. Ceftizoxime is more active than other cephalosporins and cephamycins such as cefotiam, cefamandole, cefuroxime, and cefmetazole against various gram-negative bacilli (1). It is also active against such strains that have acquired resistance to related antibiotics. The activity of ceftizoxime against a wide variety of gram-positive and gram-negative organisms is due in part to its stability to both penicillinase- and cephalosporinase-type β-lactamases. The level of its stability to β-lactamases is comparable to that of cephamycin derivatives and cefotaxime and is much superior to that of cefotiam and cefoperazone (2, 5).

We have evaluated the therapeutic effectiveness of this new antibiotic on respiratory tract infections and validated this clinical performance by a concurrent microbiological study.

The in vitro and clinical antibacterial activities of ceftizoxime are summarized in Tables 1 and 2. The geometric mean MICs of ceftizoxime at 10^6 colony-forming units per ml were as follows: 0.0186 μg/ml against ampicillin-sensitive *Haemophilus influenzae*, 0.025 μg/ml against β-lactamase–producing, ampicillin-resistant *H. influenzae*, 0.046 μg/ml against *Streptococcus pneumoniae*, $\leq$0.05 μg/ml against *Klebsiella pneumoniae*, 15.4 μg/ml against *Pseudomonas aeruginosa*, $\leq$0.05 μg/ml against *Escherichia coli*, and 0.09 μg/ml against *Enterobacter* spp. Ceftizoxime suppressed respiratory tract pathogenic bacteria as strongly as did cefotaxime. It was also as active as was cefotaxime against β-lactamase–producing *H. influenzae*, which has defied ampicillin. Clinically, ceftizoxime has successfully eradicated most organisms that are known to cause respiratory infections. It was ineffective against three exceptional strains, i.e., two strains of *P. aeruginosa* and one strain of *S. pneumoniae*. The MICs of ceftizoxime against

TABLE 1. *In vitro antibacterial activity of ceftizoxime*

Respiratory pathogen	No. of strains	Geometric mean MIC of: Ceftizoxime	Cefotaxime	Cefotiam	Cefazolin	Ampicillin
H. influenzae (ampicillin susceptible)	31	0.0186	0.0175	1.42	15.8	0.35
H. influenzae (β-lactamase producing, ampicillin resistant)	18	0.025	0.025	1.56	25	>100
S. pneumoniae	51	0.046	0.0148	0.138	0.095	0.03
K. pneumoniae	27	≦0.05	≦0.05	0.187	1.38	
P. aeruginosa	33	15.4	9.2	>800	>800	
E. coli	9	≦0.05	0.062	0.066	4.4	
Enterobacter spp.	10	0.09	0.23	1.85	66	

TABLE 2. *Clinical antibacterial activity of ceftizoxime*

Causative organism (MIC[a] before treatment)	No of patients[b]	Bacteriological effect[c]: Eradicated	Partially eradicated	Persisted
H. influenzae (0.013–≦0.025)	9	9		—
S. pneumoniae (0.05)	2	2		
H. influenzae + *S. pneumoniae*	3	2	1[d]	
P. aeruginosa (100, >100)	2			2

[a] MIC (μg/ml) at 10^6 colony-forming units per ml.

[b] The group of 16 patients consisted of 11 with chronic bronchitis, 2 with pneumonia, 2 with bronchiectasis, and 1 with chronic bronchiolitis. The causative organisms were identified by the quantitative sputum culture method.

[c] None of the patients were found to be superinfected with any of the strains tested.

[d] *H. influenzae* was eradicated, but *S. pneumoniae* which acquired resistance to ceftizoxime persisted. The MIC of ceftizoxime against *S. pneumoniae* was 0.05 μg/ml before treatment but 1.56 μg/ml after treatment.

these organisms were 200, 100, and 1.56 μg/ml, respectively.

The maximum sputum levels were 0.25 to 1.37 μg/ml, with a ratio to the peak serum concentration of 1.35 to 4.66% (mean, 2.99%) in seven patients, four of whom had chronic bronchitis, one of whom had chronic bronchiolitis, one of whom had bronchiectasis, and one of whom had pneumonia. These patients were given 0.5 to 2.0 g of ceftizoxime by intravenous drip infusion twice daily. The serum half-lives of ceftizoxime in two patients with normal renal function were 1.39 and 1.58 h.

Both the geometric mean MICs and the mean maximum sputum concentrations of four cephalosporin antibiotics, i.e., ceftizoxime, cefotaxime, cefotiam, and cefazolin, are shown in Fig. 1. The test organisms used were *H. influenzae*, *S. pneumoniae*, *P. aeruginosa*, and *K. pneumoniae*, which we have proved to account for 70% of the organisms that cause respiratory infections (3).

Cefotaxime, which is structurally similar to ceftizoxime, showed an antibacterial activity similar to that of ceftizoxime, but gave way to ceftizoxime in sputum concentration, due probably to its inferior stability resulting from the 3-position substituent, which is not found in ceftizoxime.

Consequently, ceftizoxime may well be an antibiotic exceeding cefotaxime and other currently available cephalosporins in the treatment of respiratory infections.

We gave ceftizoxime to a group of 18 patients comprised of 11 patients with chronic bronchitis, 1 with chronic bronchiolitis, 2 with bronchiectasis, 3 with pneumonia, and 1 with acute tonsillitis in daily doses of 1 to 4 g by intravenous drip infusion twice daily for 4 to 15 days. Identification of causative organisms was conducted either by the quantitative sputum culture method (4) or by the throat swab culture (in one patient with tonsillitis). The organisms were identified as *H. influenzae* in nine patients, *H. influenzae* and *S. pneumoniae* in three patients, *S. pneumoniae* in two patients, *P. aeruginosa* in two patients, mixed organisms in one patient with pneumonia and nongroup A, B, C, and G β-hemolytic *Streptococcus* in one patient with acute tonsillitis. The clinical daily doses, determined taking account of the in vitro antibacterial activity, penetration into sputum, and the serum concentrations, were as follows: 0.5 and 1.0 g in 10 and 4 patients, respectively, with *H. influenzae* or *S. pneumoniae* infections or both, 0.75 and 2.0 g in 2 patients with *P. aeruginosa* infections, one with chronic renal failure and the other with normal renal function, and 1.0 g in 2 patients with miscellaneous infections. β-Lactamase–producing, ampicillin-resistant *H. influenzae* was not isolated in this study.

The results of the treatment were as follows: 15 of the 18 patients were assessed as "excellent" or "good"; 1 was "fair," with evident eradication

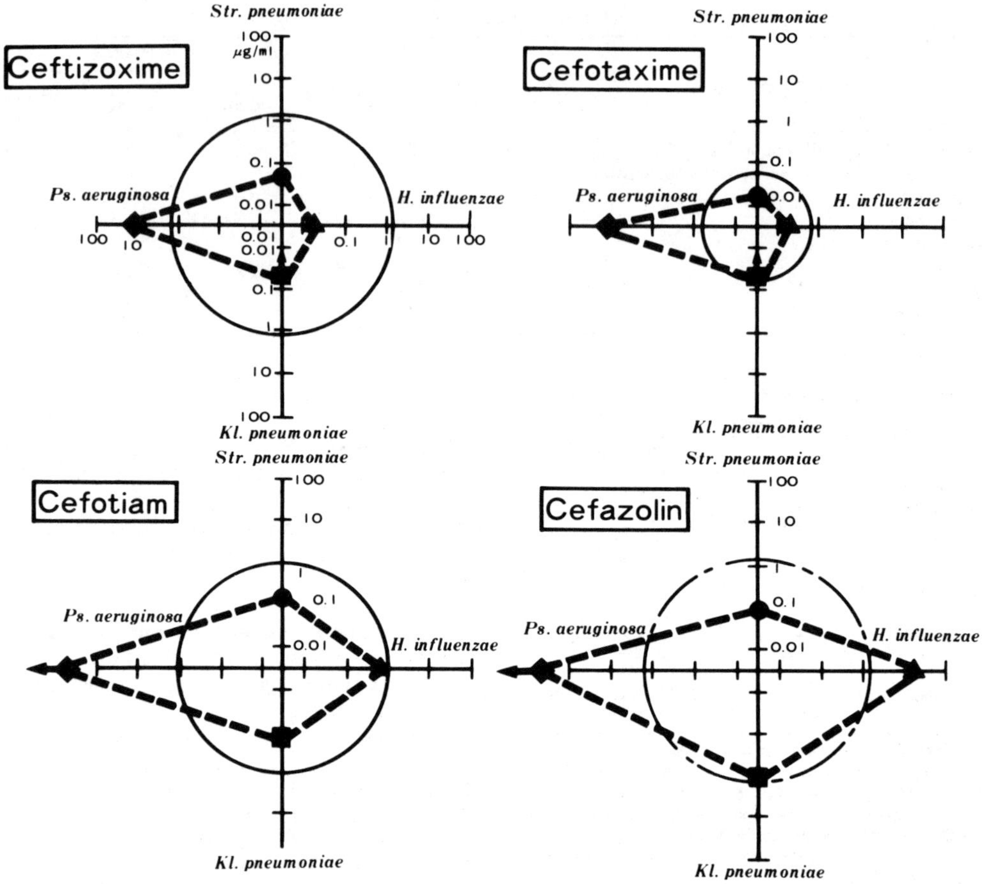

FIG. 1. *Geometric mean MICs against four major respiratory pathogens and mean of maximal sputum concentrations. Symbols represent geometric mean MICs of: S. pneumoniae (●), H. influenzae (▲), K. pneumoniae (■), and P. aeruginosa (◆). The inoculum size was 10^6 colony-forming units per ml, and the dose was 0.5 g of ceftizoxime, cefotaxime, or cefotiam (——) or 3 g of cefazolin (- - -). The large circles represent the drug concentrations in the sputum.*

of *H. influenzae*; and 2 were "poor" due to the resistance of the causative organism *P. aeruginosa*. The final rate of effectiveness was 83%. Adverse reaction occurred in only one patient who showed reversible, slight elevation of serum alkaline phosphatase.

It was concluded that ceftizoxime may well be one of the most effective and useful antibiotics for respiratory bacterial infections, particularly for those due to *H. influenzae* or *S. pneumoniae* or both.

1. **Kamimura, T., Y. Matsumoto, N. Okada, Y. Mine, M. Nishida, S. Goto, and S. Kuwahara.** 1979. Ceftizoxime (FK 749), a new parenteral cephalosporin: in vitro and in vivo antibacterial activities. Antimicrob. Agents Chemother. **16:**540–548.
2. **Kojo, H., M. Nishida, S. Goto, and S. Kuwahara.** 1979. Antibacterial activity of ceftizoxime (FK 749), a new cephalosporin, against cephalosporin-resistant bacteria, and its stability to β-lactamase. Antimicrob. Agents Chemother. **16:**549–553.
3. **Matsumoto, K., Y. Uzuka, and T. Nagatake.** 1980. Respiratory infections: the determination of causative organisms and the recent trends of respiratory infectious diseases. Infect. Inflammation Immun. **10:**359–371. (In Japanese.)
4. **Matsumoto, K., Y. Uzuka, T. Nagatake, Y. Noguchi, and H. Suzuki.** 1978. A quantitative sputum culture method: the significance of the quantity ≧10^7/ml of isolated organisms. Jpn. J. Thorac. Dis. (Nihon Kyobu Shikkan Gakkai Zasshi) **16:**77–89. (In Japanese with English abstracts.)
5. **Nishida, M., T. Kamimura, N. Okada, Y. Matsumoto, Y. Mine, and T. Murakawa.** 1979. Comparison of antibacterial activity of a new cephalosporin, ceftizoxime (FK749) with other cephalosporin antibiotics. J. Antibiot. **32:**1319–1327.

In Vitro Activity and Sensitivity to Beta-Lactamases of Cefotiam

KEVIN SHANNON,* ANNA KING, CHRISTINE WARREN, DAVID HANSLO, AND IAN PHILLIPS

St. Thomas's Hospital Medical School, London, SE1 7EH, England

The sensitivity of cefotiam to β-lactamases was assessed by the UV spectrophotometric method (2, 3). The compound, though generally more stable than cephaloridine, was hydrolyzed much more readily than cefotaxime (Table 1). However, this sensitivity to β-lactamases was not always reflected in the in vitro activity of the compound, as assessed by the determination of MICs as described before (1), since strains of *Escherichia coli* that produced plasmid-mediated β-lactamases were susceptible to the compound, as were some cephalosporinase producers (Table 1).

The activity of cefotiam against a range of clinical isolates is shown in Table 2. The compound was active against most enterobacteria, though less so than cefotaxime. Resistance to 8 μg of the compound per ml was found in 9.3% of the 400 isolates of enterobacteria (mostly *Enterobacter cloacae, Morganella morganii, Proteus vulgaris, Providencia rettgeri*, and *Serratia* spp.). Cefotiam had some activity against *Acinetobacter* spp. but no useful activity against *Pseudomonas aeruginosa* and other pseudomonads with the exceptions of *P. paucimobilis* and *P. putrefaciens* (MICs, 0.25 to 4 μg/ml). The compound was active against *Haemophilus influenzae* and *Neisseria gonorrhoeae*, including β-lactamase producers. Cefotiam was active against most staphylococci and streptococci, though less so than cephaloridine. Cefotaxime, also, was more active than cefotiam against streptococci. Both ampicillin and cefotaxime were more active than cefotiam against anaerobes.

We are grateful to Ciba-Geigy Laboratories for financial support and for providing cefotiam.

TABLE 1. *Sensitivity of cefotiam to β-lactamases*

Organism (enzyme)	MICs (μg/ml)			β-Lactamase activity			
	Cephaloridine	Cefotiam	Cefotaxime	Rate[a]	Cephaloridine	Cefotiam	Cefotaxime
Plasmid-mediated β-lactamases							
E. coli (TEM-1)	32	0.12	0.03	7.9	100	7	—[b]
E. coli (TEM-2)	64	0.5	0.06	34.7	100	10	0.2
E. coli (SHV-1)	16	0.12	0.06	0.8	100	3	—
E. coli (OXA-1)	4	0.25	0.12	0.4	100	17	45
E. coli (OXA-2)	4	0.5	0.03	0.3	100	30	—
E. coli (OXA-3)	4	0.25	0.06	0.08	100	108	—
Chromosomally determined broad-spectrum β-lactamase							
Klebsiella 1082E	>128	16	1	43.0	100	50	6
Chromosomally determined cephalosporinases							
Citrobacter freundii 11.21.75	64	0.25	0.12	1.3	100	12	—
Enterobacter cloacae P99	>128	>128	64	19.5	100	12	—
E. cloacae 4.37.76	>128	>128	16	53.5	100	64	0.3
E. coli A0211205	64	1	1	1.2	100	21	—
Morganella morganii 1036.3	128	16	0.5	17.4	100	32	—
Proteus vulgaris PC37	>128	16	1	1.2	100	108	20
Providencia rettgeri A120513	>128	16	4	18.9	100	5	0.7
P. stuartii A130118	>128	1	0.5	2.3	100	7	—
Serratia 9.2.75	>128	16	0.12	0.4	100	51	—
Pseudomonas aeruginosa 10662	>128	>128	16	1.3	100	22	—
Bacteroides fragilis 1781	>128	>64	32	23.3	100	47	31

[a] Nanokatals per milligram of protein with cephaloridine as substrate.
[b] —, Not detected.

TABLE 2. *The in vitro activity of cefotiam*

Organism (no. of isolates)	Antibiotic	MICs (μg/ml) Range	For (% of isolates) 50	75	90
Enterobacteria (400)[a]	Cefotiam	0.008 to >128	0.25	1	8
	Cefotaxime	0.004 to 128	0.06	0.12	0.25
	Cephaloridine	0.25 to >128	32	>128	>128
Acinetobacter spp. (40)	Cefotiam	0.5 to >128	8	32	64
	Cefotaxime	0.12 to >128	1	4	16
Pseudomonas aeruginosa (59)	Cefotiam	>128	>128	>128	>128
	Cefotaxime	1 to 128	8	16	64
Pseudomonas spp. (58)	Cefotiam	0.12 to >128	>128	>128	>128
	Cefotaxime	0.06 to 64	4	16	32
Haemophilus influenzae (19)	Cefotiam	0.5 to 4	1	2	2
	Cefotaxime	0.016 to 0.06	0.016	0.03	0.06
	Cephaloridine	2 to 32	8	16	16
Neisseria gonorrhoeae (39)	Cefotiam	0.016 to 2	0.06	0.12	0.5
	Cefotaxime	0.002 to 0.12	0.008	0.008	0.03
	Penicillin G	0.008 to >2	0.12	0.5	1
Staphylococcus aureus (30)	Cefotiam	0.5 to 8	1	2	4
	Cefotaxime	0.5 to 32	2	8	8
	Cephaloridine	0.016 to 1	0.06	0.25	0.5
Beta-hemolytic streptococci groups A, C, and G (40)	Cefotiam	0.016 to 0.12	0.06	0.06	0.12
	Cefotaxime	0.004 to 0.016	0.016	0.016	0.016
	Cephaloridine	0.002 to 0.008	0.004	0.008	0.008
Streptococcus agalactiae (25)	Cefotiam	0.25 to 0.5	0.25	0.25	0.25
	Cefotaxime	0.016 to.0.06	0.06	0.06	0.06
	Cephaloridine	0.008 to 0.03	0.016	0.016	0.016
Enterococci (20)	Cefotiam	64 to 128	64	64	128
	Cefotaxime	4 to >64	>64	>64	>64
	Cephaloridine	8 to >64	8	16	16
Viridans streptococci (37)	Cefotiam	0.25 to 64	0.5	2	4
	Cefotaxime	0.016 to >32	0.12	0.25	0.25
	Cephaloridine	0.002 to >1	0.03	0.06	0.12
S. pneumoniae (18)	Cefotiam	0.06 to 4	0.25	0.25	2
	Cefotaxime	0.004 to 1	0.016	0.016	0.12
	Cephaloridine	0.016 to 1	0.03	0.03	0.12
Bacteroides fragilis group (43)	Cefotiam	4 to >64	32	>64	>64
	Cefotaxime	0.12 to >64	32	64	>64
	Ampicillin	0.5 to >64	32	32	>64
Other *Bacteroides* spp. (32)	Cefotiam	0.12 to >64	2	64	>64
	Cefotaxime	0.016 to >64	0.5	2	8
	Ampicillin	0.016 to >64	0.5	4	16
Miscellaneous anaerobes (41)[b]	Cefotiam	0.016 to >64	1	8	>64
	Cefotaxime	0.016 to >64	1	2	8
	Ampicillin	0.016 to 8	0.12	0.25	8

[a] *Citrobacter freundii* (20 isolates), *C. koseri* (20 isolates), *Enterobacter aerogenes* (25 isolates), *E. cloacae* (35 isolates), *Escherichia coli* (50 isolates), *Klebsiella* spp. (65 isolates), *Morganella morganii* (20 isolates), *Proteus mirabilis* (50 isolates), *P. vulgaris* (26 isolates), *Providencia alcalifaciens* (8 isolates), *P. rettgeri* (20 isolates), *P. stuartii* (35 isolates), and *Serratia* spp. (25 isolates).

[b] *Clostridium* sp. (11 isolates), *Fusobacterium* sp. (7 isolates), *Veillonella* sp. (10 isolates), and anaerobic gram-positive cocci (13 isolates).

1. **Hanslo, D., A. King, K. Shannon, C. Warren, and I. Phillips.** 1981. *N*-Formimidoyl thienamycin (MK0787): in-vitro antibacterial activity and susceptibility to beta-lactamases compared with that of cefotaxime, moxalactam and other beta-lactam antibiotics. J. Antimicrob. Chemother. **7**:607–617.
2. **King, A., C. Warren, K. Shannon, and I. Phillips.** 1980. The *in vitro* antibacterial activity of cefotaxime compared with that of cefuroxime and cefoxitin. J. Antimicrob. Chemother. **6**:479–494.
3. **O'Callaghan, C. H., P. W. Muggleton, and G. W. Ross.** 1969. Effects of β-lactamase from gram-negative organisms on cephalosporins and penicillins, p. 57–63. Antimicrob. Agents Chemother. 1968.

Activity of Cefotiam and Other New Cephalosporins and Penicillins Against the Most Common Bacterial Pathogens

WERNER TOSCH,* HERMANN FEHLMANN, AND OTO ZAK

Research Department, Pharmaceuticals Division, CIBA-GEIGY Limited, Basel, Switzerland

Cefotiam is a potent new injectable cephalosporin antibiotic. Its inhibitory activity in vitro against the bacterial species most commonly isolated from the blood of hospitalized patients (1) was tested and compared with that of some of the newer cephalosporins and penicillins.

The minimum inhibitory concentrations (MICs) of cefotiam for 490 clinical isolates of *Escherichia coli*, *Klebsiella pneumoniae*, *Proteus mirabilis*, *Staphylococcus aureus*, *Staphylococcus epidermidis*, *Streptococcus pneumoniae* and *Streptococcus pyogenes*, derived from several hospitals in Switzerland, Germany, and the United States, were determined by the agar dilution method, using DST agar (Oxoid Ltd.) (2) and a Steers multiple-point replicator (3) with inocula of 10^4 bacteria. Ninety percent of the isolates of each species were inhibited by cefotiam at a concentration of 2 μg/ml. The streptococci proved extremely sensitive (MIC_{90} = 0.1 μg/ml) and were therefore not included in the subsequent experiments. Of each of the remaining five species, the 20 to 36 strains least susceptible to cefotiam were selected to eliminate any bias in its favor, and the MICs of cefazolin, cefamandole, cefuroxime, cefotaxime, cefoperazone, moxalactam, amoxicillin, azlocillin, and piperacillin for these strains were determined. The comparison of the numbers of strains susceptible at concentrations ≤2 μg/ml revealed that cefotiam inhibited the broadest spectrum of bacteria (Fig. 1). Cefamandole, cefazolin, and cefuroxime were relatively active against staphylococci, but only moderately so against gram-negative bacteria. Cefotaxime and moxalactam were only highly active against gram-negative bacteria. Cefoperazone, amoxicillin, azlocillin, and piperacillin inhibited only a moderate number of isolates at concentrations of up to 2 μg/ml.

To assess the activity of the antibiotics in vitro under conditions that more closely approximate their effective sojourn in the body, seven of them were incubated for short periods in a liquid medium with 32 of the least sensitive clinical isolates, including 7 strains of *Staphylococcus aureus*, 7 *Staphylococcus epidermidis* strains, 7 *E. coli* strains, 7 *K. pneumoniae* strains, and 4 *P. mirabilis* strains. The drugs were added in various concentrations to suspensions of 10^6 bacteria in 1 ml of Iso-Sensitest broth. The turbidity of the suspension was monitored at intervals of

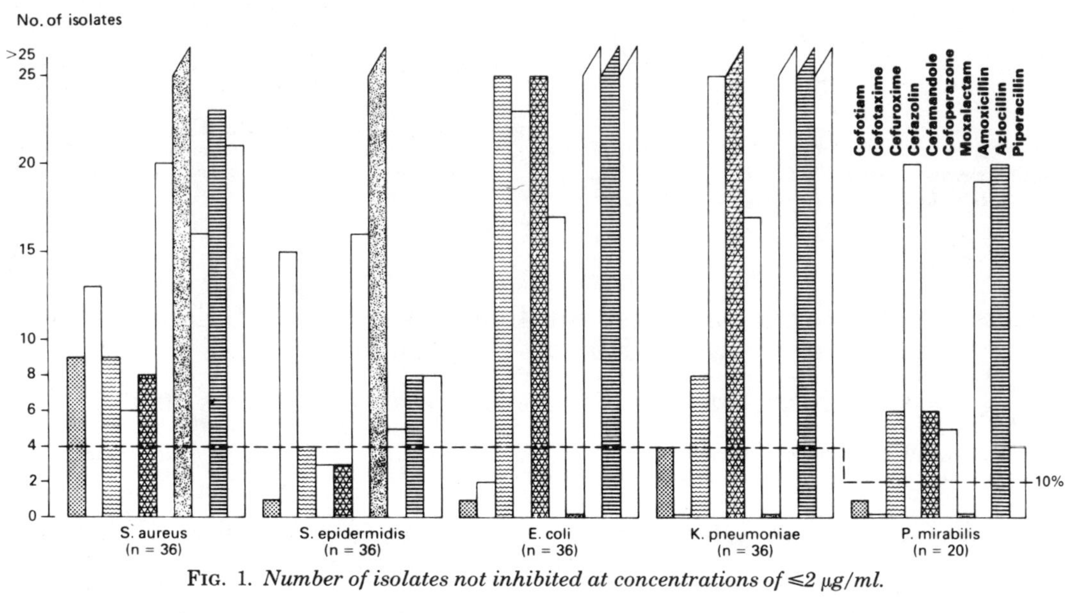

FIG. 1. *Number of isolates not inhibited at concentrations of* ≤2 μg/ml.

5 min in an Abbott MS-2 Research Device and plotted with the aid of a Hewlett-Packard HP 9825A calculator and an HP987A printer. Extinction values of ≤0.1 (approximate limit of macroscopic detectability) were taken as being indicative of growth inhibition. The minimum growth-inhibitory concentrations (MICG) for incubation times of 3, 6, and 18 h were determined graphically by measuring the retardation of growth in comparison with that of controls. The MICG at 18 h ($MICG_{18\,h}$) values were higher (generally by a factor of 2 to 10) than the MICs in the agar dilution test. Cefotiam, however, was again active against a broader spectrum of bacteria than the other drugs (Fig. 2). The comparison of the $MICG_{3\,h}$ and $MICG_{18\,h}$ values for the 32 strains showed that, in most cases, the concentrations needed to inhibit growth for 3 h were about 0.2 times those needed to inhibit growth for 18 h. It is therefore noteworthy that when MIC determinations were made in liquid medium during an incubation period of 18 h, subinhibitory concentrations down to approximately 0.2 MIC still arrested the growth of bacteria for a period of 3 h. The MICs in the agar dilution test, however, correlate fairly well with the $MICG_{3\text{-}6\,h}$ values in broth.

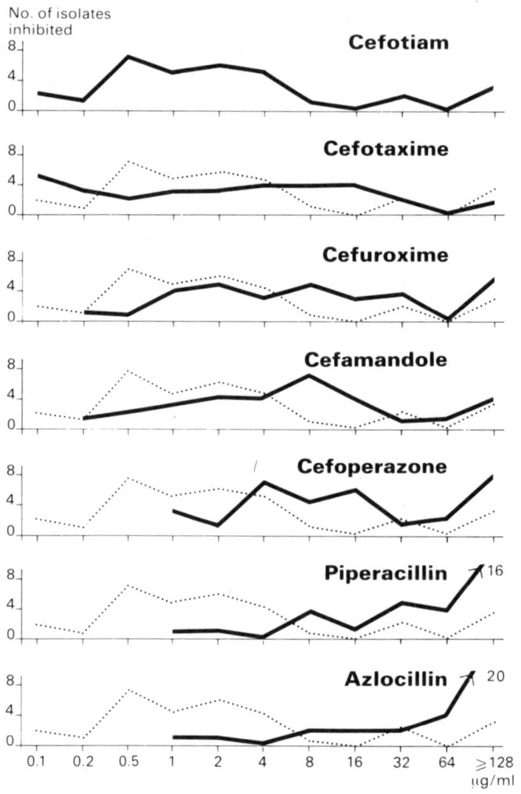

FIG. 2. *Growth inhibition of 32 clinical isolates (least sensitive to cephalosporins) after 3 h of incubation with the drugs in Iso-Sensitest broth.*

These foregoing results demonstrate that of the cephalosporins and penicillins tested in these experiments at concentrations of up to 2 μg/ml, cefotiam is active against the broadest spectrum of the most frequent pathogenic bacteria. Compared with cefazolin, cefamandole and cefuroxime, it is slightly more active against staphylococci, but distinctly so against gram-negative bacteria. Although the MICs of the newer cephalosporins cefotaxime and moxalactam for *E. coli* and *K. pneumoniae* are low, they are considerably less active against *Staphylococcus aureus* and *Staphylococcus epidermidis*, and only cefotiam was as effective as the older cephalosporins against staphylococci.

1. **Atkinson, B. A.** 1980. *In* V. Lorian (ed.), Antibiotics in laboratory medicine, p. 607–713. The Williams & Wilkins Co., Baltimore.
2. **Ericsson, M. H., and J. C. Sherris.** 1971. Antibiotic sensitivity testing. Acta Pathol. Microbiol. Scand. Sect. B, Suppl. 217 **76B:**1–90.
3. **Steers, E., E. L. Foltz, and B. S. Graves.** 1959. An inocula replicating apparatus for routine testing of bacterial susceptibility to antibiotics. Chemotherapia **9:** 307–311.

Bactericidal Potential and Post-Antibiotic Effects on Cefotiam in Broth and in Human Body Fluids

WERNER TOSCH,* FRIEDRICH KRADOLFER, OTO ZAK, AND HANS BUOL

Research Department, Pharmaceuticals Division, CIBA-GEIGY Limited, Basel, Switzerland

Cefotiam is an injectable cephalosporin that is highly active against a broad spectrum of bacteria. Its inhibitory activity was compared with that of other cephalosporins in previous studies (W. Tosch, H. Fehlmann, and O. Zak, this volume). The MICs of cefotiam were shown to be lower than those of cefazolin, cefamandole, and cefuroxime against gram-negative bacteria and lower than those of cefotaxime, cefoperazone, and moxalactam against staphylococci. The present study was carried out to assess the bactericidal potential and the post-antibiotic effects (PAEs) of cefotiam.

Viable counts of laboratory strains of *Staphylococcus aureus, Escherichia coli, Klebsiella pneumoniae* and *Proteus mirabilis* were determined after incubation of the bacteria with serial dilutions of cefotiam and cefotaxime for a defined period. A broad-spectrum β-lactamase from *Bacillus cereus* 569/H9 (Whatman, Inc.) was added to the agar plates to inactivate the drugs. Viable counts were plotted against the drug concentrations for incubation periods of 2, 4, and 6 h (Fig. 1).

The bactericidal activity of cefotiam and cefotaxime against all four species, tested in Iso-Sensitest broth, was clearly dependent on the incubation period and only to a slight extent on the drug concentration. The incubation period had only to be doubled, but the concentrations increased by more than 100-fold to induce the same bactericidal effects on *E. coli* and *P. mirabilis*. Improved bactericidal activity against *K. pneumoniae* and *S. aureus* could be achieved only through prolongation of the incubation period, and not by increasing the concentrations. When human urine (pH 7.2) from healthy volunteers was used as the medium instead of broth, a similar dependency of the bactericidal potency of cefotiam and cefotaxime against *E. coli* was evident; concentrations up to 1,024 μg/ml did not kill 2 $\log_{10}$ of cells within 2 h, but 4 μg/ml during an incubation period of 6 h did so. The same strong influence of the exposure time was demonstrable in acidified urine (pH 5.7); moreover, the bactericidal activity of the drugs diminished if the concentrations were increased above approximately 100 to 200 μg/ml. Similar conditions were found in tests with human serum from healthy volunteers: the viable count of *E. coli* and *K. pneumoniae* were scarcely influenced when the concentrations of cefotiam and cefotaxime were increased to approximately 50 μg/ml; only higher concentrations had any distinct influence on the bactericidal activity of the drugs.

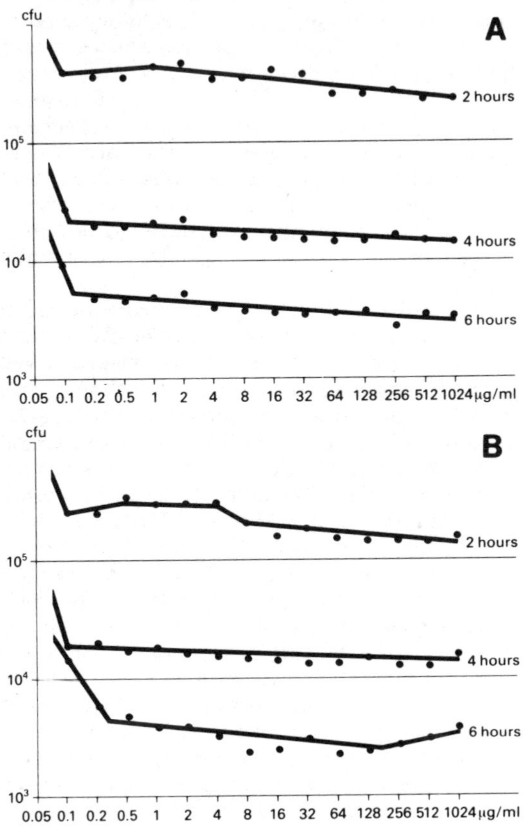

FIG. 1. *Viable counts of K. pneumoniae 327 in Iso-Sensitest broth after incubation with cefotaxime (A) and cefotiam (B). Initial CFU, 1 × 10⁶.*

Further experiments were performed to assess the PAEs, defined as the time elapsing until the viable counts increase by 1 $\log_{10}$ compared with the control culture after inactivation of the drug (1). The antibiotics were eliminated by dilution with the DST broth (Oxoid) test medium by 1:500, so that no more than approximately 0.01 × MIC was present in the culture. Significant PAEs were demonstrable with staphylococci, but not with *E. coli*. Correlations were evident between the PAEs and the preincubation time or the drug concentration. The PAEs of intraperitoneal cefotiam on *S. aureus* 2999 were 1 h after preincubation with 1 × MIC and 2 h after preincubation with 4 × MIC; it was 0.7 h after preincubation for 10 min and 1.9 h after preincubation for 90 min. The PAEs of cefotiam on two strains of *S. aureus* and two strains of *Staph-*

TABLE 1. *PAEs of cefotiam and cefotaxime on four clinical isolates of staphylococci*[a]

Organism	Drug	Concentration (μg/ml)	Postantibiotic effect (h)
S. aureus A29	Cefotiam	2	2.2
	Cefotaxime	4	1.9
S. aureus A30	Cefotiam	3	1.9
	Cefotaxime	6	1.4
S. epidermidis R14	Cefotiam	2	1.8
	Cefotaxime	4	0.6
S. epidermidis R28	Cefotiam	2	1.5
	Cefotaxime	4	0.8

[a] Concentration, 2 × MIC; preincubation time, 2 h.

ylococcus epidermidis were distinctly longer than those of cefotaxime (Table 1).

It can be concluded that the bactericidal activity of cefotiam is similar to that of cefotaxime, that incubation time has a much greater influence on the bactericidal activity of these drugs than the concentrations used, and that cefotiam exerts longer-lasting PAEs on *S. aureus* and *S. epidermidis* than does cefotaxime.

1. **McDonald, P. J., W. A. Craig, and C. M. Kunin.** 1976. Brief antibiotic exposure and effects on bacterial growth. *In* J. D. Williams and A. M. Geddes (ed.), Chemotherapy 2. Plenum Press, London.

Activity and Relative Serum and Tissue Concentrations of Cefotiam, Cefamandole, and Cephalothin in Rats with a *Klebsiella pneumoniae* Eye Infection

E. A. KONOPKA,* H. C. ZOGANAS, AND K. P. FU

Research Department, CIBA-GEIGY Corporation, Summit, New Jersey 07901, U.S.A.

Cefotiam is a new parenteral cephalosporin that is active against a broad spectrum of bacteria. The bactericidal activity of cefotiam (CT) has also been found to be more pronounced than that of either cefamandole (CM) or cephalothin (CL) against β-lactamase–producing strains of *Klebsiella pneumoniae*. At twofold multiples of the MIC, CT (2 μg/ml) produced a rapid reduction in bacteria number and total elimination upon continued exposure. CM and CL, at a concentration of 16 μg/ml, also produced a similar initial effect, but total regrowth occurred over the 24-h exposure period.

The therapeutic potential of CT was further evaluated and compared with those of CM and CL in rats infected intracorneally with a β-lactamase–producing strain of *K. pneumoniae*. All groups received intramuscular injections of 50 mg/kg twice daily for 3 days.

The therapeutic response achieved was judged on the basis of differences occurring in the gross pathology and recoveries of bacteria from the eyes of rats treated with the different antibiotics. The overall effects attained in the individual groups were also compared in relation to the antibiotic serum and eye tissue concentrations present.

Albino rats (Martland Farms), each weighing 180 to 200 g, were anesthetized before intracorneal injection with 10^3 *K. pneumoniae* cells contained in a volume of 0.025 ml. Manifestation of the infection became evident within 24 to 48 h, at which time the cornea appeared hazy and progressed to complete opaqueness and eventual necrosis.

The population densities of *K. pneumoniae* present in the infected treated eyes were determined by plating homogenates of the enucleated eyes in MacConkey agar medium (BBL Microbiology Systems).

Antibiotic serum and eye tissue levels of the infected rats were also established simultaneously on samples collected at 15, 30, 60, and 90 min after treatment.

The in vivo activities of CT, CM, and CL are shown in Fig. 1. The gross eye pathology present in each rat is illustrated in this scatter graph. The dots represent the mean pathology scores. All rats treated with CT were devoid of gross eye involvement, an effect which is associated with a complete suppression or elimination of the challenge organisms. In the CM-treated group, only 30% of the rats showed no evidence of eye pathology; the remainder exhibited a moderate to severe pathology. CL was virtually ineffective.

The therapeutic effects and the corresponding antibiotic serum and eye tissue levels reached are compared in Table 1. The response achieved with CT, based on the mean gross pathology and bacterial recoveries from the eyes, was superior to those of CM and CL. The latter compound was totally inactive. The peak serum levels attained with CT, CM, and CL, in all instances, exceeded the in vitro MIC and MBC values for the challenge organisms. The maximum eye tissue levels reached with CT and CM were approximately 1.0 μg per eye. Despite the high peak serum and measurable eye tissue levels reached with CM, the therapeutic response was less than fair. The mean eye tissue level reached in the CT-treated group was equivalent to only one MIC; the concentration was still high enough to eradicate all bacteria from the eyes of the CT-treated rats. Although CT is considered to be somewhat labile to in vitro hydrolysis by the β-lactamase of *K. pneumoniae*, CT was nevertheless superior to CM and CL in its in vitro bactericidal activity and in vivo efficacy.

The superiority of CT over CM and CL in the

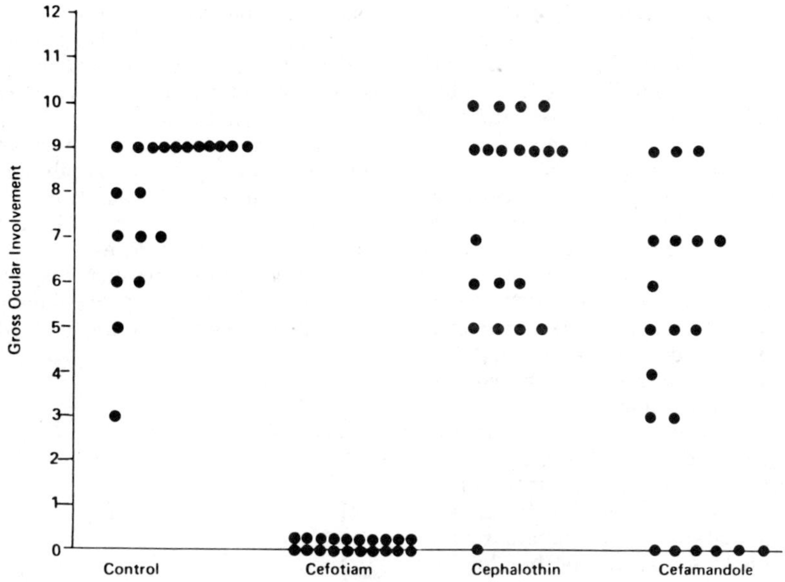

FIG. 1. *Mean gross pathology scores of individual rats treated with 50 mg/kg (intramuscularly twice daily for 3 days). The average severity (0 to a maximum of 12) represents the sum of 0 to 4+ grading (i) corneal surface showing infiltration (ii) density of infiltrate, and (iii) vascularization, hemorrhaging of the sclera, and conjunctiva.*

TABLE 1. *Comparative pharmacokinetic and therapeutic activity in rats with a K. pneumoniae eye infection*

Antibiotic	Dose (mg/kg)	Mean peak levels (μg) in: Serum	Eye	% Penetration	Gross pathology[a]	Bacterial recovery[b]
CT	50	29.1	0.8	2.8	0	1.6
CM	50	54.2	1.0	1.8	4.8	6.7
CL	50	69.5	0.3	0.4	7.4	7.9
Control	0	0	0	0	7.8	7.7

[a] Values recorded indicate the average severity of gross eye pathology. The average severity ranges from 0 to a maximum of 12.
[b] Mean $\log_{10}$ CFU recovered per eye.

K. pneumoniae rat keratitis model has been attributed to its intrinsic ability to penetrate through the outer bacterial membrane and reach effective concentrations at the target site.

Pharmacokinetics of Cefotiam in Humans

A. GERARDIN, M. C. ROUAN, J. B. LECAILLON,* F. ABADIE, A. DANIELOU, J. P. SCHOELLER, J. GUIBERT, AND J. MODAÏ

CIBA-GEIGY, Rueil-Malmaison, Hôpital Saint Joseph, Paris, and Hôpital Claude Bernard, Paris, France*

The pharmacokinetics of cefotiam was investigated in three studies during which the drug was administered as bolus intravenous doses, constant-rate infusion, and repeated doses. Blood samples and urine fractions were collected. Concentrations of cefotiam in plasma and urine were determined by high-pressure liquid chromatography. Plasma was deproteinized by adding trichloroacetic acid (3 parts of plasma and 1 part of a 10% aqueous trichloroacetic acid solution). Urine was diluted 1/10 with water. Twenty-microliter portions of these solutions were injected into a 20-cm RP 18 LiChrosorb column. The drug was eluted with the mobile phase: methanol (24%) in an aqueous solution of NaH_2PO_4 (1.4×10^{-3} mol/liter) and Na_2HPO_4 (2.5×10^{-2} mol/liter). Temperature was 40°C. The limit of sensitivity was 0.4 μmol of cefotiam per liter of plasma and 10 μmol per liter of urine.

Bolus dose study. Three healthy volunteers were given intravenously 0.5-, 1-, and 2-g bolus doses of cefotiam in a three-period cross-over design. Blood was obtained before administration and at 2, 10, 20, and 30 min and 1, 2, 4, 6, 8, and 12 h. Plasma was separated, and the samples were stored at −20°C until analysis.

Constant-rate infusion study. Six healthy volunteers participated in the study. They were given a 250-mg loading dose as an intravenous bolus injection. Immediately after, cefotiam was continously administered at a constant rate of 104 mg/h for 2.5 h. At 2.5 h, another loading dose (1,000 mg) was given, which was followed by a constant-rate infusion (703 mg/h) for an additional period of 2.5 h. Blood was collected before and at 1.5, 1.75, 2, 2.25, 2.5, 4, 4.25, 4.5, 4.75, and 5 h after the beginning of the treatment. Plasma samples obtained by centrifugation were stored at −20°C until analysis.

Repeated-dose study. Three patients with infectious diseases were given by fast intravenous injection 1 g of cefotiam every 12 h for 10 days. Concentrations in plasma and urinary excretion were studied at the beginning and at the end of the treatment. Blood was collected before and at 2, 10, 20, and 30 min and 1, 2, 4, 6, 8, and 12 h after the first and last administrations.

Pharmacokinetics. Log-linear plots of cefotiam plasma concentrations versus time showed three distinct disposition phases. The curves were not superimposable when the concentrations were normalized for a 1-g dose as cefotiam concentration/dose (grams): the 2-g dose gave rise to normalized concentrations higher than those produced by the 0.5-g dose. The area under the plasma concentration-time curve (AUC) did not vary linearly with the dose (Table 1 and Fig. 1). Consequently, the total plasma clearance (Cl_T) was not constant and decreased with the dose (Table 1). A similar variation in renal clearance (Cl_u) was observed, as the percentage of the dose excreted in urine was comparable for the three doses.

Although three distinct disposition phases were observed, these results show that a model with linear kinetics cannot be used to describe

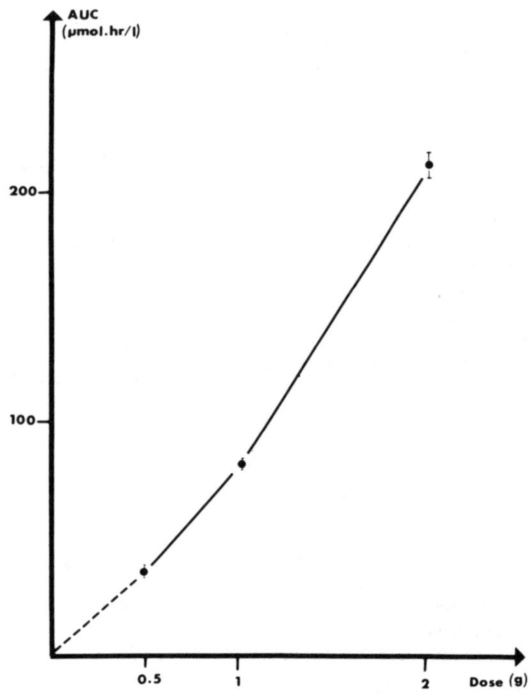

FIG. 1. *Plot of mean AUC values ± SD as a function of the administered dose.*

TABLE 1. *Mean pharmacokinetic parameters ± SD*[a]

Study	Dose (g)	AUC (μmol.h/liter)	C_{max} (μmol/liter)	$T_{1/2}$ (h)	U (% of dose)	Cl_T (liters/h)	Cl_u (liters/h)
Single dose	0.5	35.7 ± 3.4	101 ± 4	0.9 ± 0.1	56 ± 8	26.8 ± 2.7	16.0 ± 2.9
	1	83.5 ± 3.0	238 ± 14	1.1 ± 0.3	49 ± 8	22.8 ± 0.8	13.3 ± 1.4
	2	214.4 ± 10.8	467 ± 69	1.6 ± 0.6	56 ± 10	17.8 ± 0.9	11.3 ± 2.6
Constant-rate infusion	0.104/h	8.5 ± 1.8/h				23.5 ± 3.2[b]	
	0.703/h	75.2 ± 15.3/h				18.2 ± 2.8[b]	
Repeated doses, 1 g every 12 h	1 on day 1	70 ± 14	307 ± 215		51 ± 16		13.7 ± 3.1
	1 on day 10	7 ± 4	240 ± 24		56 ± 16	24.8 ± 1.3	13.8 ± 3.7

[a] Abbreviations not given in text: C_{max}, maximum plasma concentration; $T_{1/2}$, elimination half-life corresponding to the last segment of the log-linear plot of the concentration-time curve.

[b] $Cl_T = \frac{1}{C}\frac{dq}{dt}$, where C is the steady-state plasma concentration and $\frac{dq}{dt}$ is the infusion rate.

cefotiam kinetics. This was confirmed by the results of the constant-rate infusion study, since the total plasma clearance (Table 1) significantly decreased when the plasma concentration plateau increased from 8.5 to 75.2 μmol/liter (t = 5.98, $t_{crit\ 0.01}$ = 4.03).

After chronic administration of cefotiam, no accumulation of the drug was recorded since cefotiam was not detected in plasma collected just before the last dose of the treatment. AUC and urine values were similar on the 1st and 10th days of treatment (Table 1).

Penetration of Cefotiam in Urogenital Tissue

P. PEYER, M. ZAUG,* AND W. VISCHER

Cantonal and University Hospital, Department of Urological Surgery, Geneva, and CIBA-GEIGY Ltd., Basel, Switzerland*

Cefotiam (CGP 14,221, SCE-963) is a broad-spectrum cephalosporin which has high antibacterial activity against gram-positive and gram-negative bacteria. It showed better clinical results than cefazolin in urinary tract infections, especially in patients undergoing urological surgery (2). Our purpose was to determine the penetration of cefotiam in urogenital tissue when given preoperatively in patients.

Seventeen male patients undergoing urogenital operations received 1 g of cefotiam intravenously (bolus injection). The average age was 68.9 ± 18.3 years (range, 25 to 95), and the average weight was 69.5 ± 13.9 kg (range, 46 to 106). Nine patients underwent suprapubic transvesical prostatectomy, three underwent transurethral prostate resection, and seven had another type of surgery.

Nineteen tissue samples were excised at different times varying from 5 min to 2 h after injection. Of these samples, 14 were prostatic tissue, 2 were bladder tissue, 1 was kidney, 1 was perivesical tissue, and 1 was periureteral tissue.

A blood sample was taken simultaneously with each tissue specimen to compare tissue and blood levels. When cefotiam was given just before the operation, blood samples were taken once immediately after the injection and again 20 to 30 min after the injection. In some patients, cefotiam was given 1 h before the operation to ensure prostate levels at 1 to 2 h after the injection.

Plasma was obtained from the blood samples; all tissue and plasma samples were kept frozen at −20°C until analysis. The tissue samples were thawed and weighed. An equal weight of phosphate buffer (pH 7.0) was added in a Potter homogenizer, and the tissue homogenates obtained were kept at 4°C for 4 to 6 h before assay to extract cefotiam. Analysis was performed by microbiological assay, using *Bacillus subtilis* ATCC 6633 as the test organism.

The plasma concentrations were measured in nine patients at 30 min after injection. The mean plasma concentration was 34.0 ± 6.3 μg/ml.

Table 1 shows the changes in cefotiam concentrations in the prostate and serum over a period of time in different patients. In patients 10 and 14, abnormally high values were found, an occurrence probably due to urine contamination. In patients 17 (at 124 min) and 15, the size of the tissue specimen was too small to allow adequate measurement. From 15 to 37 min after injection, the concentrations in the prostate varied from 23 to 28 μg/g. After about 40 min, the concentrations decreased to less than 10 μg/ml. There were still appreciable concentrations after 2 h. The blood content was determined in six tissue samples and varied between 1 and 6%. The mean tissue/plasma ratio was 0.544 ± 0.217.

The concentrations of cefotiam in bladder, kidney, periureteral, and perivesical tissue are shown in Table 2. High levels were reached in the kidney and bladder. In perivesical and periureteral tissue, levels are quite similar to those in the prostate.

After administration of 1 g intravenously, the plasma concentrations of cefotiam found in nine elderly patients at 30 min were slightly higher than those found in volunteers. This slower elimination was probably due to the general condition and the ages of the subjects. However, the findings of the renal function tests were within the normal range.

Cefotiam penetrates rapidly into the prostatic tissue, maintaining levels above 20 μg for 0.5 h. The concentrations in the prostate of five injectable cephalosporins were measured after a dose of 2 g by the intravenous route (1). Compared with this study, cefotiam, at a dose of 1 g, reaches

TABLE 1. *Concentration of cefotiam in prostate after injection of 1 g intravenously*

Patient	Time (min)	Tissue concn (μg/g)	Plasma concn (μg/ml)	Tissue/plasma ratio
3	5	12.3	55.9	0.22
7	15	25.1	30.1	0.83
10	17	51.1	55.2 (20 min)	
14	20	102.1	38.1 (30 min)	
3	30	28.1	35.1	0.80
13	35	23.5	34.5	0.68
6	37	27.5	37.8	0.73
2	43	9.3	28.0	0.33
5	45	6.8	23.3	0.29
11	85	2.6	8.3	0.31
17	85	8.3	18.6	0.45
16	105	12.2	25.3	0.48
17	124	0.9[a]	12.9	
15	165	12.6[a]	12.6	

[a] Tissue samples weighing less than 20 mg.

TABLE 2. *Concentration of cefotiam in bladder, kidney, perivesical, and periureteral tissue after injection of 1 g intravenously*

Patient	Time (min)	Tissue type	Tissue concn (μg/g)	Plasma concn (μg/ml)	Tissue/plasma ratio
1	39	Bladder	71.7	63.3[a]	
9	105	Bladder	131.2	6.2	20.5
8	90	Kidney	315.3	15.4	20.5
12	50	Periureteral	4.2	28.8	0.15
4	55	Perivesical	11.8	31.0	0.38

[a] The patient took Bactrim 1 day before administration of cefotiam.

nearly equal levels to those of cefamandole, cefradine, and cefapirin and higher levels than those of cefacetrile and cephalothin. The tissue/plasma ratio is also higher than that of the former cephalosporins. However, this ratio is not constant and decreases in time from about 0.7 to 0.8 at 20 to 30 min to about 0.3 to 0.4 after 40 min. Not only the concentrations but also the relative proportion of cefotiam in the prostate seems to increase when the plasma concentrations are high, and afterwards, cefotiam is eliminated more rapidly from prostatic tissue than from blood.

In another study (3), the concentrations of cefotiam in the prostate were measured after 1.5 h and more. Concentrations ranged from 5.3 (1.5 h) to less than 0.2 μg/ml (4 h). The tissue/plasma ratio was 0.68, 0.15, 0.09 at 1.5, 2, and 2.5 h, respectively (mean, 0.26).

Cefotiam, like other cephalosporins, is excreted by the kidneys and reaches high levels in the kidney and bladder, as has been demonstrated in both animals (4) and humans (3). The adjacent periureteral and perivesical tissues, on the other hand, showed relatively lower concentrations.

1. **Adam, D., A. G. Hofstetter, and F. Eisenberger.** 1979. Zur Diffusion von Cefamandol in das Prostatagewebe. Med. Klin. **74**:235–238.
2. **Ishigami, J., et al.** 1979. Clinical evaluation of cefotiam in complicated urinary tract infections. A comparative study with cefazolin by a randomized double-blind technique. Chemotherapy (J) **27**(Suppl. 3):629–648.
3. **Kato, H., K. Yoneda, Y. Yamazaki, H. Urata, K. Tajima, and S. Tada.** 1979. Clinical experience with cefotiam. Chemotherapy (J) **27**(Suppl. 3):558–563.
4. **Tanayama, S., T. Kondo, and Y. Kanai.** 1978. Metabolic fate of SCE-963, a new broad-spectrum cephalosporin after parenteral administration in rats and dogs. J. Antibiot. **31**:703–711.

Pharmacokinetics and Clinical Study of Cefotiam in the Pediatric Field

TADAFUMI NISHIMURA* AND RYOCHI FUJII

Department of Pediatrics, Osaka Medical College, Takatsuki, and Department of Pediatrics, School of Medicine, Teikyo University, Tokyo, Japan*

Cefotiam is a newly developed, broad-spectrum, synthetic antibiotic of the cephalosporin series. Its antibacterial activity against gram-negative bacteria, such as *Escherichia coli*, *Klebsiella pneumoniae* and *Proteus mirabilis*, is more potent compared with the former cephalosporins, and its antibacterial spectrum has been expanded to include *Haemophilus influenzae*, *Enterobacter*, *Citrobacter*, and indole-positive *Proteus* spp. In Japan, this product has been clinically studied in adults, and its features and utility have been evaluated at the 26th Meeting of the Japan Society of Chemotherapy and in the 18th Interscience Conference on Antimicrobial Agents and Chemotherapy (ICAAC). We carried out fundamental and clinical investigations of cefotiam in the pediatric field with the cooperation of 17 institutes all over Japan. The results are presented here.

Absorption and excretion of cefotiam were

studied in six groups of 5 to 10 patients each. Doses of 10, 20, and 40 mg/kg were given by intravenous bolus injection and intravenous drip infusion over 1 h. The changes in the mean serum levels are shown in Fig. 1. With an intravenous bolus injection of 10, 20, and 40 mg/kg, the mean serum levels were 17.2, 40.3, and 125.6

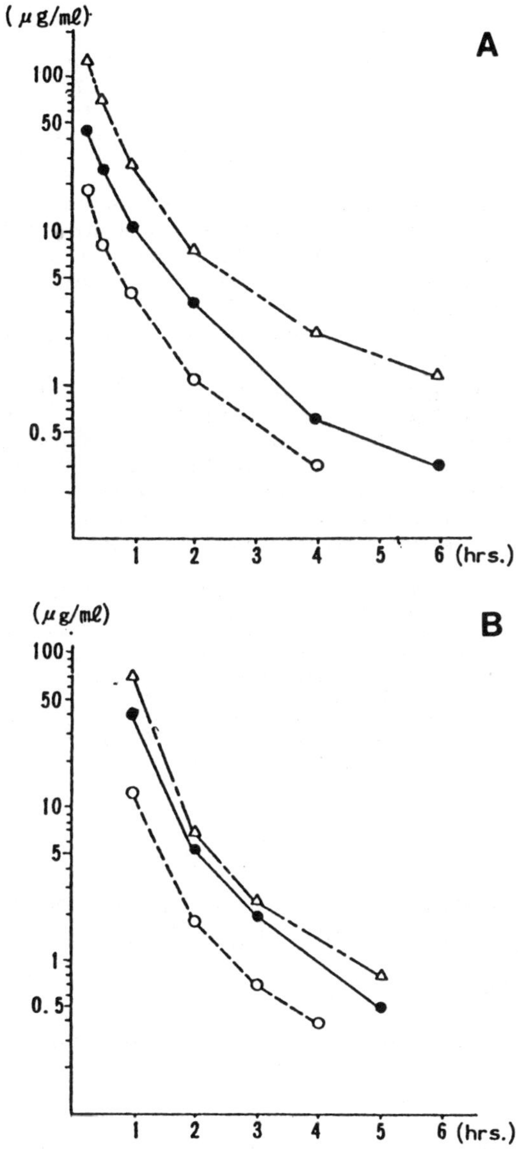

FIG. 1. *Comparison of mean serum concentrations of cefotiam given by intravenous bolus injection (A) and intravenous drip infusion (B). The drug was given in doses of:* (△) *40 mg/kg (n = 6 [A]; n = 5 [B]),* (●) *20 mg/kg (n = 10 [A]; n = 7 [B]), and* (○) *10 mg/kg (n = 5 [A]; n = 5 [B]).*

μg/ml, respectively, 15 min after injection and 8.6, 25.2, and 72.9 μg/ml, respectively, 30 min after injection. The half-lives in the serum were 0.83 h (10 mg/kg), 0.97 h (20 mg/kg), and 1.21 h (40 mg/kg). With an intravenous drip infusion over 1 h, the mean serum levels were 12.0, 39.9, and 70.0 μg/ml, respectively, at the termination of infusion in doses of 10, 20, and 40 mg/kg and 1.8, 5.3, and 6.8 μg/ml, respectively, after 1 h. The half-lives were 0.92 h (10 mg/kg), 0.90 h (20 mg/kg), and 1.01 h (40 mg/kg) (Fig. 1).

Thus, a distinct dose-response relation was seen with both modes of administration, intravenous bolus injection and intravenous drip infusion over 1 h, and there was a relatively rapid decrease. In the urine, recovery was at the rate of 50 to 70% at 0 to 6 h with each mode of administration. The greater part of the total urinary excretion was noted in 0 to 2 h. A clinical study was carried out in a group of 220 patients comprised of 125 males and 95 females; of these, 157 cases were infants, and 63 cases were school children. The dose was 41 to 100 mg/kg per day in 166 of 220 patients, and the highest dose was 375 mg/kg per day in a child with purulent meningitis. Administration was by intravenous bolus injection in 142 patients and by intravenous drip infusion in 78 patients, and the daily dose was divided into 3 to 4 doses in most cases. The clinical effect was evaluated in 180 patients in which inflammatory signs were observed and causative organisms were determined, excluding the patients in which viral and *Mycoplasma* infections were suspected. The clinical effect of diagnosis was as high as 94.4%, on the whole (Table 1). The rate of effectiveness in the main diseases was as follows: 3/3 (100%) in septicemia, 5/5 (100%) in purulent meningitis, 63/68 (93%) in pneumonia, 12/12 (100%) in bronchitis, 11/12 (91.7%) in pyelonephritis, and 27/28 (96.4%) in cystitis. Cefotiam showed a marked clinical effect in respiratory and urinary tract infections as well as in severe infections such as purulent meningitis and septicemia. To observe the bacteriological effect, the fate of the causative organism after administration of cefotiam was studied in 117 patients in which an organism was detected which could be presumed to be causative. The rate of eradication of the bacteria which were isolated in high incidences was as follows: *Staphylococcus aureus*, 18/21 (85.7%); *Streptococcus pneumoniae*, 9/11 (81.8%), and gram-positive bacteria, on the whole, 40/49 (81.6%). Of the gram-negative bacteria, *E. coli* was eradicated in 29 of 30 patients, (96.7%), *H. influenzae* was eradicated in 17 of 18 patients (94.4%), and 59 of 68 patients (81.6%) showed eradication of gram-negative bacteria, on the

TABLE 1. *Clinical effect of cefotiam classified by diagnosis*

Infection	Patient	Response			Efficacy rate (%)
		Excellent	Good	Poor	
Septicemia	3	2	1		3/3
Purulent meningitis	5		5		5/5
Tonsillitis	16	6	9	1	15/16 (93.8)
Bronchitis	12	5	7		12/12 (100.0)
Pneumonia	68	31	32	5	63/68 (92.6)
Empyema	5	1	2	2	3/5 (60.0)
Enteritis	6		6		6/6
Cystitis	28	17	10	1	27/28 (96.4)
Pyelonephritis	12	4	7	1	11/12 (91.7)
Purulent infections of soft tissue	8	2	6		8/8
Other infections	17	7	10		17/17 (100.0)

whole. It can be seen that cefotiam exerted a potent effect against gram-positive and gram-negative bacteria, and the findings corresponded well with the in vitro result (Table 1).

Examination of the clinical effect in relation to the dose revealed that cefotiam was effective in 11 of 11 patients with a dose of less than 40 mg/kg, in 58 of 62 patients (93.5%) with doses of 41 to 60 mg/kg, in 41 of 43 patients (95.3%) with 60 to 80 mg/kg, in 37 of 39 patients, (94.9%) with 81 to 100 mg/kg, in 15 of 16 patients (93.8%) with 101 to 150 mg/kg, and in 8 of 9 patients (88.9%) with a dose of more than 150 mg/kg, showing a high rate of effectiveness for each dose. Side effects and laboratory test findings were investigated in all of the 220 patients in which cefotiam was administered. As for side effects, eruption was observed in 2 patients (0.9%), and diarrhea was observed in 4 patients (1.8%). In the clinical laboratory tests, the abnormal findings included elevated serum transaminases in 7 patients (3.2%) and increased eosinophils in 8 patients (3.6%). All of these side effects and abnormal test values were transient and returned to normal at the time of the end of administration or after discontinuation of administration. No especially severe cases were encountered.

In 220 cases of children with various infections, cefotiam was administered in a daily dose of 40 to 100 mg/kg (more than 150 mg/kg in severe cases) divided into 3 to 4 times, and highly satisfactory therapeutic effects (94.9% effectiveness) were obtained. There were no cases worthy of note, in terms of safety. From the above data, cefotiam can be regarded as highly useful against various infections in the field of pediatrics.

1. **Tsuchiya, K., M. Kida, M. Kondo, S. Goto, M. Ogawa, A. Tsuji, and S. Kuwahara.** SCE-963, a new cephalosporin. II. In vitro and in vivo antibacterial activities. Program Abstr. Intersci. Conf. Antimicrob. Agents Chemother. 17th, New York, N.Y., abstr. no. 45, 1977.
2. **Shimizu, K.** Clinical studies on SCE-963, a new broad-spectrum semisynthetic cephalosporin. Program Abstr. Instersci. Conf. Antimicrob. Agents Chemother. 18th, Atlanta, Ga., abstr. no. 160, 1978.

Clinical Evaluation of Cefotiam in Pulmonary Infections: a Comparative Study with Cefazolin Using a Randomized Double-Blind Method

AKIRA SAITO* AND KEIZO MATSUMOTO

Hokkaido University School of Medicine, Sapporo, and Institute for Tropical Medicine, Nagasaki University, Nagasaki, Japan*

Cefotiam is a new semisynthetic cephalosporin antibiotic for injection which has an aminothiazole ring at the 7-position of the cephalosporin nucleus; it originated at the Central Research Division of Takeda Chemical Industries, Ltd., Osaka, Japan. Cefotiam has remarkable antibacterial activities against *Streptococcus pneumoniae*, *S. pyogenes*, *Haemophilus influenzae*, and *Klebsiella pneumoniae*, which are frequently isolated from patients with respiratory tract infections. The antibacterial potency of cefotiam has been reported to be more than 10 times greater than that of cefazolin.

The present study was performed to evaluate

the clinical effectiveness and safety of cefotiam in the treatment of bacterial pneumonia and pulmonary suppuration by double-blind comparative trials, using cefazolin as a reference drug.

The study was carried out in patients with moderate to severe bacterial pneumonia or pulmonary suppuration, because the methodology of drug evaluation has been well established for these respiratory infections and parenteral cephalosporins seemed to be best indicated. The dosage regimen was fully discussed by the physicians attending the present trials, and 2 and 4 g were chosen as the daily dosages of cefotiam and cefazolin, respectively. Each dose (in a vial) was diluted with 250 to 300 ml of physiological saline or 5% glucose solution and administered by intravenous drip infusion over approximately 1 h, twice daily, for 14 consecutive days.

Of the 122 patients admitted to the trial, 101 (48 on cefotiam and 53 on cefazolin) were eligible for evaluation of clinical efficacy. For safety evaluation, however, the data from all patients were included.

The distribution of patient characteristics (demographic and diagnostic variables) showed no significant bias between the two treatment groups except that the volume of sputum was higher in the cefazolin group than in the cefotiam group. A stratified analysis, however, revealed that this bias had virtually no influence on the assessment of clinical efficacy.

Overall clinical response was excellent in 20 patients, good in 25, and fair in 3 on cefotiam, the rate of satisfactory (excellent and good) response being 94%. For cefazolin, the response was excellent in 12 patients, good in 28, fair in 9, and poor in 4, the rate of satisfactory response being 75%. Cefotiam was significantly superior to cefazolin ($P < 0.01$). When stratified by diagnoses, cefotiam treatment was again found to be significantly superior to cefazolin treatment in patients with pneumonia, whereas the difference in effectiveness for pulmonary suppuration was not statistically significant, apparently due to the limited number of subjects (Table 1). Cefotiam treatment produced significantly greater improvement than cefazolin treatment in X-ray findings, which are considered to be objective and most important in assessment of drug efficacy in pneumonia and pulmonary suppuration.

Bacteriologically, the cefotiam group displayed a significantly higher ($P < 0.05$) rate of eradication (27 of 27, 100%) than the cefazolin group (21 of 27, 78%). With regard to *H. influenzae* especially, all isolates (5 of 5, 100%) from the cefotiam group were eradicated, whereas 40% (4 of 10) from the cefazolin group persisted after treatment.

Statistical analysis made for global safety ratings disclosed that cefotiam treatment showed a tendency ($P < 0.1$) to be safer than cefazolin treatment; the incidence of side effects were 10% (6 of 56) in the cefotiam group and 22% (14 of 63) in the cefazolin group. The most frequent side effect was elevation of transaminase in both groups.

Factor analysis was then performed to examine the basic structure of the symptoms relating to bacterial pneumonia (1). This analysis, which was done on the basis of changes in symptoms during the 2-week treatment with cefotiam or cefazolin, indicated that the symptoms might adequately be classified as follows: group I (basic symptoms)—dyspnea, rale, cyanosis, and cardiac insufficiency; group II (respiratory tract inflammation)—cough, character of sputum, and volume of sputum; group III (systemic reaction)—fever and leukocytosis; and group IV—X-ray findings and erythrocyte sedimentation rate. The changes in X-ray findings also corre-

TABLE 1. *Overall assessment of clinical responses*

Disease	Group	Excellent	Good	Fair	Poor	Total	Statistical test
Pneumonia	Cefotiam	19 (43%)	22 (93%)	3 (100%)	0	44	$Z_0=2.591^{**}$ (P<0.01)
	Cefazolin	11 (23%)	26 (77%)	8 (94%)	3	48	$\chi_0^2=3.45^{\triangle}$(P<0.1)
Pulmonary suppuration	Cefotiam	1 (25%)	3 (100%)	0	0	4	$Z_0=0.944$ (N.S.)
	Cefazolin	1 (20%)	2 (60%)	1 (80%)	1	5	$\chi_0^2=0.39$ (N.S.)
Total	Cefotiam	20 (42%)	25 (94%)	3 (100%)	0	48	$Z_0=2.764^{**}$ (P<0.01)
	Cefazolin	12 (23%)	28 (75%)	9 (92%)	4	53	$\chi_0^2=5.016^{*}$ (P<0.05)

lated with group I symptoms. The same type of classification was derived from cluster analysis.

The changes in each group of symptoms during the 2-week treatment period were investigated by "life table" analysis, using disappearance of symptoms as the endpoint instead of "death" (Fig. 1). Rates of symptom persistence in the cefotiam and cefazolin treatment groups were compared by log rank test. Cefotiam showed significantly higher efficacy in healing the group I and II symptoms than did cefazolin ($P < 0.05$).

This method of analysis, which consists of aggregation of symptoms in a few groups and comparison of the rates of symptom persistence between two treatment groups, gives us a fairly compact and reasonable summary of the test results since it focuses the results on disappearance of the symptoms, which is the most important target in chemotherapy.

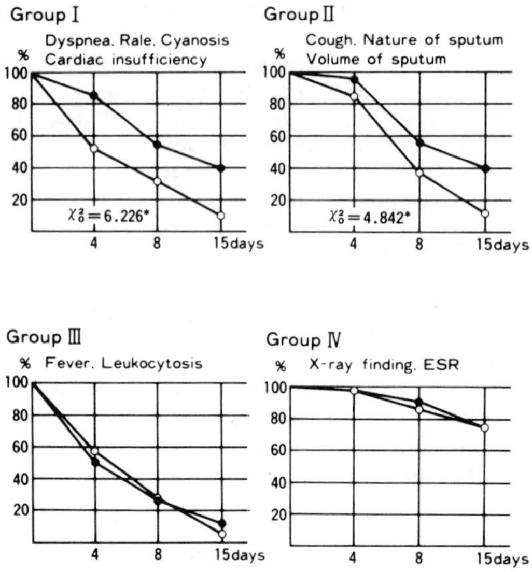

FIG. 1. *Rates of symptom persistence (life table analysis). Symbols: ○, cefotiam; ●, cefazolin; *, $P < 0.05$. ESR, Erythrocyte sedimentation rate.*

1. **Matsumoto, K., A. Saito, K. Shima, T. Kusunoki, and Y. Kosato.** 1980. A method of assessing clinical states in bacterial pneumonia (part II). Jpn. J. Clin. Pharmacol. Ther. **11**:37–47.

Treatment of Lower Respiratory Tract Infections with Cefoxitin and Cefotiam

P. VEYSSIER,* J. AUBERT, AND C. CARBON

Centre Hospitalier, Compiègne, Hôpital St. Joseph, Marseille, and Hôpital Louis Mourier, Colombes, France*

Cefotiam is a new injectable cephalosporin with excellent bactericidal activity against most gram-positive and gram-negative bacteria. In this open comparative trial, cefotiam was compared in lower respiratory tract infections with cefoxitin, an established injectable cephalosporin which shares similar kinetics with cefotiam. The patients were selected according to defined criteria and allocated at random to one of the two treatment regimens. Both treatments were given mainly by intravenous drip infusion or bolus injection.

Sixty-five patients were treated; two patients were excluded from the statistical analysis. A total of 63 patients suffering from lobar pneumonia, superinfected bronchial and lung disease, or lung abscess received either cefotiam (1 g two times a day, 31 patients) or cefoxitin (1 g three times a day, 26 patients). Two patients in the cefotiam group and four patients in the cefoxitin group received higher dosages. The mean treatment duration was 9.9 days in the cefotiam group and 10.2 days in the cefoxitin group. The clinical response was assessed on a four-scale order as excellent, good, fair, or poor. The patients were evaluated as to improvement in their clinical symptoms and signs (cough, expectorations, temperature, etc.) and by evaluation of their X rays.

Whenever possible, a bacteriological examination of the sputum was performed with isolation, identification, and a susceptibility test of the causative pathogen(s) before, during, and after treatment. The bacteriological response was assessed according to the fate of the bacteria (elimination, diminution, no change, or replacement).

The patients were watched for adverse reactions, local pain, and thrombophlebitis. Hematological and renal tolerability were checked by performing laboratory value examinations.

Tests for homogeneity of the distributions

were performed by χ^2 analysis and descriptive statistics. The level of significance was fixed at $P = 0.05$. The population was homogeneous between the two treatment groups as to sex, height, weight, body temperature before start of the trial, severity of infection, and type of infection.

The comparative efficacy of each drug was evaluated clinically, bacteriologically, and with regard to tolerability.

The clinical response is shown in Table 1. Statistical comparison of the clinical efficacy, in spite of a tendency in favor of cefoxitin, did not show any significant difference between the two groups ($\chi^2 = 0.380$ with 2 df). The improvement of signs and symptoms and stratified analysis in moderate and severe infections also did not show any difference. The decrease of body temperature was generally below 37.5°C after 3 to 5 days in both treatment groups.

Bacteriological evaluation was possible in 44 patients. There was no statistical difference between the two groups ($\chi^2 = 0.094$) in the bacteriological efficacy expressed by: (rate of disappearance + reduction)/total. Table 2 shows the bacteriological and clinical efficacy in regard to the causative agents seen at the start of the trial. The small numbers per species do not allow a conclusive statistical analysis.

Tolerability was evaluated globally by the investigator at the end of the treatment. Both treatments were evaluated as having a good tolerability. Only in one patient in the cefotiam group was tolerability moderate due to the appearance of eruption. One patient in the cefoxitin group reported mild pain at the site of injection. Treatment was not interrupted. There were laboratory findings outside the normal range in two patients in the cefotiam group (slight increase of serum creatinine, increase of metamyelocytes in a cancer patient) and in three patients in the cefoxitin group (elevation of thrombocytes [two patients], increase of SGPT). There was no evidence, based on the results of routine blood tests and urine analysis, of renal toxicity with either of the treatments.

TABLE 1. *Clinical response*

Clinical response	No. of patients	
	Cefotiam treatment (*n* = 33)	Cefoxitin treatment (*n* = 30)
Excellent	20	13
Good	8	14
Fair	3	2
Poor	2	1
Clinical efficacy (%)	28/33 (84.8)	27/30 (90.0)

TABLE 2. *Rate of clinical and bacteriological efficacy*

Causative agent	Clinical efficacy		Bacteriological efficacy	
	Cefotiam	Cefoxitin	Cefotiam	Cefoxitin
Diplococcus pneumoniae	3/3[a]	1/1	3/3	1/1
Streptococcus spp.	1/2	4/5	0/1	4/5
Haemophilus spp.	3/3	2/2	1/2	1/2
Klebsiella pneumoniae	2/2	1/1	2/2	0/1
Klebsiella oxytoca		1/1		0/1
Escherichia coli		1/1		1/1
Proteus mirabilis	2/2	1/1	2/2	1/1
Enterobacter spp.		1/1		0/1
Pseudomonas aeruginosa	1/1		1/1	
Veillonella spp.		1/1		0/1
Total monoinfections	12/13	13/14	9/11	8/14
Total mixed infections	6/28	5/6	4/8	3/6

[a] Number eradicated/number present.

Cefotiam was compared with cefoxitin in the treatment of pneumonia, bronchiectasis, severe bronchitis, or other serious lung infections. The efficacy, both clinical and, whenever possible, bacteriological, of both drugs was good. Cefotiam was usually given in a total daily dose of 2 g (1 g two times a day) in contrast to cefoxitin, which was given in a daily dose of 3 g (1 g three times a day). Although cefotiam was given at a lower dosage, no statistically significant difference was observed between the two treatment groups.

The efficacy of cefotiam at a lower dosage and a less frequent administration rate is probably due to its excellent activity against gram-positive bacteria and *Haemophilus* spp. (2), which are the main pathogens in lower respiratory tract infections, and to its excellent penetration in bronchial secretions (1). Higher dosages for both drugs were given in some severe cases. Both drugs proved safe at the dosages given.

1. **Berthelot, G., E. Bergogne-Bérézin, J. Pierre, and H. Kafé.** 1980. Pénétration des céphalosporines dans les voies respiratoires: place du cefotiam. Abstr. 134, 2nd Mediterranean Congress of Chemotherapy, Nice.
2. **Tsuchiya, K., M. Kida, M. Kondo, H. Ono, M. Takeuchi, and T. Nishi.** 1978. SCE-963, a new broad-spectrum cephalosporin: in vitro and in vivo antibacterial activities. Antimicrob. Agents Chemother. **14**:557–568.

Human Pharmacokinetics of YM09330 (Cefotetan), a New Cephamycin Antibiotic, After Parenteral Administration

AKIRA SAITO, MASAHIDE SHINOHARA,* ICHIRO NAKAYAMA, AND KEIMEI MASHIMO

The Second Department of Internal Medicine, Hokkaido University School of Medicine, Sapporo, and Tokyo Kosei Nenkin Hospital, Tokyo, Japan*

Cefotetan (YM09330) is a new parenteral cephamycin antibiotic with a broad spectrum and potent activity against gram-negative bacteria, including β-lactamase–producing strains. The activities of cefotetan against gram-negative bacteria were much higher than those of cefoxitin, cefmetazole, and cefazolin. In addition, cefotetan was not hydrolyzed by any of the β-lactamases obtained from various bacteria which were shown to produce cephalosporinases (2). Tachibana et al. (1) reported the pharmacokinetics of cefotetan in experimental animals in comparison with cefmetazole and cefazolin. Cefotetan was converted into its tautomer in the urine and bile of animals under the conditions of alkaline pH and high Mg^{2+} concentration. We determined the extent of the tautomer in human body fluids by using high-performance liquid chromatography (HPLC). The present communication describes the pharmacokinetics of cefotetan in humans after parenteral administration.

Subjects were male adult volunteers who were found to be normal in medical examinations. Cefotetan was dissolved in 20 ml of saline and administered intravenously (i.v.) to six subjects in a single dose of either 0.5 or 1 g as a slow bolus injection over 3 min. Blood samples were obtained immediately before and periodically after drug administration, and the plasma was separated by centrifugation. Urine was collected before injection and during several consecutive periods after injection. Drug concentrations in plasma and urine were determined by both bioassay and HPLC assay methods. The assay organism *Escherichia coli* NIHJ was used in bioassay. HPLC was carried out on a model ALC 202 liquid chromatograph (Waters Instruments, Inc.), using a mobile phase system of Acetnitrile-0.1 M sodium dihydrogen phosphate, pH 3.0 (8:92).

The mean plasma levels of cefotetan obtained by both bioassay and HPLC assay methods after a single i.v. administration of 0.5 or 1 g to humans are shown in Fig. 1. The plasma concentrations of cefotetan determined by the bioassay method were comparable to those estimated as the total amount of cefotetan and the tautomer determined by HPLC, since almost no tautomer was detected in the plasma specimens.

In the results obtained by bioassay, the mean plasma concentrations of cefotetan 30 min after dosing were 74.0 and 139 μg/ml for the 0.5- and 1-g i.v. bolus injections, respectively. They slowly declined to 4.1 and 9.1 μg/ml at 12 h after dosing. The plasma levels for the 1-g dosage were approximately twice as high as those for the 0.5-g dosage at every time indicated. These plasma concentration-time curves were analyzed by the two-compartment open model with first-order rate constants; the equation $C = Ae^{-\alpha t} + Be^{-\beta t}$ was used.

The values of C_0 of cefotetan in humans were 152 and 262 μg/ml for the 0.5- and 1-g intravenous injections, respectively. Respective average half-life (β) and elimination rate constant (K_{el}) were calculated to be 3.3 h and 0.55 h^{-1} for 0.5-g i.v. doses and 3.05 h and 0.45 h^{-1} for 1-g i.v. doses. These values were reflected to the area under the plasma concentration-time curves (AUC), which were 277 h.μg/ml for 0.5-g i.v. doses and 579 h.μg/ml for 1-g i.v. doses. The pharmacokinetic parameters of cefotetan analyzed in the study were comparable to those obtained in studies of this drug in 37 research

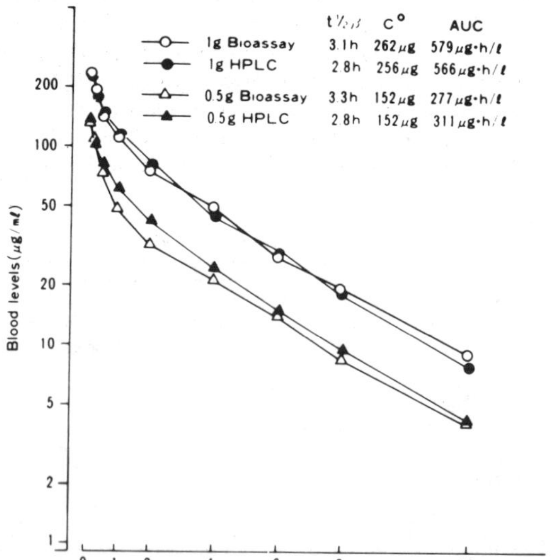

FIG. 1. *Blood levels of cefotetan after a single i.v. administration of 0.5 g (△) and 1 g (○) to healthy volunteers.*

TABLE 1. *Urinary excretion of cefotetan after a single i.v. administration of 0.5 and 1 g to healthy volunteers*

Antibiotic	Dose & Route	n	Assay method		Excretion in urine														
					0~2h		2~4h		4~6h		6~8h		8~10h		10~12h		12~24h		Total 0~24h
					µg/ml [d]	% [e]	µg/ml	%	µg/ml	%	µg/ml	%	µg/ml	%	µg/ml	%	µg/ml	%	%
Cefotetan	0.5g iv	3	Bioassay		1467 ±88	38.2 ±2.3	540 ±95	16.6 ±0.7	512 ±132	12.3 ±1.1	165 ±36	5.7 ±0.2	77 ±22	5.0 ±0.5	72 ±37	3.1 ±0.5	38 ±12	4.0 ±0.2	84.9 ±1.6
	1g iv	3	Bioassay		2667 ±1334	38.6 ±2.8	983 ±233	16.1 ±2.4	925 ±138	9.9 ±1.6	390 ±15	7.1 ±0.8	213 ±32	5.6 ±0.3	112 ±27	3.1 ±0.4	98 ±4	5.1 ±0.5	85.5 ±1.0
	0.5g iv	3	HPLC [a]	YM+T [b]	1556 ±189	40.0 ±1.2	602 ±76	17.7 ±1.0	441 ±89	10.9 ±0.9	190 ±44	6.5 ±0.3	60 ±12	4.0 ±0.5	68 ±35	2.9 ±0.4	51 ±22	5.0 ±0.6	86.8 ±4.0
				T [c]	61.9 ±14.7	1.6 ±0.2	39.5 ±15.9	1.1 ±0.3	71.9 ±19.4	1.8 ±0.5	21.0 ±4.4	0.8 ±0.2	7.1 ±0.3	0.5 ±0.1	14.3 ±10.0	0.5 ±0.2	13.3 ±8.8	1.2 ±0.5	7.5 ±1.5
	1g iv	3	HPLC	YM+T	2526 ±1095	38.8 ±0.4	1201 ±444	17.8 ±0.1	785 ±156	8.8 ±2.3	347 ±65	6.1 ±0.7	140 ±19	3.7 ±0.4	106 ±34	2.9 ±0.4	98 ±13	5.0 ±0.4	83.0 ±4.2
				T	250 ±150	4.3 ±2.7	189 ±93	4.1 ±3.0	117 ±33	1.3 ±0.3	44 ±15	0.8 ±0.3	19.2 ±3.5	0.5 ±0.1	13.3 ±6.0	0.3 ±0.1	15.6 ±5.2	1.2 ±0.6	11.8 ±6.0

a) High-performance liquid chromatography
b) Sum of YM 09330 and tautomer
c) Tautomer of YM 09330
d) Concentration of the drug in urine
e) Recovery % of the dose

institutes in Japan. In comparison with a 1-g i.v. bolus injection of cefmetazole, the half-life (β) of cefotetan was much longer than that of cefmetazole (0.92 h), and the AUC for the 1-g i.v. dose of cefotetan was also 4 times as great as that of cefmetazole. The half-life (β) and AUC values of cefotetan in humans were demonstrated to be approximately twice as great as those reported for moxalactam and cefazolin. The results indicated that the i.v. injection of cefotetan to humans not only produced high concentrations in plasma but also maintained them longer than did an injection of cefmetazole of the same dosage level.

Urinary concentrations and recoveries of cefotetan by bioassay as well as those of the total amount of cefotetan and its tautomer were determined by HPLC (Table 1). In the bioassay method, the average concentrations of cefotetan in urine were highest during the first 2 h after dosing, and they were as high as 1,500 µg/ml and over 2,500 µg/ml for the injection of 0.5 and 1 g, respectively. During 12 to 24 h after the above doses, the average levels of 38 µg/ml and 98 µg/ml of cefotetan were still present in the urine after single injections of 0.5 and 1 g. These concentrations would be sufficient for therapy of infections caused by most of the organisms susceptible to cefotetan.

Though urinary excretion of cefotetan in humans seemed to be slow, the cumulative recoveries in 24-h urine after dosing reached 84.9% of the administered dose for the 0.5-g i.v. injection and 85.5% for 1-g i.v. injection. Since the tautomer possesses a quite similar antibacterial activity to cefotetan, the results obtained by bioassay were in good agreement with those determined by HPLC as the total amounts of cefotetan and the tautomer. On the other hand, the cumulative recoveries of tautomer in urine over a period of 24 h after administration were 7.5 and 11.8% for the 0.5- and 1-g i.v. injections, respectively. The percentage of recovery for tautomer in the study was in the range of variation obtained in the urine of normal subjects in other studies for cefotetan.

Physiological examinations, serum biochemical analyses, and other laboratory tests before and after drug administration revealed no signs of toxicity. These studies demonstrated that cefotetan, a new parenteral cephamycin antibiotic, was well tolerated, and that the parenteral administration to humans resulted in high and prolonged plasma levels, with half-lives (β) of 3 h in comparison with cefmetazole, cephalothin, cefazolin, and other available cephalosporins. In addition, the concentration of cefotetan in urine was maintained at high levels, and about 85% of the administered dose was recovered during 24 h in humans.

1. **Tachibana, A., M. Komiya, Y. Kikuchi, K. Yano, and K. Mashimo.** 1980. Pharmacological studies on YM09330, a new parenteral cephamycin derivative, p. 273–275. *In* J. D. Nelson and C. Grassi (ed.), Current chemotherapy and infectious disease. American Society for Microbiology, Washington, D.C.
2. **Toda, M., T. Saito, K. Yano, K. Suzaki, M. Saito, and S. Mitsuhashi.** 1980. In vitro and in vivo antibacterial activities of YM09330, a new cephamycin derivative, p. 280–281. *In* J. D. Nelson and C. Grassi (ed.), Current chemotherapy and infectious disease. American Society for Microbiology, Washington, D.C.

Diffusion into Human Prostatic Fluids of New Cephem Antibiotic Drugs

K. SUZUKI,* Y. NAIDE, K. OKADA, M. OHKOSHI, AND Y. IKI

Department of Urology, Hiratsuka City Hospital, Kanagawa; Fujitagakuen University, School of Medicine, Nagoya; Tokai University, School of Medicine, Kanagawa; and Kanto Teishin Hospital, Tokyo, Japan*

Chronic bacterial prostatitis is encountered as the most frequent cause of recurrent urinary tract infections in adult males, and extreme difficulty is inherent in the therapeutic attempt to achieve complete eradication of bacterial pathogens in this condition.

The purpose of this study was to assess the therapeutic effect and to clarify the pharmacodynamic physiology of drugs that pass through the external membrane into the prostate gland by determinations of drug concentrations in the prostatic fluid (PF) of patients after administration of cephalosporin antibiotics. Nine cephalosporin derivatives were used in the study: cefazolin; three cephamycin antibiotics, cefoxitin, cefmetazole, and cefotetan; and five cephalosporin derivatives of the tertiary generation, cefoperazone, cefotaxime, ceftizoxime, moxalactam, and cefmenoxime.

The experimental procedures are summarized in Table 1. Cefoperazone, cefotaxime, ceftizoxime, moxalactam, and cefmenoxime were administered intravenously in doses of 1 g, whereas cefazolin, cefoxitin, and cefmetazole were given intravenously in doses of 2 g. At 1 h after injection of a drug, specimens of PF were collected by prostatic massage from patients with bacterial prostatitis at its stable stage and from those with prostatosis, care being taken to avoid admixture of urine. The PF specimens (pH 6.5 to 7.8) and serum samples were bioassayed for drug concentration, using the test organisms specified in Table 1.

The summary of nine β-lactam antimicrobial drug levels in human PF is shown in Table 2. The mean drug concentration in five PF specimens at a dose of 2 g was determined to be 5.3 μg/ml for cefazolin, 3.7 μg/ml for cefoxitin, and 0.7 μg/ml for cefmetazole. Of these three drugs, cefazolin showed the highest concentration, cefoxitin showed a slightly lower concentration, and cefmetazole yielded a concentration apparently lower than either of these. The ratio of drug concentration in PF to serum level (R value) was 0.05 for cefazolin, 0.10 for cefoxitin, and 0.01 for cefmetazole.

The mean drug concentrations in PF at doses of 1 g of the other six antibiotics were as follows (μg/ml): the highest concentration was observed with cefoperazone (2.2), followed by moxalactam (1.6), ceftizoxime (1.4), cefotaxime (1.1), cefotetan (0.8), and cefmenoxime (0.3). The PF serum drug concentration ratio of these antibiotics ranged from 0.01 to 0.12. As seen from the R values, all of the cephalosporin antibiotics tested generally showed notably lower concentrations in PF, as compared with serum levels.

These experimental results suggest that the cephalosporin antibiotics can sparingly cross the prostatic membrane into the acinus. In clinical practice, however, many investigators have reported the clinical usefulness of these drugs in the treatment of infections of the prostate by gram-negative bacilli. We have tried one of the cephalosporins described herein, ceftizoxime, in a series of 13 cases of bacterial prostatitis due to infection with gram-negative bacteria, with notably gratifying results. The treatment produced a significant clinical improvement in eight cases (61.5%).

As an index for the clinical evaluation of effectiveness of antimicrobial chemotherapeutic agents in infections of the prostate, we calculated the M value from the present data for each of the cephalosporins studied (Table 2). The M value is defined as the ratio of mean drug concentration in PF to the MIC of the respective drug against *Escherichia coli*, which is the pathogen that most frequently produces bacterial prostatitis. It represents the magnitude of antibiotic concentration yielded in PF against the commonest bacterial pathogen. The M values, determined as a therapeutic marker, show that intravenous administration of the tertiary cephalosporins, such as cefotaxime, ceftizoxime, moxalactam, and cefmenoxime, yields PF antibiotic concentrations more than 10 times as high as the respective MICs.

It is universally recognized that cephalosporin derivatives scarcely pass into the prostatic gland across its membrane and, consequently, their administration yields a drug concentration in PF that is substantially lower than the serum level. The results of the present study with nine cephalosporin antibiotics in human PF are remarkably consistent with the findings in laboratory animals reported by many other investigators, including Stamey, Winningham, and Reeves.

TABLE 1. *Nine β-lactam antibiotics used and experimental methods*[a]

No	Drug	Dose (g), route, time after dosing(h)	Assay method	Indicator strain	Lowest assayable level(ug/ml)
1	Cefazolin	2.0, i.v., 1	Bioassay, disc	B.subtilis ATCC-6633	0.1
2	Cefoxitin	2.0, i.v., 1	Bioassay, disc	S.aureus MB-2786	0.25
3	Cefmetazole	2.0, i.v., 1	Bioassay, cup plate	M.luteus ATCC-9341	0.39
4	Cefo-tetan	1.0, i.v., 1	Bioassay, cup plate	E.coli NIHJ	0.20
5	Cefo-perazone	1.0, i.v., 1	Bioassay, cup plate	M.luteus ATCC-9341	0.39
6	Cefotaxime	1.0, i.v., 1	Bioassay, disc	B.subtilis ATCC-6633	0.1
7	Ceftizoxime	1.0, i.v., 1	Bioassay, disc	B.subtilis ATCC-6633	0.1
8	Moxa-lactam	1.0, i.v., 1	Bioassay, agar well	E.coli 7437	0.1
9	Cefme-noxime	1.0, i.v., 1	Bioassay, cup plate	P.mirabilis ATCC 21100	0.1

TABLE 2. *Summary of nine β-lactam antimicrobial drug levels in human PF*

No	Drug	Dose (g)	No. of speci-mens*	Mean levels into PF (μg/ml)	(1) R.value	MIC on E.coli (μg/ml)	(2) M.value
1	Cefazolin	2.0	5	5.3	0.05	1.56~6.25	3.4~1.1
2	Cefoxitin	2.0	5	3.7	0.10	3.12~6.25	1.2~0.6
3	Cefmetazole	2.0	5	0.7	0.01	1.56~3.13	0.4~0.2
4	Cefotetan	1.0	5	0.8	0.01	0.2~0.39	4.0~2.0
5	Cefoperazone	1.0	4	2.2	0.02	0.78~1.56	2.8~1.4
6	Cefotaxime	1.0	5	1.1	0.12	≦0.1	≧10.5
7	Ceftizoxime	1.0	9	1.4	0.04	≦0.1	≧13.8
8	Moxa-lactam	1.0	5	1.6	0.04	≦0.1	≧15.9
9	Cefme-noxime	1.0	5	0.3	0.02	≦0.1	≧ 2.8

(1) PF (prostatic fluid) / plasma

(2) PF/ MIC value against E.coli strains

* pH values of the specimens were 6.5~7.8

The low concentrations in PF may be explained by the fact that these drugs are non-fat soluble and markedly ionized in the serum. In addition, such factors as the pH of PF and protein binding of drugs have also been suggested to take part in the passage of drugs through the prostatic membrane propria. No significant variation in drug concentrations in PF was observed among different pH's of PF in the present experiment.

Under the experimental conditions described, drug concentrations in PF that seem to be therapeutically sufficient especially against gram-negative bacilli causing infections of the prostate were achieved by the administration of cefotetan or cephalosporins of the tertiary generation, among other drugs tested. The administration of cefazolin or cefoxitin yielded PF drug concentrations that were somewhat borderline from the viewpoint of therapeutic effectiveness.

The present data pertain solely to PF and serum levels of drugs at 1 h after an intravenous dose of 1 or 2 g, and further detailed assessments by pharmacokinetic analyses are considered necessary for clinical application of the drugs in the treatment of chronic bacterial prostatitis. However, collection of PF specimens from humans should be preceded by voiding, from which contamination with urine is inevitable; thus, difficulty is caused in such studies.

It may be tentatively concluded that cephalosporins of the tertiary generation are useful as drugs of first choice and cefazolin and cefoxitin are useful as drugs of second choice in high-dose chemotherapy for acute exacerbation of bacterial prostatitis. Such oral preparations as co-trimethoprim and others and pipemidic acid are the drugs of choice in cases where prolonged suppressive antimicrobial therapy is needed. The data presented herein are derived from patients with chronic inflammation of the prostate, and investigation of the distribution of drugs in acute infection is yet to be pursued.

Comparative Pharmacokinetic Study of Cefotetan (YM09330) and Moxalactam

I. NAKAYAMA,* Y. AKIEDA, H. KAWAGUCHI, AND S. ISHIYAMA

Nihon University School of Medicine, Department of Surgery, 1-8-13, Surugadai Kanda, Chiyoda-ku, Tokyo, Japan

Cefotetan (YM09330), disodium 7-β-[4-(carbamoyl carboxylatomethylene)-1,3-dithietan-2-yl]carboxy-amino-7-α-methoxy-3-(1-methyltetrazol-5-yl)-thiomethyl-Δ3-cephem-4-carboxylate, is a new synthetic parenteral cephamycin antibiotic recently developed in Japan; it shows a wide spectrum against gram-positive and gram-negative bacteria, including β-lactamase-producing resistant strains.

A single dose of cefotetan (1,000 mg) or moxalactam (1,000 mg) was given intravenously by a crossover method to three healthy adult volunteers. By high-performance liquid chromatography (HPLC) and bioassay, with *Escherichia coli* NIHJ for cefotetan and *E. coli* 7437 for moxalactam as the test organisms, mean peak plasma levels of 245 and 136 μg/ml for HPLC and 217 and 126 μg/ml for bioassay were attained after administration at 5 min for cefotetan and moxalactam, respectively.

The measurable concentrations of cefotetan and moxalactam are shown in Table 1.

The average urine and plasma concentrations reached peaks of 3,705 and 3,588 μg/ml at 1 h for cefotetan and 4,600 and 4,980 μg/ml at 0.5 h for moxalactam in the HPLC and bioassay, respectively, after administration. The average peak concentrations for cefotetan were 2,177, 1,309, 748, and 446 μg/ml by HPLC and 3,588, 1,630, 736, and 429 μg/ml by bioassay at 2, 4, 6, and 8 h, respectively. For moxalactam, the average peak concentrations were 4,288, 2,984, 1,558, 637, and 315 μg/ml by HPLC and 4,530, 3,280, 1,750, 632, and 322 μg/ml by bioassay at 1, 2, 4, 6, and 8 h, respectively (Table 2).

Of the doses given, 68.7 and 68.0% of cefotetan by HPLC and bioassay, respectively, and 75.4 and 80% of moxalactam by HPLC and bioassay, respectively, were recovered from the urine within 8 h. About 5% of the cefotetan dose was detected in urine as a tautomer with the same antibacterial activities as those of cefotetan.

Metabolites of cefotetan in humans were examined by thin-layer chromatography, bioautography, and HPLC. Almost no metabolites of cefotetan were detected in the urine. It was found, however, that a small part of the cefotetan given was recovered in the urine as a biologically active tautomer of cefotetan. The tautomer has a 3-hydroxy-4-carboxyisothiazole ring at the 7-β position of the β-lactam skeleton, showed a lower R_f value and a longer retention time than cefotetan on thin-layer chromatography and HPLC, respectively, and possessed a quite similar antibacterial activity compared with cefotetan. In the investigation of the equilibrium reaction between cefotetan and its tautomer, it was concluded that cefotetan was easily converted to the tautomer by the high alkaline pH (over pH 9) and the high concentration of Mg^{2+} (about 20 mM).

An 8-h urine bioautogram was determined from human subjects for the purpose of studying the metabolites of cefotetan and moxalactam. The examination was made by thin-layer chromatography and bioautography. The adsorbent used was Merck DC-Fertigplatten Kieselgel F 254, and the solvent system was composed of $CHCl_3$:CH_3OH:HCOOH (53:45:2).

In this study, a biologically active substance

TABLE 1. *Plasma levels of cefotetan and moxalactam (crossover study)*

Antibiotic[a]	Assay	Concn (μg/ml) in plasma at (h)[b]:							
		1/12	1/4	1/2	1	2	4	6	8
Cefotetan	Bioassay	217 ± 9	151 ± 5	119 ± 2	94.3 ± 2.6	63.0 ± 2.6	38.8 ± 1.2	22.9 ± 1.4	13.9 ± 1.3
	HPLC	245 ± 13.5	176 ± 1.5	114 ± 1.5	81.5 ± 2.4	62.7 ± 2.3	35.5 ± 1.5	22.2 ± 2.1	13.4 ± 1.1
Moxalactam	Bioassay	126 ± 7.5	96.5 ± 5.8	70.8 ± 2.5	51.7 ± 1.1	32.5 ± 2.5	16.3 ± 2.0	6.8 ± 0.5	3.4 ± 0.3
	HPLC	136 ± 6.3	100 ± 1.2	78.4 ± 1.4	56.0 ± 1.5	35.6 ± 2.2	16.3 ± 1.1	7.2 ± 1.0	ND[c]

[a] Antibiotics were given intravenously at 1 g.
[b] Mean of three volunteers ± standard error of the mean.
[c] ND, Not detectable.

TABLE 2. *Urinary excretion of cefotetan and moxalactam (crossover study)*

Antibiotic[a]	Assay	% Excretion in urine at (h)[b]:					
		0–1/2	1/2–1	1–2	2–4	4–6	6–8
Cefotetan	Bioassay	14.0 ± 1.6	9.1 ± 1.4	10.6 ± 8.0	19.4 ± 1.6	8.1 ± 3.3	6.8 ± 0.2
	HPLC						
	Total[c]	14.1 ± 1.2	9.4 ± 1.8	10.9 ± 0.6	18.6 ± 1.0	8.6 ± 3.7	7.1 ± 0.5
	Tautomer	0.35 ± 0.05	0.46 ± 0.22	0.74 ± 0.23	1.35 ± 0.22	0.78 ± 0.33	0.71 ± 0.11
Moxalactam	Bioassay	20.1 ± 0.03	13.9 ± 1.8	16.2 ± 0.7	17.4 ± 2.3	7.9 ± 1.0	4.5 ± 0.3
	HPLC	18.7 ± 0.2	13.3 ± 1.5	15.3 ± 0.5	15.9 ± 1.5	7.9 ± 0.9	4.4 ± 0.3

[a] Antibiotics were given intravenously at 1 g.
[b] Mean of three volunteers ± standard error of the mean.
[c] Sum total of cefotetan and tautomer.

was found in the 8-h urine, which showed that there were no metabolites of either cefotetan or moxalactam.

A pharmacokinetic study was carried out by use of a two-compartment open model method. Pharmacokinetic parameters showed that the half-life (β) of cefotetan was 2.83 h, being 1.5-fold longer than that of moxalactam. The areas under the curve of two antibiotics in a dose of 1,000 mg given intravenously were 503 h.μg/ml for cefotetan and 208 h.μg/ml for moxalactam.

In this study, no abnormal findings in clinical signs or laboratory tests were observed in any of the subjects.

1. **Ishiyama, S., I. Nakayama, H., Iwamoto, S. Iwai, M. Okui, and T. Matsubara.** 1970. Absorption, tissue concentration, and organ distribution of cefazolin. Antimicrob. Agents Chemother. **1970**:476–480.
2. **Nakayama, I., H. Iwamoto, S. Iwai, H. Mizuashi, and S. Ishiyama.** 1978. Comparative study of CS-1170 and cefoxitin: absorption, distribution, and metabolism, p. 851–852. *In* W. Siegenthaler and R. Lüthy (ed.), Current chemotherapy, vol. 2. American Society for Microbiology, Washington, D.C.
3. **Tachibana, A., M. Komiya, Y. Kikuchi, K. Yano, and K. Mashimo.** 1980. Pharmacological studies on YM09330, a new parenteral cephamycin derivative, p. 273–275. *In* J. D. Nelson and C. Grassi (ed.), Current chemotherapy and infectious disease, vol. 1. American Society for Microbiology, Washington, D.C.

Clinical Study of Cefotetan (YM09330) in Aerobic and Anaerobic Surgical Infections

I. NAKAYAMA,* Y. AKIEDA, H. KAWAGUCHI, AND S. ISHIYAMA

Nihon University School of Medicine, Department of Surgery, 1-8-13, Surugadai Kanda, Tokyo, Japan

Cefotetan (YM09330) is a new injectable cephamycin antibiotic derivative developed in Japan and is characterized by high activity against gram-positive and gram-negative bacteria, including β-lactamase–producing bacteria.

An open clinical trial was carried out on 30 patients (22 males and 8 females) with surgical infections in our department of surgery, and the results were evaluated. The ages of patients were distributed over the range of 8 to 77 years (mean, 28.4 years).

The duration of the treatment was in the range of 4 to 17 days (mean, 6.9 days). Among 30 cases, 22 cases were distributed in the range of 4 to 6 days. In these cases, the efficacy rate was 95.5%.

Of the 30 surgical infections, 21 were peritonitis cases, 3 were soft-tissue infections, 2 were acute cholecystitis cases, 1 was a bacteremia case, 1 was a case of purulent orchitis, 1 was a respiratory tract infection, and 1 was a urinary tract infection.

The clinical efficacy rates were 90.5% for peritonitis and 100% for soft-tissue infections, acute cholecystitis, bacteremia, and purulent orchitis (Table 1).

From 30 cases, 26 strains of bacteria were isolated from surgical specimens. The most prevalent pathogen in all studies was *Escherichia coli* (5 strains); its clinical efficacy rate was 80%. *Pseudomonas aeruginosa* was the second most prevalent pathogen (10 strains). *Staphylococcus aureus, S. epidermidis, Streptococcus faecalis, Haemophilus influenzae, Klebsiella pneumoniae*, a *Citrobacter* sp., a *Pseudomonas* sp., an anaerobe, and *Bacteroides fragilis* were also isolated. *E. coli* and *B. fragilis* were isolated from four polymicrobial mixed infections, and *K. pneumoniae* and *B. fragilis* were isolated from three polymicrobial mixed infections (Table 2).

The bactericidal efficacy of clinical isolates was such that infections due to *E. coli* and polymicrobial infections responded well to cefotetan; their eradication rates were 100%. The total bacteria eradication rate was 90.5%.

Of 30 patients, 7 were given 500-mg doses twice daily, and the efficacy rate was 85.7%. Twenty-one patients were given 1,000-mg doses twice daily, with an efficacy rate of 95.2%. Two cases were given 1,000-mg doses.

As for the relation between clinical efficacy and the dose of cefotetan per day, a group of 7 patients treated with 500 mg twice daily consisted of 1 excellent result, 5 effective results, and 1 fair result. Of 21 patients treated with 1,000 mg twice daily, 2 patients showed excellent results, 18 patients showed effective results, and 1 patient failed to respond. The total clinical efficacy rate was 90%.

Patient 17, a 10-year-old male, was admitted with a high temperature, progressive abdominal pain, and tenderness in the lower abdominal region. The leukocyte count on admission was 12,400. Upon operation, a gangrenous, perforated appendix was found, with localized peritonitis.

The patient received 1 g of cefotetan per day

TABLE 1. *Clinical efficacy of cefotetan*

Disease (no. of cases)	Result			
	Excellent	Effective	Fair	Failure
Abscess (3)		3		
Purulent orchitis (1)	1			
Acute cholecystitis (2)	1	1		
Localized peritonitis (20)		19	1	
Diffuse peritonitis (1)				1
Bacteremia (1)	1			
Respiratory tract infection (1)		1		
Urinary tract infection (1)				1

intravenously for 5 days. The patient improved rapidly in his general condition, fever disappeared by 2 days, and the leukocyte count was down to 5,100 on the 5th postoperative day. Bacteriological culture showed mixed infections of *E. coli* and *B. fragilis.*

By gas-liquid chromatographic analysis of the composition of fatty acids of pus at the time of surgery, acetic acid, propionic acid, and isovaleric acid were detected. This composition pattern was that of the *Bacteroides* group, which was susceptible to cefotetan. The patient improved rapidly with appropriate surgery and antibiotic therapy which was effective against *E. coli* and *B. fragilis.*

Fatty acid patterns of the anaerobe by gas-liquid chromatography showed acetic acid-propionic acid-isovaleric acid (C_2:C_3:iC_5) as the vaporizing fatty acid pattern of the *Bacteroides* group, and lactic acid-succinic acid as the nonvaporizing fatty acid pattern of the *Bacteroides* group.

Moreover, the fluorescent-antibody test revealed the presence of the *Bacteroides* group.

Side effects were reported by four patients. Of these, 1 patient showed an increase of serum glutamic pyruvic transaminase, 1 patient showed an increase of serum glutamic oxalacetic transaminase and serum glutamic pyruvic transaminase, and 1 patient was superinfected. In this study, no abnormal findings in clinical signs or laboratory tests were observed in any of the cases.

TABLE 2. *Bacteriological efficacy of cefotetan*

Organism (no. of cases)	Result[a]		
	Eradicated	Unchanged	Unknown
Staphylococcus aureus (1)	1		
S. epidermidis (1)	1		
Streptococcus faecalis (2)		1	1
H. influenzae (1)	1		
E. coli (5)	5		
K. pneumoniae (1)	1		
Citrobacter (1)	1		
P. aeruginosa (3)		1	2
Pseudomonas sp. (1)			1
Anaerobe (1)	1		
B. fragilis (2)	1		1
E. coli + *B. fragilis* (4)	4		
K. pneumoniae + *B. fragilis* (3)	3		

[a] There was one case of superinfection with *Streptococcus faecalis.*

1. **Ishiyama, S., I. Nakayama, H. Iwamoto, S. Iwai, M. Okui, and T. Matsubara.** 1970. Absorption, tissue concentration, and organ distribution of cefazolin. Antimicrob. Agents Chemother. **1970:** 476–480.
2. **Nakayama, I., H. Iwamoto, S. Iwai, H. Mizuashi, and S. Ishiyama.** 1979. Comparative study of CS-1170 and cefoxitin: absorption, distribution, and metabolism, p. 851–852. *In* W. Siegenthaler and R. Lüthy (ed.), Current chemotherapy, vol. 2. American Society for Microbiology, Washington, D.C.

Clinical Study on YM09330 (Cefotetan) in Internal Medicine

KOHEI HARA* AND KEIMEI MASHIMO

Nagasaki University, Nagasaki, and Tokyo Kosei Nenkin Hospital, Tokyo, Japan*

Cefotetan, a new cephamycin derivative developed in Japan, has a broad spectrum and high antibacterial activity against gram-negative bacteria, including beta-lactamase-producing strains (2). The plasma half-life of cefotetan is as long as 3 h in humans, and therapeutic plasma levels are maintained for approximately 12 h (1). This report summarizes the results of a clinical study on cefotetan performed in the field of internal medicine at 41 institutions in Japan.

A total of 544 patients received the drug. However, 75 cases were excluded from analysis, because the patients in these cases also received other antibiotics or were too seriously ill. As a result, 469 cases were evaluated. The ratio of males to females was 3:2, and more than half the patients were over 60 years of age.

Most patients were administered cefotetan in a dose of 1.0 to 2.0 g twice a day by intravenous bolus injection or drip infusion. The duration of treatment was 3 to 77 days, but most patients received the drug for 5 to 14 days. The clinical results were excellent in 95 and good in 258 cases; thus, the total effective rate was 75.3% (Table 1).

Among the cases of respiratory tract infections, 21 were upper respiratory tract infections, such as tonsillitis and acute bronchitis; the effective rate in these cases was 90.5%. In 235 cases with lung parenchymal infections, such as pneumonia (including secondary pulmonary disease) and suppurative pulmonary infection, an effec-

TABLE 1. *Clinical results of cefotetan treatment*

	Sites of infection	No. of cases	Clinical effectiveness				Effective rate (%)
			Excel-lent	Good	Fair	Poor	
Respiratory tract infections	Upper respiratory tract infection						
	Tonsilitis	3	1	2			
	Acute bronchitis	18	6	10		2	88.9
	Sub total	21	7	12		2	90.5
	Lung parenchymal infection						
	Pneumonia	208	39	126	27	16	79.3
	Supparative pulmonary disease	19	4	11	2	2	78.9
	Secondary pulmonary infection	8		4	2	2	50.0
	Sub total	235	43	141	31	20	78.3
	Chronic pulmonary infection						
	Chronic bronchitis	55	5	33	9	8	69.1
	Bronchoectasis	26	1	9	12	4	38.5
	Sub total	81	6	42	21	12	59.3
	Pleura infection						
	Pleurisy	3			2	1	
	Pyothorax	7	1	4	1	1	71.4
	Sub total	10	1	4	3	2	50.0
	Total	347	57	199	55	36	73.8
Urinary tract infections	Acute						
	Cystitis	17	9	7		1	94.1
	Pyelonephritis	22	7	13		2	90.9
	Sub total	39	16	20		3	92.3
	Chronic						
	Cystitis	29	6	13	3	7	65.5
	Pyelunephritis	9	3	3	2	1	66.7
	Sub total	38	9	16	5	8	65.8
	Total	77	25	36	5	11	79.2
Biliary tract infection		22	3	16	2	1	86.4
Septicemia		8	4	2	1	1	75.0
Subacute bacterial endocarditis		2	1	1			
Miscellaneous		13	5	4	3	1	69.2
Ground total		469	95	258	66	50	75.3

tive rate of 78.3% was obtained. In contrast, the effective rate in 81 cases with chronic pulmonary infections was 59.3%, and it was only 50% in 10 cases with pleural infections, including pyothorax.

For urinary tract infections, an effective rate of 92.3% was obtained in 39 acute cases, whereas only a 65.9% effective rate was obtained in 38 chronic cases.

In 22 cases with biliary tract infections, the

TABLE 2. *Bacteriological results of cefotetan treatment in causative organisms*[a]

causative organisms

	Organisms	No. of cases	Clinical effectiveness				Effective rate (%) *
			Eliminated	Decreased	Replaced	Unchanged	
Simple infection	S. aureus	7	7				100.0
	S. epidermidis	1	1				
	β-Streptococcus	7	6		1		100.0
	Str. pneumoniae	14	9		2	3	78.6
	Str. faecalis	5	4			1	80.0
	Other GPB	3	3				
	Sub total	37	30		3	4	89.2
	E. coli	39	31	2	6		94.9
	K. pneumoniae	30	23	1	5	1	93.3
	K. oxytoca	2	1		1		
	Ps. aeruginosa	12	1	2	1	8	16.7
	P. mirabilis	7	3		4		100.0
	P. rettgeri	3	1		2		
	Enter. aerogenes	1	1				
	Enter. cloacae	5	4		1		100.0
	Ser. marcescens	5	4		1		100.0
	H. influenzae	48	39	3	5	1	91.7
	Citrobacter	1			1		
	Other GNB	3	3				
	Sub total	156	111	8	27	10	88.5
	Bacteroides	1				1	
	Total	194	141	8	30	15	88.1
Mixed infection	Pseudomonas+etc.	5	3			2	60.0
	Serratia+etc.	6	2	1	2	1	66.7
	Proteus+etc.	5	3	1	1		80.0
	Klebsiella+etc.	11	4	5	2		54.5
	E. coli+etc.	2	2				
	Miscellaneous	9	7	1	1		88.9
	Total	38	21	8	6	3	71.1
Ground total		232	162	16	36	18	85.3

$$\text{* Disappearance rate} = \frac{\text{Eliminated + Replaced}}{\text{Eliminated + Decreased + Replaced + Unchanged}}$$

[a] *Disappearance rate = [(Eliminated + replaced)/(eliminated + decreased + replaced + unchanged)]. GPB, Gram-positive bacilli; GNB, gram-negative bacilli.

effective rate was 86.4%. In 10 cases with bacteremia, including subacute bacterial endocarditis, the effective rate was 80%. Against miscellaneous infections, the effective rate was 69.2%.

As analyzed by the presence or absence of underlying diseases such as cancer, the effective rate was increased to 80.5% in 256 cases without underlying disease, and it was reduced to 69.0% in 213 patients with underlying diseases.

The bacteriological response of cefotetan was analyzed (Table 2). Of gram-positive bacteria, all strains of staphylococci and streptococci disappeared, and the disappearance rate for pneumococci and enterococci was about 80%; thus, the disappearance rate for all gram-positive bacteria was 89.2%. Among the gram-negative bacilli, *Escherichia coli* and *Klebsiella* spp. disappeared at a rate of 93 to 95%, and all strains of *Proteus* spp., *Enterobacter* spp., and *Serratia marcescens* disappeared at substantially high rates. These results are consistent with the antibacterial activity of the drug in vitro. The disappearance rate for *Haemophilus* spp. was 91.7%.

The clinical effects were classified by individual bacteria and analyzed. For gram-positive bacteria, poor results were obtained with *Streptococcus pneumoniae*, the effective rate being 61.1%. For gram-negative bacilli, an effective rate of 70 to 80% was obtained in infections due to *E. coli*, *Klebsiella* spp., *Proteus* spp., *Enterobacter* spp., and *Haemophilus* spp., as expected from the antibacterial activity of the drug. However, in infections caused by *Pseudomonas aeruginosa*, the effective rate was only 28.6%.

No correlation or dose response could be found between clinical effect and daily dosage.

Side effects were observed in 18 of the 538 cases. The symptoms were rash in six, fever in five, rash with fever in four, and face edema, nausea, and vomiting in one case each.

In clinical laboratory data, an increase in serum transaminase was observed in 22 cases (4.3%); an increase in alkaline phosphatase, in 5 (1.1%); an increase in eosinophilia, in 4 (1.0%); and a decrease in erythrocytes, leukocytes, and platelets, in 1 case each.

From these results, it has been found that cefotetan is a useful new antibiotic against various infections, especially with gram-negative bacilli, in the field of internal medicine.

1. **Tachibana, A., M. Komiya, Y. Kikuchi, K. Yano, and K. Mashimo.** 1980. Pharmacological studies on YM09330, a new parenteral cephamycin derivative, p. 273–275. *In* J. D. Nelson and C. Grassi (ed.), Current chemotherapy and infectious disease, vol. 1. American Society for Microbiology, Washington, D.C.
2. **Toda, M., T. Saito, K. Yano, K. Suzaki, M. Saito, and S. Mitsuhashi.** 1980. In vitro and in vivo antibacterial activities of YM09330, a new cephamycin derivative, p. 280–281. *In* J. D. Nelson and C. Grassi (ed.), Current chemotherapy and infectious disease, vol. 1. American Society for Microbiology, Washington, D.C.

Clinical Study on YM09330 (Cefotetan) in Urinary Tract Infection

JOICHI KUMAZAWA, SHUNRO MOMOSE,* AND KEIMEI MASHIMO

Saga Medical School, Saga; Kyushu University, Fukuoka; and Tokyo Kosei Nenkin Hospital, Tokyo, Japan*

Cefotetan, a new cephamycin derivative antibiotic, has higher antibacterial activity against gram-negative bacteria, including indole-positive *Proteus* spp., *Enterobacter* spp., *Citrobacter* spp., and *Serratia* spp., than other cephamycins commercially available (2). This report summarizes the clinical results obtained in cefotetan treatment of urinary tract infections; the study was performed in 17 institutions in Japan.

Subjects and methods. Cefotetan was administered to a total of 419 patients. Overall efficacy was confirmed in 397 cases, consisting of 317 men and 80 women, 297 of whom were aged 60 years and above.

Cefotetan was given by intravenous bolus injection or drip infusion. The daily dosage was 0.5 g in 7, 1 g in 273, and 2 g in 117 cases, whereas the number of administrations per day was once in 64, twice in 325, and four times in 8 cases. The treatment was continued for 5 days in almost all cases.

Results. The overall clinical efficacy was excellent in 81, good in 150, fair in 67, and poor in 99 cases. Classification of the results by disease revealed a very high clinical efficacy rate in the treatment of simple urinary tract infections and a fairly high rate in the treatment of pyelonephritis, a complicated urinary tract infection (Table 1).

There are criteria used for the assessment of clinical efficacy of antimicrobial agents which were set up by the Committee on Urinary Tract

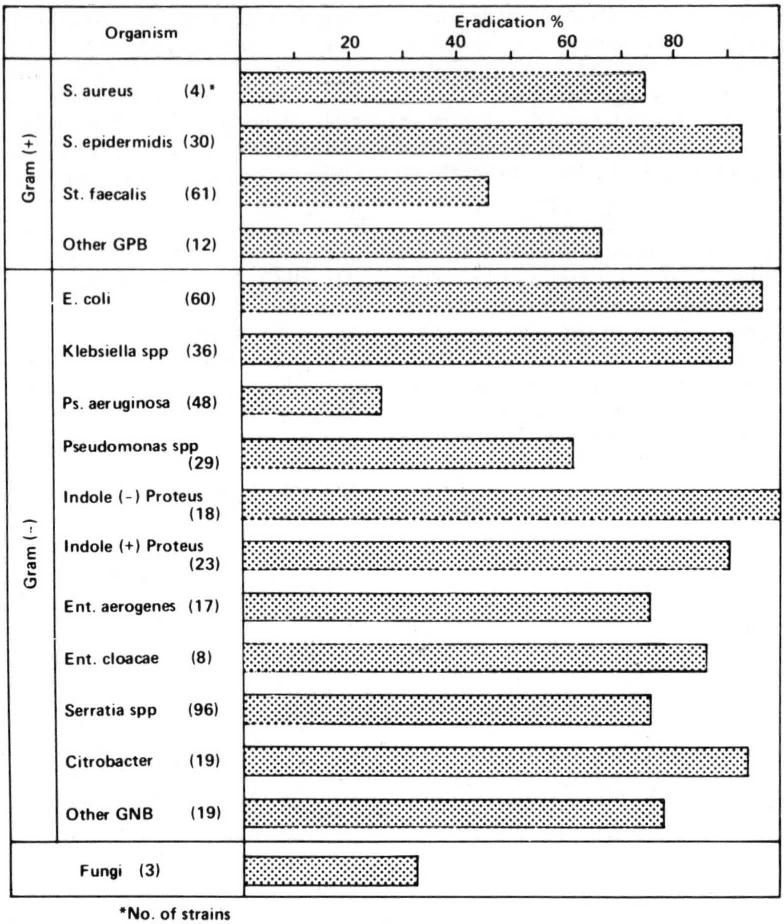

FIG. 1. *Bacteriological response of cefotetan classified by organism. GPB, Gram-positive bacilli; GNB, gram-negative bacilli.*

TABLE 1. *Clinical efficacy, by disease, of cefotetan in treatment of urological infections*

Diagnosis			No. of cases	Clinical results				Efficacy (%)
				Excel-lent	Good	Fair	Poor	
Urinary tract infections	Cystitis	Simple	5	4	1			100.0
		Complicated	267	43	96	50	78	52.1
	Pyelone-phritis	Simple	6	2	4			100.0
		Complicated	94	23	41	15	15	68.1
	Post prostatectomy		15	5	4	1	5	60.0
	Gonorrhea		3	2	1			
	Subtotal		390	79	147	66	98	57.9
Prostatitis			4	2	1	1		
Epididymitis			2		2			
Other			1				1	
Total			397	81 (20.4%)	150 (37.8%)	67 (16.9%)	99 (24.9%)	58.2

Infection in Japan (1). According to the criteria, the efficacy of antimicrobial agents can be divided into three levels, excellent, moderate, and poor; these are based on the change in organisms and the variation of leukocyte count in the urine.

The clinical efficacy of cefotetan was confirmed in 359 cases of complicated urinary tract infections according to these criteria; the efficacy was excellent in 64, moderate in 149, and poor in 146 cases, giving an efficacy rate of 59%. Bacteriuria was eliminated in 45%, decreased in 4%, and replaced in 24% of the cases, giving a bacteriological efficacy rate of 73%. Analysis of these bacteriological results with respect to individual organisms showed a high efficacy rate for most organisms, although a low eradication rate was observed for *Streptococcus faecalis* and *Pseudomonas aeruginosa* (Fig. 1). The above results conform well with the in vitro properties of cefotetan.

Side effects. Subjective side effects were reported by patients in 8 of the 419 cases. The percentage (1.9%) of revealing side effects was not high compared with that of the β-lactam derivative antibiotics now available.

The symptoms were fever in one, rash in three, nausea in three, and nausea with vomiting in one case. In four cases, administration of the drug was discontinued due to the side effects.

For abnormalities in clinical laboratory findings after administration of the drug, an increase in SGOT values was observed in 1.4% cases; an increase in SGPT, in 0.8% cases; an increase in BUN, in 0.3%; an increase in serum creatinine, in 0.3%; and an increase in eosinocytes, in 0.6%.

Conclusion. The above results show that cefotetan is a highly useful new antibiotic against both simple and complicated urinary tract infections, with the exceptions of infections caused by *S. faecalis* and *P. aeruginosa*.

1. **Ohkoshi, M., and Committee on Urinary Tract Infection in Japan.** 1980. Criteria for a drug evaluation in urinary tract infections, 2nd report. Chemotherapy (Tokyo) **28:**324–341; 1351–1358. (In Japanese)

2. **Toda, M., T. Saito, K. Yano, K. Suzaki, M. Saito, and S. Mitsuhashi.** 1980. In vitro and in vivo antibacterial activities of YM09330, a new cephamycin derivative, p. 280–281. *In* J. D. Nelson and C. Grassi (ed.), Current chemotherapy and infectious disease, vol. 1. American Society for Microbiology, Washington, D.C.

Ceftriaxone (Ro 13-9904): Evaluation In Vitro

A. ALBERTE,* R. TORIO, P. P. PASCUAL, AND A. GOMEZ

Residencia Sanitaria, Valladolid, Spain

Ceftriaxone (Ro 13-9904) is a new cephalosporin which offers undoubted advantages over the first generation of cephalosporins, such as its high mean half-life, its stability against the action of bacterial beta-lactamases, and its broad spectrum and activity in vitro against numerous species of microorganisms. For this reason, our intention was to study the activity in vitro of ceftriaxone in different strains isolated in the clinic, comparing it with that of other antimicrobial agents.

A total of 305 bacterial isolates used in the present study were obtained from clinical samples originating from patients hospitalized in the Residencia Sanitaria, Valladolid, Spain, during 1980. All of the species isolated represent clinical isolates from different patients. The bacteria tested (*n*) were: *Salmonella* spp. (85), *Serratia marcescens* (44), *Staphylococcus aureus* (47), *Pneumococcus* spp. (18), *Haemophilus influenzae* (22), *Escherichia coli* (19), *Pseudomonas aeruginosa* (19), beta-hemolytic group A and B streptococci (9), and other strains that are gentamicin resistant (39). The standardized antibiotic substance named ceftriaxone was supplied by P. Roche, and cefotaxime, cefoxitine, amikacin, gentamicin, etc., were supplied by their manufacturers. In vitro agar dilution tests were per formed in the conventional manner (6), using a Steers replicator (5). For the study of beta-lactamase production, Glaxo chromogenic cephalosporin was used (3).

A study was made of the activity of ceftriaxone, ampicillin, fosfomycin, chloramphenicol, and co-trimoxazole against strains of *Salmonella* spp. To inhibit 90% of the strains, 8 μg of ampicillin per ml was necessary, the same as for chloramphenicol, whereas for fosfomycin 128 μg/ml was needed. However, ceftriaxone inhibited 97.6% of the strains at 0.25 μg/ml, and achieved 100% inhibition with 0.5 μg/ml. Co-trimoxazole also showed good activity and required a fractionary inhibitory concentration of 0.25/32 to inhibit 90% of the strains.

At 1 μg/ml, ceftriaxone inhibited 90% of the *S. marcescens* strains, and at 8 μg/ml, it in-

TABLE 1. *Susceptibility of different clinical isolates to ceftriaxone*

Organism (no. of strains)	Cumulative % inhibited at concn (μg/ml) of:												
	≤0.06	0.12	0.25	0.5	1	2	4	8	16	32	64	128	>128
Salmonella spp. (85)	69.4		97.6	100									
S. marcescens (44)		31.8		61.3	90	94.5		100					
E. coli (19)	63.1		100										
P. aeruginosa (19)								18.1	26.3	52.6	68.4	84.1	100
H. influenzae (23)	95.6	100											
E. cloacae (2)	100												
S. aureus (47)			4.2			14.9	72.3	95.7				98	100
Pneumococcus (17)	76.4	100											
Beta-hemolytic A and B streptococci (9)	100												
Viridans streptococci (1)						100							

TABLE 2. *Susceptibility of 39 gentamicin-resistant strains to different antibiotics*

Drug	Cumulative % inhibited at concn (μg/ml) of:											
	≤0.25	0.5	1	2	4	8	16	32	64	128	256	>256
Cefoxitin					10.2	25.6			35.8		38.4	100
Cefotaxime	18.4	34.3	71.7	81.1	84.2		87.3	93.4		100		
Ceftriaxone	41	56.3	71.7	74.2	79.3	82		87		89.5		100
Amikacin		5.2	48.6	58.9	76.8			78.3	89.6	100		

hibited 100%. At a concentration of ≤0.06 μg/ml, ceftriaxone inhibited 63.1% of the *E. coli* strains and 0.25 μg/ml was required to inhibit 100%. Ceftriaxone showed less activity against *P. aeruginosa*, inhibiting 50% of the strains at a concentration 64 times greater than that required for *S. marcescens* (Table 1).

Ceftriaxone exhibited a special effect against strains of *H. influenzae*, whether producers of beta-lactamase or not; at concentrations of ≤0.06 μg/ml, it inhibited 95.6% of such strains, and no strain was isolated with a MIC above 0.12 μg/ml. However, 8 μg/ml was needed to inhibit 95.7% of *S. aureus* strains, and others were also resistant. Against penicillin-resistant strains of *Pneumococcus*, ceftriaxone showed great activity, inhibiting 76.4 and 100% of the strains at concentrations of 0.06 and 0.12 μg/ml, respectively. Ceftriaxone also inhibited 100% of the strains of beta-hemolytic A and B streptococci at a concentration of ≤0.06 μg/ml. However, inhibition of one strain of viridans streptococci required 2 μg/ml.

Finally, a study was made of the comparative activity of cefoxitin, cefotaxime, ceftriaxone, and amikacin against 39 strains resistant to gentamicin (MIC, >64 μg/ml). Taking as the susceptibility limit for the cephalosporins mentioned a concentration of ≤8 μg/ml and a concentration of ≤16 μg/ml for amikacin, it may be observed that cefoxitin inhibits 25.6% of the strains; cefotaxime, 84.2%; ceftriaxone, 82%; and amikacin, 76.8% (Table 2). In this case, cefotaxime was slightly superior to ceftriaxone, although the latter was more active against more susceptible strains.

An interesting future awaits the newly prepared ceftriaxone, stemming from its activity in vitro, where it shows good activity against *S. marcescens*, with values similar to those quoted by other authors (1) for cephalosporins such as cefotaxime and moxalactam, and surpassing the results communicated by Neu et al. (2) of the above-mentioned cephalosporins against *Salmonella*, although Shelton et al. (4) observed greater activity. Against both *E. coli* and the remaining *Enterobacteriaceae*, ceftriaxone was very active, but displayed little activity against strains of *P. aeruginosa*. Against infections due to *H. influenzae*, *Pneumococcus*, and beta-hemolytic streptococci, ceftriaxone was the antibiotic of choice, but not for *S. aureus* strains. Finally, against gentamicin-resistant hospital strains, the use of ceftriaxone may be considered an alternative, cooperating in displacing the use of aminoglycosides.

1. **Delgado, D. G., C. J. Brau, C. G. Cobbs, and W. E. Diamukes.** 1979. In vitro activity of LY 127935, a new 1-oxa cephalosporin, against aerobic gram-negative bacilli. Antimicrob. Agents Chemother. **16:**864–868.
2. **Neu, H. C., N. Aswapokee, P. Fu, and P. Aswapokee.** 1979. Antibacterial activity of a new 1-oxa cephalosporin compared with that of other β-lactam compounds. Antimicrob. Agents Chemother. **16:**141–149.
3. **O'Callaghan, C. H., A. Morris, S. M. Kirby, and A. H.**

Shingler. 1972. Novel method for detection of β-lactamases by using a chromogenic cephalosporin substrate. Antimicrob. Agents Chemother. 1:283–288.
4. Shelton, S., J. D. Nelson, and G. H. McCracken, Jr. 1980. In vitro susceptibility of gram-negative bacilli from pediatric patients to moxalactam, cefotaxime, Ro 13-9904, and other cephalosporins. Antimicrob. Agents Chemotherapy. 18:476–479.
5. Steers, E., E. L. Foltz, B. S. Graves, and J. Riden. 1959. An inocula replicating apparatus for routine testing of bacterial susceptibility to antibiotics. Antimicrob. Chemother. (Basel) 9:307–311.
6. Washington J. A., II, and V. L. Sutter. 1980. Dilution susceptibility test: agar and macro-broth dilution procedures, p. 453–458. *In* E. H. Lennette, A. Balows, W. J. Hausler, Jr., and J. P. Truant (ed.), Manual of clinical microbiology, 3rd ed. American Society for Microbiology, Washington, D.C.

In Vitro Activity of Ceftriaxone, a Novel Cephalosporin, Compared with Those of Other Cephalosporins

A. J. BINT,* P. YEOMAN, P. KILBURN, R. ANDERSON, AND E. STANSFIELD

Department of Microbiology, Royal Victoria Infirmary, Newcastle upon Tyne, U.K.

Ceftriaxone (Ro 13-9904) is a new parenteral cephalosporin with a broad spectrum of activity (3). Its activity needs to be compared with those of other recently described, high-potency cephalosporins such as cefotaxime (1) and ceftazidime (2). In this study, the in vitro activity of ceftriaxone was compared with the activities of cefoperazone, cefotaxime, cefsulodin, ceftazidime, cefuroxime, and cephalothin against 331 clinical bacterial isolates.

All bacterial strains were recent clinical isolates, identified by standard methods. The production of β-lactamase by selected strains was confirmed by the use of nitrocefin. Antibiotics were obtained from their respective manufacturers. The activities of the cephalosporins were measured by an agar plate dilution method, using Oxoid DST agar. This medium was supplemented with 5% horse blood for testing streptococci and *Bacteroides fragilis* and with 5% horse blood and 1% NAD for testing *Haemophilus influenzae*. With the exceptions of *H. influenzae* and *B. fragilis*, inocula were prepared by suspending overnight surface growth into saline (gram-negative bacilli) or Todd-Hewitt broth (staphylococci and streptococci) to achieve 10^8 colony-forming units (CFU)/ml. Inocula for *H. influenzae* were prepared by suspending surface growth into brain heart infusion broth, and for *B. fragilis* they were prepared by diluting overnight cultures in thioglycolate broth. Using a multipoint inoculator (Denley Tech Ltd.), drops containing 10^5 CFU were delivered onto antibiotic-containing agar plates. Plates were incubated at 37°C in 10% CO_2 except for *B. fragilis*, which was incubated in GasPak jars (BBL Microbiology Systems).

Inoculum effects were investigated with two strains each of *Escherichia coli* and *Staphylococcus aureus* and one strain each of *Klebsiella pneumoniae* and *Proteus mirabilis*. MICs were measured as described above but with inocula of 10^3 and 10^7 CFU tested in parallel. The MIC was defined as the concentration of antibiotic at which 99.9% of CFU were inhibited after 24 h of incubation. Measurement of MICs and MBCs was performed with and without 50% pooled human serum in Isosensitest broth (Oxoid) inoculated with 10^5 CFU/ml. Subcultures of 5 μl to plates were made after 24 h of incubation. The MBC was defined as the lowest concentration producing a 99.9% kill of the inoculum.

Table 1 summarizes the activity of ceftriaxone compared with the other cephalosporins tested against the 331 isolates. Ceftriaxone, with an MIC_{90} of 0.015 to 0.25 mg/liter, was highly active against *E. coli*, *K. pneumoniae*, *Salmonella* spp., *Enterobacter* spp., *Proteus mirabilis*, and indole-positive *Proteus* spp. The rank order of activity against these genera was generally ceftriaxone and cefotaxime as the most active, followed by ceftazidime, cefoperazone, cefuroxime, and cephalothin. Ceftriaxone inhibited *Serratia* spp., *Acinetobacter* spp., and *Citrobacter* spp. at higher concentrations (MIC_{90}, 1.0 to 4 mg/liter). Against *P. mirabilis* and indole-positive *Proteus* spp., ceftriaxone was the most active of the cephalosporins tested. Ceftriaxone was less active than ceftazidime and cefsulodin against *Pseudomonas aeruginosa*, similar in activity to cefoperazone, and more active than cefotaxime. *H. influenzae* was highly susceptible to ceftriaxone, which was the most active of the compounds tested, with an MIC_{90} of 0.015 mg/liter. In common with the other cephalosporins tested, ceftriaxone had poor activity against *B. fragilis*.

Ceftriaxone was one of the least active ceph-

TABLE 1. *Comparative activities of ceftriaxone and other cephalosporins*

Species (no. of isolates)	% Inhibited	MIC for 50 and 90% of the isolates (mg/liter)[a]						
		CFT	CTX	CFZ	CPZ	CFU	CLT	CSL
E. coli (33)	50	0.06	0.06	0.25	0.12	4	16	
	90	0.12	0.12	0.25	32	8	64	
K. pneumoniae (25)	50	0.06	0.03	0.12	2	2	8	
	90	0.12	0.06	1	16	4	32	
P. mirabilis (26)	50	0.008	0.03	0.06	1	1	8	
	90	0.015	0.06	0.12	2	4	32	
Enterobacter spp. (10)	50	0.12	0.12	0.25	0.12	4	128	
	90	0.25	0.25	0.25	0.5	8	>128	
Proteus spp. (indole positive) (10)	50	0.008	0.03	0.06	1	16	>128	
	90	0.015	0.06	0.12	2	32	>128	
Serratia spp. (40)	50	0.25	0.25	0.25	2	64	>128	
	90	4	4	1	>128	>128	>128	
Salmonella spp. (10)	50	0.06	0.06	0.25	0.12	0.5	2	
	90	0.06	0.06	0.25	0.12	1	2	
Citrobacter spp. (8)	50	0.12	0.12	0.25	0.5	2	32	
	90	1	0.5	4	>128	32	>128	
Pseudomonas aeruginosa (58)	50	8	16	2	4			1
	90	16	32	4	16			4
Acinetobacter spp. (9)	50	2	2	2	8	8	>128	
	90	4	4	2	32	8	>128	
H. influenzae (16)	50	0.008	0.015	0.12	0.03	1	8	
	90	0.015	0.06	0.25	1	4	8	
B. fragilis (6)	50	8	8	16	32	32	128	
	90	32	32	32	64	128	>128	
S. aureus (34)	50	2	1	8	1	0.5	0.25	
	90	2	2	16	4	1	0.5	
Group A streptococci (14)	50	0.03	0.015	0.12	0.06	0.015	0.12	
	90	0.03	0.015	0.12	0.06	0.015	0.12	
Group B streptococci (20)	50	0.06	0.03	0.25	0.12	0.03	0.25	
	90	0.06	0.06	0.5	0.12	0.03	0.25	
Streptococcus faecalis (12)	50	>128	>128	128	16	128	32	
	90	>128	>128	128	64	>128	64	

[a] CFT, Ceftriaxone; CTX, cefotaxime; CFZ, ceftazidime; CPZ, cefoperazone; CFU, cefuroxime; CLT, cephalothin; CSL, cefsulodin.

alosporins against *S. aureus*, being similar in activity to cefoperazone and cefotaxime. Ceftazidime was the least active against *S. aureus*. Against group A and B streptococci, ceftriaxone was one of the most active of the agents tested. In common with the other cephalosporins tested, ceftriaxone was poorly active against group D streptococci.

A comparison of the MICs and MBCs of ceftazidime and ceftriaxone and the effects of the addition of 50% human serum are shown in Table 2. There was no more than a twofold difference between MICs and MBCs of both compounds for the strains tested, both β-lactamase-positive and -negative strains. However, the addition of 50% human serum increased MICs and MBCs of ceftriaxone by a factor of 8 to 16, whereas those of ceftazidime were unaffected. The effects of increasing the inoculum size from 10^3 to 10^7 CFU on the MICs of ceftriaxone were small, the highest increase being a fourfold rise seen with β-lactamase-producing strains of *K. pneumoniae* and *Pseudomonas aeruginosa*.

This study showed that ceftriaxone is a highly active cephalosporin against the *Enterobacteriaceae*. It was as active as cefotaxime and more active than the other cephalosporins tested. The wide spectrum included such "hospital" organisms as *Serratia* spp., *Klebsiella* and *Enterobacter* spp., and *Acinetobacter* spp. Ceftriaxone was also highly active against *H. influenzae*. Against *S. aureus* ceftriaxone was less active, but the attainable serum levels should be well above MICs. *Pseudomonas aeruginosa* and *B. fragilis* can only be regarded as moderately susceptible, and it will be interesting to see how infections with these pathogens respond to therapy. The high protein binding of ceftriaxone, 95% (3), probably explains the decreased activity in the presence of human serum. It remains to be seen whether this effect will be of importance in vivo, particularly with pathogens of moderate susceptibility such as *S. aureus* and *Pseudomo-*

TABLE 2. *Comparison of MICs and MBCs and effect of 50% human serum*

Organism	Characteristic	Ceftazidime (mg/liter)		Ceftriaxone (mg/liter)	
		MIC	MBC	MIC	MBC
S. aureus	β-Lactamase negative	8	16	4	8
	β-Lactamase negative + 50% serum	8	8	64	128
	β-Lactamase positive	8	8	2	4
E. coli	β-Lactamase negative	0.5	0.5	0.06	0.06
	β-Lactamase negative + 50% serum	0.5	1.0	0.5	1.0
	β-Lactamase positive	0.25	0.5	0.12	0.12
P. aeruginosa	Carbenicillin susceptible	4	4	16	16

nas aeruginosa. In conclusion, ceftriaxone, with high activity and a very broad spectrum, warrants further investigation and clinical trials.

1. **Hamilton-Miller, J. M. T., W. Brumfitt, and A. V. Reynolds.** 1978. Cefotaxime (HR756) a new cephalosporin with exceptional broad spectrum activity *in vitro*. J. Antimicrob. Chemother. **4**:437–444.
2. **O'Callaghan, C. H., P. Acred, P. B. Harper, D. M. Ryan, S. M. Kirby, and S. M. Harding.** 1980. GR20263, a new broad-spectrum cephalosporin with anti-pseudomonas activity. Antimicrob. Agents Chemother. **17**:876–883.
3. **Wise, R., A. P. Gillett, J. M. Andrews, and K. A. Bedford.** 1980. Ro 13-9904: a cephalosporin with a high degree of activity and broad antibacterial activity: an *in vitro* comparative study. J. Antimicrob. Chemother. **6**:595–600.

Ceftriaxone (Ro 13-9904), a Long-Lasting Cephalosporin: Further Studies on the Mode of Antibacterial Action

SUSUMU MITSUHASHI, YUZURU SEKINE, MIKIO ARISAWA, MATSUHISA INOUE, JUNKO OHSHIMA, AND HIROMI B. MARUYAMA*

Gunma University, Maebashi, and Nippon Roche Research Center, Kamakura, Japan*

Ceftriaxone (CTA) is a third-generation parenteral cephalosporin with an aminothiazolylmethoxyiminoacetamide (ATMI) group as C7 side chain (3). It exhibits extraordinary antibacterial activity, especially against gram-negative bacteria. The stability to β-lactamases is also high, except to the enzymes from *Proteus vulgaris*, *P. cepacia*, and *Bacteroides fragilis*. However, the most characteristic feature of CTA is its unusually long serum half-life (1, 4; M. Arisawa et al., submitted for publication). The purpose of this study was to examine reasonable correlations between killing velocity, the morphological changes provoked in bacteria, and the pharmacokinetic properties of ATMI cephalosporins.

Growth kinetics experiments with *Escherichia coli* NIHJ showed that CTA was bactericidal, reducing the number of viable cells by 10^{-2} to 10^{-3} after 2-h treatment at 2 to 4 × MIC. No regrowth was detected within 24 h above 2 × MIC. On the other hand, cefotaxime and cefoperazone, having the same initial killing activity as CTA, allowed a regrowth even at 4 × MIC by 24 h.

An in situ study of morphological changes was carried out by monitoring bacterial morphology directly on a plate under a microscope, because it was suspected that long filaments were easily broken by shearing forces in the process of dilution or plating. The main morphological effect of CTA was filament formation, as shown in Fig. 1. CTA converted the cells into filaments at concentrations ranging from 0.5 to 32 × MIC without reducing the cell number to less than 50% within 4 h. Exactly the same dose-morphology change relationship was observed with cefotaxime. The effect of cefazolin on *E. coli* morphology was obviously different from that of ATMI cephalosporins. The concentration range at which cefazolin induced a morphological change without cell lysis was very narrow, being only at 1 × MIC. More than half of the cells were already lysed at 2 × MIC. This indicates that ATMI cephalosporins need much higher concentrations (on the basis of MIC) than cefazolin to cause the same extent of cell lysis. Actually, at 6.3 μg/ml there was no difference in the percentage of lysed cells among the three antibiotics, though cefazolin was 16 times less active by comparison of the MIC values. Figure 1 also indicates the occurrence of morphological

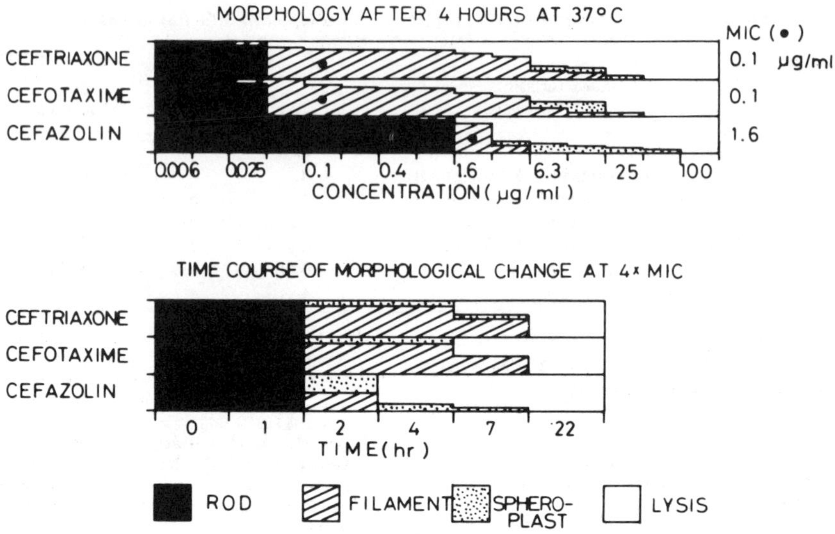

FIG. 1. *Morphological change of E. coli NIHJ as a function of drug concentration and of time. (Morphology judged from a microscopic photograph taken directly from the agar plate under phase contrast.)*

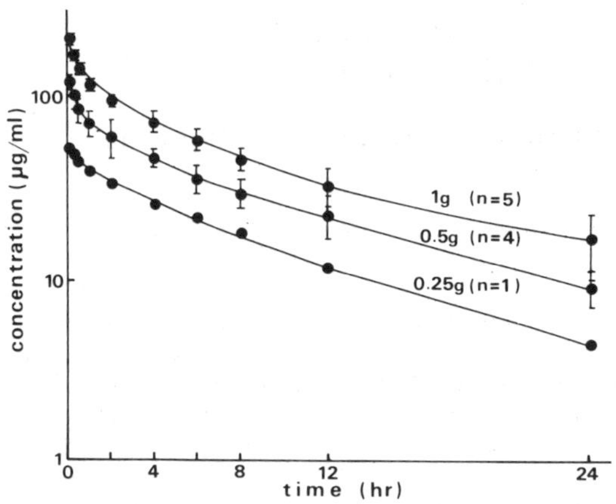

FIG. 2. *Plasma concentration-time curve of ceftriaxone measured by bioassay with E. coli NIHJ as test strain. Single doses (0.25, 0.5, and 1 g) administered to healthy volunteers. Elevenfold diluted plasma was assayed. (The concentration of CTA was estimated with the activity of CTA in 11-fold diluted human serum as the standard.)*

changes with time. All three drugs began to induce morphological changes after a 2-h treatment, but the only drug that led to cell lysis by 4 h was cefazolin. With the other two cephalosporins, CTA and cefotaxime, cell lysis was observed as late as 7 h. Needless to say, no intact cells were seen after 22 h, a common incubation period for MIC determinations. This killing velocity was significantly slower than that obtained by growth kinetics. Therefore, ATMI cephalosporins are judged to be "slow-acting" β-lactam antibiotics.

For such slow-acting cephalosporins, the serum half-life would seem to be of importance. Figure 2 shows the serum level of CTA in healthy human volunteers administered a single dose intravenously. Half-lives were 6.8, 6.9, and 7.4 h at doses of 1.0, 0.5, and 0.25 g, respectively. These values were much longer than that of cefotaxime (1.2 h at a 1-g dose; 2). Reflecting such long half-lives, serum levels at 24 h were found to be high: 17 μg/ml (1.0 g), 9 μg/ml (0.5 g), and 5 μg/ml (0.25 g). This pharmacokinetic property would lead to the maintenance of serum levels high enough and long-lasting enough to provoke complete bacterial cell lysis with a single dose.

1. **Angehrn, P., P. J. Probst, R. Reiner, and R. L. Then.** 1980. Ro 13-9904, a long-acting broad-spectrum cephalosporin: in vitro and in vivo studies. Antimicrob. Agents Chemother. **18:**913–921.
2. **Fu, K. P., P. Aswapokee, I. Ho, C. Matthijssen, and H. C. Neu.** 1979. Pharmacokinetics of cefotaxime. Antimicrob. Agents Chemother. **16:**592–597.
3. **Reiner, R., U. Weiss, U. Brombacher, P. Lanz, M. Montavon, A. Furlenmeier, P. Angehrn, and P. J. Probst.** 1980. Ro 13-9904/001, a novel potent and long-acting parenteral cephalosporin. J. Antibiot. **33:**783–786.
4. **Stoeckel, K.** 1981. Pharmacokinetics of Rocephin®, a highly active new cephalosporin with an exceptionally long biological half-life. Chemotherapy (Basel) **27**(Suppl. 1):42–46.

Effect of Ceftriaxone (Ro 13-9904) and Cefotaxime on Experimental Rat Pyelonephritis

PETER J. PROBST

Pharmaceutical Research Department, F. Hoffmann-La Roche & Company Ltd., Basel, Switzerland

A variety of different pyelonephritis models can be found in the literature. Many of them require surgical operations and a long period of treatment to obtain significant therapeutic effects. For our purposes in the screening and further evaluation of antibacterial substances, we were interested in having at our disposal a kidney infection model which is easy to induce (without surgical operations) and simple to treat, with as few administrations as possible, to save the substance. A model which was first described by Fletcher and Goldstein (2), and modified by Comber (1), appeared to be suitable for our purpose. In this model pyelonephritis is induced by concomitant administration of a parenteral iron preparation which is thought to enhance the virulence of the infective organism specifically in the kidney. Using the ampicillin-resistant strain *Escherichia coli* J44, which was originally isolated from a patient with urinary tract infection, it was possible to reduce the number of necessary iron injections from four to one. The treatment regimen, too, could be drastically reduced to only a few administrations, but still result in a significant therapeutic effect.

Female rats of 200-g body weight (Fullinsdorf specific pathogen-free) were intravenously infected with 2×10^7 colony-forming units (CFU) of *E. coli* J44, using an appropriately diluted overnight broth culture. Five hours later the rats received an intramuscular injection of 30 mg of Fe^{3+} sorbitol citrate (Jectofer, Astra) per kg. In more than 90% of the animals this procedure gave rise to localized kidney infections with macroscopic lesions in the cortex within 24 h. Bacterial counts of $>10^6$ CFU/g of tissue were found in kidney homogenates. Occasionally, some animals died from a generalized infection. In untreated rats, acute pyelonephritis persisted for at least 10 days, during which period *E. coli* was eliminated in the urine at a level of $>10^5$ CFU/ml, as examined by a dip slide method (Urotube, Roche). The optimal time for assessment in this model was found to be day 5 (96 h after infection). The animals were sacrificed, and the kidneys were aseptically removed and macroscopically examined for abscesses. The kidneys were then homogenized in phosphate buffer (pH 7), appropriately diluted, and samples were plated on McConkey agar (Difco Laboratories) for the determination of viable counts. The total body weight (decreased in untreated infected animals) and the weight of the kidneys (increased) may serve as additional parameters for evaluation of the nephritis condition.

The effect of antibiotic treatment was studied by applying three different dosage schedules, (Fig. 1): (a) a prophylactic one, consisting of a single high dose at 16 h before the infection; (b) a "simultaneous" one giving a single dose at 5 h after challenge, i.e., at the same time as the intramuscular injection of the iron sorbitol citrate; and (c) a therapeutic dosage regimen, starting at 24 h after infection. Figure 1 shows schematically the time-dependent development of the kidney infection in untreated animals and under the influence of each of the three different treatments. Both the prophylactic and the simultaneous administration of an effective drug, such as ceftriaxone (CTR), prevent to some extent the multiplication of the infective organism occurring otherwise after the injection of the iron preparation. The mode of action seems to be predominantly bacteriostatic. In the therapeutic dosage regimen, however, the antibiotic substance encounters an established infection with high levels of the pathogen within the tissue. In this case a strong bactericidal action and elevated drug concentrations at the site of infection are thought to be essential.

A comparison was made between the efficacies of CTR and cefotaxime (CTX) in this model; both antibiotics were used in equivalent doses on the basis of their free acids. For statistical evaluation, the Mann/Whitney U-test or the Tukey Quick test, respectively, was used.

In prophylactic experiments CTR at doses of 250, 125, and 62.5 mg/kg subcutaneously (s.c.) prevented the development of kidney infections in most animals so that no viable bacteria could be recovered from their kidneys at the end of the observation period. CTX at the same high dosage levels produced only a more or less pronounced reduction of the viable counts as compared with the untreated controls.

In simultaneous treatment CTR and CTX were about equally active at doses of 0.1 to 2 mg/kg. After administration of 0.4 mg of either antibiotic per kg s.c., most animals presented sterile kidneys without visible abscesses at the time of dissection on day 5.

In therapeutic treatment much higher doses

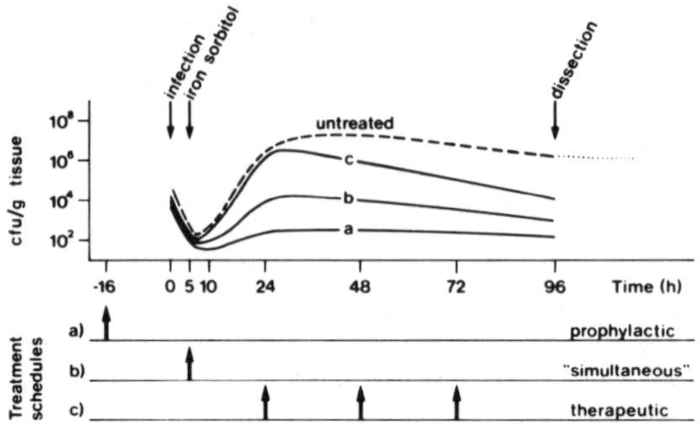

FIG. 1. *Representation of the three different treatment schedules used in this study and their influence on the time course of development of E. coli J44 pyelonephritis in rats. Number of viable bacteria (CFU) recovered from renal tissue is shown (antibiotic used was CTR).*

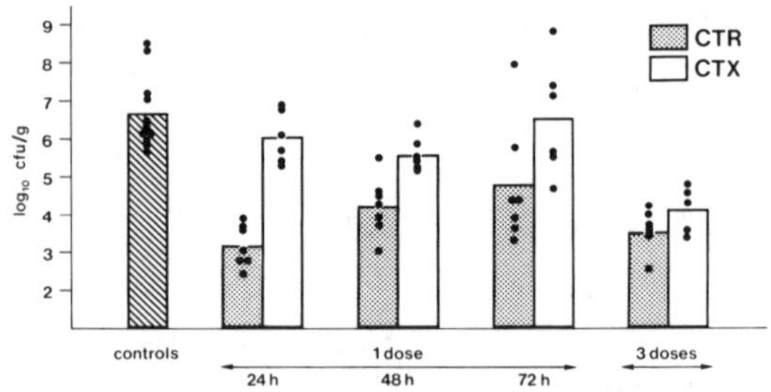

FIG. 2. *Comparative therapeutic effects of CTR and CTX on E. coli J44 nephritis in rats. Doses of 10 mg/kg s.c. were administered either as a single dose at 24, 48, or 72 h or as three repeated injections on the same occasions. Log of CFU per gram of renal tissue; each point stands for one rat (two kidneys); the height of the columns represents the mean log of the group.*

were required to obtain a significant effect. CTR given as a single dose at 10 mg/kg 24 h after infection was effective in reducing the number of CFU per gram of kidney significantly ($P < 0.001$) (Fig. 2). When the same single dose was administered as late as 48 or 72 h after infection, the reduction of viable counts was less pronounced. Analogous single-dose treatment with CTX was ineffective. Only when administered in three consecutive daily doses was a significant effect obtained with CTX. The repeated injection of CTR did not result in a stronger effect than that observed after the single dose at 24 h.

The reason for the observed superiority of CTR over CTX when administered as single doses prophylactically or therapeutically was further investigated. The in vitro intrinsic activities of the two cephalosporins in terms of MIC (0.05 μg/ml) and MBC (0.05 μg/ml) against *E. coli* J44, as well as their "killing curves," were identical. Total plasma levels of CTR in the rat, after 20 and 2 mg/kg s.c., were microbiologically determined and found to be higher and longer lasting than those of CTX. The biological half-life of CTR, which was determined to be about 40 min after intravenous dosing (CTX, about 15 min) (4), however, was considered to be too short to maintain sufficient antibacterial activity in plasma and tissues for more than 10 h. Examination of activity in renal tissue homogenate by an agar diffusion assay, however, revealed the persistence of a minimal residual activity of CTR up to 48 h after administration of 50 mg/kg s.c., which was not observed with CTX. On the other hand, CTX has been reported to have poor stability in tissue homogenates (3), which was confirmed in our experiments. The lack of activity might therefore be explained in part by this fact.

In conclusion, there is some evidence that the good activity of CTR that was demonstrated in the experimental nephritis model described in this paper is related to the unusual, but obviously favorable, pharmacokinetic properties of this new cephalosporin. In spite of its high plasma protein binding and the resulting small volume of distribution, excellent therapeutic efficacy of CTR was achieved within the tissues. Since some principal pharmacokinetic characteristics of CTR in humans are similar to those in rats, therapeutic efficacy may also be expected in clinical situations comparable to these animal experiments. The clinical results obtained so far seem to confirm this statement.

1. **Comber, K. R.** 1976. Pathogenesis of an experimental pyelonephritis model in the mouse and its use in the evaluation of antibiotics, p. 311–316. *In* J. D. Williams and A. M. Geddes (ed.), Proceedings of the 9th International Congress of Chemotherapy, London, 1975, vol. 2. Plenum Press, New York.
2. **Fletcher, J., and E. Goldstein.** 1970. The effect of parenteral iron preparations on experimental pyelonephritis. Br. J. Exp. Pathol. **51**:280–285.
3. **Murakawa, T., H. Sakamoto, S. Fukada, S. Nakamoto, T. Hirose, N. Itoh, and M. Nishida.** 1980. Pharmacokinetics of ceftizoxime in animals after parenteral dosing. Antimicrob. Agents Chemother. **17**:157–164.
4. **Reiner, R., U. Weiss, U. Brombacher, P. Lanz, M. Montavon, A. Furlenmeier, P. Angehrn, and P. J. Probst.** 1980. Ro 13-9904/001, a novel potent and long-acting parenteral cephalosporin. J. Antibiot. **33**:783–786.

Comparison of Ceftriaxone, Moxalactam, and Penicillin in the Treatment of Experimental Pneumococcal Meningitis

THOMAS R. BEAM, JR.,* DALE W. COCHRANE, THOMAS A. RAAB, AND JOSEPH M. MYLOTTE

Infectious Diseases, Buffalo VA Medical Center, and Department of Medicine, State University of New York at Buffalo, Buffalo, New York 14215, U.S.A.*

Ceftriaxone is an investigational cephalosporin with an extended spectrum of activity against both gram-negative and gram-positive bacteria, including *Streptococcus pneumoniae*. Preliminary pharmacokinetic studies in humans have revealed a serum half-life of approximately 8 h (1). Cephalosporins have generally been relegated to treatment of extracranial infections because of poor central nervous system penetration characteristics (3). However, because of its established favorable characteristics, ceftriaxone may be a promising agent for treatment of serious infections, including meningitis. In this study, we compared the central nervous system penetration and therapeutic effectiveness of ceftriaxone, moxalactam, and penicillin in rabbits with pneumococcal meningitis.

Methods have been previously described in detail (2). For the current studies the infecting organism was a type 25 pneumococcus. After removal of 0.5 ml of cerebrospinal fluid (CSF), an inoculum of 3×10^4 to 4×10^4 colony-forming units suspended in 0.5 ml of saline was injected intracisternally into New Zealand white rabbits. Sixteen hours later a single intravenous (i.v.) bolus delivered over 10 min, multiple i.v. boluses delivered over 10 min at 4-h intervals, or continuous i.v. infusion with one of the various antibiotics was begun. Bolus doses and rates of infusion were chosen to produce those drug concentrations frequently obtained in the serum of humans and considered within the therapeutic range.

Concentrations of the antibiotics in serum, CSF, and brain tissue homogenates were determined by means of an agar well diffusion technique. *Bacillus subtilis* was the reference organism for penicillin; *Providencia stuartii*, for moxalactam; and *Escherichia coli* 1346, for ceftriaxone.

The type 25 pneumococcus was passed five times intracisternally in rabbits to establish virulence. This organism produced rhinorrhea, excitability, seizures, nuchal rigidity or opisthotonos, hyperpnea, and ultimate death among untreated animals. Sixteen hours after infection but before the initiation of therapy, there was a mean $\log_{10}$ of 7.21 colony-forming units/ml of CSF among 155 animals.

Quantitative culture of the CSF 8 h after the delivery of bolus therapy revealed a mean decline in viable organisms ($\log_{10}$ colony-forming units per milliliter) of 5.9 for ceftriaxone (data pooled for 10, 20, and 30 mg/kg), 2.1 for penicillin (30 and 100 mg/kg), and 0.9 for moxalactam (20 and 50 mg/kg). A single dose of ceftriaxone (10, 20, or 30 mg/kg) produced significantly greater killing of pneumococci at 8 h whether penicillin ($P < 0.001$) or moxalactam ($P < 0.001$) was delivered as a single dose or two doses 4 h apart. Continuous infusion of ceftriaxone (−6.8 logs) or penicillin (−5.6 logs) produced similar killing over an 8-h period. Both drugs had significantly greater bactericidal effect than moxalactam (−2.7 logs; $P < 0.001$ for each) administered by continuous i.v. infusion (Table 1).

CSF concentrations of ceftriaxone and moxalactam measured 8 h after initiation of therapy exceeded the MBC of the infecting organism regardless of the dose or type of infusion (Table 1). Only if two boluses or a continuous infusion of penicillin was used could the drug be detected in CSF 8 h later. Ceftriaxone was the only drug which accumulated in the CSF over the 8-h period of continuous i.v. infusion (data not shown).

The maximal rate of killing (therapeutic effect) among various dosing schedules of ceftriaxone was achieved with a 10-mg/kg bolus. This rate of kill over 8 h was equalled but never exceeded by larger-pulse doses or continuous i.v. therapy (Fig. 1).

CSF was sterilized in 11 of 11 rabbits given a 30-mg/kg bolus of ceftriaxone 16 and 24 h after infection, when cultures were obtained 16 and 64 h after the last dose. Moxalactam, a 50-mg/kg bolus, or penicillin, a 100-mg/kg bolus, administered 16, 20, and 24 h after infection sterilized CSF in zero of six moxalactam-treated animals ($\chi^2 = 12.9$; $P < 0.001$) or one of nine penicillin-treated animals ($\chi^2 = 12.8$; $P < 0.001$) 16 h later. All moxalactam-treated animals died within 72 h after infection. Follow-up cultures 64 h after completion of therapy revealed zero of nine sterile cultures among the penicillin-treated animals.

The results obtained in this study of experimental meningitis suggest that: (i) single bolus

TABLE 1. *Results of therapy of experimental S. pneumoniae meningitis*

Drug	Infusion (mg/kg)	No. of rabbits	Concn (range) 8 h after initiation of therapy			Bacteriological status[a]
			Serum (μg/ml)	CSF (μg/ml)	Brain (μg/g)	
Ceftriaxone	10	4	0.6 (0.5–0.7)	0.9 (0.8–0.9)	0.5 (0.13–0.99)	−7.0
MIC = 0.004 μg/ml	20	10	2.3 (0.1–5.6)	0.5 (0.1–1.0)	0.3 (0.08–0.66)	−5.4
MBC = 0.004 μg/ml	30	11	5.2 (0.5–17)	3.4 (0.1–10)	0.4 (0.06–0.81)	−5.4
	20 + 6 per h	8	18.3 (10–26)	2.7 (0.9–3.6)	2.2 (1.6–2.9)	−6.8
Penicillin	30	5	0.05 (0.003–0.10)	NZ[b]	NZ	−1.6
MIC = 0.02 μg/ml	30 × 2	7	0.2 (0.004–0.5)	0.01 (0.009–0.02)	NZ	−1.7
MBC = 0.04 μg/ml	100	5	0.8 (0.3–1.8)	NZ	NZ	−2.6
	100 × 2	7	1.0 (0.5–2.3)	0.05 (0.02–0.08)	0.03	−2.6
	100 + 40 per h	8	12.3 (2.6–27.6)	0.6 (0.4–0.8)	0.1	−5.6
Moxalactam	30	12	0.4 (0.05–0.7)	0.3 (0.1–0.5)	NZ	−1.0
MIC = 0.04 μg/ml	30 × 2	11	1.0 (0.7–1.3)	1.2 (0.2–1.8)	0.5 (0.2–0.9)	−1.6
MBC = 0.04 μg/ml	50	11	1.2 (0.3–5.7)	0.4 (0.2–0.6)	NZ	−0.02
	50 × 2	9	2.7 (0.5–5.6)	5.4 (1.6–7.9)	0.4 (0.3–0.6)	−0.8
	50 + 20 per h	10	25.3 (8.6–46)	2.4 (1.2–4.2)	0.7 (0.1–1.3)	−2.7

[a] Net change in mean number of bacteria (log colony-forming units per milliliter of CSF).
[b] NZ, No measurable drug.

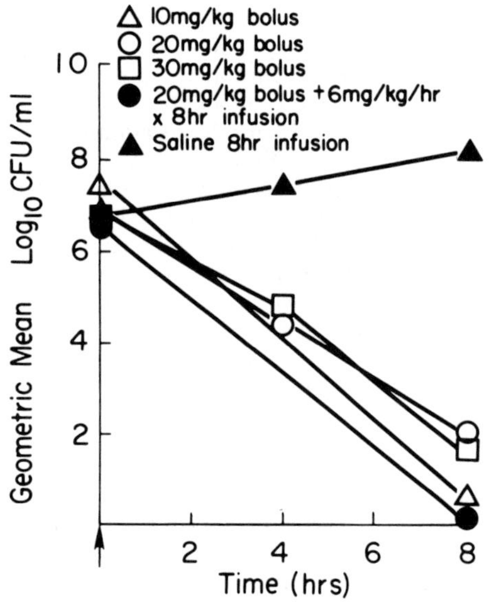

FIG. 1. *Killing effect in CSF of several dosing regimes of ceftriaxone delivered parenterally to rabbits with experimental pneumococcal meningitis. Therapy was delivered at time zero, as indicated by the arrow.*

therapy with ceftriaxone, 10, 20, or 30 mg/kg, produced significantly greater killing of pneumococci than did penicillin, 30 or 100 mg/kg, or moxalactam, 20 or 50 mg/kg; (ii) continuous infusion of ceftriaxone or penicillin produced significantly greater killing of pneumococci than moxalactam; and (iii) the therapeutic efficacy demonstrated by ceftriaxone warrants further study in animals. Clinical trials may also be indicated.

1. **Anghern, P., P. J. Probst, R. Reiner, and R. Then.** 1980. RO 13-9904, a long-acting broad-spectrum cephalosporin: in vitro and in vivo studies. Antimicrob. Agents Chemother. **18:**913–921.
2. **Beam, T. R., and J. C. Allen.** 1980. Comparison of cefamandole, cephalothin, ampicillin, and chloramphenicol in experimental *Escherichia coli* meningitis. Antimicrob. Agents Chemother. **17:**37–42.
3. **Mangi, R. J., R. S. Kundargi, R. Quintiliani, and V. T. Andriole.** 1973. Development of meningitis during cephalothin therapy. Ann. Intern. Med. **78:**374–351.

Pharmacokinetics and Efficacy of Ceftriaxone (Ro 13-9904) in Experimental *Haemophilus influenzae* Type b Meningitis in the Rat

J. CARL CRAFT* AND SHEREE H. TAN

Department of Pediatrics, Section of Infectious Diseases, Tulane University School of Medicine, New Orleans, Louisiana 70114, U.S.A.

Ceftriaxone (Ro 13-9904) is a new parenteral cephalosporin with excellent in vitro activity against both β-lactamase-negative and -positive *Haemophilus influenzae* type b. Susceptibility testing demonstrated MICs between 0.08 and 0.0008 μg/ml for all strains tested. Prior to 1974,

TABLE 1. *Serum and CSF concentrations of ceftriaxone and ampicillin in the infant rat*

Specimen	Concn (μg/ml) at:						Half-life (h)
	0.5 h	1 h	2 h	4 h	6 h	8 h	
Ceftriaxone serum							
Normal	111	103	58	53	—	22	3.3
Meningitis	96	80	65	53	—	24	3.9
Ceftriaxone CSF							
Normal	1.9	3.0	1.7	2.3	—	1.2	8.8
Meningitis	14.7	20	12.7	8.5	—	2.5	2.7
Ampicillin serum							
Normal	169	65	21	4.2	1.8	—	0.9
Meningitis	190	73	24	6.3	2.4	—	0.9
Ampicillin CSF							
Normal	2.9	2.2	1.1	0.7	0.4	—	1.9
Meningitis	20.7	4.9	2.8	0.6	0.7	—	1.2

H. influenzae type b strains were uniformly susceptible to ampicillin, but since 1974 the incidence of ampicillin-resistant strains has increased. Recently, multiply resistant *H. influenzae* type b strains have been isolated with resistance to ampicillin and chloramphenicol. Because of the increasing clinical challenge posed by multiply resistant strains, we initiated the study of ceftriaxone in the treatment of *H. influenzae* type b meningitis in the infant rat model.

Pharmacokinetic experiments were performed in 10-day-old pathogen-free Sprague-Dawley rats. Four groups of 40 rats each were used. Group 1 was treated for 24 h starting on day 9 with ampicillin, 400 mg/kg per day given every 6 h subcutaneously. Group 2 was inoculated intranasally with 7 $\log_{10}$ colony-forming units (CFU) of *H. influenzae* type b strain Eagan at 5 days of age. Cerebrospinal fluid (CSF) and blood cultures were performed on day 9, and then the rats were treated for 24 h with ampicillin, 400 mg/kg per day given every 6 h subcutaneously. Group 3 was treated for 24 h starting on day 9 with ceftriaxone, 100 mg/kg per day given every 8 h subcutaneously. Group 4 was inoculated intranasally with 7 $\log_{10}$ CFU of strain Eagan at 5 days of age. CSF and blood cultures were performed on day 9, and then the rats were treated for 24 h with ceftriaxone, 100 mg/kg per day given every 8 h subcutaneously. Ampicillin treatment groups 1 and 2 were given a fifth dose of ampicillin. CSF and serum specimens were obtained at 0.5, 1.0, 2.0, 4.0, and 6.0 h and were assayed for ampicillin by a microbioassay technique within 24 h of collection. Ceftriaxone treatment groups 3 and 4 were given a fourth dose of ceftriaxone. CSF and serum specimens were obtained at 0.5, 1.0, 2.0, 4.0, and 8 h and were assayed for ceftriaxone by a microbioassay technique within 24 h of collection.

Efficacy experiments were done with four representative strains of *H. influenzae* type b. Eagan is an ampicillin-susceptible strain with no plasmid. A-Sm is an ampicillin-resistant strain with a nonsegregating integrated 30-megadalton plasmid. PE_4 is an ampicillin-resistant strain with a segregating 30-megadalton plasmid. MG_1/E-Sm is an ampicillin- and chloramphenical-resistant strain with a nonsegregating 50-megadalton plasmid. Five-day-old infant rats were inoculated intranasally with 7 $\log_{10}$ CFU of one of the four test strains. At 9 days of age, CSF and blood specimens were obtained for quantitative bacterial culture. Animals were treated with either ampicillin, 400 mg/kg per day subcutaneously every 6 h for 7 days, or ceftriaxone, 100 mg/kg per day subcutaneously every 8 h for 7 days. CSF and blood specimens were obtained at 24-h intervals after antibiotics were started until cultures were sterile. Forty-eight hours after antibiotics were stopped, CSF and blood specimens were obtained for quantitative culture.

Results of antibiotic assay are shown in Table 1. Average ampicillin CSF/blood concentrations changed from 9.8% to 13.6% with meningitis. Average ceftriaxone CSF/blood concentrations changed from 3.5% to 17.2% and demonstrated less fluctuation in CSF levels with time. The area under the serum concentration curve for ceftriaxone was 629 μg.h/ml without inflamed meninges and 489 μg.h/ml with inflamed meninges. The volumes of distribution for ceftriaxone were 251 ml/kg and 382 ml/kg, respectively. The area under the serum concentration curve for ampicillin was 178 μg.h/ml without inflamed meninges and 206 μg.h/ml with inflamed meninges. The volumes of distribution for ampicillin were 727 ml/kg and 629 ml/kg, respectively. Blood values of both ceftriaxone and ampicillin exceeded the MIC and MBC for all strains. Minimal CSF concentrations of ceftriaxone exceeded the MIC for all strains by 100 times. Minimal CSF concentrations of ampicillin were equal to the MIC for the ampicillin-susceptible

TABLE 2. *Number of rats with meningitis or bacteremia, or both, after 24, 48, and 72 h of therapy and 48 h after stopping therapy*

Strain	Drug[a]	No.[b]	During therapy			After therapy (48 h)	Died
			24 h	48 h	72 h		
Eagan	AMP	19	1/0[c]	0/0	0/0	7/11	1
	CTA	19	0/0	0/0	0/0	0/0	0
A-Sm	AMP	18	4/3	0/0	0/0	6/12	1
	CTA	18	0/0	0/0	0/0	0/0	0
PE_4	AMP	20	1/0	0/0	0/0	1/9	0
	CTA	20	0/0	0/0	0/0	0/0	0
Mg/E-Sm	AMP	20	12/8	0/0	0/0	1/1	2
	CTA	19	0/0	0/0	0/0	0/0	0

[a] AMP, Ampicillin; CTA, ceftriaxone.
[b] Number of rats with meningitis before therapy.
[c] Meningitis/bacteremia.

strain and were greatly exceeded by the MIC for ampicillin-resistant strains.

Efficacy is defined by sterilization of the blood and CSF, at 24, 48, and 72 h of therapy and 48 h after stopping therapy, and by deaths during therapy. As shown in Table 2, sterilization of CSF and blood after 24 h and after stopping therapy were significantly ($P < 0.05$) improved in the ceftriaxone group. The increased deaths seen in the ampicillin treatment groups were not significant. Ampicillin-resistant strains were not significantly different from the ampicillin-susceptible strains.

The pharmacokinetics of ampicillin and ceftriaxone were best adapted to a one-compartment model since the early elimination phase was tempered by the absorption phase from the subcutaneous tissue. Ceftriaxone was characterized by a prolonged serum half-life and increased area under the curve when compared with ampicillin. Ampicillin pharmacokinetics were comparable to those seen in humans. Both ceftriaxone and ampicillin demonstrated improved CSF penetration with meningitis.

Ceftriaxone was significantly more efficacious in sterilizing the CSF and blood in the infant rat with meningitis. No failures were seen in the rats treated with ceftriaxone. The ampicillin-treated rats had failures with both susceptible and resistant strains. The failures with the resistant strains were expected, but the significant relapse rate was unexpected. These failures may be related to the 6-h half-life dosing schedule and prolonged periods of suboptimal CSF and blood concentrations in the ampicillin-treated animals.

Sterilization of all animals with both resistant and susceptible strains by 48 h of therapy was surprising. The cure of the majority of ampicillin-treated animals with resistant strains was unexpected. Sterilization of resistant strains treated with ampicillin has been reported in children. This may be due to the extremely high serum concentrations obtained and nearly bactericidal concentrations transiently seen in the CSF. The relapse rate for ampicillin suggests that not all organisms are eliminated by the concentrations obtainable in CSF and blood. Many animals were cured with inappropriate antibiotics, demonstrating the ability of rats to resolve infection with a minimum of assistance from the antibiotic. Another possibility for the observed cures in the ampicillin-resistant groups is related to a potential decreased virulence of the organisms with ampicillin-resistant coding plasmids.

In conclusion, ceftriaxone has satisfactory pharmacokinetics in the infant rat model of *H. influenzae* type b meningitis. The prolonged dosing interval is an additional advantage in treatment. The demonstrated efficacy of ceftriaxone against all strains tested compared with ampicillin would make ceftriaxone an excellent drug for treating *H. influenzae* type b meningitis in the infant rat.

Treatment of Experimental Syphilis in the Rabbit with Ceftriaxone (Ro 13-9904)

RUSSELL C. JOHNSON,* RUSSELL F. BEY, AND SANDRA J. WOLGAMOT

Department of Microbiology, University of Minnesota, Minneapolis, Minnesota 55455, U.S.A.

Syphilis remains one of the major sexually transmitted diseases. Since *Treponema pallidum* is exceptionally susceptible to the action of penicillin, it is the drug of choice for the treatment of this disease. The 50% curative dose (CD_{50}) for experimental syphilis in the rabbit was reported to be 1,000 to 2,000 U (0.6 to 1.2 mg) per kg (1). Since hypersusceptibilities to penicillin are not uncommon and penicillin-resistant agents of venereal disease exist, a continuing search for other effective antibiotics is necessary.

Ceftriaxone (Ro 13-9904), a new cephalosporin derivative, was evaluated for its therapeutic effectiveness for the treatment of experimental syphilis in the rabbit. Penicillin G was included in this study as the standard or reference antibiotic. The shaved backs of male rabbits were injected at each of six sites with 10^7 or more cells of *T. pallidum* (Nichols strain). This cell suspension was derived from the testes of intratesticularly infected rabbits. Treatment was initiated 7 to 10 days after infection when dark-field positive cutaneous lesions, measuring 7 to 12 mm in diameter, were present. The treatment schedule consisted of one daily intramuscular injection of an aqueous solution of the sodium salts of the test drugs for 5 days. The total drug dosage was 5, 2.5, 1.25, and 0.625 μmol/kg, which is equivalent to 3,000, 1,500, 750, and 375 U of penicillin. Animals were divided into groups of five rabbits, with nine rabbits serving as untreated controls. Cutaneous lesions were observed for regression in size and the presence of *T. pallidum*. Serological response of the animals was monitored with the rapid plasma reagin (RPR) card test. Six months after treatment, popliteal lymph node extracts of treated and untreated rabbits were transferred to the testes of normal rabbits. Recipients of the lymph nodes were monitored for antibody response with the RPR test, and testicular aspirates were examined for *T. pallidum* during the 2-month observation period.

Primary syphilitic lesions of most treated rabbits were no longer detectable 12 days after initiation of treatment. Although several rabbits required 27 days for lesion healing, this was not correlated with drug dosage. Cutaneous lesions became dark-field negative within 1 to 2 days after initiation of treatment with 5 and 2.5-μmol of the two antibiotics, whereas as long as 5 days were required for the lower drug concentrations. No relapses (secondary lesions) were observed at treatment levels of 5 and 2.5 μmol. Relapses occurred in 40% of the rabbits receiving 1.25 μmol of either antibiotic. The use of 0.625 μmol of penicillin and ceftriaxone resulted in relapses in 60% and 100% of the treated animals, respectively. Dark-field positive cutaneous lesions were observed as long as 120 days in the untreated rabbits, and all these animals experienced relapses. At 6 months posttreatment, the percentages of animals RPR positive at treatment levels of 5, 2.5, 1.25, and 0.625 μmol were 25, 0, 25, and 67 for those receiving penicillin and 67, 40, 60, and 100 for those treated with ceftriaxone. All untreated rabbits were RPR positive.

Popliteal lymph node transfers were conducted at 6 months posttreatment. Animals receiving lymph nodes from rabbits treated with 5 and 2.5 μmol of penicillin or 5 μmol of ceftriaxone remained negative to the RPR test and the presence of *T. pallidum*. Twenty percent of the recipients of lymph nodes from rabbits receiving 2.5 μmol of ceftriaxone became positive for *T. pallidum* and for the RPR test. The percentages of recipients of lymph nodes from animals treated with 1.25 and 0.625 μmol of penicillin that were positive for *T. pallidum* were 25 and 67. The percentages treated with ceftriaxone were 40 and 80. *T. pallidum* was observed in 78% of rabbits receiving lymph nodes from control animals. At all treatment levels, with the exception of 0.625 μmol of ceftriaxone, lymph node recipient rabbits which were positive for *T. pallidum* were also serologically positive. Although 100% of recipients of lymph nodes from rabbits treated with 0.625 μmol of ceftriaxone were RPR positive, spirochetes could be detected in only 80% of these animals. This is similar to what was observed with the recipients of lymph nodes from untreated rabbits. One hundred percent of these animals seroconverted, whereas 78% were positive for *T. pallidum*.

The data obtained demonstrated that the serological test was a more sensitive indicator of infection than the dark-field examination of testicular aspirates for the presence of *T. pallidum*. Accordingly, the calculation of the CD_{50} for the two antibiotics was based on serological results. The CD_{50} for penicillin G was 0.924 μmol or 0.33 mg (550 U) per kg. Ceftriaxone has a CD_{50} of 0.665 μmol or 0.40 mg per kg, indicating that it has a therapeutic effectiveness similar to that of penicillin G for experimental syphilis in the rabbit. Our results with penicillin G are comparable to those reported by Arnold et al. (1). They investigated the efficacy of penicillin G for the treatment of experimental syphilis in the rabbit and established a CD_{50} value of 1,000 to 2,000 U (0.6 to 1.2 mg) per kg.

1. **Arnold, R. C., R. A. Boak, C. M. Carpenter, A. M. Chesney, W. F. Fleming, B. Gueft, J. F. Mahoney, and P. D. Rosahn.** 1947. A joint report on a cooperative investigation of the efficacy of species of penicillin in the treatment of experimental syphilis. Am. J. Syph. Gonorrhea Vener. Dis. **31**:469–475.

Influence of Protein Binding on Pharmacokinetics of Ceftriaxone

KLAUS STOECKEL,* PATRICK J. McNAMARA, ROGER BRANDT, AND WALTER H. ZIEGLER

Pharmaceutical Research Department, F. Hoffmann-La Roche & Company, Ltd., Basel, Switzerland

Ceftriaxone (Rocephin) is a new semisynthetic parenteral cephalosporin which displays broad-spectrum activity against gram-negative and gram-positive pathogens. In its activity against *Haemophilus influenzae*, *Neisseria gonorrhoeae*, and *Neisseria meningitidis* it exceeds those of cefuroxime, cefamandole, cefoxitin, and cefazolin (1). Moreover, it is remarkably stable against various types of β-lactamase. Ceftriaxone exhibits an exceptionally long biological half-life ($t_{1/2(\beta)}$) of 8 h in comparison with other cephalosporins ($t_{1/2}$ = 0.5 to 2.7 h). In this paper we summarize the pharmacokinetics of this new investigational cephalosporin.

Basic pharmacokinetics. The basic pharmacokinetics of ceftriaxone were studied in six healthy volunteers after intravenous bolus injections of 150, 500, 1,500, and 3,000 mg. The total (bound plus unbound) plasma concentration-time data of ceftriaxone could be described satisfactorily by a two-exponential equation. The data were, however, not analyzed according to a compartment model, since the mean areas under the total (bound plus unbound) plasma concentration-time curves ($AUC_{0-\infty}$) did not increase in proportion to the dose. This non-linearity resulted in an apparent dose-dependent increase in the volume of distribution ($V_{D(\beta)}$) and total systemic clearance (Cl_S^T) values with reference to total drug concentrations (Table 1). The greatest increase in Cl_S^T occurred between the 1,500- and 3,000-mg doses (42%), being only 5% between the 150- and 500-mg doses. Hence, deviations from linear pharmacokinetics with reference to total drug are less noticeable at lower (<1,000 mg) doses. The two important pharmacokinetic parameters, $t_{1/2(\beta)}$ and fraction excreted unchanged in the urine (f_u), are, however, dose independent.

The nonlinear pharmacokinetic behavior was explained by the concentration-dependent plasma protein binding of the drug. Ceftriaxone showed a marked increase in the free fraction (ratio of concentration of free to total drug) in plasma in the concentration range above 150 μg/ml (free fraction changing from 4.4% at 150 μg/ml to 17% at 300 μg/ml). Since the Cl_S^T of ceftriaxone is subject to restricted elimination (total clearance is considerably lower than blood flow to the eliminating organ), changes in the free fraction (f_p) lead to clearance changes. The $t_{1/2}$ of ceftriaxone is, however, dose independent. This can be understood by the constant f_p (hence, clearance and volume of distribution) values at the plasma concentrations (<150 μg/ml) occurring during the terminal phase of the concentration-time curves.

The pharmacokinetics of ceftriaxone with reference to the pharmacologically relevant free (unbound) concentrations are, however, dose independent. Therefore, the pharmacokinetic parameters with reference to unbound ceftriaxone are constant and do not change with dose (Table 2).

Coadministration of probenecid. The renal clearance of ceftriaxone is almost exclusively by glomerular filtration (2). Probenecid, an effective inhibitor of renal tubular secretion, should have no influence on the clearance (hence, half-life) of ceftriaxone. Indeed, the pharmacokinetic parameters of ceftriaxone were not changed in volunteers who had received 500 mg of probenecid at 2 h and 10 min before administration of ceftriaxone.

Pharmacokinetics in functionally anephric patients. The $t_{1/2(\beta)}$ of ceftriaxone in functionally anephric patients after a single 150-mg intravenous dose was only slightly increased

TABLE 1. *Pharmacokinetic parameters with reference to total (bound + unbound) plasma concentrations of ceftriaxone after administration of four intravenous doses in healthy volunteers (n = 6)*

Dosage (mg)	Parameter		
	Cl_S^T (ml min^{-1})	$V_{D(\beta)}$ (liters)	$t_{1/2\ (\beta)}$ (h)
150	9.7	7.0	8.6
500	10.2	6.7	7.7
1,500	13.0	8.6	7.8
3,000	18.5	12.7	8.0

TABLE 2. *Pharmacokinetic parameters with reference to free (unbound) plasma concentrations of ceftriaxone after administration of four intravenous doses in healthy volunteers (n = 6)*

Dosage (mg)	Parameter				
	Cl_S^F (ml min^{-1})	Cl_{Renal}^F (ml min^{-1})	$V_{D\ (\beta)}^F$ (liters)	$t_{1/2(\beta)}^F$ (h)	f_u
150	262	152	192	8.6	0.59
150	253	162	165	7.6	0.64
1,500	249	161	162	7.6	0.65
3,000	258	170	168	7.8	0.67

compared to normal subjects (12 versus 8 h). This increase in $t_{1/2}$ was the result of an increased volume of distribution (7 versus 10 liters) rather than a decreased total body clearance (9.7 versus 10 ml/min). The decrease in renal clearance appeared to be compensated for by an increased nonrenal clearance (Cl_{NR}^T). The changes in $V_{D(\beta)}$ and Cl_{NR}^T could be explained by a decreased plasma protein binding of the drug in the anephric patients.

Possible approach for ceftriaxone dosage regime. The long $t_{1/2(\beta)}$ of ceftriaxone calls for a once-daily administration of ceftriaxone. Moreover, the data in anephric patients collected so far suggest that no dose adjustments need to be made in renally diseased patients provided that their liver functions are normal.

1. **Angehrn, P., P. J. Probst, R. Reiner, and R. L. Then.** 1980. Ro 13-9904, a long-acting broad-spectrum cephalosporin: in vitro and in vivo studies. Antimicrob. Agents Chemother. **18:**913–921.
2. **Stoeckel, K., P. J. McNamara, R. Brandt, H. Plozza-Nottebrock, and W. H. Ziegler.** 1981. Effects of concentration-dependent plasma protein binding on ceftriaxone kinetics. Clin. Pharmacol. Ther. **29:**650–657.

Single-Dose Pharmacokinetics of Ceftriaxone (Ro 13-9904) in Infants and Young Children

URS B. SCHAAD* AND KLAUS STOECKEL

Department of Pediatrics, University of Berne, Inselspital, CH-3010 Berne, and Pharmaceutical Research Department, F. Hoffmann-La Roche & Company Ltd., CH-4002 Basel, Switzerland*

Standard antimicrobial regimens for childhood bacterial meningitis consist of ampicillin, chloramphenicol, or penicillin G. The therapeutic dilemma of physicians who manage pediatric patients with bacterial meningitis includes: an increasing percentage of ampicillin-resistant *Haemophilus influenzae* type b strains, mainly due to beta-lactamase production; potential toxicity and wide variability in pharmacokinetics of chloramphenicol; recent reports of clinical isolates of *H. influenzae* type b that are resistant to chloramphenicol; experimental evidence of antagonistic action of ampicillin plus chloramphenicol against some strains of pneumococcus or meningococcus; and, finally, the emergence of pneumococcal strains that are "nonsusceptible" (MIC, 0.1 to 1 μg/ml) or resistant (MIC, >1 μg/ml) to penicillin G.

Ceftriaxone is a new semisynthetic parenteral cephalosporin antibiotic with excellent in vitro activity against the three major etiological agents of bacterial meningitis in childhood: *H. influenzae* type b, *Streptococcus pneumoniae*, and *Neisseria meningitidis* (1). A considerable penetration of ceftriaxone into cerebrospinal fluid (CSF) has been shown in experimentally infected rabbits and dogs (2). Preliminary clinical experience in children and young adults with bacterial meningitis confirmed the potential usefulness of this compound in meningitis therapy (M Cadoz et al., 2nd Mediterran. Congr. Chemother., Nice, abstr. 204, 1980). Pharmacokinetic studies in adult volunteers resulted in exceptionally long elimination half-lives of approximately 8 h (3).

The purpose of the present study was to evaluate pharmacokinetics of ceftriaxone in infants and young children and use this information to formulate dosage recommendations of this investigational antibiotic for therapy of invasive bacterial diseases, such as meningitis, in this age group.

Pharmacokinetic studies after intravenous administration over 5 min of a single 50-mg/kg dose of ceftriaxone were performed in 10 pediatric patients. There were five infants between 7 and 15 months of age (mean, 11 months) and five children between 2 and 6 years of age (mean, 3.3 years). No significant pharmacokinetic differences were observed between these two patient populations. Plasma, urine, and buffer samples were analyzed for free acid of ceftriaxone by a specific high-pressure liquid chromatographic assay (4).

The total (bound plus unbound) plasma concentration-time curves were best described in each case by a biexponential equation ($r = 0.993$ to 0.999). Mean values and ranges of observed plasma ceftriaxone concentrations are shown in Fig. 1. Mean values ± SD were 227 ± 24 μg/ml at 15 min after dosing, 46 ± 13 μg/ml at 8 h, 22 ± 6 μg/ml at 16 h, 9 ± 5 μg/ml at 24 h, and 4.3 ± 2.5 μg/ml at 32 h. The individual elimination half-lives ($t_{1/2(\beta)}$) ranged from 4.1 to 7.7 h (mean ± SD, 6.5 ± 1.1 h). This biological half-life value of ceftriaxone in pediatric patients is considerably longer than the values reported for other third-generation cephalosporins: moxalactam, 1.6 to 1.8 h; cefotaxime, 0.7 to 1 h; and cefoperazone, 1.4 h.

The upper part of Fig. 2 displays the mean ± SD of the excretion of unchanged drug in urine, expressed in cumulative percentage of dose recovered, for the 0- to 12-h period after dosing. By 12 h, 47.5 ± 7.0% of intact drug was recovered in the urine. In the lower part of Fig. 2, the mean values of total renal clearance (Cl_R^T) of ceftriaxone are given for the four 3-h periods from 0 to 12 h after dosing. The renal clearances declined from 0.71 ml/min per kg at the 0- to 3-h interval to 0.23 ml/min per kg at the 9- to 12-h interval. This pronounced influence of time on total renal clearance had been previously found in healthy adults and is due to the concentration-dependent plasma protein binding of ceftriaxone (3). These time-dependent clearance changes show why plasma concentration-time curves of ceftriaxone could not be analyzed by a simple two-compartment pharmacokinetic model.

Mean ± SD of the free fractions (ratio of unbound to total drug concentration) of ceftriaxone was 16.1 ± 3.0% in children compared to 10.0 ± 1.3% in adults (3). The lower plasma protein binding in children is probably due to the lower plasma concentrations of albumin measured in these patients compared to adults (31 versus 46 mg/ml). Consequently, at comparable total plasma concentrations, the therapeutically important free concentrations will always be higher in pediatric than in adult patients.

In comparison to adults, total systemic clearance (Cl_s^T) was about four times greater and volume of distribution ($V_{D(\beta)}$) was about three times greater: Cl_s^T, 0.71 ± 0.16 ml/min per kg in children and 0.19 ± 0.03 ml/min per kg in adults; $V_{D(\beta)}$, 394 ± 69 versus 125 ± 6 ml/kg (3). These increased values of Cl_s^T and $V_{D(\beta)}$ resulted in a slightly reduced $t_{1/2(\beta)}$ (mean) of 6.5 h in pediatric patients versus 8 h in adult patients (3). The increased $V_{D(\beta)}$ in children compared with adults is explained by lower plasma protein binding and relatively larger extracellular fluid space in this young age group. Both components of total systemic clearance of ceftriaxone, renal and nonrenal, must be larger in pediatric than in adult patients, since urine recoveries within 12 h after dosing were similar: 47% in children and 52% in adults (3).

On the basis of our pharmacokinetic data of

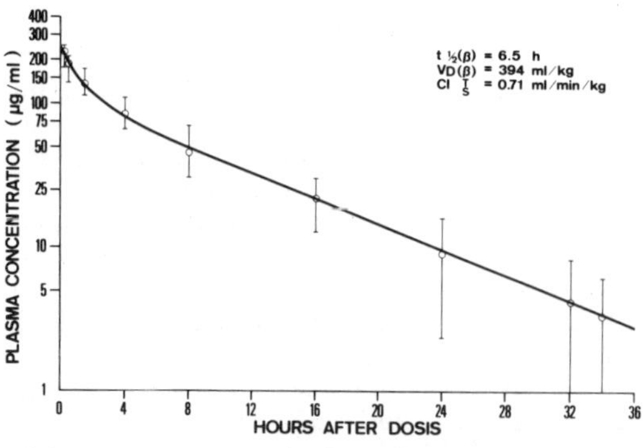

FIG. 1. *Mean plasma concentration-time curve and ranges of observed plasma concentrations of ceftriaxone (50 mg/kg intravenously) in 10 infants and young children.*

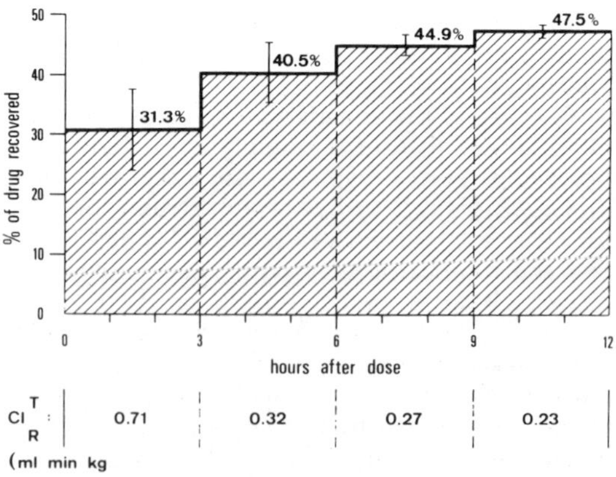

FIG. 2. *Recovery of ceftriaxone in urine. (Upper) Mean ± SD of cumulative percent excretion of ceftriaxone in urine. (Lower) Mean total renal clearances (Cl_R^T) at 0 to 3, 3 to 6, 6 to 9, and 9 to 12 h after dosing.*

ceftriaxone, the high in vitro activity of this drug against the etiological agents of childhood bacterial meningitis, and the preliminary human data on CSF penetration, the following dosage schedule for therapy of invasive bacterial diseases in pediatric patients beyond the neonatal age group is suggested: 50 mg of ceftriaxone per kg given intravenously over 5 min every 12 h. This dosage interval of about twice the elimination half-life is expected to produce plasma peak ceftriaxone concentrations of 200 to 320 μg/ml and plasma trough concentrations of 30 to 40 μg/ml. Ceftriaxone penetration into CSF trough inflamed meninges of children was reported to result in CSF levels of 5 to 10% of the concurrent plasma levels (Cadoz et al., 2nd Mediterran. Congr. Chemother., Nice, abstr. 204, 1980). It is concluded that, after 50-mg/kg doses of ceftriaxone twice daily, the ceftriaxone concentrations in both plasma and CSF will constantly exceed by severalfold the susceptibilities of the principal pathogens that cause bacterial meningitis in childhood, with MICs for 90% of these bacteria being <0.1 μg/ml (1). It must be emphasized, however, that this dosage recommendation is intended only for well-controlled clinical evaluations of this antibiotic, which is still under investigation.

1. **Neu, H. C., N. J. Meropol, and K. P. Fu.** 1981. Antibacterial activity of ceftriaxone (Ro 13-9904), a beta-lactamase-stable cephalosporin. Antimicrob. Agents Chemother. **19:**414–423.
2. **Schaad, U. B., G. H. McCracken, Jr., C. A. Loock, and M. L. Thomas.** 1981. Pharmacokinetics and bacteriologic efficacy of moxalactam, cefotaxime, cefoperazone, and rocephin in experimental bacterial meningitis. J. Infect. Dis. **143:**156–163.
3. **Stoeckel, K., P. J. McNamara, R. Brandt, H. Plozza-Nottebrock, and W. H. Ziegler.** 1981. The effects of concentration-dependent plasma protein binding on the pharmacokinetics of ceftriaxone (Ro 13-9904), a new parenteral cephalosporin. Clin. Pharmacol. Ther. **29:** 650–657.
4. **Trautmann, K. H., and P. Haefelfinger.** 1981. Determination of Ro 13-9904 in plasma, urine and bile by means of ion-pair reversed phase chromatography. J. High Resolut. Chromatogr. Chromatogr. Commun. **4:** 54–59.

Pharmacokinetics and Tissue Penetration of Ceftriaxone (Ro 13-9904) at Two Dosage Levels

RUTH M. BROWN, CHRISTOPHER D. FINDLAY, JANET E. ALLCOCK, AND RICHARD WISE*

Department of Medical Microbiology, Dudley Road Hospital, Birmingham, U.K.

Ceftriaxone is a broad-spectrum cephalosporin (3, 4) with a long serum half-life of about 8 h (2) and is about 95% bound to serum protein. When the serum concentration of ceftriaxone exceeds 150 mg/liter, protein binding decreases, and therefore administration of a larger dose of ceftriaxone than the 500 mg previously studied (2) might result in relatively higher serum levels of unbound agent and hence possibly higher tissue levels and a more rapid excretion (which are both dependent on serum-free fraction). In this study the serum pharmacokinetics, renal excretion, and tissue levels were evaluated after two dosage levels, 500 and 1,500 mg. The tissue penetration was performed with a chemically induced blister (5).

Seven healthy male volunteers, aged 24 to 40 years and with mean weight and height of 78.225 kg and 1.79 m, respectively, took part in the study; five of them participated in a crossover trial, having both doses of ceftriaxone, and the remaining two had only one dose. No volunteers had a history of allergy to β-lactam compounds. Hematological and biochemical profiles were normal in all subjects.

Stool specimens were obtained from the volunteers for 3 days before and 3 days after the administration of the higher dose of 1,500 mg. Dilutions of fecal material were made, and selective media were inoculated such that a quantitative estimation of major *Enterobacteriaceae*, anaerobes, and yeasts could be made. Also, stools from the volunteers with diarrhea were examined for *Clostridium difficile* and its toxin.

On the evening before the study two cantharides plasters (1 by 1 cm) were taped to the anterior aspect of the forearm to induce blister formation. On the morning of the study, the drug, either 500 or 1,500 mg of the hydrated disodium salt of ceftriaxone, dissolved in 5 or 10 ml of sterile water, respectively, was administered intravenously for 3 or 10 min, respectively. Blood samples were taken at 10, 20, and 40 min and at 1, 2, 3, 4, 6, 8, 10, 12, 14, 16, 26, and 31 h after the dose of ceftriaxone. Urine was collected over 48 h. Fluid was removed from the two blisters at 1, 2, 4, 6, 10, 14, and 15 h and placed onto preweighed, sterile 6-mm assay disks. The assays were performed by a routine agar plate diffusion technique using *Escherichia coli*

NCTC 10418 as indicator organism and Oxoid antibiotic medium no. 1 (pH 6.5). The pharmacokinetic analysis of the individual data was performed by standard graphical methods (1).

The concentration/tissue profiles for the two doses are shown in Fig. 1. The pharmacokinetic data for both doses are shown in Table 1. It can be seen from the graph that the serum profiles fit a two-compartment open model. After both doses, there was a fairly rapid initial distribution phase complete within 2 h and followed by a gradual and steady decline. The calculated volumes of distribution approximate to the volume of the vascular compartment. The serum half-lives after each dose were similar, being 8.8 ± 1.7 h and 7.5 ± 0.5 h for 500 and 1,500 mg, respectively; the shorter half-life after the larger dose was accompanied by an increase in urinary excretion of ceftriaxone over the first 4 h. Both the total and renal clearances over the total period of the study were very similar. Ceftriaxone penetrates blister fluid rapidly (Fig. 1). One hour after administration of ceftriaxone, the blister fluid levels were 17.2 mg/liter (500 mg) and 41.25 mg/liter (1,500 mg). The mean maximum blister levels were 32.7 mg/liter (500 mg) and 96.5 mg/liter (1,500 mg), which are similar if the 500-mg level is multiplied by three for comparison.

Two volunteers who received the 500-mg dose and four who received the 1,500-mg dose had diarrhea. This was usually two to three loose explosive stools 36 to 48 h postadministration. The stools of the volunteers who received the

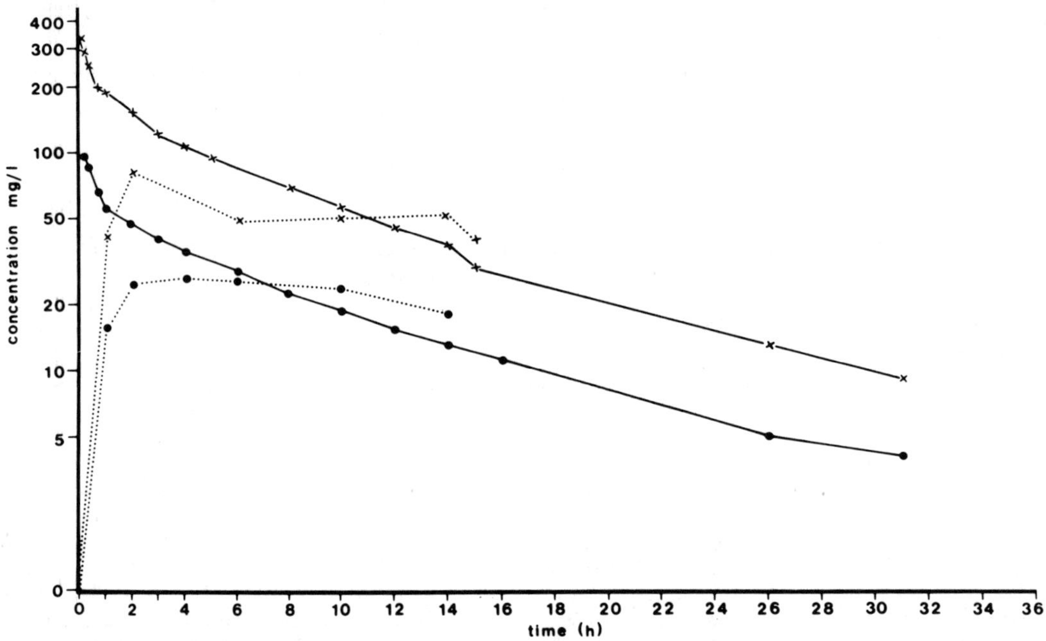

FIG. 1. *Concentration/tissue profiles for two doses of ceftriaxone:* ●*, 500 mg;* ×*, 1,500 mg. Solid lines are serum levels and dotted lines are blister fluid levels.*

TABLE 1. *Pharmacokinetic data on ceftriaxone*

Parameter	Units	500-mg dose	1,500-mg dose
K_e	h^{-1}	0.080 ± 0.013	0.093 ± 0.006
$t_{1/2}$ (half-life) in serum	h	8.8 ± 1.7	7.5 ± 0.5
C_0 (concentration of drug in serum at 0 h)	mg/liter	351 ± 42[a]	342 ± 53.3
AUC (area under concentration/time curve)	mg.h/liter	1,832 ± 368[a]	1,716 ± 175
Total clearance	ml/min	14.2 ± 3.1	14.7 ± 1.5
Renal clearance	ml/min	8.6 ± 2.2	8.4 ± 0.9
V_{ss} (volume of distribution in static state)	liters	10.7 ± 1.5	9.6 ± 1.1
V_c (apparent distribution of drug in central compartment)	liters	4.3 ± 0.6	4.5 ± 0.8
Maximum concn in blisters	mg/liter	98.3 ± 21.0[a]	96.5 ± 42.9
AUC 0–15 blister levels	mg.h/liter	325	885

[a] Actual value multiplied by 3 to allow for differences in dose.

1,500-mg dose were bacteriologically studied, and a greater fall in coliform count was noted in those with diarrhea. There was also a reduction in *Bacteroides* spp. and an increase in yeasts in all but one volunteer. There were no consistent trends associated with *Clostridium* spp., enterococci, or anaerobic streptococci. No *C. difficile* toxin was found in those volunteers with diarrhea.

The aim of this study was to see whether administration of three times the dose of ceftriaxone resulted in relatively greater tissue penetration and increased excretion due to the decrease in serum protein binding at higher serum concentrations. The results of the study show that no significant deviation from a linear dose dependency was found. The tissue penetration was not relatively greater after administration of 1,500 mg of ceftriaxone; this is shown in the 1-h blister fluid level as well as the areas under the curve for blister fluid.

The concept of increasing the dose to obtain relatively higher protein-free drug levels is of interest but is likely to be of little clinical consequence in the case of ceftriaxone.

1. **Greenblatt, D. J., and J. Koch-Weser.** 1975. Clinical pharmacokinetics. N. Engl. J. Med. **292:**702–705.
2. **Seddon, M., R. Wise, A. P. Gillett, and R. Livingston.** 1980. Pharmacokinetics of Ro 13-9004, a broad spectrum cephalosporin. Antimicrob. Agents Chemother. **18:**240–242.
3. **Shannon, K., A. King, C. Warren, and I. Phillips.** 1980. In vitro antibacterial activity and susceptibility of the cephalosporin Ro 13-9904 to beta-lactamases. Antimicrob. Agents Chemother **18:**292–298.
4. **Wise, R., A. P. Gillet, J. M. Andrews, and K. A. Bedford.** 1980. Ro 13-9904: a cephlosporin with a high degree of activity and broad antibacterial activity. J. Antimicrob. Chemother. **6:**595–600.
5. **Wise, R., A. P. Gillett, B. Cadge, S. R. Durham, and S. Baker.** 1980. The influence of protein binding on the tissue levels of 6 β-lactams. J. Infect. Dis. **142:**77–82.

Renal and Biliary Excretion of Ceftriaxone and Effect on the Normal Colon Flora

ANNIE ARVIDSSON,* GUNNAR ALVÁN, BO ANGELIN, AND CARL ERIK NORD

Departments of Clinical Pharmacology, Medicine, and Microbiology, Karolinska Institute, Huddinge University Hospital, and National Bacteriological Laboratory, Stockholm, Sweden*

The development of broad-spectrum cephalosporins with heavy side chains in positions 3 and 7 of the β-lactam ring has resulted in compounds with molecular weight in excess of 500, which increases the possibility of biliary excretion. The aim of this study was therefore to investigate the biliary excretion of ceftriaxone and the effect on the normal flora that can occur when an antibiotic is excreted in large amounts in bile. In an earlier study, we found that some cephalosporins undergo a saturable tubular reabsorption, and we were also interested in clarifying whether this was the case with ceftriaxone (1).

On the night before the experiment, a three-lumen tube was passed into the duodenum. In one of the tubes proximal to the ampulla of Vater, an amino acid-glucose solution was infused to keep the gall bladder contracted. The solution also contained sulfobromophthalein serving as a nonabsorbable marker. Aspirate was continuously collected from the other two tubes in 1-h fractions for determination of the ceftriaxone excretion rate.

Ceftriaxone was intravenously infused to give a low plasma concentration of about 5 μg/ml during the first 3 h. The infusion rate was thereafter increased to obtain a plasma steady-state level of 50 μg/ml during the next 4 h. Blood samples were drawn frequently during the experimental period. Urine and bile specimens were collected in 1-h fractions. Fecal specimens for bacteriological cultivation and ceftriaxone analyses were taken on the day before the antibiotic administration and on days 1, 3, and 10 after the experiment (2).

Five healthy volunteers participated in the study, and in four of them it was possible to study both renal and biliary clearance. The fifth volunteer did not complete the biliary part of the investigation for technical reasons. There was no tendency toward lower clearance values at the low plasma concentrations (Table 1), which would have been the case if ceftriaxone was reabsorbed in the tubuli by a saturable transport mechanism. As ceftriaxone is not metabolized, the sum of renal and biliary clearance should equal the total plasma clearance, as in subjects 1, 3, and 4. Subject 5 had high biliary and renal clearances of 14 ml/min each. The two

TABLE 1. *Plasma and fecal concentrations of ceftriaxone and renal and biliary clearance in five volunteers receiving ceftriaxone*

Subject no.	Obtained plasma concn (μg/ml)	Total plasma clearance (ml/min)	Renal clearance (ml/min)	Biliary clearance (ml/min)	Amt of dose recovered in bile (%)	Fecal concn (μg/g)
1	83.6	12	9	2	17	0
2	46.4	10	4			0
	5	8	8			
3	42.0	12	10	3	17	26
	3.6	14	6			
4	54.7	7	4	1	14	75
	4.8	10	5			
5	25.6	20	14	14	70	39
	3.2	16	12			

values exceeded the total plasma clearance of 20 ml/min. The interpretation was that ceftriaxone underwent enterohepatic recirculation in this case.

As compared with other antibiotics, an appreciable amount of ceftriaxone is excreted via the bile, at least 15% of the dose, and an effect on the colon microflora is therefore expected. Pronounced suppression of both aerobic and anaerobic colon microflora was noticed. Figure 1 shows the results from one volunteer. The number of aerobic bacteria decreased significantly, and *Escherichia coli* disappeared completely on day 3. There was no effect on the anaerobic flora in the two subjects who had no ceftriaxone concentration in feces, whereas the three volunteers with measurable concentrations showed a marked decrease in the number of anaerobic bacteria.

Since all volunteers were colonized with potentially pathogenic bacteria after a single dose of ceftriaxone, it is recommended that special attention be paid to intestinal disturbances when treating patients with ceftriaxone for a longer time period.

This study shows that there is considerable biliary excretion of ceftriaxone and that enterohepatic recirculation might occur. No evidence for saturable tubular reabsorption of ceftriaxone was found. Ceftriaxone markedly suppressed both aerobic and anaerobic normal colon microflora.

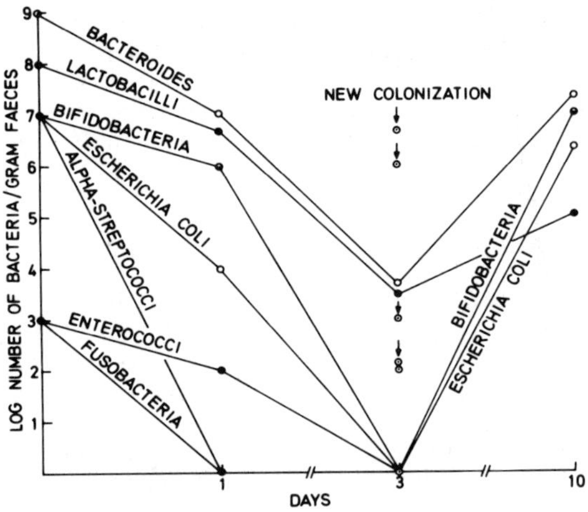

FIG. 1. *Effect of ceftriaxone on the colon microflora in one volunteer receiving ceftriaxone.*

1. **Arvidsson, A., O. Borgå, and G. Alván.** 1979. Renal excretion of cephapirin and cephaloridine: evidence for saturable tubular reabsorption. Clin. Pharmacol. Ther. **25:**870–876.
2. **Heimdahl, A., and C. E. Nord.** 1979. Effect of phenoxymethylpenicillin and clindamycin on the oral, throat and faecal microflora of man. Scand. J. Infect. Dis. **11:** 233–242.

Comparative Clinical Trial of Ceftriaxone and Doxycycline in Patients with Pneumonia

H. PICHLER,* W. VALASEK, G. KIESSLING, E. JESCHKO, AND M. ROTTER

Infectious Disease Unit, Kaiser Franz Josef-Hospital, and Institut of Hygiene, University of Vienna, 1100 Vienna, Austria*

Ceftriaxone, a new β-lactamase-stable cephalosporin belonging to the third generation, shows better antibacterial activity against *Haemophilus influenzae*, *Neisseria* spp., and *Proteus mirabilis* than cefotaxime and moxalactam. Additionally, this new compound possesses an outstanding pharmacokinetic property, namely, a plasma half-life of 8 h. The superior activity against *H. influenzae* and the long half-life, permitting a once-daily administration, led to the decision to compare ceftriaxone with doxycycline in patients with community-acquired pneumonia.

All patients admitted to the ward whose diagnosis of pneumonia had been clinically and radiologically established, and who were without prior antibiotic treatment, received at random either ceftriaxone, 2 g in 50 ml of sterile water once daily, or doxycycline, 200 mg on day 1 and 100 mg on any subsequent day intravenously during the febrile course of the disease and for an additional 3 days. The administered drug was changed in favor of the other if no significant decrease of fever could be achieved within 3 days or whenever symptoms and signs of pneumonia recurred after the end of treatment. Patients with pneumonia without fever were given the appropriate antibiotic for 7 days.

Patient exclusion criteria were known allergy to penicillins or cephalosporins, pregnancy, renal impairment (creatinine clearance, <10 ml/min), or active tuberculosis. Patients with nonbacterial pneumonia were evaluated only for side effects.

The daily clinical assessment of all patients included the recording of body temperature, pulse rate, sputum purulence, intensity of cough, physical signs of pneumonia, and drug tolerance.

Chest X ray was taken before treatment and on days 7 and 14. In case of no complete resolution of the pulmonary infiltrate on day 14, the X ray was repeated on day 21 or whenever necessary for clinical reasons. Sputum specimens were examined microscopically and bacteriologically, and antibiotic sensitivity was determined pre- and post-treatment. Blood was investigated for complete blood count, blood sedimentation rate, SGOT, SGPT, γ-GT, alkaline phosphatase, total bilirubin, electrophoresis, serum creatinine, and BUN before and after treatment, and urinalysis was done as well. In any patient serological examinations for mycoplasma chlamydia and cytomegalo-, adeno- and influenza virus infection were performed twice.

Success was defined as defervescence below 37.5°C within 3 days, marked improvement of subjective and physical signs of pneumonia on day 7, and far-reaching resolution of the infiltrate on day 14. Delayed resolution was classified as no improvement of subjective and auscultatory signs of pneumonia on day 7 and no complete resolution of the infiltrate on day 21.

Relapse was defined as a recurrence of fever after an afebrile period associated with increased lower respiratory signs and symptoms and, in the X ray, either a new infiltrate or an infiltrate in the same lobe previously involved after resolution of the infiltrate had been documented.

Fifty-one patients (29 males and 22 females) entered the study. Six patients were excluded due to evidence of mycoplasma pneumonia in four and cytomegalovirus pneumonia in two. Twenty-three patients (15 males, 8 females; mean age, 68 years [range, 33 to 86]) received ceftriaxone. Seventeen of the patients suffered from either systemic or local underlying disease. Twenty-two patients (11 males, 11 females; mean age, 61 years [range, 27 to 85]) were given doxycycline. Fourteen of 22 patients had underlying disease.

The results of sputum bacteriology in 21 patients are shown in Table 1. Of the remaining 24 patients, either normal flora was recorded or no specimen could be obtained.

Results of treatment are shown in Table 2. The defervescence times of successfully treated patients was 2.5 and 2.2 days in the ceftriaxone and doxycycline groups, respectively. The mean length of treatment with either drug was 7 days. All patients with delayed resolution had underlying diseases. In two of the three patients in the ceftriaxone group, the drug had to be changed due to persistence of fever for >3 days. Fever continued under doxycycline treatment for another 6 and 2 days, respectively, in the two patients. The third patient started with fever on day 8 after 7 days of treatment with ceftriaxone and received doxycycline for another 9 days. All

TABLE 1. *Etiological agents in 21 patients with positive cultures*

Bacterium	No. of patients (no. eliminated)	
	Ceftriaxone group	Doxycycline group
H. influenzae	3 (3)	5 (4)
Proteus mirabilis	2 (2)	0
Proteus morganii	1 (1)	0
Klebsiella oxytoca	1 (1)	0
Enterobacter cloacae	0	1 (1)
Streptococcus pneumoniae	0	2 (2)
Streptococcus faecalis	1 (0)	2 (2)
Beta-hemolytic *Streptococcus*	1 (1)	1 (1)
Staphylococcus aureus	1 (1)	1 (1)

TABLE 2. *Outcome of treatment in 45 patients with pneumonia*

Drug (no. of patients)	No. of patients			
	Success (%)	Delayed resolution	Change of drug	Relapse (days after treatment)
Ceftriaxone (23)	17 (74)	6	3	New lobe, 1 (14)
Doxycycline (22)	16 (73)	5	2	Same lobe, 3 (10, 12, 21)

three patients belonged to the group with delayed resolution. Both patients for whom doxycycline had to be changed had fever persisting for longer than 3 days. These patients continued to have fever for another 3 and 4 days, respectively. One of the two patients had a delayed resolution. One patient and three patients, respectively, in the ceftriaxone and doxycycline groups relapsed. All four patients had serious underlying disease and recovered on the alternative drug.

Side effects (namely, glossitis) in 30 patients receiving ceftriaxone for a mean length of 7 days were recorded in two patients. No side effects were observed in 30 patients receiving doxycycline for a mean length of 7 days.

Our preliminary results show that ceftriaxone is as effective as doxycycline in the treatment of community-acquired pneumonia and is very well tolerated. Whether relapses occur more frequently under treatment with doxycycline than with ceftriaxone, as observed in our series, needs further investigation with larger numbers of patients.

Ceftriaxone (Ro 13-9904), a new Third-Generation Cephalosporin for Parenteral Use in Hospitalized Patients with Sepsis

J. NAGLER* AND A. MERTENS

Medical Intensive Care Unit, Department of Internal Medicine, and Laboratory of Clinical Microbiology, Algemeen Ziekenhuis Middelheim, 2020 Antwerp, Belgium*

The clinical usefulness of ceftriaxone (Ro 13-9904), a new cephalosporin of the third generation, was investigated for treatment in sepsis. Patients suffering from septicemia hospitalized in a medical intensive care unit of a general hospital were selected for treatment with ceftriaxone according to the following criteria: (i) sepsis had to be proven by positive blood cultures; (ii) no concomitant antibiotics were administered; (iii) prior administration of antibiotics had to be discontinued for more than 48 h; (iv) patients with preexisting renal disease were excluded; and (v) women of less than 50 years of age were excluded from the study.

Susceptibility to ceftriaxone was assessed by the disk agar diffusion method (disk content, 30 μg). Strains were considered as resistant when the diameter of the inhibition zone was $\leq$14 mm; intermediate, from 15 to 17 mm; and susceptible, $\geq$18 mm. Serum levels were determined by an agar well method, using *Bacillus subtilis* as the test organism.

According to the above-mentioned criteria, 10 patients were treated with ceftriaxone. A daily dose of 2 g diluted in 150 ml of 5% dextrose was administered intravenously over a 5-min period. Initially, 1 g of ceftriaxone was administered twice daily. Later, patients received 2 g once a day, to evaluate the clinical differences of those two dose regimens. Duration of treatment varied from 5 to 8 days. If clinical deterioration occurred, the drug was discontinued after 48 h. Treatment was considered successful if infection was cured and blood cultures remained sterile for 48 h after treatment.

Table 1 summarizes the treated cases; six women and four men varying in age from 28 to 74 years were treated. Gram-negative sepsis occurred in seven cases, and gram-positive sepsis occurred in three cases.

Eight patients were considered as cured after treatment. One patient relapsed after 2 weeks with the same germ. This patient was a 59-year-old woman suffering from intracerebral hematoma. She was subcomatose and had an indwelling bladder catheter for convenience. In two patients the outcome was unfavorable. The first was a 71-year-old woman who swallowed ammonium hydroxide in a suicide attempt and developed caustic erosions in the upper gastrointestinal tract. Bronchopneumonia with septicemia developed soon after admission. After 3 days of treatment with ceftriaxone, the patient died from massive upper gastrointestinal bleeding. Necropsy confirmed the presence of florid bronchopneumonia. The second patient was a 73-year-old man hospitalized because of chronic bronchitis and intractable congestive heart failure. During admission he developed septic arthritis, with septicemia of the left shoulder. Despite repetitive arthrocentesis and administration of 2 $\times$ 1 g of ceftriaxone intravenously, synovial fluid remained infected after 8 days of treatment. Blood cultures had become negative.

Local tolerance to the drug was excellent. No patient complained of pain during or after the

TABLE 1. *Summary of the cases treated*

Case no.	Patients: Sex	Patients: Age (yr)	Underlying disease	Type of infection	Germ (susceptibility to ceftriaxone)[a]	Dose of ceftriaxone (mg/day)	Period of administration (days)	Outcome	Complications
1	F	59	Cerebral hematoma, coma, bladder catheter	Acute pyelonephritis	*Proteus mirabilis* (S)	2 × 1,000	6	Favorable (relapse after 2 wk)	
2	F	74	Angina pectoris	Cholangitis	*Klebsiella* (S)	2 × 1,000	6	Cure	
3	F	70	Diabetes mellitus, ketoacidotic coma, septic shock	Acute pyelonephritis	*E. coli* (S)	2 × 1,000	5	Cure	
4	F	71	Ammonia poisoning, caustic gastrointestinal lesions	Bronchopneumonia	*Klebsiella pneumoniae* (S)	2 × 1,000	3	Failure	
5	M	73	Chronic bronchitis, heart failure	Pyogenic arthritis	*Staphylococcus aureus* (I)	2 × 1,000	8	Failure	
6	F	67	Suicide attempt, barbiturates, coma	Decubitus ulcers	*Staphylococcus aureus* (I)	2 × 1,000	5	Cure	
7	M	76	Acute myocardial infarction	Acute pyelonephritis	*E. coli* (S)	2 × 1,000	8	Cure	
8	M	74	Nephrolithiasis	Acute pyelonephritis	*Proteus morganii* (S)	2 × 1,000	4	Cure	Generalized rash after 9,000 mg intravenously
9	M	28	Coma, cerebral hematoma, bladder catheter	Decubitus ulcers	*Staphylococcus epidermidis* (S)	2 × 1,000	5	Cure	
10	F	58	Gall stones	Cholangitis	*E. coli* (I)	1 × 2,000	5	Cure	

[a] S, Susceptible; I, intermediate.

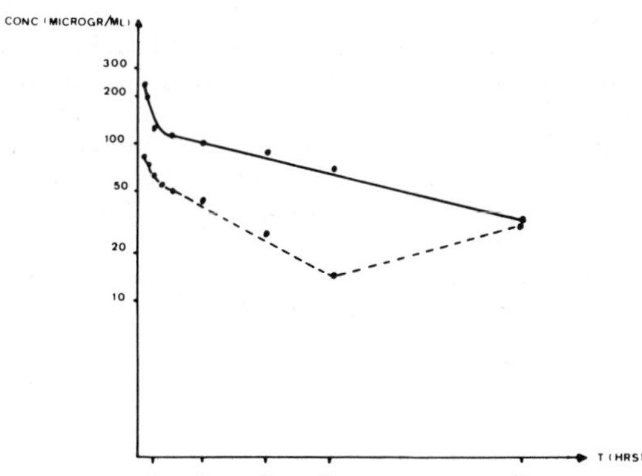

FIG. 1. *Serum levels of ceftriaxone: (——) 1 × 2 g intravenously; (- - -) 2 × 1 g intravenously at 12-h intervals.*

injection, and no induration was noticed during or after the treatment period at the injection site. One of 10 patients developed a generalized rash after administration of a total dose of 9 g. The following parameters were examined before and after treatment: (i) hematological—hemoglobin, hematocrit, leukocyte count and formula, and platelets; (ii) blood chemistry—SGOT, SGPT, alkaline phosphatase, total bilirubin, creatinine, ureum, and electrolytes; (iii) urinalysis—protein content, glucosuria, leukocytes, erythrocytes, and casts. None of these parameters revealed a significant alteration after treatment.

To evaluate the dose regimens, serum levels were determined in patients receiving different doses, namely, 2 × 1 g/day and 1 × 2 g/day. Serum levels were determined at 15, 30, 60, and

120 min and 4, 8, 12, and 24 h. The results are shown in Fig. 1.

Considering the amount of free antibiotic and the MICs for most strains as determined by others, serum levels remained sufficiently high over the 24-h period to be bactericidal in either dose regimen. Further studies will have to confirm these preliminary findings.

Our results indicate that ceftriaxone can be successfully used in treating septicemia at the indicated doses. The drug was well tolerated locally and systemically.

Ceftriaxone Pharmacokinetics in Subjects with Varying Degrees of Renal Dysfunction

NOEL WRIGHT* AND RICHARD WISE

Department of Medicine and Department of Medical Microbiology, Dudley Road Hospital, Birmingham, B18 7QH, U.K.*

Ceftriaxone is a novel, highly active cephalosporin with an antibacterial spectrum similar to that of cefotaxime. It is particularly active against *Haemophilus* spp. and *Neisseria gonorrhoeae*. Chemically it is similar to other cephalosporins except for the substituents in the 3 and 7 positions. However, it is strikingly different from other new cephalosporins in that its half-life in normal volunteers is exceptionally long (approximately 8 h) and only 60% appears in the urine of normal volunteers. Most, if not all, of the remainder is eliminated unchanged by the liver. These studies were designed to investigate the pharmacokinetics in patients with varying degrees of renal dysfunction.

All 20 subjects, including two normal volunteers, gave informed consent. There were 12 males and 8 females (mean age, 50.2 years). The causes of renal failure were various but included infection, hypertension, glomerulonephritis, and polycystic kidneys. No patient in terminal renal failure was on a chronic dialysis program, and hence the biochemical disturbance was greater in these patients than was present for comparable studies on other compounds. That is, the mean blood urea in these patients was 38 mmol/liter, whereas the blood urea in patients on chronic dialysis is usually in the region of 20 mmol.

A 0.5-g amount of ceftriaxone was given intravenously over a 5-min period. Serial drug concentrations were then obtained from blood samples taken from the contralateral arm over the succeeding 36 h. Creatinine clearances were obtained during the 24 h before the study, during the study, and then for a further 24 h afterwards. Routine toxicological screening, including hemoglobin, platelets, blood urea, and liver function tests, were performed before and after the study. Drug concentrations were measured by a microbiological assay in which *Escherichia coli* was used as the indicator organism. The 95% confidence limit of the assay was better than ±13%. A high-pressure liquid chromatography assay was also used on selected samples, and good agreement was found between the two methods. Drug elimination constants for the β phase and half-life were calculated from the slope of the line between 4 and 24 h after administration. In all cases each line had 6 or more points, and the correlation for the regression line was better than 0.95. In eight patients the α-phase elimination constant was calculated from drug measurement during the first 2 h, and the central compartment volume of distribution was calculated.

The drug half-life (Table 1) was 7.3 h in two normal volunteers and had only increased to 11.5 h when the creatinine clearance fell to 10 ml/min. However, in uremic patients the half-life became considerably extended and had a mean of 57 h.

Calculation of volume of distribution in eight patients gave a mean of 4.2/liter, and there was no evidence in the small number of patients that it increased in patients with renal failure. Surprisingly, the relationship of the elimination constant to creatinine clearance was not linear (Fig.

TABLE 1. *Mean ceftriaxone elimination constants (k) and half-lives in patients with varying degrees of renal failure*

Creatinine clearance (ml/min)	n	$k \pm$ SD	$T_{1/2} \pm$ SD
Normal	2	0.1 ± 0.02	7.3 ± 0.01
100–30	6	0.07 ± 0.16	9.7 ± 1.0
29–10	4	0.06 ± 0.01	11.5 ± 2.4
9–5	3	0.04 ± 0.14	17.6 ± 6.4
4–0	5	0.01 ± 0.01	57 ± 26.1

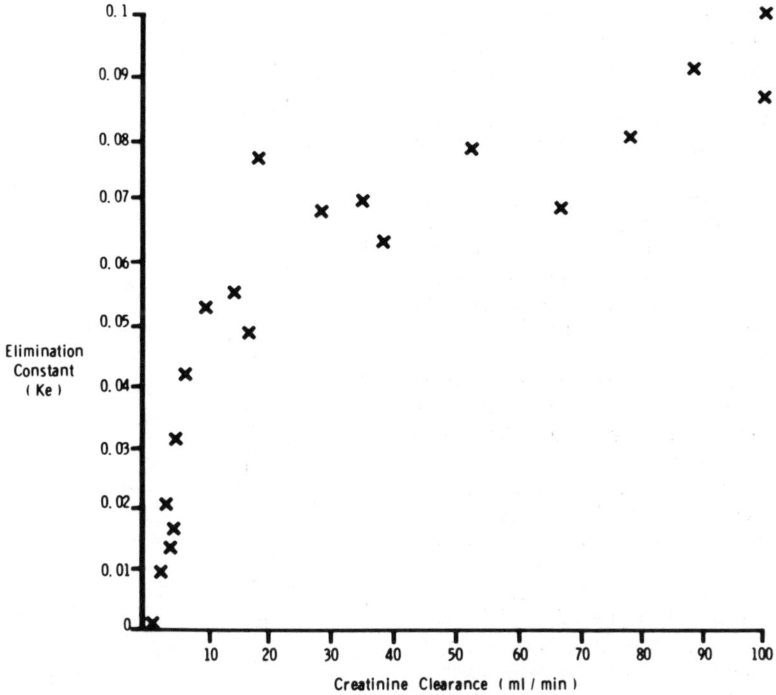

FIG. 1. *Elimination constant against creatinine clearance.*

1) but showed a disproportionate reduction in patients with severe renal failure.

There was no evidence of toxicity either with respect to symptoms or signs developed by the patient nor were any systematic changes noted in toxicological screening.

The marked increase in half-life in patients with creatinine clearances of less than 10 ml/min was a surprise. It was expected that extrarenal mechanisms would be sufficient to allow only a moderate increase in half-life. One patient with a creatinine clearance of only 3 ml/min also had liver damage and had a drug half-life of 53 h, thus implying that hepatic elimination was not contributing much. These findings suggest that dose reduction on therapy should occur when the glomerular filtration rate falls below 10 ml/min if accumulation is to be avoided. The half-life was extremely variable in patients with glomerular filtration rates of less than 5 ml/min.

Experience with Ceftriaxone in Bacterial Meningitis: Clinical, Bacteriological, and Pharmacological Results in 62 Patients

M. CADOZ,* F. DENIS, D. PEYRAMOND, AND I. DIOP MAR

Infectious Diseases Unit, Faculté de Médecine, Dakar Fann, Sénégal

The first bacteriological (2) and pharmacological (3) results obtained with ceftriaxone (Rocephin; Ro 13-9904) have led us to think that this new third-generation cephalosporin might be useful in the treatment of bacterial meningitis. The satisfactory results of a preliminary study (1) encouraged us to pursue this trial in a larger series of patients.

Ceftriaxone was used to treat 62 consecutive patients with proven meningitis due to *Haemophilus influenzae* (25 cases), *Streptococcus pneumoniae* (23 cases), *Neisseria meningitidis* (8 cases), *Serratia marcescens* (3 cases), and *Pseudomonas aeruginosa*, *Proteus mirabilis*, and *Streptococcus pyogenes* (one case each).

Patient ages ranged from 4 days to 62 years

(mean, 6.7 years); 43 patients were under 2 years of age (3 neonates), 11 were between 2 and 20, and 8 were older than 20. There were 35 males and 27 females.

Except in the three neonates, ceftriaxone was always used alone, and the daily dose ranged between 25 and 70 mg/kg of body weight (mean, 39.1 mg/kg). Three neonates with *S. marcescens* meningitis received ceftriaxone (200 mg/kg daily) in combination with intramuscular and intrathecal lividomycin. Ceftriaxone was administered intramuscularly twice daily in the first 22 patients and then only once daily in the 40 remaining patients.

Clinical results. Forty-two patients were cured: 22 of the 25 with *H. influenzae* meningitis (3 had severe neurological sequelae), 13 of the 23 with pneumococcal meningitis (1 with sequelae), 7 of the 8 with meningococcal meningitis (1 with sequelae), and 1 with *S. marcescens* (with sequelae) and 1 with *P. mirabilis* meningitis.

The mean duration of treatment in patients who were cured was 13.6 days for *H. influenzae*, 11.2 days for *S. pneumoniae*, and 4.3 days for *N. meningitidis* (2 patients were cured with a single dose of ceftriaxone).

The drug was generally well tolerated except in two of the three neonates receiving high doses of ceftriaxone in combination with lividomycin who presented with a very severe eczematous erythrodermia, which disappeared when the treatment was stopped. Watery diarrhea occurred in 10 patients and was due to the elimination of the bacterial flora susceptible to ceftriaxone.

Bacteriological results (Fig. 1). All strains except one were susceptible to ceftriaxone, and the highest MICs were 0.78 μg/ml for *H. influenzae*, 0.12 μg/ml for *S. pneumoniae*, 0.007 μg/ml for *N. meningitidis*, 0.5 μg/ml for *P. mirabilis*, 1 μg/ml for *S. pyogenes*, and 2 μg/ml for *S. marcescens*. These MICs were determined by the agar diffusion technique but seemed to be lower by the dilution technique. The *P. aeruginosa* strain was highly resistant to ceftriaxone (MIC, ⩾128 μg/ml).

Sterilization of the cerebrospinal fluid (CSF) (Table 1) was obtained within the first 24 h of treatment in all but one of the meningitis cases. Sterilization was also easily obtained in the *P. mirabilis* meningitis but was more difficult to obtain in the three neonates with *S. marcescens* meningitis. The highly resistant *Pseudomonas* strain was not eradicated from the CSF and the patient died with a positive CSF culture on day 7 after admission, when ceftriaxone had been replaced by colistin and gentamicin. This case was the only one in which the death could, at least partly, be attributed to the failure of ceftriaxone. Indeed, in the other cases death was generally due to fulminating forms or occurred later because of severe neurological damage in patients who were bacteriologically cured. Ceftriaxone levels in the CSF (Fig. 1) were determined 128 times.

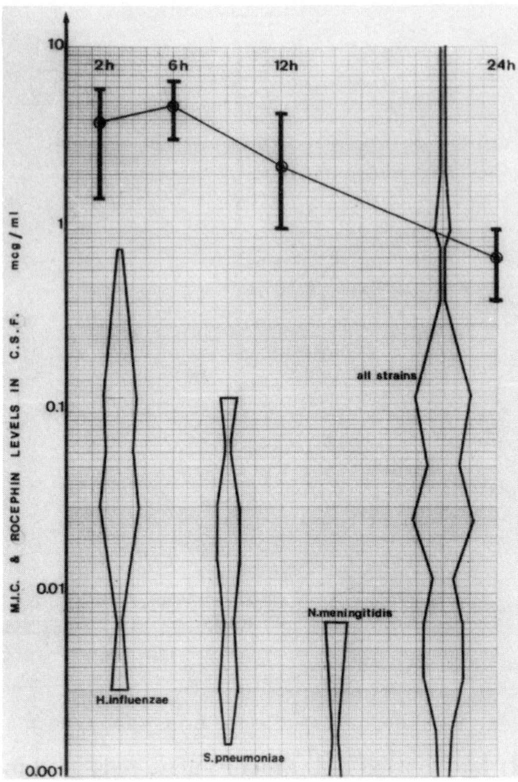

FIG. 1. *MICs for the causative strains and ceftriaxone (Rocephin) levels in the CSF.*

TABLE 1. *CSF sterilization delay after the first injection of ceftriaxone*

Organism	No. of positive cultures/no. of CSF cultures		
	2 h[a]	6 h	24 h
H. influenzae	0/5	1/21	0/23
S. pneumoniae	0/8	0/16	1/19
N. meningitidis	0/2	0/7	0/8

[a] Time after first injection.

The peak concentration generally occurred 6 h after intramuscular injection and reached 4.8 ± 1.7 μg/ml after a mean dose of 36.5 mg/kg of body weight. Furthermore, satisfactory concentrations were still obtained up to 24 h after injection, with a mean level of 0.7 ± 0.3 μg/ml, i.e., more than the MIC of 95% of the causative strains studied.

Ceftriaxone thus appears to be an adequate treatment for most forms of purulent meningitis. Its high activity against *H. influenzae* and most of the enterobacteria makes it a good alternative for the treatment of meningitis in neonates and children, and the very low MIC of *N. meningitidis* and the long duration of satisfactory concentrations in the CSF might make this also the treatment of choice for this form of meningitis.

1. **Cadoz, M., F. Denis, H. Felix, and I. Diop Mar.** 1980. Treatment of purulent meningitis with a new cephalosporin Rocephin (RO 13 9904) Clinical, bacteriological and pharmacological observations in 24 cases. Chemotherapy (Basel) **27**(Suppl. 1):57–61.
2. **Denis, F., M. Cadoz, S. Mboup, M. Pousset, and M. Prince-David.** 1981. Etude préliminaire de l'activité antibactérienne in vitro d'une nouvelle céphalosporine la ROCEPHINE (RO 13 9904). Lyon Med. **245:**765–768.
3. **Marchou, B., Tran Van Tho, and M. Armengaud.** 1980. Diffusion of Ceftriaxone (RO 13 9904) in the C.S.F. Comparison with other Bêta-Lactam antibiotics in dogs with experimental meningitis. Chemotherapy (Basel) **27**(Suppl. 1):37–41.

Prospective Comparative Evaluation of Ceftriaxone (Rocephin; Ro 13-9904) Versus Gentamicin and Cefotaxime in Chronic Urinary Tract Infections

H. GIAMARELLOU,* B. POULOPOULOS, A. AVLAMI, G. PETRIKKOS, J. TSAGARAKIS, AND G. K. DAIKOS

First Department of Propedeutic Medicine, Athens University School of Medicine, King Paul's Hospital, Athens 609, Greece

Ceftriaxone (Rocephin; Ro 13-9904) is a new broad-spectrum third-generation parenteral cephalosporin with a prolonged half-life of 8 h. Due to its stability against β-lactamase hydrolysis, it has an expanded spectrum of antimicrobial activity, including many strains of *Pseudomonas aeruginosa*, *Serratia marcescens*, and the *Enterobacter* group (Neu et al., Program Abstr. Intersci. Conf. Antimicrob. Agents Chemother. 20th, abstr. 95, 1980). Among 464 various gram-negative nosocomial isolates, Giamarellou et al. (1) found that 100% of *Escherichia coli* (105) and *Klebsiella pneumoniae* (40) strains were susceptible to $\leq$8 μg/ml, 90% of *Proteus mirabilis* (60) were susceptible to $\leq$16 μg/ml, and 70% of indole-positive *Proteus* (45) and 80% of *Enterobacter* spp. (20) were susceptible to $\leq$16 μg/ml; at a concentration of 25 μg/ml, 65 to 70% of *P. aeruginosa* (159) and *Bacteroides fragilis* (35) strains were inhibited.

In the present prospective randomized and open clinical trial, we compared the in vivo efficacy of ceftriaxone when given (i) at a dose of 500 mg intramuscularly (i.m.) every 12 h (11 patients, group 1) with the efficacy of gentamicin (12 patients, group 2) given at the conventional treatment schedule (80 mg i.m. every 8 h) and (ii) at a dose of 1,000 mg i.m. every 12 h (10 patients, group 3) compared with the efficacy of cefotaxime administered at a dose of 1 g i.m. every 8 h (10 patients, group 4). Antibiotics in all groups were given for 7 days. All 43 patients who entered the trial were suffering from chronic but symptomatic urinary tract infections (UTI). In group 1 the mean age was 51.5 ± 21.4 years; five patients had underlying kidney diseases, but without any urine flow obstruction, and six were suffering from chronic pyelonephritis, as indicated by the presence of antibody-coated bacteria (ACB) in their urine. In group 2 the corresponding mean age was 61.7 ± 20.2 years; four patients had renal underlying disease, and two had ACB. In group 3, in which ceftriaxone was given at a higher dose, the mean age was 63.0 ± 15 years; five patients had underlying kidney diseases and four had ACB in their urine. Finally, in group 4, in which cefotaxime was administered, the mean age was 55 + 13 years; six patients had underlying kidney disease and six had ACB. Mean duration of recurrent episodes of UTI in the past was 4.7 ± 3.9, 1.6 ± 0.7, 4.3 ± 3.7, and 5.1 ± 3.8 years in the respective groups.

Isolated microorganisms in urine were as follows: group 1, *E. coli* (7), *P. mirabilis* (3), and *Enterobacter cloacae* (1); group 2, *E. coli* (5), *P. mirabilis* (4), *E. cloacae* (2), and *P. aeruginosa* (1); group 3, *E. coli* (7), *P. mirabilis* (2), *Morganella* (1), and *E. cloacae* (1); and group 4, *E. coli* (5), *P. mirabilis* (1), *E. cloacae* (3), and *S. epidermidis* (1).

Before starting treatment and on the last day of treatment, hematology tests, liver and renal toxicity tests, and urine cultures were performed.

TABLE 1. *Ceftriaxone versus gentamicin in chronic symptomatic UTI without urine flow obstruction*[a]

Drug	Outcome			
	Clinical success	Eradi-cation	Super-infec-tion	Re-lapse
Ceftriaxone (n = 11)	11	11	2	1
with ACB (n = 6)			2	1
Gentamicin (n = 12)	11	10	1	2
with ACB (n = 2)			1	1

[a] Long-term follow-up relapse: ceftriaxone, four of nine (two with ACB); gentamicin, four of five (two with ACB). There were no failures with either drug.

TABLE 2. *Ceftriaxone versus cefotaxime in chronic symptomatic UTI without urine flow obstruction*

Drug	Outcome				
	Clinical Success	Eradi-cation	Fail-ure	Rein-fec-tion	Re-lapse
Ceftriaxone (n = 10)	10	10		2	
with ACB (n = 4)				1	
Cefotaxime (n = 10)	9	10			2
with ACB (n = 6)					2

Urine cultures were thereafter followed each week for another 21 days after treatment discontinuation.

Clinical and bacteriological results are shown in Tables 1 and 2. Adverse reactions included only local pain at the site of i.m. injection in 7 out of 11 patients in group 1, in 7 of 12 patients in group 2, in 9 of 10 patients in group 3, and in 10 of 10 patients in group 4. However, duration and intensity of pain were worst in the cefotaxime group.

From this study, we conclude that (i) ceftriaxone, cefotaxime, and gentamicin are equally effective considering clinical and bacteriological results during treatment of chronic UTI; (ii) there is no difference in the activity of ceftriaxone when given at a daily dose of 500 mg or 1,000 mg every 12 h; (iii) ceftriaxone and cefotaxime, when considering long-term follow-up results, particularly in the presence of ACB, are superior to gentamicin. However, on a weight basis and considering local muscular tolerance and the advantage of administering the new antibiotic once or twice daily, ceftriaxone should be preferable to cefotaxime. Finally, in the presence of ACB, a more prolonged treatment course with either ceftriaxone or cefotaxime seems necessary to avoid recurrences.

1. **Giamarellou, H., B. Poulopoulos, A. Katsabas, G. Petrikkos, M. Papapetropoulou, and G. K. Daikos.** 1981. Antibacterial activity of Ro 13-9904 and preliminary experience in gonorrhoea and chronic urinary tract infections. Chemotherapy **27**(Suppl. 1):70–74.

Pharmacokinetics of Ceftriaxone in Cystic Fibrosis

MARI VANGDAL, TOM BERGAN,* HELGE MICHALSEN, AND AUD SALVESON

Department of Microbiology, Aker Hospital, Department of Microbiology, Institute of Pharmacy, University of Oslo, and Department of Pediatrics, Aker Hospital, Oslo, Norway*

Chemical modifications of the cephalosporin molecule have led to ceftriaxone, which has a wide antibacterial spectrum (1). It exhibits the unique pharmacokinetic property that its serum half-life ($t_{1/2}$) is some three to four times longer than that of other β-lactam antibiotics (3, 4, 6).

Patients with cystic fibrosis (CF) eliminate β-lactam antibiotics (3) more rapidly than normal individuals or non-CF patients. Doses must thus be increased to produce therapeutic serum levels. On the other hand, pharmacokinetics of aminoglycosides are similar in CF patients and normal individuals (5). Therefore, antibiotics must be studied in CF to ensure correct dosage in this particular patient group. This study presents the pharmacokinetics of ceftriaxone in CF.

Included in the study were eight patients (two female and six male) with CF studied for one to three courses; their mean age (± SD) was 10.1 (±4.8) years. Their renal function was normal. A total of 14 doses were studied.

The patients received ceftriaxone for therapeutic reasons, and the guardians consented to participation in the pharmacokinetic study. The doses were 50 mg/kg of body weight and were given as a 3-min intravenous bolus injection.

The samples were assayed by both microbiological assay and high-pressure liquid chromatography (HPLC). The agar well diffusion method using Antibiotic Medium No. 1 (Oxoid Ltd.) and *Escherichia coli* 1346 (from Hoffmann-La Roche, Basel, Switzerland) was employed for the microbiological assay, with a lower sensitivity limit of 0.4 mg/liter. The HPLC proceeded as ion pair chromatography with Lichrosorb RP8, 5 μm (E. Merck), as material in a column with an inner diameter of 4.5 mm and a length of 15 cm. The eluant was a mixture of 150 ml of methanol and 850 ml of a solution consisting of 0.1 M tetrabutyl-ammonium hydrogen sulfate and 0.09 M tripotassium phosphate at a flow rate of 1 ml/min and a pressure of 2,050 lb/in^2. The lower limit of sensitivity was 0.01 mg/liter and the SD 3% of the spiked level was within the range 6 to 200 mg/liter.

HPLC of the urine failed to detect biotransformation products of ceftriaxone. Accordingly, pharmacokinetic assessments (by AUTOAN 2/NONLIN) are based on the microbiological assay data. The mean serum concentrations are shown in Fig. 1. All curve regressions followed the two-compartment equation. The pharmacokinetic characteristics are shown in Table 1. A high total area under the serum curve of 1,177.6 mg.h/liter was seen, but with a high coefficient of variation (CV), 0.52. The difference between the k_{12} and k_{21} was not statistically significant (Wilcoxon nonparametric test). The $t_{1/2}$ was long, 7.09 h, with a CV of 0.58. The distribution volume coefficient (distribution volume per kilogram) CV was 0.79 and that of the total body clearance 0.67 liter/h.

Ceftriaxone is active against both *Pseudomonas* and staphylococci, which are responsible for most of the recurrent infections of the respiratory tract in patients with CF (3, 5). The long $t_{1/2}$ observed previously in normal adults (6) was also observed in our patients with CF. The patients with CF, consequently, have the same advantage as normal subjects regarding the prolonged $t_{1/2}$. This factor would be instrumental in governing the extravascular penetration of the antibiotic relative to that of other β-lactam antibiotics, which have a three to four times faster rate of elimination. For instance, the $t_{1/2}$ of other recent parenteral cephalosporins is 2.7 for moxalactam and 1.3 h for cefotaxime (4).

The concentration reached and the duration of antibacterial levels are a function of and are proportional to the area under the serum concentration curves (2). The prolonged $t_{1/2}$, accordingly, would possibly allow a reduction of total dose, longer intervals between doses, and, consequently, relative ease of administration.

It is of considerable interest that the CF patients have a $t_{1/2}$ similar to that in non-CF subjects. To our knowledge, pharmacokinetic assessment has not so far been published either on this category of patients or with a dosage of 50 mg/kg twice daily in children. It is notable, though, that the response in a study on healthy normal volunteers, given an average of 6.3938 mg/kg, resulted in an area under the serum curve of 95.40 mg.h/liter when normalized to a dose of 1 mg/kg (6) compared with our value of 23.55 mg.h/liter for 1 mg/kg. Our clearance was 29.5 ml/min compared with 14.2 ml/min in healthy adult volunteers (6). Compared with healthy individuals, therefore, lower serum levels were observed in our patients, and the elimination rate was somewhat faster, although the rate of serum elimination was of the same order as in normal subjects. However, final conclusions have to be postponed until data from non-CF children receiving the same doses are available; this is particularly important since dose-dependent pharmacokinetics has been demonstrated for this antibiotic (data on file, Hoffmann-La Roche, Basel and Nutley, N.J.).

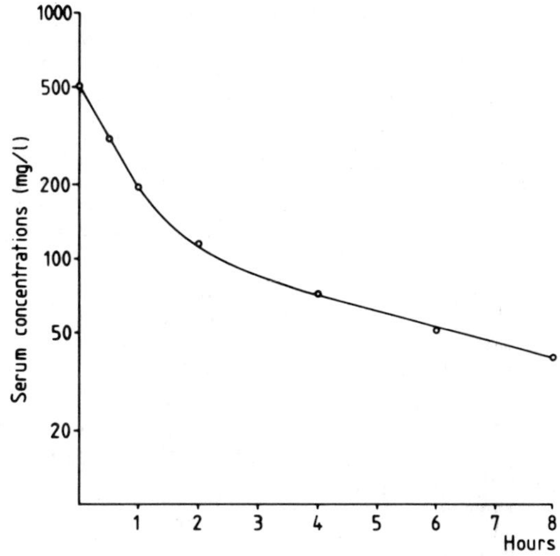

FIG. 1. *Mean serum concentrations (and SD) in patients with CF after single doses of 50 mg of ceftriaxone per kg as rapid intravenous bolus injections.*

The present data demonstrate that the dosage of ceftriaxone may proceed at 12-h or even 24-h intervals in CF patients as in non-CF individuals. The serum levels were high compared with the in vitro susceptibility of even the relatively more resistant species like *Pseudomonas* and *Serratia*. The trough levels were exceeded by 90% of the MICs for *Serratia* and other enterobacteria, but *Enterobacter* MICs (1) were exceeded by a factor of 10 to 20. The relatively higher MIC for *Pseudomonas*, *Enterobacter*, and staphylococci would indicate that the dose of 50 mg/kg or higher should be used in the treatment of res-

TABLE 1. *Pharmacokinetic characteristics of ceftriaxone in patients with cystic fibrosis after the first dose of 14 courses with 50 mg/kg as intravenous bolus injections*[a]

Result	k_{21} (h^{-1})	k_{12} (h^{-1})	k_E (h^{-1})	c_0 (mg/liter)	F (mg.h/liter)	$t_{1/2}$ (h)	$V_{d,\beta}$ (liters)	$\Delta_{d,\beta}$ (liters/kg)	Cl_B (liters/h)
Mean	0.413	0.689	0.437	500.1	1,177.6	7.09	18.26	0.56	1.77
SD	0.221	0.232	0.057	232.6	607.8	4.12	16.81	0.44	1.19

[a] Symbols: k_{21} and k_{12}, transfer rate constants between compartments; k_E, elimination rate constant; c_0, initial hybrid serum concentration at time zero; F, area under the serum curve; $V_{d,\beta}$, volume of distribution; Cl_B, total body clearance.

piratory tract infections in patients with CF, but this point needs clinical elucidation. At any rate, the penetration of ceftriaxone has been shown to be good (6).

Limited or no adjustment of the dose being necessary in CF patients, ceftriaxone can consequently, in principle, be administered as in non-CF subjects.

1. **Angehrn, P., P. J. Probst, R. Reiner, and R. L. Then.** 1980. Ro 13-9904, a long-acting broad-spectrum cephalosporin: in vitro and in vivo studies. Antimicrob. Agents Chemother. **18**:913–921.
2. **Bergan, T.** 1981. Pharmacokinetics of tissue penetration of antibiotics. Rev. Infect. Dis. **3**:45–66.
3. **Bergan, T., and H. Michalsen.** 1979. Pharmacokinetics of azlocillin in children with cystic fibrosis. Arzneim. Forsch. **29**:1955–1957.
4. **Lüthy, R., R. Münch, J. Blaser, H. Bhend, and W. Siegenthaler.** 1979. Human pharmacology of cefotaxime (HR-756), a new cephalosporin. Antimicrob. Agents Chemother. **16**:127–133.
5. **Michalsen, H., and T. Bergan.** 1981. Pharmacokinetics of netilmicin in children with and without cystic fibrosis. Antimicrob. Agents Chemother. **19**:1029–1031.
6. **Seddon, M., R. Wise, R. P. Gillett, and R. Livingston.** 1980. Pharmacokinetics of Ro 13-9904, a broad-spectrum cephalosporin. Antimicrob. Agents Chemother. **18**:240–242.

Treatment of Severe Gram-Negative Infections with Ceftriaxone

J. D. BAUMGARTNER, J. P. BERNARD, AND M. P. GLAUSER*

Division des Maladies Infectieuses, Départment de Médecine, Centre Hospitalier Universitaire Vaudois, 1011 Lausanne, Switzerland

Ceftriaxone, a new cephalosporin antibiotic with a high intrinsic antimicrobial activity against most gram-negative microorganisms, is unique in having an extremely long serum half-life in humans. We treated 58 patients for 61 episodes of severe gram-negative infections, using a twice or once a day schedule.

Three hundred forty-three gram-negative strains were isolated from blood cultures from 1979 to 1981 at the Centre Hospitalier Universitaire Vaudois and identified at the Institute of Microbiology of the University of Lausanne. The strains were kept frozen at −80°C in lysed horse blood until tested for antimicrobial susceptibility. MICs of various β-lactam antibiotics were determined by use of a microtiter system and standard laboratory procedures (1).

As shown in Table 1, ceftriaxone was more active than the other cephalosporins tested and was more active than ticarcillin against *Escherichia coli*, *Klebsiella pneumoniae*, indole-positive and -negative *Proteus*, and *Serratia marcescens*. Ceftriaxone, like cefoperazone and cefotaxime, showed activity similar to that of ticarcillin against *Pseudomonas aeruginosa*.

Serum levels of ceftriaxone were determined by the agar diffusion technique, with *Bacillus subtilis* as the test microorganism (2). In 13 patients with normal renal function, serum levels after 1.5 g intravenously (i.v.) were 149 μg/ml (range, 100 to 225 μg/ml) 1 h after rapid infusion, 52 μg/ml (40 to 90 μg/ml) after 12 h, and 27 μg/ml (13 to 43 μg/ml) after 24 h (trough levels). Thus, 24 h after injection of 1.5 g of ceftriaxone, serum levels were between 10 and 100 times above the MICs for all gram-negative microorganisms tested, with the exception of *P. aeruginosa*.

Synovial fluid collected by drains over a 24-h period in three patients showed a mean ceftriaxone concentration (five measurements) of 58 μg/ml (range, 40 to 72 μg/ml) after 2 g i.v. per 24 h.

Ceftriaxone was administered to 58 patients for 61 episodes of severe gram-negative infections. Ceftriaxone in a dose of 1.5 g was given i.v. twice daily during acute infection; after dis-

TABLE 1. *In vitro susceptibility to various β-lactam antibiotics of 343 gram-negative microorganisms isolated from blood cultures (expressed as cumulative percentage of susceptible strains)*

Organism and drug (no. of strains)	MIC (μg/ml)																	
	<0.04	0.004	0.008	0.016	0.032	0.064	0.125	0.25	0.5	1	2	4	8	16	32	64	128	>128
E. coli																		
Ceftriaxone (157)	4	4	6	11	32	72	89	93	96	99	100							
Cefoperazone (137)							6	26	51	73	85	93	93	96	96	97	97	100
Cefamandole (70)								1	6	60	74	83	91	96	97			
Ticarcillin(157)							10	25	36	43	59	68	71	71	72	73		
K. pneumoniae																		
Ceftriaxone (35)				3	31	71	89	97	100									
Cefotaxime (35)			3	14	63	86	89	97	100									
Cefoperazone (42)							2	29	38	55	69	86	86	88	95	98	100	
Cefamandole (35)									17	60	69	77	80	80	91			
Ticarcillin (35)																20		
P. mirabilis																		
Ceftriaxone (25)	36	36	92	100														
Cefotaxime (24)	4	4	38	63	83	100												
Cefoperazone (24)								4	46	92	96	96	96	96	96	100		
Cefamandole (15)									13	53	73	80	80	87	93			
Ticarcillin (25)										80	88	96	96	96	96	96		
Proteus, indole-positive																		
Ceftriaxone (13)				31	69	92	92	92	100									
Cefotaxime (13)			8	38	62	77	92	92	100									
Cefoperazone (13)									8	85	92	92	100					
Cefamandole (8)														13	25			
Ticarcillin (13)										31	38	54	77	92	100			
S. marcescens																		
Ceftriaxone (32)						44	91	97	97	97	97							
Cefotaxime (32)							13	84	97	97	97	97						
Cefoperazone (41)									2	5	15	15	24	88	95	100		
Cefamandole (32)														3	16	47		
Ticarcillin (32)												6	6	6	6	6	6	100
P. aeruginosa																		
Ceftriaxone (65)										5	5	5	18	82	92	98	100	
Cefotaxime (65)										3	8	15	25	88	94	98	100	
Cefoperazone (65)												5	82	97	98	100		
Ticarcillin (62)										6	6	6	10	27	81	94	95	100

appearance of fever or symptoms, this was followed by a single daily dose of 2.0 g i.v. Three patients received the drug intramuscularly in 1% lidocaine. Treatment usually lasted for 2 to 3 weeks (mean, 18 days; range, 1 day to 26 weeks), but seven patients with deep-seated infection received the drug for 4 weeks or more.

Eleven patients (among them seven with septicemia and two with osteoarticular infections) were treated at home, nine of them after initial therapy in the hospital.

Infection was microbiologically documented in 53 cases and clinically documented in 8 cases. Thirty patients were bacteremic at the time of presentation. The infection was of urinary origin in 23 patients, catheter associated in 10, abdominal or gynecological in 10, pulmonary in 6, and in the soft tissues in 5 patients. Furthermore, there were 2 patients with posttraumatic gram-negative osteoarticular infections, 2 patients with meningitis, and 3 patients with neutropenia and fever. The predominant microorganism were *E. coli* (21 cases), *S. marcescens* (10 cases), *P. aeruginosa* (7 cases), and *K. pneumoniae* (5 cases). In 32 patients treatment with ceftriaxone

TABLE 2. *Side effects*[a]

Effect	No. of reactions in 58 patients
Necessitating discontinuation of treatment	
Leukothrombopenia (reversible)	1
Cutaneous reactions	2
Diarrhea, vomiting	1
Total	4 in 4 patients (7%)
Mild, no discontinuation of treatment	
Symptomatic	
Cutaneous reactions	2
Diarrhea	1
Phlebitis	1
Fever	1
Total	5 in 5 patients (9%)
Asymptomatic	
Eosinophilia (>400/mm^3)	12
Abnormal liver function tests	7
Resistance to dicumarol	1
No side effect	33 patients

[a] No increases in blood creatinine were observed in 11 patients who received concomitant aminoglycoside antibiotics (tobramycin, 6 patients; gentamicin, 4 patients; amikacin, 1 patient) for 3 to 47 days (mean, 11.2 days).

was started after failure of another antibiotic, or a combination of antibiotics, to eradicate infection. In 2 patients, ceftriaxone was administered immediately after severe allergic reactions to penicillins.

Complete cure was achieved in 45 patients (75%) and improvement resulted in 5 (8%). The clinical outcome was not assessable in 6 patients (10%). Relapse of infection occurred in 2 patients (3.2%). One patient with a transplanted kidney was successfully treated for a bacteremic urinary infection, but suffered a relapse in the form of an asymptomatic bacteriuria 1 week posttreatment. One patient presented with *S. marcescens* meningitis 6 months after 2 weeks of ceftriaxone for *S. marcescens* septicemia due to an infected i.v. line. Failure was observed in 3 patients (4.9%), all of whom had *P. aeruginosa* infections (MIC = 128 μg/ml for the three strains) either in the lung (2 patients) or during severe neutropenia (1 patient).

One patient with stercoral peritonitis due to ceftriaxone-susceptible *E. coli*, *K. pneumoniae*, and *P. aeruginosa* developed a symptomatic superinfection with septicemia due to a ceftriaxone-resistant *K. pneumoniae* 2 days after ceftriaxone treatment ended.

Asymptomatic colonization with ceftriaxone-resistant organisms was observed in 12 patients (*Candida albicans* in 9 cases, *P. aeruginosa* in 3 cases).

Reversible side effects (Table 2) necessitating discontinuation of treatment were observed in four patients. All other side effects detected were mild or asymptomatic. Eleven patients had concomitant aminoglycoside administration and no nephrotoxicity was observed.

Because of its unique pharmacological properties and its high in vitro activity, ceftriaxone might be successfully used as a single daily dose in the treatment of severe infections due to susceptible organisms. This opens up new possibilities for treating patients parenterally at home.

1. **Gavan, T. L., and A. L. Barry.** 1980. Microdilution test procedures, p. 459–462. *In* E. H. Lennette, A. Balows, W. J. Hausler, Jr., and J. P. Truant (ed.), Manual of clinical microbiology, 3rd ed. American Society for Microbiology, Washington, D.C.
2. **Sabath, L. D., and J. P. Anhalt.** 1980. Assay of antimicrobics, p. 485–490. *In* E. H. Lennette, A. Balows, W. J. Hausler, Jr., and J. P. Truant (ed), Manual of clinical microbiology, 3rd ed. American Society for Microbiology, Washington, D.C.

Treatment of Hepatic and Other Intraabdominal Abscesses and Septicemia with Ceftriaxone

W. GRANINGER,* T. EGGER, R. LENZHOFER, S. BREYER, E. DIEM, AND K. CZECH

Department of Chemotherapy, First Department of Dermatology, Department of Anaesthesia and General Intensive Care, University of Vienna, Vienna, Austria

Ceftriaxone is a highly protein-bound parenteral cephalosporin derivative with an average plasma elimination half-life of 8 h. The excretion of the drug is via the urinary (56%) and biliary tracts (44% in feces) (1, 2). We tested the in vitro activity of ceftriaxone against cephalothin-resistant bacterial strains and compared it with the activity of cefamandole, cefuroxime, cefoxitin, cefoperazone, and cefotaxime. Susceptibility testing was carried out by the agar diffusion technique using 30-μg disks. An inhibition zone greater than 18 mm indicated susceptibility for all compounds except cefotaxime, for which a 25-mm diameter was the breakpoint. Ceftriaxone exhibited a spectrum of antibacterial activity similar to that of cefotaxime. Its activity against *Staphylococcus aureus* strains was less than that of cefamandole (59% susceptible strains versus 93%, $n = 112$). Recently isolated strains of *Proteus mirabilis* ($n = 35$), indole-positive *Proteus* species ($n = 25$), *Serratia marcescens* ($n = 33$), and *Acinetobacter cloacae* exhibited a high percentage of susceptibility (97, 92, 94, and 97%, respectively). The activity of ceftriaxone, cefotaxime, and cefoperazone exceeded by far that of cefamandole and cefoxitin. Relatively weak activity was recorded against strains of *Enterobacter cloacae* (66% of strains susceptible compared with 82% susceptible to cefoperazone).

The excellent antibacterial activity of ceftriaxone and its remarkable pharmacokinetic properties prompted us to test it as a sole medication in patients with severe nosocomial infections. Forty adult patients with an average age of 52 (19 to 72) years and average weight of 75 (62 to 85) kg were treated. All patients were referred to us because the infection did not respond to commercially available β-lactam agents including cefamandole and cefoxitin or to aminoglycosides. Indications for treatment with ceftriaxone included hepatic abscesses (n = 13), abscesses after abdominal and vascular reconstructive surgery (n = 10), septicemia (n = 11), acute pyelonephritis (n = 4), and pneumonia (n = 2). Ceftriaxone was administered intravenously in a dose of 2 g every 12 h except in patients with urinary tract infections, who received 2 g only once daily. Two patients, one 35-year-old man and one 2-year-old child, received 200 mg/kg per day. Therapy was given for 6 to 25 days (median, 11 days) depending on clinical effect and severity of disease. Frequent clinical assessment and determination of renal, hepatic, and hematological parameters were performed. The criteria for cure were the disappearance of the causative pathogen and the improvement or disappearance of clinical symptoms.

The bacteriological results are shown in Table 1. Clinically favorable results were seen in these refractory cases. The therapeutic evolution in patients with hepatic abscesses was favorable in 9 of 13 cases. In four patients with infections caused by *Staphylococcus aureus* (n = 2), *Pseudomonas aeruginosa*, and *Enterobacter cloacae*, the pathogens could not be eradicated. Four patients who had undergone hemihepatectomy responded initially but died of hepatic failure. Among the 10 patients with mostly mixed intraabdominal infections, eight showed satisfactory progress. In one patient with pancreatic abscess caused by *P. aeruginosa*, the pathogen could not be eliminated. The other patient had undergone open heart surgery and developed a substernal abscess due to *S. marcescens*. Because of multiple treatment failures with other cephalosporins and aminoglycosides, he was treated with 6 g of ceftriaxone twice a day, but without any effect. Superinfection with *Streptococcus faecalis* occurred. In 7 of the latter 10 patients, superinfections with resistant *S. aureus* (2 cases), *P. aeruginosa* (5 cases), and *S. faecalis* (2 cases) occurred which had no evident clinical effect. In septicemia 9 of 11 patients showed a favorable outcome. Among these favorable results the cases with *Acinetobacter* species (n = 3) and *Serratia* species are particularly interesting. One result, however, should be assessed as only fair. A 2-year-old child had developed septicemia due to *S. marcescens* after open heart surgery (Fig. 1). After starting treatment with 3 mg/kg twice daily, the patient seemed to improve but developed meningitis after 2 days. The dose was increased to 120 mg/kg per day, and gentamicin was administered intrathecally. Surprisingly, the organism could be grown in blood cultures on day 8. The dose of ceftriaxone was further increased to 200 mg/kg per day, and gentamicin was administered parenterally and intrathecally. The patient recovered, but with the sequela of bilateral blindness. Cerebrospinal fluid cultures had always been sterile. In three burn patients, septicemia due to resistant *S. aureus* and *P. aeruginosa* (n = 2) occurred. All patients with acute pyelonephritis were cured by a dosage of 2 g of ceftriaxone per day. The two patients with suppurative pneumonia due to *S. aureus* improved slowly.

The systemic tolerance of ceftriaxone was satisfactory in 32 of 42 patients. Side effects recorded were elevation of alkaline phosphatase in three patients, a macular rash in three patients, loose stool in two, and severe colitis in two patients. The elevation of alkaline phosphatase was not clearly related to ceftriaxone because it occurred only in patients with liver disease. The colitis lasted for 10 days in both patients, who had received 2 g per day for their urinary tract

TABLE 1. *Bacteriological response to ceftriaxone treatment*

Species	Hepatic and postoperative wound abscesses			Septicemia, pyelonephritis		
	n	Elimination	Persistence	n	Elimination	Persistence
Staphylococcus aureus	6	4	2	3	3	
Anaerobic streptococci	1	1		1	1	
Streptococcus faecalis	1	1		0		
Escherichia coli	5	5		4	4	
Citrobacter spp.	1	1		0		
Klebsiella pneumoniae	8	8		2	2	
Enterobacter cloacae	2	1	1	1	1	
Serratia spp.	2	1	1	3	3	
Proteus mirabilis	2	2		1	1	
Pseudomonas aeruginosa	4	2	2	1	1	
Acinetobacter spp.				3	3	
Total	32	26	6	19	19	0

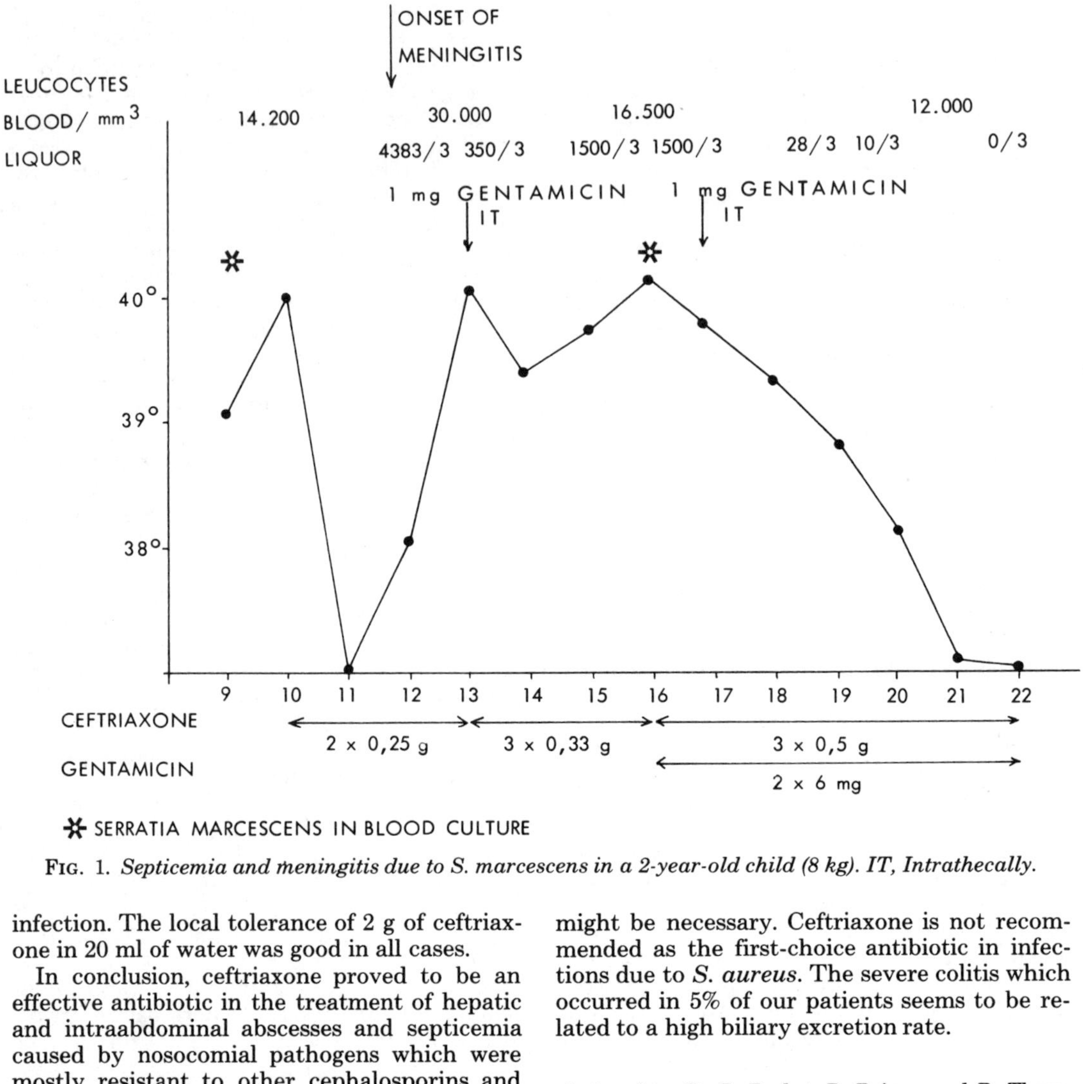

FIG. 1. *Septicemia and meningitis due to S. marcescens in a 2-year-old child (8 kg). IT, Intrathecally.*

infection. The local tolerance of 2 g of ceftriaxone in 20 ml of water was good in all cases.

In conclusion, ceftriaxone proved to be an effective antibiotic in the treatment of hepatic and intraabdominal abscesses and septicemia caused by nosocomial pathogens which were mostly resistant to other cephalosporins and aminoglycosides. A dosage of 2 g every 12 h seems to be sufficient. A dosage of 2 g once a day is suitable for the treatment of pyelonephritis. In infections due to moderately susceptible organisms such as *S. marcescens* and *P. aeruginosa*, doses up to 150 to 200 mg/kg per day might be necessary. Ceftriaxone is not recommended as the first-choice antibiotic in infections due to *S. aureus*. The severe colitis which occurred in 5% of our patients seems to be related to a high biliary excretion rate.

1. **Angehrn, P., P. Probst, R. Reiner, and R. Thern.** 1980. Ro 13-9904, a long acting broad-spectrum cephalosporin: in vitro and in vivo studies. Antimicrob. Agents Chemother. **18:**914–921.
2. **Seddon, M., R. Wise, A. Gillett, and R. Livingston.** 1980. Pharmacokinetics of Ro 13-9904, a broad-spectrum cephalosporin. Antimicrob. Agents Chemother. **18:**240–242.

Ceftazidime, a New Antipseudomonal Antibiotic: Introduction

P. W. MUGGLETON* AND G. W. ROSS

Glaxo Group Research Ltd., Greenford, Middlesex, England

Ceftazidime (6R,7R)-7-[(Z)-2-(2-aminothiazol-4-yl)-2-(2-carboxyprop-2-yloxyimino) acetamido]-3-(pyridinium-1-ylmethyl)ceph-3-em-4-carboxylate, is derived from cephalosporin C and has the structure shown in Fig. 1. The compound was discovered, developed, and evaluated in our research laboratories at Greenford, Middlesex, England. It is a colorless crystalline solid which, as the monosodium salt, is highly soluble in water. One gram will readily dissolve in 3 ml of water for injection.

The study which has led to the discovery of ceftazidime started when the earlier β-lactamase–sensitive cephalosporins (exemplified by cephaloridine, cephalothin, and cefazolin) were succeeded by a "second series" of agents that included cefuroxime, cefoxitin, and cefamandole. These newer compounds had various degrees of stability to β-lactamases produced by gram-negative bacteria and thus a considerably widened spectrum. Lack of activity against *Pseudomonas aeruginosa* was, however, a common characteristic, and they thus could not be regarded as completely acceptable replacements for the aminoglycoside antibiotics, the use of which is increasingly being questioned on the grounds of resistance development and potential toxicity. A β-lactam antibiotic with its characteristic low toxicity and an antibiotic spectrum equivalent to the aminoglycosides was required. Activity against *P. aeruginosa* was seen as the key to the problem.

Infections with *P. aeruginosa,* together with those caused by other organisms such as the indole-positive *Proteus* spp., are frequently encountered in immunocompromised patients, e.g., those with severe burns, the elderly, or those undergoing cancer chemotherapy. It follows that, for an antibiotic to be fully effective in such cases, it must possess a long list of favorable properties and not be deficient in any of them. Among recently announced β-lactam antibiotics, a number are claimed to have practical activity against *Pseudomonas* infections. These include cefotaxime, moxalactam, ceftriaxone, cefoperazone, and cefsulodin. Some of these are less effective than others because they lack one or more key properties.

The essential properties are as follows:

Efficient penetration of the bacterial cell. Antibiotics which fail to penetrate the cell or which penetrate only slowly are unlikely to be effective. It is widely accepted that the major reason for the resistance of *P. aeruginosa* to many antibiotics is a high crypticity barrier for that organism.

Resistance to bacterial enzyme degradation. Most of the more difficult gram-negative organisms produce one or more intracellular β-lactamases. Resistance to these is a necessity.

High intrinsic activity at the bacterial cell target. Studies with penicillin-binding proteins (PBPs) have shown that different cephalosporin and other β-lactam antibiotics have different affinities for the different PBPs. It seems likely that the most efficient action is for the inactivation of PBPs 1a, 1b, 2, and 3. PBPs 4, 5, and 6 appear to be nonessential, and activity against them may be wasted. An appropriate target enzyme pattern is therefore required for optimal antibacterial potency.

A broad spectrum of activity. P. aeruginosa or indole-positive *Proteus* spp. are often present in mixed infections. It follows that it may be a marked disadvantage if the activity is predominantly of narrow spectrum against *P. aeruginosa* only.

Toxicology. It is evident that, since compounds of this type may need to be given in high doses in very difficult cases, low toxicity is essential.

Pharmacokinetics. Most serious infections with *P. aeruginosa* will be treated by injection, rather than orally, and thus absorption from the injection site into the blood should be rapid and complete so as to give high serum levels. These will be maintained only if the rate of excretion is not too great. It is also desirable that losses via the bile should be low, as this might lead to very high levels of antibiotic in the intestine with undesirable effects on the bacterial flora.

Tissue penetration. Pseudomonas and *Proteus* infections are often encountered in sites where the blood supply is low (burn sloughs, fistulae, lung cavities, etc.), and good penetrability from the blood into the infected tissues is especially important.

Metabolic stability. Some cephalosporin compounds such as cephalothin or cefotaxime are susceptible to attack by tissue esterases in the body, which results in the removal of their ester-linked 3′ position substituent. This de-esterification occurs to an unpredictable extent from

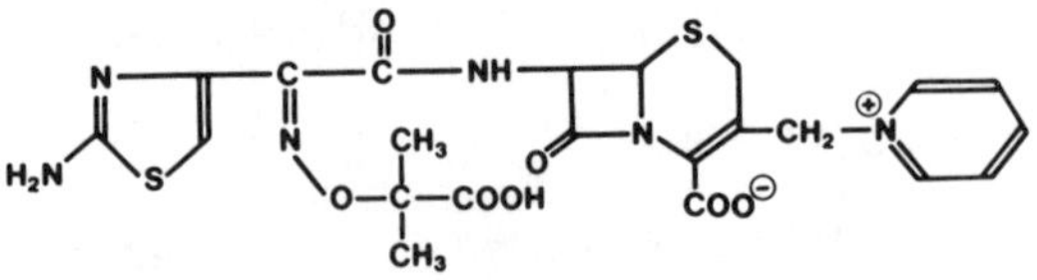

(6R, 7R) - 7 - [(Z) - 2 - (2 - AMINOTHIAZOL - 4 - YL) - 2 - (2 - CARBOXYPROP - 2 - YLOXYIMINO) ACETAMIDO] - 3 - (PYRIDINIUM - 1 - YLMETHYL) CEPH - 3 - EM - 4 - CARBOXYLIC ACID

FIG. 1. *Chemical structure of ceftazidime.*

patient to patient and is undesirable because the resulting hydroxy acid is reduced in activity and will have an altered antibacterial spectrum. The efficacies of such antibiotics are therefore to some extent unpredictable, and in infections with *P. aeruginosa,* such diminution of activity may lead to treatment failure.

Serum protein binding. It is generally agreed that a very high serum protein binding rate may diminish the amount of unbound, active antibiotic that reaches the tissues.

A β-lactam antibiotic that has favorable properties in each of the areas listed will have the best chance of being active against serious infections, even in immunocompromised patients, that are due to organisms such as *P. aeruginosa.* Later papers will deal in detail with the properties of ceftazidime in comparison with other recent β-lactam antibiotics. They will show that the antibiotic has favorable properties in each area and that it is not seriously deficient in any. For this reason, it seems likely that the very good protective effect of ceftazidime which has been found in animals with a wide range of experimental infections will be reflected in high effectiveness in patients, and preliminary results available from clinical trials so far appear to confirm this prediction.

Agar Disk Diffusion Method for Determination of Susceptibility of Bacteria to Ceftazidime

CLYDE THORNSBERRY,* RONALD N. JONES, AND ARTHUR L. BARRY

Centers for Disease Control, Public Health Service, Department of Health and Human Services, Atlanta, Georgia 30033; Kaiser Foundation Regional Laboratory, Clackamas, Oregon 97015; and University of California, Davis Medical Center, Sacramento, California 95817, U.S.A.*

Ceftazidime (formerly GR 20263) is one of the newer semisynthetic β-lactam antibiotics that belongs to the "third-generation" cephalosporins. It has a wide spectrum of antibacterial activity, including the *Enterobacteriaceae, Pseudomonas* spp., *Acinetobacter* spp., *Haemophilus* spp., *Neisseria* spp., and gram-positive cocci, except for enterococci (1). It is stable to β-lactamase and has favorable pharmacological properties. These characteristics indicated to us that we should investigate an agar disk diffusion method for determining the susceptibility of appropriate bacterial species to ceftazidime. This is a report of those studies.

For this study, we used a challenge set of 420 bacterial strains comprising 14 genera recently selected from several laboratories in the United States. These strains included *Enterobacteriaceae,* nonfermentative, gram-negative bacilli, and gram-positive cocci. An additional 177 strains, selected for their resistance factors or because they were not tested by the disk diffusion method, were added for cross-resistance studies in the MICs.

Antimicrobial susceptibility tests were performed by the standard methods of the National Committee for Clinical Laboratory Standards (NCCLS) (3, 4). The disk diffusion test was performed on Mueller-Hinton agar with an inoculum of 10^8 colony-forming units (CFU) per ml, incubated for approximately 18 h at 35°C. Interpretations of susceptibility were based on zone size as described in the NCCLS disk diffusion standard (3). The MICs were performed by microdilution in Mueller-Hinton broth supplemented with calcium and magnesium as described in the NCCLS dilution test standard (4).

The cross-resistance data for ceftazidime, cefotaxime, and cefoperazone are shown in Table 1. In previous studies, we had shown that the cross-resistance data for cefotaxime, moxalactam, cefmenoxime, and ceftizoxime were nearly the same, but that cefoperazone was different. Therefore, we chose cefotaxime (a representative of the first group) and cefoperazone for a cross-resistance comparison with ceftazidime. As an example of what the data in Table 1 show, 75% of the organisms that were susceptible to ceftazidime were susceptible to cefotaxime, and 83.1% were susceptible to cefoperazone. Of particular interest are the major (resistant to ceftazidime and susceptible to the other drug) and

TABLE 1. *Cross-resistance data for ceftazidime, cefotaxime, and cefoperazone*

Antibiotic MIC breakpoint (μg/ml)		Ceftazidime MICs (μg/ml)[a]		
		≤8 (S)	16 (I)	>16 (R)
Cefotaxime				
≤8	S	75.0%	4.7%	0.5%[b]
16–32	I	10.5	0.5	0.5
>32	R	2.4[c]	0.3	5.7
Cefoperazone				
≤16		80.7	4.7	2.4
≤32	S	83.1	5.0	5.0[d]
64	I	1.8	0.2	0.8
>64	R	2.8[e]	0.3	0.8

[a] S, Susceptible, I, indeterminate; R, resistant.
[b] Major discrepancies: *S. faecalis* (1), Meth-R *S. aureus* (1).
[c] Very major discrepancies: *P. aeruginosa* (12), *P. fluorescens* (1), *P. maltophilia* (1).
[d] Major discrepancies: Enterococci (23), *Pseudomonas* sp. (3), *Enterobacter* sp. (2), Meth-R *S. aureus* (2).
[e] Very major discrepancies: *Acinetobacter* (7), β-lac+ *Enterobacteriaceae* (10).

very major (susceptible to ceftazidime and resistant to the other drug) discrepancies. Only 0.5% major discrepancies were found between ceftazidime and cefotaxime (one methicillin-resistant [Meth-R] *Staphylococcus aureus* and one enterococcus). If ≤32 μg/ml is used as the breakpoint for cefoperazone, there were 5% major discrepancies with this drug, mostly enterococci. The very major discrepancies are more serious because of the clinical consequence of using a drug to which the infecting organism is resistant. Therefore, we consider the very major discrepancies between ceftazidime and cefotaxime (2.4%) and cefoperazone (2.8%) to be of concern. The organisms involved in most of the very major discrepancies between ceftazidime and cefotaxime are *P. aeruginosa,* because of the greater activity of ceftazidime on these organisms. This is not the case, however, with cefoperazone, because the activity of both drugs on *P. aeruginosa* is similar. The groups of organisms involved in the very major discrepancies with cefoperazone are certain β-lactamase-producing *Enterobacteriaceae* (because of the greater stability of ceftazidime to β-lactamases)

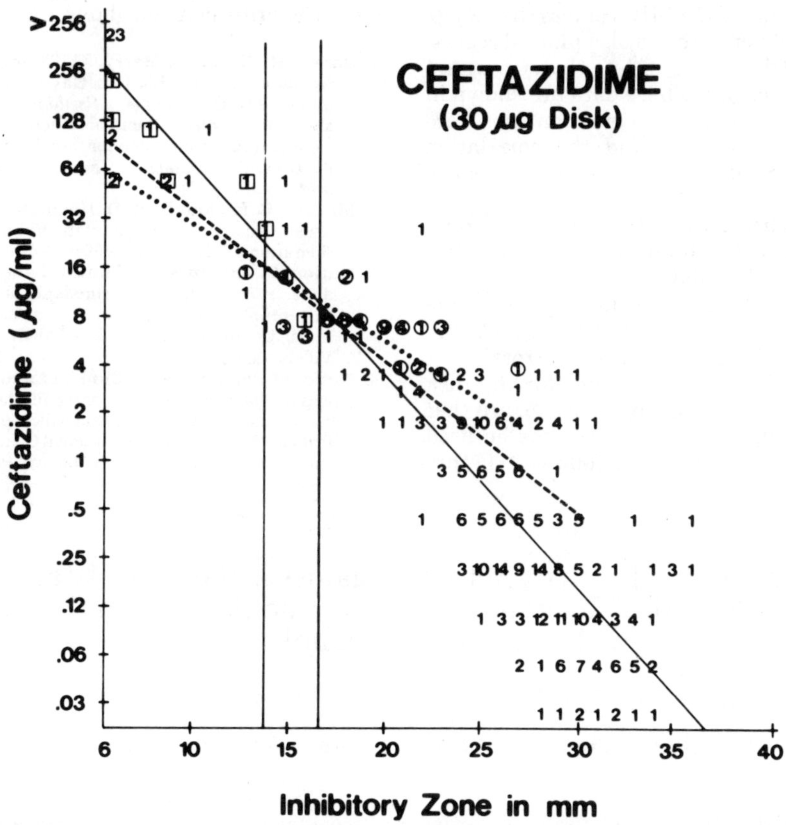

FIG. 1. *Regression lines obtained with disks containing 30 μg of ceftazidime. ——, Regression line with all MICs; -----, regression line with MICs of ≥0.5 μg/ml; ····, regression line with MICs of ≥2 μg/ml.*

TABLE 2. *Tentative interpretive zone criteria for third-generation cephalosporins (NCCLS method)*

Antibiotic	Disk (μg)	Zone breakpoints (mm)[a]			MIC breakpoints (μg/ml)		
		R	I	S	R	I	S
Ceftazidime	30	≤13	14–16	≥17	>16	16	≤8
Cefotaxime	30	≤14	15–22	≥23	>32	16–32	≤8
Moxalactam	30	≤14	15–22	≥23	>32	16–32	≤8
Cefoperazone	75	≤14	15–17	≥18	>64	64	≤32
Ceftizoxime	30	≤10	11–19	≥20	>32	16–32	≤8
Cefmenoxime	30	≤14	15–21	≥22	>32	16–32	≤8

[a] R, Resistant; I, indeterminate; S, susceptible.

and *Acinetobacter* (because of the greater activity of ceftazidime on the bacteria in this genus).

These cross-resistance data indicate that moxalactam, cefmenoxime, and ceftizoxime might be represented by a single disk for diffusion testing and could include ceftazidime if cross-resistance among *Enterobacteriaceae* were analyzed. If, however, non-*Enterobacteriaceae* and gram-positive cocci are included, ceftazidime and cefoperazone need separate disks.

In the diffusion studies, the organisms were tested with disks containing 10, 30, and 75 μg of ceftazidime. As with other similar β-lactam antibiotics, there is a significant parabolic effect on the regression line when MICs of less than 2 μg/ml were used. Therefore, we also plotted regression lines omitting MICs of less than 0.5 μg/ml and less than 2 μg/ml. These data are shown in Fig. 1. The slopes for these regression lines were −0.44, −0.32, and −0.24, and the correlation coefficients were 0.85, 0.83, and 0.83, respectively.

The data indicate that the 30-μg disk would be the most efficacious for diffusion testing. With the regression line data and the error-rate bounded method (2), the interpretive zone breakpoint for susceptibility would be ≥17 mm, which would yield ≤1% very major errors.

Our tentative recommendations for the disk diffusion test, as described by NCCLS, are that a disk containing 30 μg of ceftazidime be used and that the breakpoints be as follows: ≥17 mm indicates susceptible (≤8 μg/ml), 14 to 16 mm indicates indeterminate (16 μg/ml), and ≤13 mm indicates resistant (>16 μg/ml). These tentative breakpoints and those for other third-generation cephalosporins are shown in Table 2.

In conclusion, ceftazidime is a new cephalosporin with a wide spectrum of activity that cannot be represented by first-, second-, or other third-generation cephalosporins, if we include nonenteric, gram-negative bacilli and gram-positive cocci. For the NCCLS method of disk diffusion testing, we recommend that a disk containing 30 μg of ceftazidime be used and that the interpretation of susceptibility be made according to the criteria listed above.

1. **Jones, R. N., A. L. Barry, C. Thornsberry, E. H. Gerlach, P. C. Fuchs, T. L. Gavan, and H. M. Sommers.** 1981. Ceftazidime, a *Pseudomonas*-active cephalosporin: in vitro antimicrobial activity evaluation including recommendations for disc diffusion susceptibility tests. J. Antimicrob. Chemother. **8**(Suppl. C), in press.
2. **Metzler, C. M., and R. M. DeHaan.** 1974. Susceptibility tests of anaerobic bacteria: statistical and clinical considerations. J. Infect. Dis. **130**:588–594.
3. **National Committee for Clinical Laboratory Standards.** 1979. Performance standards antimicrobic disc susceptibility tests. Approved standard M2-A2. National Committee for Clinical Laboratory Standards, Villanova, Pa.
4. **National Committee for Clinical Laboratory Standards.** 1980. Standard methods for dilution antimicrobial susceptibility tests for bacteria which grow aerobically. Proposed standard M7-P. National Committee for Clinical Laboratory Standards, Villanova, Pa.

Ceftazidime: In Vitro Activity Against Isolates Resistant to Aminoglycoside or β-Lactam Antibiotics and Activity in Combination with Antibiotics in Clinical Use

ANNE M. HARRIS,* P. B. HARPER, S. J. PLESTED, AND ELENA BENIACOVA

Glaxo Group Research Ltd., Greenford, Middlesex, England

Ceftazidime (CAZ) is one of the most active of the new cephalosporins and has potent activity against strains which are resistant to aminoglycosides or to other β-lactam antibiotics. In this study, CAZ MICs were determined against antibiotic-resistant *Enterobacteriaceae, Acine-*

tobacter, and *Pseudomonas* strains of clinical origin by using the agar dilution method and inocula of 10^5 colony-forming units as previously described by O'Callaghan et al. (2). A total of 515 strains were examined.

CAZ showed very little cross-resistance with other new cephalosporins and with gentamicin (Table 1). A high proportion of *Serratia* spp. (86%), indole-positive *Proteus* spp. (91%), *Enterobacter* spp. (75%), *Klebsiella* spp. (51%), and *Acinetobacter* spp. (100%) were cephalothin resistant; many of these strains (58%) were also resistant to cefamandole. All of these isolates were highly susceptible to CAZ, with geometric mean (GM) MICs below 1 μg/ml for *Enterobacteriaceae* and 6.7 μg/ml for *Acinetobacter* strains.

Fewer strains were resistant to cefoxitin, cefotiam, cefmetazole, and cefoperazone, but these organisms were also susceptible to CAZ at GM MICs in the range of 0.06 to 2.1 μg/ml for *Enterobacteriaceae.*

Among the *Enterobacter* strains, nine cefotaxime-resistant isolates occurred; these had CAZ MICs in the range of 4 to 62 μg/ml. Seven of the strains were also resistant to other new cephalosporins, ceftizoxime, cefmenoxime, and moxalactam. These were the only organisms exhibiting cephalosporin cross-resistance.

Gentamicin-resistant strains were susceptible to CAZ at GM MICs in the range of 0.1 to 1.0 μg/ml for *Enterobacteriaceae.* Approximately 30% of *Serratia, Klebsiella,* and indole-positive *Proteus* strains had gentamicin MICs of ≥16 μg/

TABLE 1. *Ceftazidime (CAZ) in vitro activity against antibiotic-resistant, gram-negative strains*

Antibiotic	CAZ GM MICs (μg/ml) against antibiotic-resistant isolates[a]				
	Serratia spp.	Indole-positive *Proteus* spp.	*Enterobacter* spp.	*Klebsiella* spp.	*Acinetobacter* spp.
Cephalothin	0.1 (88)	0.07 (120)	0.5 (77)	0.4 (75)	6.7 (32)
Cefamandole	0.1 (80)	0.07 (69)	0.8 (48)	0.5 (71)	6.7 (32)
Cefoxitin	0.1 (58)	0.3 (11)	0.4 (69)	0.6 (38)	6.7 (32)
Cefotiam	0.1 (36)	0.06 (29)	1.2 (29)	0.2 (14)	7.8 (27)
Cefmetazole	0.2 (30)	0.7 (3)	0.4 (59)	0.5 (4)	7.8 (27)
Cefoperazone	0.2 (19)	0.3 (16)	2.1 (22)	0.4 (55)	7.8 (27)
Cefotaxime	—[b] (0)	— (0)	14.6 (9)	— (0)	8.0 (27)
Ceftizoxime	— (0)	— (0)	28.0 (7)	— (0)	11.3 (10)
Cefmenoxime	— (0)	— (0)	34.6 (7)	— (0)	8.2 (26)
Moxalactam	— (0)	— (0)	28.4 (7)	— (0)	8.5 (23)
Gentamicin	0.1 (32)	0.2 (42)	1.0 (16)	0.5 (34)	7.7 (20)

[a] Ceftazidime GM MICs (μg/ml) for unselected isolates (number tested): *Serratia,* 0.1 (102); *Proteus,* 0.07 (132); *Enterobacter,* 0.3 (103); *Klebsiella,* 0.3 (146); *Acinetobacter,* 6.7 (32). Parentheses in table indicate number of strains tested (MICs of ≥16 μg/ml for the antibiotics listed).

[b] —, No resistant strains tested.

TABLE 2. *Ceftazidime in vitro activity in combination with other antibiotics*[a]

Organism (no. of strains)	CAZ combined with:	Activity of antibiotics alone and in combination			Antibiotic interaction (no. of strains)	
		CAZ	Other	CAZ + other	Additive	Synergy[b]
Bacteroides fragilis (25)	Metronidazole	11.4	0.5	3.9 + 0.2	23	2
Clostridium spp. (12)	Metronidazole	17.1	0.4	3.6 + 0.09	9	3
Staphylococcus aureus (15)	Flucloxacillin	4.0	0.13	2.0 + 0.06	15	0
S. aureus (15)	Erythromycin	7.3	1.4	2.9 + 0.6	15	0
Streptococcus faecalis (24)	Ampicillin	19.5	0.4	0.3 + 0.3	24	0
S. faecalis (24)	Piperacillin	19.5	1.5	1.5 + 1.5	24	0
S. faecalis (24)	Mezlocillin	19.5	0.7	0.5 + 0.5	24	0
Pseudomonas spp. (26)	Gentamicin	1.7	5.5	1.1 + 0.3	26	0
Pseudomonas spp. (26)	Tobramycin	1.7	3.6	0.9 + 0.2	25	1
Pseudomonas spp. (26)	Amikacin	1.7	10.1	1.5 + 0.4	26	0
Pseudomonas spp. (26)	Sisomicin	1.2	2.5	0.4 + 0.4	13	13
Pseudomonas spp. (26)	Netilmicin	1.2	4.7	0.6 + 0.6	22	4

[a] Antibiotics were tested either by isobologram or in fixed ratios. Results are the mean of the most effective combinations against each strain.

[b] Synergy, Fractional inhibitory concentration of <0.5.

ml. CAZ was at least 5 times more active than gentamicin on a weight basis in MIC test comparisons.

Pseudomonas strains included strains resistant to gentamicin (50), amikacin (58), carbenicillin (132), piperacillin (12), cefoperazone (33), and cefsulodin (27). Resistant strains had MICs of ≥16 μg/ml for aminoglycosides and cephalosporins; carbenicillin and piperacillin MICs were ≥62 μg/ml. CAZ was active against all of these isolates at concentrations of 8 μg/ml or less. GM MICs for CAZ against cefulsodin- and cefoperazone-resistant strains were 1.6 and 2.7 μg/ml, respectively, compared with a GM MIC of 1.3 μg/ml for unselected isolates. This finding suggests minimal cross-resistance between CAZ and the most active of the new cephalosporins with antipseudomonal activity. Gentamicin- and amikacin-resistant strains were highly susceptible to CAZ, with GM MICs of 1.4 and 1.3 μg/ml, respectively. Carbenicillin- and piperacillin-resistant strains showed similar susceptibility to CAZ at 1.6 and 1.7 μg/ml, respectively. These findings confirm those of Verbist and Verhaegen (3), Wise et al. (4), and Bauernfeind (1), all of whom reported CAZ to be highly active against *Pseudomonas* species, including antibiotic-resistant isolates.

Compatibility of CAZ with other antibiotics was tested by using isobolograms or mixtures of fixed ratios of CAZ with other antibiotics in agar. CAZ was usually additive in combination with other antibiotics (Table 2), and two- to fourfold reductions in MICs of CAZ or the other antibiotic used in combination were commonly achieved. Synergy was defined by using the fractional inhibitory concentration, and statistically significant synergy was recorded when the fractional inhibitory concentration was <0.5. CAZ and sisomicin in combination were synergistic against about 50% of the *Pseudomonas* species tested, but with other antibiotics, synergistic interactions with CAZ were less common. The spectrum of CAZ can be augmented to cover *Streptococcus faecalis* by using ampicillin, mezlocillin, or piperacillin. Anaerobic activity can be enhanced by using metronidazole, as CAZ was invariably additive when used with metronidazole. In combination with flucloxacillin, erythromycin, cephalothin, or other cephalosporins, CAZ activity against *Staphylococcus aureus* was usually enhanced. MICs of both CAZ and antistaphylococcal agents were reduced at least twofold for almost all strains. No clinically significant instances of antagonism were observed for CAZ in combination with other antibiotics. The findings show that the broad spectrum of CAZ, which extends to many antibiotic-resistant isolates, should be wide enough for the antibiotic to be used alone in most cases. If specific clinical circumstances indicate combined therapy, in vitro findings show that CAZ may be used with a wide range of other antibiotics to achieve an additive effect.

1. **Bauernfeind, A.** 1981. New β-lactam antibiotics for the treatment of *Pseudomonas aeruginosa* infections. *In* C. Grassi and L. Sabath (ed.), New trends in antibiotics: research and therapy: Proceedings of the Symposium on New Trends in Antibiotics: Research and Therapy, October 1980, Milan, Italy.
2. **O'Callaghan, C. H., P. Acred, P. B. Harper, D. M. Ryan, S. M. Kirby, and S. M. Harding.** 1980. GR20263: a new broad-spectrum cephalosporin with antipseudomonal activity. Antimicrob. Agents Chemother. **17**:867–883.
3. **Verbist, L., and J. Verhaegen.** 1980. GR20263: a new aminothiazolyl cephalosporin with high activity against *Pseudomonas* and *Enterobacteriaceae*. Antimicrob. Agents Chemother. **17**:807–812.
4. **Wise, R., J. M. Andrews, and K. A. Bedford.** 1980. Comparison of in vitro activity of GR20263, a novel cephalosporin derivative, with activities of other betalactam compounds. Antimicrob. Agents Chemother. **17**: 884–889.

In Vitro Activity of Ceftazidime Compared with That of Other β-Lactam Antibiotics and Gentamicin Against Pseudomonads and Enterobacteria

IAN PHILLIPS,* ANNA KING, KEVIN SHANNON, CHRISTINE WARREN, AND DAVID HANSLO

St. Thomas's Hospital Medical School, London, England

We compared the in vitro activity of ceftazidime with that of other β-lactam antibiotics and gentamicin against members of the *Enterobacteriaceae* family and *Pseudomonas aeruginosa* by determination of MICs. Agar dilution was used for *P. aeruginosa,* but broth dilution, with an MIC 2000 dispenser and inoculator (Dynatech Laboratories Ltd., Billingshurst, West Sussex, England), was used for enterobacteria as described before (1).

Ceftazidime was highly active against *P. aeruginosa,* three-quarters of the isolates being inhibited by 2 μg/ml and all being inhibited by 8 μg/ml (Table 1). The activity of ceftazidime

TABLE 1. *In vitro activity of ceftazidime*

Organism (no. of isolates)	Antibiotic	MICs (μg/ml)			
		Range	For (% of isolates)		
			50%	75%	90%
P. aeruginosa (59)	Ceftazidime	0.25–8	1	2	4
	Cefsulodin	0.5–64	2	8	16
	Cefotaxime	1–128	8	16	64
	Moxalactam	1–>32	8	16	32
	Azlocillin	2–>128	8	32	64
	Carbenicillin	16–>4,096	64	512	4,096
	N-Formimidoyl thienamycin	0.5–8	2	4	8
	Gentamicin	0.12–128	1	1	2
Other species of *Pseudomonas* (58)[a]	Ceftazidime	0.12–128	1	2	4
	Cefsulodin	8–>512	128	256	256
	Cefotaxime	0.06–64	4	16	32
	Moxalactam	0.25–>32	16	>32	>32
	Azlocillin	0.5–64	8	16	32
	Carbenicillin	2–2,048	256	1,024	2,048
	N-Formimidoyl thienamycin	0.12–>128	1	2	>128
	Gentamicin	0.12–>128	1	128	>128
Enterobacteriaceae[b]					
Ampicillin and cephaloridine susceptible (84)	Ceftazidime	0.008–0.5	0.06	0.12	0.25
	Cefotaxime	0.004–0.12	0.03	0.06	0.06
	Moxalactam	0.016–0.5	0.12	0.12	0.25
	N-Formimidoyl thienamycin	0.03–8	0.25	2	8
	Gentamicin	0.03–16	0.5	1	2
Ampicillin resistant, cephaloridine susceptible (75)	Ceftazidime	0.008–1	0.12	0.12	0.25
	Cefotaxime	0.004–0.5	0.03	0.06	0.06
	Moxalactam	0.03–0.5	0.12	0.12	0.25
	N-Formimidoyl thienamycin	0.06–4	0.25	0.25	1
	Gentamicin	0.06–16	0.5	1	1
Ampicillin susceptible, cephaloridine resistant (25)	Ceftazidime	0.06–2	0.25	0.25	0.5
	Cefotaxime	0.004–0.5	0.12	0.12	0.25
	Moxalactam	0.03–4	0.12	0.12	0.5
	N-Formimidoyl thienamycin	0.12–4	0.5	1	2
	Gentamicin	0.25–64	0.5	0.5	4
Ampicillin and cephaloridine resistant (216)	Ceftazidime	0.03–128	0.12	0.25	1
	Cefotaxime	0.008–128	0.12	0.25	0.25
	Moxalactam	0.016–32	0.12	0.25	0.5
	N-Formimidoyl thienamycin	0.06–8	1	2	4
	Gentamicin	0.12–>128	0.5	2	16

[a] *P. acidovorans* (11 isolates), *P. cepacia* (8 isolates), *P. fluorescens* (8 isolates), *P. maltophilia* (10 isolates), *P. pseudoalcaligenes* (1 isolate), *P. putida* (12 isolates), *P. putrefaciens* (2 isolates), *P. stutzeri* (3 isolates), and *P. thomasii* (1 isolate).

[b] *Citrobacter freundii* (20 isolates), *C. koseri* (20 isolates), *Enterobacter aerogenes* (25 isolates), *E. cloacae* (35 isolates), *Eschericia coli* (50 isolates), *Klebsiella* sp. (65 isolates), *Morganella morganii* (20 isolates), *Proteus mirabilis* (50 isolates), *P. vulgaris* (26 isolates), *Providencia alcalifaciens* (8 isolates), *P. rettgeri* (20 isolates), *P. stuartii* (35 isolates), and *Serratia* sp. (25 isolates).

exceeded that of *N*-formimidoyl thienamycin, cefsulodin, cefotaxime, moxalactam, azlocillin, and carbenicillin. MICs of ceftazidime were poorly correlated with those of carbenicillin for *P. aeruginosa* as a whole (correlation coefficient = 0.14); however, if results for highly carbenicillin-resistant isolates (MICs > 1,024 μg/ml) that produced β-lactamase constitutively were excluded, correlation was good (correlation coefficient = 0.88). Thus, the mechanism that gives

TABLE 2. *Sensitivity of ceftazidime to β-lactamases*

Organism (enzyme)	MICs (mg/liter)			β-Lactamase activity[a]	Hydrolysis relative to cephaloridine (100)		
	Ceftazidime	Cefotaxime	Moxalactam		Ceftazidime	Cefotaxime	Moxalactam
Plasmid-mediated β-lactamases							
E. coli (TEM-1)	0.25	0.03	0.06	7.9	—[b]	—	—
E. coli (TEM-2)	0.5	0.06	0.06	34.7	—	0.2	—
E. coli (SHV-1)	0.25	0.06	0.12	0.8	—	—	—
E. coli (OXA-1)	0.25	0.12	0.12	0.4	—	45	—
E. coli (OXA-3)	0.25	0.06	0.12	0.3	—	—	—
P. aeruginosa (PSE-1)	2	16	16	0.5	—	—	—
P. aeruginosa (PSE-2)	2	16	16	0.02	—	—	—
P. aeruginosa (PSE-3)	2	16	16	0.04	—	—	—
P. aeruginosa (PSE-4)	1	8	8	1.4	—	—	—
Chromosomally determined broad-spectrum β-lactamase							
Klebsiella 1082E	0.5	1	0.12	43.0	—	6	—
Chromosomally determined cephalosporinases							
C. freundii 11.21.75	0.12	0.12	0.06	1.3	—	—	—
E. cloacae 4.37.76	32	16	16	53.5	0.2	0.3	—
E. cloacae P99	32	64	8	19.5	—	—	—
E. coli AO21205	2	1	0.25	1.2	—	—	—
M. morganii 1036.3	0.5	0.5	0.25	17.4	—	—	—
P. vulgaris PC37	0.03	1	0.25	1.2	—	20	—
P. rettgeri A120513	0.12	4	0.12	18.9	—	0.7	—
P. stuartii A130118	1	0.5	0.06	2.3	—	—	—
Serratia sp. strain 9.2.75	0.25	0.12	0.25	0.4	—	—	—
P. aeruginosa 10662	1	16	8	1.3	—	—	—

[a] Nanokatals per milligram of protein with cephaloridine as substrate.
[b] Not detected.

rise to moderate resistance to carbenicillin also reduces susceptibility to ceftazidime, though the effect is small. On a weight basis, gentamicin was more active than ceftazidime against gentamicin-susceptible isolates, but this is offset by the greater toxicity and, consequently, lower doses of the aminoglycoside.

Ceftazidime was also the most active β-lactam antibiotic tested against other *Pseudomonas* species (Table 1). It was highly effective against *P. acidovorans* (MICs, mostly 0.12 to 2 μg/ml), *P. cepacia* (MICs, 1 to 2 μg/ml), *P. maltophilia* (MICs, 1 to 4 μg/ml), *P. paucimobilis* (MICs, 2 μg/ml), *P. pseudoalcaligenes* (MIC, 4 μg/ml), *P. putrefaciens* (MICs, 0.12 to 0.25 μg/ml), and *P. stutzeri* (MICs, 0.25 to 0.5 μg/ml), but it was less active against *P. fluorescens* (MICs, 0.25 to 8 μg/ml) and *P. putida* (MICs, 2 to 16 μg/ml). Only two *Pseudomonas* isolates were resistant to ceftazidime: one each of *P. acidovorans* (MIC, 128 μg/ml) and *P. thomasii* (MIC, 32 μg/ml).

Ceftazidime was only slightly less active than cefotaxime and moxalactam against enterobacteria (Table 1) and was more active than *N*-formimidoyl thienamycin and gentamicin against most isolates. Isolates that were resistant (MICs $\geq$ 16 μg/ml) to ampicillin, cephaloridine, or both compounds were slightly less susceptible to ceftazidime than were fully susceptible isolates, but the differences were small (Table 1).

The UV spectrophotometric method (2, 4) was used to study the sensitivity of ceftazidime to β-lactamases. Results are shown in Table 2, where the enzymes are classified by the system of Sykes and Matthew (5). Ceftazidime was resistant to all the β-lactamases except for a trace of activity by the enzyme from *Enterobacter cloacae* 4.37.76. This enzyme is notable for its activity against cefoxitin, which is hydrolyzed at about 1.7% of the rate of hydrolysis of cephaloridine. Moxalactam possesses the 7-α-methoxy group characteristic of cephamycins, so it was not surprising that hydrolysis of this compound was not detected. Cefotaxime was attacked by several enzymes, notably OXA-1, the enzyme from *Klebsiella* 1082E and the cephalosporinase from *Proteus vulgaris*; however, this activity was not sufficient to confer resistance to cefotaxime, except possibly to a small extent in *Klebsiella* 1082E.

Our results confirm previous reports of the

high activity of ceftazidime against enterobacteria and pseudomonads (3, 6, 7) and its resistance to β-lactamases (3).

We are grateful to Glaxo Group Research for providing ceftazidime and for financial support.

1. **Hanslo, D., A. King, K. Shannon, C. Warren, and I. Phillips.** 1981. *N*-Formimidoyl thienamycin (MK 0787): in-vitro antibacterial activity and susceptibility to beta-lactamases compared with that of cefotaxime, moxalactam and other beta-lactam antibiotics. J. Antimicrob. Chemother. **7**:607–617
2. **King, A., C. Warren, K. Shannon, and I. Phillips.** 1980. The in vitro antibacterial activity of cefotaxime compared with that of cefuroxime and cefoxitin. J. Antimicrob. Chemother. **6**:479–494.
3. **O'Callaghan, C. H., P. Acred, P. B. Harper, D. M. Ryan, S. M. Kirby, and S. M. Harding.** 1980. GR 20263, a new broad-spectrum cephalosporin with antipseudomonal activity. Antimicrob. Agents Chemother. **17**:876–883.
4. **O'Callaghan, C. H., P. W. Muggleton, and G. W. Ross.** 1969. Effects of β-lactamase from gram-negative organisms on cephalosporins and penicillins, p. 57–63. Antimicrob. Agents Chemother. 1968.
5. **Sykes, R. B., and M. Matthew.** 1976. The β-lactamases of Gram-negative bacteria and their role in resistance to β-lactam antibiotics. J. Antimicrob. Chemother. **2**: 115–157.
6. **Verbist, L., and J. Verhaegen.** 1980. GR 20263: a new aminothiazolyl cephalosporin with high activity against *Pseudomonas* and *Enterobacteriaceae*. Antimicrob. Agents Chemother. **17**:807–812.
7. **Wise, R., J. M. Andrews, and K. A. Bedford.** 1980. Comparison of in vitro activity of GR 20263, a novel cephalosporin derivative, with activities of other betalactam antibiotics. Antimicrob. Agents Chemother. **17**: 884–889.

Antibacterial Activity of Ceftazidime (GR 20263) and Other Cephalosporins Against Highly Resistant Strains of *Enterobacteriaceae* and *Pseudomonas aeruginosa*

D. A. LEIGH,* D. NISBET, J. M. MARRINER, AND M. OSBORNE

Department of Microbiology, Wycombe General Hospital, High Wycombe, Buckinghamshire HP11 2TT, England

Ceftazidime (GR 20263) is the latest compound in the range of parenteral cephalosporins with enhanced antibacterial activity due to β-lactamase resistance and stability. It has a wide spectrum of activity which includes most strains of the *Enterobacteriaceae* family, streptococci, *Haemophilus influenzae*, and *Neisseria* species. Unlike other β-lactamase–stable cephalosporins except cefsulodin, it shows significant activity against *Pseudomonas aeruginosa* comparable to that of the aminoglycoside antibiotics. It is relatively inactive against *Staphylococcus aureus* and *Bacteroides fragilis* and is ineffective against *Streptococcus faecalis*.

A laboratory assessment of the antibacterial activity of ceftazidime was carried out for susceptible and multiply resistant strains of *Escherichia coli*, *Klebsiella aerogenes*, and *Enterobacter cloacae*, and this was compared with activities of cefotaxime, cefuroxime, and cefamandole. Comparative antibacterial activities of ceftazidime, cefotaxime, several penicillins, and aminoglycosides were determined for hospital strains of *P. aeruginosa*.

All bacterial strains had been isolated from routine hospital specimens from patients considered to have an infection. Most commonly used antibiotics were active against susceptible strains, but the typical antibiogram for resistant strains showed susceptibility to amikacin and colistin only, with variable resistance to tobramycin, gentamicin, and the β-lactamase–stable cephalosporins. The MICs were determined by a solid agar method, and inoculation was carried out with a multipoint inoculator using a bacterial count of 10^5 to 10^6 organisms per ml. The rate of killing with ceftazidime and tobramycin was compared for a susceptible strain of *P. aeruginosa* in nutrient broth with an antibiotic concentration equal to five times the MIC.

Comparative MICs for susceptible strains of *E. coli*, *K. aerogenes*, and *E. cloacae* are shown in Table 1. The MICs of ceftazidime for all three bacterial species were between 0.06 and 2 mg/liter, with mean MICs of 0.20, 0.26 and 0.25 mg/liter, respectively. Cefuroxime and cefamandole were considerably less active, with mean MICs between 2.14 and 58 mg/liter, but cefamandole showed comparable activity against strains of *E. coli*, with a mean MIC of 0.90 mg/liter. The MICs of ceftazidime against the resistant strains (Table 2) showed a two- to fourfold rise, but for cefuroxime and cefamandole these were considerably raised, particularly with strains of *E. cloacae*, for which the mean MICs were 59.8 and 109.2 mg/liter, respectively. Cefotaxime was four

TABLE 1. *Comparative MICs for susceptible strains of Enterobacteriaceae*

Organism	Drug[a]	MIC (mg/liter)									Mean MIC
		0.06	0.12	0.25	0.5	1	2	4	8	16	
E. coli (25 strains)	CFZ	3	11	10	—	1	—	—	—	—	0.20
	CXM	—	—	—	—	2	12	10	1	—	2.96
	CMD	—	—	4	12	7	1	1	—	—	0.80
K. aerogenes (22 strains)	CFZ	2	10	8	1	—	1	—	—	—	0.26
	CXM	—	—	—	—	9	9	3	1	—	2.14
	CMD	—	—	1	5	3	6	5	2	—	2.44
E. cloacae (20 strains)	CFZ	1	7	10	1	1	—	—	—	—	0.25
	CXM	—	—	—	—	—	4	9	5	2	5.80
	CMD	—	—	—	—	7	5	4	2	2	4.85

[a] CFZ, Ceftazidime; CXM, cefuroxime; CMD, cefamandole.

TABLE 2. *Comparative MICs for resistant strains of Enterobacteriaciae*

Organism	Drug[a]	MIC (mg/liter)											Mean MIC
		0.06	0.12	0.25	0.5	1	2	4	8	16	32	64	
E. coli (35 strains)	CFZ	5	9	13	4	—	—	2	2	—	—	—	0.90
	CTX	28	2	1	—	—	4	—	—	—	—	—	0.28
	CXM	—	—	—	—	1	7	18	3	2	3	1	8.7
	CMD	—	—	—	—	3	4	7	9	7	4	1	11.9
K. aerogenes (34 strains)	CFZ	6	10	9	4	4	—	1	—	—	—	—	0.41
	CTX	29	1	1	2	1	—	—	—	—	—	—	0.10
	CXM	—	—	—	—	1	18	8	2	2	3	—	6.3
	CMD	—	—	—	3	1	6	4	2	3	5	10	32.0
E. cloacae (31 strains)	CFZ	—	—	3	8	18	1	1	—	—	—	—	0.93
	CTX	1	2	4	5	13	5	1	—	—	—	—	0.99
	CXM	—	—	—	—	—	1	1	3	4	5	17	59.8
	CMD	—	—	—	—	—	—	—	1	1	3	26	109.2

[a] CFZ, Ceftazidime; CTX, cefotaxime; CXM, cefuroxime; CMD, cefamandole.

times as active as ceftazidime against *E. coli* and *K. aerogenes*, but it was marginally less active against *Enterobacter* strains.

Ceftazidime showed activity comparable to that of tobramycin against strains of *P. aeruginosa*, with mean MICs of 1.8 and 1.1 mg/liter, respectively. Cefotaxime (mean MIC, 14.6 mg/liter) was less active, as were gentamicin (22 mg/liter), amikacin (3.1 mg/liter), and the antipseudomonal penicillins mezlocillin (41.3 mg/liter), ticarcillin (53.4 mg/liter), and carbenicillin (72.6 mg/liter). The rate of killing by ceftazidime for a strain of *P. aeruginosa* was slower than that of tobramycin, which achieved a total kill of the bacterial inoculum in 60 min whereas with ceftazidime viable bacteria were still present after 4 h.

Ceftazidime shows a marked degree of antibacterial activity against most strains of commonly isolated pathogens which is superior to that of cefuroxime and cefamandole and comparable to that of cefotaxime. Although there are deficiencies in its spectrum of activity, particularly against *B. fragilis* and *S. aureus*, it is highly effective against strains of *P. aeruginosa*. Despite the slower rate of killing which was observed for a susceptible strain, the mean MIC (1.8 mg/liter) is comparable to that of tobramycin (1.1 mg/liter) and suggests that ceftazidime will be valuable for the treatment of infection caused by *P. aeruginosa*.

During the last 3 years in the Wycombe District, there have been many infections due to multiresistant strains of *E. coli*, *K. aerogenes*, and *E. cloacae*. Although there has been evidence of cross-infection with the same strain, many serotypes have been isolated. This suggested plasmid-mediated resistance, which has been confirmed by therapeutic success with treatment with amoxicillin/clavulanic acid (1). The multiresistance has included such commonly prescribed antibiotics as tobramycin, gentamicin, carbenicillin, ticarcillin, and the β-lactamase–stable cephalosporins cefuroxime and cefamandole. The activity of ceftazidime against these resistant strains was satisfactory although the MICs were two to four times higher than for susceptible hospital and domiciliary strains. A previous report on some of these strains (2) suggested greater resistance, but reexamination of the strains did not confirm the high MICs. Ceftazidime is generally less active than cefotaxime against the resistant strains of *E. coli* and *K. aerogenes*, but comparable activity was found with *E. cloacae*.

The antibacterial activity of ceftazidime suggests that it will have a significant place in the treatment of serious infections due to β-lactamase–producing bacteria. However, when there is an anaerobic component in the infection, it will be necessary to prescribe an antimicrobial agent, such as metronidazole, with selective activity against *B. fragilis*.

D. Nisbet, M. Osborne, and J. M. Marriner are in receipt of research grants from Beechams Pharmaceuticals and I.C.I. Ltd.

1. **Leigh, D. A., K. Bradnock, and J. M. Marriner.** 1981. Augmentin (amoxycillin and clavulanic acid) therapy in complicated infections due to β lactamase producing bacteria. J. Antimicrob. Chemother. **7**:229–236.
2. **Leigh, D. A., and D. Nisbet.** 1981. Antibacterial activity of ceftazidime (GR 20263) against routine hospital isolates and highly resistant strains of *Enterobacteriaceae* and *Pseudomonas aeruginosa*. J. Antimicrob. Chemother. **8**(Suppl. B):107–110.

Bactericidal Activity of Ceftazidime Against Cephalothin-Resistant, Gram-Negative Clinical Isolates

R. VANHOOF,* H. COIGNAU, G. STAS, B. GORDTS, AND J. P. BUTZLER

St. Pieters Hospital and Institute Pasteur, 1040 Brussels, Belgium*

Ceftazidime is a new semisynthetic cephalosporin with exceptional in vitro activity against a wide range of pathogenic microorganisms. We studied the bactericidal activity of this compound against different cephalothin-resistant, gram-negative clinical isolates.

The following microorganisms were used in this study (number of strains): *Acinetobacter anitratus* (26), *Enterobacter cloacae* (27), *Escherichia coli* (115), *Klebsiella pneumoniae* (43), *Proteus mirabilis* (16), *Proteus* spp., indole positive (47), *Providencia stuartii* (19), *Pseudomonas aeruginosa* (172), and *Serratia marcescens* (13).

All strains were isolated from clinical material and routinely identified in our laboratory. The cephalothin resistance of the strains was defined by the disk susceptibility test of Bauer et al (1). The following antimicrobial agents were included in the study: ceftazidime, cefuroxime (Glaxo), cefoperazone (Pfizer), moxalactam, cefamandole (Eli Lilly), cefotaxime (Hoechst-Roussel), cefoxitin (Merck Sharp & Dohme), azlocillin (Bayer), carbenicillin, and ticarcillin (Beecham). The MICs of the different compounds were determined by using a Cooke-Dynatech MIC 2000 dispenser and inoculator. The final inoculum was approximately 10^5 colony-forming units per ml. The antibiotic solutions were prepared in Mueller-Hinton broth in microtiter plates. MICs were recorded as the lowest concentrations inhibiting visible growth. To measure the MBC, the MIC plates were subcultured on a solid medium without any antibiotics. A reduction of at least 99% of the initial inoculum of the strain was regarded as evidence of bactericidal activity.

Table 1 summarizes the geometric mean MBCs of the different antibiotics.

Ceftazidime had high bactericidal activity against all of the strains and had the best killing effect on *A. anitratus* and *Pseudomonas aeruginosa* (range, ≤0.097 to 12.5 μg/ml). The range of bactericidal activity of ceftazidime on the other strains varied from ≤0.097 to 12.5 μg/ml, except for one strain of *Enterobacter cloacae* that required 50 μg/ml to be killed (MIC, 25 μg/ml) and one strain of *Serratia marcescens* (MBC, 25 μg/ml; MIC, 12.5 μg/ml). Cefotaxime, ceftazidime, and cefoperazone also had an excellent killing effect on strains of *Enterobacter cloacae*, *Escherichia coli*, and *Providencia stuartii*. The bactericidal activities of cefotaxime, moxalactam, and ceftazidime against *K. pneumoniae*, *Proteus mirabilis*, indole-positive *Proteus* strains, and *Serratia marcescens* were comparable. Against *Pseudomonas* strains, ceftazidime had the best bactericidal activity and was more active than cefoperazone and azlocillin, an antipseudomonal penicillin.

The differences between the MICs and MBCs for the different antibiotics we investigated are listed in Table 2. For most of the strains the MIC and MBC of ceftazidime were identical,

TABLE 1. *Geometric mean MBCs of different beta-lactam antibiotics*[a]

Strains	MBC (μg/ml)									
	CAZ	CPZ	CXM	MOX	CTX	CMD	CFX	AZL	CAR	TIC
Acinetobacter anitratus	2.15	24.33	16.76	13.90	3.04	39.33	30.94	ND	ND	ND
Enterobacter cloacae	0.17	0.16	7.01	0.13	0.13	1.84	45.70	ND	ND	ND
Escherichia coli	0.38	0.72	4.98	0.13	0.16	3.13	6.12	ND	ND	ND
Klebsiella pneumoniae	0.15	3.88	3.30	0.16	0.09	8.02	4.21	ND	ND	ND
Proteus mirabilis	0.08	1.26	0.85	0.08	0.08	1.37	1.43	ND	ND	ND
Proteus spp., indole positive	0.09	0.28	4.35	0.11	0.08	1.22	2.11	ND	ND	ND
Providencia stuartii	0.20	3.55	2.65	0.08	0.09	1.91	1.84	ND	ND	ND
Serratia marcescens	0.14	0.94	8.30	0.11	0.09	5.47	4.19	ND	ND	ND
Pseudomonas aeruginosa	0.61	2.99	ND	6.85	6.74	ND	ND	6.17	42.06	18.55

[a] Abbreviations: CAZ, ceftazidime; CPZ, cefoperazone; CXM, cefuroxime; MOX, moxalactam; CTX, cefotaxime; CMD, cefamandole; AZL, azlocillin; CAR, carbenicillin; TIC, ticarcillin; ND, not determined.

TABLE 2. *Comparison of MICs and MBCs of different beta-lactam antibiotics from gram-negative isolates*

Species	No. tested	Ceftazidime			Cefoperazone			Cefuroxime			Moxalactam			Cefotaxime			Cefamandole			Cefoxitin		
		ID[a]	2×[b]	4×[b]	ID	2×	4×	ID	2×	4×	ID	2×	4×	ID	2×	4×	ID	2×	4×	ID	2×	4×
Acinetobacter anitratus	26	12[c]	12	2	22	4		16	8	2	17	9		20	5		23	3		15	11	
Enterobacter cloacae	27	24	3		25	2		19	8		25	2		23	4		22	5		21	6	
Escherichia coli	115	105	10		101	14		104	11		109	6		106	9		107	8		72	42	1
Klebsiella pneumoniae	43	36	7		38	5		31	11	1	35	8		42	1		39	4		34	8	1
Proteus mirabilis	16	16			16			15	1		15	1		15	1		15	1		15	1	
Proteus spp., indole positive	47	46	1		44	3		32	15		44	3		45	2		39	8		40	7	
Providencia stuartii	19	17	2		16	3		15	4		18	1		17	2		17	2		15	4	
Serratia marcescens	13	10	3		5	6	2	5	6	2	5	8		10	3		7	5	1	7	5	1
		Ceftazidime			Cefoperazone			Moxalactam			Cefotaxime			Azlocillin			Carbenicillin			Ticarcillin		
		ID	2×	4×	ID	2×	4×	ID	2×	4×	ID	2×	4×	ID	2×	4×	ID	2×	4×	ID	2×	4×
Pseudomonas aeruginosa	127	128	39	5	129	37	6	133	37	2	129	40	3	138	31	3	146	20	6	140	30	2

[a] ID, Identical.
[b] 2×, 4× = MBC greater by two- or fourfold.
[c] Number of strains.

and only seven strains (two *A. anitratus* and five *Pseudomonas aeruginosa*) required a fourfold increase of ceftazidime for killing. For cefotaxime, moxalactam, and cefoperazone the bactericidal concentrations were identical to the MICs or fell within a twofold dilution.

In conclusion, it can be said that ceftazidime has excellent bactericidal activity against a wide range of gram-negative pathogenic microorganisms and that its activity against the *Enterobacteriaceae* is comparable to those of moxalactam and cefotaxime. Thus, ceftazidime might be useful in the treatment of serious infections due to cephalothin-resistant clinical pathogens.

1. **Bauer, A. W., W. M. M. Kirby, J. C. Sherris, and M. Turck.** 1966. Antibiotic susceptibility testing by a standardized single disk method. Am. J. Clin. Pathol. **45:** 493–496.

Antibacterial Activity of Ceftazidime (GR 20263) Against Hospital Strains

P. ORSOLINI, P. L. XERRI, B. CARO, E. ERANI, AND G. COPPI

Glaxo S.p.A., Verona, Italy

Ceftazidime (GR 20263) is a new broad-spectrum, injectable β-lactam antibiotic, characterized by high resistance to β-lactamase. In the present study we evaluated its in vitro activity against freshly isolated strains from one Italian hospital in comparison with the activity of other β-lactam and aminoglycoside antibiotics.

The results in Table 1 show that *Escherichia coli*, *Klebsiella* spp., and *Salmonella* spp. were the most susceptible genera. In fact, most of the strains were inhibited by 0.48 to 0.96 μg of ceftazidime per ml. Cefotaxime was slightly more active, and gentamicin was definitely less active. Against the more resistant genus *Serratia*, the activity of ceftazidime was similar to that against the previous group, and most of the strains were inhibited by 1.9 μg/ml. *Citrobacter* spp. revealed some strains resistant to all the antibiotics. *Acinetobacter* spp. were less susceptible to the antibiotics; ceftazidime, however, proved to be the most active even in comparison with gentamicin, which was incapable of inhibiting one of the five strains tested. *Staphylococcus aureus* proved less susceptible to ceftazidime than did gram-negative bacteria, but nevertheless all the strains were inhibited by 15.6 μg/ml.

Table 2 shows that *Enterobacter* spp. were very susceptible to ceftazidime, most of the strains being inhibited by 0.96 μg/ml. Only 2 strains of 13 needed 62 μg/ml to be inhibited. Two strains were completely resistant to cefotaxime, four to gentamicin, and one to sisomicin. No strain was resistant to tobramycin or amikacin. Among *Proteus* spp., the majority of the strains were susceptible to very low levels of ceftazidime and cefotaxime, with only two strains resistant to both antibiotics. Gentamicin, sisomicin, and tobramycin were characterized by poor activity, with a large number of strains completely resistant. Amikacin was the best among the aminoglycoside group, but needed relatively high levels to inhibit the strains as compared with the β-lactam group. Against indole-negative *Proteus*, the two β-lactams were very active, but resistant strains were observed in the case of the aminoglycosides gentamicin and sisomicin.

Against *Pseudomonas* spp. strains (Table 3) ceftazidime proved to be the best antibiotic as compared with the other β-lactams and aminoglycosides, and it was the only drug effective against all the strains at concentrations easily

TABLE 1. *In vitro activity of ceftazidime, cefotaxime, and gentamicin against recently isolated strains*

Microorganism	Antibiotic	No. of strains	No. of microorganisms with MIC (μg/ml):											
			≤0.06	0.12	0.24	0.48	0.96	1.9	3.9	7.8	15.6	31.2	62.5	≥125
S. aureus	Ceftazidime	27					1		6	14	6			
	Cefotaxime	27			3	7	8	6	3					
	Gentamicin	27	6	1	5	10	5							
E. coli	Ceftazidime	15	1	1	9	2		2						
	Cefotaxime	15	4	6	4		1							
	Gentamicin	15					1	7	7					
Klebsiella spp.	Ceftazidime	18	9	4	4		1							
	Cefotaxime	18	6	11	1									
	Gentamicin	18			1		12	3					1	1
Serratia spp.	Ceftazidime	10	1		1	4	1	2	1					
	Cefotaxime	10	1		2	3	4							
	Gentamicin	10					2	3	2	2				1
Citrobacter spp.	Ceftazidime	11		1	1	3	1	2		1				2
	Cefotaxime	11		1	6	1					1	1		1
	Gentamicin	11				1	1	1	3					5
Acinetobacter spp.	Ceftazidime	5							2	2	1			
	Cefotaxime	5								1	4			
	Gentamicin	5						1	3					1
Salmonella spp.	Ceftazidime	8			1	3	4							
	Cefotaxime	8		2	5	1								
	Gentamicin	8					4	2	2					

TABLE 2. *In vitro activity of ceftazidime, cefotaxime, and aminoglycoside antibiotics against recently isolated strains*

Microorganism	Antibiotic	No. of strains	No. of microorganisms with MIC (μg/ml):											
			≤0.06	0.12	0.24	0.48	0.96	1.9	3.9	7.8	15.6	31.2	62.5	≥125
Enterobacter spp.	Ceftazidime	13			4	5	1			1			2	
	Cefotaxime	13	1		6	2						1	1	2
	Gentamicin	13				1	3		1	2	1		1	4
	Sisomicin	13			2	3	2	1	1			1	2	1
	Tobramycin	13			1	5	1	2		1	3			
	Amikacin	13				6	6			1				
Proteus spp., indole positive	Ceftazidime	27	10	3	4	1		3	4					2
	Cefotaxime	27	12	2	2	3	2	2	1				1	2
	Gentamicin	27			1	2	2	1	4		2	1	1	13
	Sisomicin	27					2	8			2		2	13
	Tobramycin	27					2	7	2	2	3	5		6
	Amikacin	27				1		10	8	4	1	1	2	
Proteus mirabilis	Ceftazidime	15	13	2										
	Cefotaxime	15	14	1										
	Gentamicin	15					8		4					3
	Sisomicin	15					1	5	5					4
	Tobramycin	15						2	9		1	2	1	
	Amikacin	15						2	6	7				

TABLE 3. *In vitro activity of ceftazidime against Pseudomonas spp. strains in comparison with β-lactam and aminoglycoside antibiotics*

Antibiotic	No. of strains	No. of microorganisms with MIC (μg/ml):											
		≤0.06	0.12	0.24	0.48	0.96	1.9	3.9	7.8	15.6	31.2	62.5	≥125
Ceftazidime	39				1	10	11	8	7	2			
Cefotaxime	39								6	5	12	10	6
Cefsulodin	36					3	15	5	5	2		2	4
Azlocillin	36					1		7	14		9	1	4
Mezlocillin	36									9	12	3	12
Carbenicillin	36										2	5	29
Gentamicin	39			1	3	8	9	2	3	2		2	9
Sisomicin	37		2	4	8	2	11	2	2			1	5
Tobramycin	37	1	3	6	1	16	1				7	1	1
Amikacin	36			2	4	4	13	8	2	1		2	

achievable in humans. The ranking order for the β-lactam group was the following: ceftazidime, cefsulodin, azlocillin, cefotaxime, mezlocillin, and carbenicillin. For the aminoglycoside group it was ceftazidime, amikacin, sisomicin, tobramycin, and gentamicin.

In the in vivo protection test, ceftazidime and cefsulodin revealed the best activity against *P. alcaligenes* 1, followed by azlocillin, tobramycin, and sisomicin. All the other antibiotics were less active. Against *P. putida* 14, ceftazidime, cefsulodin, and all four aminoglycosides were characterized by the same degree of activity. The other antibiotics were not active. Against *P. aeruginosa* 588, ceftazidime showed the best activity, followed by cefsulodin. None of the other β-lactam or aminoglycoside antibiotics was active.

In conclusion, the data show the high activity of ceftazidime against 188 strains; in fact, only 6 strains needed concentrations of 15.6 μg/ml for inhibition. Thirty-six strains proved resistant to cefotaxime and 43, to gentamicin. About 90% of gram-negative isolates, including *Pseudomonas* spp., were inhibited by ceftazidime at 3.9 μg/ml. Similar activity was achieved with cefotaxime at 62.5 μg/ml and with gentamicin at 125 μg/ml. Against *S. aureus*, the activity of ceftazidime was lower than against gram-negative bacteria, but 100% of the strains were inhibited by 15.6 μg/ml. When sisomicin, amikacin, and tobramycin were included in the comparison, in the case of *Enterobacter* spp. and *Proteus* spp., ceftazidime revealed similar or higher activity. For *Pseudomonas* spp., the in vitro results showed the highest activity for ceftazidime, a finding confirmed by the in vivo protection test.

In Vitro Activity of Cefuroxime and Ceftazidime Against Anaerobic Bacteria

ANTHONY W. CHOW,* KAREN H. BARTLETT, AND MARIE J. GRIBBLE

Division of Infectious Disease, Department of Medicine, University of British Columbia, and Vancouver General Hospital, Vancouver, British Columbia V5Z 1M9, Canada*

Infections originating from the oropharynx, skin, and soft tissues, the female genital tract, and the intestinal tract are usually caused by a mixed flora of both aerobes and anaerobes. The new β-lactam antibiotics cefuroxime and ceftazidime have broad-spectrum in vitro activity and are potential candidates as single-agent therapy for some of these infections. Their comparative in vitro activity against clinically important obligate anaerobes, however, has not been extensively studied. We therefore evaluated the in vitro activity of cefuroxime and ceftazidime against 586 clinical isolates of anaerobic bacteria by an agar dilution technique and compared the results with cefoxitin.

The 586 anaerobic isolates examined were obtained from inpatients of Harbor-UCLA Medical Center during 1975 through 1978. Identification to species level was determined in prereduced anaerobically sterilized (PRAS) differential media by the method of Holdeman, Cato, and Moore (1). Isolates were stored in 20% skim milk and frozen at −75°C until ready for antibiotic susceptibility testing. Susceptibility to cefuroxime, ceftazidime, and cefoxitin was determined simultaneously by an agar dilution technique on Wilkins-Chalgren media supplemented with hemin (5 μg/ml) and vitamin K_1 (10 μg/ml) by the method of Sutter et al. (2). Twofold serial dilutions of cefuroxime (Glaxo), ceftazidime (Glaxo), or cefoxitin (Merck Sharp & Dohme) sensitivity powder were added. A 48-h subculture of the test organism in PRAS thioglycolate broth was adjusted to a McFarland no. 1 nephelometer standard previously determined to approximate 10^6 to 10^7 organisms per ml by colony count in roll tubes and PRAS media. Inocula (0.0025 ml) were delivered with a Steers replicator. Plates were incubated at 37°C in anaerobic jars after air had been evacuated and replaced with a gas mixture containing 80% nitrogen, 10% hydrogen, and 10% carbon dioxide. Anaerobic, microaerophilic (incubated in candle jars), and aerobic plates without antibiotics were used for controls, and two reference strains (*Bacteroides fragilis* 3186 and *Clostridium perfringens* 3000) with known MICs were included in each test for reproducibility. All results were read at 48 h, and the MIC was recorded as the lowest antibiotic concentration which yielded no visible growth.

MICs of control strains (*B. fragilis* 3186 and *C. perfringens* 3000) determined in 17 separate tests agreed with the modal MIC ± 1 $\log_2$ dilution from 94 to 100% for all three antibiotics studied, confirming the reproducibility of the test method. The antibiotic concentrations required to inhibit 50% (MIC_{50}) and 90% (MIC_{90}) of strains, and the cumulative percentage of these 586 clinical isolates of anaerobic bacteria inhibited by the study antibiotics at 16, 32, and 64 μg/ml are summarized in Table 1. Comparative in vitro activity of these agents was determined by analysis of geometric mean MICs for each genus and species of anaerobic bacteria studied by the Student *t* test (two tailed) with a significance level of $P < 0.01$, and important differences are summarized in Table 2.

Overall, cefuroxime and cefoxitin were comparable in activity, and both were significantly more active than ceftazidime ($P < 0.001$). At 32 μg/ml, 83% of all isolates were inhibited by cefuroxime, compared with 86% by cefoxitin and 70% by ceftazidime. Considerable variation in susceptibility was observed among different genera or species of anaerobes tested. Among gram-negative anaerobes, the geometric mean MIC for cefoxitin was significantly lower than that for both ceftazidime ($P < 0.001$) and cefuroxime ($P < 0.005$). This difference reflects the relative lack of activity of both cefuroxime and ceftazidime against the *B. fragilis* group compared with that of cefoxitin. Against gram-positive anaerobes, cefuroxime had the lowest geometric mean MIC compared with both ceftazidime ($P < 0.001$) and cefoxitin ($P < 0.025$). The enhanced activity of cefuroxime was particularly striking for microaerophilic streptococci (*Streptococcus intermedius* and *S. constellatus*) and lactobacilli, against which cefuroxime was significantly more active than cefoxitin ($P < 0.005$ and $P < 0.001$, respectively) as well as ceftazidime ($P < 0.001$ and $P < 0.001$, respectively).

These data indicate that, with the exception of *B. fragilis*, cefuroxime has a wide spectrum of activity against anaerobic bacteria, and its overall activity is comparable to that of cefoxitin. Cefuroxime appears particularly active against

TABLE 1. *Comparative in vitro activity of cefuroxime, ceftazidime, and cefoxitin against anaerobic bacteria*

Organism (no. tested)	Antibiotic	MIC_{50} (μg/ml)	MIC_{90} (μg/ml)	Cumulative % inhibited at: 16 μg/ml	32 μg/ml	64 μg/ml
Bacteroides fragilis group (92)	Cefuroxime	81	>128	21	30	45
	Ceftazidime	67	>128	1	18	48
	Cefoxitin	14	86	59	76	86
Other *Bacteroides* spp. (69)	Cefuroxime	5	>128	72	79	84
	Ceftazidime	5	>128	57	66	76
	Cefoxitin	4	51	79	85	92
Fusobacterium spp. (14)	Cefuroxime	4	102	85	85	85
	Ceftazidime	16	>128	50	78	85
	Cefoxitin	6	51	71	85	92
Veillonella spp. (22)	Cefuroxime	1.5	8	90	100	100
	Ceftazidime	11	64	63	86	90
	Cefoxitin	0.4	8	100	100	100
Peptococcus spp. (92)	Cefuroxime	<0.25	4	98	100	100
	Ceftazidime	2	17	89	96	98
	Cefoxitin	<0.25	2.3	97	100	100
Peptostreptococcus spp. (30)	Cefuroxime	0.3	3	100	100	100
	Ceftazidime	1	8	90	96	100
	Cefoxitin	0.2	2	100	100	100
Streptococcus spp. (20)	Cefuroxime	0.4	8	100	100	100
	Ceftazidime	3	16	90	95	100
	Cefoxitin	5	12	100	100	100
Clostridium perfringens (28)	Cefuroxime	1.7	4	96	96	100
	Ceftazidime	7	22	85	96	100
	Cefoxitin	1.1	3	96	100	100
Other *Clostridium* spp. (33)	Cefuroxime	7	>128	63	66	69
	Ceftazidime	54	>128	33	39	54
	Cefoxitin	6	53	66	75	96
Actinomyces spp. (10)	Cefuroxime	1.5	8	100	100	100
	Ceftazidime	6	48	60	80	100
	Cefoxitin	1	48	70	80	100
Eubacterium spp. (25)	Cefuroxime	1.5	24	84	96	100
	Ceftazidime	12	>128	60	68	68
	Cefoxitin	1.8	20	88	96	100
Bifidobacterium spp. (7)	Cefuroxime	6	20	85	100	100
	Ceftazidime	10	>128	71	85	85
	Cefoxitin	20	>128	42	71	85
Lactobacillus spp. (42)	Cefuroxime	6	32	80	90	95
	Ceftazidime	72	>128	21	28	45
	Cefoxitin	>128	>128	16	16	23
Propionibacterium spp. (94)	Cefuroxime	<0.25	0.5	100	100	100
	Ceftazidime	4	13	96	100	100
	Cefoxitin	0.2	1	100	100	100
Miscellaneous (8)[a]	Cefuroxime	<0.25	9	100	100	100
	Ceftazidime	2	76	75	87	87
	Cefoxitin	0.2	9	100	100	100
Total isolates (586)	Cefuroxime	1.4	107	79	83	87
	Ceftazidime	8	>128	60	70	80
	Cefoxitin	1.5	56	80	86	91

[a] Includes *Ruminococcus* (six), *Megasphaera* (one), *Selenomonas* (one).

gram-positive anaerobes, especially microaerophilic streptococci and lactobacilli. Cefuroxime may be useful as single-agent treatment of mixed infections, particularly of the oropulmonary tract, in which *B. fragilis* is infrequently involved. Controlled clinical trials are indicated. Ceftazidime, however, only has moderate activity against anaerobic bacteria, and its overall

TABLE 2. *Comparative in vitro activity against 586 anaerobic bacteria*

Organism	No. tested	Geometric mean MIC ± SD (μg/ml)		
		Ceftazidime	Cefuroxime	Cefoxitin
Gram-positive anaerobes	387	7.3 ± 4.3	1.1 ± 5.9	1.6 ± 8.8
		← $P < 0.001$[a] →	← NS[b] →	
		←	$P < 0.001$	→
Streptococcus	20	4.5 ± 3.8	0.8 ± 3.6	4.0 ± 3.8
		← $P < 0.001$ →	← $P < 0.005$ →	
		←	NS	→
Lactobacillus	42	57 ± 4.5	7.7 ± 4.2	91 ± 7.3
		← $P < 0.001$ →	← $P < 0.001$ →	
		←	NS	→
Gram-negative anaerobes	199	26 ± 14.6	16 ± 9.7	8.9 ± 6.1
		← NS →	← $P < 0.005$ →	
		←	$P < 0.001$	→
Bacteroides fragilis group	92	95 ± 2.5	68 ± 4.4	21 ± 3.2
		← NS →	← $P < 0.001$ →	
		←	$P < 0.001$	→
Veillonella	22	10 ± 5.5	2.1 ± 4.0	1.0 ± 3.9
		← $P < 0.005$ →	← NS →	
		←	$P < 0.001$	→
Overall	586	11 ± 7.8	2.8 ± 10.2	2.9 ± 9.1
		← $P < 0.001$ →	← NS →	
		←	$P < 0.001$	→

[a] Significant difference by Student *t* (two-tailed) analysis.
[b] No significant difference ($P > 0.01$).

activity is inferior to that of both cefoxitin and cefuroxime.

1. **Holdeman, L. V., E. P. Cato, and W. E. C. Moore.** 1977. Anaerobe laboratory manual, 4th ed. Virginia Polytechnic Institute Anaerobe Laboratory, Blacksburg.
2. **Sutter, V. L., A. L. Barry, T. D. Wilkins, and R. J. Zabransky.** 1979. Collaborative evaluation of a proposed reference dilution method of susceptibility testing of anaerobic bacteria. Antimicrob. Agents Chemother. **16:**495–502.

Comparative Activity of Ceftazidime (GR 20263) in Experimental Urinary Tract Infections

P. ACRED,* D, M. RYAN, AND ANGELA E. COLLARD

Glaxo Group Research Ltd., Greenford, Middlesex, United Kingdom

Ceftazidime (GR 20263) is a new cephalosporin with very high intrinsic activity against members of the *Enterobacteriaceae* family, combined with stability to almost all known β-lactamases. A feature which distinguishes ceftazidime from other recently introduced cephalosporins is its high activity against *Pseudomonas aeruginosa*. There have been many reports of the in vitro (2, 5, 6) and in vivo (1, 3) antibacterial characteristics of ceftazidime. The potential effectiveness of a new antibacterial agent can be assessed either in experimental septicemia in animals or in models of specific infections such as endocarditis or meningitis. We have investigated the activity of ceftazidime in comparison with the related aminothiazolyl cephalosporin cefotaxime and the aminoglocoside gentamicin in experimental urinary tract infections in rats.

An ascending pyelonephritis was established by inoculating 0.05 ml of an overnight culture of the test organism, diluted to contain 10^5 to 10^6 colony-forming units per ml, into the urinary bladder, in which a 1-cm length of braided nylon thread had been implanted. The presence of a

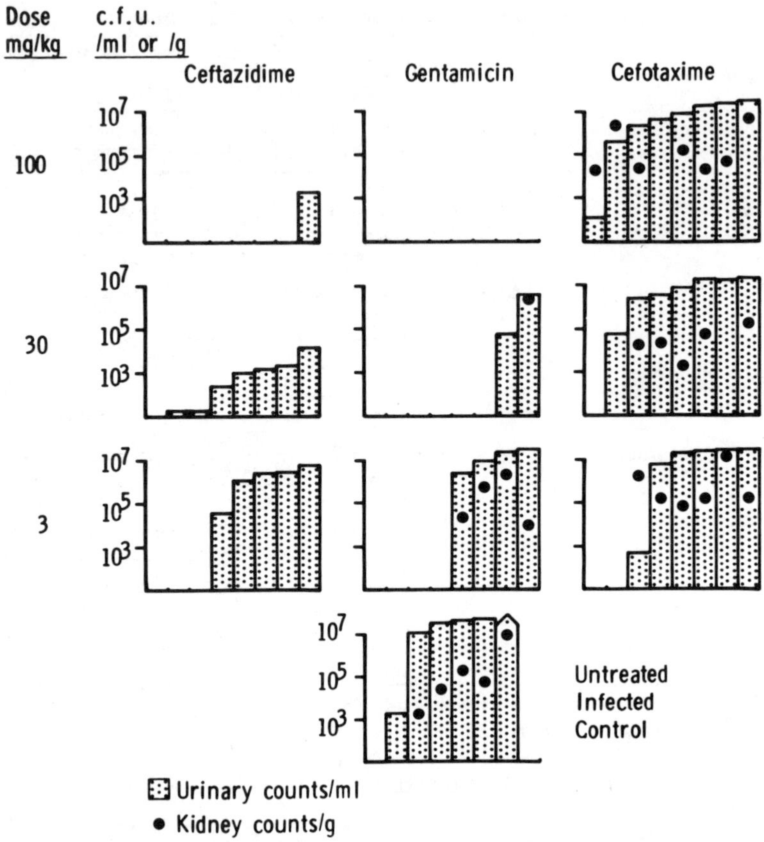

FIG. 1. *Therapeutic activity of ceftazidime, cefotaxime, and gentamicin in experimental P. aeruginosa 1911E urinary tract infections in rats. Columns indicate viable bacterial counts in urine and kidneys of individual rats in each dose group on day 4 of the experiment.*

TABLE 1. *Therapeutic activity of ceftazidime, cefotaxime, and gentamicin against gram-negative experimental urinary tract infections in rats*[a]

Organism	Therapeutic dose (mg/kg)					
	Ceftazidime		Gentamicin		Cefotaxime	
	Urine	Kidney	Urine	Kidney	Urine	Kidney
P. aeruginosa 1911E	9.3	<3	5.8	<3	>100	>100
P. aeruginosa 1912E	13.0	<3	11.5	3.6	>100	>100
E. coli 2025E	0.3	0.008	>0.3	>0.3	>0.3	>0.3
E. cloacae 2010E	0.6	0.4	1.1	<0.3	8.1	<0.3
K. pneumoniae 2011E	4.0	1.6	0.8	0.6	1.6	<0.3
P. vulgaris 1356E	3.5	1.2	3.8	1.6	129.	12.9

[a] The results are expressed as the dose (milligrams per kilogram) that reduced the bacterial count in urine and homogenized kidney to 10^3 colony-forming units per milliliter or gram.

foreign body in the bladder is essential for the establishment of the urinary tract infection (for full details of the experimental model, see reference 4). The six test organisms used were *P. aeruginosa* 1911E and 1912E, *Escherichia coli* 2025E, *Enterobacter cloacae* 2010E, *Klebsiella pneumoniae* 2011E, and *Proteus vulgaris* 1356E. The three antibiotics were tested in parallel against each of the six test organisms. Groups of eight female Sprague-Dawley rats weighing 100 to 120 g were dosed subcutaneously, the first dose being given 24 h postinfection. Three dose levels were used for each antibiotic, the rats being dosed on three occasions on days 1 and 2 and two occasions on day 3. Animals were sacrificed on day 4, and bacterial counts of urine and homogenized kidney samples were carried out.

The three antibiotics showed dose-related activity in controlling infections in urine and kidney tissue, with the higher doses being the most active. For example, against infections induced with *P. aeruginosa* 1911E, ceftazidime and gentamicin showed good activity at doses of 100 and 30 mg/kg; the counts in the urine and renal tissue were significantly lower than the corresponding counts in the untreated control rats. Animals treated with the lowest dose (3 mg/kg) remained infected, but in the case of ceftazidime the infection was seen only in bladder urine. Rats treated with cefotaxime were not protected from infection even with the highest dose (100 mg/kg) used (Fig. 1). The good dose-related therapeutic effect seen with ceftazidime against *P. aeruginosa* 1911E was repeated with the other organisms tested. The response for each organism was quantified by calculating the dose needed to reduce the geometric mean bacterial counts of urine and renal tissue to an arbitrarily chosen figure of 10^3 colony-forming units per ml or g. As can be seen in Table 1, ceftazidime proved as active as gentamicin in the treatment of the *P. aeruginosa*, *E. cloacae*, and *P. vulgaris* infections; it was more effective than gentamicin against the *E. coli* infection but less effective against the *K. pneumoniae* urinary tract infection. Cefotaxime was inactive against the *P. aeruginosa* infections and was less effective than ceftazidime in eliminating the other four test organisms from the urine. However, cefotaxime was more effective than ceftazidime in reducing infection in the kidneys of rats infected with *E. cloacae* and *K. pneumoniae*, in the latter case proving more active than gentamicin.

The results of these experiments indicate that bacterial counts of urinary tract pathogens are significantly reduced by low doses of ceftazidime. Furthermore, the results show that ceftazidime is as effective as the aminoglycoside gentamicin and more effective than the related aminothiazolyl cephalosporin cefotaxime. Ceftazidime should be a valuable antibiotic for the treatment of urinary tract infections. These results, together with the low toxicity of ceftazidime compared with gentamicin, indicate this new cephalosporin as a useful alternative to aminoglycoside therapy.

1. **Acred, P., and D. M. Ryan.** 1980. In vivo properties of GR 20263, p. 271–273. *In* J. D. Nelson and C. Grassi (ed.), Current chemotherapy and infectious disease. American Society for Microbiology, Washington, D.C.
2. **Harper, P. B., S. Kirby, and C. H. O'Callaghan.** 1980. In vitro properties of GR 20263—a highly active broad-spectrum cephalosporin with antipseudomonal activity, p. 269–271. *In* J. D. Nelson and C. Grassi (ed.), Current chemotherapy and infectious disease. American Society for Microbiology, Washington, D.C.
3. **O'Callaghan, C. H., P. Acred, P. B. Harper, D. M. Ryan, S. M. Kirby, and S. M. Harding.** 1980. GR 20263, a new broad-spectrum cephalosporin with anti-pseudomonal activity. Antimicrob. Agents Chemother. **17**:876–883.
4. **Ryan, D. M.** 1970. A method for inducing experimental urinary tract infections in the rat and its use in experimental chemotherapy. Postgrad. Med. J. Suppl. **46**:19–24.
5. **Verbist, L., and J. Verhaegen.** 1980. GR 20263: a new aminothiazolyl cephalosporin with high activity against *Pseudomonas* and *Enterobacteriaceae*. Antimicrob. Agents Chemother. **17**:807–812.
6. **Wise, R., J. M. Andrews, and K. A. Bedford.** 1980. Comparison of in vitro activity of GR 20263, a novel cephalosporin derivative, with activities of other β-lactam compounds. Antimicrob. Agents Chemother. **17**: 884–889.

Treatment of Urinary Tract Infections Due to *Pseudomonas aeruginosa*: Ceftazidime Versus Netilmicin

W. GRANINGER,* C. P. SCHMIDBAUER, U. GANZINGER, R. LENZHOFER, I. HO, AND K. H. SPITZY

Department of Chemotherapy, University of Vienna, and Urological Department, Allgemeine Poliklinik der Stadt Wien and Ludwig Boltzmann-Research Institute for Tumors and Infections of the Urinary Tract, Vienna, Austria

Gram-negative bacteria are responsible to a great extent for nosocomial infections. With a 40% rate of nosocomial infections, urological departments are an important source for these infections in hospitals.

Pseudomonas aeruginosa is the etiological agent in 8.5% of all nosocomial urinary tract infections (UTI) (1). Primary infection with this organism is uncommon. *Pseudomonas* enters the urinary tract when catheters or other urological instruments are introduced for diagnostic or therapeutic reasons. By avoiding invasive preoperative diagnostic measures and refraining from uncontrolled general antibacterial prophylaxis, we were able to lower the incidence of *P. aeruginosa* infections after suprapubic prostatectomy from 55% in 1974 to 5% in 1979 (3).

In patients with "obstructive uropathy" or with paraplegia, genitourinary infection with *P. aeruginosa* occurs frequently. If urosurgical repair is not possible and urostasis persists, these infections are uncurable or recurrent.

Ceftazidime is a new semisynthetic cephalosporin with pronounced activity against *P. aeruginosa* (5), which shows increasing rates of resistance against the former highly effective aminoglycosides as a result of uncritical use. The lack of toxicity and applicability to penicillin-allergic patients, together with the activity against strains of *P. aeruginosa*, render this cephalosporin suitable for clinical study.

In an open trial, the efficacy and safety of ceftazidime was compared with that of netilmicin. Netilmicin is an aminoglycoside with antibacterial activity comparable to that of gentamicin, but with apparent lower toxicity (2).

Forty patients were selected and, by means of a randomization schedule, were allocated to one of two groups, each consisting of 20 patients. All these infections were subsequent to urological catheterization or surgery. Most of the patients had suffered from their UTI for many years, with an average of 30 months. There was no significant difference between the two groups with respect to age, weight, and duration of disease. The kidney function was decreased in both groups. The average creatinine clearance in the ceftazidime group was 68 ml/min; in the netilmicin group it was 55 ml/min. Patients in the ceftazidime group received 1 g of the drug twice daily by the intramuscular or intravenous route. Netilmicin was administered at a dose of 100 mg twice a day. Duration of treatment was 10 days in both groups. Indications for the treatment of UTI due to *P. aeruginosa* were fever in 13 cases, loin pain in 9, and dysuria in 15 patients. Nine patients who were asymptomatic but showed a positive test for antibody-coated bacteria were also treated.

Criteria for inclusion in the study were significant bacteriuria, significant elevation of leukocyte-excretion count in urine, and symptoms of UTI as mentioned before.

Urinary cultures were obtained before therapy, on day 3, at the end of therapy, and at weekly intervals up to 6 weeks. Routine tests of renal, hepatic, and hematopoietic functions were carried out before, during, and after therapy.

All bacterial isolates were identified by the usual techniques. For susceptibility testing a modified Kirby-Bauer technique on diagnostic sensitivity test agar was used; 30-μg disks of ceftazidime and netilmicin were used. Susceptibility was assumed if the zone of inhibition exceeded 18 mm. Antibody-coated bacteria were detected by the immunofluorescence technique described by Thomas et al. (4).

A classification of UTIs is important for the evaluation of the efficacy of a drug. We usually classify UTI in three stages. In grade I, more commonly known as uncomplicated UTI, no obstruction or predisposing factors, e.g., bladder dysfunction or metabolic disorders, can be demonstrated. UTI grade II is complicated by obstruction without evident kidney damage. Radiological renal lesions are evident in grade III; the infection is supported by predisposing factors, e.g., staghorn stones, drug abuse, neoplastic disease.

The efficacy was judged on the basis of the microbiological findings as eradication when the urine showed no significant bacterial growth during and at the end of treatment. Cure was assumed if urine samples remained sterile during a follow-up of 6 weeks.

According to these criteria the following clinical results were obtained. In 17 of 20 patients in the ceftazidime group, the organism was eradicated, as compared with 12 of 20 patients in the netilmicin group. The difference is not significant because there were more patients with severe renal lesions in the netilmicin group (Table 1). This must also be taken into consideration regarding the cure rate. As anticipated, the cure

TABLE 1. *Results of treatment of UTIs*

UTI	Effect of therapy							
	Eradication during therapy				Cure rate			
	Ceftazidime group		Netilmicin group		Ceftazidime		Netilmicin	
	Total	Eradicated	Total	Eradicated	Total	Cured	Total	Cured
Grade I	4	4	3	3	4	2	3	2
Grade II	12	10	11	6	12	6	11	0
Grade III	4	3	6	3	4	1	6	1
Total	20	17	20	12	20	7	20	3

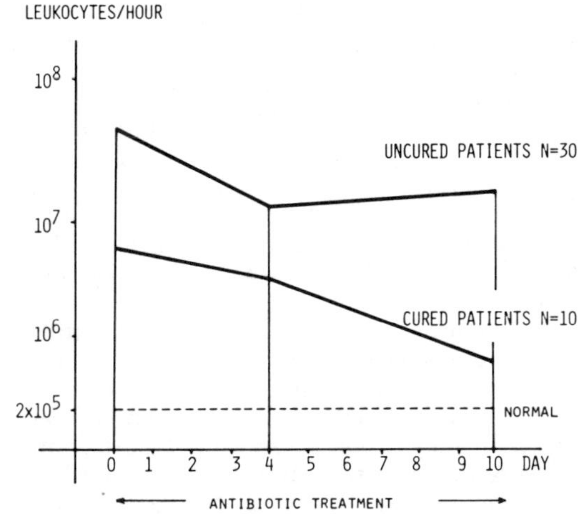

FIG. 1. *Leukocyte excretion rate in UTI due to P. aeruginosa.*

rate in uncomplicated UTI was high. The three patients who had a relapse within 6 weeks suffered from extensive leukoplakia of the bladder mucosa, recurrent superficial carcinoma of the bladder, and severe interstitial cystitis, respectively. Patients with UTI grade II of the ceftazidime group showed a remarkable cure rate, whereas no cure could be obtained with netilmicin. Equal efficacy was seen in patients with severe renal lesions (Table 1).

In summary, the therapeutic result was good considering the chronic nature and severity of these infections. The dynamics of the quantitative leukocyte count (Addis count) is a valuable tool in predicting the success of antibacterial therapy. Cured patients showed slow normalization of the leukocyte excretion rate; patients who did not respond to therapy showed an initial decline and remained stable on high urinary leukocyte values throughout therapy and follow-up (Fig. 1).

Adverse reactions were minimal. Local tolerance of both intravenous and intramuscular application was well tolerated in all patients. In the ceftazidime group one patient developed mild diarrhea which did not cause cessation of therapy, and another patient had a macular rash at the end of therapy. Transient nausea in one patient was the only side effect in the netilmicin group.

The aim of this study was to investigate the efficacy and safety of ceftazidime compared with that of an aminoglycoside. Ceftazidime at a dosage of 1 g twice a day was at least as efficient as netilmicin at 100 mg twice daily and might be sufficient as a monotherapeutic agent in severe UTI due to *P. aeruginosa*. Ceftazidime seemed to be slightly more efficient than netilmicin; however, superiority cannot be concluded from this study because of too few patients and diversity of the underlying diseases.

1. **Center for Disease Control.** 1977. National nosocomial infections surveillance, annual summary 1975. Center for Disease Control, Atlanta, Ga.
2. **Fu, K. W., and A. C. Neu.** 1976. In vitro study of netilmicin compared with other aminoglycosides. Antimicrob. Agents Chemother. **10:**526.
3. **Schmidbauer, C. P., and P. Porpàczy.** 1981. Consequences of a changed antibiotic strategy in an urological department—a six year follow up, p. 343–346. *In* G. G. Grassi and L. D. Sabath (ed.), New trends in antibiotics: research and therapy. Elsevier/North-Holland Biomedical Press, Amsterdam.
4. **Thomas, V., A. Shelokov, and M. Forland.** 1974. Proteinuria and antibody coated bacteria in the urine. N. Engl. J. Med. **290:**588.
5. **Verbist, L., and J. Verhaegen.** 1980. GR 20263: a new aminothiazolyl cephalosporin with high activity against *Pseudomonas* and *Enterobacteriaceae*. Antimicrob. Agents Chemother. **17:**807–812.

Clinical Pharmacology of Ceftazidime

STUART M. HARDING

Glaxo Group Research Ltd., Greenford, Middlesex UB6 0HE, U.K.

Ceftazidime (CAZ) is a new broad-spectrum and antipseudomonal cephalosporin. It has been given to both volunteers and patients, and data are accumulating to allow a preliminary review of the clinical pharmacology of this drug to be made.

Of 67 healthy adult male volunteers given CAZ by the parenteral route, the average 24-h urinary excretion of drug was 83% (1). Serum from a number of these volunteers was examined by high-pressure liquid chromatography under a variety of different conditions, and no metabolite peaks were detected. Urine was subjected to chromatography and bioautography, and no activity other than that associated with CAZ was present. In rats, the biliary excretion of CAZ was <1%, and, in humans, concentrations in T-tube bile after a 2-g intravenous (i.v.) injection reached a peak of 36.4 mg/liter 1.5 h after injection and averaged 9.4 mg/liter 8 h after injection (4); these figures again suggest <1% biliary excretion.

There was no indication that hepatic metabolism of CAZ occurred: after 5 h of incubation with 10% human liver homogenate at 37°C, 88% unchanged CAZ could be recovered and no microbiologically active degradation products could be detected by chromatography and bioautography. The apparent lack of complete urinary recovery of CAZ is probably explained by its instability in biological fluids before assay.

The serum protein binding of CAZ was low: equilibration dialysis performed with radiolabeled CAZ at three concentrations (1.4, 16, and 58 mg/liter) gave 5% binding or less, independent of concentration. The ultimate serum half-life ($t_{1/2}$) of CAZ averaged 1.8 in volunteers (1) which is long for a beta-lactam antibiotic with low protein binding. Probenecid had no effect on the rate of elimination of drug from the serum (Fig. 1), indicating that no net renal tubular secretion occurred.

On the assumption that the volume of distribution of CAZ is unaffected by impaired renal function, estimations of rates of elimination over a range of glomerular filtration rates (GFR) can be made (2). Preliminary data from P. Gower and R. Norrby (personal communication) support this assumption and the estimations made. They are that k_N (rate of elimination from the serum in normal renal function) is 0.39 h^{-1} and k_{nr} (rate of nonrenal elimination) is 0.04 h^{-1}. With a linear relationship between rate constant and GFR, the $t_{1/2}$ of CAZ can be calculated for any value of GFR. Examples are: GFR, 80 ml/min, and $t_{1/2CAZ}$, 2.2 h; GFR, 50 ml/min, and $t_{1/2CAZ}$, 3.3 h. Only when GFRs of <30 ml/min occur should a reduction in dose or frequency be necessary: i.e., 15 to 30 ml/min, reduce dosing from every 8 h to every 12 h; below 15 ml/min, reduce to once daily dosing. At the end of hemodialysis or peritoneal dialysis, an extra dose should be given since CAZ is removed by these procedures.

With normal renal function, accumulation did not occur when doses of 1 or 2 g were given every 8 h for 10 days (Fig. 1 and 2). This supports the hypothesis that there is no deep compartment for CAZ and that CAZ, like other beta-lactams, has a fairly small total apparent volume of distribution (average, 17.61 ± 3.41 SD from 22 volunteers given bolus i.v. injections) which can be summarized in kinetic terms as comprising a central compartment (volume, 8.9 ± 1.71) and a peripheral compartment (volume, 8.7 ± 2.81). Kinetic studies involving eight volunteers given 1 g of CAZ i.v. and having simultaneous samples taken from blood, subcutaneous cotton threads, suction blisters, and cantharidin blisters highlighted the problems in interpretation of single peripheral models since the kinetics of distribution and elimination from each of these fluids differed, although in none of these compartments was elimination prolonged. Possibly because of the low protein binding of CAZ, high concentrations of drug were reached, with an overall average ratio of areas under fluid level/time curves to serum level/time curves being

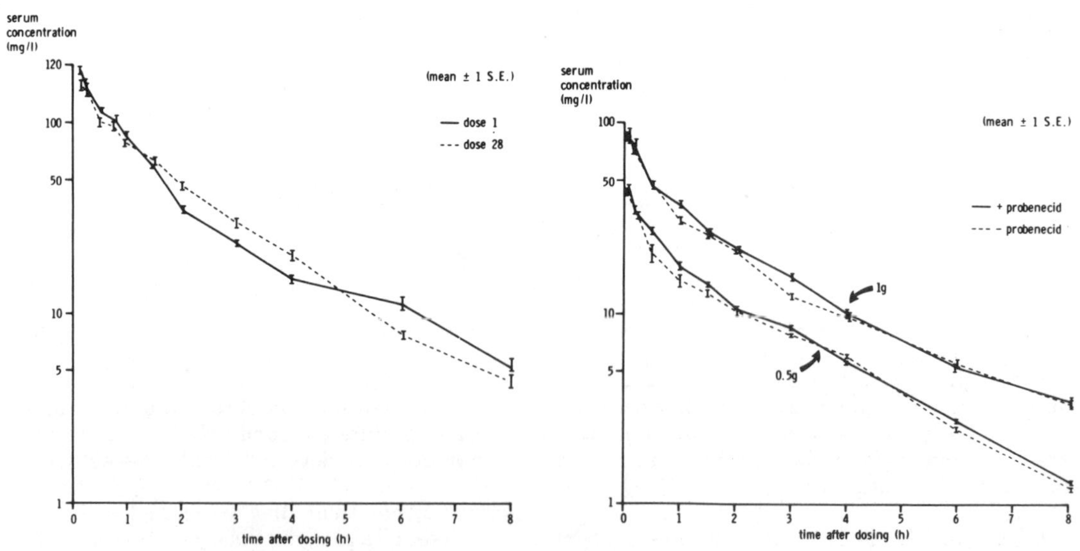

FIG. 1. *Serum level/time curves for CAZ after i.v. injection of: (left) 1 and 28 2-g doses of CAZ to eight male volunteers; (right) 1 g of CAZ with and without probenecid to four male volunteers.*

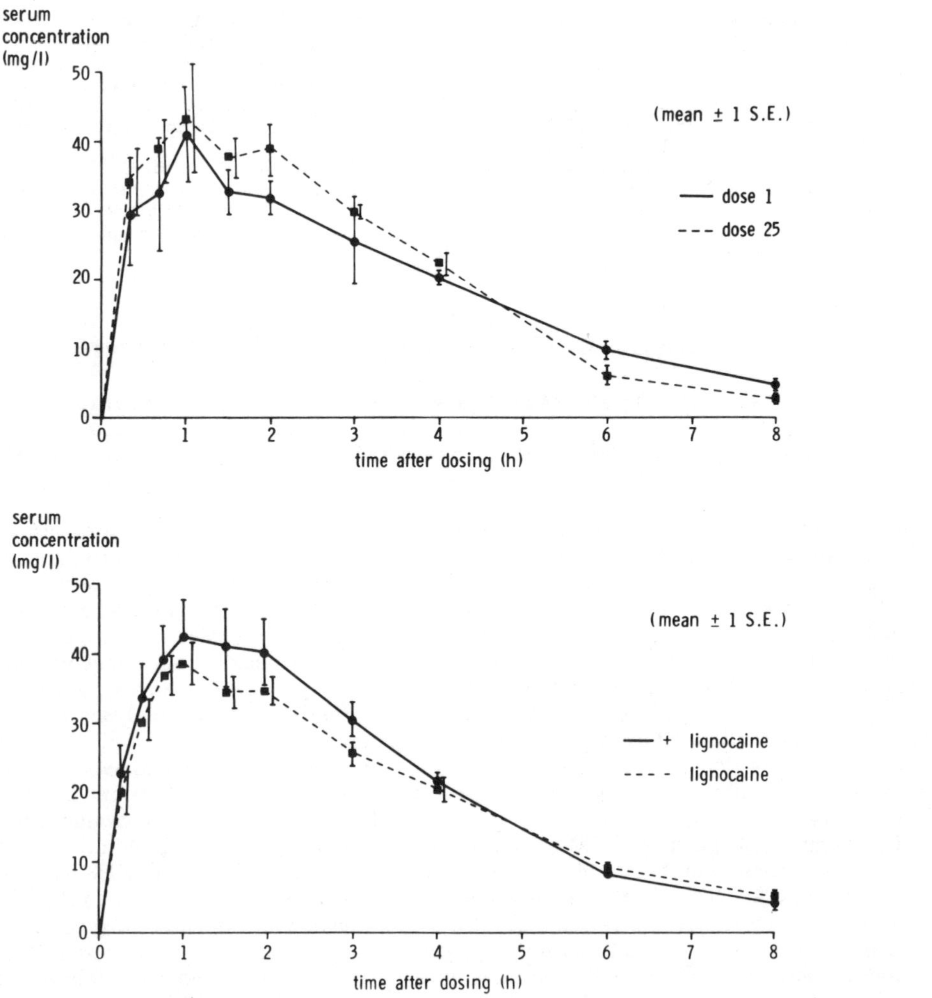

FIG. 2. *Serum level/time curves for CAZ after i.m. injection of: (top) 1 and 25 1-g doses of CAZ to four male volunteers; (bottom) 1 g of CAZ with and without 1% lignocaine to six male volunteers.*

0.8. Peak concentrations of CAZ from samples obtained from various tissues or fluids from patients were as follows: T-tube bile, 36.4 mg/liter; inorganic bone, 24.1 mg/liter; periprosthetic hip replacement fluid, 25.6 mg/liter; peritoneal drain fluid, 27.6 mg/liter; psoas abscess pus, 17.5 mg/liter; sputum 12 mg/liter; cerebrospinal fluid, 11.8 mg/liter; aqueous humor, 4 mg/liter. These are preliminary data only and are from small numbers of patients. However, the levels mostly exceeded the MIC (8 mg/liter) for 88% of 12,986 organisms obtained clinically (3). As can be seen from Fig. 1 and 2, such a level was exceeded in the serum for many hours after i.v. or intramuscular (i.m.) doses ranging from 0.5 to 2 g.

Injections of CAZ i.m. were well tolerated. Peak serum concentrations were reached about 70 min after injection and were 17.5 ± 2.5 (SD) mg/liter after 500-mg doses and 38.8 ± 4.5 mg/liter after 1-g doses. In a repeat-dose study (Fig. 2), peak values were 33.0 mg/liter after a first dose of 1 g and 36.6 mg/liter after 25 doses given three times daily. The use of 1% lignocaine did not alter the kinetics (Fig. 2): peak values were 44.3 (no lignocaine) and 38.9 (with lignocaine) mg/liter.

In summary, the kinetics of CAZ are straightforward. There is no metabolism, negligible protein binding, and <1% biliary excretion. Elimination is by glomerular filtration only; dose intervals have to be increased when the GFR falls. The serum level profile fits a two-compartment model after i.v. dosing and a one-compartment model after i.m. dosing. The levels are unaltered by probenecid, repeated dosing, or lignocaine (i.m. dosing). Tissue or fluid levels from a number of compartments exceed the MIC_{90} for a wide variety of clinical isolates.

1. **Acred, P., S. M. Harding, and D. M. Ryan.** 1981. The in vivo properties of GR 20263 (ceftazidime), a highly active broad-spectrum cephalosporin with anti-pseudomonal activity. Drugs Exp. Clin. Res. **7**:189–199.
2. **Dettli, L.** 1976. Drug dosage in renal disease. Clin. Pharmacokinet. **1**:126–134.
3. **Jones, R. N., A. L. Barry, C. Thornsberry, E. H. Gerlach, P. C. Fuchs, T. L. Gavan, and H. M. Sommers.** 1981. Ceftazidime: a pseudomonas-active cephalosporin: in vitro antimicrobial activity evaluation including recommendations for disc diffusion susceptibility tests. J. Antimicrob. Chemother. **8**(Suppl. B):187–211.
4. **Wittmann, D. H., H. H. Schassan, and F. Kohler.** 1981. Pharmacokinetic studies of ceftazidime in serum, bone, bile, tissue fluid and peritoneal fluid. J. Antimicrob. Chemother. **8**(Suppl. B):293–297.

Kinetics of Ceftazidime in Renal Impairment

PETER E. GOWER, PATRICIA M. HOBBS,* AND STUART M. HARDING

Charing Cross Hospital, London, and Glaxo Group Research Ltd., Greenford, Middlesex, England*

Ceftazidime is a new broad-spectrum and antipseudomonal cephalosporin with a high activity against gram-negative organisms (3). It is likely to be used in various life-threatening situations including infections in patients with renal failure. A study was undertaken to investigate the kinetics of ceftazidime in 14 patients with renal failure (average age, 49 years; average weight, 64 kg), 6 of whom were on hemodialysis, and to compare the data obtained with those from 8 healthy subjects (average age, 35 years; average weight, 78 kg).

Ceftazidime was given as a 1.0-g intravenous bolus, and timed samples of blood and urine were obtained at intervals after its administration. Patients on dialysis were studied both on and between dialysis. Renal function was measured by either a ^{51}Cr-EDTA clearance (patients) or by creatinine clearance (volunteers). Routine hematological, biochemical, and urinary microscopic analyses were undertaken to monitor possible toxic effects.

Ceftazidime was assayed by high-pressure liquid chromatography, and best fit serum level/time curves were obtained by computerized exponential regression. Kinetic calculations, including estimation of fictive serum concentration at time zero, serum elimination rate constant, serum half-life, area under the serum level/time curve to infinity, and volume of distribution during the postdistributive phase, and predictions concerning accumulation were carried out by standard methods (2).

Mean peak serum concentrations of 66 mg/liter at 1 h declined to 50 mg/liter at 6 h in patients requiring dialysis, compared with 40 and 5 mg/liter at 1 and 6 h, respectively, in normal controls. Mean maximum urine levels of ceftazidime varied between 211 mg/liter at 0 to 6 h for patients with a glomerular filtration rate (GFR) of less than 5 ml/min and 835 mg/liter in a patient with a GFR of 88 ml/min. Mean minimum urine levels at 12 to 24 h were 142 mg/liter and 30 mg/liter, respectively. Only 6% of the 1.0-g dose was recovered at 24 h from patients in advanced renal failure compared with approximately 90% in control subjects. The pharmacokinetic data are shown in Table 1, and the relationship between half-life and GFR is shown in Fig. 1. No hematological, biochemical, or urinary microscopic abnormalities were found.

These results obtained from patients with renal failure confirm the known pharmacokinetics of ceftazidime in normal subjects: the drug is largely excreted by the kidney, and renal

TABLE 1. *Average pharmacokinetic parameters after 1 g of ceftazidime intravenously*[a]

Group	C_0 (mg/liter)	AUC_T (mg.h/liter)	β (h^{-1})	$t\frac{1}{2}\beta$ (h)	$V_{D\beta}$ (liters)	U_R (%)	GFR (ml/min)
Volunteers	108	152	0.378	1.9	17.8	88	115
Patients	70	1,360	0.061	16.7	19.2	24	12
Patients during dialysis	82	292	0.176	4.6	22.2	0	—

[a] C_0, Fictive serum concentration at time zero; AUC_T, area under the serum level/time curve to infinity; β, serum elimination rate constant; $t\frac{1}{2}\beta$, serum half-life; $V_{D\beta}$, volume of distribution during the postdistributive phase; U_R, urinary recovery over 24 h.

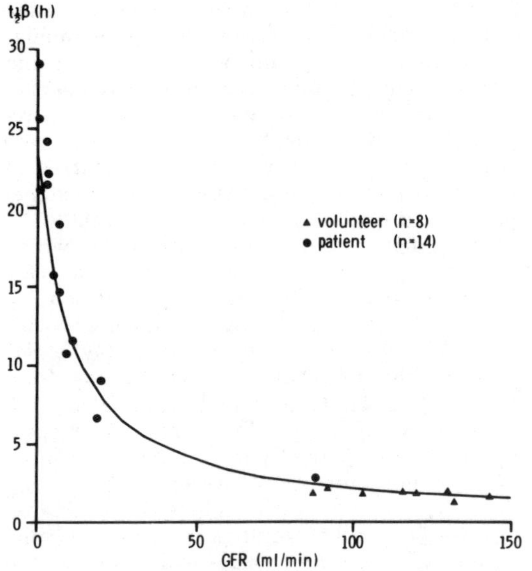

FIG. 1. *Relationship between serum elimination half-life of ceftazidime and GFR.*

failure will greatly prolong the half-life. No metabolites were detected in the urine of either patients or volunteers, and it is assumed that the amount of drug not accounted for was lost by natural breakdown in the serum or excretion by nonrenal routes. Defining dosage is difficult from the curvilinear relationship between half-life and GFR, and more information can be gained from the linear relation between the serum elimination rate constant and GFR (1). Using the confirmed assumption that the volume of distribution during the postdistributive phase was not significantly different in the patients with renal failure and control subjects, one obtains a series of breakpoints beyond which accumulation is likely to occur and lengthening of dosing intervals will be required. These points were found at a GFR of 5, 20, and 40 ml/min, and it is suggested that the dosing frequency of every 8 h in normal subjects be reduced to every 12 h at a GFR between 20 and 40 ml/min, to every 24 h at a GFR between 5 and 20 ml/min, and to every 36 h with a GFR below 5 ml/min. Patients on hemodialysis should be given an extra dose at the end of dialysis, since the half-life during hemodialysis was reduced from 24 h to 4.6 h.

1. **Dettli, L.** 1976. Drug dosage in renal disease. Clin. Pharmacokinet. **1:**126–134.
2. **Gibaldi, M., and D. Perrier.** 1975. Pharmacokinetics. Marcel Dekker Inc., New York.
3. **O'Callaghan, C. H., P. Acred, P. B. Harper, D. M. Ryan, S. M. Kirby, and S. M. Harding.** 1980. GR 20263, a new broad-spectrum cephalosporin with antipseudomonal activity. Antimicrob. Agents Chemother. **17:**876–883.

Ceftazidime, a New Broad-Spectrum Antipseudomonal Cephalosporin: In Vitro Activity, Human Pharmacokinetics, and Therapeutic Efficacy

GEORGE K. DAIKOS,* JOHN KOSMIDIS, CHARALAMPOS STATHAKIS, HELEN GIAMARELLOU, EMMANUEL DOUZINAS, AND SERAFIM KASTANAKIS

First Department of Propedeutic Medicine, Athens University School of Medicine, King Paul's Hospital, Athens 609, Greece

In severe gram-negative infections, especially when complicated by septicemia, a bactericidal antibiotic with activity against most gram-negative bacteria, including *Pseudomonas* species, is necessary. To date, only the aminoglycosides meet this need, and they are extensively used in spite of their toxicity and the need for monitoring serum levels.

Ceftazidime (GR 20263) is a new cephalosporin that may offer the advantages of the aminoglycosides without danger of toxicity. It has an exceptionally high, broad-spectrum bactericidal activity that covers most gram-negative bacteria, including *P. aeruginosa* (1), and exhibits high stability to a wide range of bacterial β-lactamases. Its pharmacokinetic behavior in animals and volunteers is quite satisfactory.

Fifty-nine patients (24 females and 35 males) were treated with ceftazidime given intramuscularly (i.m.) or intravenously (i.v.): those suffering from urinary infection received 500 mg or 1 g every 12 h in a randomized fashion; those with lower respiratory infection similarly received either 500 mg or 1 g every 8 h based on a different set of random numbers; patients with serious infections, regardless of system affected, received higher dosages, ranging from 2 to 6 g daily, divided into two or three doses, according to the nature and severity of the infection and whether *P. aeruginosa* was present, in which case higher doses were given. The patients' ages ranged from 2 to 81 years, but 35 were aged between 51 and 80 years.

In a total of 32 patients, one or more aggravating factors were present, including renal stone in 10, other anatomical urinary abnormality in 10, hydronephrosis in 2, renal failure in 4, hemodialysis in 1, diabetes in 3, malignancy in 4, agammaglobulinemia in 1, etc.

The number of patients suffering from each infection and the dosages are given in Table 1.

Pathogens included *Escherichia coli* in 26 patients, *Klebsiella pneumoniae* in 9, other *Enterobacteriaceae* in 7, *P. aeruginosa* in 24, and others in 2. Of the above 68 strains, 56 were resistant to ampicillin, 41 to carbenicillin, 38 to cephalothin, 28 to cefamandole, and 23 to gentamicin. In particular, 17 of the 24 *P. aeruginosa* strains were resistant to carbenicillin, 16 to gentamicin, and 8 to amikacin.

Clinical and bacteriological results of treatment are presented in Table 1.

Fifty-five patients (93%) were completely cured clinically, and the remainder improved. This result is extremely satisfactory in view of the severity of the illness in many patients, the presence of aggravating factors, and the resistance pattern of the pathogens. All patients with pyelonephritis were cured, even with a dose of 500 mg every 12 h. In 8 patients the organisms persisted or relapsed in spite of clinical cure in 6. These were mostly patients with acute or recurrent pyelonephritis in the presence of kidney stone, where sterilization of urine is not expected.

Some patients had severe infections due to an organism resistant to all commercially available antibiotics and responded to ceftazidime promptly and steadily. In this category are included patients with osteomyelitis, pneumonia, septicemia, cellulitis, and a case of iatrogenic meningitis due to multiresistant *P. aeruginosa*.

The only side effect was epigastric pain reported by two patients. The injections were painless, and no thrombophlebitis occurred in any patient. One patient with acute pyelonephritis had a fall in leukocytes from 5,800 (54% neutrophils) to 2,800 (68% neutrophils), which rose during continued treatment to 4,200 (68% neutrophils) and after stopping treatment to 5,600 (56% neutrophils). Another patient with pyelonephritis and septicemia developed a rise of serum glutamic oxalacetic transaminase from 19 to 55 U and in lactic dehydrogenase from 170 to 700 U, which reverted to 21 and 350, respectively, after stopping treatment. No other laboratory abnormality was observed.

In vitro activity of ceftazidime was evaluated against 275 recent multiresistant nosocomial strains of *Enterobacteriaceae* in comparison with cephalothin, cefoxitin, and cefotaxime. In addition, 150 strains of *P. aeruginosa* were tested against ceftazidime, cefoperazone, cefotaxime, ceftriaxone, cefsulodin, and moxalactam. MICs were determined by the standard microtiter broth dilution method in tryptose phosphate broth (Difco Laboratories) with an inoculum size of 10^5 colony-forming units per ml, after dilution of an overnight culture. The MIC was defined as the concentration of antibiotic giving no visible growth after 24 h of incubation. The results in Table 2 show that ceftazidime was definitely superior to any of the antibiotics with which it was compared, with the exception of cefsulodin, which had an activity against *P. aeruginosa* comparable to that of ceftazidime.

From six patients successive specimens of serum and urine were taken after the first dose,

TABLE 1. *Therapeutic results with ceftazidime in 59 patients*[a]

Diagnosis	Daily dose (g)	No. of pts	Clinical result			Bacteriological result			
			Cure	Imp	Fail	Erad	Part erad	Pers or Rel	NA
Acute or recurrent pyelonephritis	0.5 × 2	17	17	—	—	15	—	2	—
Acute or recurrent pyelonephritis	1 × 2	18	18	—	—	17	—	1	—
Acute or recurrent pyelonephritis	Other	4	4	—	—	2	—	2	—
Exacerbated chronic bronchitis	0.5–1 × 3	3	3	—	—	1	2	—	—
Pneumonia	0.5–2 × 3	6	5	1	—	3	—	2	1
Chronic otitis media	1 × 2	1	—	1	—	1	—	—	—
Malignant otitis externa	2 × 3	1	—	1	—	—	—	1	—
Cellulitis—abscess	1 × 3	2	2	—	—	2	—	—	—
Osteomyelitis	2 × 3	3	2	1	—	3	—	—	—
Cholangitis	1–2 × 3	2	2	—	—	1	—	—	1
Meningitis, iatrogenic	2 × 3	1	1	—	—	1	—	—	—
Septicemia	2 × 3	1	1	—	—	1	—	—	—
Total		59	55	4	—	47	2	8	2

[a] Pts, Patients; Imp, improvement; Fail, failure; Erad, eradication; Part erad, partial eradication; Pers or Rel, persistence or relapse; NA, not assessable (organism not isolated).

TABLE 2. *Comparative activity of ceftazidime and various β-lactam antibiotics against 425 strains of gram-negative microorganisms*

Species (no. of isolates)	Antibiotic	Percent inhibited[a]	Inhibitory concn (mg/liter)		
			MIC_{50}	MIC_{90}	Range
E. coli (60)	Cephalothin	27	32	125	0.25->500
	Cefoxitin	89	2	16	0.12-250
	Cefotaxime	100	0.06	4	0.006-8
	Ceftazidime	100	0.25	1	<0.03-16
K. pneumoniae (60)	Cephalothin	25	32	125	0.5->500
	Cefoxitin	83	0.25	32	0.25-250
	Cefotaxime	97	0.25	8	0.003-32
	Ceftazidime	100	0.25	0.5	<0.03-8
P. mirabilis (60)	Cephalothin	35	250	>500	0.5->500
	Cefoxitin	62	8	250	0.5->500
	Cefotaxime	88	0.25	64	<0.03-250
	Ceftazidime	95	0.25	1	<0.03-64
Proteus, indole positive (45)	Cephalothin	17	250	>500	0.5->500
	Cefoxitin	55	32	>500	0.25->500
	Cefotaxime	78	0.25	64	0.03-125
	Ceftazidime	98	0.25	0.25	0.03-32
Enterobacter spp. (50)	Cephalothin	12	>500	>500	0.5->500
	Cefoxitin	40	125	>500	8->500
	Cefotaxime	80	0.5	64	0.03->500
	Ceftazidime	88	0.25	16	0.03-125
P. aeruginosa (150)	Cefotaxime	45	25	50	1.5-200
	Cefoperazone	70	6	50	1.5-200
	Ceftriaxone	67	8	64	1.5-200
	Moxalactam	85	6	50	1.5-100
	Cefsulodin	98	3	12	<1.5-25
	Ceftazidime	91	1.5	12	0.03-100

[a] At ≤16 mg/liter.

and ceftazidime concentrations were measured with an agar plate assay method, using *Proteus morgani* 235 as indicator organism for serum and *Bacillus subtilis* 1904 E for the urine assays. Mean serum concentrations after 500 mg and 1 g i.m. reached a peak of 15.1 and 33 mg/liter, respectively at 2 h. At 4 h levels were 7.3 and 16.3 mg/liter, at 6 h 5.1 and 13.7 mg/liter, and at 12 h 2.8 and 8.5 mg/liter. Half-life measured up to 6 h averaged 2.6 h, but the still high levels at 12 h indicate the presence of a γ-phase. After a 2-g i.v. bolus, levels were as follows: 15 min, 210 mg/liter; 30 min, 113 mg/liter; 1 h, 62 mg/liter; 2 h, 41 mg/liter; 3 h, 31 mg/liter; 4 h, 20 mg/liter; 6 h , 8.5 mg/liter; and 12 h, 2.1 mg/liter. Half-life at β-phase was calculated as 1.6 h, and evidence of γ-phase was again present with an apparent half-life of 3 h.

Urine levels after 500 mg i.m. were 2,100 mg/liter at 0 to 2 h, 1,740 mg/liter at 2 to 4 h, 375 mg/liter at 4.8 h, and 180 mg/liter at 8 to 12 h. Total recovery was 79% of dose. After 1 g i.m. mean levels at 0 to 2, 2 to 4, 4 to 8, and at 8 to 12 h were 4,950, 3,109, 987, and 490 mg/liter, respectively, with a total urinary recovery of 85% of dose. Finally, after 2 g i.v. urine levels were 12,000, 3,900, 1,750, and 610 mg/liter at 0 to 2, 2 to 4, 4 to 8, and 8 to 12 h, respectively, with a total recovery of 92% of dose.

Ceftazidime proved very effective in the treatment of a variety of infections which were often severe in the presence of aggravating factors and multiresistant pathogens, including *P. aeruginosa*. Tolerance and safety of the drug were excellent. In vitro studies confirmed the excellent properties of ceftazidime, and pharmacokinetic studies gave very satisfactory results.

For the treatment of urinary tract infections, 0.5 g every 12 h is adequate. In infections caused by *P. aeruginosa*, 1 g every 12 h may be indicated, however. For respiratory infections not due to *P. aeruginosa*, 0.5 g every 8 h is probably sufficient, but whenever this organism is involved 3 g or more daily is indicated. In serious, life-threatening infections 3 to 6 g should be given, according to severity and the presence or absence of *P. aeruginosa*.

1. **O'Callaghan, C. H., P. Acred, P. B. Harper, D. M. Ryan, S. M. Kirby, and S. M. Harding.** 1980. GR 20263, a new broad-spectrum cephalosporin with antipseudomonal activity. Antimicrob. Agents Chemother. **17**:876–883.

Comparative Penetration of Ceftazidime, Cefotaxime, and Gentamicin into Specific Naturally Occurring Tissue Fluid Compartments in Rabbits

D. M. RYAN, URSULA A. MASON, AND P. ACRED*

Glaxo Group Research Ltd., Greenford, Middlesex, U.K.

It is important to measure concentrations of antibiotics at extravascular sites since these are the regions where bacterial infections are normally located. Under normal conditions, extravascular fluids, of a nonexcretory nature, are generally present in small volumes in virtually inaccessible sites. To obtain sufficient volumes for assay, methods have been used to collect tissue fluid in specially created reservoirs, e.g., tissue cages or blisters on the surface of the skin. We have conducted antibiotic experiments in rabbits in which the fluids from naturally occurring compartments were sampled in situ (e.g., peritoneal, pleural, pericardial, and subcutaneous fluids, and aqueous humor). To measure the distribution of the antibiotics ceftazidime, cefotaxime, and gentamicin, each drug was dosed intramuscularly (25 mg/kg) to rabbits, and samples of serum and selected tissue fluids were removed at the following times: 0.08, 0.25, 0.5, 1.0, 2.0, 3.0, and 4.0 h. Six rabbits were killed at each time interval, and the fluids were sampled immediately. Peritoneal, pleural, and pericardial fluids were aspirated in 25-μl volumes and impregnated onto paper assay disks; subcutaneous fluid was absorbed directly onto thin paper disks (average volume taken up, 3 μl); and 0.1-ml volumes of aqueous humor were aspirated with a syringe. Concentrations of antibiotic in the various fluids were measured by large-plate microbiological assay, using suitably susceptible assay organisms. Cefotaxime concentrations were assayed with a *Proteus morganii* mutant which is resistant to desacetyl cefotaxime, the primary metabolite of cefotaxime.

For all three antibiotics, the serum levels rose quickly to achieve peak levels of 72 to 92 μg/ml within 5 to 15 min of dosing. There was then a short distributive phase followed by the elimination (β) phase. Serum concentrations of all three antibiotics at 4 h after dosing were ≤5 μg/ml. All three antibiotics were detected in the various fluids, the concentrations achieved depending on the compartment sampled and the antibiotic administered. The average peak levels of ceftazidime and gentamicin in peritoneal, pericardial, pleural, and subcutaneous fluids were 24 and 31 μg/ml, respectively. The corresponding value for cefotaxime in these fluids was only 14 μg/ml despite the fact that it had the highest peak serum level (92 μg/ml). Antibiotic concentrations in subcutaneous and peritoneal fluids were generally higher than the concurrent concentrations in pleural and pericardial fluids, probably because there was a more rapid exchange of antibiotic between these compartments and the serum. All three antibiotics gave relatively poor levels in aqueous humor. The peak values of ceftazidime, cefotaxime, and gentamicin in the various fluids are shown in Table 1. The concentration-time profiles seen for the antibiotics in the fluids, although similar in shape to the serum level profiles, were generally lower in both the peak levels attained and the areas under the curves (AUCs). The penetration of the antibiotics into the various compartments was determined by comparing the AUCs of the tissue fluids with the AUCs for their corresponding serum levels (Table 2). Gentamicin showed good penetration into peritoneal, pericardial,

TABLE 1. *Peak concentrations of ceftazidime, cefotaxime, and gentamicin achieved in various tissue fluid compartments after a single intramuscular injection (25 mg/kg) to rabbits*

Tissue fluid	Peak concn (μg/ml)		
	Ceftazidime	Cefotaxime	Gentamicin
Serum	73	92	72
Peritoneal	30	15.8	29
Pericardial	18.6	9.7	16.4
Pleural	16.1	14.3	40
Subcutaneous	31	14.8	39
Aqueous humor	0.3	1.2	4.1

TABLE 2. *Penetration of ceftazidime, cefotaxime, and gentamicin into various tissue fluid compartments after a single intramuscular injection (25 mg/kg) to rabbits*

Tissue fluid	% Penetration[a]		
	Ceftazidime	Cefotaxime	Gentamicin
Peritoneal	61	36	61
Pericardial	53	26	53
Pleural	33	31	86
Subcutaneous	38	17	48
Aqueous humor	1.0	1.7	11.0

[a] Penetration = (AUC, tissue fluid/AUC, serum) × 100.

pleural, and subcutaneous fluids, with an average penetration of 62%. Ceftazidime had an overall penetration value of 46% in the same fluids, whereas cefotaxime showed relatively poor penetration, the average being 28%. The difference in the 62% penetration seen with gentamicin and the 46% value for ceftazidime was largely due to the high degree of penetration (86%) of gentamicin into pleural fluid. Ceftazidime and cefotaxime showed relatively poor penetration into aqueous humor (1 to 2%), and the penetration of gentamicin was 11% (Table 2). However, it is likely that the concentrations of antibiotics in inflamed eyes will be somewhat higher. Data on the penetration of ceftazidime into the subcutaneous compartment in humans are available (Ryan, J. Antimicrob. Chemother., in press) and confirm the results obtained in rabbits in that ceftazidime rapidly distributes into subcutaneous tissue fluid and achieves a concentration-time profile similar to that seen in the serum, with a percent penetration of 54.

We have demonstrated that ceftazidime, cefotaxime, and gentamicin distribute into a variety of naturally occurring tissue fluid compartments in rabbits after intramuscular injection. The peak levels and AUCs attained depend on the compartment sampled and the antibiotic administered. We conclude that ceftazidime penetrates as readily as gentamicin and to a greater extent than cefotaxime. Ceftazidime has the potential to be an effective chemotherapeutic agent in treating bacterial infections located in extravascular sites.

Comparative Study of the Concentration of Cefoperazone and Ceftazidime in Bone

BASIL PAPATHANASSIOU,* JOHN KOSMIDIS, AND GEORGE K. DAIKOS

First Department of Propedeutic Medicine, Athens University School of Medicine, King Paul's Hospital, Athens 609, Greece

A very important factor for success in chemotherapy of osteomyelitis and chemoprophylaxis after orthopedic operations is concentration of the antibiotic in bone. Two methods of processing the bone specimen have been used: (i) immersion in buffer with agitation for several hours and (ii) pulverization followed by suspension in buffer. The first technique may result in incomplete elution of the drug, and destruction of the antibiotic may occur during the second procedure. It is recommended, therefore, that both techniques be performed and both results be reported.

Treatment of osteomyelitis due to *Pseudomonas aeruginosa*, which often complicates an open fracture, is a difficult task. Aminoglycosides are active in vitro, but the large dosages that are necessary for weeks or months for the successful treatment of osteomyelitis cannot be administered as a result of the danger of toxicity. Two new cephalosporins with broad spectrum and good antipseudomonal activity, ceftazidime (2) and cefoperazone (1), have offered new prospects and hopes for the treatment of *Pseudomonas* osteomyelitis.

We have studied the bone concentrations of these agents, and the results are reported here.

Twenty-two patients (9 males and 13 females) were studied. They were aged from 60 to 80 years and were all suffering from hip fractures. No pathology other than degenerative disease was present in their bones. They had not been treated with antibiotics or other substances interfering with cephalosporin kinetics in the recent past, and their renal functions were normal. The antibiotics were administered intramuscularly at a dosage of 1 or 2 g every 12 h for 1 or 3 full days before operation. The last injections were planned so that they were administered at various times before sampling. Two pieces of cancellous bone were removed, briefly washed with phosphate-buffered saline, pH 7.4, weighed, and then treated in two different ways. One piece was immersed in 1 ml of the above buffer and was agitated for 18 h at 4°C. The next day the concentration of the antibiotic in the buffer was measured and converted into bone concentration as micrograms per gram. The second piece was dried overnight at 4°C with a vacuum pump and then crushed with mortar and pestle into a pulp which was subsequently suspended in 1 ml of buffer. Assay of antibiotic was then performed in the suspension, and bone levels were calculated. A simultaneous specimen of blood was obtained with every bone specimen.

Assays were performed by using an agar cup plate technique with *Proteus morgani* 235 as assay organism for ceftazidime and *Bacillus subtilis* for cefoperazone.

Results are shown in Tables 1 and 2. Ceftazi-

TABLE 1. *Concentrations of ceftazidime in bone of 14 patients*

Daily dose (g)	Days of therapy	Hours after dose	Concn (μg/g)	
			Eluate	Crushed
1 × 2	1	2	0.1	0.3
1 × 2	1	2	0.7	2.8
1 × 2	1	3	1.4	2.2
1 × 2	1	4	0.6	0.8
1 × 2	1	6	0.2	0.0
1 × 2	3	2	3.5	3.0
1 × 2	3	4	0.3	0.8
1 × 2	3	6	3.3	11.0
2 × 2	1	2	0.2	0.2
2 × 2	1	4	1.2	1.6
2 × 2	1	6	2.4	6.2
2 × 2	3	2	12.4	15.6
2 × 2	3	4	12.6	12.5
2 × 2	3	6	7.2	6.2

TABLE 2. *Concentrations of cefoperazone in bone of eight patients*

Daily dose (g)	Days of therapy	Hours after dose	Concn (μg/g)	
			Eluate	Crushed
1 × 2	1	2	0.0	0.0
1 × 2	1	4	0.8	1.0
1 × 2	1	6	1.0	0.8
1 × 2	3	4	0.4	1.0
1 × 2	3	6	3.6	8.0
2 × 2	1	2	0.6	0.6
2 × 2	1	6	1.1	2.3
2 × 2	3	4	10.2	9.0

dime concentrations reached levels around 3 μg/g after 3 days of 1 g every 12 h, but were much higher, 6.2 to 15.6 μg/g, after 3 days of 2 g every 12 h. The latter values are quite satisfactory in view of the fact that the MIC_{90} of ceftazidime for *P. aeruginosa* is usually about 4 mg/liter (2). Concentrations of cefoperazone were somewhat lower, but they, too, reached levels of 9 to 10 μg/g after 3 days of therapy with 2 g every 12 h. However, in view of the higher MIC of cefoperazone for *P. aeruginosa*, MIC_{50} of 6.2 mg/liter and MIC_{90} of 50 mg/liter (1), these concentrations may not be adequate.

From the above data it can be concluded that ceftazidime should be a very effective drug for the treatment of osteomyelitis due to *P. aeruginosa* and, of course, other susceptible organisms. Indeed, results of treatment of *Pseudomonas* osteomyelitis have been excellent in our hands (G. K. Daikos, J. Kosmidis, C. Stathakis, H. Giamarellou, E. Douzinas, and S. Kastanakis, this volume). Cefoperazone is also well concentrated in bone, but in view of its lesser activity against *Pseudomonas*, it is not as good a choice for *Pseudomonas* osteomyelitis, unless the MIC for the infecting organism has been measured and found to be 4 mg/liter or lower. We have treated three such cases with good results (J. Kosmidis et al., unpublished data). Naturally, osteomyelitis due to other, more susceptible organisms can safely be treated with cefoperazone.

1. **Neu, H. C., K. P. Fu, N. Aswapokee, P. Aswapokee, and K. Kung.** 1979. Comparative activity and β-lactamase stability of cefoperazone, a piperazine cephalosporin. Antimicrob. Agents Chemother. **16:**150–157.
2. **O'Callaghan, C. H., P. Acred, P. B. Harper, D. M. Ryan, S. M. Kirby, and S. M. Harding.** 1980. GR 20263, a new broad-spectrum cephalosporin with antipseudomonal activity. Antimicrob. Agents Chemother. **17:**876–883.

Single- and Repeat-Dose Studies on Ceftazadime

DAVID PRATT, KEITH CAPEL-EDWARDS, AND MALCOLM TUCKER

Glaxo Group Research Ltd., Ware, Hertfordshire, England

The following program of tests was undertaken prior to initial administration of ceftazidime to humans.

Single-dose studies. The intravenous LD_{50} for mice was 7.1 g/kg in males and 6.3 g/kg in females. In tolerance studies a dose of 5 g/kg was given to mice (intravenously, subcutaneously, orally), rats (subcutaneously, intravenously), dogs (intravenously), and monkeys (intravenously); death occurred in 4 of 20 mice dosed orally and 1 of 12 rats dosed intravenously; no specific cause of death was established. All other animals were in good condition 7 days after dosing, and the only change found on microscopic examination of the major organs was slight dilatation of the renal tubules in rats.

The intramuscular irritancy of 1 ml of a 20% solution of ceftazidime injected into the sacrospinalis muscles of rabbits was mild and was less than that produced by a similar injection of benzylpenicillin.

Nephrotoxicity studies. Specific tests for

nephrotoxicity, as judged by the occurrence of proximal tubular necrosis 48 h after subcutaneous or intramuscular injection, showed that ceftazidime had a low potency in relation to cephaloridine. In mice, ceftazidime at its smallest nephrotoxic dose of 8 g/kg caused less damage than a 1.1-g/kg dose of cephaloridine. In rats a 2-g/kg dose of ceftazidime was not nephrotoxic, and the renal damage produced by a 4-g/kg dose was similar to that following a 4-g/kg dose of cefuroxime or a 2-g/kg dose of cephaloridine. In rabbits the maximum dosage was limited by the adverse effects resulting from the antibiotic alteration of gut flora, but a dose of 0.5 g of cefazidime per kg was not nephrotoxic, whereas 0.14 g of cephaloridine per kg had a marked effect.

Immediately after 10 days of treatment with a nephrotoxic dose (4 g/kg per day), rats had only residual signs of previous renal damage.

Studies in combination with other drugs that might be given concurrently with ceftazidime showed that in single-dose tests in mice furosemide or probenecid had little or no effect but respectively enhanced and diminished the nephrotoxic effect of cephaloridine. The nephrotoxic effect of 10 days of treatment of rats with gentamicin was reduced by concurrent administration of ceftazidime.

Repeat-dose studies. A total of 144 rats and 48 dogs were treated once daily for 30 days. Intravenous and subcutaneous or intramuscular administration was studied, and some animals were allowed a recovery period on completion of 1 month of treatment. Rats were given 0.1, 0.3, 0.9, 2.7, or 8.1 g/kg per day. There were no pathological changes at the lowest two dosages, though at 0.1 g/kg per day serum alanine transaminase was reduced and at 0.3 g/kg per day serum cholesterol was increased and liver and kidney weights were increased. At 0.9 g/kg there were the first signs of a mild anemia of uncertain origin and an increased urinary excretion of epithelial cells and protein. Larger doses produced a number of nonspecific abnormalities reflecting mainly stress and electrolyte disturbances. Bolus intravenous injection was immediately lethal to two rats given 2.7 g/kg and all those given 8.1 g/kg. Females tolerated both these dosages given subcutaneously, and males tolerated 2.7 g/kg per day. Males given 8.1 g/kg per day were killed after 3 days because of massive renal damage.

In dogs there was no specific toxicity at any dosage (0.06, 0.18, or 0.54 g/kg per day).

There were no differences between the effects of intravenous and subcutaneous administration, and all effects regressed soon after cessation of treatment.

Reproductive studies. Treatment during organogenesis had no teratogenic effects in mice or rabbits at the maximum dosages of 6.5 g/kg per day subcutaneously and 0.2 g/kg per day intramuscularly, respectively: in mice the young produced grew normally to weaning. In a fertility study in mice, treatment of both sexes before mating for the maturation period of their germ cells and of the females throughout pregnancy had no adverse effects except that at the maximum dosage of 6.5 g/kg per day subcutaneously the weight gain of the F_1 and F_2 generations may have been slightly affected.

Conclusions. In no test were significant toxic signs elicited except at dosages between 10 and 80 times the proposed maximum therapeutic dose of 6 g per day (about 0.1 g/kg per day). Ceftazidime, therefore, promises to be among the safest of the cephalosporin antibiotics.

In Vitro Quantitative Evaluation of Ceftazidime Compared with Cefamandole, Gentamicin, and Other Antimicrobics: a Collaborative (Four Medical Centers) Study of 7,435 Clinical Isolates and Other Special Organism Populations

RONALD N. JONES,* ARTHUR L. BARRY, CLYDE THORNSBERRY, AND THOMAS L. GAVAN

Kaiser Foundation Regional Laboratory, Clackamas, Oregon 97015, University of California, Davis, Medical Center, Sacramento, California 95871, Centers for Disease Control, Atlanta, Georgia 30333, and The Cleveland Clinic Foundation, Cleveland, Ohio 44106, U.S.A.*

Ceftazidime (CTAZ; formerly GR 20263) is an investigational semisynthetic cephalosporin with very broad spectrum of antimicrobial activity that includes the *Enterobacteriaceae* family, most species of gram-positive cocci, *Acinetobacter*, and *Pseudomonas* spp. This potent inhibition appears to be similar to that of several other new cephalosporins, and the antipseudomonal activity is comparable to that of cefsulodin (CSUL) and cefoperazone (CFOP) (2–5). CTAZ possesses clinical qualities that combine an intrinsic antimicrobial effect with β-lactamase stability and an extended serum half-life. In this evaluation we compared CTAZ to commonly prescribed parenteral drugs in the United States, cefamandole (CMAN) and gentamicin (GENT), using the reference broth microdilution method (6) in three large clinical microbiology facilities. Additional studies were performed on a subset of recently isolated bacteria pooled from six geographical locations. These strains were tested against new β-lactam compounds that included CMAN, CFOP, CSUL, cefotaxime (CTAX), cefoxitin (CFOX), ceftizoxime (CTIZ), cephalothin (CEPH), cefmenoxime (CMEN), and moxalactam (MOXA).

A total of 7,435 isolates were tested by the reference broth microdilution method (6) at The Cleveland Clinic Foundation, Kaiser Foundation Laboratories, and the University of California, Davis, Medical Center. The isolates were consecutive clinical strains from patients' infections detected over a 45- to 60-day interval (December 1980–January 1981). Most of these bacteria are tabulated in Tables 1 and 2, with others noted in the text. Another 597 bacteria were collected from the four participating laboratories, plus others contributed by P. C. Fuchs (Portland, Oregon), E. H. Gerlach (Wichita, Kansas), and H. M. Sommers (Chicago, Illinois). The breakdown of these strains is given in Tables 1 and 2 or cited in the text. The strains of β-lactamase-producing and -deficient *Haemophilus influenzae* and *Neisseria gonorrhoeae* were recent referrals to the Centers for Disease Control (C. Thornsberry).

The susceptibility test used in this protocol was the National Committee for Clinical Laboratory Standards reference broth microdilution technique (6) with divalent cation-supplemented Mueller-Hinton broth (Difco Laboratories, Detroit, Mich.). The major technical steps included: an inoculum of 5×10^5 colony-forming units per ml; 15- to 18-h incubation; 35°C incubator temperature; ambient air (except some fastidious streptococci); three observer readings; and the use of five quality control strains that included *Escherichia coli* ATCC 25922, *Staphylococcus aureus* ATCC 25923, *Pseudomonas aeruginosa* ATCC 27853, *Streptococcus faecalis* ATCC 29212, and *S. aureus* ATCC 29213. All quality control results were within the preestablished limits for the investigational and reference drugs.

TABLE 1. *In vitro activity of CTAZ, CMAN, and GENT against Enterobacteriaceae clinical isolates and selected challenge strains tested against seven other antimicrobics*

Organism	Source (no.)[a]	Median MIC (μg/ml) of:									
		CTAZ	CMAN	GENT	CFOP	CMEN	CTAX	CTIZ	MOXA	CFOX	CEPH
Citrobacter diversus	C (31)	≤0.12	0.5	0.5	—	—	—	—	—	—	—
	S (10)	0.25	1.0	0.5	0.12	0.06	0.12	0.12	0.12	2.0	4.0
C. freundii	C (59)	0.5	2.0	0.5	—	—	—	—	—	—	—
	S (11)	0.5	2.0	1.0	0.5	0.25	0.25	0.12	0.25	64	>64
Enterobacter aerogenes	C (94)	≤0.12	1.0	0.5	—	—	—	—	—	—	—
	S (21)	0.25	2.0	0.5	0.25	0.06	0.06	0.06	0.25	>64	>64
E. cloacae	C (181)	0.5	4.0	0.5	—	—	—	—	—	—	—
	S (18)	0.12	4.0	0.5	0.5	0.12	0.25	0.06	0.12	>64	>64
Escherichia coli	C (2275)	≤0.12	0.5	0.5	—	—	—	—	—	—	—
	S (25)	0.12	0.5	1.0	0.12	0.06	0.06	0.03	0.12	2.0	8.0
Klebsiella spp.	C (537)	≤0.12	1.0	0.5	—	—	—	—	—	—	—
	S (25)	0.12	1.0	0.5	0.25	0.06	0.06	0.06	0.12	2.0	4.0
Morganella morganii	C (97)	≤0.12	8.0	0.5	—	—	—	—	—	—	—
	S (10)	0.12	16	2.0	1.0	0.06	0.06	0.5	0.25	8.0	>64
Proteus mirabilis	C (372)	≤0.12	0.5	1.0	—	—	—	—	—	—	—
	S (25)	0.06	0.5	0.5	0.5	0.01	0.01	0.12	0.25	2.0	4.0
P. vulgaris	C (30)	≤0.12	>32	0.5	—	—	—	—	—	—	—
	S (10)	0.06	>64	1.0	1.0	0.12	0.06	0.25	0.25	2.0	>64
Providencia spp.	C (70)	≤0.12	0.5	2.0	—	—	—	—	—	—	—
	S (29)	0.5	8.0	8.0	4.0	0.12	0.25	0.25	0.25	4.0	>64
Serratia spp.	C (268)	≤0.12	>32	0.5	—	—	—	—	—	—	—
	S (25)	0.25	>64	1.0	2.0	0.12	0.5	0.5	0.5	32	>64

[a] C, Clinical isolates; S, selected challenge strains.

TABLE 2. *In vitro activity of CTAZ, reference β-lactam, and GENT against commonly isolated nonfermentative gram-negative bacilli, S. aureus, and streptococci*

Organism	No. clinical/ no. selective challenge	Agent[a]	Clinical isolates		Stock strains	
			MIC_{50}	MIC_{90}	MIC_{50}	MIC_{90}
Acinetobacter calcoaceticus subsp. *anitratus*	56/15	CTAZ	4.0	8.0	8.0	16
	120/15	CTIZ	4.0	32	8.0	16
	132/15	CTAX	8.0	32	16	16
	56/15	GENT	0.5	8.0	1.0	4.0
Pseudomonas aeruginosa	759/50	CTAZ	2.0	4.0	2.0	4.0
	520/50	CSUL	4.0	16	2.0	4.0
	718/50	CFOP	4.0	16	4.0	8.0
	718/50	GENT	4.0	8.0	4.0	16
Pseudomonas spp.	85/30	CTAZ	2.0	32	4.0	64
	16/30	CFOP	2.0	64	16	128
	146/30	CTAX	8.0	>32	16	256
	85/30	GENT	1.0	>32	0.5	>64
Staphylococcus aureus	1,161/50	CTAZ	8.0	8.0	8.0	16
	924/50	CEPH	≤0.25	1.0	≤0.25	0.5
	936/50	CMAN	≤0.5	1.0	≤0.25	1.0
	1,161/50	GENT	0.5	8.0	0.25	0.5
Streptococcus faecalis	683/25	CTAZ	>32	>32	>256	>256
	588/25	CFOP	64	64	32	32
	680/25	CMAN	32	>32	32	32
	683/25	GENT	32	32	32	32
S. pneumoniae	2/20	CTAZ	—	—	0.25	0.5
	100/20	CTAX	≤0.5	≤0.5	0.01	0.06
	17/20	CFOP	≤0.25	1.0	0.12	0.25
	19/20	GENT	≤0.25	8.0	0.5	8.0
Beta-hemolytic *Streptococcus* spp.	37/20	CTAZ	≤0.12	0.5	0.12	0.12
	81/20	CTAX	≤0.5	≤0.5	≤0.008	0.03
	84/20	CFOP	≤0.25	1.0	0.12	0.12
	37/20	GENT	4.0	32	8.0	16

[a] Clinical series data for CTAX, CFOP, CEPH, CSUL, and MOXA taken from references (1–5). Only the CTAZ data, the other two most active β-lactam antimicrobics, and GENT are shown from this protocol.

An agar dilution method was used to determine MICs for *N. gonorrhoeae* (1). Fildes' peptic digest of horse cells was added to the inoculum (5%) for the broth testing of *N. meningitidis*, *S. pneumoniae*, *S. pyogenes*, and other fastidious streptococci. The antimicrobics were obtained from the appropriate pharmaceutical companies, which included: Glaxo Research Group, Hoechst-Roussel Pharmaceuticals, Eli Lilly Research Laboratories, Pfizer Inc., Abbott Laboratories, Merck Sharp & Dohme, Schering Corp., and Smith Kline & French.

Table 1 summarizes the *Enterobacteriaceae* results that show little variation between CTAZ, CMAN, and GENT against clinical and stock organism populations. CTAZ median (MIC_{50}) values range from 0.12 to 1.0 μg/ml. Only *Citrobacter freundii* and *Enterobacter aerogenes* showed MIC_{90}s of CTAZ >8 μg/ml. CTAZ was markedly superior to CMAN (MIC_{90} range, 2 to >32 μg/ml) and GENT (MIC_{90} range, 1 to 32 μg/ml). CTAZ inhibited >77% of *C. freundii* isolates and >98% of all enteric bacilli at ≤8 μg/ml (MIC_{50} = 0.5 μg/ml). A similarly excellent spectrum against the stock strains was found for CFOP, CMEN, CTAX, CTIZ, and MOXA. CTAX and CTIZ seem most potent among the "third-generation" drugs, with CTAZ and CMEN intermediate and MOXA and CFOP least inhibitory. All of these agents inhibited >95% of enteric bacilli at ≤8 μg/ml. The most resistant species for all third-generation drugs were *C. freundii*, *E. aerogenes*, and *E. cloacae* (5 to 18% resistant).

Table 2 shows the in vitro results against nonfermentative gram-negative bacilli and gram-positive cocci. CTAZ was the most active cephalosporin tested against *Acinetobacter* (MIC_{50} and MIC_{90}, 4 and 8 μg/ml). The next most active β-lactams were CTIZ and CTAX. CTAZ was also the most effective broad-spectrum cephalosporin against *P. aeruginosa* (median MIC, 2 μg/ml) and *Pseudomonas* spp. (median MIC, 2 μg/ml). Only CSUL and CFOP had comparable MICs against the *P. aeruginosa* isolates (medians of 4 μg/ml). CTAZ was excellent against all *Pseudomonas* spp. except *P. maltophilia*, against which MOXA and CFOP were slightly more effective. Most new cephalosporins are *not* comparable to CEPH or CMAN in anti-staphylococcal effect. The MIC_{50} and MIC_{90} of CTAZ against *S. aureus* were 8 μg/ml. None of the cephalosporins or aminoglycosides was active on enterococci or methicillin-resistant *S. aureus*. The methoxyimino compounds had very low MICs against *H. influenzae* (CTAZ MIC range, 0.015 to 0.25), *N. gonorrhoeae* (CTAZ range, ≤0.008 to 0.12), *N. meningitidis* (CTAZ range, ≤0.008 to 0.03), *S. pyogenes* (CTAZ range, 0.06 to 0.12), and pneumococcus (CTAZ range, 0.12 to 4). The highest MIC of CTAZ against *S. pneumoniae* was with a penicillin-resistant isolate (penicillin G MIC, 8 μg/ml).

CTAZ was found to be bactericidal, minimally influenced by inoculum concentration increases (some strain variation), and would inhibit 71% of CEPH/CMAN-resistant isolates (≤8 μg/ml). In a group of 50 strains resistant to aminoglycosides, 88% were inhibited by CTAZ at ≤8 μg/ml, compared with 80% for CFOP and 74% for MOXA.

We conclude that CTAZ is a very promising new cephalosporin with a spectrum of use that includes nearly all commonly isolated facultative species. Only enterococci, some *P. maltophilia* isolates, and methicillin-resistant *S. aureus* were routinely CTAZ resistant.

1. **Baker, C. N., C. Thornsberry, and R. N. Jones.** 1980. In vitro antimicrobial activity of cefoperazone, cefotaxime, moxalactam (LY127935), azlocillin, mezlocillin, and other beta-lactam antibiotics against *Neisseria gonorrhoeae* and *Haemophilus influenzae*, including beta-lactamase-producing strains. Antimicrob. Agents Chemother. **17**:757–761.
2. **Barry, A. L., R. N. Jones, and C. Thornsberry.** 1981. Cefsulodin: antibacterial activity and tentative interpretive zone standards for the disk susceptibility test. Antimicrob. Agents Chemother. **20**:525–529.
3. **Fuchs, P. C., A. L. Barry, C. Thornsberry, R. N. Jones, T. L. Gavan, E. H. Gerlach, and H. M. Sommers.** 1981. Cefotaxime: in vitro activity and tentative interpretive standards for disk susceptibility testing. Antimicrob. Agents Chemother. **18**:88–93.
4. **Jones, R. N., P. C. Fuchs, A. L. Barry, T. L. Gavan, H. M. Sommers, and E. H. Gerlach.** 1980. Cefoperazone (T-1551), a new semisynthetic cephalosporin: comparison with cephalothin and gentamicin. Antimicrob. Agents Chemother. **17**:743–749.
5. **Jones, R. N., P. C. Fuchs, H. M. Sommers, T. L. Gavan, A. L. Barry, and E. H. Gerlach.** 1980. Moxalactam (LY127935), a new semisynthetic 1-oxa-beta-lactam antibiotic with remarkable antimicrobial activity: in vitro comparison with cefamandole and tobramycin. Antimicrob. Agents Chemother. **17**:750–756.
6. **National Committee for Clinical Laboratory Standards.** 1980. Standard methods for dilution antimicrobial susceptibility tests for bacteria which grow aerobically. Proposed Standard, M7-P, National Committee for Clinical Laboratory Standards, Villanova, Pa.

Investigations on the In Vitro Antibacterial Activity of Cefsulodin

GEORG PETERS* AND GERHARD PULVERER

Hygiene-Institut der Universität, Cologne, Federal Republic of Germany

Infections caused by *Pseudomonas aeruginosa*, especially when they occur as nosocomial infections, are often characterized by a strong clinical course and difficult therapeutic problems. The number of antibiotics effective against *Pseudomonas* is very small because of its multiple drug resistance. The new cephalosporin cefsulodin has been reported to be very active against *P. aeruginosa* and *Pseudomonas* group bacteria (4, 5). The mean serum concentration reached 10 min after intravenous injection of 1,000 mg of cefsulodin is 90 to 130 mg/liter and is about 20 mg/liter after 2 h (1; W. Glöckner and G. Peters, unpublished data). Furthermore, this substance seems to be very stable to various β-lactamases from gram-negative and gram-positive bacteria (2).

We examined the in vitro antibacterial activity of cefsulodin against 144 *P. aeruginosa* strains in comparison with that of azlocillin, ticarcillin, piperacillin, and cefoperazone. Cefsulodin was also tested against 102 other gram-negative rods and 60 gram-positive cocci. All strains were freshly isolated and expecially selected on the basis of their clinical importance. Their identification and differentiation were performed according to *Bergey's Manual*, 8th edition. The MICs were determined by the agar dilution test recommended by an international collaborative study as previously described (3). Mueller-Hinton broth and Mueller-Hinton agar were used as test media. The inoculation was carried out with a multipoint inoculator; the inoculum was adjusted to 10^5 colony-forming

TABLE 1. *Comparative activity of cefsulodin against P. aeruginosa (n = 144)*

Antibiotic	MIC (mg/liter)								
	0.78	1.56	3.12	6.25	12.5	25	50	100	>100
Ticarcillin				1[a]	17	66	74	85	100
Azlocillin			2	13	55	74	83	86	100
Piperacillin			11	56	72	82	86	94	100
Cefoperazone			4	37	76	85	91	94	100
Cefsulodin		11	51	74	83	90	92	97	100

[a] Cumulative percentage of strains inhibited.

TABLE 2. *Comparative activity of cefsulodin against 37 azlocillin-resistant P. aeruginosa strains*

Antibiotic	MIC (mg/liter)							
	1.56	3.12	6.25	12.5	25	50	100	>100
Azlocillin						35[a]	43	100
Ticarcillin			3	8	16	19	43	100
Piperacillin			3	11	32	46	76	100
Cefoperazone			3	35	51	65	78	100
Cefsulodin	3	22	30	49	68	73	86	100

[a] Cumulative percentage of strains inhibited.

units. Positive and negative controls, and also three activity controls (*Staphylococcus aureus* ATCC 25923, *Escherichia coli* ATCC 25922, *P. aeruginosa* ATCC 27853), were always included.

Cefsulodin was inactive against all strains examined of *E. coli*, *Klebsiella* spp., *Citrobacter* spp., *Enterobacter* spp., *Serratia* spp., and *Proteus* spp. Within the group of gram-positive cocci, all strains of *Streptococcus faecalis* were resistant to cefsulodin. With staphylococci and micrococci, MICs of 1.56 to 12.5 mg/liter were found, and with *S. pyogenes*,, *S. agalactiae*, and *S. pneumoniae* they ranged from 0.78 to 12.5 mg/liter. Although cefsulodin showed some activity against staphylococci and streptococci, its clinical importance has to be doubted because of the availability of other, more effective drugs.

In contrast to this statement, cefsulodin demonstrated a very remarkable activity range against *P. aeruginosa*. In comparison with azlocillin, ticarcillin, piperacillin, and cefoperazone, cefsulodin was the most active antipseudomonal drug tested (Table 1). Eighty-three percent of all strains tested were inhibited by cefsulodin concentrations of 1.56 to 12.5 mg/liter, and 90% were inhibited at 25 mg/liter. Only 8% of 144 strains remained resistant to cefsulodin. No cross-resistance of cefsulodin with the other antibiotics tested could be observed. Table 2 shows the comparative activity of cefsulodin against 37 azlocillin-resistant *P. aeruginosa* strains. Forty-nine percent of those strains were inhibited by cefsulodin concentrations of 1.56 to 12.5 mg/liter, and about 70% were inhibited by 25 mg/liter. Here again, cefsulodin was the most active substance tested.

In conclusion, we can state that cefsulodin is the first cephalosporin with significant activity against *P. aeruginosa*. Pharmacological investigations and clinical experience are now needed to confirm the very positive bacteriological results.

1. **Mashimo, K., T. Taguchi, Y. Nakano, T. Yamamoto, and N. Yamaguchi.** 1978. Pharmacology of SCE-129, a new cephalosporin antibiotic, in human volunteers, p. 841–842. *In* W. Siegenthaler and R. Lüthy (ed.), Current chemotherapy, vol. 2. American Society for Microbiology, Washington, D.C.
2. **Okonogi, K., M. Kida, M. Yondea, Y. Itoh, and S. Mitshuhashi.** 1978. In vitro characterization of CGP 7174/E, a cephalosporin active against *Pseudomonas*, p. 838–841. *In* W. Siegenthaler and R. Lüthy (ed.), Current chemotherapy, vol. 2. American Society for Microbiology, Washington, D.C.
3. **Peters, G., and G. Pulverer.** 1980. Comparative in vitro activity of cefotaxime (HR 756). Chemotherapy (Basel) **26**:177–183.
4. **Tsuchiya, K., M. Kondo, and H. Nagatomo.** 1978. SCE-129, antipseudomonal cephalosporin: in vitro and in vivo antibacterial activities. Antimicrob. Agents Chemother. **13**:137–145.
5. **Ullmann, U.** 1979. Bacteriological studies with cefsulodin (CGP 7174/E), the first antipseudomonal cephalosporin. J. Antimicrob. Chemother. **5**:563–567.

In Vitro Susceptibility of *Pseudomonas aeruginosa* and Other Nonfermentative Gram-Negative Bacilli to Cefsulodin and Nine Other Antibiotics: a Multicenter Study

K. MACHKA,* U. ULLMANN, W. RITZERFELD, G. RUCKDESCHL, H. KNOTHE, AND I. BRAVENY

Institute of Medical Microbiology, Technical University of Munich, D-8000 Munich 80, Federal Republic of Germany

The in vitro activity of cefsulodin, a new semisynthetic sulfacephalosporin, was compared with that of three other cephalosporins (cefotaxime, moxalactam, and cefoperazone), two penicillins (azlocillin and piperacillin), and four aminoglycosides (gentamicin, tobramycin, amikacin, and netilmicin) against recently obtained isolates of *Pseudomonas aeruginosa* and other nonfermentative gram-negative bacilli. The isolates were collected consecutively over a period of 3 weeks in various university hospitals (Kiel, Munich, Muenster, and Frankfort).

The strains were identified by normal bacteriological techniques, by pigment formation, and biochemically by API 20. *P. aeruginosa* strains were serotyped by agglutination slide screening according to O antigens, using commercially available antisera. The MIC determinations were performed by the microdilution technique, using Mueller-Hinton broth supplemented with 0.5% glucose and 0.002% phenol red. The inoculum was adjusted to 10^5 colony-forming units per ml. The limits of susceptibility were defined as 16 mg/liter for the cephalosporins, piperacillin, and amikacin, as 4 mg/liter for the other aminoglycosides, and as 64 mg/liter for azlocillin. To determine the MBC, 10 μl was taken from each well of the microtiter plate showing no visible growth. Each 10-μl sample was then subcultivated on antibiotic-free Mueller-Hinton agar.

Pseudomonas spp. were most frequently cultured from midstream urine, wound, and ear swabs. The proportion of *Pseudomonas* spp. isolated from tracheal secretion and sputum varied from city to city. In Frankfort no strains were found in tracheal secretions whereas in Muenster 18% and in Kiel 20% of the *Pseudomonas* strains were isolated from tracheal secretions. Only three *P. aeruginosa* strains were isolated from blood. In the case of 39 strains, duplicates of the strains were isolated.

We found 25 strains (7.9%) of different nonfermentative gram-negative bacilli within the 318 recently isolated strains. The isolates belonged to the species *P. cepacia*, *P. fluorescens*, *Alcaligenes* spp., *P. maltophilia*, *P. stutzeri*, *Achromobacter*, *Acinetobacter calcoaceticus*, and *P. paucimobilis*. The most frequently occurring *P. aeruginosa* O serotype was type 6 followed by types 11, 5, and 16. Statistical calculation of percentage distribution of the *P. aeruginosa* serotypes most frequently encountered in the specimens collected was impossible because of the wide scattering of serotypes and sources.

The susceptibility of *P. aeruginosa* to the antibiotics tested is shown in Table 1. Cefsulodin demonstrated better antibacterial activity than the new broad-spectrum cephalosporins tested, inhibiting 95% of the *P. aeruginosa* strains (2). Cefotaxime and moxalactam inhibited 76 and 77% of these strains, respectively, and cefoperazone inhibited 84%. Azlocillin and piperacillin inhibited nearly the same percentage of *P. aeruginosa* strains as cefoperazone. The aminoglycoside amikacin inhibited 98% of the strains, the highest percentage of inhibition of all drugs tested, whereas the other three aminoglycosides inhibited nearly 90% of the strains at a concentration of 4 mg/liter.

Cefsulodin was also active against the nonfermentative bacilli except some strains of *P. fluorescens*, *Alcaligenes* spp., *P. cepacia*, and *Achromobacter*. These results agree with those of Shannon et al. (1).

There were local variations in the percentages resistant to the various drugs. Whereas in Frankfort all *P. aeruginosa* strains were susceptible to cefsulodin and 97% were susceptible to azlocillin, in Munich only 91% were susceptible to cefsulodin, and in Kiel only 81% were susceptible to azlocillin. For the aminoglycosides the reverse was true, the percentage of strains resistant to gentamicin, amikacin, and netilmicin being higher in Frankfort than in the other three cities.

We established the MBC of each drug (Table 2). The MBC of cefsulodin was the same as the MIC in 60% of the 50 strains investigated. In 38% of the strains, the MBC was twice as high as the MIC. Piperacillin showed the lowest percentage of concordance between MBC and MIC; gentamicin and tobramycin showed the highest percentage (70%).

We found 27 *P. aeruginosa* strains resistant

TABLE 1. *Susceptibility of P. aeruginosa to 10 antibiotics*

Antibiotic	Geometric mean	Cumulative % of inhibition with given MIC (mg/liter)									
		≤0.25	0.5	1	2	4	8	16	32	64	≥128
Cefsulodin	3.1		4	19	62	77	91	95	96	97	100
Cefotaxime	11.6			1	2	21	32	76	89	97	100
Moxalactam	10.7		1	1	9	29	53	77	90	97	100
Cefoperazone	7.2		1	2	13	55	73	84	91	95	100
Azlocillin	16.0		0.5	1	2	12	50	69	84	88	100
Piperacillin	8.6		0.5	1	5	49	70	83	90	93	100
Gentamicin	3.0	13	61	78	86	90	91	92	93	94	100
Tobramycin	0.5	60	83	89	91	92	94	95	97	99	100
Amikacin	2.0	1	5	39	73	87	95	98	99	100	
Netilmicin	1.3	3	20	64	79	90	95	96	97	100	

TABLE 2. *Percentage of MBCs equaling MICs for Pseudomonas spp. (n = 50)*

Antibiotic	% MBC = MIC	% MBC = 2× MIC	% MBC = 4× MIC
Cefsulodin	60	38	2
Cefotaxime	65	32	2
Moxalactam	64	32	4
Cefoperazone	64	32	4
Azlocillin	64	30	6
Piperacillin	44	40	16
Gentamicin	70	28	2
Tobramycin	70	26	4
Amikacin	64	34	2
Netilmicin	56	40	4

to gentamicin. Cefsulodin inhibited 79% of these strains. Cefsulodin also inhibited 79% of the strains resistant to the other cephalosporins tested; 74% of the strains resistant to azlocillin were susceptible to cefsulodin.

The good in vitro activity of cefsulodin indicates that the drug may be useful in the therapy of infections caused by *P. aeruginosa* and some of the other nonfermentative gram-negative bacilli.

1. **Shannon, K., A. King, and I. Phillips.** 1980. In vitro antibacterial activity of cefsulodin, an antipseudomonal cephalosporin, p. 188–190. *In* Current chemotherapy and infectious disease. American Society for Microbiology, Washington, D.C.
2. **Tsuchiya, K., M. Kondo, and H. Nagotoma.** 1978. SCE-129, antipseudomonal cephalosporin: in vitro and in vivo antibacterial activities. Antimicrob. Agents Chemother. **13:**137–145.

Cefsulodin and *Pseudomonas aeruginosa*: the Influence of β-Lactamases

R. LABIA,* R. BEGUIN, J. M. MASSON, AND A. KAZMIERCZAK

CNRS-CERCOA, 94320 Thiais, and Faculté de Médecine, 21033 Dijon, France*

Cefsulodin (6) is a new cephalosporin that is highly active against *Pseudomonas aeruginosa*. This bacterial species is usually resistant to a large number of antibiotics, including many β-lactam compounds. *P. aeruginosa* resistance to β-lactam antibiotics is very often related to β-lactamase production. Thus, it was interesting to study the behavior of cefsulodin toward the usual β-lactamases of this bacterial species, in comparison with some other β-lactam antibiotics which are also known for their antibacterial activity against *P. aeruginosa*.

A large variety of β-lactamases can be produced by *P. aeruginosa* strains. They can be classified into two main groups: penicillinases and cephalosporinases. The penicillinases which may be R-factor mediated include the TEM-type enzymes, such as the TEM-1 and TEM-2, and carbenicillinases, such as CARB-1 (also named PSE-4), CARB-2 (also named PSE-1), and CARB-3, and some other enzymes (1, 3). These β-lactamases have a common property: they confer to the producing strains a high level of resistance to carbenicillin and probably to all of the other anti-*P. aeruginosa* penicillins. On the other hand, *P. aeruginosa* strains usually produce a chromosomally mediated, and inducible, cephalosporinase. A large number of these enzymes are known, but apart from their various isoelectric points and levels of production or biosynthesis, these enzymes present very closely related biochemical properties. The best-known cephalosporinase is probably the one produced by the NCTC 8203 strain, the so-called Sabath and Abraham's enzyme (5).

Kinetic constants. After bacterial culture, extraction of β-lactamases by established methods (e.g., ultrasound), and various purifications, the kinetic constants were determined by on-line computerized microacidimetry (3). Table 1 shows that, with the TEM-1 and CARB-2 enzymes, cefsulodin appears to be a "bad substrate." This point is characterized by a very low V_m, associated with a low affinity for the enzymes: high K_m.

This double aspect is relevant, as a given molecule can be considered resistant to hydrolysis only if it shows a high ratio $\tau = K_m/V_m$, which is directly proportional to the half-life of the antibiotic in the presence of the β-lactamase (3). For these two enzymes, we can see a quite similar situation for cefotaxime and moxalactam, which are extremely resistant to these enzymes. Cefoperazone is moderately hydrolyzed, particularly by the TEM-1. With the CARB-2 enzyme, which is a true penicillinase, it is surprising to see that cefoperazone is the antibiotic which presents the best affinity (lower K_m or K_i). Thus, all of the penicillins tested are extremely susceptible to hydrolysis.

Sabath and Abraham's cephalosporinase (5) shows almost no degradation of cefsulodin: poor affinity and low hydrolysis. On the other hand, the action of this enzyme is difficult to quantify in the particular case of cefotaxime, in relation with its very good affinity constant (low K_i). Moxalactam shows a similar situation, but this molecule can also act as a cephalosporinase inactivator (R. Labia, unpublished data). This cephalosporinase also has a moderate activity against cefoperazone. It is possible to classify the penicillins tested into two groups: the carboxypenicillins (carbenicillin and ticarcillin), which appear resistant to hydrolysis, and the ureidopenicillins (azlocillin, mezlocillin, and piperacillin), which are more readily hydrolyzed.

Masuda's double disk technique. To confirm or refute the analysis of the kinetic constants and to clarify the results for the antibiotics which were resistant to hydrolysis, we used the very sensitive bacteriological double-disk technique described by Masuda et al. (4). Figure 1 shows the action of penicillinases TEM-1 (A) and CARB-2 (B) and of the cephalosporinases produced by strains NCTC 8203 (C) and NCTC 10701 (D). This last strain is identical to NCTC 10490. The antibiotics tested were cefsulodin and five other β-lactam antibiotics selected from the various classes of antibiotics previously studied.

In the first instance, we can see that, on the whole, the two penicillinases (A and B) present the same action, as do the two cephalosporinases (C and D). With the two penicillinases cefsulodin shows a slight hydrolysis, which probably is more important than the kinetic constants would suggest. Nevertheless, its resistance to the cephalosporinases appears excellent. Carbenicillin is a carboxypenicillin which is very sensitive to penicillinases, but also extremely resistant to the action of cephalosporinases. Azlocillin, a ureidopenicillin, shows a sensitivity to penicillinases comparable to that of carbenicillin, but it is more sensitive to the action of cephalosporinases. Cefoperazone is subject to some degradation by both types of enzymes. Cefotaxime and moxalactam, which are extremely resistant to the action of the penicillinases, show an unsuspected slight sensitivity to cephalosporinases, which is probably more important with cefotaxime than with moxalactam.

In conclusion, we have observed that there is no β-lactam antibiotic totally resistant to the action of β-lactamases. However, in comparison

TABLE 1. *Kinetic constants of β-lactamases*

Antibiotic	TEM-1			CARB-2			Cephalosporinase		
	K_m (μM)	V_m[a]	τ[a]	K_m (μM)	V_m	τ	K_m (μM)	V_m	τ
Penicillin G	22	100	100	7.2	100	100	3.0	100	100
Carbenicillin	13.6	10.6	583	67.5	318	295	0.06	ND	—
Ticarcillin	9.7	9.6	459	17.7	238	103	0.03	ND	—
Azlocillin	35	60	257	5	50	129	0.45	5.4	277
Mezlocillin	253	102	1,127	14	83	234	1.25	2.8	1,490
Piperacillin	66	120	250	3.7	11	470	1.1	2.5	1,470
Cefoperazone	270	40	3,070	0.1	<1	—	160	9	60,000
Cefotaxime	>3,000	ND	—	>1,000	ND	—	0.13	ND	—
Moxalactam	>2,000	ND	—	>1,000	ND	—	0.2	ND	—
Cefsulodin	2600	<1	—	>600	5	—	120	≃1	400,000

[a] V_m and τ are expressed as a percentage of the corresponding values for penicillin G. ND, Not determined.

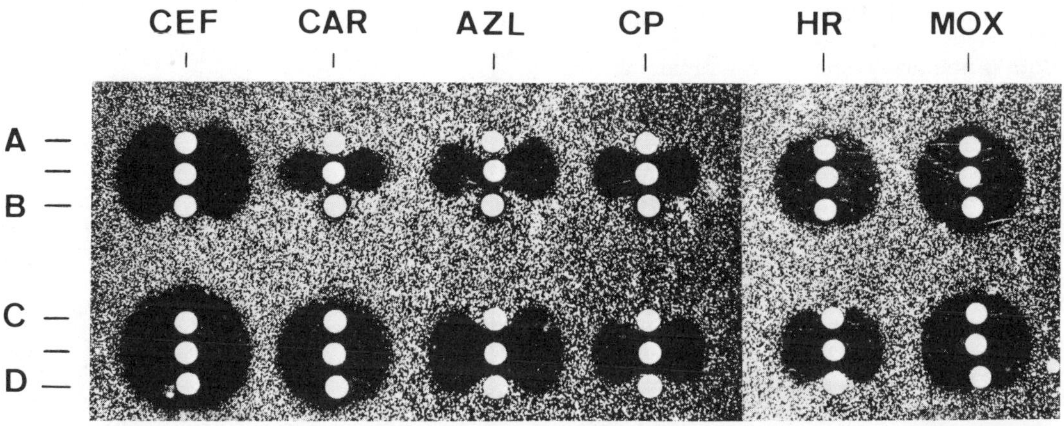

FIG. 1. *Masuda's double disk technique. The enzymes are penicillinases TEM-1 (A) and CARB-2 (B) and cephalosporinases from P. aeruginosa strains NCTC 8203 (C) and 10701 (D). Antibiotics: CEF = cefsulodin, CAR = carbenicillin, AZL = azlocillin, CP = cefoperazone, HR = cefotaxime, and MOX = moxalactam. Indicator organism: susceptible P. aeruginosa strain.*

with other β-lactam antibiotics that are active against *P. aeruginosa* strains, cefsulodin shows a slight sensitivity to the action of penicillinases but an excellent resistance to the action of cephalosporinases.

1. **Jacoby, G. A., and M. Matthew.** 1979. The distribution of β-lactamases genes on plasmids found in *Pseudomonas*. Plasmid **2:**41–47.
2. **Jacoby, G. A., and L. Sutton.** 1979. Activity of β-lactam antibiotics against *Pseudomonas aeruginosa* carrying R-plasmid determining different β-lactamases. Antimicrob. Agents Chemother. **16:**243–245.
3. **Labia, R., M. Guionie, M. Barthélémy, and A. Philippon.** 1981. Properties of three carbenicillin-hydrolysing β-lactamases (CARB) from *Pseudomonas aeruginosa*: identification of a new enzyme. J. Antimicrob. Chemother. **7:**49–56.
4. **Masuda G., S. Tomioka, and M. Hasegawa.** 1976. Detection of β-lactamase production by gram-negative bacteria. J. Antibiot. **29:**662–664.
5. **Sabath, L. D., M. Jago, and E. P. Abraham.** 1965. Cephalosporinase and penicillinase activities of a β-lactamase from *Pseudomonas pyocyanea*. Biochem. J. **96:**739–752.
6. **Tsuchiya K., M. Kondo, and H. Nagatomo.** 1978. SCE 129 antipseudomonal cephalosporin, in vitro and in vivo antibacterial activities. Antimicrob. Agents Chemother. **13:**137–145.

Killing Kinetics of Cefsulodin, Ceftazidime, and Gentamicin in *Pseudomonas aeruginosa*

B. L. SINGLETON

The London Hospital Medical College, London, U.K.

The efficacy of cefsulodin against *Pseudomonas aeruginosa* was adequately demonstrated in studies of MICs and MBCs reported at the 11th International Congress of Chemotherapy. Goto et al. (1) suggested that it was as effective as gentamicin. Tsuchiya et al. (2) found a killing effect at the MIC, with an inoculum of 10^5 organisms.

In this study the killing activity of cefsulodin was compared with that of gentamicin and also ceftazidime, another cephalosporin active against *Pseudomonas aeruginosa*. Combinations of both cephalosporins with gentamicin were studied for a possible synergistic effect.

Three strains of *P. aeruginosa*, R20, R29, and R70, were used, against which MICs of cefsulodin were 2, 8, and 64 μg/ml, respectively. R29 produced PSE-1 β-lactamase, and R70 showed barried-mediated resistance. The MICs of gentamicin were 2, 1, and 0.5 μg/ml, and those of ceftazidime were 1, 1, and 16 μg/ml, respectively.

The studies were performed with shaking cultures in Oxoid No. 2 nutrient broth, the antibiotics being added during the logarithmic phase of growth. Viable counts were performed on nutrient agar, and morphology was assessed with phase-contrast microscopy.

With inocula of 10^2 to 10^3 organisms of the

susceptible strain R20 per ml, cefsulodin, at the MIC, reduced the viable count to zero in 6 h. Both gentamicin alone and gentamicin in combination with cefsulodin killed in 4 h. Regrowth occurred in all cultures between 8 and 24 h.

With R20 inocula of 10^8 organisms per ml, neither cefsulodin nor gentamicin, alone or in combination, had an effect on growth at the MIC or four times the MIC.

With R20 inocula of 10^6 organisms per ml, both cefsulodin and ceftazidime at the MIC and four times the MIC held the viable count to an increase of within 1 log throughout 24 h. Gentamicin at the MIC had a similar effect but showed marked killing at the higher concentration, with regrowth between 8 and 24 h.

Both cefsulodin and ceftazidime showed a similar lack of effect against strain R70 at the MIC and four times the MIC. However, viable counts at 24 h were reduced to 10^5 with the higher concentration. Gentamicin showed greater activity but again allowed regrowth between 8 and 24 h.

Against the β-lactamase-producing strain, both cephalosporins again showed a "static" effect up to 8 h, with a subsequent increase in viable count. Gentamicin behaved as previously.

At the MIC, both cefsulodin and ceftazidime appeared to show synergy with gentamicin only against the susceptible R20 strain. This effect was more pronounced with ceftazidime (Fig. 1).

Both cefsulodin and ceftazidime produced marked filamentation, apparently in proportion to their concentrations and not to their relative efficacies. Small "bud-shaped" projections were observed on some filaments. Combination of either cephalosporin with gentamicin at the MIC produced filaments of up to 25 μm in length, with no apparent relationship to killing activity. At 24 h, a mixture of "ghost" filaments and normal-sized rods or short filaments of two or three elongated cells was observed.

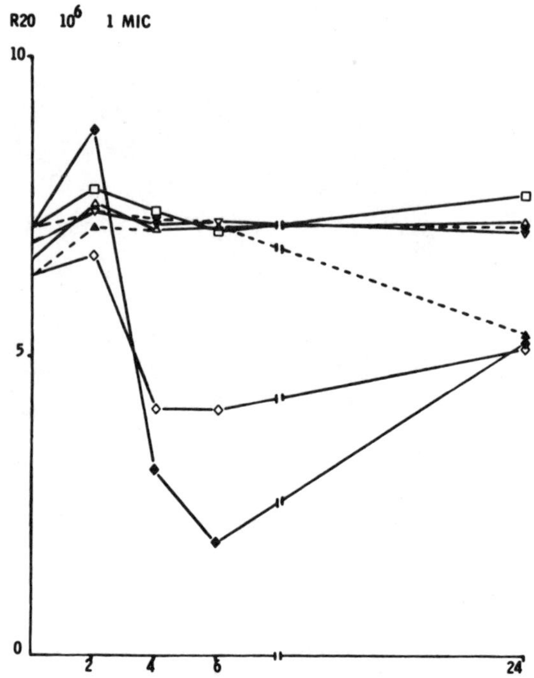

FIG. 1. *Synergy of cefsulodin and ceftazidime with gentamicin against strain R20. Symbols:* □, *gentamicin;* △, *cefsulodin;* ▽, *ceftazidime;* ◇, *gentamicin plus cefsulodin;* ◆, *gentamicin plus ceftazidime;* ▲, *cefsulodin × 4 MIC;* ▼, *ceftazidime × 4 MIC.*

1. **Goto, S., M. Ogawa, Y. Kaneko, et al.** SCE-129, a new antipseudomonal cephalosporin: in vitro and in vivo antibacterial activity, p 835–838. *In* W. Siegenthaler and R. Lüthy (ed.), Current chemotherapy, vol. 2. American Society for Microbiology, Washington, D.C.
2. **Tsuchiya, K., M. Kondo, and A. Nagatomo.** 1978. SCE-129, antipseudomonal cephalosporin: in vitro and in vivo antibacterial activities. Antimicrob. Agents Chemother. **12:**137–145.

Early Response of *Pseudomonas aeruginosa* Growth Curve to Cefsulodin and *N*-Formimidoyl Thienamycin

E. YOURASSOWSKY, M. P. VAN DER LINDEN, M. J. LISMONT, AND F. CROKAERT*

Department of Microbiology, Brugmann University Hospital, Brussels, Belgium

Cefsulodin and *N*-formimidoyl thienamycin are particularly active in vitro against *Pseudomonas aeruginosa* in terms of MIC. Indeed, 4 μg or less per ml inhibited the growth of the majority of the clinical strains. The aim of this study was to compare the activity of the two antibiotics with regard to the following parameters: (i) the microscopic appearance of the bacteria and (ii) the growth curve pattern, particularly the early response (within the first 2 h) when the morphological modifications of bacteria exposed to an antibiotic are the most specific.

We used eight strains of *P. aeruginosa* of different biotypes isolated from clinical specimens. The MICs for these strains were from 0.4 to 3.12 μg/ml for *N*-formimidoyl thienamycin and cefsulodin. The MS-2 system (Abbott Laboratories, Diagnostic Division, Dallas, Tex.) equipped with research cuvettes was used for the study of the growth curves (medium, Iso-Sensitest, Oxoid; inoculum, 10^5 colony-forming units per ml).

Graphs showed the relationship between the logarithm n of the increase in optical density related to the initial point and time. If β-lactamase was introduced at time zero (together with the antibiotic), all the growth curves would have been identical to the control curve. After 2 and 22 h, phase-contrast microscopy was used for the study of microbial morphology.

Figure 1 shows the effect of cefsulodin and *N*-formimidoyl thienamycin on *P. aeruginosa* growth curves. An inhibitory effect on growth was observed with cefsulodin at all concentrations above 2 μg/ml (Fig. 1, left side). An increase in optical density was observed within the first 2 h at all concentrations, including 125 μg/ml (50 times the MIC). The maximum residual growth (early response of the growth curve) in an antibiotic-treated culture was hardly influenced by the initial cefsulodin concentrations. Phase-contrast microscopy after 2 h showed filamentous forms. With *N*-formimidoyl thienamycin (Fig. 1, right side) all concentrations equal to or greater than 1 μg/ml inhibited the growth, but neither filamentous forms nor residual growth was observed.

Figure 2 shows the growth curve patterns in the β-lactamase–treated culture. A brief contact (30 min) of cefsulodin and culture before addition of β-lactamase showed practically no antibacterial effect (expressed by the delay of regrowth). If the contact between cefsulodin and bacteria had been longer, the regrowth delay would also have been longer, but the relationship between concentrations and lag or regrowth was very poor. In contrast, the regrowth delay in the *N*-formimidoyl thienamycyn-treated culture was not only dependent on time of contact with the active drug but was also dependent on initial concentrations. So far, a relationship might be established between the early responses of the growth curves and the lag of regrowth in the postantibiotic phase (concentration dependent for *N*-formimidoyl thienamycin but not for cefsulodin). The last seven strains of *P. aeruginosa* showed the same pattern during the early phase of growth.

Thus, two major differences between these two drugs can be observed by this technique. First, with cefsulodin the early response of the growth curve (within the first 2 h) showed an increase in the optical density and filament formation practically independent of the concen-

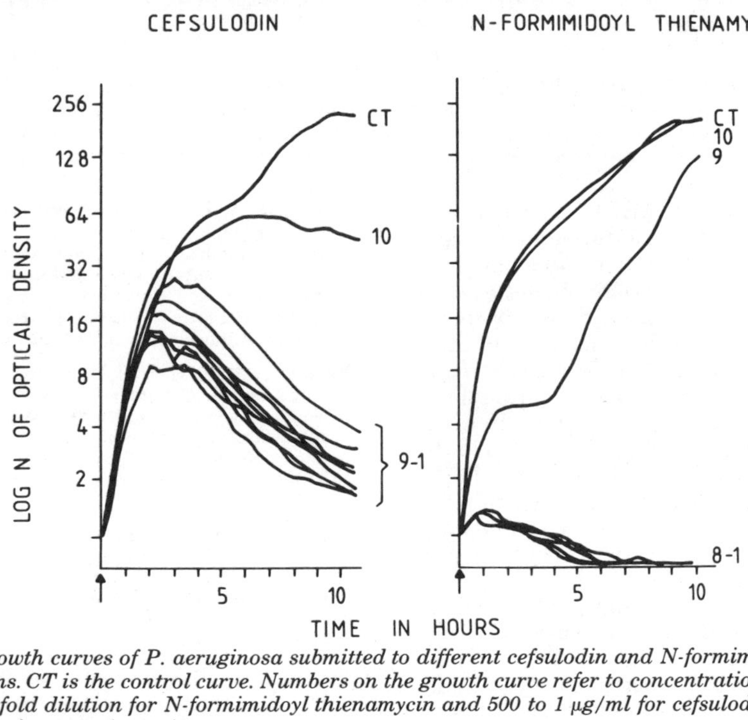

FIG. 1. *Growth curves of P. aeruginosa submitted to different cefsulodin and N-formimidoyl thienamycin concentrations. CT is the control curve. Numbers on the growth curve refer to concentrations from 125 to 0.25 μg/ml by twofold dilution for N-formimidoyl thienamycin and 500 to 1 μg/ml for cefsulodin. Antibiotics are introduced at time zero (arrow).*

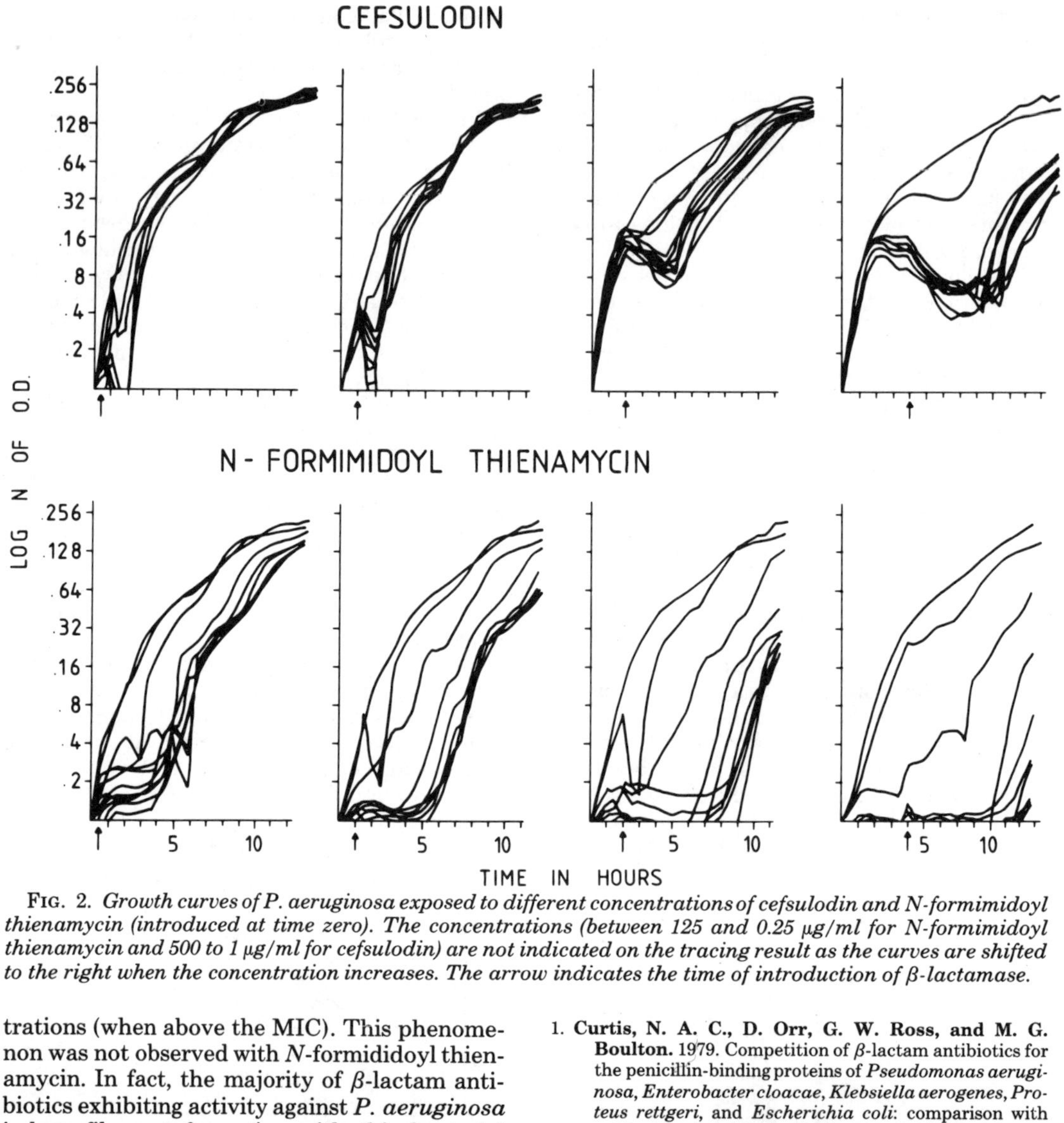

FIG. 2. *Growth curves of P. aeruginosa exposed to different concentrations of cefsulodin and N-formimidoyl thienamycin (introduced at time zero). The concentrations (between 125 and 0.25 μg/ml for N-formimidoyl thienamycin and 500 to 1 μg/ml for cefsulodin) are not indicated on the tracing result as the curves are shifted to the right when the concentration increases. The arrow indicates the time of introduction of β-lactamase.*

trations (when above the MIC). This phenomenon was not observed with *N*-formididoyl thienamycin. In fact, the majority of β-lactam antibiotics exhibiting activity against *P. aeruginosa* induce filament formation with this bacterial species (1–3) despite the fact that some of them are rapidly lytic when used against *Escherichia coli* (4). From this point of view, *N*-formimidoyl thienamycin appears to be different from its congeners. Second, the delay of regrowth in the postantibiotic period also appeared poorly dependent on the concentration of cefsulodin but concentration dependent for *N*-formimidoyl thienamycin. This observation might be predicted by the study of the early response of the growth curves. A relationship with penicillin-binding proteins might be established (E. Yourassowsky, M. P. Van der Linden, M. J. Lismont, and F. Crokaert, 3rd International Symposium on Rapid Methods and Automation in Microbiology, Washington, D.C., 1981, abstr. 166).

1. **Curtis, N. A. C., D. Orr, G. W. Ross, and M. G. Boulton.** 1979. Competition of β-lactam antibiotics for the penicillin-binding proteins of *Pseudomonas aeruginosa, Enterobacter cloacae, Klebsiella aerogenes, Proteus rettgeri*, and *Escherichia coli*: comparison with antibacterial activity and effects upon bacterial morphology. Antimicrob. Agents Chemother. **16**:325–328.

2. **Ellis, L. F., D. K. Herron, D. A. Preston, L. K. Simmons, and R. A. Schlegel.** 1976. Evaluation of antibiotic efficacy using electron microscopy: morphological effects of guanylureido cephalosporin, chlorobenzoylureido cephalosporin, BL-P1654, and carbenicillin on *Pseudomonas aeruginosa*. Antimicrob. Agents Chemother. **9**:334–342.

3. **Lorian, V., B. A. Atkinson, and L. Amaral.** 1980. Effect of subminimum inhibitory concentrations of antibiotics on *Pseudomonas aeruginosa*: the MIC/MAC ratio, p. 193–205. *In* L. D. Sabath (ed.), *Pseudomonas aeruginosa*, the organism, diseases it causes, and their treatment. Hans Huber Publishers, Bern.

4. **Spratt, B. G., V. Jobanputra, and W. Zimmerman.** 1977. Binding of thienamycin and clavulanic acid to the penicillin-binding proteins of *Escherichia coli* K-12. Antimicrob. Agents Chemother. **12**:406–409.

Synergistic Effect of Cefsulodin and Cefotiam Against *Serratia marcescens*

K. TSUCHIYA* AND M. KONDO

Takeda Chemical Industries, Ltd., Osaka, Japan

Serratia marcescens is frequently responsible for hospital-acquired infections that present serious therapeutic problems because of the low susceptibility of the organism to many antibiotics and the high frequency of strains resistant to certain effective antibiotics. Cefsulodin is active against *Pseudomonas aeruginosa* and some gram-positive cocci (5). Treatment of *P. aeruginosa* infections with cefsulodin has produced a high incidence of eradication of *P. aeruginosa* in various clinical specimens from patients, but in some cases other bacterial species such as *S. marcescens*, *Enterobacter cloacae*, and *Proteus* spp. appear in place of *P. aeruginosa*. Cefotiam, a broad-spectrum cephalosporin, has been used in the therapy of various kinds of infection (4). Previously, a synergistic effect was reported for the combination of cefsulodin and mecillinam against *S. marcescens* (2). This paper examines the effect of combinations of cefsulodin and cefotiam on in vitro and in vivo activities against *S. marcescens*.

Test organisms were laboratory strains and recent clinical isolates of *S. marcescens*. The MIC was determined by the agar dilution method, using Trypticase soy agar (BBL Microbiology Systems). The MIC was defined as the lowest concentration of antibiotic that prevented visible growth after overnight incubation at 37°C. Bactericidal effect was evaluated by the method of time-kill curve in Trypticase soy broth (BBL). The effect of the combination was tested by the checkerboard dilution method, the fixed combination method, and the killing kinetic method. The protective effect against systemic infection was tested in Slc:ICR mice infected with *S. marcescens* TN66. Mice were infected intraperitoneally with 1×10^3 to 3×10^3 colony-forming units (CFU) in 0.5 ml of 5% mucin (Difco Laboratories) per mouse. All experiments were repeated five times. The ED_{50} (in milligrams per kilogram) was calculated by the probit method from the survival rate, recorded 5 days after infection (3). The effect of the combination was tested by the checkerboard dilution method. To compare the effect of cefsulodin plus cefotiam with each of the two antibiotics individually, the fractional inhibitory concentration (FIC) and FIC index were calculated according to the method reported by Elion et al. (1); to assess the protective effect of the combination of the two antibiotics, the fractional effective dose (FED) and FED index were used as substitutes for the FIC and FIC index.

The FIC and FIC index values of the combination of cefsulodin and cefotiam, using the checkerboard dilution method on *S. marcescens* IFO12648, TN66, and TN73, are summarized in Table 1. A synergistic effect was observed and was more distinct with an inoculum size of 10^8 CFU/ml than with 10^6 CFU/ml. Against 36 clinical isolates of *S. marcescens*, cefsulodin and cefotiam alone and the fixed combination of cefsulodin and cefotiam (1:1 and 1:2) were examined with inoculum sizes of 10^8 and 10^6 CFU/ml. About half of the strains were resistant to cefotiam used alone or in combination with cefsulodin. These strains were classified as indifferent. With the larger inoculum, the combination of cefsulodin and cefotiam had a synergistic effect against many cefotiam-susceptible strains; with the smaller inoculum, the synergistic effect of the combination was slightly weak. The bactericidal activity of cefsulodin in combination with cefotiam against *S. marcescens* IFO12648 was compared with that of the antibiotic alone. The combination of cefsulodin and cefotiam showed a synergistic effect. The FED and FED index values (Table 2) were calculated from the survival rates of mice treated with cefsulodin, cefotiam, or both. The optimal combination ratio was 1:1. With this ratio, the FED index was 0.438 and the ED_{50} value was 9.71 mg/kg. This ratio of combination was similar to the ratio of the dose of each antibiotic used clinically.

Over the past decade, *S. marcescens* infections have increased and are now a cause of serious nosocomial infections. The organism was considered relatively insusceptible to antibiotics. Aminoglycosides have a potent activity against *S. marcescens*; however, clinical use of aminoglycosides is limited by their serious side effects, and recently the number of aminoglycoside-resistant strains of *S. marcescens* has increased. A synergistic effect was found with combinations of cefsulodin and cefotiam against *S. marcescens*. A synergistic effect is the outcome of one or more steps in a complex series of events, such

TABLE 1. *Effect of the combination of cefsulodin and cefotiam against S. marcescens*

Strain	10^8 CFU/ml[a]			10^6 CFU/ml		
	FIC		FIC index	FIC		FIC index
	Cefsulodin	Cefotiam		Cefsulodin	Cefotiam	
IFO12648	0.03 (100/3.13)[b]	0.03 (>100/6.25)	0.06	0.03 (100/3.13)	0.13 (6.25/0.78)	0.16
TN66	0.02 (>100/3.13)	0.06 (50/3.13)	0.08	0.25 (>100/25)	0.25 (1.56/0.39)	0.50
TN73	0.06 (>100/12.5)	0.02 (>100/3.13)	0.08	0.02 (100/3.13)	0.19 (6.25/0.78)	0.19

[a] Inoculum size was one loopful of bacterial suspension.
[b] Numbers in parentheses indicate MIC of first cephalosporin alone/MIC of first cephalosporin in combination with second cephalosporin.

TABLE 2. *Effect of the combination of cefsulodin and cefotiam on mice infected with S. marcescens*[a]

Ratio, cefsulodin/cefotiam	ED_{50} (mg/kg)	FED		FED index
		Cefsulodin	Cefotiam	
Alone/0	149 (127–176)[b]			
0/alone	12.0 (9.45–15.2)			
64:1	110 (84.1–130)	0.725 (149/108)[c]	0.140 (12.0/1.69)	0.865
32:1	66.2 (54.1–80.6)	0.431 (149/64.2)	0.167 (12.0/2.00)	0.599
16:1	49.4 (39.9–61.1)	0.312 (149/46.5)	0.242 (12.0/2.90)	0.554
8:1	35.4 (27.6–45.2)	0.212 (149/31.5)	0.328 (12.0/3.90)	0.540
4:1	22.8 (16.4–31.0)	0.123 (149/18.2)	0.380 (12.0/4.60)	0.503
2:1	14.7 (10.6–20.5)	0.066 (149/9.80)	0.409 (12.0/4.90)	0.475
1:1	9.71 (6.57–14.0)	0.033 (149/4.85)	0.405 (12.0/4.85)	0.438
1:2	11.7 (8.69–15.1)	0.027 (149/3.90)	0.650 (12.0/7.80)	0.683
1:4	8.26 (4.93–11.8)	0.011 (149/1.56)	0.551 (12.0/6.61)	0.562
1:8	10.2 (5.71–14.2)	0.008 (149/1.13)	0.756 (12.0/9.07)	0.764

[a] Mice were infected intraperitoneally with *S. marcescens* TN66 (10^3 CFU/mouse) in 0.5 ml of 5% mucin. Cephalosporins were administered subcutaneously at 0 h after infection.
[b] Numbers in parentheses are 95% confidence limits.
[c] Numbers in parentheses indicate ED_{50} of first cephalosporin alone/ED_{50} of first cephalosporin in combination with second cephalosporin.

as increased permeation of the antibiotics into the organism, prevention of inactivation of one antibiotic by the other, and action by the antibiotics at two different points in a biochemical pathway. *S. marcescens* is a constitutive producer of cephalosporinase (Richmond's type Ia). Cefotiam is sensitive to hydrolysis by this enzyme, and cefsulodin is resistant to it. However, because the affinity of cefsulodin for the β-lactamases is remarkably low, a synergistic effect of the combination of cefsulodin and cefotiam may not depend on the inhibition of *S. marcescens* β-lactamase by cefsulodin. The effect of cefsulodin and cefotiam on permeability and target enzymes will be investigated subsequently.

The optimal ratio of the combination of cefsulodin and cefotiam was almost the same in the two test systems (in vitro susceptibility test and protective test in mice), but the optimal ratio of the combination of cefsulodin and mecillinam was markedly different in the two test systems

(3). These results suggest that the effect of a combination must be tested in vitro and then confirmed in vivo.

1. **Elion, G. B., S. Singer, and G. H. Hitchings.** 1954. Antagonists of nucleic acid derivatives. J. Biol. Chem. **208**:477–488.
2. **Kondo, M., and K. Tsuchiya.** 1981. Effect of combination of cefsulodin and mecillinam. J. Antibiot. **34**:727–738.
3. **Litchfield, J. T., and F. Wilcoxon.** 1949. A simple method of evaluating dose effect experiments. J. Pharmacol. Exp. Ther. **96**:99–113.
4. **Tsuchiya, K., M. Kida, M. Kondo, H. Ono, M. Takeuchi, and T. Nishi.** 1978. SCE-963, a new broad-spectrum cephalosporin: in vitro and in vivo antibacterial activities. Antimicrob. Agents Chemother. **14**:557–568.
5. **Tsuchiya, K., M. Kondo, and H. Nagatomo.** 1978. SCE-129, antipseudomonal cephalosporin: in vitro and in vivo antibacterial activities. Antimicrob. Agents Chemother. **13**:137–145.

Pseudomonas-Active Cephalosporins in Animal Experiments

ANNA BURGHELE* AND WOLFGANG RITZERFELD

Ciba-Geigy Ltd., Frankfurt am Main, and Institute of Hygiene, University of Münster, Münster, Federal Republic of Germany*

The etiological significance of *Pseudomonas* in human infections is quite remarkable. In his paper presented at the International Symposium in Boston, Sabath said, "*Pseudomonas aeruginosa* is currently one of the most important pathogens responsible for infections in hospitalized patients. Despite the fact that during the last decade much more has become known about this organism and the diseases it causes, *Pseudomonas* infections remain difficult to treat" (4).

Of 10,253 pathogens isolated in the University Hospital in Münster during the first six months of 1981, 1,136 were *Pseudomonas* strains. The percentage of the total figure was 8.1% *P. aeruginosa* and 3% other *Pseudomonas* species.

The antimicrobial susceptibility of the isolated *Pseudomonas* strains was very unfavorable. Many of the strains proved resistant to most of the penicillin derivatives, cephalosporins, and some aminoglycosides. These facts emphasize the need for cephalosporin derivatives with high antipseudomonal activity, favorable pharmacokinetic properties, and a low incidence of side effects.

The antipseudomonal activity of the new cephalosporin derivatives cefsulodin, ceftazidime, and ceftriaxone is well established. Cefsulodin, a narrow-spectrum antibiotic, is highly active against *Pseudomonas.* Ceftazidime is a broad-spectrum cephalosporin with anti-pseudomonal activity similar to that of cefsulodin (3), and ceftriaxone is likewise a broad-spectrum antibiotic with good activity against *Pseudomonas* and a very long half-life of 3.5 h (5).

We have tested the efficacy of these agents in reducing bacterial counts in the experimental model of acute occlusive *Pseudomonas* pyelonephritis in rats. Earlier studies had shown that even small doses of cefsulodin (10 mg/kg of body weight three times daily) produced a reduction in bacterial counts (1). Thus, pyelonephritis due to *Pseudomonas* could be affected more favorably by cefsulodin than by any other antibiotic agent tested so far.

In the present study the experiments were carried out by an already-published method using albino rats (2). The main steps of the procedure are as follows. The left kidney of albino rats is predamaged by ligature of the ureter for 4 h. This is followed 1 h after removal of the ligature by intraurethral injection of 1 ml of freshly isolated *P. aeruginosa* A 9532 (suspension of 1.5×10^9 viable organisms; the MICs of the substances for the *P. aeruginosa* strain were 1 μg/ml). Treatment with the test antibiotics was started 6 h after infection and was continued on days 2, 3, and 4. Because of the longer half-life of ceftriaxone, two treatment groups were studied with treatment started at 6 and 14 h after infection. Dosage was 50 mg/kg three times daily for cefsulodin and ceftazidime, and 25 mg/kg three times daily for ceftriaxone.

Days 5 and 6 were treatment free. On day 7, the animals were sacrificed, and the kidneys and urine samples (aseptically obtained by puncture of the bladder) were used for microbiological cultures. The untreated control animals received 0.5 ml of physiological saline three times daily.

Bacteria from the culture plates were identified by immune sera in agglutination tests. The Wilcoxon test was used to evaluate the significance of differences in bacterial counts.

Figure 1 shows the results obtained with cefsulodin and ceftazidime (50 mg/kg three times

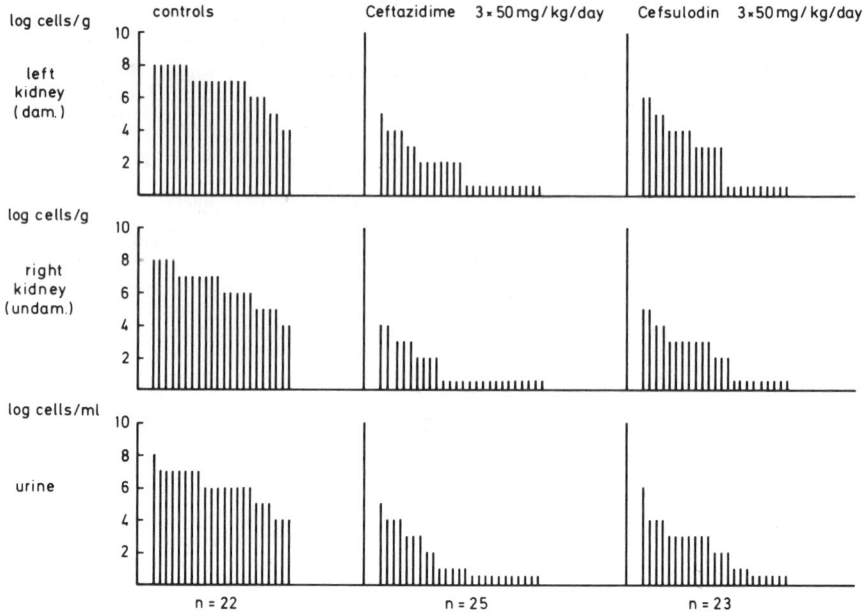

FIG. 1. *Experimental Pseudomonas pyelonephritis in rats: results (bacterial cell counts) with cefsulodin and ceftazidime after P. aeruginosa A 9532 infection.*

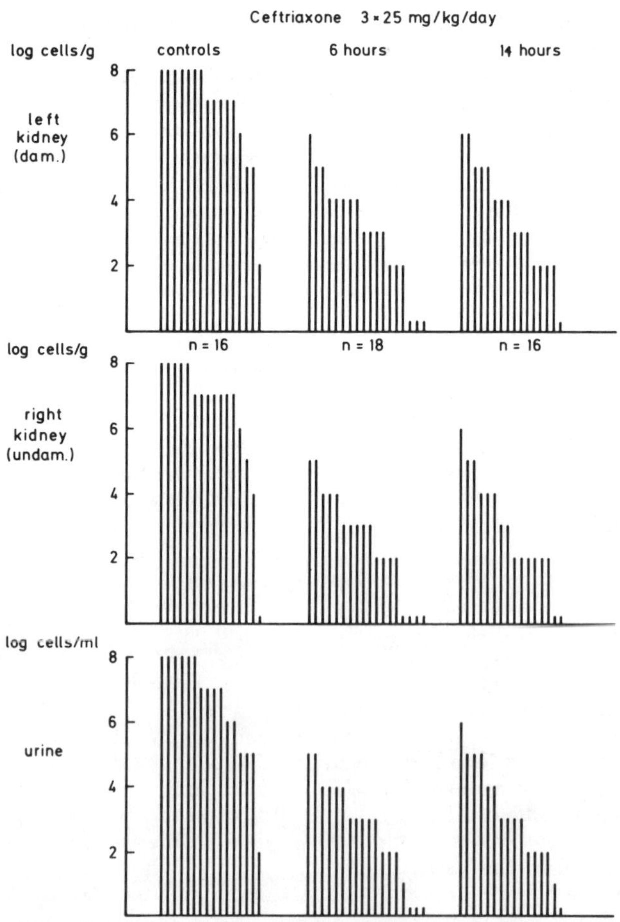

FIG. 2. *Experimental Pseudomonas pyelonephritis in rats: results (bacterial cell counts) with ceftriaxone 6 and 14 h after P. aeruginosa A 9532 infection.*

daily). In the upper part of the figure, the numbers of viable bacteria (colony-forming units) found in the left (damaged) kidneys of the treated animals and the untreated control animals are given. Beneath these are the corresponding numbers of cells isolated from the right (undamaged) kidneys. In the lower part of the figure, the bacterial counts in the urine are given. The reduction in bacterial counts caused by cefsulodin and ceftazidime at a dosage of 50 mg/kg three times daily versus the untreated control group was statistically significant. This was true for the left predamaged as well as for the right undamaged kidney and for the urine sample. No difference in activity between these two cephalosporins was seen.

Figure 2 illustrates the results obtained with ceftriaxone administered at a dosage of 25 mg/kg three times daily on three consecutive days. Two treatment groups were used: in group 1 treatment was started at 6 h after infection; in group 2 therapy was delayed for 14 h. Because of the longer time interval elapsed between infection and start of treatment, higher bacterial counts were to be expected in the second group. Ceftriaxone significantly reduced the number of pathogens at a dose of 25 mg/kg three times daily when therapy was started at 6 h after infection. With therapy started at 14 h after infection, reduction in bacterial counts was less pronounced but still significant in comparison with the control animals. Even under these aggravated experimental conditions, ceftriaxone clearly exhibited its antibacterial activity.

In conclusion, we can say that in these animal experiments the *Pseudomonas*-active cephalosporins cefsulodin, ceftazidime, and ceftriaxone proved to be highly effective at relatively low doses.

1. **Balacescu, A., and W. Ritzerfeld.** 1980. Efficacy of cefsulodin in experimental *Pseudomonas* pyelonephritis in rats, p. 185–186. *In* J. D. Nelson and C. Grassi (ed.), Current chemotherapy and infectious disease. American Society for Microbiology, Washington, D.C.
2. **Ritzerfeld, W.** 1981. Ceftazidime activity in experimental Pseudomonas pyelonephritis in rats. J. Antimicrob. Chemother. **8**(Suppl. B), in press
3. **Ritzerfeld, W., R. Koschmieder, and W. Drees.** 1975. Animal experiments on current antibiotics, p. 281–287. *In* Proceedings of the 9th International Congress of Chemotherapy, London.
4. **Sabath, L. D.** 1980. Pseudomonas aeruginosa. An International Symposium, Boston, 1 October 1979. Hans Huber Publishers, Bern.
5. **Stoeckel, K., P. J. McNamara, R. Brandt, H. Plozza-Nottebrock, and W. H. Ziegler.** 1980. Pharmacokinetics of RO 13-9904 (Rocephin), a highly active new semisynthetic cephalosporin with an exceptionally long biological half-life. Abstr. 2nd Mediterranean Congr. Chemother., Nice, October, abstr. no. 472.

Protein Binding of Cefsulodin and Cefotiam in Human Serum

RUDOLF SONAK,* WOLFGANG RITZERFELD, AND GERD SCHMITZ

Hygiene Institut der Westfälischen Wilhelms-Universität and Zentrallaboratorium der Universitätskliniken, Münster, Federal Republic of Germany*

The biological significance of protein binding of antibiotics has been clarified only to some extent. It is generally assumed that only the antibiotics not bound to the protein can exert antibacterial activity in the organism. The data from experiments on the binding of antibiotics to proteins, carried out mainly by an in vitro equilibrium dialysis, differ greatly according to the method used. Conceptions about the mechanism and the significance of the protein binding of antibiotics are contradictory and confusing (3). It seems, therefore, to be desirable to verify these conceptions, especially with regard to the recent knowledge on the physiological functions of the serum proteins and their interactions with microorganisms.

We assume that the binding of antibiotics to proteins represents a transport mechanism important for antibacterial activities produced by the antibiotics. According to this assumption, the binding of antibiotics to proteins takes part in the following three main functions: (i) transport of the antibiotic from the intestinal tract or the interstitial tissue into the circulation, i.e., resorption of the antibiotic substance; (ii) transport to the target organ with an infectious lesion; and (iii) transport into the target cell, i.e., up to the part of the bacterial cell (organelle) in which the antibiotic substance carries out the antibacterial activity.

In the course of our studies on the pharmacokinetics of some cephalosporins, we summarized the data on their protein-binding capacity. In spite of a great variability of the values, clear differences in the protein-binding capacity of individual cephalosporins could be found (2).

First of all, we wanted to know the fraction or fractions of human serum to which cephalosporins are bound and the nature of the binding. In our preliminary experiments with sera of two volunteers with concentrations of resorbed cephalexin, 46 and 44 μg/ml, determined by a diffusion method in vitro, we detected the antibacterial activity only in the low-molecular-weight fractions following the albumin peak, after the sera had been separated by gel column chromatography. There was no activity in any protein fraction of serum—immunoglobulin M, immunoglobulin G, albumin. The same results were obtained in in vitro experiments with a higher concentration of antibiotic. Here 5 mg of cephradine was incubated for 60 min at 4°C with 1 ml of human serum. The serum was later separated by gel column chromatography. The antibacterial activity was again only in the low-molecular-weight fractions. In addition, in the same fractions a peak of the unbound cephalosporin was recorded.

The question arose of whether in the inactive protein fractions of the serum—immunoglobulin M, immunoglobulin G, albumin—some antibiotic yet occurred that could not be detected by an in vitro diffusion test because of the binding of the antibiotic to proteins. To answer this question, experiments with radioactively labeled antibiotics seemed to be the only adequate method.

Because of our technical limitations we at first labeled cefsulodin and cefotiam with radioactive iodine, ^{125}I. The labeling was performed by the McFarlane iodination method. The unbound part of the ^{125}I was removed by gel filtration on PD-10 columns. We were conscious of the possibility of damaging the molecular structure of the antibiotics by the iodination method. The introduction of radioactive carbon, ^{14}C, into the molecules of the two cephalosporins is without doubt a more reliable method, but it requires much more equipment and remains for the further experiments in our laboratories. One milliliter of the labeled cephalosporin was incubated for 60 min at 4°C with 1 ml of human serum. The separation of serum proteins was carried out by gel filtration on a Sephacryl S-300 column (26 by 950 mm) in 0.5 M NaCl solution at pH 8.0. All fractions were photometrically recorded at 280 nm. The ^{125}I activity was determined with a gamma counter.

The results of our experiments with the two labeled cephalosporins are given in Fig. 1 and 2. The experiment with the labeled cefsulodin clearly showed that the greater part of the antibiotic was physically dissolved in the serum (Fig. 1). The main radioactivity could be detected in the same low-molecular-weight fractions following the albumin peak as in our preliminary experiments dealing with the antibacterial activity of unlabeled cephalosporins. A small part of the labeled cefsulodin was bound to the serum albumin fraction.

Nearly the same results were obtained with the labeled cefotiam (Fig. 2). In experiments with cefotiam, a larger amount of the labeled antibiotic was used, but without any influence on the protein binding. It can, therefore, be assumed that the saturation of the activity bound to the albumin is achieved already by the low counts.

In addition, the results of our experiments were underlined by the fact that only a negligible quantity of the free ^{125}I remained in the antibiotic solution. The influence of iodination on the antibacterial activity of the tested substances has not been investigated.

To avoid any change or damage of the molecular structure of the cephalosporins by the radioactive labeling procedure, we performed an analysis of cefotiam protein binding by a spectrofluorometric method without labeling the molecule (1). The results of our preliminary

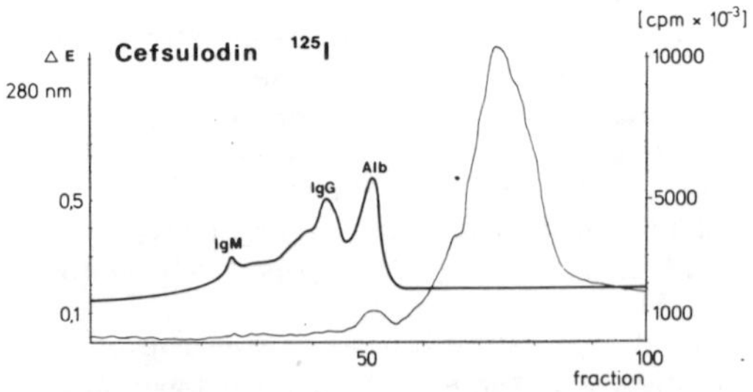

FIG. 1. *Binding of labeled cefsulodin to human serum protein.*

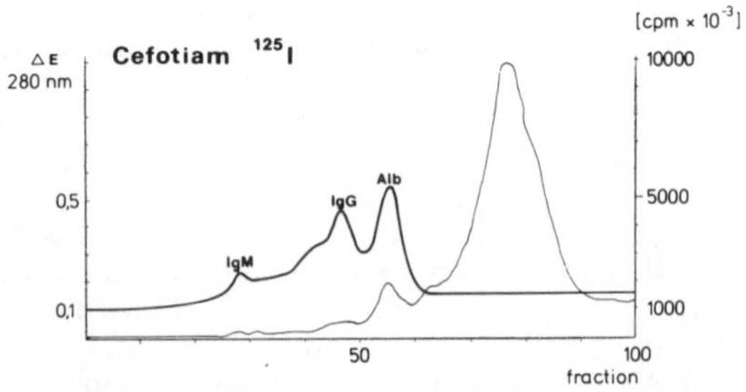

FIG. 2. *Binding of labeled cefotiam to human serum protein.*

experiments seem to be quite encouraging. They let us hope that we will be able to report our results of protein binding of a series of cephalosporin derivatives in the near future.

Summing up, it can be said that, after incubation with human serum, cefsulodin and cefotiam remained physically dissolved in the serum. Only a small part was bound to the albumin fraction. To detect responsibly the real nature and the biological significance of this binding, suitable methods avoiding any possibility of molecular damage to antibiotics should be used.

1. **Aikawa, R., M. Nakano, and T. Arita.** 1976. Fluorometric determination of cephalexin in urine. Chem. Pharm. Bull. **24:**2350–2355.
2. **Brogard, J. M., F. Compte, and M. Pinget.** 1978. Pharmacokinetics of cephalosporin antibiotics. Antibiot. Chemother. **25:**123–162.
3. **Scholtan, W.** 1978. Bestimmungsmethoden und Gesetzmäßigkeiten der Serumproteinbindung von Arzneimitteln. Arzneim. Forsch. **28:**1037–1047.

Metabolism and Excretion of Carbon-14–Labeled Cefsulodin in Human Subjects

DAVID J. ANDERSON, BARBARA A. BOPP, ILMAR MERITS, BEVERLY A. WYNNE, AND JOHN F. A. VANCE

Abbott Laboratories, North Chicago, Illinois 60064, U.S.A.

Cefsulodin sodium is a semisynthetic cephalosporin antibiotic that is active against *Pseudomonas* organisms. Studies with the carbon-14–labeled drug in rats and dogs have indicated that the compound is primarily excreted unchanged in the urine after parenteral administration (1). The purpose of this study was to investigate the disposition of intramuscularly administered cefsulodin sodium in humans through the use of the radiolabeled compound.

Cefsulodin sodium was labeled with carbon-14 in the sulfophenylacetamide group. The specific activity of this material was 0.053 μCi/mg, and it was at least 94% radiochemically pure, as determined by high-pressure liquid chromatography (HPLC).

Three healthy, adult male volunteers were each given a 0.5-g dose of cefsulodin, containing 24 to 25 μCi of carbon-14, intramuscularly in the upper, outer quadrant of the buttock. Heparinized venous blood samples were withdrawn at selected times after dosing. The blood samples were centrifuged as soon as possible, and a 2-ml portion of each plasma sample was then diluted with an equal volume of 1 M phosphate buffer (pH 6) and frozen. All urine and fecal samples were collected as excreted during a 5-day period after drug administration and were frozen individually.

Total radioactivity was determined in the plasma, urine, and fecal samples by oxidation and liquid scintillation spectrometry. Correction for quenching was made by automatic external standardization. Ultrafiltrates of the buffered plasma samples were analyzed for cefsulodin by an HPLC assay with UV detection. Metabolic patterns were determined in the 0- to 12-h and 12- to 24-h urine samples by HPLC with a μ-Bondapak C_{18} analytical column and a mobile phase of 0.02 M ammonium formate, containing 2% acetonitrile and adjusted to pH 4.3 with formic acid. Sequential fractions of the eluate were collected and assayed for radioactivity by liquid scintillation counting.

Both the levels of total radioactivity and cefsulodin in plasma peaked by 1.0 h after dosing at concentrations of 27.7 μg equivalents/ml and 19.0 μg/ml, respectively. Thereafter, the levels of carbon-14 declined slowly, falling to 17.6, 9.3, and 5.1 μg equivalents/ml at 3, 6, and 12 h, respectively. Low levels of radioactivity (2 to 3 μg equivalents/ml) remained in the plasma for the duration of the 5-day study period. In contrast, the cefsulodin concentrations decreased rapidly, with a half-life of approximately 2.0 h.

Initially at 0.25 h, unchanged drug accounted for an average of 80% of the total radioactivity in the plasma. The percentage of parent drug gradually decreased so that cefsulodin represented only about half of the total radioactivity in the plasma by 3 to 4 h, and less than 10% by 12 h. Since the cefsulodin assay was performed on ultrafiltrates of the plasma samples, it was of interest to determine whether the rest of the radioactivity was free in the plasma or was bound to the plasma proteins. Therefore, the levels of radioactivity in the filtrates were determined and compared with those in the respective plasma samples.

At 15 min, 74% of the radioactivity in the plasma was free and 26% was bound. However, by 12 h, only 22% of the total radioactivity in the plasma was free and 78% was bound. During the first 3 h, cefsulodin accounted for virtually all of the free radioactivity in the plasma, but by 12 h the parent drug represented only 39% of the free radioactivity.

An average of 37.9% of the ^{14}C dose was excreted in the urine within the first 2 h after intramuscular administration, and by 4 h 53.0% of the dose had been eliminated from the body. Urinary excretion accounted for 80.8 and 84.5% of the administered radioactivity at 12 and 24 h, respectively. Small and decreasing amounts of carbon-14 were excreted in the urine during the next 4 days, and a total of 87.3% of the administered radioactivity was recovered in the urine by the end of the 5-day study. Only about 1% of the dose was eliminated in the feces, indicating that biliary secretion was not a significant factor in the disposition of cefsulodin. The total recoveries averaged 88.4% and ranged from 95.7 to 83.3% in the three subjects.

HPLC analysis of the 0- to 12-h and 12- to 24-h urine samples resolved the radioactivity into at least five zones. Cefsulodin exhibited chromatographic behavior similar to zone 5 and was well separated from the unknown labeled species in zones 1, 2, 3, and 4. An average of 63.8% of the dose was eliminated in the first 12 h as the unchanged drug, and the labeled metabolites or decomposition products accounted for 16.9% of the ^{14}C dose. Between 12 and 24 h, only 1.0% of the ^{14}C dose was excreted in the urine as the parent drug, and the four unidentified labeled metabolites or decomposition products comprised 2.5% of the dose.

Cefsulodin is known to be unstable in aqueous solution at physiological pH, and a considerable amount of chemical degradation was observed when labeled cefsulodin was incubated at 37°C in freshly voided urine. After incubation for 18 h, only 72% of the cefsulodin was intact, and after 90 h, less than 30% of the parent drug was unchanged. Only one major labeled reaction product was produced, and it chromatographed in zone 2 of the HPLC system previously described. These results indicated that the biotransformation of cefsulodin in humans may, in part, be due to chemical reaction, rather than enzyme-catalyzed metabolism.

1. **Tanayama, S., K. Yoshida, and Y. Kanai.** 1978. Metabolic fate of SCE-129, a new antipseudomonal cephalosporin, after parenteral administration in rats and dogs. Antimicrob. Agents Chemother. **4:**137–143.

Pharmacokinetics of Cefsulodin After Single and Chronic Intravenous Administration to Humans

W. VISCHER, A. GERARDIN, G. HUMBERT, J. B. LECAILLON,* J. P. SCHOELLER, AND W. THEOBALD

Ciba-Geigy, Basle, Switzerland; Ciba-Geigy, Rueil-Malmaison, France; and Hôpital Charles Nicolle, Rouen, France*

The pharmacokinetics of cefsulodin was studied in humans after single and chronic administrations. Blood samples and urine fractions were collected in each study. The concentrations in plasma and urine samples of the single-dose study were determined both microbiologically (MB) and by high-pressure liquid chromatography (HPLC). Good agreement between the two assay techniques was recorded. The parameters of the regression lines and the correlation coefficients (r) obtained from the plot of the MB versus HPLC results in plasma and urine were, respectively, MB = 1.00 HPLC + 3.6 ($r = 0.985$) and MB = 0.96 HPLC + 11 ($r = 0.992$). The sensitivity was slightly better with the MB method in urine and with the HPLC method in plasma. The samples derived from the chronic-treatment study were assayed by HPLC only.

Single-dose study. Twelve healthy male volunteers ranging from 26 to 49 years of age and from 66 to 92 kg of body weight participated in the study after a two-period balanced incomplete block design. The doses (0.5, 1, and 2 g) were administered to the fasted subjects in 4 min.

The mean pharmacokinetic parameters (±SD) derived from plasma and urine data are given in Table 1. The cefsulodin body clearance continued similarly when the dose varied from 0.5 to 2 g (mean value ± SD = 144 ± 21 ml/min). As a result, the area under the concentration-time curve (AUC) plotted versus dose showed a linear relationship: AUC = 114 × dose + 4 ($n = 24$; $r = 0.934$). The elimination half-life was not changed by the dose administered. The main elimination pathway was renal elimination,

TABLE 1. *Mean cefsulodin parameters (±SD)*

Dose (g)	Maximum plasma concn (μg/ml)	AUC (μg.h/ml)	$t_{1/2}$ (h)	Total clearance (ml/min)	Excretion in urine (% of dose)	Renal clearance (ml/min)
0.5	51 ± 14	61 ± 8	2.0 ± 0.7	139 ± 19	72 ± 6	100 ± 18
1	82 ± 20	117 ± 15	1.8 ± 0.2	145 ± 18	72 ± 9	107 ± 8
2	194 ± 59	231 ± 47	1.9 ± 0.3	149 ± 27	67 ± 11	97 ± 20

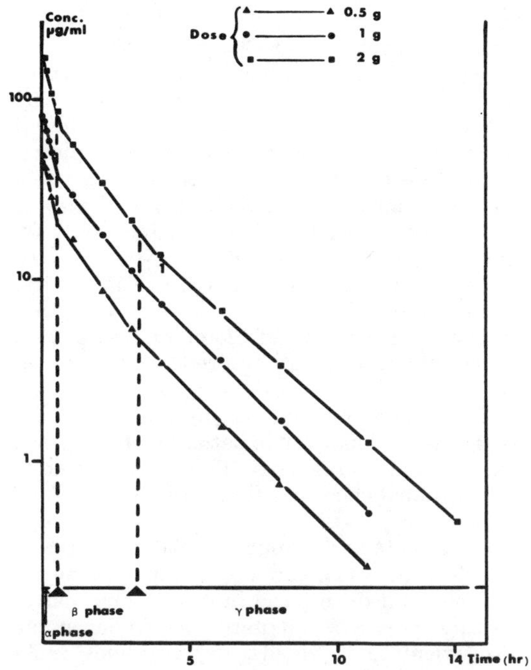

FIG. 1. *Mean concentrations in plasma (eight volunteers).*

since 70% of the dose, as a mean, was excreted in urine as unchanged drug over 24 h. The renal clearance calculated for each urine fraction did not seem to be time dependent and did not vary largely during the experiment.

The cefsulodin plasma concentrations plotted versus time as log-linear graphs decreased according to three phases (Fig. 1) that could be shown by using the back projection technique. Nine sets of data out of 24 were fitted by nonlinear regression analysis. The criteria of selection were an α-phase defined by at least two data points and a constant decay of concentration as the time increased. The resulting equations were used to define the parameters of the simplest three-compartment open model. The apparent volume of distribution was low: 254 ± 41 ml/kg. If the drug had been homogeneously distributed, this volume would have been slightly higher than that of the extracellular fluids (20% of body weight). As a mean, the volume of the central compartment, 121 ± 41 ml/kg, amounted to half the value, the rest being equally divided between the other two compartments.

Chronic-administration study. Four patients, two males and two females ranging from 18 to 64 years of age and from 31 to 61 kg of body weight, were given intravenously 1 g of cefsulodin every 12 h over 10 days.

The mean AUC values on days 1 and 10 were, respectively, 144 ± 47 and 161 ± 53 μg.h/ml. The elimination half-lives were, respectively, 1.5 ± 0.4 and 1.6 ± 0.5 h, and the urinary excretion values were 49 ± 20 and 57 ± 34% of the dose. These results, similar at days 1 and 10, indicated that the pharmacokinetic parameters were not modified at the end of the chronic treatment. These results are consistent with those previously reported (1) after intramuscular administration of four consecutive doses to healthy subjects. The SDs of the pharmacokinetic data of our study were large, mainly due to variations in the physical and pathological states of the patients. No accumulation of cefsulodin was recorded in the plasma of these patients at the end of the treatment, since the concentration curves after the first and the last dose of the treatment were almost superimposable.

1. **Ahrens, T., W. Vischer, P. Imhof, J. Füllhaas, O. Zak, and F. Kradolfer.** 1979. Human pharmacology of CGP 7174/E (SCE-129) and initial results of clinical trials in Europe. Drugs Exp. Clin. Res. **5**:61–70.

Pharmacokinetics of Cefsulodin in Patients with Renal Insufficiency

J. P. SCHOELLER,* J. P. FILLASTRE, G. HUMBERT, AND J. B. LECAILLON

Ciba-Geigy, Rueil-Malmaison; Hôpital de Bois Guillaume, Rouen; and Hôpital Charles Nicolle, Rouen, France*

Cefsulodin is a semisynthetic cephalosporin with marked antibacterial activity against *Pseudomonas aeruginosa.* Pharmacokinetics were compared between renal-insufficient patients and normal subjects. The subjects were divided into six groups according to creatinine clearance (Cl_{cr}) (Table 1). The 27 males and 9 females ranged from 22 to 77 years of age and from 44 to 98 kg of body weight. One gram of cefsulodin was administered as an intravenous bolus dose to the six healthy volunteers with Cl_{cr} higher than 100 ml/min and to the 30 patients with impaired renal functions. The six patients of group 5, undergoing dialysis, received the cefsulodin solution at the beginning of dialysis.

Blood samples were collected just before injection and at times ranging from 10 to 48 h, increasing with the degree of renal impairment. In dialyzed patients, blood was collected at the same time on the arterial and venous sides of the dialyzer. Urine fractions were collected from 0 to 2, 2 to 4, 4 to 6, 6 to 8, and 8 to 24 h for healthy subjects and from 0 to 6, 6 to 12, 12 to 24, and 24 to 48 h for patients of groups 1, 2, and 3.

In dialyzed patients, the dialysis fluid was collected before injection and over intervals of 0 to 1, 1 to 2, 2 to 3, 3 to 4, 4 to 5, and 5 to 6 h.

The concentrations of cefsulodin in plasma, urine, and dialysis solution were determined by a high-pressure liquid chromatography method. A Hewlett-Packard model 1081 instrument and a LiCrosorb RP8 (Merck) 15-cm-long column were used. The mobile-phase composition was 15% methanol in aqueous solution (tetrabutylammonium hydrogen sulfate, 10^{-1} M; K_3PO_4, 9.10^{-2} M). The detector was UV 254 nm. Then 10 to 20 μl of deproteinized plasma (1 part of methanol, 2 parts of plasma, and centrifugation) or 20 μl of 1:10 urine diluted with water were injected. The limit of sensitivity was 0.5 μg per ml of plasma or dialysis solution and 50 μg per ml of urine.

The mean (±SD) pharmacokinetic parameters of cefsulodin derived from plasma, urine, and dialysis solution are given in Table 1. A linear relationship was recorded between the total clearance of cefsulodin (Cl_t) and Cl_{cr}: $Cl_t = 1.06\ Cl_{cr} + 8$ ($r = 0.986$; $n = 24$). A good correlation was obtained between the elimination rate constant and Cl_{cr} ($r = 0.96$; $n = 24$). The urinary clearance, Cl_u, was also well correlated with Cl_{cr} ($r = 0.977$; $n = 24$). For each group, the back projection technique was applied to mean plasma concentrations plotted versus time as log-linear profiles: the decrease in concentration corresponded to three phases. As the degree of renal insufficiency increased, the elimination rate decreased; however, the total apparent volume of distribution (Table 1) did not seem to vary.

The elimination of cefsulodin proceeded from renal elimination, largely predominant for patients with a low degree of renal impairment; and from nonrenal elimination, whose contribution became important in patients suffering from severe renal insufficiency. This was revealed by the nonrenal clearance (Cl_m) reported in Table 1.

In patients undergoing dialysis, 45 ± 10% of the dose of cefsulodin was eliminated by the dialysis fluid during the first 6 h. The dialysis clearance (58 ± 20 ml/min) was similar among the patients and seemed to depend almost exclusively on the dialysis conditions (dialyzer, blood, and dialysis flows). The dialysis elimination was similar to the renal excretion recorded for patients of group 1 (Cl_{cr}, 80 to 30 ml/min). From plasma data, the area under the concentration-time curve (AUC) and $t_{1/2}$ were also similar in group 1 and in dialyzed patients.

The adjustment of the dose of cefsulodin in renal-insufficient patients could be estimated from the mean plasma concentrations calculated at steady state by the superposition method for each group of subjects. Dettli (1) and Fabre and Balant (2) recommended using the maximum plasma concentrations of antibiotics as a reference parameter over AUC, $t_{1/2}$, or minimum plasma concentrations to achieve the best therapeutic effect. The dose in percentage of that for a subject with normal renal function (assuming the same C_{max}) was calculated for patients whose Cl_{cr} range was 100 to 2.5 ml/min (Table 2). The dose was adjusted for different time intervals between administrations. The choice of the time interval between two doses should take into account the elimination rate of the drug, which

TABLE 1. *Mean (±SD) pharmacokinetic parameters of cefsulodin*[a]

Group (mean of 6 subjects)		Plasma					Urine			Dialysis solution	
No.	Cl_{cr} (ml/min)	C_{max} (μg/ml)	AUC_{∞} (μg.h/ml)	$t_{1/2}$ (h)	Cl_t (ml/min)	V_d (ml/kg)	UE (% of the dose)	Cl_u (ml/min)	Cl_m (ml/min)	DE (% of the dose)	Cl_D (ml/min)
0	130	109	115	1.8	148	287	66.5	93.7	54.1		
	±12	±23	±18	±0.1	±13		±7.2	±21.8	±7.8		
1	50	143	304	3.1	57.6	250	59.6	32.2	25.4		
	±27	±40	±80	±0.4	±11.2		±10.2	±11.7	±5.9		
2	17	98	685	8.1	25.3	271	33.5	8.91	16.4		
	±3	±23	±146	±0.6	±6.0		±6.1	±1.78	±5.2		
3	8	85	885	12.1	19.1	290	18.2	3.78	15.3		
	±2	±13	±99	±1.0	±2.3		±7.2	±1.70	±2.6		
4	<5	111	935[b]	9.3[b]	20.3	301					
		±37	±348	±1.8	±8.2						
5	<5	178[c]	247[d]	2.6[d]	68.6[d]					45.1	50
		±103	±38	±0.3	±11.0					±10.2	±18[e]
											66
											±21[f]

[a] Abbreviations: Cl_{cr}, creatinine clearance without correction for body area; C_{max}, maximum of plasma concentration; AUC_{∞}, area under the plasma concentration-time curve extrapolated to infinite time; $t_{1/2}$, apparent elimination half-life calculated from the last log-linear segment of the plasma concentration-time curve; Cl_t, total plasma clearance (dose/AUC); V_d, total apparent volume of distribution; UE, total urinary excretion; Cl_u, renal clearance (ΔUE/ΔAUC); Cl_m, nonrenal clearance (Cl_t-Cl_u); DE, elimination by the dialysis solution.

[b] The cefsulodin concentrations were determined up to 6 or 8 h for that group; thus, AUC_{∞} and $t_{1/2}$ may be slightly underestimated.

[c] Mean of three values.

[d] Calculated from concentration values corresponding to plasma samples collected on the arterial side of the dialyzer.

[e] ΔDE/ΔAUC.

[f] [(Plasma concentration on arterial side − plasma concentration on venous side)/plasma concentration on arterial side] × blood flow.

TABLE 2. *Adjusted cefsulodin doses in renal-insufficient patients in percentage of dose for a subject with normal renal function*

Cl_{cr} (ml/min)	% of dose at given time interval (h) between doses				
	6	8	12	24	48
100	99	100	100	100	100
90	98	99	100	100	100
80	97	98	100	100	100
70	95	97	99	100	100
60	92	98	98	100	100
50	88	93	97	100	100
40	82	88	93	99	100
30	76	81	89	97	100
20	66	73	83	95	100
15	61	68	77	93	99
10	54	63	73	90	98
5	45	54	65	84	95
2.5	40	47	59	79	92

should lead to increasing this interval for patients with severe renal impairment. To obtain rapidly the same C_{max} as in normal subjects, a loading dose equal to the individual dose given to a normal subject should be given first.

In dialyzed patients, the elimination of cefsulodin in dialysis fluid suggests giving a normal dose (not adjusted) at the start of the dialysis period and again at the end.

1. **Dettli, L.** 1976. Drug dosage in renal disease. Clin. Pharmacokin. **1:**126–134.
2. **Fabre, J., and L. Balant.** 1976. Renal failure, drug pharmacokinetics and drug action. Clin. Pharmacokin. **1:**99–120.

Treatment of *Pseudomonas* Infections with Cefsulodin: Results of a Multicenter Clinical Trial in Europe

THEODOR AHRENS

Research Department, Pharmaceuticals Division, Ciba-Geigy, Ltd., Basel, Switzerland

Cefsulodin underwent an extensive multicenter clinical trial from mid-1977 to mid-1980 in Europe. The trial design was open and noncomparative, adhering to a standard protocol, but allowing for adaptation of the dosage and duration of treatment to the individual needs of the patients.

Altogether, 347 patients (231 male, 116 female) suffering from various *Pseudomonas* infections were treated in 56 hospitals in Austria, Denmark, France, the Federal Republic of Germany, Greece, Sweden, Switzerland, and the United Kingdom. Figure 1 shows the distribution of this population according to age and sex.

The types of *Pseudomonas* infection for which cefsulodin was given included urinary tract infections in 155 patients (44.7%), respiratory tract infections in 111 (32.0%), bone and soft tissue infections in 45 (13.0%), septicemia in 30 (8.6%), and meningitis in 6 (1.7%). More than half of the patients with respiratory tract infections (n = 59) were suffering in addition from cystic fibrosis.

Bacteriological examinations before treatment revealed that *Pseudomonas* was the only infecting agent in 273 (78.7%) of the patients, the remainder having mixed infections. *Pseudomonas* was considered fully susceptible if the inhibition zone diameter was ≥19 mm, and this criterion was met by 92% of the strains isolated (n = 137); of the remaining strains, 3.6% were of intermediate susceptibility (18 mm) and 4.4% were resistant (≤17 mm). Determinations of the MICs showed full susceptibility (≤16 μg/ml) in 91.5% of the strains (n = 106), intermediate susceptibility (32 μg/ml) in 6.6%, and resistance (>32 μg/ml) in 1.9%.

Cefsulodin was administered intramuscularly in 154 patients, by intravenous injection in 141, and by drip infusion in 52. It was given as monotherapy to 263 patients (75.8%) and as part of an antipseudomonal drug combination in 84 (24.2%). In adults (n = 310), the daily doses ranged from 1 to 9 g: 68.4% received up to 3 g, 30.0% up to 6 g, and 1.6% more than 6 g. In children and adolescents (n = 37), the daily dosages were <10 to 100 mg/kg. The duration of treatment ranged from 3 to 48 days; it lasted up to 10 days in 35.0%, up to 20 days in 42.0%, and more than 20 days in 23.0%. Treatment was discontinued prematurely in 27 patients, but on account of side effects in only 12 of these, corresponding to 3.5% of the total patient population.

The results of cefsulodin treatment in terms of the elimination of *Pseudomonas* and clinical improvement are illustrated in Table 1. The average success rate in the whole patient population, both bacteriologically and clinically, was about 70%. In cystic fibrosis there was a striking discrepancy between the good clinical improvement and the relatively low elimination rate of *Pseudomonas*. The same tendency was also evident in the patients with respiratory tract infection not suffering from cystic fibrosis. In septicemia, *Pseudomonas* persisted in 12 patients, in the blood in three of them and in nine other patients in secretions, smears, etc.; in the latter, however, the general condition of the patients improved. In urinary tract infection, follow-up results were available for 123 of the 138 patients in whom *Pseudomonas* had been eliminated by treatment. In 61 of these (49.6%) the *Pseudomonas* infection had relapsed, in most instances within 3 weeks of the end of treatment.

The clinical evolution of urinary tract infection was assessed in only 112 patients, since the remainder were asymptomatic from the beginning. Generally speaking, the condition of patients showing no improvement remained unchanged; exacerbations were seen in only six patients and were probably due to the underlying disease (pneumonia, neoplasms, burns).

Local pain after intramuscular injection was reported by 40 of 154 patients (25.9%); it was relieved by the subsequent injection of a local anaesthetic together with cefsulodin, and no tissue damage was observed. Intravenous injection was painful in 10 of 193 patients (5.2%), 2 of whom also showed signs of phlebitis.

Systemic adverse reactions were observed in 37 patients (10.7% of the total), 9 of whom were receiving combined chemotherapy. The reactions were unspecific (dizziness, headache, somnolence, malaise) in 16 of these patients. Allergic phenomena (rash, edema, accompanied with fever in 4 and oliguria in 1) occurred in 15 patients. Gastrointestinal signs and symptoms were reported in 13, and exacerbations of arthralgia and neuralgic pains, in 4 patients. Six patients com-

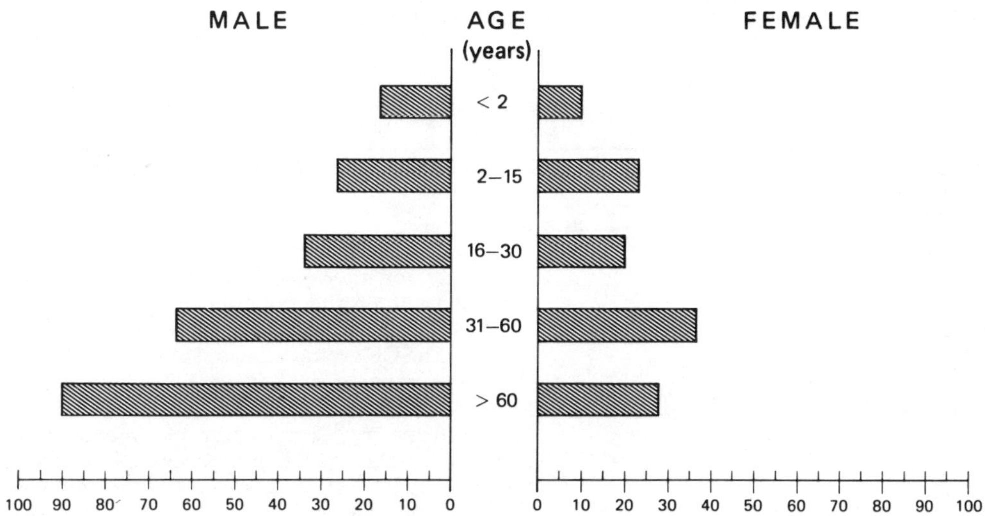

FIG. 1. *Age and sex distribution of 347 patients with Pseudomonas infections.*

TABLE 1. *Bacteriological and clinical results of cefsulodin treatment in 347 patients with Pseudomonas infections*

Indication	No. of patients	No. with elimination of *Pseudomonas*	No. with clinical improvement
Urinary tract infection	155	138 (89.0%)	83 (74.1%)[a]
Respiratory tract infection	52	33 (63.5%)	44 (84.6%)
Respiratory tract infection in cystic fibrosis	59	14 (23.7%)	43 (72.9%)
Bone and soft tissue infection	45	36 (80.0%)	41 (91.1%)
Septicemia	30	18 (60.0%)	23 (76.7%)
Meningitis	6	5 (83.3%)	4 (66.7%)
Total	347	244 (70.3%)	238 (68.6%)

[a] Of a total of 112 patients.

plained of paresthesia, tinnitus, drug smell of perspiration, and hoarseness.

Changes in laboratory data were found in 50 patients (14.4% of the total). These included eosinophilia in 14, decreases or increases in blood cell counts in 6, and increases in transaminases in 19, in alkaline phosphatase in 6, and in bilirubin in 1. Granular casts were observed in 1 patient. The serum creatinine, urea, or blood urea nitrogen values increased in 12 patients. The overall tolerability, assessed in 333 patients, was excellent in 151 (45.3%), good in 154 (46.3%), fair in 19 (5.7%), and poor in 9 (2.7%) patients.

Effect of Cystic Fibrosis on the Pharmacokinetics of Cefsulodin (CGP 7174/E)

HELGE MICHALSEN* AND TOM BERGAN

Departments of Pediatrics and Microbiology, Aker Hospital, and Institute of Pharmacy, Oslo, Norway*

Cefsulodin is a new cephalosporin derivative with pronounced activity against *Pseudomonas* (3). Since many patients suffering from cystic fibrosis (CF) harbor chronic respiratory tract infections with *Pseudomonas aeruginosa*, this compound was thought to be of interest in this group of patients.

Patients with CF eliminate beta-lactam anti-

TABLE 1. *Pharmacokinetic characteristics of cefsulodin in CF patients and in non-CF controls*[a]

Group	AUC (μg.h/ml)	$t_{1/2}$ (h)	$\Delta V_{d\beta}$ (liters/kg)	Cl_B (liters/h)
CF	193.6 ± 54.9	1.16 ± 0.30	0.342 ± 0.080	5.34 ± 1.65
Non-CF	409.3 ± 155.4	1.46 ± 0.30	0.245 ± 0.084	5.46 ± 2.70

[a] AUC, Area under curve; $t_{1/2}$, serum half-life; $\Delta V_{d\beta}$, distribution volume coefficient; Cl_B, total body clearance. Data are mean ± SD.

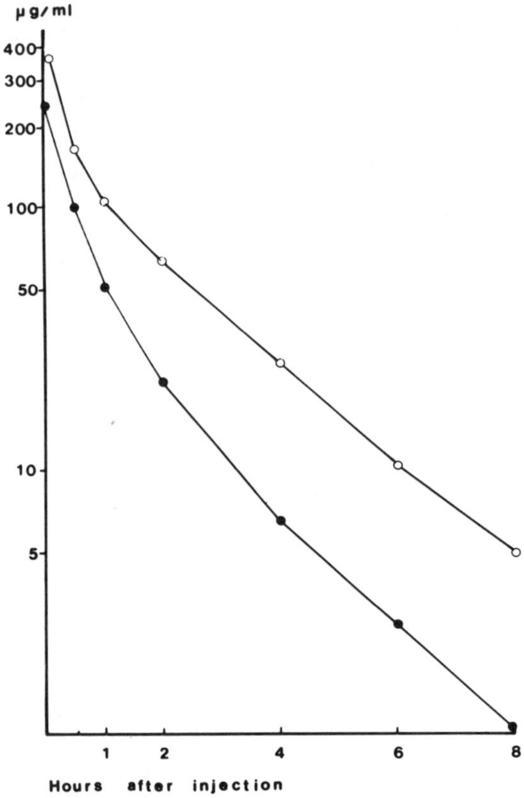

FIG. 1. *Comparison of the mean serum concentrations after an intravenous bolus dose of 40 mg/kg in the CF group (●) and in the non-CF group (○).*

biotics faster than children without CF (1), whereas the pharmacokinetics of aminoglycosides are similar in these two groups (2). Before their use in patients with CF, antibiotics must accordingly be studied in these special patients to be sure that the dosage renders the intended serum concentrations of the antibiotic in question.

We studied the pharmacokinetic characteristics of cefsulodin during 11 courses of therapy in 7 patients with CF. Four children without CF served as normal controls. The drug was used only for therapeutic purposes. The informed consent of the patients or their parents was obtained before the patients joined the study.

The CF group consisted of three girls and four boys ranging in age from 1.5 to 15 years (mean, 10.5). The control group consisted of three girls and one boy, 12 to 15 years old (mean, 13.4). The patients in the CF group were treated for respiratory tract infections caused by *P. aeruginosa*. The non-CF group was treated for various gram-negative multiresistant infections. Cefsulodin was administered via indwelling venous catheters as bolus injections during 3 to 5 min in doses of 40 mg per kg of body weight every 8 h.

The mean serum concentrations of cefsulodin in the two groups are demonstrated in Fig. 1. The pharmacokinetic characteristics are shown in Table 1. The control group of non-CF children was small, but the differences in serum concentrations in the two groups were highly significant. The remaining differences between the groups were not significant.

Our preliminary conclusions, awaiting further data from the non-CF group, are as follows: (i) serum concentrations are significantly lower in children with CF than in non-CF children when equivalent doses are administered; (ii) serum half-life is slightly, but not significantly, lower in CF than in non-CF subjects; (iii) the distribution volume coefficient is higher in CF than in non-CF subjects; and (iv) cefsulodin doses must be increased in children with CF to achieve serum concentrations equivalent to those obtained in non-CF children.

1. **Bergan, T., and H. Michalsen.** 1979. Pharmacokinetics of azlocillin in children with cystic fibrosis. Arzneim. Forsch. **29:**1955–1957.
2. **Michalsen, H., and T. Bergan.** 1981. Pharmacokinetics of netilmicin in children with and without cystic fibrosis. Antimicrob. Agents Chemother. **19:**1029–1031.
3. **Shannon, K., A. King, and I. Phillips.** 1980. In vitro activity of cefsulodin, an antipseudomonal cephalosporin, p. 188–190. *In* J. D. Nelson and C. Grassi (ed.), Current chemotherapy and infectious disease. American Society for Microbiology, Washington, D.C.

Penetration and Therapeutic Efficacy of Cefsulodin and Gentamicin in a Rat Abscess Model

ETHAN RUBINSTEIN, JOSEPH WEISS, ZEEV DREZNIK, AND ZIVA MARK

The Infectious Diseases Unit, Chaim Sheba Medical Center, Tel-Aviv University School of Medicine, Tel-Hashomer, Israel

The penetration of an antibiotic into the site of infection is of great therapeutic interest. Since most bacterial infections are tissue infections, the concentration of an antibiotic in the interstitial fluid and the infected fluid are of greater interest than the antibiotic concentrations in serum. We have previously reported that both cefsulodin and gentamicin obtain adequate interstitial fluid concentrations in rats (1, 3). In a foreign body-induced abscess model, gentamicin concentrations in the abscess fluid were adequate; however, the drug failed to sterilize the abscess, probably because low local Po_2 inhibited gentamicin uptake by the susceptible test microorganism (2).

In the present study the penetration and therapeutic efficacy of cefsulodin and gentamicin in foreign body-induced *Pseudomonas aeruginosa* abscesses were investigated. Abscesses were induced in rats by the subcutaneous implantation of six to eight dialysis tube units filled with 10^3 to 10^4 *P. aeruginosa* organisms. The outer surface of the dialysis bag was contaminated with 0.1 ml containing 10^5 *P. aeruginosa* organisms. The MIC of cefsulodin for the strain used was 3.7 μg/ml and that of gentamicin was 0.78 μg/ml. This procedure resulted in the development of abscesses in all control animals with intraabscess bacterial counts of 10^8 to 10^9/ml.

Cefsulodin and gentamicin serum and abscess fluid concentrations were measured at 0, 30, 60, 120, 240, and 360 min after the last administration of each of the antibiotics. Blood was obtained from the tail vein, and abscess fluid was obtained by the removal of a dialysis unit from its implantation site and aspiration of the fluid (ultrafiltrate) from the dialysis bag. Both antibiotic concentrations were determined in a microbiological assay with the disk diffusion technique. For gentamicin determination *Staphylococcus epidermidis* on Mueller-Hinton agar was used, and for cefsulodin determinations, *P. aeruginosa* NCTC 10701 on brain heart infusion agar was used. Standards were performed by dissolving gentamicin and cefsulodin in pooled rat serum for blood determinations and in phosphate-buffered saline, pH 7.2, for abscess fluid determinations. All results were obtained in triplicate and then averaged. Bacterial counts were performed by the pour-plate technique with nutrient agar. The pH, Po_2, and Pco_2 were determined in a blood gas analyzer. Cefsulodin, 100 mg/kg, administered intramuscularly once daily for 4 days, starting immediately after the implantation in 15 animals, resulted in a mean peak serum concentration after the last dose of 124.4 ± 58.8 μg/ml (Table 1).

Mean peak concentrations of cefsulodin in abscess fluid were 38.7 ± 17.4 μg/ml and were obtained 120 min after the administration. Cefsulodin persisted in the abscess for a longer period than in the blood. The cefsulodin half-life in blood was 58 min and in the abscess was 105 min. Blood area under the curve was 28.7 μg/ml per min and abscess fluid area under the curve was 25.2 μg/ml per min.

Forty-eight implants in 8 rats showed no bacterial growth, and 10 abscesses in five animals had a mean bacterial count of $3.5 \times 10^6 \pm 4 \times 10^4$, whereas the controls had bacterial counts of 10^8 to 10^9 ($P \leq 0.01$); thus, 61.5% of the animals were cured and 82.7% of the induced abscesses were eradicated.

The characteristics of pH, Po_2, and Pco_2 are shown in Table 2, the most significant being a Po_2 of 22 mm of Hg in the abscess fluid.

Thirty animals infected in the same fashion

TABLE 1. *Blood and abscess fluid concentrations of cefsulodin and gentamicin*[a]

Drug	No. of animals	Time (min)	Concn (μg/ml) in: Blood	Concn (μg/ml) in: Abscess fluid
Cefsulodin	15	0	0	0
		30	124.4 ± 58.8	24.0 ± 22.9
		60	77.0 ± 43	35.6 ± 8.5
		120	23.3 ± 16.0	38.7 ± 17.4
		240	2.13 ± 2.13	17.6 ± 10.6
		360	0.4	4.9 ± 2.7
Gentamicin	30	0	0	0
		30	20.5 ± 2.0	0.4 ± 0.2
		60	17.1 ± 4.9	6.0 ± 2.1
		120	7.1 ± 3.0	14.9 ± 5.1
		240	1.8 ± 1.1	4.9 ± 2.1
		360	0	2.8 ± 1.2

[a] Doses of cefsulodin (100 mg/kg) and gentamicin (10 mg/kg) were administered intramuscularly for 4 days, starting immediately after the induction of abscesses. Results are given as the mean ± SD.

TABLE 2. *Bacterial count, pH, and gas results of blood and abscess fluid in rats treated with cefsulodin and gentamicin*

Factor	Cefsulodin	Gentamicin	Control
Infected animals	5/13 (38.5%)	30/30 (100%)	10/10 (100%)
Sterile animals	8/13 (61.5%)	0/30 (0%)	0/10 (0%)
Abscesses	10/58 (17.3%)	60/60 (100%)	20/20 (100%)
Sterile implant	48/58 (82.7%)	0/60 (0%)	0/10 (0%)
Blood			
pH	7.4 (±0.2)	7.41 (±0.2)	
Po_2	85.6 (±10.0)	88.0 (±12.0)	
Pco_2	37.0 (±6.6)	38.0 (±7.2)	
Abscess fluid			
pH	7.13 (±0.3)	7.4 (±0.18)	
Po_2	22.2 (±8.6)	18.4 (±2.4)	
Pco_2	40.4 (±15.2)	40.4 (±3.7)	

received gentamicin, 10 mg/kg intramuscularly daily for 4 days, starting immediately after the implantation. The procedure for sample collection and assay was similar. Blood and abscess fluid concentrations of gentamicin are shown in Table 1. The mean peak concentration of gentamicin in blood occurred at 30 min and was 20.5 μg/ml. That in abscess fluid occurred at 120 min and was 14.9 (±5.1) μg/ml. Gentamicin persisted significantly longer in the abscess fluid than in blood; at 360 min, no gentamicin was detected in blood but the abscess fluid still contained 2.8 μg/ml. The half-life of gentamicin in abscess fluid was significantly longer than the corresponding half-life in blood; the area under the curve in blood was 6.32 μg/ml per min, and that in the abscess was 7.38 μg/ml. These results suggest that abscesses act as a "trap" or "third space" for gentamicin.

Unlike cefsulodin-treated animals, all gentamicin-treated animals developed marked abscesses despite adequate gentamicin concentrations in the abscess fluid. The explanation for the occurrence of abscesses despite gentamicin therapy probably lies in the observation that the Po_2 in the abscess fluid was low. Low oxygen tension and high CO_2 tension have been shown to decrease the antibacterial activity of aminoglycosides because these agents need an oxygen-dependent transport mechanism for bacterial penetration. Conversely, cell wall-active antibiotics such as cefsulodin can exert their antibacterial activity in a reduced milieu as well. This is supported by the view that the gentamicin MBC for the test organism was increased from 0.78 μg/ml in aerobic conditions to 62.0 μg/ml in anaerobic conditions and that of cefsulodin was unchanged.

In addition, killing curves of the test organism in the presence of 10 μg of cefsulodin per ml revealed that under aerobic conditions both agents achieved a complete kill by the end of 24 h of incubation; however, under anaerobic conditions gentamicin did not reduce the bacterial count whereas cefsulodin reduced the inoculum 100-fold.

In conclusion, both gentamicin and cefsulodin penetrate well into foreign body-induced abscesses in the rat model, the concentrations in the abscess fluid being similar to simultaneous serum concentrations. Unlike gentamicin, cefsulodin was efficacious in sterilizing the abscesses. This is probably due to the ability of cefsulodin to act in an anaerobic milieu. This observation may be important in the prophylaxis and therapy of *P. aeruginosa* infections associated with the presence of foreign bodies.

1. **Dan, M., H. Halkin, and E. Rubinstein.** 1981. Interstitial fluid concentrations of aminoglycosides. J. Antimicrob. Chemother.
2. **Dreznik, Z., R. Schwartzkopf, I. T. Wolfstein, and E. Rubinstein.** 1980. Gentamicin penetration into abscesses, p. 649–650. *In* J. D. Nelson and C. Grassi (ed.), Current chemotherapy and infectious diseases. American Society for Microbiology, Washington, D.C.
3. **Landau, Z., H. Halkin, and E. Rubinstein.** 1981. Interstitial fluid concentrations of cefsulodin, azlocillin and carbenicillin. Scand. J. Infect. Dis. **13**:1–5.

Treatment of Pulmonary *Pseudomonas aeruginosa* Infection in Cystic Fibrosis with Cefsulodin Combined with Tobramycin

NIELS E. MØLLER,* CHRISTIAN KOCH, NIELS HØIBY, AND KLAUS JENSEN

Pediatric Department TG, Danish Cystic Fibrosis Center, Rigshospitalet, Statens Seruminstitut, Rigshospitalet, and Hvidovre Hospital, Copenhagen, Denmark*

Cystic fibrosis (CF) is the most frequent inborn error of metabolism, affecting 1 of 2,000 newborns.

The bronchopulmonary infections are the most important reasons for the short life expectancy in CF patients. Since the introduction of effective antibiotics against *Haemophilus influenzae* and *Staphylococcus aureus* and regular controls together with daily lung physiotherapy, the life expectancy has increased. The main problem now is infections with *Pseudomonas aeruginosa*.

When patients are colonized with *P. aeruginosa*, there will be signs of infection after a few months, with a steadily increasing number of precipitins against *P. aeruginosa* in serum (1) as well as in tracheal secretions (5). In spite of successful chemotherapy, the patients after a short while will harbor the same or a new strain of *P. aeruginosa* (4). The chronically infected patients are characterized by elevated numbers of precipitins, immunoglobulin G, albumin concentration, and proteolytic activity in tracheal secretions, erythrocyte sedimentation rate, leukocyte count, percentage of neutrophils, and by diminished forced vital capacity and peak flow. The last six parameters are partly affected by chemotherapy, whereas the first three are unaffected (4).

At the Danish CF center the patients are regular treated every third month with a 2-week course of antibiotics against *P. aeruginosa*, most often carbenicillin, 500 mg/kg per day, combined with tobramycin, 10 mg/kg per day (efficacy [E] in 82% decreasing to 23% of patients). The same dose of tobramycin has also been used alone (E = 11%) or combined with piperacillin (E = 33%) or azlocillin (E = 28%). Development of allergic or toxic reactions to the penicillins or poor clinical response to the previous treatment encouraged us to initiate in vitro studies followed by clinical investigations with cefsulodin (Monaspor). This paper reports on our results with cefsulodin.

In vitro study. Initially, 170 strains of *P. aeruginosa* collected from CF patients (1975–1977) were tested. Susceptibility to cefsulodin was determined by a method previously described (3).

The results from the study are given in Fig. 1. The geometric mean of the IC_{50} (50% inhibitory concentration) was found to be 1.4 μg/ml, and only 2 of the strains were resistant ($IC_{50} \geq 16$ μg/ml).

Serum concentration. The serum concentrations of cefsulodin after single intravenous (i.v.) injections of 100 mg/kg per day were measured in the first 11 CF patients receiving cefsulodin. The agar-cup method was used (horse blood agar, 10%), and the test strain was *P. ellesworth.*

The peak concentration in serum was found to be about 150 μg/ml, and the 8-h level was about 5 μg/ml (3).

Efficacy. A total of 60 courses of cefsulodin were given to 42 CF patients, 25 males and 17 females. The mean age was 14.3 (3 to 29) years, and the mean number of previous anti-*Pseudomonas* courses was 8.8 (1 to 19). Cefsulodin was given i.v. in doses of 100 to 150 mg/kg per day in three divided doses combined with tobramycin, 10 mg/kg per day.

One patient discontinued treatment prematurely as a result of urticaria. At the end of treatment, *P. aeruginosa* was eradicated after 14 of the 59 courses (E = 24%). The chance of eradication was greater when the number of precipitins was below 20 ($P < 0.002$), and the erythrocyte sedimentation rate was below 10 ($P < 0.05$), as shown in Fig. 2. Eradication was obtained in 7% of the patients harboring mucoid *P. aeruginosa* ($n = 14$), 17% of patients with partly mucoid types ($n = 23$), and 41% with solely nonmucoid types ($n = 22$).

When only considering changes above 20%, an increase in forced vital capacity and peak flow was found in 51% and 51% of the courses, and 45% and 47%, respectively, were unchanged. The leukocyte count and erythrocyte sedimentation rate decreased in 66% and 46% of the courses and were unchanged in 32% and 41% of the courses, respectively; for all four parameters the differences were found to be statistically significant ($P < 0.01$).

Tolerability. In 22 courses (37%) the patients complained of moderate to severe nausea, vertigo, and headache in direct relation to the bolus injection of cefsulodin. This complaint dimin-

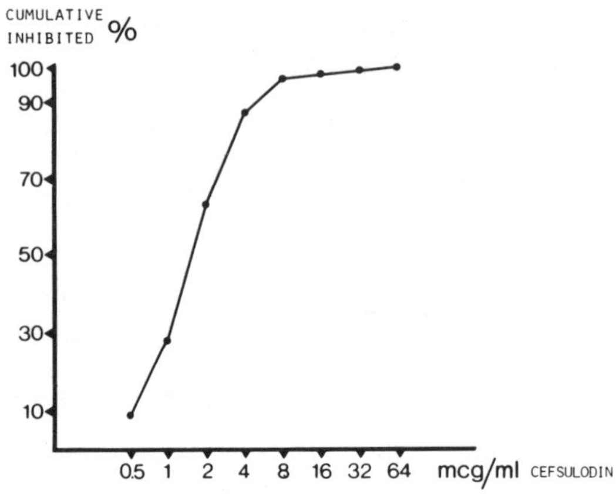

FIG. 1. *IC_{50} values for cefsulodin for 170 clinical isolates of P. aeruginosa from CF patients.*

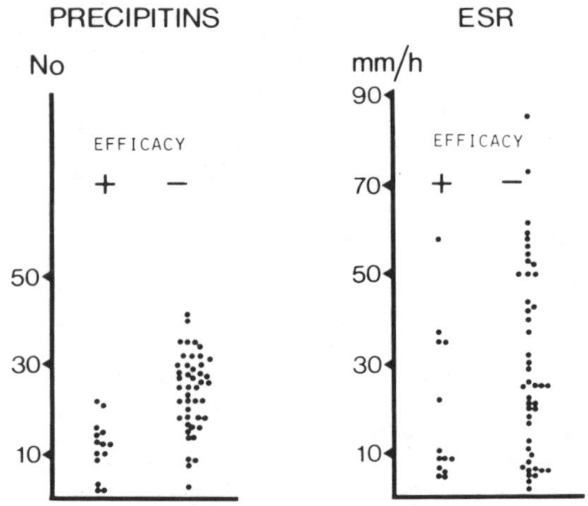

FIG. 2. *Eradication of P. aeruginosa after treatment in relation to number of precipitins and erythrocyte sedimentation rate before treatment.*

ished during the treatment and might be due to possible acute vestibular toxicity (3).

Four patients developed allergic reactions (6%), characterized by local hives in three and generalized urticaria in one patient. The 10 patients with allergic reactions to carbenicillin tolerated cefsulodin, and so did four patients previously reacting to carbenicillin with trigonourethritis.

Liver enzymes increased reversibly during 14 courses (24%), a reaction also seen when tobramycin is administered alone.

One girl developed acute interstitial nephritis leading to uremia, which was treated with peritoneal dialysis. This girl also received cloxacillin for *Staphylococcus aureus*. In no other case were found any significant differences in blood urea nitrogen, serum creatinine, or 24-h creatinine clearance, but in seven patients hyaline casts were found in the urine during treatment.

Since treatment with cefsulodin was initiated in the department 2 years ago, 90 strains of *P. aeruginosa* have been examined. The geometric mean of the IC_{50} for these strains was found to be 0.3 μg/ml and for 2% of the strains the IC_{50} was above 32 μg/ml (A. M. Heilesen, unpublished data).

Conclusions. We found that cefsulodin combined with tobramycin is as effective as the previously given treatments in eradication of *P. aeruginosa* and is superior to tobramycin alone. The patients in this study were more heavily infected (mean number of precipitins, 21) than those in previous studies and had previously received more treatment courses, and this explains the somewhat lower percentage of eradication.

Patients intolerant to carbenicillin seem to tolerate cefsulodin, and the number of side effects is comparable to that reported earlier for the other combinations. The development of interstitial nephritis may be due to cloxacillin, but we recommend following parameters of renal function during treatment. It is uncertain whether cefsulodin alone could be just as effective as in combination with tobramycin, but we will now look at this possibility.

Even though cefsulodin and other antibiotics possess bacteriological and clinical efficacy, the *P. aeruginosa* infections in CF patients still cannot be controlled satisfactory with these short-term i.v. courses. The possibilities for giving long-term treatment courses, preferably with peroral medication, should be looked for. The raised proteolytic activity in the tracheal secretions might be a potent factor in the lung destruction, and treatment with antiproteolytic drugs should be examined further.

Until more safe, long-term treatments can be used, we recommend the use of frequent courses of antibiotics, and here cefsulodin often will be the drug of choice.

1. **Høiby, N.** 1977. Pseudomonas aeruginosa infection in cystic fibrosis. Acta Pathol. Microbiol. Scand. Sect. C Suppl. 262.
2. **Møller, N. E., and N. Høiby.** 1981. Antibiotic treatment of chronic Pseudomonas aeruginosa infection in cystic fibrosis patients. Scand. J. Infect. Dis. Suppl.
3. **Møller, N. E., C. Koch, S. Vesterhauge, and K. Jensen.** 1981. Treatment of pulmonary Pseudomonas aeruginosa infections in cystic fibrosis with a new cephalosporine: cefsulodin. Scand. J. Infect. Dis., in press.
4. **Møller, N. E., K. Riewerts Eriksen, C. Feddersen, E. W. Flensborg, N. Høiby, S. Norn, K. Rosendal, P. O. Schiøtz, and P. Stahl Skov.** 1981. Anti-Pseudomonas treatment in cystic fibrosis. Eur. J. Resp. Dis., in press.
5. **Schiøtz, P. O.** 1981. Local humoral immunity and immune reactions in the lungs of patients with cystic fibrosis. Acta Pathol. Microbiol. Scand. Sect. C Suppl. 276.

Clinical Study of Cefsulodin in Respiratory Tract Infections and Soft Tissue Infections Due to *Pseudomonas aeruginosa*

K. MASHIMO,* K. HARA, AND J. YURA

Tokyo Kosei Nenkin Hospital, Tokyo; Second Department of Internal Medicine, Nagasaki University, Nagasaki; and First Department of Surgery, Nagoya City University, Nagoya, Japan*

We report the results of continuing investigations on cefsulodin (CFS) treatment of respiratory tract and soft tissue infections.

CFS sputum levels and bacteriological response in sputum. The results suggest that at any dose level within single dosage from 0.5 to 2.0 g, CFS can produce a favorable clinical response when the peak sputum levels are almost equal to or slightly higher than the MIC against *Pseudomonas aeruginosa*.

CFS levels in wound exudates. CFS levels in the exudates from wounds were similar to serum levels.

Clinical results. The subjects were adult patients suffering from either chronic respiratory tract or soft tissue infections, with *P. aeruginosa* isolated as the pathogen. Of a total of 113 cases, 79 with isolated *P. aeruginosa* were statistically analyzed for clinical and bacteriological responses. Clinically, CFS had a response rate of 71% in 79 cases, with excellent response in 14, good in 42, fair in 14, and poor in 9. Bacteriologically, *P. aeruginosa* was eradicated in 70% of the cases, with elimination in 29, decrease in 15, replacement in 26, and no change in 9 (Tables 1 and 2). Side effects were observed in three cases (2.7%).

TABLE 1. *Clinical and bacteriological effects of CFS treatment in respiratory tract infections with P. aeruginosa*

Diagnosis	No. of cases	Clinical response: Excellent	Good	Fair	Poor	Clinical response rate[a] (%)	Bacteriological effects: Eliminated	Decreased	Replaced	Persisted	Bacteriological response rate[b] (%)
Pneumonia	9	4		2	3	44	4	2	1	2	56
Bronchopneumonia	4	1	3			100	2		2		100
Chronic bronchitis	12	1	8	2	1	75	4	2	4	2	67
Diffuse bronchiolitis	3			1	2	0		1		2	33
Bronchiectasis	7		5	1	1	71	3	3		1	43
Total	35	6	16	6	7	63	13	8	7	7	57

[a] (Number of excellent + good responders/total number of patients studied) × 100.
[b] (Number of strains eliminated + replaced/total number of isolates) × 100.

TABLE 2. *Clinical and bacteriological effects of CFS treatment in soft tissue infections with P. aeruginosa*

Diagnosis	No. of cases	Clinical response: Excellent	Good	Fair	Poor	Clinical response rate[a] (%)	Bacteriological response: Eliminated	Decreased	Replaced	Persisted	Bacteriological response rate[b] (%)
Postoperative wound infection	15	2	10	2	1	80	5	2	8		87
Postburn infection	6		4	2		67	4	2			67
Abscess	7	2	4	1		86	3	1	2	1	71
Ulcerative skin infection	4	1	3			100	2	1	1		75
Postdecubital infection	8	2	3	2	1	63	1	1	5	1	75
Others	4	1	2	1		75	1		3		100
Total	44	8	26	8	2	77	16	7	19	2	80

[a,b] See Table 1.

Comparative Pharmacology of Moxalactam and the Third-Generation Cephalosporins

H. LODE,* G. BELMEGA, T. JENDROSCHEK, B. KEMMERICH, K. BORNER, AND P. KOEPPE

Medical and Biochemical Departments of Klinikum Steglitz, Freie Universität Berlin, 1000 Berlin 45, Federal Republic of Germany

Moxalactam (LY) is a newly developed cephalosporin antibiotic with high antibacterial activity and a broadened range of action. In the present study, the pharmacokinetic parameters of LY were compared with cefoperazone (CPZ; T-1551) and cefotaxime (CTX) after a single intravenous bolus injection. In a randomized cross-over study, 10 healthy test persons (5 females, 5 males; mean body weight: 66.7 ± 5.3 kg; mean age 32 years; range, 21 to 51 years) received a 3-min intravenous bolus injection of 1,000 mg of LY, CPZ, and CTX. The intervals between the single test days were 7 to 14 days. Serum concentrations were measured before and after the injection for a period of 12 h; fractional urine samples were collected before and after injection in four periods up to 24 h. Antibiotic concentrations in serum and urine were assayed by an agar diffusion method with *Bacillus subtilis* (ATCC 6633), *Sarcina lutea* (ATCC 9341), and *Escherichia coli* (V6311/65) as test strains (7). The lowest detectable antibiotic activities were 0.15 mg/liter in serum and 0.15 mg/liter in urine for LY, 0.6 mg/liter in serum and 0.15 mg/liter in urine for CPZ, and 0.3 mg/liter in serum and 0.15 mg/liter in urine for CTX.

CTX and desacetylcefotaxim (DACM) concentrations were determined in addition in five volunteers with high-performance liquid chromatography (HPLC) method using reversed-phase chromatography (1). Relevant pharmacokinetic parameters were determined by the least-squares method with the use of a digital computer and Fortran programs (4, 9). The programs are based on a two- as well as a three-compartment, open-system kinetic model (2, 3). The calculated values of pharmacokinetic constants were corrected for a mean body weight of 70.0 kg, which means an average dose of 14.3 mg/kg of body weight.

The serum concentrations of LY were 95.3 ± 21.1 mg/liter after 5 min, 29.4 ± 4.5 mg/liter after 2 h, 14.6 ± 1.7 mg/liter after 4 h, and finally 1.8 ± 0.9 mg/liter after 12 h. The serum concentration courses of CTX and DACM demonstrated the quick elimination of CTX with a short biological half-life, whereas DACM had a significantly longer elimination with a mean biological half-life of 103 min.

The comparative curves of the mean serum concentrations of the three antibiotics (Fig. 1) underline the fact that LY and CPZ result in higher serum concentrations than CTX throughout the entire examination period.

The urine recovery data showed a significantly higher elimination via the kidneys of CTX (53.3 ± 9.1%) and LY (61.0 ± 9.2%) in comparison to CPZ with 25.1 ± 8.1%. The total urine recovery of CTX and DACM during 24 h was 83.8% of the applied doses, CTX 54.7%, and DACM 29.1%.

A comparison of important concentration and pharmacokinetic data is demonstrated in Table 1. Trough concentrations at 12 h, elimination half-lives, volumes of distribution, and serum clearances of LY and CPZ are very similar; differences between these two substances could be seen in renal elimination, with a high extrarenal excretion of CPZ. Neu and co-workers (8) determined nearly the same pharmacokinetic data after 1,000 mg in a 30-min infusion and after 1,000 mg intramuscularly.

Protein binding in serum of the new cephalosporin antibiotics are remarkably different: LY 45 to 51%, CPZ 87 to 94%, and CTX 27 to 50%.

As a result of their characteristic renal and extrarenal eliminations, the biological half-lives in renal insufficiency are distinctly different. LY has a half-life in terminal renal insufficiency ($C_{CR} < 7$ ml/min) of 30 h, whereas CPZ has one

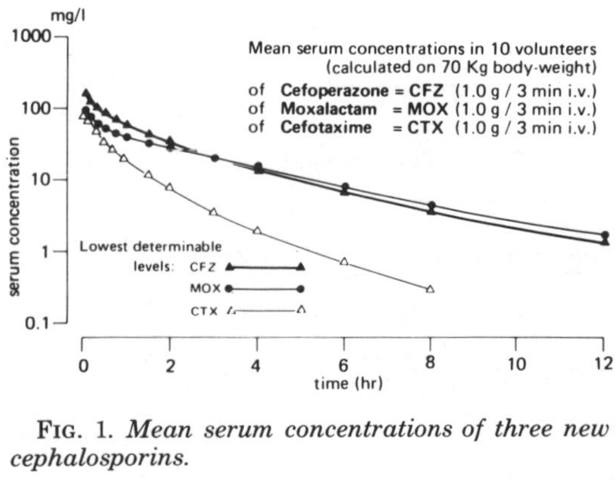

FIG. 1. *Mean serum concentrations of three new cephalosporins.*

TABLE 1. *Comparative concentrations and pharmacokinetics of three new cephalosporins after 1,000 mg intravenously*

	Moxalactam	Cefoperazone	Cefotaxime
Mean peak serum level (5 min after i.v., mg / l)	93 ± 21	158 ± 40	87 ± 19
Serum level (mg / l) at h			
2	28,3 ±4,5	36,2 ± 9	7,5 ± 4,2
6	8,3 ±1,7	6,9 ± 4,5	0,7 ± 0,4
12	1,8 ±0,9	1,3 ± 1,2	---
Biological termin. half life (h)	2,5	2,4	1,3
Vol. of distribut. (l / 100 kg)	19,6	14,9	18,2
Serum clearance (ml / min)	88	71	238
Renal clearance (ml / min)	54	18	127
Urinary levels, 0 - 6 h (mg / l)	1511	547	1559
Mean urinary excret., 0 - 24 h (%)	61	25	53

of 2.2 to 4.2 h and CTX one of 2.7 h (DACM: 8 to 12 h!). During hemodialysis there was a reduction of all biological half-lives with 4 h for LY, 1.8 h for CPZ, and 2.5 h for CTX.

Conclusions. On the basis of our studies and data from the literature, we conclude the following: (i) LY and CPZ have a similar serum concentration course with high serum levels of long duration; (ii) CTX possesses a more rapid elimination characteristic; the metabolite DACM offers a slower decrease of serum concentration with a longer biological half-life; (iii) the pharmacokinetic parameters of the new cephalosporins can be calculated with an open three- or two-compartment model; (iv) elimination via the kidneys is low with CPZ (20 to 30%); in LY and CTX, the urine recovery lies between 50 and 80%; (v) protein binding in serum of LY and CTX is moderate (30 to 50%), whereas CPZ has a high protein binding (>80%); (vi) for clinical practice, we can conclude that CPZ and LY can be applied two times daily; CTX should be given three times per day.

1. **Borner, K., and H. Lode.** 1980. Determination of cefotaxime and desacetylcefotaxime in serum and urine by high performance liquid chromatography. J. Clin. Chem. Clin. Biochem. **18:**719.
2. **Dost, F. M.** 1968. Grundlagen der Pharmakokinetik. Georg Thieme Verlag, Stuttgart.
3. **Greenblatt, D. J., and J. Koch-Weser.** 1975. Clinical pharmacokinetics. N. Engl. J. Med. **293:**702–705, 964–970.
4. **Kienl, G.** 1976. Vergleich der Pharmakokinetik von Epicillin und Ampicillin. Arzneim. Forsch. **26:**781–786.
5. **Lam, M., C. V. Manion, and A. W. Czerwinski.** 1981. Pharmacokinetics of moxalactam in patients with renal insufficiency. Antimicrob. Agents Chemother. **19:**461–464.
6. **Lode, H., B. Kemmerich, P. Koeppe, D. Belmega, and H. Jendroschek.** 1980. Comparative pharmacokinetics of cefoperazone and cefotaxime. Clin. Ther. (special issue) **3:**80–88.
7. **Reeves, D. S., and M. J. Bywater.** 1976. Assay of antimicrobial agents, p. 21–78. *In* J. de Louvois (ed.), Selected topics in clinical bacteriology. Balliere Tindall, London.
8. **Srinivasan, S., K. P. Fu, and H. C. Neu.** 1981. Pharmacokinetics of moxalactam and cefazolin compared in normal volunteers. Antimicrob. Agents Chemother. **19:**301–305.
9. **Wagner, J. G.** 1971. Biopharmaceutics and relevant pharmacokinetics. Hamilton, Illinois.

Pharmacokinetic Studies with Moxalactam

K. KANELLAKOPOULOU, J. TSAGARAKIS, H. GIAMARELLOU,* V. PAPATHANASSIOU, AND G. K. DAIKOS

First Department of Propedeutic Medicine, Athens University School of Medicine, King Paul's Hospital, Athens 609, Greece

In recent years, considerable effort has been given to developing improved β-lactam antibiotics showing resistance, if possible, to all β-lactamases, and at the same time possessing a strong bactericidal activity and satisfactory pharmacokinetic properties. Moxalactam (LY127935), a member of a new class of oxy-β-lactam antibiotics, seemed from preliminary studies to have these features (1). Among 47 patients with life-threatening gram-negative infections given moxalactam by our group, excellent clinical response was observed in 74.5%, with improvement in the remaining patients and eradication of the pathogen in 54.3% of them (H. Giamarellou et al., Prog. Abstr. Intersci. Conf. Antimicrob. Agents Chemother. 20th, New Orleans, 22–24 September 1980, abstr. no. 364). In the present study, results on moxalactam pharmacokinetics in various body compartments after at least 24 h of treatment in 43 patients are discussed.

Blood and urine specimens were collected at suitable intervals after 1 g intramuscularly (i.m.) every 8 h in 8 patients and a 2-g 30-min intravenous (i.v.) infusion every 8 h in 12 patients. Kinetic studies thereafter were always performed after a dosage schedule of 2 g by 30-min i.v. infusion every 8 h. Gall bladder bile was collected from four patients during cholocystectomy. It should be noted that three of four patients were jaundiced. Eight-hour bronchial secretion levels of moxalactam were measured in seven patients with chronic bronchitis in exacerbation. Three of them were intubated; in the other four cases, sputum was collected by expectoration. Sputa were homogenized in a Sorvall homogenizer before assay. Aqueous humor was taken from four patients during elective cataract extraction. Cerebrospinal fluid (CSF) was taken from three patients, in two with inflamed and in one with noninflamed meninges. Pieces of cancellous bone were removed during operation for hip fracture. Fragments of bone were assayed as follows. A piece of bone was washed with phosphate buffer (pH 6.4) to remove excess blood, weighed, and dried overnight at −20°C. The following day it was crushed and pulverized with mortar and pestle. From two patients, pleuritic and prostatic fluid specimens were also taken. On all occasions a blood specimen was withdrawn simultaneously. All specimens of serum, urine, sputum, bile, CSF, aqueous humor, bones, pleuritic fluid, and prostatic fluid were either assayed immediately after collection or frozen and assayed within one week.

Concentrations of moxalactam were measured by an agar well plate technique with Mueller-Hinton agar (BBL Microbiology Systems) and a very susceptible strain of *Escherichia coli* (ATCC 4157) as the indicator organism.

Serum kinetics after a 2-g dose are described in Table 1. In contrast to these results, after a 1-g i.m. dose, mean levels at 0.5, 1, 2, 4, 6, and 8 h postdose were 5.5, 15, 22.2, 24.6, 15.5, 10, and 4.5 μg/ml, respectively, with a mean terminal half-life of 2.3 (± 0.4) h. The long serum terminal half-life of moxalactam when given either i.v. or i.m. indicates that this new antibiotic, unlike related compounds, could be administered, at least in common enterobacterial infections, every 12 h.

Moxalactam mean urine concentrations after a 2-g i.v. dose at collection periods of 0 to 2, 2 to 4, 4 to 6, and 6 to 8 h were found to be 468.3, 427.7, 165.2, and 166.2 mg, respectively, with a mean recovery rate of 63.3 ± 12.1%. The corresponding mean urine values after 1-g i.m. dose were 216.7, 179.7, 133.1, and 98.3 mg, with a mean recovery rate of 69.3 ± 2.7%. As the renal route accounted for 50.5 to 74.5% of the drug excretion, we feel that modification of the dose regimen may be necessary for patients with renal insufficiency.

Kinetic results in various body compartments are shown in Table 2. It is obvious that moxalactam produced satisfactory levels in gall bladder bile (with and without jaundice), bronchial

TABLE 1. *Moxalactam serum concentrations after a 30-min infusion of three 2-g doses every 8 h*

	Concn (μg/ml) at indicated time (h)							$t_{1/2}$ (h)
	0	0.5	1	2	4	6	8	
	7		115	42.5	27.5	15	7	2
	3.3	100		70	17.5	12.5	14	2.2
	6.5	125	120	40	25	20.5	9.5	2
	9.5	95	52.5	30	22.5	5.5	3.3	2.5
	10		67.5	30	20.5	11.9	7.5	2.3
	6		59	49.5	28.5	11.3	8.7	2.9
	13		100	52.5	24.3	18	11	3.2
	22		97.5	60	39	28	22.2	4.2
	6.8		80	65	14.4	12		
		170	105	60	30	13.8	7.5	2.2
		160	47.5	35	17.5	8.5	5.3	2.2
			40	23	15	5	3.3	2.3
Mean	9.3	130	80.4	54.8	23.5	13.5	9	2.5
SD	5.5	34.1	28.6	30.9	7.2	6.4	5.4	0.67

TABLE 2. *Moxalactam kinetics in various body compartments in 23 patients*

Source	No. of patients	Moxalactam level (μg/ml)	Indicated time after 2-g dose (h)
Gall bladder	4	11.5,[a] 15.0,[a] 16.25,[a] 13.0	1.5, 2, 3.5, 6
Sputum	4	1.2, 1.0, 1.3, 7.5	8-h collection
Bronchial secretions	3	6.4, 19.5, 39.6	8-h collection
Aqueous humor	4	3.3, 2.5, 3.0, 9.5	3, 4, 4.5, 5
CSF	3	1.0,[b] 4.0, 4.5	4, 4, 4
Bone	3	0.47/79,[c] 1.9/40, 0.36/120	2.5, 5.5, 6
Prostatic fluid	1	28.0	4
Pleuritic fluid	1	6.5	4

[a] Presence of jaundice.
[b] Noninflamed meninges.
[c] Micrograms per milligram of bone weight.

secretions, inflamed and noninflamed CSF, aqueous humor, prostatic gland fluid, and pleuritic fluid, therefore predicting a satisfactory clinical response in relevant infections. On the other hand, kinetic results in bone were rather unsatisfactory but also not sufficient to draw final conclusions, since moxalactam's very low MIC of <0.25 μg/ml against the enterobacteriaceae may counterbalance the low local concentrations. It is also probable that during inflammation local bone kinetics will be more promising. On the other hand, considering the quite high MICs of moxalactam against *P. aeruginosa*, it should be kept in mind that in relevant infections a correlation between the estimated MICs and the expected local concentrations is necessary before one decides on administering the new antibiotic.

1. **Yoshida, T., S. Matsuura, M. Mayama, Y. Kameda, and S. Kuwahara.** 1980. Moxalactam (6059-S), a novel 1-oxa-β-lactam with an expanded antibacterial spectrum: laboratory evaluation. Antimicrob. Agents Chemother. **17**:302–312.

Moxalactam Plasma-Urine Kinetics and Antibacterial Activity After Single Intramuscular or Intravenous Doses

ROBERT L. PERKINS,* JOSEPH F. PLOUFFE, ROBERT J. FASS, RICHARD B. PRIOR, BARRY BERNSTEIN, AND KARL A. DE SANTE

Division of Infectious Diseases, The Ohio State University, Columbus, Ohio 43210, and Lilly Research Laboratories, Indianapolis, Indiana 46206, U.S.A.*

The purpose of this study was to define the pharmacokinetic properties and antibacterial activity obtained from intravenous (i.v.) and intramuscular (i.m.) administration of moxalactam in volunteers. Single doses of 250, 500, 1,000, and 2,000 mg were given to groups of four normal volunteers in 20-min and 5-min constant i.v. infusions, using a Harvard pump, and as i.m. injections. Blood samples for assays were drawn at 5, 20, and 30 min and at 1, 2, 4, 6, 8, and 12 h. Urine collections were obtained 0 to 1, 1 to 6, and 6 to 12 h after doses.

Plasma and urine concentrations of moxalactam were determined by a disk plate assay procedure, using *Escherichia coli* ATCC 10536 as the test organism and antibiotic medium 1 (Difco Laboratories, Detroit, Mich.). Standard curves were made in pooled normal human plasma and phosphate buffer, pH 6.0, for plasma and urine assays, respectively. Minimum susceptibility was approximately 0.5 μg/ml. The pharmacokinetic data were fitted by means of the NONLIN computer program, using equations suggested by Wagner (1, 2). Antibacterial activity (ABA) of plasma and urine samples was determined by microdilution methods. Dilutions of samples from 1:2 to 1:2,048 were made in cation-supplemented Mueller-Hinton broth (Difco) for testing against facultative and aerobic organisms and in Schaedler broth for *Bacteroides fragilis*. Final test inocula of 1×10^5 to 5×10^5 colony-forming units of the following pathogens per ml (moxalactam MIC given in micrograms per milliliter) were used: *E. coli*,

≤0.125; *Proteus vulgaris*, ≤0.125; *Enterobacter aerogenes*, 16; *Serratia marcescens*, 8; *Pseudomonas aeruginosa*, 16; and *B. fragilis*, 0.25. Plates were incubated at 37°C for 18 h (48 h in an anaerobic chamber for *B. fragilis*); endpoints were the highest dilutions completely inhibiting visible growth. ABA titers were expressed as $\log_2$ values: 1:2 = 1, 1:128 = 7, etc.

Mean plasma concentrations are shown in Table 1. Peak concentrations were observed immediately at the end of the i.v. infusions, but peaks ranged from 1 to 2 h after i.m. dosing. Definite dose linearity in the plasma levels was noted for peak values and areas under the curves. A biexponential decay was evident immediately after cessation of the i.v. infusions. Mean $t_{1/2\beta}$ were 2.4 and 2.2 h for the 5- and 20-min i.v. infusions, respectively, and 2.8 h for the i.m. route. Renal clearances were approximately 50% of expected normal creatinine clearance values. The mean volume of distribution was similar for i.v. and i.m. routes, approximately 0.30 liter/kg; the volume of the central compartment was 50% of the total volume of distribution.

Urinary recovery (percentage) of moxalactam (means of recovery for 250-, 500-, 1,000-, and 2,000-mg doses combined) during 0 to 1-, 1 to 6-, and 6 to 12-h periods were, respectively, 22.5, 25, and 7 (total, 54%) after 5-min i.v. infusions, 25, 34, and 9 (total, 68%) after 20-min i.v. infusions, and 12, 41, and 11 (total, 64%) after i.m. injections.

In vitro ABA of plasma and urine samples against six clinical bacterial isolates is shown in Table 2. Only peak values and declining activity during elimination phases after 250- and 2,000-mg doses are depicted for plasma and are expressed as $\log_2$ dilutions (1:2 = 1; 1:128 = 7, 1:2,048 = 11). Against highly susceptible strains (*E. coli* and *P. vulgaris*, MIC ≤ 0.125), peak plasma ABA after 2,000 mg i.v. exceeded 1:2,048 dilutions and remained at significant levels even at 12 h; the 250-mg i.v. dose resulted in lower peak inhibition (1:256 to 1:1,024) and considerably lower values at 8 and 12 h for those isolates. Against the less susceptible strains tested (*S. marcescens*, MIC = 8; *P. aeruginosa*, MIC = 16), markedly lower plasma ABA was noted after i.v. administration but was highest initially after 5-min infusions of 2,000 mg; thereafter, ABA declined at 8 and 12 h to nearly base-line values. The 250-mg i.v. dose caused little inhibitory effect against the *S. marcescens* and *P. aeruginosa* strains tested. Initial peak plasma ABA against the highly susceptible strains after i.m. administration of 2,000 mg was only one dilution lower than after i.v. doses and showed slightly greater sustained activity at 8 and 12 h. The 250-mg i.v. dose resulted in significant inhibition of the susceptible pathogens by early plasma samples, but ABA declined markedly at 12 h; no additional inhibition over base-line predosing values (1:2 to 1:4) was observed with early plasma samples against the *Pseudomonas* strain.

In vitro urinary ABA of 0 to 1 and 1 to 6-h samples after 2,000 mg i.v. exceeded 1:2,048 dilutions against *E. coli*, *P. vulgaris*, *E. aerogenes*, and *B. fragilis*: most 6- to 12-h samples showed similar activity. The *P. aeruginosa* and *S. marcescens* strains were also inhibited at slightly lower dilutions. The 250-mg i.v. dose resulted in inhibition at ≥1:2,048 dilutions against *E. coli* and *P. vulgaris* but lesser effect against other

TABLE 1. *Moxalactam plasma concentrations and kinetics after 5- and 20-min i.v. infusions and i.m. injections in volunteers*

Dose (g)	Plasma concn (μg/ml)[a]							$t_{1/2}$ (h)	Plasma clearance (liters/kg per h)	Renal clearance (liters/kg per h)	Vol of distribution (liters/kg)
	5 min	20 min	30 min	1 h	2 h	8 h	12 h				
5-min i.v.											
0.25	23			8	6	<1	<1	2.4	0.10	0.06	0.33
0.5	49			19	10	2	<1	2.5	0.13	0.06	0.36
1	104			41	22	4	1	2.3	0.09	0.05	0.26
2	200			80	49	7	3	2.4	0.10	0.07	0.29
20-min i.v.											
0.25		17		7	5	3	<1	2.1	0.11	0.09	0.30
0.5		35		18	10	1	<1	1.9	0.13	0.06	0.34
1		95		53	30	5	1	2.6	0.09	0.07	0.24
2		233		120	56	11	4	2.5	0.09	0.06	0.25
i.m.											
0.25			9	9	7	2	<1	2.8	0.08	0.03	0.30
0.5			18	20	17	4	2	3.1	0.07	0.05	0.30
1			39	40	38	7	3	2.8	0.07	0.05	0.26
2			28	60	81	17	7	2.6	0.05	0.03	0.18

[a] Mean of four volunteer samples.

TABLE 2. *Plasma and urinary antibacterial activity after single 5- and 20-min i.v. infusions and i.m. injections in volunteers*[a]

Dose and species	Plasma									Urine							
	i.m.			5-min i.v.			20-min i.v.			i.m.			5-min i.v.			20-min i.v.	
	1 h	8 h	12 h	5 min	8 h	12 h	20 min	8 h	12 h	0–1 h	1–6 h	6–12 h	0–1 h	1–6 h	6–12 h	0–1 h	1–6 h
250 mg																	
E. coli	7	4	2	9	3	2	8	4	2	≥11	≥11	10	≥11	≥11	10	≥11	≥11
P. vulgaris	8	7	3	10	4	2	9	4	1	≥11	≥11	11	≥11	≥11	10	≥11	≥11
E. aerogenes	3	1	4	5	2	1	4	2	1	8	8	5	7	7	5	8	8
S. marcescens	2	4	4	2	4	4	2	1	1	5	6	3	5	5	2	6	5
P. aeruginosa	2	2	1	2	2	2	2	2	2	4	4	2	4	4	2	5	4
B. fragilis	5	2	2	4	1	4	4	1	1	10	11	8	9	8	6	10	9
2,000 mg																	
E. coli	10	8	6	≥11	7	6	≥11	7	5	≥11	≥11	≥11	≥11	≥11	≥11	≥11	≥11
P. vulgaris	≥11	9	7	≥11	7	6	11	8	6	≥11	≥11	≥11	≥11	≥11	≥11	≥11	≥11
E. aerogenes	5	4	2	8	3	2	6	3	2	≥11	≥11	≥11	≥11	≥11	8	≥11	9
S. marcescens	3	2	2	5	2	1	4	1	1	8	8	6	10	8	5	7	7
P. aeruginosa	3	3	2	4	2	2	3	2	2	9	8	7	8	7	5	6	6
B. fragilis	7	5	4	9	3	2	8	3	1	≥11	≥11	≥11	≥11	≥11	10	≥11	≥11

[a] Results are expressed as $\log_2 N$ dilution (1:2 = 1, 1:128 = 7, ≥1:1,028 = ≥11); mean of four volunteer samples.

strains tested. Overall, the i.m. route tended to produce equally or slightly more sustained ABA in 1 to 6- and 6 to 12-h collections as compared with i.v. administration.

In summary, 5- and 20-min i.v. infusions of moxalactam produced high mean peak plasma concentrations and area under the curve and showed linear relationships to dosage. The i.m. route resulted in similar kinetics. The long $t_{1/2\beta}$ of 2.2 to 2.4 h for i.v. and 2.8 h for i.m. administration were consistent with the relatively low renal clearances. Mean urinary recovery in 12 h ranged from 54 to 68%. The highest in vitro plasma ABA, especially against the less susceptible organisms tested, was observed after the 5-min (bolus-like) 2,000-mg i.v. infusions; however, significant decline in ABA against those organisms occurred within 8 h and was minimal at 12 h. In contrast, urinary ABA against even *P. aeruginosa* and *S. marcescens* after i.v. administration of 2,000 mg remained high (≥1:32) through the 6 to 12-h sample (one portion) and was extremely high through 0 to 12 h for the *E. coli* and *P. vulgaris* strains. The i.m. route produced effectively high ABA, even with the smaller 250-mg dose. These in vitro results suggest that moxalactam dosage and intervals of administration in patients with normal renal function should possibly be chosen according to the relative susceptibility of the infecting organism(s) and the body site of involvement. Dosage at 12-h intervals could prove feasible for most uncomplicated urinary tract infections due to susceptible organisms.

1. **Metzler, C. M., G. L. Elfring, and A. J. McEwen.** 1974. A users manual for NONLIN and associated programs. The Upjohn Co., Kalamazoo, Mich.
2. **Wagner, J. G.** 1976. Linear pharmacokinetic equations allowing direct calculations of many needed pharmacokinetic parameters from the co-efficients and exponents of poly-exponential equations which have been fitted to the data. J. Pharmacokinet. Biopharm. **4**:443–467.

Penetration of Moxalactam and Cefoperazone into Cerebrospinal Fluids

CHIEN LIU, FONG-WEN SHI, JANE L. HARMS, AND DANIEL R. HINTHORN

Division of Infectious Diseases, University of Kansas Medical Center, Kansas City, Kansas 66103, U.S.A.

The need for an antimicrobial for treatment of gram-negative bacterial central nervous system infections is obvious. Aminoglycosides and existing cephalosporins do not cross the blood-brain barrier well. The present report describes the results of studies determining the penetration of moxalactam and cefoperazone into the cerebrospinal fluids (CSF) in human subjects with normal noninflamed meninges.

Selection of participants. Forty hospitalized patients or healthy volunteers participated in this study. After informed consent was obtained, the participants were equally divided, 20 in each study, to receive moxalactam or cefoperazone. The demographic characteristics of the studied subjects are as follows: in the moxalactam group there were 16 males and 4 females with mean ages of 38.7 ± 18.1 years (range, 23 to 72); in the cefoperazone group there were 11 males and 9 females with mean ages 35.2 ± 19.6 years (range, 19 to 76). Two subjects in each group had an Ommaya reservoir implanted 5 to 6 years previously for therapeutic reasons.

Before administration of antibiotics, each participant was given a physical examination and a set of laboratory tests was performed. The laboratory tests included a complete blood count, urinalysis, blood urea nitrogen, serum creatinine, alkaline phosphatase, and serum glutamic oxalacetic transaminase. At 24 to 48 h after receiving the antibiotics, another set of similar laboratory tests was again performed.

Drug administration and specimen collection. A total of 2 g of moxalactam or cefoperazone was dissolved in 50 ml of 5% dextrose in water and was infused intravenously over a period of 15 to 30 min. Half of the participants in each study received a single dose and the other half in each study received three multiple doses at 8-h intervals. At 1 or 3 h after infusion with the single dose or the last multiple dose, five individuals in each subgroup were subjected to lumbar puncture or aspiration via Ommaya reservoir for collection of CSF. The two subjects with Ommaya reservoir had both 1-h and 3-h CSF collection after receiving the antibiotics. A simultaneous blood sample was obtained. A portion of the CSF sample was sent for cell count, glucose, and protein determinations. The remaining CSF and serum after separation from blood by centrifugation were frozen at −70°C until assay.

Bioassay. Serum and CSF concentrations of moxalactam and cefoperazone were determined by bioassay with agar well diffusion method. For moxalactam, *Escherichia coli* (ATCC 10536) was used and for cefoperazone, *Sarcina lutea* (ATCC 9341) was the assay organism.

Results. With a single dose of 2 g of moxalactam, mean serum levels at 1 and 3 h after infusion were 65.2 ± 28.7 μg/ml and 35.7 ± 11.2 μg/ml, respectively. However, no detectable CSF moxalactam penetration (<1.25 μg/ml) was found in any of the subjects. After multiple doses of moxalactam administration, mean serum level at 1 h after infusion was 101.6 ± 28.4 μg/ml, and three of the five participants had detectable CSF levels with a mean of 1.72 ± 0.12 μg/ml. Serum moxalactam level after multiple dosing at 3 h after infusion was 42.6 ± 9.9 μg/ml, and all five subjects had detectable CSF levels with a mean of 1.44 ± 0.15 μg/ml.

In the cefoperazone study, the mean serum levels at 1 and 3 h after a single-dose infusion were 122.0 ± 48.8 μg/ml and 43.3 ± 35.3 μg/ml, respectively. One subject had detectable CSF level at 1 and 3 h after a single-dose cefoperazone administration. This individual had an Ommaya reservoir implanted in his cerebral ventricles. However, none of the other subjects had detectable cefoperazone levels (<0.62 μg/ml) in CSF samples collected either at 1 h or at 3 h after receiving multiple doses of cefoperazone (Table 1).

Discussion. From our data, a single 2-g dose of moxalactam or cefoperazone given intravenously did not penetrate into the CSF in individuals with normal noninflamed meninges either at 1 or 3 h after intravenous infusion. With multiple doses, moxlactam appeared to penetrate into CSF more predictably than cefoperazone, with all five subjects having detectable CSF levels 3 h after infusion. Once penetrated into the CSF, moxalactam seemed to maintain its CSF levels while the serum concentrations decreased. This resulted in a more favorable CSF/serum moxalactam ratio at 3 h than at 1 h postinfusion. Kaplan et al. (1) have reported that moxalactam adequately penetrates into the CSF of 39 children with bacterial meningitis after repetitive 50-mg/kg doses. In seven adult patients with bacterial meningitis, Landesman et al. (2) found that with 2 g of moxalactam given intravenously every 8 h, peak CSF levels

TABLE 1. *Penetration of moxalactam and cefoperazone into human CSF*

Dose and drug [a]	No. of penetrations	Mean ± SD and ranges of drug concentrations in:	
		Serum (μg/ml)	CSF (μg/ml)
Single (1 h)			
MO	0/5	65.2 ± 28.7 (26.8–107.0)	<1.25
CE	1/5	122.0 ± 48.8 (78.0–205.0)	0.76
Single (3 h)			
MO	0/5	35.7 ± 11.2 (31.0–55.0)	<1.25
CE	1/5	43.3 ± 35.3 (17.5–104.0)	1.25
Multiple (1 h)			
MO	3/5	101.6 ± 28.4 (66.0–132.0)	1.72 ± .12 (1.6–1.9)
CE	0/5	105.4 ± 17.5 (87.5–127.5)	<0.63
Multiple (3 h)			
MO	5/5	42.6 ± 9.9 (29.0–56.0)	1.44 ± 14 (1.3–1.6)
CE	0/5	32.8 ± 13.9 (21.5–56.0)	<0.63

[a] MO, Moxalactam; CE, cefoperazone.

ranged from 25 to 39 μg/ml, which occurred 2.5 h after infusion. In our laboratory study in rabbits infected experimentally with *E. coli* or pneumococcal meningitis, we have found cefoperazone penetrated inflamed meninges very readily to reach good therapeutic levels and sterilized the CSF *E. coli* or pneumococci within 8 h after intramuscular injections (F. W. Shi, G. W. Mitchell, N. Marshall, D. R. Hinthorn, and C. Liu, Abstr. Annu. Meet. Am. Soc. Microbiol. 1981, A25, p. 5). In comparing several antibiotics for treatment of experimental bacillary meningitis, Schaad et al. reported moxalactam to be statistically more effective than ampicillin or netilmicin in treatment of gram-negative meningitis (3). Extension of the present study to investigate the penetration of these antibiotics into human CSF in individuals with inflamed meninges is currently underway.

1. **Kaplan, S. L., E. O. Mason, Jr., H. Garcia, S. J. Kvernland, E. M. Loiselle, D. C. Anderson, A. A. Mintz, and R. D. Feigin.** 1981. Pharmacokinetics and cerebrospinal fluid penetration of moxalactam in children with bacterial meningitis. J. Pediatr. **98**:152–157.
2. **Landesman, S. H., M. L. Corrado, C. C. Cherubin, M. Gompert, and D. Cleri.** 1980. Diffusion of a new beta-lactam (LY 127935) into cerebrospinal fluid. Implications for therapy of gram-negative bacillary meningitis. Am. J. Med. **69**:92–98.
3. **Schaad, U. B., G. H. McCracken, Jr., C. A. Loock, and M. L. Thomas.** 1980. Pharmacokinetics and bacteriological efficacy of moxalactam (LY127935), netilmicin, and ampicillin in experimental gram-negative enteric bacillary meningitis. Antimicrob. Agents Chemother. **17**:406–411.

Comparison of Moxalactam and Cefotaxime Concentrations in Ventricular Cerebrospinal Fluid

OSWALD BRÜCKNER* AND HARTMUT COLLMANN

Department of Internal Medicine and Neurosurgical Department of Klinikum Charlottenburg, Freie Universität Berlin, West Berlin, Federal Republic of Germany

Treatment of gram-negative bacillary meningitis has remained unsatisfactory as regards mortality rates, particularly in neonates but also in older children and adults. Mortality rates could be reduced only to a minor extent, although recommendations for therapeutic regimens changed from chloramphenicol and kanamycin to ampicillin in combination with newer aminoglycosides given systemically, topically, or both into the cerebrospinal fluid (CSF), preferably by the intraventricular route. After systemic application alone, aminoglycosides are transported to the CSF compartment in amounts exceeding MICs of most *Enterobacteriaceae* in only a few patients, even in the presence of severe meningeal inflammation. Additional intraventricular application of aminoglycosides does not seem to be without hazards, at least for neonates (6).

Beta-lactam antibiotics others than ampicillin, which has been rendered ineffective in the past decade because of rapidly growing numbers of highly resistant *Enterobacteriaceae* and some strains of *Haemophilus influenzae*, have been instituted in several instances instead of ampicillin. Results with cephalosporins and recent synthetic penicillins have been disappointing in the majority of trials for treatment of meningitis due to enteric bacilli. The outcome of these trials has remained unreliable.

Thus, there has been a need for other safe, nontoxic drugs combining properties such as high activity against enteric bacilli and good penetrability into the CSF compartment with long-lasting high levels. Some of the cephalosporin compounds with extremely extended activity against *Enterobacteriaceae* have recently become available and are likely to fulfill these conditions.

Moxalactam (1-oxa-cephalosporin; MOX) and cefotaxime (CTX) have been evaluated in treatment of gram-negative bacillary meningitis, including cases due to *H. influenzae*, in investigations in a lapine or rat model (2, 8, 9) as well as in a limited number of patients (1, 3–5). *Escherichia coli*, *Klebsiella oxytoca*, and *Serratia marcescens* could be eradicated as causative organisms in bacterial meningitis (3, 5). Results reported on these patients and on investigational trials in rabbits with experimental meningitis revealed CSF concentrations of MOX exceeding by far the MICs of most *Enterobacteriaceae.* In fact, the penetration ratios (concentration in CSF/concentration in serum) of MOX were higher than were ratios of other cephalosporin compounds (9).

The purpose of our investigation was to determine CSF concentrations of this drug in patients with no or only slight impairment of the blood-CSF barrier as seen in neurosurgical patients at least 2 days after neurosurgical procedures with insertion of an external ventricular drain. Drawing ventricular CSF from the drain gave us the chance to gather serial CSF samples after one dose of 2 g intravenously (i.v.). Determinations of MOX levels were performed by the bioassay method, using Mueller-Hinton agar and *E. coli* ATCC 10536 as the test strain. Standard regression curves were established by preparing six different concentrations in pooled CSF and serum, respectively, being without antibacterial activity before dilution. Each determination was done in duplicate or triplicate.

Two serial determinations could be performed after the first and the fourth applications in one patient (Fig. 1) and after the third and the sixth applications of 2 g in two other patients. Measurable amounts of the drug in CSF after the first dose of 2 g were detected only in the 4-h sample, not in the 1- and 2-h samples. The drug probably accumulated within the CSF compartment, since the CSF concentration determined

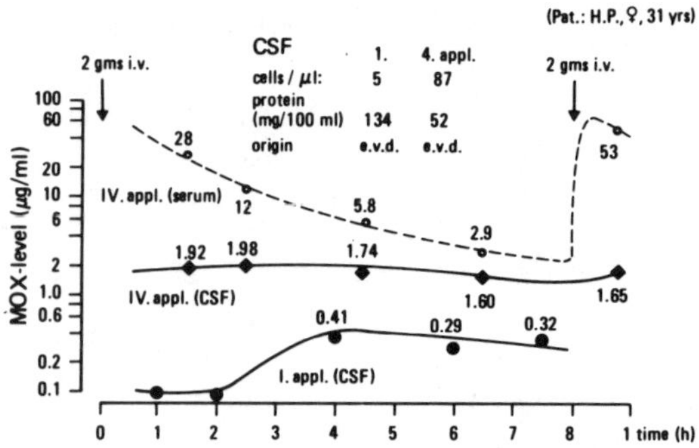

FIG. 1. *Determination of MOX and CSF levels after first and fourth applications.*

after the fourth application of 2 g was much higher than after the first application. We also noted that CSF drug levels in the other two patients were higher after the sixth application (3.45 to 5.05 μg/ml in one patient; 1.31 to 2.20 μg/ml in the other patient) than after the third application as well (1.08 to 1.71 μg/ml in one patient; 1.34 to 1.72 μg/ml in the other patient). Highest levels were usually seen between 2 and 4 h after one distinct application.

CSF concentrations of MOX in patients with inflamed meninges (Table 1) ranged from 1 to 2.30 μg/ml in one patient with meningeal inflammation after neurosurgical procedures, without identification of the causative organism, and 7.20 to 16.0 μg/ml in lumbar CSF of another patient with *Staphylococcus epidermidis* shunt-associated meningitis.

CTX levels determined by bioassay using *E. coli* 6311/65 as the test organism in lumbar or ventricular CSF of six patients with meningitis are demonstrated for the purpose of comparison (Table 1). CTX levels in CSF ranged from 1.1 to 16.0 μg/ml, but there was no correlation with the amount of CSF protein or CSF cell counts.

Excellent therapeutic success with CTX alone in three patients with meningitis showed CTX levels in CSF to be higher than the MICs of the infecting organisms (*E. coli*, MIC of CTX, 0.06 μg/ml; *Streptococcus pneumoniae*, MIC of CTX, 0.25 μg/ml; and *H. influenzae*, which was not assayed for MIC, but was treated insufficiently in a 7-month-old child by ampicillin and chloramphenicol before CTX). Serial tests in two neurosurgical patients with only slight impairment of the blood-CSF barrier ranged from <0.1 to 3.07 μg/ml of CTX, indicating CTX to be of good value in prophylaxis and therapy of meningeal infection in neurosurgical patients. Highest CSF levels were found 1 to 4 h after a distinct systemic CTX application of 2 g.

Comparing the two compounds MOX and CTX, the latter is of advantage in therapy of

TABLE 1. *CSF levels of MOX and CTX*[a]

patient	application number	CSF protein (mg/100 ml)	CSF cells/µl	CSF origin	drug conc. µg/ml serum	CSF	interval from last application	creatinine in serum (mg/100 ml)
Serial determinations of MOX in ventricular CSF of neurosurgical patients after 2 gms i.v.								
1. ♀, 32 yrs	7	35	18	e.v.d.	38.0	2.25	1 h 00′	0.4
					30.0	2.94	2 h 00′	
					7.5	2.97	4 h 15′	
					5.6	2.20	6 h 00′	
					2.1	1.23	8 h 00′	
2. ♂, 23 yrs	3	115	10	e.v.d.	25.0	2.18	1 h 20′	0.8
					16.0	1.71	2 h 15′	
					7.5	2.50	4 h 30′	
					2.9	1.23	6 h 15′	
					1.5	1.20	8 h 10′	
MOX levels in CSF of patients with meningeal inflammation after 2 gms i.v.								
2. 23 yrs	14	49	710	e.v.d.	54.0	1.58	2 h 00′	1.0
					20.0	2.30	4 h 15′	
					11.0	1.45	6 h 00′	
					4.8	1.10	8 h 00′	
3. ♂, 61 yrs	3	165	130	lumbar	52.0	7.20	2 h 15′	0.7
				lumbar	30.0	7.90	4 h 15′	
	8	166	93	lumbar	38.0	16.00	4 h 00′	0.7
	20	143	12	lumbar	53.0	8.04	2 h 30′	0.8
CTX levels in CSF of patients with meningeal inflammation after 2 gms i.v.								
4. ♂, 38 yrs		n.d.	4600	lumbar	3.8	1.5	3 h 30′	0.5
		n.d.	1664	e.v.d.	10.7	1.1	2 h 00′	0.6
5. ♂, 41 yrs		308	6530	lumbar	50.2	2.9	1 h 15′	1.1
		88	900	lumbar	25.9	4.3	1 h 45′	1.1
6. ♂, 59 yrs		384	230	lumbar	n.d.	7.1	3 h 30′	0.6
		371	143	lumbar	5.1	5.3	3 h 30′	0.6
7. ♀, 47 yrs		57	619	lumbar	67.9	5.4	2 h 20′	0.8
8. ♂, 61 yrs		506	2048	lumbar	2.0	4.7	4 h 15′	0.8
9. ♀, 51 yrs		220	658	e.v.d.	2.8	2.8	7 h 00′	0.4
		115	9	e.v.d.	44.0	16.0	?	0.6
Serial CTX determinations in ventricular CSF of neurosurgical patients after 2 gms i.v.								
10. ♂, 72 yrs		n.d.	20	e.v.d.	52.4	3.07	1 h 00′	
					6.7	1.93	4 h 00′	1.1
					3.2	1.78	6 h 00′	
					1.8	1.67	7 h 45′	
4. ♂, 38 yrs		n.d.	n.d.	e.v.d.	42.0	0.19	2 h 00′	
					3.8	0.21	4 h 00′	
					1.0	0.10	6 h 00′	0.9
					<0.1	<0.10	8 h 00′	
					122.0	0.23	0 h 15′	

[a] Abbreviations: i.v., intravenously; e.v.d., external ventricular drain; n.d., not done.

patients with meningitis of unknown bacterial origin (1), since its antibacterial activity includes many gram-positive cocci such as pneumococci (7), but MOX seems to be more active in proven cases of meningitis due to enteric bacilli (9).

1. **Belohradsky, B. H., K. Bruch, D. Geiss, D. Kafetzis, W. Marget, and G. Peters.** 1980. Intravenous cefotaxime in children with bacterial meningitis. Lancet **i**:61–63.
2. **Cordera, C. S., and R. S. Pekarek.** 1980. Treatment of experimental *Haemophilus influenzae* type B meningitis with 1-oxa-β-lactam (LY 127935). Antimicrob. Agents Chemother. **17**:258–262.
3. **Fisher, J. F., M. J. Carter, J. Parsons, and J. P. Rissing.** 1981. Moxalactam (LY 127935) in treatment of meningitis due to gram-negative bacilli. Antimicrob. Agents Chemother. **19**:218–221.
4. **Kaplan, S. L., E. O. Mason, H. Garcia, S. J. Kvernland, E. M. Loiselle, D. C. Anderson, A. A. Mintz, and R. D. Feigin.** 1981. Pharmacokinetics and cerebrospinal fluid penetration of moxalactam in children with bacterial meningitis. J. Pediatr. **98**:152–157.
5. **Landesman, S. H., M. L. Corrado, C. C. Cherubin, M. Gombert, and D. Cleri.** 1980. Diffusion of a new betalactam (LY 127935) into cerebrospinal fluid. Implications for therapy of gram-negative bacillary meningitis. Am. J. Med. **69**:92–98.
6. **McCracken, G. H., S. G. Mize, and N. Threlkeld.** 1980. Intraventricular gentamicin therapy in gram-negative bacillary meningitis of infancy. Report of the Second Neonatal Meningitis Cooperative Study Group. Lancet **i**:787–791.
7. **Neu, H. C., N. Aswapokee, P. Aswapokee, and K. P. Fu.** 1979. HR 756, a new cephalosporin active against gram-positive and gram-negative aerobic and anaerobic bacteria. Antimicrob. Agents Chemother. **15**:273–281.
8. **Schaad, U. B., G. H. McCracken, C. A. Loock, and M. L. Thomas.** 1980. Pharmacokinetics and bacteriological efficacy of moxalactam (LY 127935), netilmicin, and ampicillin in experimental gram-negative enteric bacillary meningitis. Antimicrob. Agents. Chemother. **17**: 406–411.
9. **Schaad, U. B., G. H. McCracken, C. A. Loock, and M. L. Thomas.** 1981. Pharmacokinetics and bacteriologic efficacy of moxalactam, cefotaxime, cefoperazone, and rocephin in experimental bacterial meningitis. J. Infect. Dis. **143**:156–163.

Cefazolin and Moxalactam Pharmacokinetics After Simultaneous Intravenous Infusion

RON E. POLK,* BERRY J. KLINE, AND SHELDON M. MARKOWITZ

Schools of Pharmacy and Medicine, Medical College of Virginia, Virginia Commonwealth University, Richmond, Virginia 23298, U.S.A.

Early investigations indicated that serum samples containing both moxalactam and cefazolin could be assayed simultaneously by high-pressure liquid chromatography, since both compounds had similar but distinct retention times (Fig. 1). This suggested that a comparative pharmacokinetic study could be performed by simultaneously administering both drugs. Thus, the objective of this study was to determine whether the kinetic behaviors of both agents were independent of each other after intravenous infusion.

Six healthy adult volunteers (three males) with no history of penicillin allergy gave informed consent. Serum biochemical studies obtained before drug administration yielded normal values for each subject. The mean age was 27 years (range, 22 to 35). Subjects were instructed to refrain from strenuous physical activity or alcohol ingestion during each study period. A 30-min infusion of 10 mg of cefazolin sodium per kg (Eli Lilly and Co., Indianapolis, Ind.; lot 3TU66A) dissolved in 50 ml of normal saline was administered via an IVAC 530 constant-infusion pump. Two days after administration of cefazolin, each subject received an infusion of 10 mg of moxalactam disodium per kg (lot CT-4765-OM). Two days after the administration of moxalactam, each subject received a simultaneous 30-min infusion of moxalactam and cefazolin (10 mg of each per kg), both dissolved in 50 ml of normal saline. Blood was obtained at the following times (hours) postinfusion for all three studies: 0 (contralateral arm), 0.25, 0.5, 1, 2, 4, 6, 9, 12, and 24. Since statistical analysis indicated moxalactam and cefazolin to be pharmacokinetically independent (see below), six additional normal volunteers (four males, mean age of 28 years) received a single simultaneous infusion of both cefazolin and moxalactam, with sampling and processing as described above.

A two-compartment open model with parameters obtained from the Statistical Analysis Service nonlinear regression program using all data points was found to characterize the serum concentration curves for each antibiotic. Student's *t*-test for paired observations was used to test for significant differences. A P value of <0.05 (two tails) was considered to be statistically significant.

The serum concentrations of cefazolin alone compared with cefazolin when given with moxalactam revealed no significant differences at any time. Likewise, a comparison of the moxalactam serum concentrations when administered alone compared with values obtained when administered with cefazolin revealed no significant differences. The computer-derived serum concentration versus time profiles for moxalactam and cefazolin after simultaneous administration to the 12 normal subjects are compared in Fig. 2. Cefazolin serum concentrations were significantly greater than moxalactam concentrations from 0 through 4 h. The differences were not significant for the remaining times. Only one subject (receiving moxalactam) had a measurable concentration (>1.0 μg/ml) at 24 h. The area under the curve for cefazolin was significantly greater than that for moxalactam (211 ± 0.7 versus 152 ± 19 μg.h/ml, respectively). The terminal half-life of moxalactam was signifi-

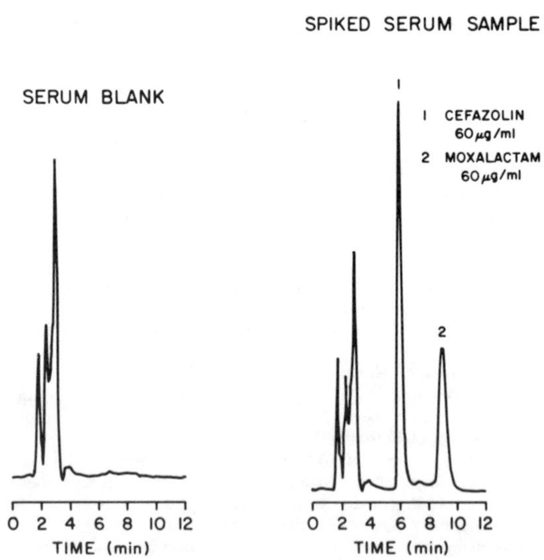

FIG. 1. *Typical chromatograms of serum containing cefazolin and moxalactam.*

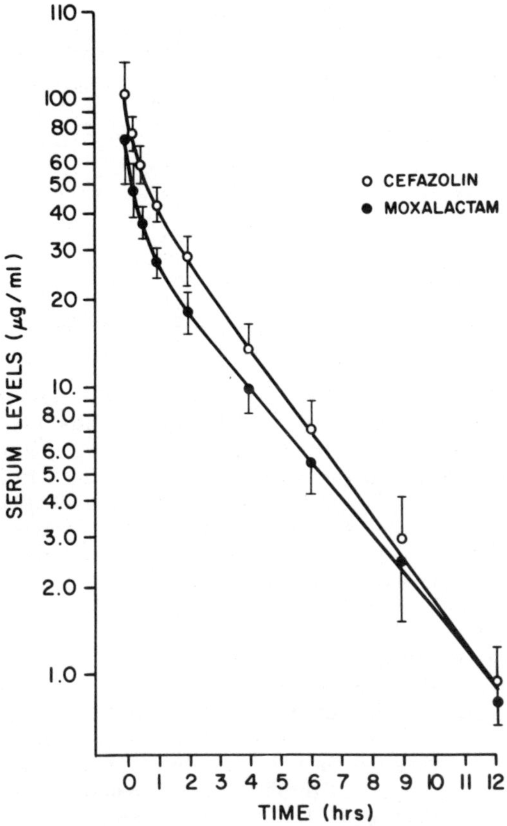

FIG. 2. *Mean (±SD) serum levels of cefazolin compared with moxalactam in 12 normal volunteers after a 30-min infusion of 10 mg of each agent per kg. Cefazolin levels are significantly greater than moxalactam levels from 0 through 4 h.*

cantly longer than that of cefazolin (2.2 ± 0.7 versus 1.9 ± 0.5 h, respectively). These findings are similar to those previously reported by Srinivasan et al. (2) and Scheld et al. (1).

The technique of simultaneous administration to determine the relative pharmacokinetics of two antibiotics apparently has not been described previously. The method described here would appear to offer a significant advantage over the conventional randomized two-group design in studies of comparative tissue penetration since simultaneous administration of the study antibiotics would require half as many patients to arrive at the same number of data points, and paired statistical tests could be used to improve the ability to detect significant differences in tissue concentrations. In addition, since tissue for antibiotic penetration studies is commonly obtained from surgical specimens after prophylactic administration of the study drug, the simultaneous administration method would allow for study of an antibiotic which is relatively inactive against potential pathogens, since an effective prophylactic agent could be administered at the same time.

1. **Scheld, W. M., D. A. Spyker, G. R. Donowitz, W. K. Bolton, and M. A. Sande.** 1981. Moxalactam and cefazolin: comparative pharmacokinetics in normal subjects. Antimicrob. Agents Chemother. **19:**613–619.
2. **Srinivasan, S., K. P. Fu, and H. C. Neu.** 1981. Pharmacokinetics of moxalactam and cefazolin compared in normal volunteers. Antimicrob. Agents Chemother. **19:** 302–305.

Penetration of Moxalactam (LY127935) into Cerebrospinal Fluid in Children with Meningitis

M. C. GARCÍA-IGLESIAS, J. AZNAR, A. ALEJO, AND E. J. PEREA*

Departments of Microbiology and Pediatrics, University Hospital, School of Medicine, University of Seville, Seville-8, Spain*

Moxalactam was administered intravenously to twenty-five children with meningitis, each of whom had been receiving adequate antibiotic therapy and had shown favorable response. The children were classified into two groups: group 1 comprised 15 children with lymphocytic meningitis, whose ages ranged from 4 months to 9 years. Group 2 comprised 10 children with meningococcal meningitis, whose ages ranged from 2 months to 7 years, with a mean of 3 years and 1 month. Diagnoses were made on clinical grounds and were confirmed by biochemical, cytological, and bacteriological tests when the children were admitted to the University Hospital of Seville.

All of the children received 100 mg of moxalactam per kg of body weight, intravenously; 22 received a single dose, and the other 3 (2 in

TABLE 1. *Clinical data of eight children in whom moxalactam was detected in CSF*

Patient no.	Age	Albumin (mg%)	Glucose (mg%)	Leukocyte count (lymphocytes %) ml	Moxalactam levels (μg/ml)		
					CSF	Serum	CSF/Serum %
1[a]	4 mo	18	56	380 (78)	0.5	110	0.5
2	1 yr	15	63	3 (100)	0.5	51	1
3	3.5 yr	39	59	1,024 (80)	2.4	33	7
4	5 yr	28	56	2 (100)	2.6	28	9
5	5.5 yr	19	60	2 (100)	1.2	36	3.5
6	2 mo	41	40	0 (0)	0.5	45	1.2
7[a]	3 mo	54	59	64 (0)	0.7	102	0.7
8	2 yr	49	60	2 (0)	1.8	11	16

[a] Four doses.

group 1 and 1 in group 2) received four doses 24, 18, and 6 h earlier. Blood and cerebrospinal fluid (CSF) specimens for determination of levels of moxalactam were taken 150 min after administration of the antibiotic and in three cases after the last dose. Serum and CSF levels of moxalactam were determined by microbiological assay by the agar diffusion method with *Escherichia coli* ATCC 25922 used as the assay organism on Mueller-Hinton medium (3).

The serum levels of moxalactam in the 25 children ranged from 5.5 to 110 μg/ml with a mean value of 36 μg/ml in group 1 and 25 μg/ml in group 2. Levels of moxalactam in the CSF were detected in 5 of the 15 children in group 1, and 3 of the 10 in group 2, with mean values of 1.44 and 1 μg/ml, respectively. The ratio of CSF/serum levels in the eight children in whom CSF levels were detected ranged from 0.5 to 16%, with a mean value of 5% (Table 1). Of these eight children, two had received four doses and were very young children (3 months and 4 months) who still had raised cell counts in the CSF. In one child, who had also received four doses, no CSF levels of moxalactam were detected. The highest levels found in CSF were 2.4 and 2.6 μg/ml, and both of these children had received a single dose of moxalactam.

Dividing the children according to age we find that six children were aged less than 1 year, and in four (67%) of these children CSF levels of moxalactam were detected. There were 19 children aged over 1 year and in only five (26%) of them were CSF levels of moxalactam detected. Only 1 of 25 children, a child diagnosed as having purulent meningitis, had a really elevated CSF albumin level in the first sample (221 mg%), and in the second sample (41 mg%) taken on day 7 of illness. This child had detectable levels (0.5 μg of moxalactam per ml) in CSF. Thirty percent of the cases studied in both groups had detectable levels of moxalactam in the CSF. The ratio of CSF/serum had a mean value of 5%.

Comparing our results with those reported by others authors (1, 2), we see that the levels reached in CSF are lower than those reported. Also, the ratio of the levels in CSF compared with the levels in serum differ slightly; our results were 0.5 to 16% and those of the other authors were 5.4 to 9%. This discrepancy could be due to the fact that, except in three cases, we administered only one dose and other authors have administered two or four doses. Also they determined the CSF levels at 75 to 90 min after the last dose and we systematically made our determinations by drug levels at 150 min afterwards, which is twice the time interval of these authors.

1. **Landesman, S. H., M. L. Corrado, C. C. Cherubin, M. Gombert, and D. Cleri.** 1980. Difusión de un nuevo betalactámico (LY-127935) al líquido cefalorraquídeo. Implicaciones para la terapéutica de las meningitis por bacilos gram negativos. Am. J. Med. **12:**77. (In Spanish.).
2. **Schaad, U. B., G. H. McCracken, Jr., N. Threlkeld, and M. L. Thomas.** 1981. Clinical evaluation of a new broad-spectrum oxa-beta lactam antibiotic, moxalactam, in neonates and infants. J. Pediatr. **98:**129–36.
3. **Washington, J. A. II.** 1976. Bacteriology procedure manual. Rochester, Minnesota.

Pharmacokinetics of Moxalactam in Children

MARIO F. ROMAGNOLI,* KERRIE FLYNN, GEORGE SIBER, AND DONALD GOLDMANN

Children's Hospital Medical Center and Harvard Medical School, Boston, Massachusetts 02116, U.S.A.*

Moxalactam (1-oxa cephalosporin, 6059-S, LY127935) was administered as perioperative prophylaxis to 11 normal children undergoing appendectomy and to 17 other children with medical and surgical infections at a dose of 50 mg/kg as a timed 30-min infusion. Blood samples were obtained at 5, 30, 120, 240, and 480 min after completion of the infusion. No significant difference in the drug disappearance curves was noted between the prophylactic and therapeutic groups, so data were combined for further analysis.

Drug assay was performed by reverse-phase high-pressure liquid chromatography (procedure developed by J. F. Erickson and A. N. Karabelas, Massachusetts College of Pharmacy, Boston), with total drug content being measured spectrophotometrically at 270 nm by peak height ratio analysis, using cefamandole as an internal standard. All sera were stored at −20°C until assayed (within 10 days of collection).

Pharmacokinetic analysis was performed using a single-compartmental analysis due to the insufficient number of data points available for valid pharmacokinetic analysis of the early distribution phase. The K_D and $T_{1/2}$ were calculated using the equations: $\ln C = \ln C'_o - K_D t$ and $\beta = -K_D$, when C'_o = Y-intercept, representing the concentration at zero time (end of infusion), β = slope of the line resulting when data points are plotted semilogarithmically, and K_D = disposition constant. C_o was corrected for the 30-min infusion time using the formula (1):

$$C_o = \left(\frac{K_D \cdot T_{inf}}{1 - e^{-K_D \cdot T_{inf}}}\right) C'_o,$$

when T_{inf} = infusion time in hours.

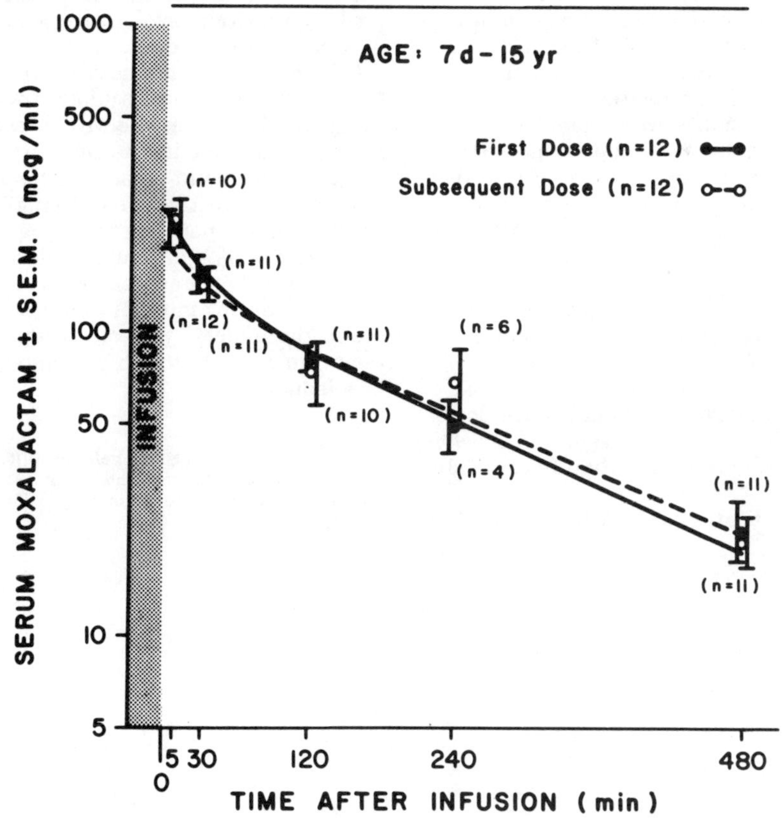

FIG. 1. *Moxalactam pharmacokinetics: multiple dose study.*

TABLE 1. *Age-related changes in pharmacokinetics*

Age	Moxalactam concn ($\mu g/ml$)		Parameter	
	Mean 30-min peak (range)	Mean 480-min trough (range)	$T_{1/2}$ (h)	V_D (liter/kg)
<1 yr	76.8	21.8	3.77	0.568
(n = 5)	(42–103)	(5.3–55.3)	(1.75–7.96)	(0.235–0.97)
1–9 yr	161[a]	17.7	2.20[b]	0.256[c]
(n = 9)	(103–275)	(5–42.8)	(1.04–3.74)	(0.10–0.311)
≥10 yr	224[d]	16.0	2.12[e]	0.228[f]
(n = 14)	(123–450)	(2.7–39.7)	(0.552–4.46)	(0.090–0.415)

[a] Difference from <1-year group, $P < 0.01$.
[b] Difference from <1-year group, not significant.
[c] Difference from <1-year group, $P < 0.01$.
[d] Difference from <1-year group, $P < 0.05$.
[e] Difference from <1-year group, $P < 0.1$.
[f] Difference from <1-year group, $P < 0.001$.

Patients ranged in age from 7 days to 16 years and had the following diagnoses: acute appendicitis, 9; fever/neutropenia, 5; intraabdominal abscess/peritonitis, 3; central nervous system infection, 3; skin/soft tissue infection, 3; biliary infection, 2; empyema, 1; urinary tract infection, 1; ruptured corpus luteum cyst, 1; malrotation of midgut, 1. Seven of these patients were bacteremic with their primary infections.

First-dose studies were completed in 28 patients; mean serum concentrations in $\mu g/ml$ were: 5 min, 247; 30 min, 177; 120 min, 82.2; 240 min, 49.3; 480 min, 17.5. Mean $T_{1/2}$ was 2.44 h, and mean V_D was 0.298 liter/kg.

Multiple-dose studies were completed in 12 patients; Figure 1 shows the superimposed time-concentration curves for this group; first dose (subsequent dose) values in $\mu g/ml$ were: 5 min, 217 (225); 30 min, 155 (139); 120 min, 82.1 (73); 240 min, 48.9 (68.3); 480 min, 22.2 (20.3). Mean $T_{1/2}$ was 3.02 (3.14); mean V_D was 0.327 (0.354). These data suggest that, in the absence of renal failure or insufficiency, there is no accumulation of moxalactam after multiple doses.

In the group of patients less than 1 year of age, mean peak levels (30-min) were lower, whereas $T_{1/2}$ and V_D values were higher when compared with children older than 1 year (Table 1).

Our study indicates that, in the presence of normal renal function, the single-dose pharmacokinetics of moxalactam in normal children undergoing appendectomy were identical to the pharmacokinetics of children with acute bacterial infections, including some with serious underlying medical problems. There was no observed change in $T_{1/2}$, V_D, or mean peak blood levels with multiple doses, nor was accumulation of the drug observed over a 3- to 5-day study period. Children under 1 year of age had a lower peak moxalactam level, a larger V_D, and longer $T_{1/2}$ than older children.

On the basis of this study, we feel that in order to achieve a 30-min postinfusion serum level of 64 $\mu g/ml$ (four times the MIC breakpoint of 16 $\mu g/ml$) or greater in the majority of patients, moxalactam should be administered as follows: infants less than 1 year old: 50 mg/kg per dose; children older than 1 year: 25 mg/kg per dose. Because the $T_{1/2}$ in young children is slightly longer (based on small numbers of patients), an 8- to 12-h dosing interval would seem appropriate in the under-1-year-old group; in older patients, an every 6- to 8-h dosing regimen would be adequate.

1. **Loo, J. C. K., and S. Riegelman.** 1970. Assessment of pharmacokinetic constants from post-infusion blood curves obtained after i.v. infusion. J. Pharm. Sci. **59:**53–55.

Therapeutic Trial of Moxalactam in Intraabdominal Sepsis and Gynecological Infections

JOHN G. BARTLETT

Department of Medicine, Johns Hopkins University School of Medicine, Baltimore, Maryland 21205, U.S.A.

Moxalactam is a relatively new beta-lactam antimicrobial which shows an excellent spectrum of in vitro activity against both aerobic and anaerobic bacteria. This report summarizes a collaborative clinical trial from 12 participating hospitals in which moxalactam was used for the treatment of intraabdominal sepsis and infections of the female genital tract.

Study design. The report is based on review of investigators' records. Criteria for inclusion were: (i) clinical evidene for infection supported by the recovery of a potential pathogen from the infected site and (ii) treatment with moxalactam as a single agent for at least 3 days. In vitro susceptibility testing was performed for moxalactam activity against most isolates using ≤16 μg/ml to indicate susceptibility, 32 μg/ml for "moderate susceptibility," and 64 μg/ml or greater to indicate resistance. Evaluation of outcome was according to the judgment of the investigator on the basis of clinical observations and follow-up cultures.

Types of infections. There were 90 patients who satisfied the criteria for inclusion with intraabdominal sepsis, including 69 with peritonitis, 19 with intraabdominal abscesses, 12 with biliary tract infections, and 5 with a ruptured appendix. (Some patients had both generalized peritonitis and intraabdominal abscesses.) There were 246 patients with infections of the female genital tract. These included 137 with endometritis, 43 with pelvic cellulitis, 40 with gonococcal salpingitis, 24 with nongonococcal salpingitis, and 2 with pelvic abscesses.

Moxalactam regimens. The group with intraabdominal sepsis received a mean total daily dose of 4.4 g for an average of 11 days (range of 1.5 to 9 g/day for 5 to 20 days). The group with gynecological infections received a mean dose of 4.8 g daily for an average of 5.9 days (range of 3 to 12 g/day for 3 to 13 days).

Bacteriological findings. Cultures of the infected site from 90 patients with intraabdominal sepsis showed aerobic bacteria only in 40 (44%), anaerobic bacteria only in 9 (10%), and a mixture of aerobic and anaerobic isolates in 41 (46%). Blood cultures showed 17 (19%) of these patients had bacteremia involving aerobic bacteria isolated from 12 and anaerobic bacteria from 5. The predominant isolates recovered from the infected site were *Escherichia coli* (51 isolates), the *Bacteroides fragilis* group (36), group D streptococci (29), clostridia (19), peptostreptococci (18), *Pseudomonas aeruginosa* (17), and klebsiella (16). Bacteriological studies in female genital tract infections are less conclusive due to the inclusion of cultures from many sites in which contamination from the normal flora could not be excluded. The major anaerobic isolates in this group were peptostreptococci (69 isolates), peptococci (52), *B. fragilis* (35), *B. melaninogenicus* (33), *B. bivius* (28), and clostridia (23). The major aerobic bacteria in this group were *E. coli* (47), group D streptococci (43), and group B streptococci (29).

In vitro susceptibility tests. One hundred and one isolates of anaerobic gram-negative bacilli from patients with intraabdominal sepsis were examined. Three (3%) proved resistant to moxalactam at >16 μg/ml; all three were strains of *P. aeruginosa* with MIC values of 50 μg/ml (Table 1). The major resistant aerobic isolates in patients with intraabdominal sepsis were group D streptococci. Among 104 anaerobic isolates, 11 were resistant at 16 μg/ml and 10 (10%) were resistant at 32 μg/ml. Resistant strains included *B. fragilis* (3), *B. thetaiotaomicron* (1), *Fusobacterium symbiosum* (1), *F. varium* (1), *Clostridium innocuum* (1), *C. paraputrificum* (1) and peptostreptococci (2). Bacteria tested from patients with gynecological infections showed 3 of 89 strains of aerobic gram-negative bacilli were resistant at 16 μg/ml, and 1 strain (*Enterobacter agglomerans*) was resistant at 32 μg/ml (Table 1). Again, the major resistant isolates were group D streptococci. Testing was performed on 305 strains of obligate anaerobes. Eighteen of these (6%) were resistant at 16 μg/ml and three were resistant at 32 μg/ml. Highly resistant strains included *B. fragilis* (1), *B. ochraceus* (1), and peptostreptococci (1). Combined data from both patient populations show 4 of 190 gram-negative bacilli and 13 of 409 anaerobic isolates resistant at 64 μg/ml. The most common resistant isolates were 33 strains of group D streptococci.

Response. The response to treatment was judged "satisfactory" in 92% of patients with intraabdominal sepsis and 91% of patients with gynecologic infections (Table 2). Review of rec-

TABLE 1. *In vitro susceptibility tests of clinical isolates*

Isolate	Intraabdominal sepsis: No. tested	Intraabdominal sepsis: No. resistant[a]	Gynecologic: No. tested	Gynecologic: No. resistant[a]
Aerobic				
E. coli	47	0	44	0
Klebsiella	14	0	15	0
P. aeruginosa	16	3	14	0
GNB (other)[b]	24	0	26	1
Streptococci				
Group D	23	14	40	19
Other	6	0	39	3
Anaerobic bacteria				
B. fragilis group	31	4	33	1
B. bivius	0	0	28	0
GNB (other)[b]	17	2	89	1
Gram-positive cocci	24	2	117	1
Clostridia	16	2	23	0

[a] Resistance defined as MIC >32 μg/ml.
[b] GNB, Gram-negative bacteria.

ords from 23 patients with an "unsatisfactory" response and 7 who had a "recurrence" following treatment showed moxalactam-resistant organisms had been recovered in the original culture from 5 (17%). Resistant strains included three group D streptococci, one *B. fragilis*, and one *P. aeruginosa*. The isolation rate of moxalactam-resistant group D streptococci was 10% both for patients with a satisfactory response and those with a less favorable outcome. Thus, resistance to the therapeutic agent does not provide an explanation for the majority of patients who either failed to respond or had recurrent infections.

TABLE 2. *Response to treatment*

Response rating	Intraabdominal sepsis	Gynecologic
Satisfactory	83 (92%)	223 (91%)
Unsatisfactory	3 (3%)	20 (8%)
Recurrence	4 (4%)	3 (1%)

Summary. The results with moxalactam treatment are reviewed for 90 patients with intraabdominal sepsis and 246 with infections of the female genital tract. Bacteriology studies in these patients showed most had polymicrobial infections with the dominant isolates being coliforms and anaerobes. In vitro suseptibility tests indicated 4 of 190 (2%) aerobic gram-negative bacilli and 13 of 409 (3%) anaerobic bacteria were resistant to moxalactam at 64 μg/ml. Evaluation of clinical outcome showed 92% of patients had a satisfactory response. It is concluded that moxalactam appears to be effective as a single agent in the treatment of intraabdominal sepsis and infections of the female genital tract.

Clinical Experiences with Moxalactam in the Therapy of Severe Intraabdominal Infections

HANS R. GONZENBACH* AND WOLFGANG SONNABEND

Department of Surgery, Kantonsspital St. Gallen, and Institute of Medical Microbiology, St. Gallen, Switzerland*

Clinical experiences with moxalactam in patients hospitalized with complicated intraabdominal infections are rare (2). Therefore, we evaluated the therapeutic efficacy of moxalactam in patients suffering from serious intraabdominal infections. Clinical cure, improvement, or failure and bacteriological eradication, persistence, or superinfection were recorded.

Between April and October 1980, 35 patients were treated with moxalactam at the surgical clinic of the Kantonsspital St. Gallen in Switzerland. Most of the patients had an intraabdominal infection and were treated surgically in combination with moxalactam alone. A total of 290 different bacteria could be isolated in specimens obtained before and during moxalactam treatment from the 35 patients. Mixed cultures of aerobes and anaerobes were recovered often; 220 of the isolates were aerobes, and 70 were anaerobes. The clinical efficacy of moxalactam in monotherapy was surprisingly good. The overall efficacy of moxalactam was assessed to be excellent in almost 90%. Treatment failed in two patients, and in two other cases assessment was impossible (1).

We have to stress that an antibiotic is quite difficult to evaluate in surgical patients because the overall therapy consists of a combination of surgery and antibiotics. We measure the efficacy of not only the antibiotic, but also the surgeon.

TABLE 1. *Moxalactam treatment in 23 patients with various intraabdominal infections*

Diagnostic group	No.
Postoperative peritonitis	3
Empyema of the gall bladder	4
Hepatic abscess	1
Perforation of stomach or small bowel	5
Perforated appendicitis	9
Perforation of colon	1

One might even say that the surgeon could probably do without the antibiotic, but it would certainly not work the other way around.

In this study, 23 patients were treated for complicated intraabdominal infections (Table 1). Half of the patients were over 70 years old and suffered from serious underlying diseases. Therapy with moxalactam was started at operation, and the dosage was usually 2 g every 8 h given as 20-min intravenous infusions. Half of the patients were treated for fewer than 10 days, but four patients were treated for more than 3 weeks. One patient received 162 g of moxalactam. Side effects were minimal and included one episode of rash, one short episode of diarrhea, and some changes in laboratory values such as eosinophilia and rise in alkaline phosphatase. No impairment of renal function was found. We had two patients whose renal function became normal while treated with a reduced dosage of moxalactam.

We placed special emphasis on the problem of moxalactam-resistant *Streptococcus faecalis* (enterococci) and the effect of moxalactam on *Candida albicans*. It seemed to us essential to complete this study by establishing whether moxalactam exerted any adverse effects, and particularly whether it produced any changes in the normal flora.

S. faecalis is primarily resistant to moxalactam. Only two patients had no enterococci at all (Table 2). Enterococci were subsequently recovered from different specimens during moxalactam treatment. Nevertheless, we had no clinical problems except in one patient who developed a subphrenic abscess after a gastric perforation. Bacteriological examination of the juice in the peritoneal cavity at the time of the gastric operation showed growth of *Klebsiella pneumoniae* and *S. faecalis*. The culture results were of course not known at that time, and moxalactam treatment was started and continued for 15 days. Seventeen days later the patient was due to go home, and a day before leaving the hospital the old penrose canal showed some purulent discharge. The subphrenic abscess was drained, and a few days later the patient went home. No bacteria were seen by microscopic examination of the pus of the abscess, but cultures showed growth of *S. faecalis*. No patient in this clinical trial had to have an additional antibiotic for enterococci. The problem is quite different in a patient who has no septic focus that can be cleared surgically. An antibiotic therapy directed against *S. faecalis* must be started in cases of positive blood cultures or of high colony counts in the urine or in the rare occasion of meningitis.

TABLE 2. *Qualitative and quantitative effects of moxalactam treatment on S. faecalis and C. albicans in 23 patients*

Determination	*S. faecalis*	*C. albicans*
Not tested	0	2
Present before treatment	8	4
Isolated during treatment	13	12
Abdominal drainage	6	5
Feces	10	11 (>10^5/g)
Urine	2	3 (>10^6/ml)
Others	3	3
Never present	2	5

Another interesting feature we encountered was the growth of *C. albicans* (Table 2). In the beginning of the clinical trial, we did not look for *C. albicans* in two patients. In four patients *C. albicans* was already present in the abdomen at the time of operation, before antibiotic therapy was started. In 12 patients the organism appeared during therapy in high quantities in the feces (>10^5/g of stool) and in urine (>10^6/ml of urine). Antibody titers to *C. albicans* were never elevated at the beginning of moxalactam therapy but were found to be elevated in four patients later on, indicating serologically a mucosal infection in two and a systemic mycosis in two others. Although these findings were astonishing, there was no clinical correlation, and we never had to start a specific antimycotic therapy.

Although we cannot present any statistical data, the overall clinical impression of moxalactam was very favorable. From the clinical standpoint, the most surprising fact was that we did not see any subcutaneous wound infections. In many patients, especially in cases of perforated appendicitis, pus fled the wound when the abdominal cavity was opened. We expected wound infections in some of the patients but they never occurred, even though drug treatment was never started before the operation.

We can recommend moxalactam as a true alternative to the antibiotic combinations, especially in patients with uncertain renal function.

1. **Gonzenbach, H. R., and W. Sonnabend.** 1981. Moxalactam—ein Beta-Laktam-Antibiotikum in Monotherapie bei schweren Infektionskrankheiten in der Chirurgie—Klinischbakteriologische Studie an 35 Patienten. Schweiz. Med. Wochenschr. **111**:1169–1183.
2. **Moxalactam: Clinical Studies.** Session 35. Program Abstr. Intersci. Conf. Antimicrob. Agents Chemother. 20th, 22–24 September 1980, New Orleans, La.

Moxalactam Therapy of Pelvic Inflammatory Disease and Pelvic Infections

RONALD S. GIBBS

The University of Texas Health Science Center, San Antonio, Texas 78284, U.S.A.

Genital tract infection is a common and occasionally severe complication of gynecological surgery and of childbirth. In addition, pelvic inflammatory disease (PID) is a major health problem, leading to both immediate and remote sequelae. Because these infections are often polymicrobial and because therapy is usually initiated before the availability of cultures, broad-spectrum agents are commonly used.

In view of its wide antibacterial activity, moxalactam was used as a single agent in the therapy of a variety of female genital tract infections. In this multicenter trial, patients were eligible if they had a clinical diagnosis of PID or genital tract infection after hysterectomy or after childbirth. Specimens for aerobic and anaerobic culture were obtained from the peripheral venous blood and the infected site. MICs were determined for most anaerobes, and disk susceptibility tests were performed for most aerobes. Response to moxalactam was considered either satisfactory or unsatisfactory depending upon the need for additional major therapy (surgical drainage or other antibiotics). If signs and symptoms of infection had not resolved within 3 days, then the course was considered unsuccessful.

From seven institutions, there were 172 evaluable cases, some of which have been reported previously (1, 2). The initial dose was usually 3 to 6 g intravenously daily. When there was a prompt clinical response, the dose was often decreased to 1.5 g intramuscularly daily. In cases with satisfactory responses, the course of therapy ranged from 5 to 10 days intravenously. The clinical diagnoses were: uterine infection, mostly after cesarean section, 119; pelvic cellulitis after hysterectomy, 32; PID, 19; pelvic abscess, 1; and intraamniotic infection, 1. Of the 19 cases of PID, 5 were gonococcal, 13 were nongonococcal, and 1 was a tuboovarian abscess.

Genital cultures revealed 446 potentially pathogenic isolates (average 2.6/patient). Anaerobes were present solely in 75 of the 172 specimens (43.5%), whereas aerobes were present solely in 4 (2.5%). In 93 specimens (54%), both aerobes and anaerobes were present.

A total of 45 isolates (10%) showed MICs ≥ 32 μg/ml or zone diameters <18 mm. The most common isolate of these were group D streptococci (17), *Bacteroides* other than fragilis group (9), *B. fragilis* group (7), and peptostreptococci (6). Only three of these were isolated from patients with unsatisfactory responses. MICs for selected organisms are shown in Table 1. All of the nine group B streptococci tested were susceptible, but the MIC_{90} was approximately 8 μg/ml. Of six isolates of *Neisseria gonorrhoeae*, two were tested for susceptibility. Both were highly susceptible. Of 83 patients from whom blood cultures were reported, 8 (9.6%) were bacteremic (group B streptococci, 1; other streptococci, 2; *Staphylococcus aureus*, 1; *Escherichia coli*, 1; *Enterobacter aerogenes*, 1; peptococci, 1; and *Bacteroides ruminicola*, 1).

The clinical response was satisfactory in 155 cases (90%). Among patients with PID, only one patient, who had nongonococcal disease, had an unsatisfactory response. Among the 17 patients with unsatisfactory responses, there were identifiable causes in 5. Three had abscesses, and two had resistant isolates (*B. fragilis* MIC = 32 and *Clostridium innocuum* MIC > 16). One patient with an abscess also had a *B. fragilis* isolate with an MIC of 64. All eight patients with bacteremia had good responses.

For postoperative and postpartum infection there may be an effective dose of moxalactam. Of 31 patients who were initially treated with 3 g/day, there were 4 failures (12.9%), but 2 of these developed abscesses. In comparison, of 122 initially treated with ≥ 6 g/day, there were 12 failures (9.8%), but none developed abscesses. While these differences are not statistically significant, this observation is interesting to note.

Antimicrobial therapy for genital tract infection must often be initiated before culture results are available. Accordingly, most regimens are broad spectrum (1, 2). Combination therapy of

TABLE 1. *MICs of moxalactam for selected organisms*

Species (no. of isolates tested)	MIC (μg/ml)	
	MIC ≥ 32	MIC ≤ 16
Bacteroides fragilis group (26)	7	19
Bacteroides bivius (27)	1	26
Bacteroides melaninogenicus (23)	3	20
Enterobacter spp. (10)	1	9
Peptostrepto-peptococci (108)	6	102
Group D streptococci (25)	17	8
Group B streptococci (9)	0	9

penicillin and aminoglycoside has generally been satisfactory in 71 to 78% of cases, while therapy with cefamandole or cefoxitin has been curative in 83 to 94%. Initial therapy with clindamycin plus gentamicin may be effective in 95% of cases. Thus, most regimens have produced good response rates and have generally been well tolerated. However, response certainly depends upon the type of infection being treated, the severity of the infection, criteria for cure or failure, and adverse effects. Single-agent therapy with moxalactam produced results which appear superior to those of penicillin-aminoglycoside combination and compare favorably with those of cefoxitin and clindamycin-gentamicin. Because of its longer half-life and infrequent adverse effects, moxalactam may have advantages compared with these regimens. Comparative trials are appropriate.

1. **Cunningham, F. G., D. L. Hemsell, R. T. DePalma, S. Kappus, M. Roark, and B. Nobles.** 1981. Moxalactam for obstetrics and gynecologic infections. Am. J. Obstet. Gynecol. **139**:915–921.
2. **Gibbs, R. S., J. D. Blanco, Y. S. Castaneda, and P. J. St. Clair.** 1980. Therapy of obstetrical infections with moxalactam. Antimicrob. Agents Chemother. **17**:1004–1007.

Moxalactam Therapy of Serious Systemic Infections

J. E. PENNINGTON* AND R. PLATT

Harvard Medical School, Boston, Massachusetts 02115, U.S.A.

Serious systemic infections are often treated with beta-lactam or aminoglycoside antibiotics. In choosing between these classes of drugs, three major considerations are important. These include spectrum, toxicity, and efficacy. The choice of a beta-lactam agent is often tempting because of the lower toxicity of this class, but the limited spectrum of this class, particularly against *Pseudomonas aeruginosa* (cephalosporins) or *Klebsiella* spp. (carbenicillin–ticarcillin group), has necessitated the use of the more toxic aminoglycoside group for empirical coverage of suspected sepsis. The advent of moxalactam, and other so-called "third-generation" cephalosporins, presents a new and unique ther apeutic potential. By virtue of an extended spectrum, several of these new beta-lactam agents provide coverage for many of the more resistant gram-negative bacilli, including *P. aeruginosa*. Thus, there exists the possibility for providing an aminoglycoside-like spectrum with a safer class of drug. In this setting one concern then becomes paramount: clinical efficacy. Is either class intrinsically more efficacious for a pathogen susceptible to both classes, or are beta-lactams and aminoglycosides of equal efficacy for similarly susceptible pathogens? Can beta-lactam antibiotics be used alone against serious systemic infection? The present report begins, but by no means completes, an analysis of these questions.

We have evaluated the clinical efficacy of moxalactam for two serious systemic infections, bacteremia and pneumonia, at our own institution, and also by a review of the cumulative clinical data for use of this drug in the United States. Five patients with bacteremia were treated at our institution, three caused by *Serratia marcescens* and two by group B streptococci. All five were successfully treated, as defined by clinical resolution of fever and eradication of bacteria from the bloodstream.

One patient was of particular interest. He was a 56-year-old male, who was 2-weeks post-dacron aortic graft implant. Blood cultures obtained because of fever grew *S. marcescens* which was susceptible to cefoxitin, moxalactam, and amikacin, but resistant to gentamicin and tobramycin, as well as all other conventional beta-lactam antibiotics. The patient received cefoxitin plus amikacin over a 3-week period, during which time fever continued and 31 of 48 blood cultures were positive for *S. marcescens*. On day 21 of therapy, cefoxitin was discontinued, and moxalactam (1.5 g/24 h) was begun. Amikacin was continued. The patient promptly de-

TABLE 1. *Moxalactam therapy of bacteremias (cumulative data–U.S.)*

Pathogenic isolate	No. of cases	Satisfactory response (%)
Gram-positive cocci	60	95
S. aureus	21	100
S. epidermidis	5	80
Streptococcus spp.	13	85
S. pneumoniae	18	100
Other	3	100
Gram-negative enteric bacilli	154	95
E. coli	76	96
Klebsiella spp.	14	100
Proteus spp.	10	100
Enterobacter spp.	8	88
P. aeruginosa	25	84
S. marcescens	21	90
Bacteroides fragilis	5	100
H. influenzae	6	100
Miscellaneous	17	82

TABLE 2. *Moxalactam therapy of pneumonias (cumulative data–U.S.)*

Pathogenic isolate	No. of cases	Satisfactory response (%)
Gram-positive cocci	151	95
S. pneumoniae	134	98
S. aureus	17	71
Gram-negative enteric bacilli	98	72
Klebsiella spp.	24	83
E. coli	19	100
S. marcescens	14	57
P. aeruginosa	39	60
H. influenzae	56	96
Miscellaneous	58	86
Multiple isolates	99	85

fervesced, and, over the ensuing month, 22 consecutive blood cultures were negative. The patient was discharged after 40 days of moxalactam plus amikacin. At this time, 2 years later, he is alive and well. Why did the switch to moxalactam help this patient? Despite similar susceptibilities, moxalactam may have been intrinsically more effective for this particular bacteremia than either cefoxitin or amikacin. Another possibility is that moxalactam, but not cefoxitin, was synergistic with amikacin. In any event, we were impressed that moxalactam offered a new and life-saving therapy for an isolate that was also susceptible to other available drugs.

The efficacy of moxalactam as single-drug therapy for bacteremia has been evaluated in 242 patients in the U.S. In 147 cases, the source of bacteremia could be identified (urinary tract, most common), and in 95 cases no source was found. Dosages ranged from 1 to 3 g/24 h (48%), 3 to 6 g/24 h (42%), and 6 to 12 g/24 h (10%). The overall efficacy, defined as eradication of bacteria from the blood, was 94%. Table 1 depicts the efficacy of moxalactam according to bacterial isolates. Of considerable interest was success in all 21 *Staphylococcus aureus* bacteremias, including one case of endocarditis. Three of the four failures among the 25 cases with *P. aeruginosa* were in patients with hematological neoplasia. Nine patients with bacteremia had associated endocarditis, and moxalactam was successful in treating six (two *Streptococcus* spp.; one *S. aureus*; one *Haemophilus parainfluenzae*; one *Bacteroides fragilis*; and one *P. aeruginosa*). Two failures were reported with streptococcal species, and one for *Alcaligenes* spp. The drug was discontinued prematurely in the latter case, due to an allergic reaction.

The usefulness of moxalactam in serious pneumonia (gram-negative) was evaluated in eight patients at our institution. Clinical success, defined as clearance of pulmonary infiltrate, as well as resolution of fever and purulent sputum, was observed in two of four *P. aeruginosa*, one of two *S. marcescens*, and two of two *Klebsiella* pneumonias. The efficacy of moxalactam as single-drug therapy for pneumonia has been evaluated in 462 patients in the U.S. Dosages ranged from 1 to 3 g/24 h (15%), 3 to 6 g/24 h (76%), and 6 to 12 g/24 h (9%). Overall, satisfactory clinical responses (defined above) were noted in 87% of cases. Table 2 depicts the efficacy of moxalactam for pneumonia according to bacterial isolates. While the mortalities for gram-negative pneumonias were higher than for gram-positive, these response rates compare favorably to those previously reported for gram-negative pneumonia (1, 3). In particular, the 60% success in treating 39 cases of *P. aeruginosa* pneumonia is quite acceptable, considering previously reported mortalities for this pathogen ranging from 50 to 80% (1–3).

In summary, moxalactam, as single-drug therapy, has proven successful in 94% of 242 reported cases of bacteremia, and in 87% of 462 cases of pneumonia. It is concluded that moxalactam is efficacious for serious systemic infections caused by a wide variety of bacterial pathogens. Furthermore, this agent may be used successfully for certain pathogens which have previously been unresponsive to agents of the cephalosporin class.

1. **Graybill, J. R., L. W. Marshall, P. Charache, C. K. Wallace, and V. B. Melvin.** 1973. Nosocomial pneumonia, a continuing problem. Am. Rev. Respir. Dis. **108:**1130–1140.
2. **Pennington, J. E., H. Y. Reynolds, and P. P. Carbone.** 1973. Pseudomonas pneumonia: a retrospective study of 36 cases. Am. J. Med. **55:**155–160.
3. **Stevens, R. M., D. Teres, J. J. Skillman, and D. S. Feingold.** 1974. Pneumonia in an intensive care unit, a 30 month experience. Arch. Intern. Med. **134:**106–111.

Clinical Efficacy and Kinetic Study of Moxalactam in Children

DIMITRIS A. KAFETZIS,* VASSILIKI MATSOUKA, CONSTANTINE A. SINANIOTIS, AND CONSTANTINE J. PAPADATOS

The University of Athens, Second Department of Pediatrics, Athens, Greece

Moxalactam, a new semisynthetic oxacephalosporin, was found to be highly resistant to gram-negative-produced β-lactamases. Of particular interest is its activity against *Haemophilus influenzae*, *Enterobacteriaceae*, and gram-negative anaerobic bacteria (1). This compound has been found effective and safe in adult patients, and its pharmacokinetic properties permit twice a day administration (H. Giamarellou, J. Tsagarakis, and G. K. Daikos, Program Abstr. Intersci. Conf. Antimicrob. Agents Chemother. 20th, New Orleans, La., abstr. no. 364, 1980). It was also found to penetrate effectively inflamed meninges of animals and humans (U. B. Schaad and G. H. McCracken, 20th ICAAC, abstr. no. 563). The purpose of our study was to evaluate the efficacy and safety of moxalactam and to study its pharmacokinetics when used in infants and children.

After informed parental consent, moxalactam was administered to 18 patients treated in the "Aglaia Kyriakou" Children's Hospital in Athens. Three of these patients were infants (1 boy and 2 girls), and 15 were children aged 14 months to 11 years (11 boys and 4 girls). Infections treated are shown in Table 1. Appropriate cultures were obtained from all patients before, during, and after therapy. All pathogens isolated from our patients were tested for susceptibility to antibiotics by use of the Bauer-Kirby disk-agar diffusion method, and the drug was continued only if the pathogen was susceptible to moxalactam or the patient was improving clinically. Pathogens isolated are also shown in Table 1.

Fourteen out of the 18 patients included were under previous unsatisfactory antibacterial therapy. Moxalactam was used as monotherapy in 15 patients, and as combination with another antibiotic in 3. Dosage used was 30 mg/kg per dose repeated every 12 h. The drug was administered intravenously in all patients. Duration of therapy ranged from 3 to 22 days, but most patients were treated for 10 to 15 days. All patients were carefully observed for side effects, and suitable laboratory tests were performed before and after therapy to detect hemopoietic, hepatic, and renal toxicity. The pharmacokinetic study was performed in nine patients from whom blood was drawn by venipuncture or heel prick, before and at 5 min, 0.5, 1, 2, 4, 6, 8, and 12 h after the first or second dose of the drug. Urine samples were collected in plastic bags from five children for the 8 h following the dose, at 2-hour intervals. Concentrations of moxalactam were bioassayed by using a strain of *Escherichia coli* as the indicator organism.

All *Enterobacteriaceae* and *H. influenzae* were found to be highly susceptible to moxalactam; one strain of *Pseudomonas aeruginosa* and the three strains of *Staphylococcus aureus* were found to be moderately susceptible (MIC $\geq$ 8 μg/ml). The *Bacteroides fragilis* strains were not tested for susceptibility.

Clinical and bacteriological results are shown in Table 1. Fourteen out of the 18 patients were cured and the pathogens were eradicated. One 14-month-old boy with hypsarrhythmia suffering from pneumonia died after completion of 3 days of treatment with moxalactam monotherapy. This boy was under previous unsatisfactory antibacterial therapy with a combination of amoxicillin plus amikacin. *Klebsiella* sp. was still isolated from bronchial aspiration 7 days after initiation of the combination. One 6-year-old boy with infected burns improved clinically. Nontheless skin lesions were still colonized by the causative pathogens 18 days after the start of therapy. In a 25-day-old girl with dacryocystitis, treatment with moxalactam failed. This girl was under unsatisfactory therapy with cephalexin. *S. aureus* was isolated 4 days after initia-

TABLE 1. *Summary of results with moxalactam therapy*

Diagnosis	Pathogen	Previous treatment	Concomitant treatment	Duration of treatment (days)	Outcome[a]	
					Clinical	Bacteriological
Peritonitis	*E. coli* (3) *E. coli* + *B. fragilis* (1) *Klebsiella* spp. + *B. fragilis* (1)	Ampicillin + gentamicin (2) Clindamycin + gentamicin (1) None (2)	None (5)	9 to 15	5C	5E
Pneumonia	*Klebsiella* spp.	Amoxicillin + amikacin		3	D	U
	H. influenzae	Ampicillin + gentamicin	None (3)	15	C	E
	None	Amoxicillin		10	C	E
Infected burns	*Enterobacter* spp.	Ampicillin + gentamicin	Amikacin	17	C	E
	P. mirabilis + *S. aureus*	Dicloxacillin + gentamicin	None	18	I	P
Pleural effusion	*Klebsiella* spp.	None	None	14	C	E
Compound fracture-osteomyelitis	*E. coli*	Ampicillin + gentamicin	None (2)	15	C but R	New pathogen
	E. coli + *P. mirabilis*	Ampicillin + amikacin		13	C	E
Cellulitis	None	Penicillin + methicillin	None	12	C	E
	S. aureus + *B. fragilis*	Dicloxacillin + gentamicin	Dicloxacillin	10	C	E
Dacryocystitis	*S. aureus*	None	None	6	F	P
Pyelonephritis	*E. coli*	Cefamandole + gentamicin	None	14	C	E
Meningitis	*P. aeruginosa*	Carbenicillin + amikacin	Amikacin	22	C	E

[a] C, Cured; E, eradicated; D, died; U, unknown; I, improved; R, recurrence of infection; F, failed.

TABLE 2. *Mean serum and urine concentrations of moxalactam in infants and children after intravenous injection of 30 mg/kg*

Time after injection (h)	Mean serum concn (μg/ml ± SD)	Time interval (h)	Mean urine concn (μg/ml)
5 min	149.0 ± 46.0	0–2	4,740
0.5	60.4 ± 35.2		
1	38.8 ± 19.1	2–4	1,998
2	23.4 ± 14.8		
4	10.3 ± 8.8	4–6	1,617
6	4.1 ± 3.5		
8	1.9 ± 1.6	6–8	610
12	ND[a]–1.2		

[a] ND, Nondetectable.

tion of moxalactam therapy. The patient responded excellently to dicloxacillin. A 9-year-old boy developed osteomyelitis after a car accident and a compound fracture of the left femur. He showed an excellent response to the drug under study. Although blood and pus were sterile after completion of therapy, 1 week later the boy was readmitted and a new pathogen was isolated from pus.

Moxalactam was very well tolerated. No toxic effects were noticed in any of the patients. A transient increase in platelet count from 300,000/mm^3 to 700,000 or 800,000/mm^3 related to the treatment was noticed in three patients.

Serum concentrations of moxalactam in infants and children after intravenous injection are shown in Table 2. Peak blood levels were obtained 5 min after injection and ranged from 82 to 180 μg/ml. At 2 h they ranged from 8.4 to 54.0 μg/ml, and at 12 h they ranged from nondetectable to 1.2 μg/ml. These blood levels are considered bactericidal for most susceptible pathogens for at least 8 h after injection. Serum half-life calculated at the elimination phase ranged from 1.2 to 2.03 (mean, 1.61 ± 0.28 h). Urinary excretion of moxalactam averaged 38.6% of the intravenously injected amount 8 h after administration. Urine concentrations (Table 2) were highly bactericidal for the whole 8-h period studied.

This study has shown that moxalactam, with its high antibacterial activity against bacteria commonly affecting pediatric patients, its clinical effectiveness, its very low incidence of side effects, and its pharmacokinetic properties suitable for treatment in pediatrics, is a promising new cephalosporin to be used in pediatric infectious diseases. However, its lack of activity against *S. aureus* should be kept in mind, and this compound should not be used alone in cases where this pathogen is likely to be the causative agent.

1. **Hall, W. H., B. J. Opfer, and D. N. Gerding.** 1980. Comparative activities of the oxa-β-lactam LY127935, cefotaxime, cefoperazone, cefamandole, and ticarcillin against multiply resistant gram-negative bacilli. Antimicrob. Agents Chemother. **17:**273–279.

Moxalactam Effectiveness in Human Purulent Infection: Laboratory Studies and Clinical Observations

RICHARD E. BRYANT,* ALAN I. HARTSTEIN, THOMAS T. WARD, MICHAEL J. MILLER, AND STEPHEN M. JONES

Oregon Health Sciences University, Portland, Oregon 97201, U.S.A.

Previous studies have shown that microbial β-lactamase can impair local activity of enzyme-sensitive antibiotics in experimental animals and that pus from some patients with polymicrobial suppurative infection contains β-lactamase (1, 2). Thus β-lactamase activity within abscesses may limit the effectiveness of enzyme-sensitive β-lactam antibiotics in the treatment of suppurative infection. The present studies were designed to evaluate the antimicrobial activity of moxalactam, cefotaxime, and cefoperazone in the suppurative environment in an attempt to determine whether the abscess milieu impaired the bactericidal activity of these new agents.

Each drug was tested against 10 clinical isolates of *Klebsiella pneumoniae* and eight clinical isolates of *Bacteroides fragilis*. MICs of these agents for *K. pneumoniae*, using a 10^{-4} dilution of an overnight broth culture, revealed median MIC values as follows: cefoperazone, ~0.39 μg/ml; cefotaxime, 0.05 μg/ml; and moxalactam, 0.01 μg/ml. All strains had MIC values of ≤1.56 μg/ml. The bactericidal activity of these agents against 10^7 colony-forming units (CFU) of *K. pneumoniae* suspended in pus is shown in Table 1. Sealed dialysis bags containing bacteria in pus were incubated for 18 h in test tubes containing 5- to 10-μg/ml concentrations of antibiotics in serum or serum free of antibiotics before bacteria in pus were quantitated. Moxalactam and cefotaxime caused a 100-fold reduction in CFU. Cefoperazone reduced CFU of one strain in pus by 1,000-fold. Colony counts of all other strains remained stable or increased 10-fold greater than the original inoculum when incubated with cefoperazone. Bacteria in pus exposed to tobramycin in serum and antibiotic-free serum had comparable growth. Failure of cefoperazone to kill *Klebsiella* strains may have been due to inactivation by microbial β-lactamase and to the high bacterial inoculum tested, because comparable results were observed when 10^7 to 10^8 *Klebsiella* organisms were added to agar plates containing 10 to 100 μg of cefoperazone per ml.

Moxalactam, cefotaxime, and cefoperazone were also tested against *B. fragilis*. Ten microliters of an 18-h broth culture of *B. fragilis* was added to agar plates containing 10% human pus and 1, 10, or 100 μg of antibiotics per ml. Moxalactam at 100 μg/ml suppressed growth of all *B. fragilis* strains, and seven of nine strains were suppressed by 10 μg/ml. Cefotaxime produced intermediate results in this system that in part reflected high MIC values of that drug for *B. fragilis* strains. Cefoperazone at 10 μg/ml did not inhibit *B. fragilis* strains in pus, even though MIC values of six strains varied from 0.195 to 3.12 μg/ml. The inhibitory effect of pus on cefoperazone activity seemed best explained by the presence of β-lactamase. To test this more directly, antibiotic degradation in clinical specimens of bacteria-free pus was examined. Pus containing no β-lactamase activity caused little change in drug concentrations after incubation at 37°C for various periods. A specimen of antibiotic-free pus containing β-lactamase caused a marked reduction in cefoperazone and cefotaxime (Table 2). Antibiotic activity of those agents was reduced to low levels at 6 h and was virtually abolished by 24 h. Moxalactam activity was only slightly reduced at 6 h and had modest activity after 24 h of incubation in pus containing β-lactamase.

Clinical observation of four patients with suppurative infection revealed a good clinical response to moxalactam therapy. A child was cured of multiple large *Citrobacter diversus* brain abscesses after failure to respond to 4 weeks of chloramphenicol and gentamicin. Furthermore, the prompt response to moxalactam obviated the need for further aspiration or surgical drainage. A patient with polymicrobial empyema complicating lung cancer had *K. pneumoniae* and *B. melaninogenicus* eradicated from empyema fluid but had persistent concomitant pleural infection with methicillin-resistant *Staphylococcus aureus* despite vancomycin therapy. A patient with diverticulitis, abscess, and peritonitis growing *C. freudii*, beta-hemolytic streptococcus, *B. fragilis*, *B. ruminicola*, and *Pseudomonas aeruginosa* was cured with surgical drainage and parenteral moxalactam. A fourth patient with *P. aeruginosa* pneumonia and lung abscess had a good response to moxalactam and tobramycin. Unfortunately, he subsequently died of a massive aspiration pneumonia after extubation. Suppurative infection in these patients responded well to moxalactam therapy.

Clinical observations of these and other pa-

TABLE 1. *Comparison of moxalactam, cefotaxime, cefoperazone, and tobramycin against 10 clinical isolates of K. pneumoniae in pus*[a]

Antimicrobial agent	Concn (μg/ml)	Bacterial counts at 18 h	
		Median CFU/ml	Range
Moxalactam	10	1×10^5	5×10^3–4×10^7
Cefotaxime	10	2×10^5	5×10^1–2×10^7
Cefoperazone	10	1.5×10^8	2.0×10^4–3.3×10^8
Tobramycin	5	1.4×10^8	2×10^7–3.8×10^8
Control	0	4.8×10^8	1.8×10^8–2×10^9

[a] Inoculum of 10^7 CFU/ml.

TABLE 2. *Effect of human pus supernatant containing β-lactamase on stability of moxalactam, cefotaxime, and cefoperazone*

Incubation time at 37°C (h)	Concn (μg/ml)[a]		
	Cefoperazone	Cefotaxime	Moxalactam
0	96.2 ± 3	70 ± 13.6	103 ± 2
1	75.5 ± 8.5	35 ± 8	102.5
4	21.7 ± 6.4	3.1 ± 1	84
6	8.7 ± 1	1.5 ± 0.2	73
24	<0.78	<0.78	15.4 ± 3.6

[a] Mean ± SD of study done in triplicate.

tients and studies demonstrating that moxalactam achieves good tissue levels, is active against inocula of bacteria comparable to those present in abscesses, and is resistant to microbial β-lactamase, suggest that moxalactam is especially well suited for treatment of suppurative infection. On the other hand, β-lactamase-sensitive cephalosporins may be destroyed by enzymatic digestion within polymicrobial abscesses and thereby precluded from killing organisms that are otherwise quite susceptible to them.

1. **Bryant, R. E., A. L. Rashad, J. A. Mazza, and D. Hammond.** 1980. β-Lactamase activity in human pus. J. Infect. Dis. **142**:594–601.
2. **O'Keefe, J. P., F. P. Tally, M. Barza, and S. L. Gorbach.** 1978. Inactivation of penicillin G during experimental infection with *Bacteroides fragilis*. J. Infect. Dis. **137**:437–442.

Moxalactam (LY127935): Clinical Study in the Treatment of Serious Infections

ZELMA Z. FUXENCH-CHIESA,* CARLOS H. RAMÍREZ-RONDA, AND RAMÓN H. BERMÚDEZ-DEL VALLE

Infectious Disease Program, University of Puerto Rico School of Medicine and Veterans Administration Medical Center; Departments of Research and Medicine, Veterans Administration Medical Center; and Department of Medicine, University of Puerto Rico School of Medicine, San Juan, Puerto Rico 00936, U.S.A.*

Moxalactam is a new semisynthetic beta-lactam antibiotic with activity against aerobic gram-positive cocci and aerobic and anaerobic gram-negative bacilli, including *Pseudomonas* and *Bacteroides fragilis* (1, 3, 5). In addition, its activity against multiple-antibiotic-resistant isolates of *Serratia marcescens*, *Pseudomonas aeruginosa*, and *Enterobacter* spp. has been demonstrated by several investigators (2, 4). Most of the *Enterobacteriaceae* are inhibited at a concentration of ≤1 μg/ml, staphylococci are inhibited at 4 to 8 μg/ml, and many strains of *P. aeruginosa* are inhibited at 16 μg/ml or less. Knowing the wide spectrum of activity and potential lack of serious adverse effects, a study was designed to evaluate the effectiveness and safety of moxalactam in the treatment of hospitalized patients with serious lower respiratory tract and soft tissue infections caused by susceptible organisms. The study was open in design and conducted between July and December 1980 in the medical and surgical services of the Veterans Administration Hospital (San Juan, P.R.). The criteria for patient inclusion were: (i) patient of either sex with documented soft tissue or lower respiratory tract infection, and (ii) informed written consent from the patient. Patients were excluded from the protocol if: (i) the use of a second antimicrobial agent was necessary, (ii) there was a history of use of antimicrobial agents within 3 days of initiation of therapy, (iii) pregnancy was present or probable, (iv) there was a history of allergic reaction to penicillin or cephalosporins, or (v) there was evidence of concomitant infection. A total of 34 patients met the criteria for the study, 12 (35%) with soft tissue infections and 22 (65%) with lower respiratory tract infections. All patients were men with an age range of 42 to 95 years and a mean age of 65 years. A complete clinical evaluation including medical history and physical examination, blood cultures, cultures of infected site, hematological studies, liver and renal function tests, and radiological studies was performed as indicated before, during, and after therapy.

The clinical condition of the patients pretherapy was as follows. The 12 patients with soft tissue infection and 6 with lower respiratory tract infection were in fair condition. The condition of the other patients with lower respiratory tract infection was serious in 12 and critical in 4. Thirty patients (88%) suffered from underlying diseases: diabetes in 13, chronic obstructive pulmonary disease in 10, alcoholism in 7, heart disease in 5, tuberculosis in 3, carcinoma in 3, and renal failure in 2. More than half of the patients with diabetes belonged to the soft tissue infection group, and all patients with chronic obstructive pulmonary disease and tuberculosis were in the lower respiratory tract infection group.

All patients were treated with moxalactam intravenously, 500 mg every 8 h for those with soft tissue infections and 2 g every 8 h for those with lower respiratory tract infections. The mean duration of treatment was 8.5 days (range, 7 to 10 days) for patients with soft tissue infection and 11 days (range, 10 to 12 days) for patients with lower respiratory tract infection. According to the clinical response, the patients were classified as satisfactory, satisfactory with relapse, failure, or indeterminate. Bacteriological response was classified as eradication, recurrence, or persistence. The drug was discontinued if the pathogen was not susceptible to the study drug, if there was evidence of adverse effects, or if there was evidence of therapeutic failure.

Specimens obtained for culture were processed by routine microbiological techniques. Organisms recovered from cultures were identified by standard microbiological methods. Susceptibility studies were done by disk diffusion methods and by microdilution methods, using the MIC-2000 system (Dynatech Laboratories).

The organisms recovered from the patients in each group are presented in Table 1. All of the organisms recovered were susceptible to moxalactam. The MIC needed to inhibit 100% of the gram-positive cocci strains was ≤8 μg/ml; 86% of the *Enterobacteriaceae* strains were inhibited by ≤0.5 μg/ml, and all of the *Pseudomonas* isolates recovered were inhibited by ≤16 μg/ml.

The response of patients with soft tissue infections was as follows. Of 12 patients with soft tissue infection, 9 had a satisfactory bacteriological response and there were 2 failures, a bacteriological relapse and a failure to eradicate the organism, both with *P. aeruginosa*. One patient had no growth on cultures before treatment and therefore could not be evaluated bacteriologically. Eleven patients had a satisfactory clinical response, and there was one clinical failure. The response of the patients with lower respiratory tract infections was as follows. Twenty-one of 22 patients had a satisfactory bacteriological response. One patient who failed was diagnosed as having a superinfection with *Enterococcus* after a successful treatment of pneumonococcal pneumonia. Clinical response was satisfactory in the 22 patients.

The overall response was 10 of 12 (83%) in the soft tissue infection group and 21 of 22 (95%) in the lower respiratory tract infection group. There were four (18%) deaths, all in the lower respiratory tract infection group, associated with the underlying diseases. There were three therapeutic failures. The analysis of the failures is as follows. The first case was a diabetic male with a leg ulcer from which *P. aeruginosa* was recovered; the patient was subsequently diagnosed as having osteomyelitis. The organism was never

TABLE 1. *Susceptibility and outcome by clinical condition and pathogen of patients with soft tissue and lower respiratory tract infections treated with moxalactam*

Microorganism	No. of isolates	MIC range (μg/ml)	Outcome success
Soft tissue infections			
Staphylococcus aureus	5	4–8	5/5
Streptococcus spp.	2	4	2/2
Citrobacter diversus	2	0.0625	2/2
Pseudomonas aeruginosa	2	8	0/2
Lower respiratory tract infections			
Klebsiella pneumoniae	7	0.025–0.5	7/7
Streptococcus pneumoniae	4	2–8	3/4
Pseudomonas aeruginosa	3	4–8	3/3
Escherichia coli	3	0.0625	3/3
Staphylococcus aureus	2	4–8	2/2
Pseudomonas fluorescens	1	8	1/1
Enterobacter cloacae	1	0.0625	1/1
Serratia marcescens	1	8	1/1

eradicated, even though the MIC was 8 μg/ml. The second case was a diabetic male with a plantar ulcer from which *P. aeruginosa* was recovered. There was clinical and bacteriological response to therapy, but the infection reoccurred soon after treatment was stopped. The organism was susceptible to moxalactam with an MIC of 8 μg/ml; the relapse organism remained susceptible to moxalactam. The third case was an elderly diabetic male with bilateral bronchopneumonia associated with *Streptococcus pneumoniae*; he responded to therapy both clinically and bacteriologically. The pathogen was susceptible to moxalactam with an MIC of 4 μg/ml. Twenty-four hours after the discontinuation of the antibiotic, the patient reaspirated, and *Enterococcus* was recovered from sputum and blood.

Concentrations in both plasma and serum were determined by microbiological methods, using *Escherichia coli* ATCC 10536. The mean peak moxalactam serum level for patients receiving 500 mg every 8 h was 21.1 μg/ml, with a range of 18 to 30 μg/ml; for patients receiving 2.0 g every 8 h, the level was 86.4 μg/ml, with a range of 67 to 90 μg/ml. The mean trough levels were 2.3 μg/ml (range, 2.1 to 6.5 μg/ml) for the lower dose and 9.4 μg/ml (range, 8.0 to 15 μg/ml) for the higher dose. Peak serum levels were determined 30 min after the end of a 30-min intravenous infusion, and trough levels were determined before the next dose. All serum levels were measured after the third and before the ninth intravenous doses.

A drug-related rash was observed in one patient, and hypoprothrombinemia was observed in another. No serious adverse effects were noted during the study period. No hepatic, renal, or alcohol intolerance adverse effects were documented. The side effects described did not change the administration of the drug.

From this study, we concluded that moxalactam is a valuable, effective, and well-tolerated agent for the treatment of patients with severe soft tissue and lower respiratory tract infections caused by susceptible organisms.

1. **Fass, R. J.** 1977. In vitro activity of LY127935. Antimicrob. Agents Chemother. **16**:503–509.
2. **Hall, W. H., B. J. Opfer, and D. N. Gerding.** 1980. Comparative activities of the oxa-β-lactam LY127935, cefotaxime, cefoperazone, cefamandole, and ticarcillin against multiple resistant gram-negative bacilli. Antimicrob. Agents Chemother. **117**:273–279.
3. **Jorgensen, J. H., G. A. Alexander, and S. A. Crawford.** 1980. Comparison of LY127935 and cefotaxime (HR-756) for in vitro activity against anaerobic bacteria, p. 79–81. *In* Current chemotherapy and infectious disease. American Society for Microbiology, Washington, D.C.
4. **Neu, H. C., N. Aswapokee, K. P. Fu, and P. Aswapokee.** 1979. Antibacterial activity of a new 1-oxa-cephalosporin compared with that of other β-lactam compounds. Antimicrob. Agents Chemother. **16**:141–149.
5. **Trager, G. M., G. W. Whide, V. M. Zimelis, and A. P. Panwalker.** 1979. LY127935: a novel β-lactam antibiotic with unusual antibacterial activity. Antimicrob. Agents Chemother. **16**:297–300.

Moxalactam Therapy of Serious Bacterial Infections

RICHARD D. MEYER,* GLENN E. MATHISEN, J. MARK THOMPSON, AND SYDNEY M. FINEGOLD

Infectious Disease Section, Research and Medical Service, Veterans Administration Wadsworth Medical Center, and the Department of Medicine, University of California School of Medicine, Los Angeles, California 90073, U.S.A.*

Moxalactam, a 1-oxa-cephalosporin, has a broad spectrum of activity against many anaerobes and many aerobic gram-positive and gram-negative bacilli (2), including most of our own nosocomial isolates resistant to cephalothin and aminoglycosides (1). The extended spectrum of activity and pharmacokinetic data indicate that this agent may be useful in the therapy of mixed infections as well as for those caused by single pathogens. We evaluated the efficacy and toxicity of moxalactam in a therapeutic trial.

Patients and bacteriology. Forty-two courses of therapy were given to 41 patients (henceforth referred to as 42 patients). All patients were hospitalized and had infections caused by a pathogen susceptible to moxalactam by disk testing (≥22-mm disk diameter) or had mixed flora with multiple pathogens of which the preponderance were susceptible. Agar dilution susceptibility testing was performed subsequently. All patients were febrile and had clinical signs and symptoms of infection. Forty were men and two were women; 19 were in serious condition when entered into the study and 23 in fair condition. Nineteen had just received other antimicrobial therapy and failed to respond.

TABLE 1. *Summary of results of moxalactam therapy*

Site of infection	No. of patients	Response				
		Total favorable (cured + improved)	Cured	Cured with clinical superinfection	Improved	Failure
Septicemia	9	7	7	0	0	0
Pleuropulmonary	8	7	4	1	2	1
Febrile UTI	5	5	3	2	0	0
Soft tissue–bone joint	16	12	3	1	8	4
Intraabdominal	4	4	4	0	0	0

Those agents were usually cefazolin, cefoxitin, or erythromycin. The patients suffered from a wide variety of underlying medical and/or surgical diseases.

Doses. The usual dose of moxalactam for patients with a normal serum creatinine level (≤1.4 mg/dl) was 2 g intravenously given every 8 or 12 h. Dose adjustments were made for renal insufficiency. No other antimicrobial was given except in two patients who received erythromycin to treat Legionnaires disease. Duration of therapy was from 4 to 65 days.

Serum levels. Mean serum levels in patients with normal serum creatinine concentrations were 36.8 μg/ml 1 h after intravenous dose (peak) and 8.1 μg/ml 7.5 h later (trough).

Results. Table 1 shows the types of infection and response rates. The majority of infections were caused by *Enterobacteriaceae* alone or mixed with anaerobes. Anaerobes included *Peptococcus* spp. and *Bacteroides* spp., including *Bacteroides fragilis* in four instances as part of mixed flora. *Pseudomonas aeruginosa* infections were also treated but with higher doses in the latter part of the study. The sources of the nine instances of septicemia were intravenous cannulas (two), urinary bladder (two), and one each of osteomyelitis, pneumonia, pancreatic pseudocyst, aortic valve, and probable gastrointestinal tract. Efficacy was evaluated for septicemia, although many of these patients also had infections at another primary site.

The high response rate is notable and complete clinical and bacteriological cure was achieved in half the patients. Failure was noted with a susceptible (MIC = 0.12 μg/ml) *Haemophilus parainfluenzae* aortic valve endocarditis case treated with 12 g/day. In other cases it was generally related to adverse local host factors and in some instances to emergence of moxalactam-resistant (MIC ≥ 64 μg/ml) organisms, e.g., a *P. aeruginosa* empyema with a mixed population of organisms that originally tested as susceptible.

Emergence of resistance. Resistant organisms such as *P. aeruginosa*, enterococci, and *Candida* spp. arose in 12 patients and were clinically important in 8. One patient had empyema caused by a susceptible *Moraxella* sp. but then suffered bacteremia after therapy with a resistant *Moraxella* sp. isolate.

Side effects. Twelve patients had side effects or adverse reactions. These were usually minor, such as phlebitis, eosinophilia, or rash, and, in one instance, reversible neutropenia. One other patient developed hypoprothrombinemia and bleeding from a gastric ulcer and required replacement therapy, transfusions, and surgery. No nephrotoxicity or antibiotic-associated diarrhea was noted.

Conclusion. Moxalactam is useful and effective in the therapy of a variety of infections caused by susceptible pathogens, but our results and others indicate that for therapy of serious *P. aeruginosa* infections it may not suffice as a single agent (D. J. Winston, R. W. Busuttil, T. O. Kurtz, and L. S. Young, Arch. Intern. Med., in press) and that emergence of resistant enterococci acting either as pathogens or colonizers may be noted (3). Administration of prophylactic vitamin K appears justified at the beginning of treatment courses in many patients.

1. **Louie, M. H., R. D. Meyer, and K. A. Pasiecznik.** 1980. In vitro susceptibility of cephalothin-resistant Enterobacteriaceae and *Pseudomonas aeruginosa* to a one-oxa cephalosporin (LY 127935 or moxalactam), amikacin, and selected cephalosporins. Curr. Microbiol. **3:** 301–304.
2. **Neu, H. C., A. Aswapokee, K. P. Fu, and P. Aswapokee.** 1979. Antibacterial activity of a new 1-oxa cephalosporin compared with that of other β-lactam compounds. Antimicrob. Agents Chemother. **16:**141–149.
3. **Yu, V. L.** 1981. Enterococcal superinfection and colonization after therapy with moxalactam, a new broad-spectrum antibiotic. Ann. Int. Med. **94:**784–785.

Clinical Efficacy and Pharmacokinetics of Moxalactam in Infants and Children

ABDUL J. KHAN, MATHEW VARGHESE, URMILLA PATEL, KUSUM KUMAR, AND HUGH E. EVANS

Department of Pediatrics, Jewish Hospital and Medical Center of Brooklyn, State University of New York Downstate Medical Center, Brooklyn, New York 11238, U.S.A.

Moxalactam is a new broad-spectrum semisynthetic antibiotic of the cephalosporin group. In addition to such common bacterial pathogens as *Streptococcus pneumoniae*, *Staphylococcus aureus*, *Haemophilus influenzae* type b, and *Escherichia coli*, the spectrum of this drug includes *Pseudomonas aeruginosa*, *Serratia marcescens*, and *Proteus* spp. (indole negative and positive) (1, 3, 4, 6). In recent studies of young infants and children with meningitis, a single dose of this drug crossed the blood-brain barrier in high concentrations (2, 5), suggesting a potential advantage in treatment of meningitis.

The efficacy, safety, and pharmacokinetics of this drug were evaluated in 21 inpatients ranging in age from 1 to 13 years (mean, 4.1 years). Sixteen were admitted for clinical pneumonia which was confirmed by roentgenogram. The other five were treated for urinary tract infection (UTI) documented by two consecutively positive urine cultures. Moxalactam was administered parenterally in the dose of 45 mg/kg of body weight (range, 25 to 50 mg/kg) in three divided doses every 8 h for an average duration of 9.5 days. Safety was monitored by serial evaluation of complete blood count, including platelet count, liver function tests (serum glutamic oxalacetic and pyruvic transaminases, bilirubin, and alkaline phosphatase), and renal function tests including urinalysis, blood urea nitrogen, and serum creatinine performed before, during, and after treatment. In patients with UTI, urine culture was repeated within 3 to 4 days after starting the therapy and 24 h, 2 weeks, and 4 to 6 weeks after stopping.

Pharmacokinetics were evaluated in 16 patients. Five to six specimens of blood were collected at different time intervals over a period of 8 h after a test dose (Table 1). Serum was separated and frozen at −20°C. One random urine specimen was also collected after the dose and kept frozen. Bioassay was performed with an agar diffusion method utilizing trypticase soy agar and *E. coli* (ATCC 12936) as the test organism. The serum half-life ($t_{1/2}$) was determined by using the formula $t_{1/2} = \ln 2/K$, where K is the elimination rate constant, represented by the slope of the regression line determined by plotting the log of drug concentration against time.

All patients with pneumonia became afebrile within 2 to 4 days after initiation of therapy and had complete clinical and radiological resolution at the end of therapy. Blood cultures were sterile in 15 patients with pneumonia. *H. influenzae* type b resistant to ampicillin but susceptible to moxalactam was isolated from the blood culture in one patient. Nasopharyngeal cultures revealed *S. pneumoniae* in 3 patients, *H. influenzae* in 5 patients, and *S. aureus* in 1 patient. Susceptibility of isolates from the nasopharynx was not determined. *E. coli*, the primary pathogen in all UTI cases, susceptible to moxalactam was eradicated by 2 to 3 days. Subsequently, urine cultures remained sterile for 4 to 5 weeks after therapy.

The drug was well tolerated by all patients. None developed skin rashes, bleeding diathesis, gastrointestinal symptoms, or other clinical evidence of toxicity. Six patients (28%) developed transient mild elevations of serum glutamic oxalacetic transaminase and alkaline phoshatase levels. Five patients had transient platelet count elevation with the mean increasing from $3.15 \times 10^5/m^3$ to $5.5 \times 10^5/m^3$ ($P > 0.05$). No changes were observed in blood urea nitrogen or serum creatinine values. Mean blood levels of moxalactam were higher in the intravenous and intramuscular group given 17 mg at 0.5, 1, and 2 h, but the differences were not significant ($P < 0.05$ in each instance). Half-lives and mean urinary concentrations were comparable in the intravenous and intramuscular groups at each dose level. Peak blood levels were severalfold higher than the reported MICs for commonly encountered pathogens, including those we isolated. Even trough levels observed at 8 h (2 to 3 μg/ml; Table 1) were about eightfold higher than the reported MIC for 100% of strains of *H. influenzae* type b (4). The latter levels were about 8 to 20 times higher than required to inhibit 90% of strains of *E. coli*, *K. pneumoniae*, and *Proteus*, and were a little more than sufficient to inhibit 90% of strains of pneumococcus and *S. marcescens*.

Our observations suggest that moxalactam is

TABLE 1. *Blood levels, half-life, and urinary concentration of moxalactam*

Dose (mg/kg)[a]	Blood levels (μg/ml)[b] at: 0.25 h	0.5 h	1 h	2 h	4 h	8 h	Half-life (min)[b]	Urinary concn (μg/ml)[b]
17 i.m. (8)		17.65	18	11.68	4.8	3.2	124.3[c]	223.76[d]
		(3.46)	(7.14)	(2.3)	(1.12)	(1.18)	(12.09)	(114.66)
17 i.v. (5)	65.26	48.4	35.72	28.76	9.8	2.8	95.108[c]	552.12[d]
	(20.48)	(21.72)	(17.55)	(18.12)	(4.37)	(2.02)	(24.49)	(199.9)
8 i.v. (2)	19	12.9	6.6	6.6	1.4	0.75	72.5	67
	(0)	(7.1)	(3.4)	(3.4)	(0.4)	(0.25)	(4.5)	(33)
8 i.m. (1)		10	10	10	2.5	0.4	102	120

[a] Administered intramuscularly (i.m.) or intravenously (i.v.) to the number of patients shown in parentheses.
[b] Mean with SE given in parentheses.
[c] $P > 0.05$.
[d] $P > 0.05$.

an effective antibiotic for infants and children but do not permit conclusions about the efficacy in well-documented bacterial pneumonia. Although pathogens including pneumococcus and *H. influenzae* type b were isolated from the upper respiratory tract in most cases, nasopharyngeal cultures correlate poorly with the bacterial etiology of pneumonia. Bacteriological efficacy, however, was well documented in the patient whose blood culture grew *H. influenzae* type b resistant to ampicillin. Successful eradication of urinary tract pathogens suggests that the drug could be used whenever the parenteral route is indicated for the treatment of UTI, especially if the infection is caused by unusual organisms, including *Pseudomonas.*

It appears that a useful drug has been added to the treatment of systemic bacterial infections including pneumonia and UTI, for older infants and children. Since it does not have significant activity against group B *Streptococcus,* a major cause of neonatal sepsis/meningitis, the drug cannot be recommended as the initial agent in therapy of neonates. Further studies are needed as to its efficacy in the therapy of meningitis.

1. **Fass, R. J.** 1979. In vitro activity of LY 127935. Antimicrob. Agents Chemother. **16:**503–509.
2. **Kaplan, S. L., E. O. Mason, H. Garcia, S. J. Kvernland, E. M. Loiselle, D. C. Anderson, A. A. Mintz, and R. D. Feigin.** 1981. Pharmacokinetics and cerebrospinal fluid penetrations of Moxalactam in children with bacterial meningitis. J. Pediatr. **98:**152–157.
3. **Lang, S. D. R., D. J. Edwards, and D. T. Durack.** 1980. Comparison of cefoperazone, cefotaxime, and moxalactam (LY 127935) against aerobic gram-negative bacilli. Antimicrob. Agents Chemother. **17:**488–493.
4. **Mason, E. O., S. L. Kaplan, D. C. Anderson, D. B. Hinds, and R. D. Feigin.** 1980. In vitro susceptibility of 104 clinical isolate of *Haemophilus influenzae* to moxalactam (LY 127935), ampicillin, chloramphenicol, and ticarcillin. Antimicrob. Agents Chemother. **17:**470–473.
5. **Schaad, U. B., G. H. McCracken, N. Threlkeld, and M. L. Thomas.** 1981. Clinical evaluation of a new broad-spectrum Oxa-Beta-Lactam antibiotic, Moxalactam, in neonates and infants. J. Pediatr. **93:**129–136.
6. **Wise, R., J. M. Andrews, and K. A. Bedford.** 1979. LY 127935, a novel oxa-β-lactam: an in vitro comparison with older β-lactam antibiotics. Antimicrob. Agents Chemother. **16:**341–344.

Clinical Use of Moxalactam in Hospitalized Patients with Severe Infections

P. CIA,* R. GOMEZ-LUS, A. MILLASTRE, M. C. RUBIO-CALVO, I. SANCHEZ-MIRET, G. RODRIGO, G. PACHECO, AND E. CIVEIRA

Catedra de Patologia Medica A and Department of Microbiology, School of Medicine, Zaragoza, Spain*

Moxalactam (LY127935) is a new beta-lactam, containing unusual substitutions both within and around its ring structure. This antibiotic is structurally similar to cefamandole, yet differs in the 4-hydroxy of the phenyl ring, a 7-methoxy group, and the substitution of an oxygen for the 1-sulfa in the cephem. Moxalactam is reported to have a broad spectrum and a potent activity against a variety of gram-positive and gram-negative bacteria, including *Enterobacteriaceae, Pseudomonas,* streptococci, and staphylococci, as well as several species of anaerobic bacteria (1–5).

The 22 patients studied were hospitalized

mainly in the Intensive Care Unit (Internal Medicine Department of the University Hospital, Zaragoza). The investigations were initiated 3 December 1980 and were completed 16 April 1981. Initial selection was made in each case on the basis of clinical findings and in the presence of bacteria susceptible to moxalactam. The following were also taken into account as criteria for selection: (i) radiological diagnosis in the case of pneumonias and bronchopneumonias; (ii) nonadministration of concomitant antimicrobial therapy; (iii) exclusion of pregnant patients and patients hypersensitive to cephalosporins; (iv) bacteriological controls, performed day 3 or 4 of treatment, at the end of it, and 4 weeks after in cases of urinary tract infections; (v) laboratory control (blood and urinalysis), conducted to evaluate the evolution of the process and renal and hepatic functions; and (vi) a moxalactam assay. For this assay, blood specimens were obtained immediately after the end of infusion or 1 h after intramuscular injection; serum assays were performed by an agar well method, with *Escherichia coli* ATCC 10536 as the test organisms.

Moxalactam was administered intramuscularly or intravenously in a dosage of 3.0 g per day in divided doses every 8 h for 5 to 12 days. Summary of patients' sex and age, diagnosis, underlying conditions, etiology, and results of therapy with moxalactam is presented in Table 1. Patients who died from any cause during

TABLE 1. *Results of therapy with moxalactam*

Case	Sex	Age (yr)	Diagnosis	Organism	Outcome
1	M	66	Chronic bronchitis, bronchiectasis	*P. aeruginosa, A. calcoaceticus*	Failure (died)
2	F	50	Bronchopneumonia, left heart failure	*Klebsiella pneumoniae*, group B streptococci	Cure
3	F	72	Pneumonia, cor pulmonale, respiratory failure, arterial hypertension	*H. influenzae*, group C streptococci, *Staphylococcus epidermidis*	Cure
4	M	62	Chronic bronchitis, cor pulmonale, respiratory failure	*Streptococcus pneumoniae*, group B streptococci	Cure
5	M	82	Pneumonia, respiratory failure, atrial fibrillation, dehydration	*S. pneumoniae, Proteus mirabilis*	Cure
6	F	70	Chronic bronchitis, pulmonary fibrosis	*P. aeruginosa, S. pyogenes*	Cure
7	M	73	Bronchopneumonia, arterial hypertension, atrial fibrillation, cerebrovascular accident	*H. influenzae, K. pneumoniae*	Cure
8	M	76	Pneumonia, respiratory failure, pneumothorax, urinary tract infection	*P. aeruginosa, S. epidermidis, E. coli*	Cure
9	M	62	Pneumonia, respiratory failure, ischemic myocardiopathy, pyopneumothorax	*H. influenzae*	Cure
10	M	59	Bronchopneumonia, cor pulmonale, pulmonary emphysema, pulmonary fibrosis, diabetes	*S. pneumoniae, E. coli*	Cure
11	M	52	Pneumonia, cor pulmonale, manic-depressive psychosis, dehydration	*S. pneumoniae, K. pneumoniae, Citrobacter freundii*	Failure (died)
12	M	51	Pneumonia, urinary tract infection, bacteremia, myocardial infarction	*S. pyogenes, E. coli*	Cure
13	M	76	Bronchopneumonia, urinary tract infection	*S. pneumoniae, E. coli*	Failure (died)
14	M	52	Bronchopneumonia, multiple sclerosis, respiratory failure	*H. influenzae, A. calcoaceticus*	Cure
15	M	80	Pneumonia, respiratory failure, myocardial infarction	*S. pneumoniae, S. aerogenes*	Cure
16	F	22	Bronchopneumonia, coma, intoxication, chronic alcoholism	*S. pyogenes, S. marcescens*	Cure
17	M	41	Pneumonia, bacteremia, septic shock	*H. influenzae*	Cure
18	M	62	Soft tissue infection, bacteremia, leukemia	*B. fragilis, P. aeruginosa, S. marcescens*	Failure (died)
19	F	69	Pyelonephritis, bacteremia	*E. coli*	Cure
20	M	61	Urinary tract infection, benign prostatic hypertrophy	*Enterobacter cloacae*	Cure
21	M	70	Pyelonephritis, bacteremia	*E. coli, S. marcescens*	Cure
22	F	53	Urinary tract infection, postprostatectomy	*P. aeruginosa*	Cure

therapy were classified as failures. Cures were clinical recovery and elimination of pathogens from relevant specimens.

Respiratory tract infections. Eight patients had pneumonia, seven had bronchopneumonia, and two had chronic bronchitis in exacerbation. Of the eight patients with pneumonia, seven were clinically cured. Follow-up sputum cultures were obtained in six patients; susceptible pathogens were eradicated in all six cases. The treatment failure occurred in a 52-year-old male patient (case 11), who was admitted to the Intensive Care Unit with serious pneumonia, cor pulmonale, manic-depressive psychosis, and dehydration. Seven patients presented bronchopneumonia; six of them achieved cure and one died. The failure occurred in a 76-year-old male patient (case 13), who was admitted to the Intensive Care Unit with bronchopneumonia caused by *Streptococcus pneumoniae* and urinary tract infection caused by *E. coli*. During 5 days a satisfactory clinical and radiological evolution was achieved, but 24 h later the patient presented severe renal failure and died. Two patients presented chronic bronchitis with exacerbation; one of them was cured and one died. Case 1 was a 66-year-old male, who presented with chronic bronchitis and bronchiectasis; *Pseudomonas aeruginosa* and *Acinetobacter calcoaceticus* were isolated from secretions of the respiratory tree. The patient's condition was extremely severe; treatment with moxalactam was started, and during 6 days the response to treatment was satisfactory. However, the patient finally died from renal failure.

Urinary tract infections. All four patients with urinary tract infection were clinically and bacteriologically cured. Two patients (cases 19 and 21) presented with pyelonephritis and bacteremia; samples of both urine and blood were obtained for culture, and treatment with moxalactam was started at a dosage of 3 g per day, intramuscularly. Cure was achieved with negative blood culture 24 h after the initiation of treatment. Urine cultures immediately and 4 months after therapy were sterile.

Soft tissue infection. Case 18 was a 60-year-old leukemic male, who presented with soft tissue infection and bacteremia. *Bacteroides fragilis*, *P. aeruginosa*, and *Serratia marcescens* were isolated both from blood and exudate. The patient's condition improved satisfactorily during 5 days, but he died from cardiorespiratory failure. Mean serum levels after a 1-g infusion ranged from 64.5 to 76.4 μg/ml. Intramuscular doses of 1 g produced a mean level of 49.5 μg/ml at 1 h.

In summary, moxalactam was used in a group of severely ill patients. Of the 22 cases, moxalactam cured 18 (81.81%). On the basis of this preliminary study we conclude that moxalactam is a promising drug for the treatment of serious gram-negative and gram-positive infections.

1. **Baker, C. N., C. Thornsberry, and R. N. Jones.** 1980. In vitro antimicrobial activity of cefoperazone, cefotaxime, moxalactam (LY127935), azlocillin, mezlocillin, and other β-lactam antibiotics against *Neisseria gonorrhoeae* and *Haemophilus influenzae*, including β-lactamase-producing strains. Antimicrob. Agents Chemother. **17**:757–761.
2. **Jones, R. N., P. C. Fuchs, H. M. Sommers, T. L. Gavan, A. L. Barry, and E. H. Gerlach.** 1980. Moxalactam (LY127935), new semisynthetic 1-oxa-β-lactam antibiotic with remarkable antimicrobial activity: in vitro comparison with cefamandole and tobramycin. Antimicrob. Agents Chemother. **17**:750–756.
3. **Jorgensen, J. H., S. A. Crawford, and G. A. Alexander.** 1980. Comparison of moxalactam (LY127935) and cefotaxime against anaerobic bacteria. Antimicrob. Agents Chemother. **17**:901–904.
4. **Rubio-Calvo, M. C., and R. Gomez-Lus.** 1980. In vitro antibacterial activity of cefoperazone and LY127935 against aerobic isolates, p. 67–69. *In* J. D. Nelson and C. Grassi (ed.), Current chemotherapy and infectious disease. American Society for Microbiology, Washington, D.C.
5. **Yoshida, T., S. Matsuura, M. Mayama, Y. Kumeda, and S. Kuwahara.** 1980. Moxalactam (6059-S), a novel 1-oxa-β-lactam with an expanded antibacterial spectrum: laboratory evaluation. Antimicrob. Agents Chemother. **17**:302–312.

Moxalactam Therapy for Serious Infections

P. VAN DER AUWERA,* N. CLUMECK, Y. VAN LAETHEM, R. VAN HOOF, J. C. LEGRAND, G. LIGNY, AND J. P. BUTZLER

Hospital St. Pierre, Brussels, and Hôpital Civil de Charleroi, Charleroi, Belgium*

Moxalactam is a semisynthetic beta-lactam antibacterial agent which is extremely active in vitro against gram-positive and gram-negative aerobes and anaerobes. The striking activity against classical cephalosporin-resistant organisms such as *Enterobacter*, indole-positive *Proteus*, *Serratia*, *Klebsiella*, *Escherichia coli*, and *Pseudomonas aeruginosa* makes this drug promising for in vivo use (1–3).

Therefore, we have undertaken a clinical

study with moxalactam in serious infections, most of them caused by multiresistant organisms. Twenty-four patients were included in this study. All of them had clinical evidence of serious infection; they did not receive any other effective antibiotic before or during the trial. Moxalactam dosage varied from 3 to 12 g a day depending on clinical situation, suspected organism, and renal function. The drug was administered in 50 ml of 5% glucose during 20 min for intravenous infusion and reconstituted with sterile water for intramuscular injection. MICs were measured by the agar dilution method in Mueller-Hinton agar for aerobes and Columbia agar for anaerobes. Inoculum size was 10^4 colony-forming units/spot for aerobes and 10^6 for anaerobes. Moxalactam serum assays were performed in triplicate in large plates (36 by 36) with *Bacillus subtilis.*

Clinical and bacteriological results are summarized in Table 1. Clinical cure was considered when a complete resolution of the signs and symptoms of infection occurred. A significant response with normalization of the temperature was considered improvement. Clinical failure was defined as no change or a worsening of the clinical situation. Bacteriological cure was when primary pathogens were eradicated. Bacteriological failure was persistence of primary pathogens. Superinfection was defined as a new infection occurring either in the primary site or elsewhere caused by an organism other than the primary pathogen. Colonization was appearance of microorganisms resistant to 50 μg of moxalactam per ml regardless of clinical significance. Seventeen patients had severe underlying diseases considered to impair the normal response towards bacterial pathogens.

Two failures were observed. The first failure

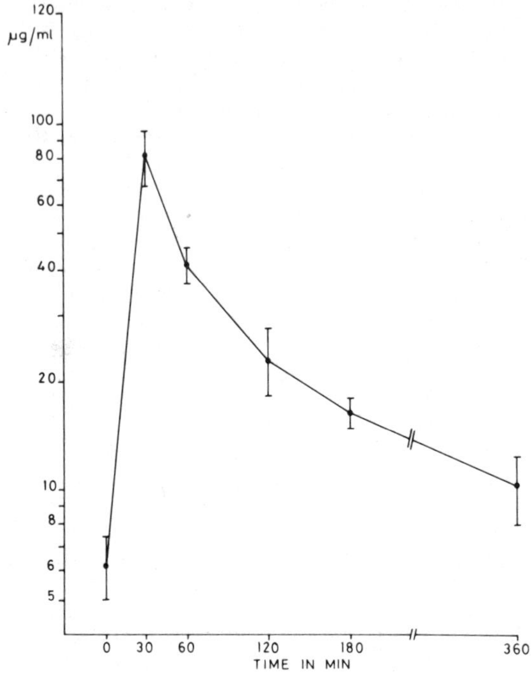

FIG. 1. *Serum moxalactam level after 1-g intravenous infusion in 30 min: 15 patients.*

TABLE 1. *Clinical and bacteriological results with intravenous moxalactam*

	CLINICAL				BACTERIOLOGICAL			
	NUMBER	CURED	IMPROVED	FAILURE	CURED	FAILURE	COLONISATION	SUPERINFECTION
ALL POPULATION	24 (17)	15 (10)	7 (5)	2 (2)	23 (16)	1 (1)	3 (3)	5 (5)
SEPTICEMIC PATIENTS	19 (14)	12 (8)	6 (5)	1 (1)	19 (14)	0	3 (3)	5 (5)
NON SEPTICEMIC PATIENTS	5 (3)	3 (2)	1 (0)	1 (1)	4 (2)	1 (1)	0	0
UTI	6 (4)	5 (3)	0	1 (1)	5 (3)	1 (1)	0	0
PULMONARY ABSCESSES	4 (4)	2 (2)	1 (1)	1 (1)	4 (4)	0	1 (1)	0
SEPTIC THROMBO-PHLEBITIS	5 (3)	5 (3)	0	0	5 (3)	0	0	2 (2)
MISCELLANEOUS INFECTIONS	10 (7)	4 (3)	6 (4)	0	10 (7)	0	2 (2)	3 (3)

: ONE PATIENT PRESENTED UTI AND PULMONARY ABSCESS.

( ) INDICATES NUMBER OF PATIENTS WITH MULTI R ORGANISMS

occurred in a neutropenic patient with necrotizing pneumonia with septicemia due to *Klebsiella pneumoniae* (MIC, 1.2 μg/ml) despite 11 days of therapy with 4.5 g/day intravenously. The second failure occurred in a patient with *P. aeruginosa* urinary tract infection (MIC, 5 μg/ml) despite 7 days of therapy with 3 g/day intravenously. Adverse reactions were observed in seven patients (29%) and consisted of three transient eosinophilias, three transient hepatic alterations (rises in serum glutamic oxalacetic and pyruvic transaminases and alkaline phosphatase), and one generalized maculopapular rash. Serum levels of moxalactam in 15 patients given 30-min intravenous infusions are shown in Fig. 1.

In conclusion, 88% of our patients were cured or improved with moxalactam therapy despite severe infections and underlying diseases. Most of the pathogens were multiresistant.

1. **Barza, M., F. P. Tally, N. V. Jacobus, and S. L. Gorbach.** 1979. In vitro activity of LY127935. Antimicrob. Agents Chemother. **16**:287–292.
2. **Flournoy, D. J., and F. A. Perryman.** 1979. LY127935, a new beta-lactam antibiotic, versus *Proteus, Klebsiella, Serratia,* and *Pseudomonas.* Antimicrob. Agents Chemother. **16**:641–643.
3. **Hall, W. H., B. J. Offer, and D. N. Gerding.** 1979. Comparative activities of the oxa-beta-lactam LY127935, cefotaxime, cefoperazone, cefamandole, and ticarcillin against multiply resistant gram-negative bacilli. Antimicrob. Agents Chemother. **16**:141–149.

Moxalactam Therapy in Seriously Ill Hospitalized Patients

BURT R. MEYERS,* GARY P. WORMSER, AND SHALOM Z. HIRSCHMAN

Department of Medicine, The Mount Sinai School of Medicine of the City University of New York, New York, New York 10029, U.S.A.

Moxalactam is a new oxycephalosporin derivative with a broad spectrum of antimicrobial activity against a wide variety of gram-positive and gram-negative bacteria. Studies in vitro have shown moxalactam to be exquisitely active against strains of *Enterobacteriaceae* and *Haemophilus influenzae. Pseudomonas aeruginosa* and *Bacteroides fragilis* strains are also inhibited by this compound (1, 2). It is stable to beta-lactamase produced by these species (4); many strains resistant to second-generation cephalosporins and aminoglycosides are susceptible in vitro to moxalactam. Moxalactam can be administered either intravenously or intramuscularly, and pharmacokinetic studies have shown that very high drug levels are achieved in the serum after administration by either route (5, 6).The efficacy and safety of moxalactam in the treatment of a variety of infections in hospitalized, seriously ill patients was investigated in this study.

Moxalactam was administered intrasmucularly in doses ranging from 3 to 12 g given over 4 to 6 h. Informed consent was obtained from each patient according to the institutional policy. Cultures were taken from appropriate sites before therapy and processed by the diagnostic microbiology laboratory of The Mount Sinai Hospital. MICs and MBCs of moxalactam for the isolates were determined by microtiter broth dilution. Susceptibility to moxalactam by disk diffusion test was determined by use of a 30-μg disk. Moxalactam serum levels were measured by the well diffusion bioassay method, with *Escherichia coli* ATCC 10536 as the test organism.

An evaluable case had to meet the following criteria: (i) a bacterial pathogen was isolated before therapy; (ii) the bacterial isolate was susceptible to moxalactam (at least one in a mixed infection); (iii) moxalactam parenteral therapy was given for a minimum of 5 days; (iv) proper clinical evaluation was carried out (i.e., temperature response, etc.); (v) posttherapy follow-up cultures were evaluated. Bacteriological response to moxalactam was considered satisfactory when, on post-treatment cultures, the causative organism had been eradicated, unless surgery was needed. The clinical response was considered satisfactory when, on clinical examination, the infection had either improved or completely cleared. Colonization was defined as the presence of a new organism during or after therapy without clinical signs. Superinfection was defined as the presence of a new organism which developed during or after treatment with concomitant clinical symptoms or signs.

Sixty-seven patients with 69 documented systemic infections were treated with moxalactam at The Mount Sinai Medical Center. Of these, 54 patients were evaluated clinically and 46 patients were evaluated bacteriologically. The mean age in years of patients treated was 60 (SD, 18.44), with a range from 18 to 93 years. There were 50 males and 17 females evaluated.

Most (56 of 67) of the patients had underlying disease. The most common of these were diabetes mellitus (17 patients); neoplasia (14 patients); cardiovascular (10 patients); neurological disease (9 patients); renal failure (5 patients); myeloproliferative diseases (5 patients); and drug addiction (3 patients). One hundred and four gram-negative microorganisms were isolated from the patients (Table 1). Thirty-three gram-positive isolates were isolated. Moxalactam was given either intravenously or intramuscularly for 1 to 45 days, with a mean of 13.6 days (SD, 10 days). The mean total daily dose was 5.3 g per day, with a range from 3 to 12 g.

There were 13 patients with urinary tract infections. Eleven had *P. aeruginosa* isolated, 2 had *Proteus* species, and 1 had *Klebsiella pneumoniae.* Bacteriological response by organism was satisfactory in 9 of 11 isolates of *P. aeruginosa* (82%). The overall bacteriological response rate was 86%. The overall clinical response was 85%. Many of the patients had a prior history of repeated urinary tract infection as well as underlying diseases of the urinary tract (i.e., stones, malformation, and surgery). Of note is the fact that 12 of 13 patients evaluated with moxalactam were males.

Fourteen patients with bacteremia were included in the study. Microorganisms evaluated included *E. coli* in three patients, *Proteus mirabilis* in two, *Staphylococcus aureus* in two, and *Klebsiella* in one. Bacteriological response was favorably noted in 75%, and a favorable clinical response rate noted in 66%. Five patients were nonevaluable either bacteriologically or clinically.

There were 11 patients with osteomyelitis evaluated with moxalactam. Microorganisms included *P. aeruginosa*, indole-positive *Proteus* spp., and *Acinetobacter* spp. There was a favorable bacteriological response with 78% of the organisms. A favorable clinical response (11 of 12) was noted.

Twenty-three patients were evaluated with soft tissue infections from a wide range of microorganisms, including *P. aeruginosa, E. coli, Proteus* spp., *S. aureus*, group A hemolytic streptococci, and other strains. The satisfactory bacteriological response and clinical response were identical (74%).

Eight patients were treated with moxalactam for respiratory tract infection. The bacteriological response was favorable in 80% (four of five) of the organisms, and the clinical response was 89% (eight of nine).

The overall clinical patient response to moxalactam is given in Table 2. The overall bacteriological response for the five clinical conditions was 80% (Table 2). The corresponding favorable clinical response was 76%. Of 69 patients, 23 (33%) were nonevaluable bacteriologically, and 15 of 69 (21.7%) were not evaluable clinically.

Members of the family *Enterobacteriaceae* were exquisitely susceptible to moxalactam. The mean MIC for *E. coli* (10 strains) was 0.75 μg/ml. All strains were inhibited by 3.1 μg/ml. *Proteus* species, including both indole-positive and indole-negative, had mean MICs of 0.72 and 0.98 μg/ml, respectively. The MIC to kill 90% of the strains (MIC_{90}) was 1.56 μg/ml. *K. pneumoniae* strains had an MIC_{90} of 0.78 μg/ml. Four of five strains of *Serratia marcescens* were exquisitely susceptible to this compound. There were 50 isolates of *P. aeruginosa* with a mean MIC of 29.5 μg/ml. When six resistant *P. aeruginosa* strains were deleted, the mean MIC (44 strains) was 20 μg/ml. Gram-positive microorganisms were less susceptible to this compound. The mean MIC_{50} for six strains of *S. aureus* was 6.2

TABLE 1. *MICs of moxalactam for gram-negative clinical isolates*

Organism	No. of isolates	MIC (μg/ml) Mean (SD)	MIC (μg/ml) Range	MIC_{50} (μg/ml)	MIC_{90} (μg/ml)
Pseudomonas aeruginosa	50[a]	29.5 (29.5)	0.39–100	12.5	100
	44	19.9 (14.4)	0.39–50	12.5	50
Klebsiella pneumoniae	6	2.3 (5.0)	0.1–12.5	0.1	0.78
Proteus mirabilis	11	0.98 (1.8)	0.1–6.25	0.39	1.56
Indole-positive *Proteus*	3	0.72 (0.74)	0.39–1.56	0.39	1.56
Enterobacter spp.	12	14.8 (30.8)	0.1–100	0.39	25
Escherichia coli	10	0.75 (0.9)	0.1–3.12	0.39	0.78
Serratia marcescens	5	10.4 (22.1)	0.2–50	0.78	50
Citrobacter spp.	4	6.3 (7.2)	0.1–12.5	0.1	12.5
Haemophilus influenzae	2	0.83 (1.03)	0.1–1.56	0.1	1.56
Providencia sp.	1	0.39 (0)	0	0.39	0.39

[a] Includes six resistant strains.

μg/ml. Group A beta-hemolytic streptococci had an MIC_{90} of 0.78 μg/ml. One strain of group B (*S. agalactiae*) was less susceptible (12.5 μg/ml). All 14 strains of enterococci were highly resistant to this compound, with MICs of greater than 100 μg/ml.

The concentration of moxalactam in the serum of treated patients was determined at both peak and trough intervals. A mean concentration of 105.3 μg of moxalactam was noted 0 to 2 h postinfusion in 26 patients; a trough level 4 to 8 h postinfusion of 25 μg/ml was noted in 28 patients. The dosages ranged from 1 to 2 g administered between 4 and 12 h.

Side effects were noted in 12 of 69 patients (17%). There were four patients with diarrhea, two with skin rash, one with phlebitis, two with eosinophilia, one with leukopenia, two with creatinine elevation, and one with ecchymosis. One patient with skin rash was receiving concomitant therapy with hydrochlorithiazide. All effects were transient and returned to normal after moxalactam therapy was concluded. Drug therapy was discontinued in three patients, all after at least 14 days of therapy.

Moxalactam was an effective agent in the treatment of 67 seriously ill patients, 56 of whom had severe underlying disease. A wide range of microorganisms were treated with this compound, including both gram-positive and gram-negative bacteria. Serum levels with a peak of 105 μg/ml and trough of 25 μg/ml would be inhibitory for greater than 50% of all the strains isolated except for the enterococci. The peak level would be greater than the MIC_{90} of all microorganisms with the exception of *Streptococcus faecalis*. The trough level of 25 μg/ml would be inhibitory for all gram-negative isolates with the exception of a few strains of *P. aeruginosa* and one *Serratia* strain.

A large number of patients were not evaluable because of strict adherence to guidelines for admission into the study. Side effects were minimal with this compound. Colonization occurred in 9 of 69 patients (13%). Five (7.2%) of the patients had enterococci, and three (4.3%) had *Candida albicans*. The development of superinfection with enterococci in 2 of 69 patients (2.9%) is in agreement with data presented at a recent symposium by Moellering, which revealed an incidence of 2.1% (3). The development of resistance in 1 of 137 strains (0.7%) is encouraging indeed. Tofle et al. (7) recently reported a cure rate of 91% in infections treated with moxalactam; however, only 3 patients were seriously ill.

TABLE 2. *Overall patient clinical and bacteriological response to moxalactam*[a]

Patient group	Cure	Failure	Nonevaluable
Clinical			
Soft tissue	14/17 (82)	3/17	6/23
Osteomyelitis	9/10 (90)	1/10	1/11
Bacteremia	6/9 (66.6)	3/9	5/14
Urinary tract	9/11 (82)	2/11	2/13
Respiratory	6/7 (86)	1/7	1/8
Overall response	41/54 (76)	13/54 (24)	15/69 (22)
Bacteriological			
Soft tissue	13/16 (81)	3/16	7/23
Osteomyelitis	5/6 (83)	1/6	5/11
Bacteremia	6/8 (75)	2/8	6/14
Urinary tract	10/12 (83)	2/12	1/13
Respiratory	3/4 (75)	1/4	4/8
Overall response	37/46 (80)	9/46 (20)	23/69 (33)

[a] Numbers in parentheses are percentages.

Moxalactam appears to be a safe, well-tolerated beta-lactam derivative with a broad spectrum of antibacterial activity. It can be administered either intramuscularly or intravenously to seriously ill hospitalized patients. Its broad spectrum of activity suggests that it may be effective initial therapy in a wide variety of clinical infections. Further clinical studies against combination chemotherapy are necessary to substantiate its use as monotherapy.

1. **Barza, M., F. P. Tally, N. V. Jacobus, and S. L. Gorbach.** 1979. In vitro activity of LY 127935. Antimicrob. Agents Chemother. **16**:287–292.
2. **Fass, R. J.** 1979. In vitro activity of LY 137935. Antimicrob. Agents Chemother. **16**:503–509.
3. **Moellering, R.** 1981. Symposium on the new generation of beta lactam antibiotics. London, England, 7–8 May.
4. **Richmond, M. H.** 1980. The beta lactamase stability of a novel beta lactam antibiotic containing a 7 α-methoxyoxacephem nucleus. J. Antimicrob. Chemother., in press
5. **Scheld, W. M., D. A. Spyker, G. R. Donowitz, W. K. Bolton, and M. A. Sande.** 1981. Moxalactam and cefazolin: comparative pharmacokinetics in normal subjects. Antimicrob. Agents Chemother. **19**:613–619.
6. **Srivanivasan, S., E. Francke, and H. Neu.** 1981. Pharmacokinetics of moxalactam and cefazolin compared in normal volunteers. Antimicrob. Agents Chemother. **19**: 302–305.
7. **Tofle, R. W., J. Rofschafer, J. Solliday, and K. B. Crossley.** 1981. Moxalactam therapy for a wide spectrum of bacterial infections in adults. Antimicrob. Agents Chemother. **19**:740–744.

Mechanism of Antibacterial Activity of Cefroxadine (CGP 9000) on *Escherichia coli*

TAKESHI NISHINO,* HIROYUKI OHWAKI, TADASHI YOSHIMOTO, MASAKO OHTSUKI, AND TERUO TANINO

Department of Microbiology, Kyoto College of Pharmacy, Kyoto, Japan

Cefroxadine (CGP 9000) is a new orally active cephalosporin developed by Ciba-Geigy (2). This drug, like other cephalosporins such as cephalexin and cefradine, has a broad antibacterial spectrum against both gram-positive and gram-negative organisms. We were interested in the strong antibacterial action of cefroxadine and carried out a study on the mechanism of its activity against *Escherichia coli* in regard to morphology and penicillin-binding proteins (1).

We first studied the effect of cefroxadine on the growth curve of *E. coli* K-12. At an inoculum size of about 10^6 cells per ml, all the cephalosporins studied, that is, cefroxadine, cefradine, and cephalexin, showed bactericidal activity at drug concentrations equal to their MICs. As shown in Fig. 1, however, at an inoculum size of 10^8 cells per ml, a cephalexin concentration of 100 μg/ml was not able to produce any bactericidal action; only a bacteriostatic effect was observed. On the other hand, significant bactericidal activity was seen with 100 μg of cefroxadine per ml, and it was recognized that cefroxadine has excellent bactericidal activity compared with cephalexin and cefradine.

In our second experiment on cefroxadine, the morphological changes of organisms were observed by use of a phase-contrast microscope and a scanning electron microscope. At a concentration of 100 μg/ml, cefroxadine caused spheroplast formation, without the organism undergoing the filamentation process in most strains, and finally caused bacteriolysis. Cephalexin and cephradine caused only elongation with little evidence of bacteriolysis.

In general, the following three factors are presumed to be mainly involved in the antibacterial actions of β-lactam antibiotics against gram-negative organisms: permeability into the outer membrane of the cell wall, stability to β-lactamases, and affinity for penicillin-binding proteins.

To analyze the mechanism of the potent antibacterial action of cefroxadine, we investigated each of these factors. As for permeability into the outer membrane, cefroxadine was inferior to cephalexin. Analysis of the stability to β-lactamases revealed that cefroxadine, like cephalexin, is hydrolyzed. Cefroxadine and CGP 3940 showed higher affinity for penicillin-binding protein 1Bs than cephalexin and cephradine, as shown in Table 1.

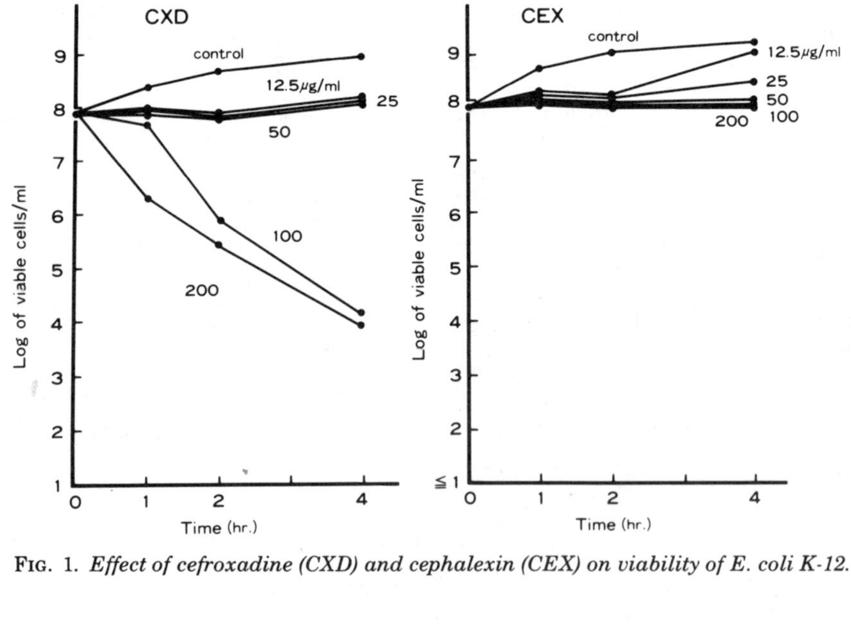

FIG. 1. *Effect of cefroxadine (CXD) and cephalexin (CEX) on viability of E. coli K-12.*

TABLE 1. *Competition of antibiotics with ^{14}C-labeled penicillin G for binding to penicillin-binding proteins (PBPs) in cytoplasmic membranes of E. coli K-12 in vitro.*

PBP	Concentration* of			
	CXD	CED	CEX	CGP-3940
1A	<0.20	0.23	<0.20	<0.20
1Bs	2.9	>25	5.6	2.8
2	4.2	>25	7.9	9.0
3	0.6	0.9	0.52	0.25
4	1.4	2.3	0.68	0.74
5/6	>25	>25	>25	>25

* Concentration, as a molar ratio, of ^{14}C-labeled penicillin G required for 50% inhibition of binding of labeled penicillin G. CXD, Cefroxadine; CED, cefradine; CEX, cephalexin.

From the above evidence, the fact that cefroxadine has strong antibacterial action in spite of the fact that its permeability into the outer membrane is inferior to that of cephalexin can be ascribed partly to its higher affinity for penicillin-binding proteins. The relationship between the strong bacterial activity of cefroxadine and autolysin is noteworthy, and we are currently investigating this.

1. **Spratt, B. G.** 1975. Distinct penicillin binding proteins involved in the division, elongation, and shape of E. coli K-12. Proc. Natl. Acad. Sci. U.S.A. **72**:2999–3003.
2. **Zak, O., W. A. Visher, C. Schenk, W. Tosch, W. Zimmermann, J. Regos, E. R. Suter, F. Kradolfer, and J. Gelzer.** 1976. CGP-9000, a new orally active, broad-spectrum cephalosporin. J. Antibiot. **29**:653–655.

Antibacterial Effects of Cefroxadine and Cephalexin in a Kinetic In Vitro System

PETER SCHNEIDER, WERNER TOSCH,* MAX MAURER, OTO ZAK AND MARIA BÄNZIGER

Research Department, Pharmaceuticals Division, CIBA-GEIGY Limited, Basel, Switzerland

A pharmacokinetic in vitro test system has been devised which permits evaluation of the action of antibiotics at constantly varying concentrations exactly simulating human serum levels. Our system has two advantages over previous models described in the literature in that the drug is continuously added and diluted, but not the bacterial suspension.

The system consists of a reservoir (R) containing the test medium, a compartment (A) containing the antibiotic in the test medium, and a compartment (B) containing the bacteria in the test medium (Fig. 1). A constant flow (F) of the medium from R to A through Teflon tubing is maintained by a pump (Labotron LDP 21) and from A to B by the pressure in flask A. The same flow as from R to A and B is maintained by another pump from B into an overflow (C). Compartment B is surrounded by a water jacket to keep the temperature of the medium constant at 37°C. A magnetic stirrer over the filter (0.45-μm pore size) prevents obstruction of the filter by bacteria. Any biexponential concentration curve can be simulated in the system on the principle of exponential dilution of the drug A, transfer of a constant volume of the diluted drug from A to B, and exponential dilution of the drug in B by the constant flow from B into the overflow. A given plasma profile of an antibiotic in humans can be reproduced in the test system by mathematical transformation of the pharmacokinetic parameters. The slope and intercept of the elimination and absorption curves of the serum concentrations (k_e, E, k_a, A) were determined in a one-compartment model with first-order absorption kinetics. The equations for flow rate, volumes, and doses of the drug in the system are the follows: flow F $= k_e \cdot$volume B $= k_a \cdot$volume A and dose d $= E \cdot$volume B. If vB is arbitrarily fixed at a volume suitable for the capacity of compartment B, flow rate, volume A, and the dose of the drug in A can be determined.

The tests were performed with cefroxadine and cephalexin in DST broth (Oxoid). The data on serum profiles of the antibiotics were taken from Bergan (1) and Hirtz et al. (2). The turbidity of the suspension in compartment B was monitored continuously, and samples were drawn from B at various times for viable cell count. The growth of *Escherichia coli* 205 was inhibited by cefroxadine for more than 2 h longer than by cephalexin after exposure to concentrations corresponding to the plasma concentration-time curve produced by a single oral dose of 250 mg in humans. If the concentrations of cephalexin were increased to levels corresponding to a single oral dose of 500 mg, the antibacterial effects were similar to those of cefroxadine, whether determined turbidimetrically or by viable cell counts (Fig. 2). Replicate experiments with *Staphylococcus aureus* 14 Smith, *Proteus mirabilis* 564 and E30, and *Salmonella typhi-*

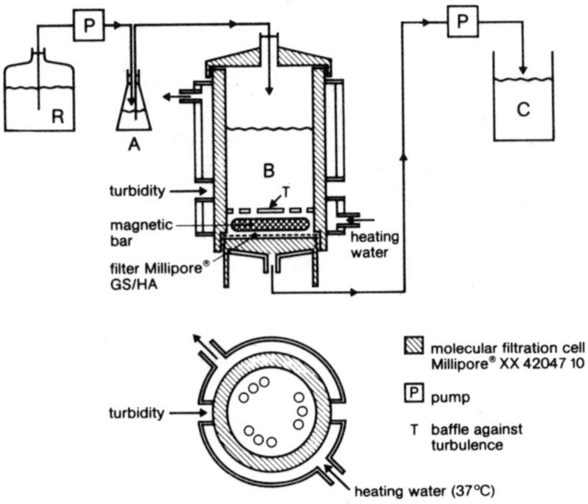

FIG. 1. *Scheme of the kinetic system.*

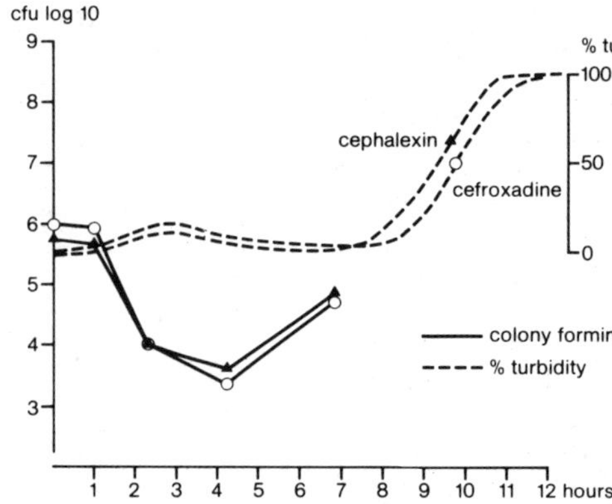

FIG. 2. *Growth kinetics of E. coli 205 after exposure to concentrations corresponding to the plasma concentration-time curves produced by a single oral dose of 250 mg of cefroxadine and 500 mg of cephalexin.*

murium 277 confirmed the equal effectiveness of cefroxadine at concentrations corresponding to those after single oral doses of 250 mg and cephalexin at concentrations twice as high (500 mg).

Additional experiments were performed to investigate the sub-MIC effects of the two drugs. To inactivate the antibiotics, β-lactamase from *Enterobacter cloacae* B99 was added to the bacterial suspensions at the time when the concentrations were not higher than about 1 MIC. A clear-cut sub-MIC effect of cefroxadine was evident from the fact that the viable cell count increased distinctly after the addition of the β-lactamase, but not at all without β-lactamase. No significant sub-MIC effect of cephalexin was found.

Since the MICs of the two drugs were equal for many strains, it can be assumed that they exert similar inhibitory effects at constant concentrations over an incubation period of 18 h. Under dynamic conditions, however, when the concentrations of the drugs decreased below the MIC after a few hours, the effects of cefroxadine were clearly longer lasting, so that cefroxadine seems to be more effective than cephalexin at sub-MIC levels.

1. **Bergan, T.** 1980. Pharmacokinetics of a new cephalosporin CGP 9000 (cefroxadine) in healthy volunteers. Chemotherapy **26:**225–230.
2. **Hirtz, J., J. B. Lecaillon, W. Theobald, and W. A. Vischer.** 1980. Comparative kinetics of CGP 9000 and cephalexin after simultaneous administration in humans, p. 215–217. *In* J. D. Nelson and C. Grassi (ed.), Current chemotherapy and infectious disease. American Society for Microbiology, Washington, D.C.

Evaluation of Cefroxadine in Acute Tonsillitis, Acute Suppurative Otitis Media, and Acute Exacerbation of Chronic Otitis Media: a Comparative Double-Blind Study Versus Cephalexin

S. BABA,* B. SANBE, AND S. KAWAMURA

Nagoya City University, Nagoya, Kanto Teishin Hospital, Juntendo University, Japan*

A double-blind controlled trial of cefroxadine, a new orally active cephalosporin, was undertaken to determine its efficacy and tolerability as compared with cephalexin in the treatment of acute tonsillitis, acute suppurative otitis media, and acute exacerbation of chronic suppurative otitis media.

The patients admitted in the study were adults over 15 years old suffering from one of these infections. The dosage was 250 mg three times per day, totaling 750 mg, for cefroxadine and 250 mg four times per day, totaling 1,000 mg, for cephalexin. The drugs were administered orally for 6 consecutive days. For the cefroxadine group, the dosage schedule was designed to include one placebo as the after-dinner dose, so that the four times per day regimen would be obtained as in the case of cephalexin treatment.

A total of 344 patients, including 174 in the cefroxadine group and 170 in the cephalexin group, were studied; 303 cases, 154 in the cefroxadine group and 149 in the cephalexin group, were evaluated for clinical efficacy (all of the drop-outs were excluded). For evaluation of adverse reactions, a total of 333 cases, including 168 in the cefroxadine group and 165 in the cephalexin group, were admitted. There were no significant biases of distribution between the two drug groups of each disease in regard to the number of patients and various factors of the patient background.

We had two types of efficacy evaluations, one by the attending physicians and the other by the evaluation committee based on uniform criteria (Fig. 1). First, in the evaluations by the committee, for the severity of clinical symptoms, the major symptoms of tonsillitis and otitis media were converted separately into rating scores, and the total scores were used to indicate the severity of each disease. Then the severity before the treatment was compared with that after 3 and 6 days of treatment, and the improvement rate was determined based on the severity after 3 and 6 days. The final overall efficacy for each infection was evaluated with both excellent and good responses defined as effectiveness of the treatment. In acute tonsillitis, cefroxadine was effective in 80.3% of the patients, and cephalexin was effective in 84.8%. In otitis media, cefroxadine was effective in 69.9%, and cephalexin was effective in 68.7%. There were no significant differences in therapeutic efficacy between the two groups in both infections.

Next, the overall efficacy between acute suppurative otitis media and acute exacerbation of chronic otitis media was compared. In acute otitis media, cefroxadine was effective in 75.9% of the cases, and cephalexin was effective in 79.2%. In acute exacerbation of chronic suppurative otitis media, cefroxadine had an efficacy rate of 58.6%, and cephalexin had a rate of 54.3%. No significant differences between the two drug groups was observed in the therapeutic effectiveness in both infections.

The assessments by the attending physicians showed results similar to the committee evaluations. Marked and moderate improvements were defined as improvement. In tonsillitis, the cefroxadine group showed 93.0% improvement, and the cephalexin group had a 95.5% improvement. In otitis media, the former group had 79.5% and the latter group had 78.3%. Again, there were no significant differences between the two drug groups.

As in the case of committee evaluation, the improvement rates in the two different forms of otitis media were not significantly different between the two drug groups. In acute otitis media, the cefroxadine group had 83.3% improvement, and the cephalexin group had 85.4% improvement. In acute exacerbation of chronic otitis media, the former group had 72.4% and the latter group had 68.6% improvement.

Adverse reactions occurred in 4 of 168 patients

1. Severity and scores of main symptoms

1) Tonsillitis

Pharyngalgia	++(3) +(2) ±(1) -(0)
Tonsillar redness	++(3) +(2) ±(1) -(0)
Coating	++(2) + ±(1) -(0)

2) Otitis media

Otalgia	++(2) + ±(1) -(0)
Redness of tympanic membrane	++(3) +(2) ±(1) -(0)
Volume of otorrhea	++(3) +(2) ±(1) -(0)

2. Global severity rate by total scores of main symptoms

+++ : 6 - 8
++ : 3 - 5
\+ : 2 - 1*
± : 1**

1* : . Only pharyngalgia or coating(1)
. Only volume of otorrhea(1)
1**: . Only tonsillar redness(1)
. Only redness of tympanic membrane(1)

4. Improvement rate by global severity rate before and after days 3 and 6

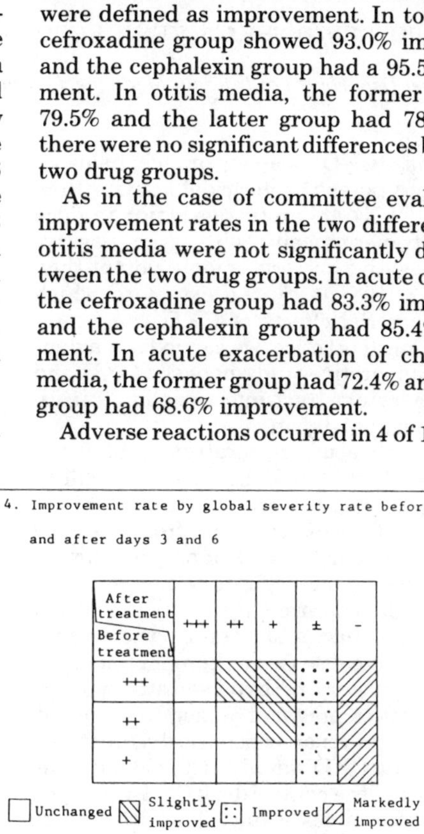

5. Overall efficacy rate by improvement rate at days 6

Excellent : "Markedly improved"(However, the cases of "Markedly improved" at days 6 but "Unchanged" at days 3 should be included in Category "Good".)
Good : "Improved"
Fair : "Slightly improved"
Poor : "Unchanged"

FIG. 1. *Criteria for overall efficacy rate by evaluation committee.*

in the cefroxadine group and 2 of 165 patients in the cephalexin group. All of them were, however, mild forms of gastric disorders, and there was no need to discontinue the treatment. The incidence of adverse reaction was not significantly different between the two drug groups.

The above evidence showed that cefroxadine is effective in the treatment of tonsillitis and otitis media. The notable finding obtained from this trial was that a daily cefroxadine dose of 750 mg was equally as effective as 1,000 mg of cephalexin.

1. **Hondoh, J., S. Baba, and T. Sekiya.** 1980. Laboratory and clinical studies on cefroxadine (CGP-9000) in otorhinolaryngological field. Chemotherapy (Tokyo) **28**(S-28):496–507.
2. **Sambe, B., S. Kawamura, and H. Miyake.** 1980. Experimental and clinical studies of cefroxadine (CGP-9000) in otorhinolaryngological field. Chemotherapy (Tokyo) **28**(S-28):482–495.

Comparative Test of the Effectiveness of Cefroxadine and Cephalexin in Acute Respiratory Tract Infections by Double-Blind Method

FUMIO MIKI, KENZO SHIOTA, KENJI KUBO, MASAKAZU KOHNO, AND KENJI TAKAMATSU

The First Department of Internal Medicine, Osaka City University Medical School, Osaka, Japan

Cefroxadine (CXD) is a new oral cephalosporin with more potent bactericidal activity than cephalexin (CEX). Its protective action in mice infected intraperitoneally with gram-positive and gram-negative bacteria is more potent than that of CEX. To clarify the extent to which these antibacterial effects of CXD can be reflected in clinical practice, we carried out a double-blind comparative study between CXD and CEX in respiratory tract infections in 30 institutions throughout Japan.

Patients with acute respiratory tract infections such as acute bronchitis, acute tonsillitis, and acute pharyngitis were chosen as subjects for the study. Patients excluded from the trial were children under 15 years of age, patients in whom the presence of respiratory tract infection was not initially confirmed, patients previously treated with antibacterial agents, patients with severe underlying diseases or complication, patients with a history of hypersensitivity to β-lactam antibiotics, pregnant or lactating women, and patients with renal or hepatic dysfunction.

The test drug CXD was given at 250 mg three times a day, and the control drug CEX was given at 250 mg four times a day. The drugs were administered orally for 7 days. To make the two therapeutic regimens indistinguishable, one placebo was given as the dose after dinner for CXD.

To evaluate efficacy and tolerability of the drugs, various parameters such as body temperature, cough, sputum volume, dyspnea, chest pain, and sore throat were followed daily. Sputum appearance, chest rales, tonsil swelling, hyperemia, and coating of the throat were examined on the first, third, and seventh days. Symptoms such as loss of appetite, nausea, vomiting, diarrhea, abdominal pain, exanthem, and other remarkable symptoms and signs were also observed. Bacteriological examinations and the laboratory investigations for erythrocyte sedimentation rate, CRP, leukocyte count and differential leukocytes, erythrocyte count, hemoglobin, hematocrit, platelet count, urinary protein, urinary sediment, serum glutamic oxaloacetic and pyruvic transaminase, alkaline phosphatase, serum creatinine, and blood nitrogen were also performed before and after treatment.

A committee comprising nine experienced doctors from eight institutions evaluated the severity of infection and clinical and bacteriological effectiveness. The severity of each infection was determined as marked, moderate, or mild, according to the degree of severity of each symptom. In bronchitis, for example, the severity was determined on the basis of such factors as body temperature, cough, volume of sputum, chest pain, rales, and dyspnea. The clinical effectiveness was evaluated as excellent, good, fair, or poor by the number of days required for each of these symptoms to heal or improve. The assessments for acute tonsillitis and acute pharyngitis were based on the respective criteria for evaluating their severity and therapeutic responses.

A total of 329 patients were treated with either CXD or CEX. The therapeutic efficacy was analyzed statistically on 275 patients (134 on CXD and 141 on CEX) by excluding the following cases: infection unconfirmed, markedly severe underlying disease, and treatment violating the protocol. The 275 patients included acute bronchitis in 165, acute tonsillitis in 67, acute pharyngitis in 34, and pneumonia in 9. Side effects and laboratory abnormalities were also analyzed statistically in 314 patients on whom assessment was possible (154 on CXD and 160 on CEX) (Table 1).

There were no significant biases between the two groups in regard to sex, age, and severity of infection. However, a significant intergroup bias was observed in the type of infections, the CEX group having more patients with acute tonsillitis. Because of the larger number of tonsillitis cases in the CEX group, significant biases were noted in regard to the various symptoms accompanying acute tonsillitis such as tonsil hyperemia, white coating, and purulent plugs. However, there were no differences between the two groups in body temperature, leukocytes, erythrocyte sedimentation rate, CRP, sore throat, swallowing pain, hyperemia of pharynx, tonsil swelling, dyspnea, chest pain, and rales.

The gram-positive organisms isolated as pathogens from 26 patients on CXD and 19 patients on CEX were *Staphylococcus aureus*, *Streptococcus pneumoniae*, and *S. pyogenes*. The gram-negative rods isolated from 8 patients on CXD and 10 on CEX were *Haemophilus influenzae* strains. Polymicrobial infection was observed in 3 patients in each group. In the remaining 207, the causative organisms were not clear.

Table 2 shows the clinical results in the total 275 patients (134 on CXD and 141 on CEX) comprising 165 with acute bronchitis (85 on CXD and 80 on CEX) and 67 with acute tonsillitis (28 on CXD and 39 on CEX) and also 34 with acute pharyngitis (13 on CXD and 21 on CEX). It is noteworthy that, at three-fourths of CEX doses, CXD was comparable to CEX in therapeutic effectiveness.

The intergroup comparison of improvements after 3 and 7 days of treatment was obtained from the rate of patients improved to the total number of patients studied. The patients asymptomatic before and throughout the treatment were excluded from analysis. CEX had a higher improvement rate in sore throat, swallowing pain, and hyperemia of pharynx. For the cough, volume and appearance of sputum, dyspnea, chest pain, and rales, however, CXD proved more effective. The improvement rate for chest pain after 7 days of CXD was significantly higher than that of CEX.

Acute bronchitis was the infection in the largest number of patients, with the smallest intergroup bias in the patient population. As for the improvements in acute bronchitis, the CXD group had a higher improvement rate in all parameters concerning this infection, such as temperature, cough, sputum volume, appearance of sputum, dyspnea, chest pain, and rales. The improvement of chest pain after 7 days was significantly higher with CXD.

Some side effects and laboratory abnormalities were observed in 22 patients on CXD and 27 on CEX. However, no serious reactions developed in either group. Six patients on CXD and 3 patients on CEX were discontinued because of side effects. The incidence rate was not significantly different between the two drugs in terms of both side effects and laboratory abnormalities.

The above comparative study between CXD and CEX in clinical use has shown that the therapeutic effectiveness of 750 mg of CXD daily is comparable to that of 1,000 mg of CEX daily in respiratory tract infections. CXD is thus considered one of the clinically useful drugs for the treatment of acute respiratory tract infections.

TABLE 1. *Distribution of patients*

No. of patients	CXD	CEX
Total	163	166
Followed for side effects	154	160
Included in evaluation	134	141
No. with:		
Acute bronchitis	85	80
Acute tonsillitis	28	39
Acute pharyngitis	13	21
Pneumonia	8	1

TABLE 2. *Clinical effectiveness*[a]

Diagnosis	Drug	Excellent	Good	Fair	Poor	Unclear	Total
Total cases	CXD	19 (14.2)	66 (49.3)	25 (18.7)	21 (15.7)	3	134
	CEX	14 (9.9)	83 (58.9)	23 (16.3)	16 (11.3)	5	141
Acute bronchitis	CXD	14 (16.5)	38 (44.7)	14 (16.5)	16 (18.8)	3	85
	CEX	6 (7.5)	44 (55.0)	13 (16.3)	14 (17.5)	3	80
Acute tonsillitis	CXD	2 (7.1)	17 (60.7)	4 (14.3)	5 (17.9)	0	28
	CEX	5 (12.8)	25 (64.1)	6 (15.4)	2 (5.1)	1	39
Acute pharyngitis	CXD	1 (7.7)	8 (61.5)	4 (30.8)	0	0	13
	CEX	3 (14.3)	13 (61.9)	4 (19.0)	0	1	21

[a] None of the results was statistically significant. Numbers in parentheses are percentages.

1. **Shiota, K., F. Miki, et al.** 1975. Comparative test of the effectiveness of cephradine and cephalexin on pneumonia by double blind method. Chemotherapy (Tokyo) **23:**2525–2545.

2. **Zak, O., W. A. Visher, C. Schenk, W. Tosch, W. Zimmermann, J. Regos, E. R. Suter, F. Kradolfer, and J. Gelzer.** 1976. CGP-9000, a new orally active, broad-spectrum cephalosporin. J. Antibiot. **29:**653–655.

Double-Blind Test of Cefroxadine (CGP 9000) Versus Cephalexin in Acute Skin Infections

NOZOMI NOHARA* AND JIRO ARATA

Department of Dermatology, Okayama University Medical School, Okayama, and Department of Dermatology, Kochi Medical School, Nangoku, Japan*

A multicenter double-blind controlled test of cefroxadine and cephalexin was done. Patients admitted to the study were limited to the following diseases: furuncle, carbuncle, furunculosis, folliculitis (except acne), cellulitis, and lymphangitis. The patients were aged over 12 years or weighed more than 25 kg. The drugs to be administered after meals in the morning and the evening were in white capsules, and those to be administered after meals at noon and at bedtime were in orange-colored capsules. The orange-colored capsules in the cefroxadine group contained a placebo. Both capsules in the cephalexin group contained active drug. Thus, cefroxadine was administered at the dosage of 250 mg two times a day, and cephalexin was administered at the dosage of 250 mg four times a day. Incision and drainage were restricted to the minimum. Combination with other antimicrobial agents or anti-inflammatory drugs was avoided. The patients on the treatment were followed up for symptoms and side effects on the third, fifth, and seventh days. Pain, redness, and edema were the main symptoms checked. No patient was treated longer than 8 days.

The total number of patients was 77 for cefroxadine and 75 for cephalexin. Seven patients in the cefroxadine group and 9 in the cephalexin group were excluded. There were 8 dropouts in the cefroxadine group and 1 in the cephalexin group. Thus, 127 patients, 62 on cefroxadine and 65 on cephalexin, were submitted to clinical evaluation. Side effects were analyzed statistically in 143 patients, 69 on cefroxadine and 74 on cephalexin.

The overall efficacy was evaluated subjectively by attending doctors. Taking into consideration the time needed for marked improvement and the severity of the disease, the attending doctors graded the results as excellent, good, fair, or poor. Patients evaluated as excellent were 28 of 62 (45.2%) in the cefroxadine group and 28 of 65 (43.1%) in the cephalexin group. Total patients evaluated as better than "good" were 90.3% for cefroxadine and 87.7% for cephalexin. The difference between the two drugs was not statistically significant.

Attending doctors also evaluated the degree of improvement on each follow-up observation day as markedly improved, improved, slightly improved, and not changed. We found no statistically significant difference between the two drugs as to any grade of improvement at any evaluation day.

Usefulness was evaluated by attending doctors as excellent, satisfactory, good, dissatisfactory, and very dissatisfactory. Results better than "satisfactory" were obtained in 87.1% of cefroxadine patients and in 83.1% of cephalexin patients. Usefulness was not significantly different between the two drugs.

We standardized the evaluation of the efficacy by totaling the differences of points for pain, redness, and edema, which were calculated by subtracting the grade number at each observation day from the grade number at the first visit. Pain, redness, and edema were graded as 3 at the first visit. An absent symptom was graded as 0. The follow-up grading was done in comparison with the grades at the first visit as follows: no improvement, 3; slightly improved, 2; improved, 1; and disappearance of the symptom, 0. If a symptom was aggravated, the corresponding grade number was marked with a double circle, and on evaluation we subtracted 1 point from the total score. Total scores and the correspond-

TABLE 1. *Total scores for standardized evaluation*

Efficacy	Total scores		
	3 symptoms	2 symptoms	1 symptom
Excellent	9–8	6	3
Good	7–5	5–4	2
Fair	4–2	3–2	1
Poor	1–0	1–0	0

TABLE 2. *Standardized evaluation of efficacy*

Day	Drug	Excellent	Good	Fair	Poor	Total	Statistical test[a]
7	Cefroxadine	35 (57.4%)[b]	24 (96.7%)	2 (100%)	0	61	$X_0^2 = 1.875$
	Cephalexin	37 (56.9%)	22 (90.8%)	5 (98.5%)	1 (100%)	65	$Z_0 = 0.335$
5	Cefroxadine	16 (26.2%)	32 (78.7%)	11 (96.7%)	2 (100%)	61	$X_0^2 = 0.393$
	Cephalexin	19 (29.2%)	35 (83.1%)	10 (98.5%)	1 (100%)	65	$Z_0 = 0.621$
3	Cefroxadine	5 (9.4%)	21 (49.1%)	20 (86.8%)	7 (100%)	53	$X_0^2 = 3.774$
	Cephalexin	7 (12.1%)	32 (67.2%)	15 (93.1%)	4 (100%)	58	$Z_0 = 1.820$

[a] No differences were significant.
[b] Percentages indicate cumulative rate.

ing evaluations are shown in Table 1. The results thus obtained are shown in Table 2. The difference between the two drugs was not statistically significant as to any grade of effectiveness at any evaluation day.

Among the stratified analyses, those cases in which *Staphylococcus aureus* was isolated are important for the present study. In those cases no significant difference was present between the two drug groups by any evaluation method at any evaluation time.

Incidence of side effects was 2 of 69 patients (2.9%) in the cefroxadine group and 8 of 74 patients (10.8%) in the cephalexin group. Side effects were mostly of gastrointestinal origin. Though the incidence was slightly higher in the cephalexin group, this difference was not statistically significant.

The bactericidal activity of cefroxadine was more potent than that of cephalexin. MICs of cefroxadine against clinical isolates of *S. aureus* were slightly lower than those of cephalexin. Tokuda et al. (1) and we (2) showed that in rats and rabbits the skin concentration after oral administration was maintained longer in the cefroxadine group than in the cephalexin group. Our experiments in golden hamsters showed that the effectiveness of an antibiotic against experimentally induced staphylococcal skin infection does not always rise with an increase in frequency of administration. Skin repair activity seems higher than the repair activity of other tissues, and an antibiotic could give a good clinical effect at a lower concentration than the MIC against causative organisms by static action on their growth to help the repair process. Our preliminary open trial (2) showed that cefroxadine was satisfactorily effective against acute skin infections at the dosage of 500 mg in two divided doses a day. On the basis of these facts and considerations, we carried out the present double-blind controlled test. In conclusion, 250 mg of cefroxadine two times a day was considered to be as effective as 250 mg of cephalexin four times a day against acute skin infections. Further studies will be necessary.

1. **Tokuda, Y., H. Shibata, C. Azuma, K. Yumoto, S. Sano, and K. Kimura.** 1980. Basic and clinical studies of cefroxadine (CGP-9000) in the treatment of pyoderma. Chemotherapy (Tokyo) **28**(S-3):515–520.
2. **Yamamoto, Y., H. Akiyama, N. Kashiwa, M. Suwaki, J. Arata, and N. Nohara.** 1980. Cefroxadine in the field of dermatology. Chemotherapy (Tokyo) **28**(S-3): 521–525.

Fundamental and Clinical Studies of Cefotaxime in Pediatrics

TAKASHI MOTOHIRO* AND FUMIO YAMASHITA

Department of Pediatrics, Kurume University School of Medicine, Fukuoka, Japan

Cefotaxime, a newly synthesized cephalosporin, was administered to four children in doses of 25 or 50 mg/kg by intravenous injection. Blood levels, urinary levels and recovery rate, cerebrospinal fluid levels in three patients with meningitis, and pleural drainage fluid levels in one patient with pyothorax were measured. In addition, 36 patients with various infections were administered a mean daily dose of 117 mg/kg for an average of 10 days. Except for one patient each receiving cefotaxime by continuous intravenous (i.v.) drip infusion, i.v. injection three times daily, and i.v. injection six times daily, all others were treated by i.v. injection four times daily.

An analysis of bioassay results by the two-compartment model revealed the following: Cefotaxime, 25 and 50 mg/kg i.v., produced serum concentrations of 81.4 and 143.9 μg/ml after 15 min and half-lives of 1.36 and 0.93 h, respectively. On the other hand, cephalothin, 20 mg/kg i.v., produced a lower serum concentration of 53.5 μg/ml after 15 min and far shorter half-life of 0.31 h.

About 80% of the administered dose of both antibiotics was recovered from the urine in 6 h. The urinary recovery rate was favorable.

In patients with bacterial meningitis, passage into the cerebrospinal fluid was relatively good in the presence of marked signs of inflammation, but poor in cases of mild inflammation or aseptic meningitis. Pleural fluid levels were higher than serum levels, except during one period, and were well maintained.

Among the 36 patients with various infections, cefotaxime was clinically effective in 72%. Among eight cases in which the bacteriological efficacy of cefotaxime was determined, the drug was assessed to be excellent in three, good in one, and poor in four.

As adverse reactions, phlebitis occurred in one patient, abnormal serum glutamic oxalacetic and serum glutamic pyruvic transaminases appeared in one patient, and abnormal lactate dehydrogenase appeared in four patients.

In conclusion, cefotaxime was found to be a highly effective and safe antibiotic. It is hoped that cefotaxime can soon be used in the field of pediatrics.

Pharmacokinetics of Cefotaxime and Desacetyl Cefotaxime in Normal Subjects and Patients with Impaired Renal Function

M. OHKAWA,* I. MOTOI, S. TOKUNAGA, R. SHODA, S. KAWAGUCHI, M. SAWAKI, S. SHIMAMURA, A. OKASHO, S. HIRANO, E. NAKASHITA, K. KURODA, AND S. AWAZU

Department of Urology, School of Medicine, Kanazawa University, Kanazawa, and Department of Biopharmacy, Tokyo College of Pharmacy, Tokyo, Japan*

The pharmacokinetics of cefotaxime was studied in 7 healthy volunteers and 23 patients with various degrees of renal dysfunction. Endogenous creatinine clearance (Ccr) corrected for 1.73 m^2 of body surface area was used as an indicator of renal function. The subjects were divided into five groups according to the severity of renal dysfunction: group 1, seven healthy volunteers with Ccr of 118.2 to 137.2 ml/min; group 2, seven patients with Ccr of 61.3 to 94.7 ml/min; group 3, seven patients with Ccr of 38.8 to 58.7 ml/min; group 4, four patients with Ccr of 12.0 to 29.9 ml/min; and group 5, five hemodialysis patients with Ccr of 0 to 6.8 ml/min.

All subjects were given a single 1-g intramuscular injection of cefotaxime. Blood samples were obtained, in principle, just before and 5, 15, and 30 min and 1, 1.5, 2, 2.5, 6, and 24 h after injection. Urine samples were collected 0 to 2, 2 to 4, 4 to 6, 6 to 8, and 8 to 24 h after injection. All five patients in group 5, treated by periodic hemodialysis, were studied between dialysis sessions. In addition, serum concentrations were determined during hemodialysis in three of the five patients by administering 1 g of cefotaxime. Each hemodialysis session lasted over 6 h.

Serum and urinary concentrations of cefotaxime and desacetyl cefotaxime were determined simultaneously by high-pressure liquid chromatography. The detection limits of cefotaxime and desacetyl cefotaxime were 0.1 μg/ml in serum and 2 μg/ml in urine, respectively. The pharmacokinetic parameters based on a one-compartment open model were calculated by using a maximum-slope method.

Table 1 shows the mean serum concentrations of cefotaxime and desacetyl cefotaxime in each group. Peak serum concentrations of cefotaxime, generally attained 30 min to 1 h after administration, tended to increase in patients with reduced renal function ($P < 0.05$). Peak serum concentrations of desacetyl cefotaxime, attained later than those of cefotaxime, tended to be higher in patients with impaired renal function, showing particularly high values in group 5, consisting of dialysis cases.

The mean 24-h urinary recovery of cefotaxime in group 1, consisting of healthy volunteers, was 52%. Urinary recovery decreased in parallel with reduction in renal function, being 3% in group 5. The mean 24-h urinary recovery of desacetyl cefotaxime was 26% in normal subjects and decreased with reduced renal function, being 9% in dialysis patients.

The pharmacokinetic parameters of the parent compound (cefotaxime) in each group are summarized in Table 2. A significant correlation ($P < 0.0001$) was obtained when the individual

TABLE 1. *Serum concentrations of cefotaxime and desacetyl cefotaxime after a single 1-g intramuscular injection*

Group	Cefotaxime (desacetyl cefotaxime) concn (μg/ml ± SE) at time:								
	5 min	15 min	30 min	1 h	1.5 h	2 h	2.5 h	6 h	24 h
1	11.0 ± 1.2	25.1 ± 2.7	26.3 ± 2.4	17.4 ± 1.6	11.8 ± 1.2	8.4 ± 0.8	5.9 ± 0.5	1.3 ± 0.2	0[a]
	(0)	(0.1 ± 0.1)	(1.4 ± 0.1)	(2.8 ± 0.4)	(3.2 ± 0.4)	(3.2 ± 0.3)	(2.9 ± 0.2)	(0.5 ± 0.2)	(0)
2	10.7 ± 3.0	18.2 ± 5.1	22.6 ± 3.7	23.8 ± 2.8	—[b]	16.2 ± 2.6	11.0 ± 2.1	2.4 ± 0.6	0
	(0)	(0.7 ± 0.5)	(0.4 ± 0.4)	(1.3 ± 0.7)	—	(2.2 ± 0.9)	(1.8 ± 2.2)	(1.3 ± 0.7)	(0)
3	14.2 ± 3.2	26.1 ± 4.1	32.4 ± 4.8	31.5 ± 3.8	—	21.2 ± 2.6	—	4.6 ± 0.5	0
	(3.4 ± 2.1)	(5.2 ± 2.9)	(4.1 ± 1.6)	(5.1 ± 2.0)	(—)	(5.6 ± 1.5)	(—)	(3.7 ± 1.0)	(0)
4	11.8 ± 3.3	28.5 ± 6.9	37.7 ± 7.7	35.1 ± 5.3	—	29.7 ± 4.8	—	8.2 ± 1.5	1.9 ± 0.8
	(5.3 ± 3.2)	(7.7 ± 5.1)	(8.0 ± 5.4)	(6.6 ± 3.8)	(—)	(7.0 ± 3.2)	(—)	(7.5 ± 3.0)	(2.5 ± 2.9)
5	11.8 ± 4.2	21.2 ± 4.7	28.4 ± 3.5	33.0 ± 3.6	—	31.2 ± 3.7	—	10.0 ± 1.8	0.1 ± 0.1
	(3.2 ± 3.2)	(5.6 ± 3.4)	(6.2 ± 3.8)	(6.9 ± 3.8)	(—)	(11.9 ± 4.5)	(—)	(22.0 ± 7.3)	(14.2 ± 5.4)

[a] 0, Below detection limit.
[b] —, Not done.

TABLE 2. *Pharmacokinetic parameters of cefotaxime after a single 1-g intramuscular injection*[a]

Group	Creatinine clearance (ml/min per 1.73 m^2)	Absorption rate constant (h^{-1})	Elimination rate constant (h^{-1})	Half-life (h)	Apparent vol of distribution (% of body wt)	Body clearance (ml/min per 1.73 m^2)	Renal clearance (ml/min per 1.73 m^2)	Area under the serum cn curve (μg.h/ml)
1	126.9 ± 2.7	9.66 ± 2.36	0.811 ± 0.018	0.86 ± 0.02	21.2 ± 3.7	272.8 ± 43.9	164.7 ± 13.3	72.5 ± 15.6
2	82.0 ± 4.8	4.26 ± 1.86	0.568 ± 0.040	1.26 ± 0.09	28.6 ± 4.2	286.3 ± 47.5	181.5 ± 30.2	79.3 ± 18.9
3	46.9 ± 2.8	6.44 ± 2.89	0.436 ± 0.032	1.65 ± 0.13	23.0 ± 1.9	194.3 ± 24.1	51.5 ± 7.7	107.7 ± 12.3
4	21.9 ± 3.7	4.39 ± 1.00	0.303 ± 0.033	2.37 ± 0.25	22.4 ± 5.0	134.9 ± 21.2	27.1 ± 14.5	177.2 ± 43.4
5	4.4 ± 1.9	1.58 ± 0.10	0.300 ± 0.020	2.35 ± 0.15	24.7 ± 2.1	129.8 ± 9.3	7.3 ± 5.6	141.4 ± 16.8

[a] Values are mean ± SE.

elimination rate constant was plotted against Ccr. The curve for individual serum half-life plotted against Ccr was hyperbolic. The mean serum half-life, 0.86 h in normal subjects, was prolonged to 2.35 h in hemodialysis patients. The mean apparent volume of distribution in normal subjects was 21 liters, or 33% (liters/body weight). The renal clearances were corrected for 1.73 m^2 of body surface area. The mean body clearance and renal clearance of cefotaxime in normal subjects were 273 and 165 ml/min, respectively, and decreased with reduced renal function. The results demonstrated significant correlations between the body clearance of cefotaxime and Ccr ($P < 0.001$), the renal clearance of cefotaxime and Ccr ($P < 0.0001$), and the body clearance and the renal clearance ($P < 0.01$). The area under the serum concentration curve of cefotaxime was 73 μg.h/ml in normal subjects. A gentle hyperbolic relation was seen between the area under the serum concentration curve and Ccr. In three dialysis patients, the mean elimination rate constant of cefotaxime was 0.305 h^{-1} when patient was out of hemodialysis and 0.432 h^{-1} during hemodialysis, whereas the mean half-life of cefotaxime was 2.37 h out of hemodialysis and 1.61 h during hemodialysis.

The peak serum concentrations of cefotaxime increased as renal function declined, but the increase was small compared with those of other cephalosporins. The mean half-life of cefotaxime in normal subjects was shorter than that of cefotaxime determined with bioassay by other authors (1, 2). Although the serum half-life of cefotaxime was prolonged with reduction in renal function, even in dialysis cases its prolongation did not exceed 2.4 times that in normal subjects. The prolongation of the half-life of cefotaxime in the present study was small compared with previously reported values for cefotaxime, determined by bioassay, and other cephalosporins.

However, the serum half-life of the drug, including the desacetyl metabolite, in patients with severe renal dysfunction approximated that reported by other investigators. These results suggested that the desacetylation of the drug was chiefly responsible for its pharmacokinetic characteristics. Namely, it was postulated that in cases with renal dysfunction the concentration of the parent compound itself did not rise so high, since part of the cefotaxime retained in the blood owing to delayed renal excretion was gradually metabolized into desacetyl cefotaxime, and as a result the half-life of cefotaxime was not prolonged greatly.

The pharmacokinetic data of cefotaxime in patients with renal insufficiency showed only a slight difference between patients with moderate renal impairment and normal subjects, indicating that dosage modification is probably unncessary in patients with Ccr of more than 30 ml/min. However, dose reduction, prolongation of dosage interval, or both, may be appropriate in patients with severe renal dysfunction to avoid excessive serum concentrations of the drug and its metabolites.

1. **Esmeu, F., J. Guibert, H. C. Rosenkilde, I. Ho, and A. Le Go.** 1980. Pharmacokinetics of cefotaxime in normal human volunteers. J. Antimicrob. Chemother. **6**(Suppl. A):83–92.
2. **Neu, H. C., P. Aswapokee, K. P. Fu, I. Ho, and C. Matthijssen.** 1980. Cefotaxime kinetics after intravenous and intramuscular injection of single and multiple doses. Clin. Pharmacol. Ther. **27**:677–685.

Determination by High-Pressure Liquid Chromatography of Cefotaxime and Desacetyl Cefotaxime Concentrations in Cerebrospinal Fluid of Adults with Bacterial Meningitis

A. KAZMIERCZAK,* H. PORTIER, C. CHANDESRIS, P. POTHIER, AND R. LABIA

Faculté de Médecine, 21033 Dijon, and CNRS-CERCOA, 94320 Thiais, France*

When a new antibiotic shows significant antimicrobial activity, its use in human therapeutics is in relation to its pharmacological properties, which are first investigated on animals and later on human volunteers. In studying antibiotic penetration into human cerebrospinal fluid (CSF), even if there were volunteers the investigation would not be significant because the antibiotic penetration into normal CSF is very low through the noninflamed meninges. Therefore, the only significant investigation concerns human bacterial meningitis. In compliance with medical ethics, we investigated the penetration of cefotaxime into the CSF during bacterial meningitis in eight human adults. In a preliminary study in vitro, we found that cefotaxime and amoxicillin in combination were not antagonistic in their antimicrobial effects on *Neisseria meningitidis*, *Streptococcus pneumoniae*, *Listeria monocytogenes*, *Staphylococcus aureus*, *Escherichia coli*, and *Klebsiella pneumoniae*.

Six adults with bacterial meningitis (*N. meningitidis*, *S. pneumoniae*, and *L. monocytogenes*) were treated with amoxicillin (25 mg/kg intravenously [i.v.] over 0.5 h, every 6 h) and in addition received cefotaxime (25 mg/kg i.v. over 0.5 h) on the 2nd day of the disease; moreover, four of these six patients received the same dosage of cefotaxime on the 4th day. Two other patients (*K. pneumoniae* and *S. aureus* meningitis) were treated and cured with cefotaxime only (25 mg/kg i.v. over 0.5 h, every 6 h).

After injection of cefotaxime, CSF specimens were collected after 2 h (four patients) or 3 h (four patients) for assays and determination of the concentrations of antibiotic by high-pressure liquid chromatography (HPLC).

HPLC was performed by using a Waters Associates liquid chromatograph with a model 6000

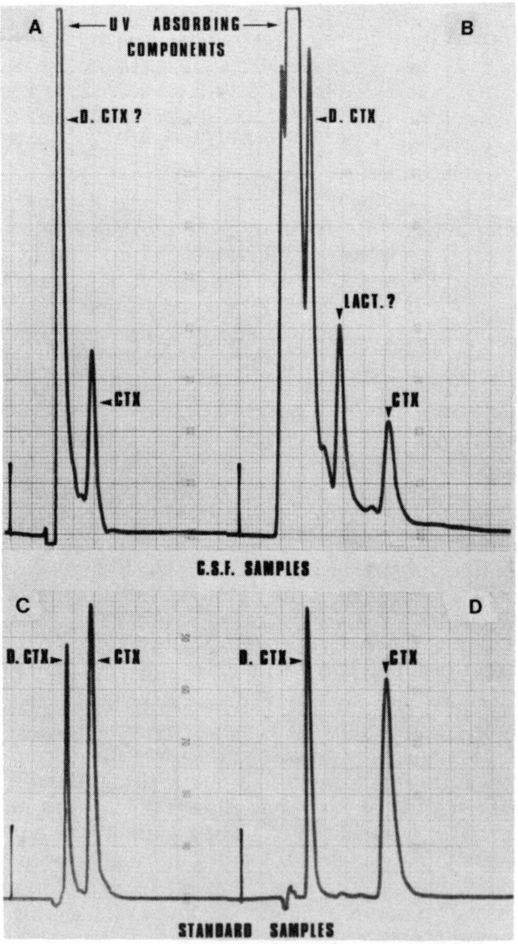

FIG. 1. *HPLC of CSF from patient with bacterial meningitis and treated with cefotaxime (CTX). D. CTX, Desacetyl cefotaxime; LACT, lactone.*

TABLE 1. *Concentrations of cefotaxime (CTX) and desacetyl cefotaxime (D-CTX) in CSF from patients with bacterial meningitis*

CSF collection	Subject		Infecting bacteria	Day 2			Day 4		
	Sex	Age (yr)		CTX (μg/ml)	D-CTX (μg/ml)	Ratio, D-CTX/CTX	CTX (μg/ml)	D-CTX (μg/ml)	Ratio, D-CTX/CTX
2 h after CTX infusion (0.5 h)	M	21	*N. meningitidis*	1.22	0.88	0.72	1.60	0.97	0.60
	M	19	*N meningitidis*	1.38	0.99	0.27	1.0	0.34	0.34
	F	51	?	1.52	10.6	6.9			
	F	55	*L. monocytogenes*	1.60	6.6	4.1	1.04	5.6	5.4
3 h after CTX infusion (0.5 h)	M	31	*S. pneumoniae*	0.40	4.8	12.0	0.5	5.8	11.6
	M	17	*N. meningitidis*	1.15	7.5	6.5			
	M	24	*K. pneumoniae*	4.25	5.75	1.3			
	M	20	*S. aureus*	5.8	12.6	2.2	4.5	11.1	2.4

A pump, a U6K universal injector, and a model 440 UV detector with a 254-nm filter. A Microbondapak C_{18} reverse-phase column (4-mm ID by 30 cm) was used with a guard column (C_{18} Corasil). After some experiments, a solution of acetate buffer (pH 4.8) and methanol in a ratio of 7:3 or 8:2 was adopted as mobile phase, with a flow rate of 1.5 ml/min at a pressure of about 150 bars. Under these experimental conditions, the untreated CSF specimens were injected into the HPLC apparatus. Good separation of cefotaxime was obtained with 30% methanol in the mobile phase (Fig. 1A, 1C). For desacetyl cefotaxime, adequate separation from UV-absorbing components of CSF occurred only with 20% methanol in the mobile phase (Fig. 1B, 1D). As for other metabolites of cefotaxime (1, 2), particularly lactone, we had no corresponding standards to indicate their place in the chromatogram and consequently their concentrations were not calculated. It should be pointed out that the presence of amoxicillin in the CSF specimens did not interfere with the HPLC assay.

Table 1 shows the results of the study. On the 2nd day, the mean levels of cefotaxime were 1.43 μg/ml (range, 1.22 to 1.60 μg/ml) after 2 h and 2.90 μg/ml (range, 0.40 to 5.8 μg/ml) after 3 h; for desacetyl cefotaxime, the mean levels were 4.74 μg/ml (range, 0.88 to 10.5 μg/ml) after 2 h and 7.66 μg/ml (range, 4.8 to 12.6 μg/ml) after 3 h. The findings from CSF specimens collected from five patients on the 2nd and 4th days showed that the ratio of the concentrations (desacetyl cefotaxime to cefotaxime) varied from one patient to another (range, 0.3 to 12.0), but this ratio appeared to remain steady for each patient. Moreover, the concentrations of desacetyl cefotaxime were not in relationship to the number of erythrocytes in the CSF specimens.

In conclusion, the presence of desacetyl cefotaxime in the CSF could result from the blood supply or from an alteration of cefotaxime in situ. In any case, cefotaxime showed high antibacterial activity, including effects against the strains which produce a β-lactamase, and it penetrated into the CSF in sufficient amounts to give therapeutic concentrations allowing the cure of bacterial meningitis.

1. **Reeves, D. S., L. O. White, H. A. Holt, D. Bahari, M. J. Bywater, and R. P. Bax.** 1980. Human metabolism of cefotaxime. J. Antimicrob. Chemother. **6**(Suppl. A): 93–101.
2. **White, L. O., H. A. Holt, D. S. Reeves, M. J. Bywater, and R. P. Bax.** 1980. Separation and assay of cefotaxime (HR-756) and its metabolites in serum, urine, and bile, p. 153–154. *In* J. D. Nelson and C. Grassi (ed.), Current chemotherapy and infectious diseases, vol. 1. American Society for Microbiology, Washington D.C.

Cerebrospinal Penetration of Cefotaxime in Experimental Meningitis

HARRY ROSIN* AND JOSEPH BRUCKERT

Institute for Medical Microbiology and Virology, University of Düsseldorf, D-4000 Düsseldorf, Federal Republic of Germany

Cephalosporins are not considered the preferred drugs for meningitis therapy. The lack of effectiveness of the older cephalosporins may be attributed to irregular penetration into the cerebrospinal fluid (CSF) or failure to penetrate in concentrations needed to inhibit growth of the infecting bacteria. In contrast to this, the very new cephalosporins, in particular cefotaxime

(CTX) and moxalactam, are clearly regarded as suitable for the treatment of meningitis. This recommendation is based on the high antibacterial activity and on the concentrations measured in the CSF, as well as on several therapeutic results. Shah et al. (6), Roos et al. (4), and Brückner et al. (2) published data on CTX concentrations in the CSF of patients. The concentrations varied widely. Armengaud et al. (1) and Morikawa et al. (3) quoted peak levels of CTX in experimental *Staphylococcus* meningitis.

We investigated the penetration of CTX into the CSF by means of our model of experimental meningitis in rabbits. The following points are some of the features of this model. (i) The head of the rabbits is not fixed in a stereotaxic frame, as employed by Sande et al. (5). Continuous anesthesia is avoided. The withdrawal of CSF occurs under a short 10-min anesthesia. (ii) Since CTX is a drug for the treatment of enterobacterial infections, we induced the experimental meningitis with an *Escherichia coli* strain. (iii) According to the conditions as in neonatal meningitis, we favored medium-grade inflammatory reactions of the meninges. (iv) The blood levels of CTX in the test animals were adjusted according to the pharmacokinetics in humans being administered therapeutic doses.

The concentration measurements, made by a standard agar diffusion method, were always carried out directly after the sampling. The *E. coli* test strain employed was very susceptible to CTX, but less susceptible to desacetyl CTX. The influence this desacetyl metabolite might have exerted on our measurements was excluded by examining random samples with a second, desacetyl CTX-nonsusceptible *Proteus morganii* strain.

Figure 1 shows serum and CSF concentrations of CTX after a single administration. By treating the rabbits with probenecid, the pharmacokinetics of CTX in the serum of the animals could be adjusted to the levels found in humans after intravenous injection of 2 g of CTX. The resulting CSF concentrations varied between 0.4 and 10 μg/ml. This spread of concentrations is similar to that found in patients, as mentioned before. Low degrees of infection resulted in low and slowly increasing concentrations in the CSF and vice versa.

A more reliable insight into the penetration of a drug into the CSF can be gained under steady-state conditions. The left side of Fig. 2 shows the results of two series of tests. In each case 11 rabbits received a continuous infusion after a quick initial intravenous injection, resulting in

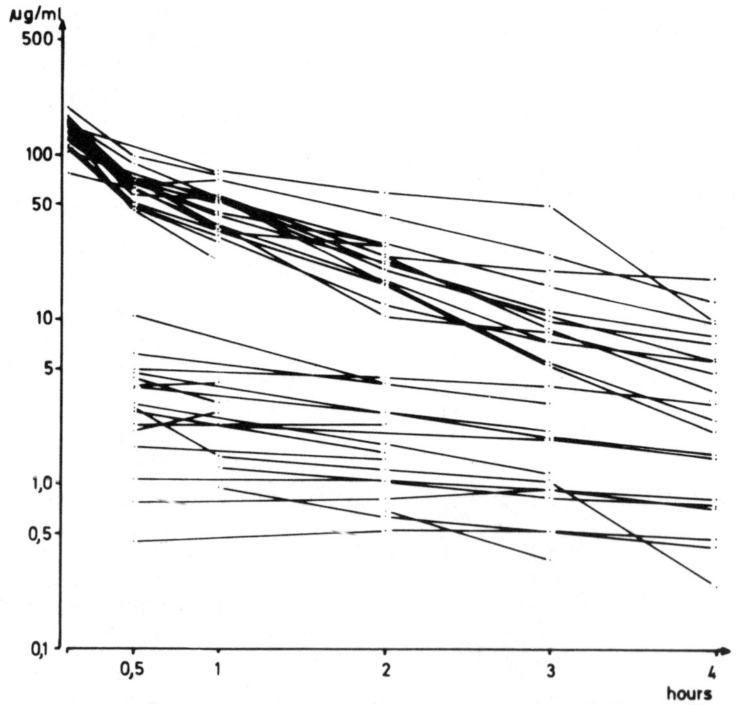

FIG. 1. *Blood levels of cefotaxime, adjusted according to the pharmacokinetics in humans under a 2-g CTX injection, and resulting CSF levels in rabbits with experimental E. coli meningitis.*

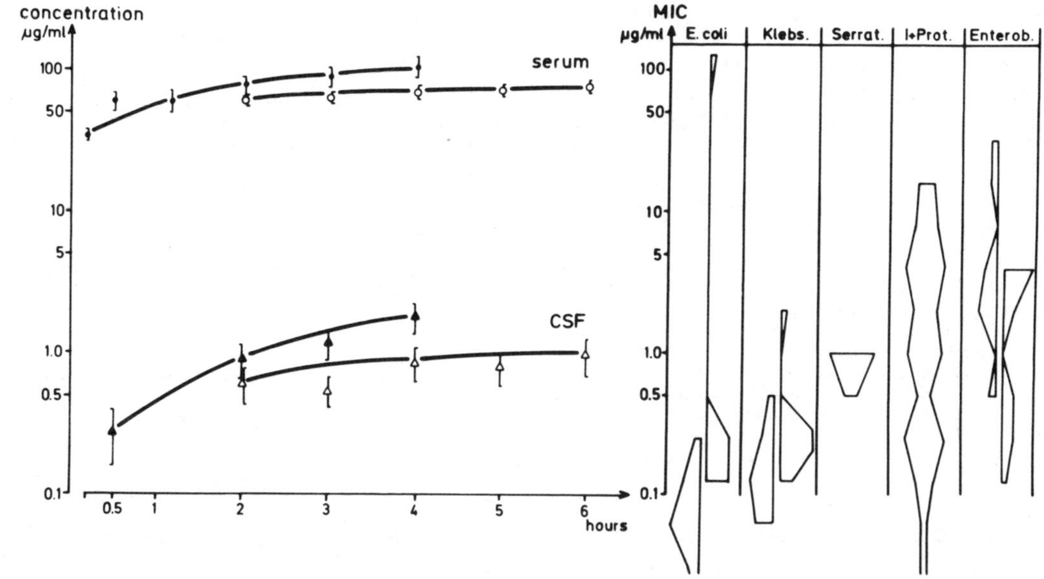

FIG. 2. *Mean concentrations and SD of CTX in blood and CSF during continuous infusion of CTX in rabbits with medium-grade experimental E. coli meningitis, in comparison with the antibacterial activity of CTX.*

serum levels remaining at approximately 50 µg/ml. The dots represent the mean concentrations; the vertical lines, their SD. The degree of infection was comparable to the conditions found in neonatal bacterial meningitis. Mean leukocyte numbers amounted to 2,100 cells per ml; mean protein content was 165 mg/100 ml. The mean CSF levels under these conditions were approximately 1 µg/ml, with a mean penetration rate of 1.7%.

To check the dependence of the drug permeation upon the degree of infection, we correlated the penetration rates with the protein contents of the CSF specimens which we obtained 4 h after continuous infusion. Although this test series consisted mainly of medium-grade infections of the meninges, the correlation coefficient of 0.78 shows reasonably well a dependence of the penetration rate upon the degree of infection. In Fig. 2 the above-mentioned mean concentration curves are compared with the MIC values which we obtained for CTX with *Enterobacteriaceae*. The antibacterial activity was studied according to the broth dilution method following the recommended procedure of the International Collaborative Study. In the broth the bacteria have good growth conditions similar to those in the CSF. The distribution of the MIC values is illustrated in the form of a spindle. Some of the spindles are split. The left half of each spindle includes the MIC values of gentamicin-susceptible and the right half of gentamicin-resistant strains of *E. coli*, *Klebsiella*, and *Enterobacter*, each of which is also a strong β-lactamase producer. Figure 2 shows that even with medium-grade inflammation of the meninges, the CTX concentrations in the CSF would be effective against most of the *E. coli* and *Klebsiella* strains. Also, for the treatment of *Serratia* meningitis, CTX will be very useful. However, CTX will not always be sufficiently effective against indole-positive *Proteus* and *Enterobacter* strains. To this enumeration of bacteria one might add ampicillin-resistant *Haemophilus influenzae* strains which are inhibited by CTX even at 0.01 to 0.03 µg/ml. On the other hand, CTX is not indicated in infections caused by *Pseudomonas*.

Our initial experiences in treating patients with meningitis with CTX correspond with our findings made in the animal investigations. Thus, the following conclusions can be made. (i) The permeation of CTX into the CSF is not extraordinary; rather, it is equivalent to that of other cephalosporins. (ii) Since one can no longer expect to regularly find ampicillin-susceptible *E. coli* when treating meningitis of the newborn infant, we recommend the use of CTX in combination with an aminoglycoside antibiotic for the primary treatment of neonatal meningitis until an antibiogram is available. (iii) The same recommendations can be applied to posttraumatic meningitis caused by gram-negative bacilli. (iv) CTX will be effective in the treatment of meningitis caused by an ampicillin-resistant *Haemophilus* strain in cases in which chloramphenicol cannot be applied. (v) For the treatment of meningitis caused by meningococcus or pneumococcus or by ampicillin-susceptible *Haemophilus* strains, we do not consider CTX indicated.

1. **Armengaud, M., J.-C. Auvergnat, R. Le Net, P. Massip, and Tran Van Tho.** 1979. Des concentrations des antibiotiques dans le LCR au cours des traitements des méningites bactériennes aiguës. Conséquences pratiques. Med. Hyg. **37**:394–400.
2. **Brückner, O., H. Collmann, and H. Hoffmann.** 1980. Concentrations of three β-lactam-antibiotics in human brain abscess fluids and of cefotaxime in CSF of patients with inflamed and uninflamed meninges. International Symposium on New Trends in Antibiotics: Research and Therapy, Milan, 29–31 October.
3. **Morikawa, Y., T. Haruta, and Y. Kobayashi.** 1980. Half-lives of penicillins and cephalosporins in the cerebrospinal fluid of rabbits with staphylococcal meningitis, p. 640–641. *In* J. D. Nelson and C. Grassi (ed.), Current chemotherapy and infectious disease. American Society for Microbiology, Washington, D.C.
4. **Roos, R., W. Marget, H. Trujillo, D. A. Kafetzis, C. J. Papadatos, H. M. v. Hattingberg, B. H. Belohradsky, and K. Bruch.** 1980. Multizentrische Studie über Cefotaxim bei Meningitis und Sepsis im Kindesalter. Klinische Ergebnisse, Serum-Pharmakokinetik und Liquorspiegel. Infection **8**(Suppl. 4):S501–S505.
5. **Sande, M. A., R. J. Sheretz, O. Zak, R. G. Dacey, J. A. Bodine, and L. J. Strausbaugh.** 1978. Factors influencing the penetration of antimicrobial agents into the cerebrospinal fluid of experimental animals. Scand. J. Infect. Dis. Suppl. **14**:160–163.
6. **Shah, P. M., E. B. Helm, and W. Stille.** 1979. Klinische Erfahrungen mit Cefotaxim, einem neuen Cephalosporin-Derivat. Med. Welt **30**:298–301.

Tissue Concentrations of Cefotaxime During Pacemaker Implantation

B. STECKMEIER,* D. ADAM, A. SCHAUDIG, AND M. ZIMMERMANN

Maria Theresia Hospital, Munich, Federal Republic of Germany

In the literature, wound infection is reported to occur in 0.5 to 13% of pacemaker procedures (3). Infected pacemaker pockets can imply serious complications and lead to sepsis and even death. Some authors demonstrated the benefit of prophylactic antibiotics in controlled prospective randomized studies to diminish infection of pacemaker systems significantly (1). Although most infections are caused by skin microbes such as *Staphylococcus aureus* and *S. epidermidis* (5), a certain number of inflammations are due to hospital-associated gram-negative bacilli, e.g., *Escherichia coli* and *Proteus*. When the subcutaneous fat tissue layer covering the pacemaker is flimsy and the pocket is too small for the generator, ischemia and necrosis of the skin may occur, which can lead to extrusion of the battery with subsequent mixed bacterial colonization. Most of the bacteria cultured from infected generator pockets produce β-lactamases and are resistant to penicillin. Thus, the antibiotic prophylaxis can be effective only when a drug is chosen that is not destroyed by β-lactamases. On the other hand protein binding capacity should be low because exudates of infected tissues tend to have a high concentration of protein that could reduce the activity of the drug at the site of infection. This fact is not always considered when MIC or MBC tests of antibiotics give good results in vitro (4). Moreover the possibility of infection implies the need for a maximal bactericidal activity as the pacemaker is implanted. Whatever agents are used, the dosage regimen must be adjusted to give adequate blood and, most of all, tissue levels; on the other hand, excessive dosage should be avoided to minimize adverse secondary effects.

The goal of this study was to evaluate the concentration of cefotaxime (CTX) in pacemaker pocket tissues in relation to different time intervals after application. For this reason a single intravenous dose of 2 g of CTX was administered to 30 patients in a bolus injection before pacemaker implantation. The generator was implanted subcutaneously in the right prepectoral area; the transvenous electrodes were applied via the cephalic or jugular veins (Fig. 1). Specimens of skin and subcutaneous fat were collected every 15 min after the application of CTX. The samples were freed from visible blood with a dry sterile swab. Serum samples were taken before the administration of CTX and simultaneously with the tissue removal. All samples were immediately frozen at −20°C, and the serum and tissue levels of CTX were determined by a biological assay using the agar diffusion method.

As shown in Fig. 2, the serum concentration of CTX was found to be between 180 and 20 μg/ml in the first time period shortly after the injection until 2.5 h afterward. Later on, serum levels of CTX diminished more slowly and reached minimal values 8 h after administration. The course of CTX concentrations in skin and

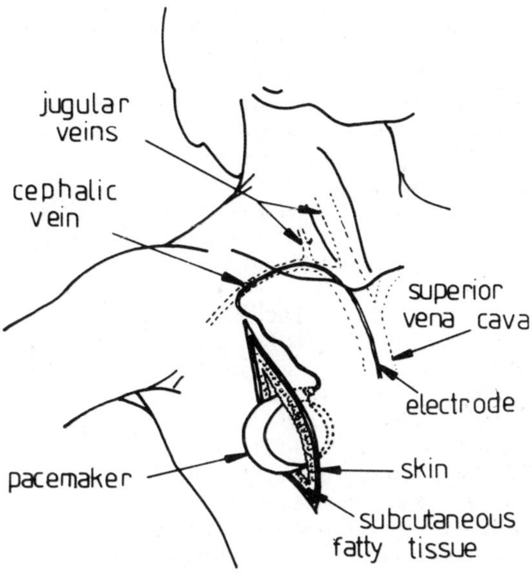

FIG. 1. *Subcutaneous pacemaker implantation in the right prepectoral area.*

subcutaneous fat is also shown in Fig. 2. Peak concentrations of CTX in the skin and fat of pacemaker pockets were measured 30 min after the CTX injection to be 4 and 3.5 μg/g, respectively. After 1 h, the skin and fat levels of CTX had fallen 30 and 50%, respectively; 60 min later, the fat concentration of CTX was equal to zero whereas in the skin CTX could be found up to 3.5 h after administration.

It is well known that foreign material in the human body, such as a pacemaker system, predisposes to infection. Despite great efforts to improve the preoperative procedure and surgical technique, we have not been able to prevent infections. Among 946 permanent transvenous cardiac pacemaker implantations performed at the Maria Theresia Hospital from May 1977 to April 1981, the incidence of infection in our own patients was 0.74%. From clinical (6) and exper-

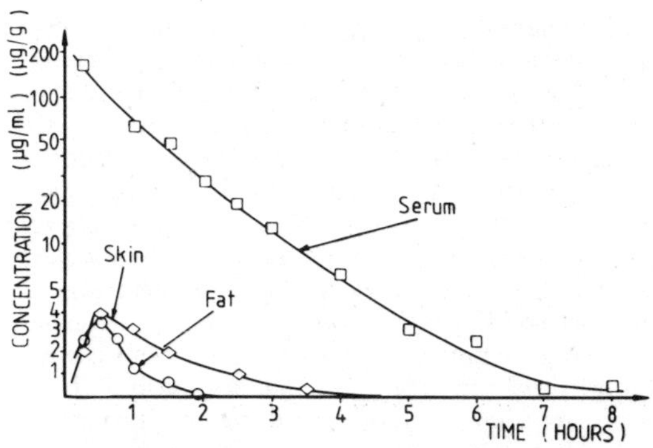

FIG. 2. *Subcutaneous fat (○), skin (◇), and serum (□) concentrations of CTX after a single dose of 2 g.*

imental (2) studies, it seems to be important to start administration of antibiotics preoperatively to reach adequate tissue levels at the time of surgery. Our results suggest that, if CTX is used as a prophylactic agent to prevent infections in pacemaker surgery, it must be administered in a time period between 30 and 60 min before onset of the implantation procedure.

1. **Bluhm, G., B. Jackobsson, I. Inlander, M. Levander-Lindgren, and C. Olin.** 1979. Antibiotic prophylaxis at pacemaker operations. Proceedings of the VIth World Symposium on Cardiac Pacing, Montreal, 2–5 October, chapter 14–7.
2. **Burke, J. F.** 1961. The effective period of preventive antibiotic action in experimental incisions and dermal lesions. Surgery **50**:161–168.
3. **Firor, W. B., J. F. Lopez, E. M. Nanson, and M. Mori.** 1968. Clinical management of the infected pacemaker. Ann. Thorac. Surg. **6**:431–436.
4. **Selwyn, S.** 1978. Microbiological basis for the rational choice of a cephalosporin. Chemother. Antimicrob. **3**: 12–22.
5. **Steckmeier, B., and A. Schaudig.** 1980. Infektionsrisiko bei Herzschrittmacherträgern. Herzmedizin. Z. Kardiol. Klin. Praxis. **4**:178–184.
6. **Stone, H. H., C. A. Hooper, L. D. Kolb, C. E. Geheber, and E. J. Dawkins.** 1976. Antibiotic prophylaxis in gastric, biliary and colonic surgery. Ann. Surg. **184**:443–452.

Placental Transfer of Cefotaxime in Late Pregnancy

EUGÉNIE BERGOGNE-BEREZIN,* JOSIANE PIERRE, JACQUES-HENRI RAVINA, AND DINA VERNANT

Department of Microbiology, and Department of Obstetrics, Bichat Hospital, 75877 Paris Cedex 18, France*

Cephalosporins are usually well accepted for treatment of infections occurring during pregnancy (6). Cefotaxime (CTX), a new semisynthetic cephalosporin with an extended bacterial spectrum and an improved stability against β-lactamases (12), is expected to be effective in treating most obstetrical infections. Knowledge concerning placental transfer of antibiotics remains fragmentary, and very few studies provide information about the passage of drugs through the placenta (5). Preliminary studies did not show either teratogenicity (3) or severe side effects in neonates and children (9), and a recent study (7) showed that cefotaxime produces bactericidal concentrations in fetal tissues and body fluids. Therefore, the objective of our study was to evaluate the transplacental penetration of cefotaxime. We measured the concentrations of the drug achieved in the maternal blood, cord blood, and amniotic fluid at successive times with the view of obtaining data on the rate of placental passage of the drug. Such information can provide a basis for the rational use of cefotaxime in obstetrics.

The study group consisted of 19 women at the end of pregnancy and undergoing a cesarean section; they all voluntarily agreed to participate in the trial and gave informed consent. All received a single intramuscular injection of 1 g of cefotaxime. Maternal blood and amniotic fluid samples were taken 0.5 h before delivery and at delivery time, 1, 2, 3, and 4 h after administration of the drug, in groups I, II, III, and IV, respectively (each group consisting of four or five patients) (Table 1). Umbilical cord blood samples were collected simultaneously at the moment of birth. In all samples the determination of CTX was carried out by means of a microbiological assay procedure (MAP) and a high-pressure liquid chromatography (HPLC) method (method AB 1003 A; the HPLC estimations were carried out at Roussel Laboratories, Swindon, U.K., by Geoffrey Ward) which resolves CTX and its three metabolites: the desacetyl metabolite (DES-CTX) of CTX and two unknown peak (UP_1/UP_2) concentrations (calculated as microgram per milliliter equivalents of DES-CTX).

No detectable concentrations of CTX were measured by either method in maternal blood samples taken as a control before the injection of the drug. In all maternal sera, amniotic fluid, and cord blood samples, measurable amounts of CTX were found by the MAP; although cefotaxime is converted to DES-CTX, data obtained by the MAP can be interpreted as CTX concentrations as a result of the lower susceptibility of the reference strain to DES-CTX. These results were confirmed by HPLC, which provided figures quite similar to those obtained by means of the MAP (Table 1). However, the concentrations of CTX and DES-CTX found in four amniotic fluid samples by HPLC assay were zero. This was contradictory to the MAP, which showed a measurable amount of activity in these samples. The limit of detection for the HPLC assay is 0.5 μg/ml, and there is also a large interfering peak, close to the desacetyl retention time, which occurs in most of the amniotic fluid samples. These two factors make low levels of both CTX and DES-CTX difficult to detect in amniotic fluids, but on the whole there was good agreement between CTX concentrations measured by MAP and HPLC; the difference was not statistically significant for most of the samples. Variable amounts of DES-CTX (Table 1) were measured, varying according to the patients; they did not correlate either with sampling times or with simultaneous concentrations of the parent compound. The unknown peaks (UP_1 and UP_2, now known as M_2 and M_3) were not detected in most of the samples, except for one patient: in samples of maternal blood taken 1.5 and 2 h after administration of the

TABLE 1. *Mean concentrations of cefotaxime in maternal blood, amniotic fluid, and fetal cord blood, measured by two methods*[a]

Sampling time	Maternal blood			Amniotic fluid			Fetal cord blood		
	MAP	HPLC		MAP	HPLC		MAP	HPLC	
		CTX	DES-CTX		CTX	DES-CTX		CTX	DES-CTX
Group I									
0.5 h[b]	11.6 ± 4.6	13.2 ± 6.6	7.7 ± 5.2	0.6 ± 0.6	0.92 ± 1.2	0.46 ± 0.6			
1 h[c]	9.7 ± 3.17	14.3 ± 5.6	9.2 ± 3.5	0.86 ± 0.73	1.1 ± 1.35	0.72 ± 1.05	3.8 ± 1.07	5.5 ± 4.7	4.5 ± 2.9
Group II									
1.5 h	8.0 ± 0.9	9.35 ± 5.9	10.9 ± 6.1	0.98 ± 0.8	0.6 ± 0.7	0.75 ± 1.5			
2 h	6.4 ± 3.2	11.0 ± 2.7	8.4 ± 1.7	2.1 ± 1.1	0.4 ± 0.4	2.0 ± 4.0	3.7 ± 0.5	3.0 ± 1.7	5.7 ± 3.4
Group III									
2.5 h	5.6 ± 1.5	5.46 ± 1.9	5.62 ± 1.8	3.0 ± 1.1	1.5 ± 0.2	2.5 ± 0.65			
3 h	4.5 ± 1.1	5.42 ± 2.9	5.3 ± 1.5	3.6 ± 1.7	3.2 ± 2.4	5.9 ± 5.6	3.3 ± 2.5	2.84 ± 1.3	4.5 ± 1.5
Group IV									
3.5 h	3.0 ± 1.1	2.36 ± 0.87	2.84 ± 1.32	2.0 ± 1.1	1.76 ± 0.7	1.32 ± 1.3			
4 h	2.1 ± 1.27	2.24 ± 1.3	1.98 ± 1.6	2.3 ± 1.3	2.2 ± 0.52	2.45 ± 1.3	2.2 ± 0.7	2.52 ± 1.64	3.96 ± 1.9

[a] Mean concentrations (micrograms per milliliter) ± SD are presented.
[b] Samples taken 30 min before delivery.
[c] Samples taken at delivery time.

drug, 1.1 and 1.3 μg of M_2, respectively, and 1.2 and 1.2 μg of M_3, respectively, were measured.

The collection of samples of maternal blood, cord blood, and amniotic fluid at various intervals in the different patients allowed us to follow approximately the kinetics of cefotaxime in the maternal blood and the fetal compartment. The maternal peak serum concentration averaged 11.6 μg/ml 30 min after the injection and the serum concentrations decreased slowly and regularly, remaining detectable (2.1 μg/ml) 4 h after administration. The kinetics of CTX concentrations in maternal blood measured by HPLC paralleled those determined by MAP (Fig. 1). Cord blood levels of CTX averaged 3.8 μg/ml by MAP and 5.5 μg/ml by HPLC, at the first hour, remained stable at the second hour, and decreased extremely slowly until the fourth hour of the trial (Table 1 and Fig. 1). In the amniotic fluid, the concentrations of CTX increased slowly, reaching a peak at the third hour of 3.6 μg/ml measured by MAP and 3.2 μg/ml by HPLC (DES-CTX averaged 5.9 μg/ml at the peak time). The concentrations of CTX measured in the amniotic fluid remained noticeable (2.3 μg/ml) 4 h after administration of the drug and were similar by both methods.

In our study it was noticed that the maternal peak serum concentrations were distinctly lower than those in normal subjects, in whom previous studies (4) showed a peak averaging 22 to 24 μg/ml after 1 g of CTX intramuscularly. These data are in accordance with other studies (2, 8), which indicated that in pregnant women the pharmacokinetic parameters are modified, especially during late pregnancy; alteration in volume of distribution with increase in plasma protein concentrations possibly modifies the protein binding of drugs and an increase in renal plasma flow, glomerular filtration, etc. may occur (10, 11). On the whole, our results showed: a rapid diffusion of CTX into the fetal compartment, with early and worthwhile concentrations in the fetal cord blood; a progressive penetration of the drug in the amniotic fluid and a delayed peak level reached at the third hour, which is an expected result according to previous studies with other cephalosporins (1, 2); variable amounts of DES-CTX which did not correlate with CTX concentrations; and an overall good agreement between the figures obtained by both methods used in the study.

In conclusion, the results of the study showed a significant placental transfer of CTX, achieving therapeutic concentrations likely to be active against pathogenic species responsible for obstetrical infections.

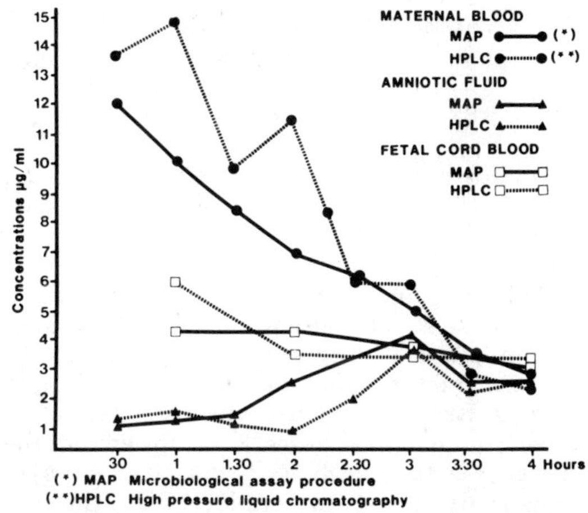

FIG. 1. *CTX kinetics in maternal blood, amniotic fluid, and cord blood: comparison of the results obtained by MAP and HPLC.*

1. **Bergogne-Berezin, E., N. Lambert-Zechovsky, and J. L. Rouvillois.** 1979. Etude du passage transplacentaire des bêta-lactamines. J. Gynecol. Obstet. Biol. Reprod. **8:**359–364.
2. **Bergogne-Berezin, E., J. Pierre, J. L. Rouvillois, and Y. Dumez.** 1980. Placental transfer of cefuroxime, p. 1168–1169. *In* J. D. Nelson and C. Grassi (ed.), Current chemotherapy and infectious disease. American Society for Microbiology, Washington, D.C.
3. **Doerr, B. I., R. Glomot, H. Kief, M. Kramer, and T. Sakaguchi.** 1980. Toxicology of cefotaxime in comparison to other cephalosporins. J. Antimicrob. Chemother. **6:**(Suppl. A):79–82.
4. **Esmieu, F., J. Guibert, H. C. Rosenkilde, I. Ho, and A. Le Go.** 1980. Pharmacokinetics of cefotaxime in normal human volunteers. J. Antimicrob. Chemother. **6:**(Suppl. A):83–92.
5. **Ginsburg, X.** 1971. Placental drug transfer. Annu. Rev. Pharmacol. **11:**387–408.
6. **Hirsch, H. A.** 1971. The use of cephalosporin antibiotics in pregnant women. Postgrad. Med. J. **47**(Suppl.):90–93.
7. **Kafetzis, D. A., C. V. Lazarides, C. A. Siafas, P. A. Georgakopoulos, and C. J. Papadatos.** 1980. Transfer of cefotaxime in human milk and from mother to foetus. J. Antimicrob. Chemother. **6:**(Suppl. A)**:**135–141.
8. **Leng, B. M., J. J. Leng, M. C. Saux, C. de Vedrinne, G. Gouday, J. P. Dubecq, and J. Latrille.** 1978. Etude de l'amoxicilline chez la femme enceinte. Passage transplacentaire et utilisation de cet antibiotique dans les ruptures prématurées des membranes et certaines infections obstétricales. Med. Mal. Infect. **8:**459–467.
9. **Lopez, E. L., N. F. Bonesana, E. Rubeglio, A. Schugurensky, G. Sommersguter, and S. Grinstein.** 1980. Cefotaxime therapy in children with serious infections associated with reduced host defense mechanisms. J. Antimicrob. Chemother. **6:**(Suppl. A)**:**249–253.
10. **Mirkin, B. L.** 1975. Perinatal pharmacology: placental transfer, fetal localization and neonatal disposition of drugs. Anesthesiology **43:**156–170.
11. **Philipson, A.** 1979. Pharmacokinetics of antibiotics in pregnancy and labour. Clin. Pharmacol. **4:**297–309.
12. **Richmond, M. H.** 1980. β-Lactamase stability of cefotaxime. J. Antimicrob. Chemother. **6:**(Suppl. A)**:**13–17.

Combinations of Cefotaxime, Moxalactam, and Cefoperazone with Gentamicin in Strains of *Klebsiella* spp.

CHRISTIAN TAUCHNITZ* AND RUDOLF EZOLD

Evangelisch-Lutherisches Diakonissenhaus and Institut für Medizinische Mikrobiologie der Karl-Marx-Universität, Leipzig, German Democratic Republic*

The introduction of antibacterial drugs for clinical use should raise the question of combination effects if they are used simultaneously with other drugs, especially one of the aminoglycosides. Extensive studies which we have done during more than 12 years (3, 4) showed that the newer β-lactam antibiotics very often act synergistically against susceptible strains if they are combined with an aminoglycoside, very similar to the long-known synergism of penicillin and streptomycin. The latter, for instance, proved to be very important for the successful therapy of streptococcal endocarditis.

Unfortunately, there are no general rules about frequency and intensity of synergism. Therefore, each single combination must be tested individually. The main questions are: Against how many strains of a species does a given combination act synergistically? How many strains show indifference? Are there examples of antagonism? How large is the degree of synergism regarding bacteriostatic and bactericidal activities?

We compared MICs and MBCs of cefotaxime, moxalactam, and cefoperazone, which had been tested singly and in combination with a subinhibitory concentration of gentamicin. Thirty strains of *Klebsiella* spp. were used which had been isolated recently from clinical specimens, especially urine samples. The investigations were done as tube dilution tests. In one row, concentrations of the β-lactam antibiotic varied according to geometric steps of dilution. In parallel, a second row contained the same concentrations in addition to gentamicin, 0.25 mg/liter. MICs and MBCs of gentamicin, determined previously, varied from 0.5 mg/liter to ≥8 mg/ml (MIC: 6 strains, 0.5; 15 strains, 1.0; 4 strains, 2.0; and 5 strains, ≥8 mg/liter, MBC: 4 strains, 0.5; 15 strains, 1.0; 6 strains, 2.0; and 5 strains, ≥8 mg/liter).

Technical details of our modification in combination tests have been described elsewhere (3). The inoculum dose was about 10^5 bacteria/ml. The tubes with the inoculated nutrient broth were stored for 18 h at 37°C. Subcultures were done from all clear tubes on solid media (Endo substrate) for determination of MBC.

The results are summarized in Table 1. The MICs of cefotaxime varied from 0.03 to 0.25 mg/liter; the MBCs varied from 0.06 to 1 mg/liter. Subinhibitory concentrations of the aminoglycoside reduced MICs and MBCs of cefotaxime considerably. Now, MICs varied from 0.0038 to 0.12 mg/liter, and MBCs varied from 0.0075 to 0.25 mg/liter. This correlates with a diminution of 1.73 geometric steps for the MBC and 1.76 steps for the MIC (arithmetic mean). The geometric mean of all the MBCs fell from 0.16 to 0.044 mg/liter, and that of the MICs fell from 0.13 to 0.038 mg/liter. Four strains showed indifference regarding MBC, and five strains showed indifference regarding MIC. The strongest reductions were five steps for MBC and six steps for MIC, one strain each.

For moxalactam, the MICs varied from 0.12 to 1.0 mg/liter, and the MBCs varied from 0.12 to 2 mg/liter. In 24 strains, MICs and MBCs were identical. In four strains the difference was one step; in two strains, it was two steps. Subinhibitory concentrations of gentamicin failed to reduce MICs and MBCs in most of the strains. The geometric mean of MBCs fell from 0.47 to 0.34 mg/liter, and that of MICs fell from 0.4 to 0.31 mg/ml. Eighteen strains showed indifference regarding MBC, and 20 strains showed indifference regarding MIC. Reduction was one geometric step in 10 strains for MBC and in 9 strains for MIC. A difference of two steps was found in two strains only for MBC and in one strain for MIC. This correlates with a reduction of 0.46 steps for MBC and 0.36 for MIC (arithmetic mean) (Table 2).

For cefoperazone, MICs and MBCs ranged from 0.12 to >32 mg/liter. Subinhibitory concentrations of gentamicin reduced MICs and MBCs for the majority of strains. Seven (MIC) and eight (MBC) strains remained resistant, defining 32 mg/liter as the breakpoint of susceptibility. Of the susceptible strains, only three (MBC) or two (MIC) showed indifference; all of the others showed synergism of one or more geometric steps. The reduction in MIC (without the resistant strains) was 1.4 steps; that of MBC was 2.0 steps (arithmetic mean). Including the resistant strains, the geometric mean of MBC fell from 5.27 to 1.82 mg/liter, and that of MIC fell from 3.24 to 1.55 mg/liter, the resistant strains defined

TABLE 1. *MBCs and MICs of cefotaxime, moxalactam, and cefoperazone singly and in combination with gentamicin (0.25 mg/liter) in 30 strains of Klebsiella spp.*

Drug	MIC and MBC with given concn (mg/liter)									Geometric mean
Cefotaxime	0.0038	0.0075	0.015	0.03	0.06	0.12	0.25	0.5	1.0	
Alone										
MBC					5	11	12	1	1	0.16
MIC				1	6	11	12			0.13
+ Gentamicin										
MBC		2	4	6	12	5	1			0.044
MIC	1	3	2	8	10	6				0.038

Drug								Geometric mean
Moxalactam	0.06	0.12	0.25	0.5	1.0	2.0	4.0	
Alone								
MBC		1	12	7	9	1		0.47
MIC		1	15	7	7			0.40
+ Gentamicin								
MBC		5	13	7	4			0.34
MIC		5	14	8	3	1		0.31

Drug												Geometric mean
Cefoperazone	0.06	0.12	0.25	0.5	1.0	2	4	8	16	32	<32	
Alone												
MBC		1		6	5	2	3	1	1		11	5.27
MIC		1		9	8	1			1	2	8	3.24
+ Gentamicin												
MBC	1	1	8	8	1		1	1	1		8	1.82
MIC	1	1	13	3	1		2		1	1	7	1.55

TABLE 2. *Reduction in MBCs and MICs (geometric steps) by subinhibitory concentrations of gentamincin (0.25 mg/liter) in 30 strains of Klebsiella spp.*

Drug Combination	Geometric step							Arithmetic mean
	±0	−1	−2	−3	−4	−5	−6	
Cefotaxime + gentamicin								
MBC	4	7	14	4		1		1.73
MIC	4	7	13	2	2		1	1.76
Moxalactam + gentamicin								
MBC	18	10	2					0.46
MIC	20	9	1					0.36
Cefoperazone + gentamicin								
MBC	3	7	4	3	5			1.53 (2.0)[a]
MIC	2	12	8		1			1.06 (1.39)[b]

[a] Without eight resistant strains (MBC > 32 mg/liter).

[b] Without seven resistant strains (MIC > 32 mg/liter).

as having an MIC at 64 mg/liter. Antagonism was not seen at all.

In comparison with results we obtained by the same method (cefamandole/tobramycin in *Escherichia coli*, *Proteus mirabilis*, and *Klebsiella* spp. [5] and cefotaxime/sisomicin against indole-positive *Proteus* spp. [6], for example), cefotaxime/gentamicin and cefoperazone/gentamicin showed an intermediate synergism against *Klebsiella* spp. Nevertheless, these combinations should be used in clinical chemotherapy, especially in treating bacterial endocarditis, septicemia, or other life-threatening or chronic infections. The reduction in MBCs may be important for eradicating persisters. According to Weinstein (8), combinations of a semisynthetic penicillin and gentamicin, or of cephalothin and gentamicin (or tobramycin), are among those currently in use in the United States for the initial therapy of severe infections. Cefotaxime and gentamicin as well as cefoperazone and gentamicin may be used in the same manner.

Moxalactam, on the other hand, seems to be the first β-lactam antibiotic without a distinct synergism with gentamicin. This combination cannot be recommended, in our opinion, for clinical use, because there is no convincing superiority in vitro. Monotherapy should be preferred considering the costs and side effects of aminoglycosides. This behavior of moxalactam was unexpected and somewhat surprising to us. It may be connected with the chemical structure of moxalactam, which is a cephalosporin-like compound, a 1-oxacephem (7), or 1-oxacephalosporin (2). It should be mentioned that in indole-positive strains of *Proteus* spp. moxalactam did not show synergism with gentamicin (C. Tauchnitz and R. Ezold, unpublished data). Furthermore, investigations are needed to confirm these findings, because Brier et al. (1) found synergistic responses in combinations of moxalactam and tobramycin as well as moxalactam and amikacin.

1. **Brier, G. L., H. R. Black, R. S. Griffith, and J. D. Wolny.** 1980. Synergy of LY 127935 (Shinogi compound 6059-S) with aminoglycoside and β-lactam antibiotics against multiple-antibiotic-resistant gram-negative isolates, p. 62–63. *In* J. D. Nelson and C. Grassi (ed.), Current chemotherapy and infectious disease. American Society for Microbiology, Washington, D.C.
2. **Fu, K. F., and H. C. Neu.** 1980. Comparative β-lactamase resistance and inhibitory activity of 1-oxacephalosporin, cefoxitin, and cefotaxime, p. 73–75. *In* J. D. Nelson and C. Grassi (ed.), Current chemotherapy and infectious disease. American Society for Microbiology, Washington, D.C.
3. **Tauchnitz, C.** 1974. Untersuchungen über synergistische Antibiotikakombinationen. Promotion-B-Schrift, Leipzig.
4. **Tauchnitz, C.** 1980. Rationelle antimikrobielle Chemotherapie. 2. Aufl. J. A. Barth, Leipzig.
5. **Tauchnitz, C., and R. Ezold.** 1978. In-vitro-Untersuchungen zum Synergismus von Cefamandol/Tobramycin. Infection **6**(Suppl. 2):223–225.
6. **Tauchnitz, C., and R. Ezold.** 1980. Synergism of mezlocillin or cefotaxime with sisomicin in strains of indole-positive *Proteus* spp., p. 481–484. *In* J. D. Nelson and C. Grassi (ed.), Current chemotherapy and infectious disease. American Society for Microbiology, Washington, D.C.
7. **Verbist, L.** 1980. Antibacterial activity of 6059-S, a new 1-oxacephem, against clinical isolates of *Enterobacteriaceae* and nonfermenters, p. 65–67. *In* J. D. Nelson and C. Grassi (ed.), Current chemotherapy and infectious disease. American Society for Microbiology, Washington, D.C.
8. **Weinstein, A. J.** 1977. Principles of concomitant antibiotic therapy. Med. J. Aust. Spec. Suppl. **2**:19–22.

Hydrolysis of Cefotaxime and Some Related Cephalosporins

W. DÜRCKHEIMER* AND H. SELIGER

Hoechst AG, Frankfurt/Main, Federal Republic of Germany

Cefotaxime (compound **1**), also known as HR-756, represents the first member of a new generation of injectable cephalosporins, developed in a joint venture by Hoechst AG and Roussel Uclaf (1). It possesses an excellent antibacterial spectrum, especially against *Enterobacteriaceae*, and a high stability against β-lactamases of gram-negative and gram-positive bacteria. These properties are due to a favorable conjunction of a new type of 7-acyl side chain, namely, the 2-aminothiazol-4-yl-2-syn-methoximino-acetyl group, and 7-aminocephalosporanic acid, the same skeleton as in the natural cephalosporin C.

This investigation was undertaken with the hope that a quantitative study of the hydrolysis of cefotaxime (**1**) and some model compounds in alkaline medium would help to answer some questions which have been raised in connection with the surprisingly high antibacterial properties of cefotaxime (**1**).

(i) Has the β-lactam ring in cefotaxime (**1**) higher chemical reactivity than in classical cephalosporins, e.g., cephalothin (compound **4**)? Several investigators have assumed that the biological activity of cephalosporins is related to the chemical reactivity of the β-lactam carbon-nitrogen bond (3).

(ii) Does the *syn* configuration of the methoximino group in the side chain of cefotaxime (**1**) influence the chemical reactivity of the β-lactam ring by steric hindrance?

(iii) Which is the most sensitive site in cefotaxime for nucleophilic attack?

(iv) Can desacetyl cefotaxime (compound **3**) be prepared by direct hydrolysis of cefotaxime (**1**)?

We have followed the alkaline hydrolysis of cefotaxime (**1**) and the model compounds **2**, **3**, and **4**. The anti-isomer (**2**) differs from cefotaxime (**1**) in the configuration of the methoximino group. Desacetyl cefotaxime (**3**) is the main metabolite of cefotaxime (**1**) in humans and other animals (2).

Cephalothin was chosen as a prototype of a 3′-acetoxycephalosporin, which differs from compound **1** only by the 7-acyl side chain.

Previous studies by G. Nebel at Hoechst have already demonstrated that cefotaxime (**1**) possesses optimal stability in water in the pH range 4 to 7. In strong acidic medium desacetyl cefotaxime lactone is formed, whereas in alkaline solution two sites of attack of hydroxide ions have to be envisaged: ester cleavage of the 3′-acetate and the β-lactam opening. The 7-acyl side chain remains intact.

In our study the rate of hydrolysis of compounds **1** to **4** in water in the pH range 9 to 13 was followed at constant pH and 25°C under a

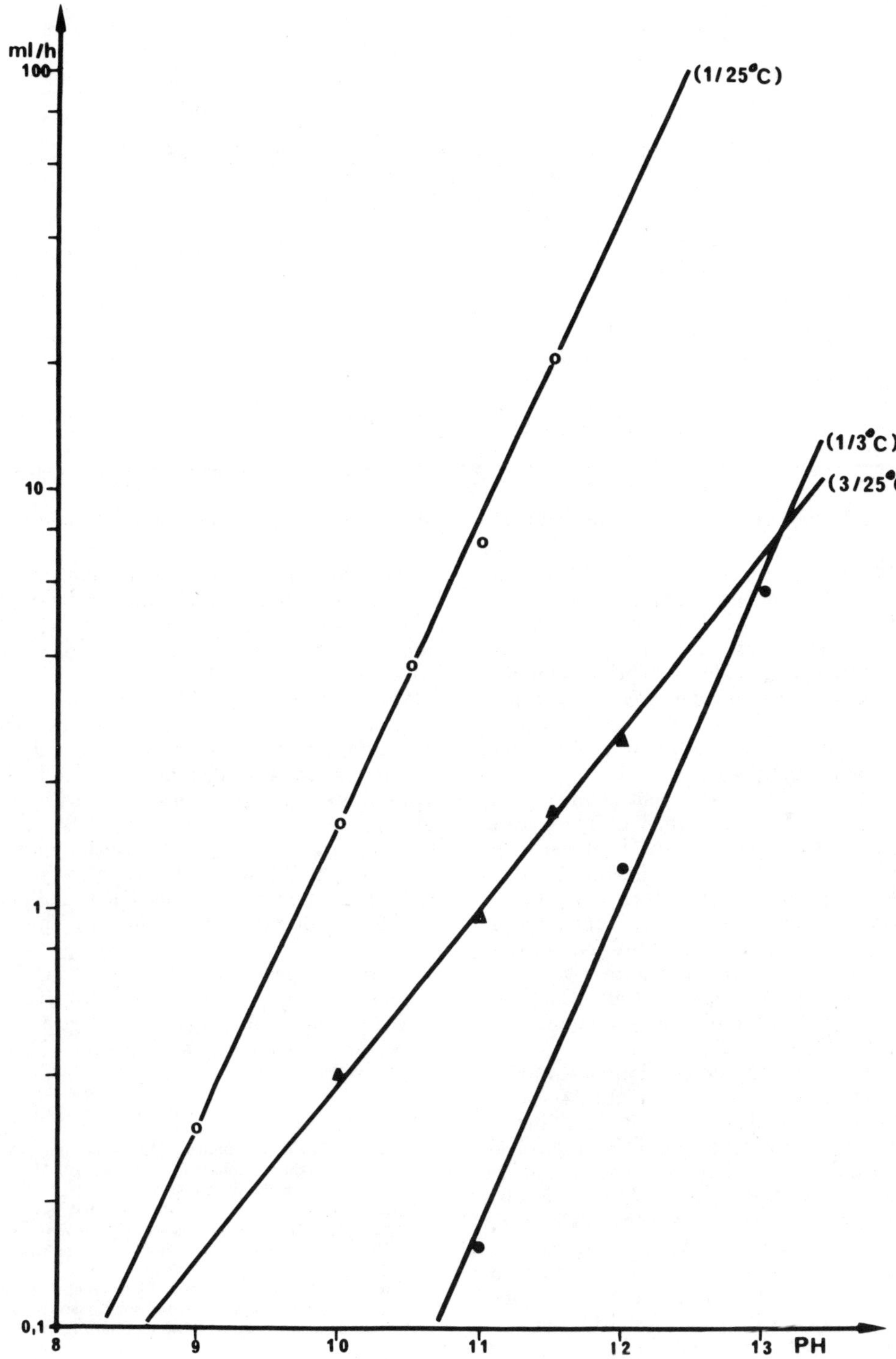

FIG. 1. *Initial rate of hydrolysis of cefotaxime* (**1**) *at 25 and 3°C and of desacetyl cefotaxime* (**3**) *at 25°C as a function of pH.*

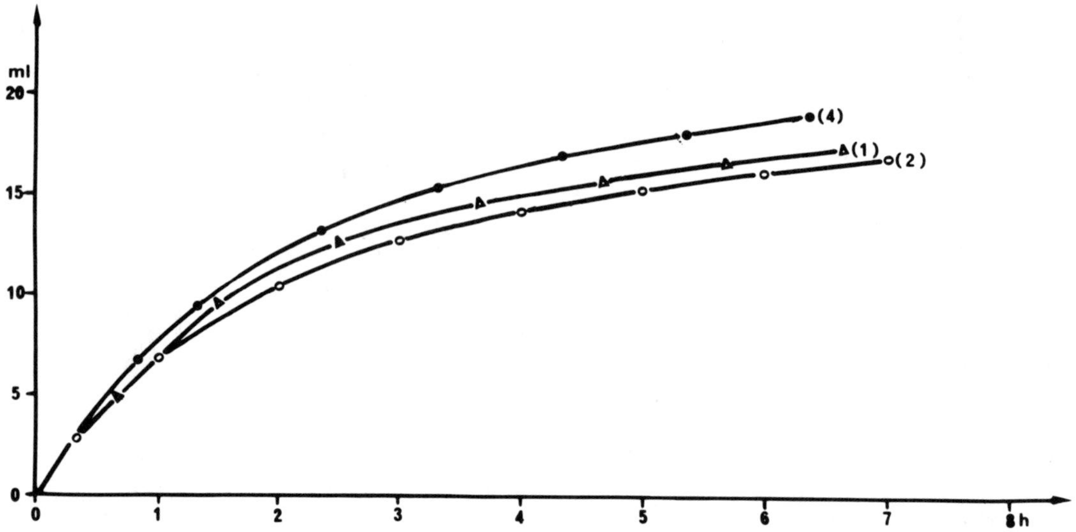

FIG. 2. *Alkaline hydrolysis of cefotaxime* (**1**), *its anti-isomer* (**2**), *and cephalothin* (**4**) *at 25°C and pH 11.*

nitrogen atmosphere; compound **1** was also followed at 3°C. The initial concentration was 1 mmol in 25 ml of water. The pH was controlled by a glass electrode and kept constant by automatic addition of 0.1 N NaOH. The consumption of the base was determined as a function of time. Compounds **1**, **2**, and **4** consume two equivalents and compound **3** consumes one equivalent of base for complete hydrolysis.

The rate of hydrolysis for cefotaxime (**1**) was followed from pH 9 to 11.5 at 25°C. The hydrolysis at pH 9 was very slow, the turnover being about 5% within the first 5 h. The initial hydrolysis rate was proportional to the hydroxide concentration and increased by a factor of 5 per pH unit (Fig. 1). The influence of the temperature on the rate can be estimated from Fig. 1. The rate of hydrolysis of compound **1** at 3°C and pH 11, 12, and 13 was diminished by a factor of 40 compared with that at 25°C.

A comparison of the degradation of cefotaxime (**1**), its anti-isomer (**2**), and cephalothin (**4**) at pH 11 and 25°C is depicted in Fig. 2. The *syn* and anti-isomer gave almost identical hydrolysis curves. This finding supports our view that the α-substituent neither protects nor significantly activates the β-lactam ring by steric or electronic effects. Therefore, it is not surprising that the hydrolysis curve of cephalothin (**4**) (with no α-substituent) and of compound **1** differ only slightly. Cephalothin (**4**) is hydrolyzed 10% faster than cefotaxime at equal pH.

The side chain of cefotaxime seems to play a very specific role in the binding and irreversible acylating step with the target enzymes. These steps cannot be simulated by a chemical model reaction.

Whereas in compound **1** both β-lactam opening and 3′-ester cleavage can take place, the β-lactam fission in compound **3** is the only base-consuming reaction. The initial rate of hydrolysis (milliliters per hour) is shown in Fig. 1 as a function of pH for compound **1** at 25 and 3°C and for compound **3** at 25°C. Both compounds gave straight lines, but the slope for β-lactam hydrolysis (compound **3**) was much smaller than that for cefotaxime (**1**), indicating that in a strong alkaline medium ester cleavage becomes the dominating reaction. This surprising finding led to a simple procedure for the preparation of pure desacetyl cefotaxime (**3**) by treatment of cefotaxime with an excess of aqueous 1 N NaOH (3 to 4 mol) for about 1 hour at 0 to 3°C.

1. **Bucourt, R., D. Bormann, R. Heymes, and M. Perronnet.** 1980. Chemistry of cefotaxime. J. Antimicrob. Chemother. **6**(Suppl. A): 63–67.
2. **Chamberlain J., J. D. Coombes, D. Dell, J. M. Fromson, R. J. Ings, C. M. MacDonald, and J. McEven.** 1980. Metabolism of cefotaxime in animals and man. J. Antimicrob. Chemother. **6**(Suppl. A):69–78.
3. **Yamana, T., and A. Tsuji.** 1976. Comparative stability of cephalosporins in aqueous solutions: kinetics and mechanisms of degradation. J. Pharm. Sci. **65**:1563–1574.

Clearance of Newly Developed Cephalosporins by Artificial Kidneys

S. SIMONIAN,* J. H. MEIJER, W. ALLON, D. M. McLAREN, J. VERHOEF, AND P. L. OE

Free University, Amsterdam, and State University, Utrecht, The Netherlands*

An increasing number of gram-negative bacilli are resistant to many of the currently used antibiotics. Therefore, to date, severe infections need to be treated by potentially toxic antimicrobials such as aminoglycosides. Newly developed cephalosporins such as moxalactam (Lilly), cefotaxime (Roussel), cefsulodin (Ciba-Geigy), ceftazidime (Glaxo), and cefotiam (Ciba-Geigy) offer a potential safe alternative treatment of serious infections because, with the exception of cefsulodin, they all have a very broad antibacterial spectrum and are highly resistant to the β-lactamases of gram-negative bacteria. Some of these cephalosporins (moxalactam, ceftazidime, and cefsulodin) are even highly active against *Pseudomonas aeruginosa*. Cefotaxime, moxalactam, and ceftazidime are also superior to the older cephalosporins in activity against *Haemophilus influenzae*.

Pharmacokinetic data on the newest cephalosporins in patients with terminal renal failure undergoing hemodialysis are limited. Therefore, this study was undertaken to determine the pharmacokinetics of these antibiotics in a short connected artificial kidney circuit in order to predict, from the clearance (Cl) thus obtained, the dosage adjustment factor for patients on hemodialysis.

Human blood was propelled by a roller pump through a hollow fiber dialyzer (Gambro GF 120 L) with a constant flow rate of 200 ml/min. Since uremic patients have a low hematocrit (Ht), the Ht of the blood was adjusted to $\simeq$0.20 by mixing erythrocytes with plasma. The total volume (V_{dis}) of the short connected circuit was about 200 ml. The dialysate had a constant flow of 500 ml/min, and the temperature of the circuit was kept at 37°C. The antibiotics were injected into the venous tubing; plasma concentrations of antibiotics in samples drawn from the venous tubing were determined by a microbiological assay, with *Escherichia coli* as test organism for moxalactam, cefotaxime, and ceftazidime and *Bacillus subtilis* for cefotiam. *P. aeruginosa* was used to assay cefsulodin. The Ht was monitored at regular time intervals. To study the effect of protein binding on the Cl, control experiments were carried out in physiological saline. The Cl of the antibiotic was calculated according to the formula Cl = $V_{dis} \times (1 - \text{Ht}) \times 0.693$/half-life ($t_{1/2}$) in blood. The $t_{1/2}$ was calculated from the washout curves. The Cl was corrected for ultrafiltration. Triplicate experiments were carried out. The pharmacokinetic parameters measured for the studied antibiotics are given in Table 1. The Cl of the antibiotics from blood varied from 21.4 ± 0.7 ml/min for moxalactam to 38 ± 1.8 ml/min for cefsulodin. Differences in Cl may be explained by the degree of protein binding because an appreciable difference between the Cl from blood and that from physiological saline for each antibiotic was found. Furthermore, the Cl from blood tended to be inversely correlated with the extent of protein binding known from the literature. The observed $t_{1/2}$ and Cl for moxalactam in physiological saline differed greatly from those of the other antibiotics. This indicates that, apart from the extent of protein binding, the physicochemical properties of moxalactam influence its Cl from the dialyzer more than those of the other antibiotics.

When it is assumed that the dialyzer is practically the only route of excretion and the antibiotics are metabolically stable, the $t_{1/2}$ of these antibiotics in patients with terminal renal failure may be determined from the observed Cl shown

TABLE 1. *Pharmacokinetic parameters of the newest cephalosporins in the artificial kidney circuit in vitro*

Antibiotic	% Protein binding[a]	$t_{1/2}$ (min)[b]		Cl (ml/min)[b]	
		PS	Blood	PS	Blood
Moxalactam	50.7	4.5 ± 0.2	4.4 ± 0.10	27.3 ± 1.4	21.4 ± 0.7
Cefotiam	40	ND	4.4 ± 0.08	ND	22.4 ± 0.6
Cefotaxime	30–40	2.7 ± 0.3	4.1 ± 0.18	46.0 ± 5	23.2 ± 1.3
Cefsulodin	15–30	2.3 ± 0.3	2.8 ± 0.10	50.6 ± 7	38.0 ± 1.8
Ceftazidime	17	2.4 ± 0.3	3.5 ± 0.17	50.4 ± 7	30.0 ± 1.8

[a] According to the literature (data from the manufacturers for cefotiam and moxalactam [2, 4, 6]).

[b] Means ± SD. $t_{1/2}$ values were calculated from the washout curves, and Cl's were calculated by the formula given in the text. PS, Physiological saline; ND, not done.

TABLE 2. *Theoretical $t_{1/2}$ values and dosage adjustment factors for the newest cephalosporins in patients with terminal renal failure*

Antibiotic	$t_{1/2}$ (h) in normal subjects[a]	$t_{1/2}$ (h) in patients:		$t_{1/2}$ disease/$t_{1/2}$ normals
		Off hemodialysis[a]	On hemodialysis[b]	
Moxalactam	2–2.5	Unk	6.0 (Unknown)	2.4–3
Cefotiam	0.8	8	5.8 (1.5)	See text
Cefotaxime	1.4 ± 0.45	9 ± 6.5	5.5 (2 ± 0.7)	See text
Cefsulodin	1.5	Unk	3.4 (Unknown)	2.3
Ceftazidime	1.8	Unk	4.3 (Unkown)	2.4

[a] According to the literature (1, 2–4, 8).
[b] Calculated (theoretical); the real values according to the literature (2, 7) are given in parentheses.

in Table 1, using the formula mentioned above. The calculated $t_{1/2}$ according to this formula for a fictitious patient weighing 70 kg with a V_{dis} of 20% of the body weight (14 liters) and with an Ht of 0.20 are shown in Table 2. The $t_{1/2}$ values derived from the literature are given also. Since moxalactam, cefatizidime, and cefsulodin are metabolically stable and are excreted almost exclusively via the kidneys (1, 3, 4), the calculated $t_{1/2}$ values in Table 2 may be considered to reflect those determined in patients. The calculated $t_{1/2}$ for cefotaxime deviates widely from the real value in patients. This can be explained by the extensive metabolism and the large V_{dis} (35 liters) of this antibiotic (5). A similar explanation may hold true for cefotiam.

The dosage adjustment factor for patients on dialysis, expressed as the quotient of $t_{1/2}$ in patients with terminal renal failure on hemodialysis and $t_{1/2}$ in subjects with normal renal function, for the first three antibiotics (moxalactam, cefsulodin, and ceftazidime) are also given in Table 2. For cefotaxime and cefotiam, this factor should be calculated from the real $t_{1/2}$ observed in patients and subjects with normal renal function and is 1.4 and 1.9, respectively (data from the literature). Dividing the normal dosage by the appropriate adjustment factor, the dosage for the patients on hemodialysis is obtained. These patients will certainly need smaller doses of the antibiotics when they are off hemodialysis.

Clinical studies are currently under way that might confirm our in vitro findings.

1. **Ahrens, T., W. Vischer, P. Imhof, J. Füllhaas, O. Zak, and F. Kradolfer.** 1979. Human pharmacology of CGP 7174/E (SCE 129) and initial results of clinical trials in Europe. Drugs Exp. Clin. Res. **5:**61–70.
2. **Fillastre, J. P., A. Leroy, G. Humbert, and M. Godin.** 1980. Pharmacokinetics of cefotaxime in subjects with normal and impaired renal function. J. Antimicrob. Chemother. **6**(Suppl. A):103–111.
3. **Kurihara, J., K. Matsumoto, Y. Uzuka, H. Shishido, T. Nagatake, et al.** 1980. Human pharmacokinetics of 6059-S, p. 110–111. *In* J. D. Nelson and C. Grassi (ed.), Current chemotherapy and infectious disease. American Society for Microbiology, Washington, D.C.
4. **O'Callaghan, C. H., P. Acred, P. B. Harper, D. M. Ryan, S. M. Kirby, and S. M. Harding.** 1980. GR 20263, a new broad-spectrum cephalosporin with antipseudomonal activity. Antimicrob. Agents Chemother. **17:**876–883.
5. **Reeves, D. S., L. O. White, H. A. Holt, D. Bahari, M. J. Bywater, and R. P. Bax.** 1980. Human metabolism of cefotaxime. J. Antimicrob. Chemother. **6**(Suppl. A): 93–101.
6. **Tosch, W., F. Kradolfer, E. A. Kanopka, J. Regs, W. Zimmermann, and O. Zak.** 1978. In vitro characterization of CGP 7174/E, a cephalosporin active against *Pseudomonas*, p. 843–844. *In* W. Siegenthaler and R. Lüthy (ed.), American Society for Microbiology, Washington, D.C.
7. **Usuda, Y., O. Sekin, N. Aoki, T. Shimuzu, N. Wakabayashi, S. Hayashi, and K. Watanabe.** 1979. Clinical studies on cefotiam. Chemotherapy (Tokyo) **27**(Suppl. 3):297–303.
8. **Yamamoto, T., I. Kuwahara, Y. Adachi, and N. Yamaguchi.** 1979. Clinical phase I studies on cefotiam. (SCE-963). Chemotherapy (Tokyo) **27**(Suppl. 3):172–180.

Penetration of Cefotaxime into Various Human Tissues During Gallbladder Operations

DIETER ADAM* AND BERND STECKMEIER

Childrens Hospital of the University of Munich and Maria-Theresia Clinic, Munich, Federal Republic of Germany*

Perioperative antibiotic prophylaxis is widely used in gastric and colonic surgery to prevent postoperative bacterial infections. Gallbladder operations can be classified as a type of the so-called "clean-contaminated" operations, in which entry is made into tracts that have an abundant resident flora and minor spillage is difficult to avoid, even with the most scrupulous technique.

The rationale for the use of antimicrobial agents is either to reduce the resident flora before surgery to such a low level that normal host defenses can handle the number of organisms involved in minor spillage without the occurrence of clinically obvious infection, or to have adequate drug levels in tissue at the time of surgery to kill any organisms gaining entry to normally sterile sites. Experimental studies have shown that the antimicrobial agent must be present in the vulnerable tissue at the time of contamination or very shortly afterwards for prophylaxis to be effective (1, 2).

In most cases, the first dose of the antibiotic is administered before the operation is started and subsequent doses are given in intervals of 8 h for the day of operation. Since with clean and clean-contaminated wounds, sterile tissue generally is exposed to contamination only during the surgery itself, adequate tissue levels of the antimicrobial agent probably need to be maintained only for the duration of the operation.

The present study examines the characteristics of the penetration of cefotaxime into various tissues (muscle, fat, fascia, skin, gallbladder) of patients who underwent gallbladder operations and provides data concerning the most appropriate time to administer the drug to ensure adequate intraoperative levels.

A total of 50 patients, 40 females and 10 males, who underwent gallbladder operations were the subjects of this study. Their ages ranged from 30 to 77 years, with a mean of 56 years. The average weight was 67 kg, the range being from 48 to 100 kg. All of the patients who participated in the study had normal clinical and laboratory values. All patients received a single dose of 2 g of cefotaxime by rapid intravenous injection (5 min) at various times between 15 and 110 min before the removal of the materials. Before treating the materials in a Stomacher no. 80 (A. J. Seward & Co., Ltd., London), the tissue samples were freed from visible blood with a dry sterile swab and dipped into a sterile glucose solution. Serum samples were collected before the administration of the antibiotic as control (in no case was antimicrobial activity detectable) and at the time of tissue removal. The centrifuged serum and the tissue samples were stored at −30°C until analyzed. Antibiotic concentrations were determined by the agar diffusion method, using punched holes, with *Escherichia coli* 6311/65 as the test organism. Excess drug concentration due to contamination with blood was found to be 5% of the measured total drug levels in tissue. Correction of this amount of contamination was thought to be insignificant.

At 15 to 20 min after a 2-g i.v. bolus injection of cefotaxime, the mean concentration in serum was about 145 μg/ml, ranging from 123 to 164 (standard deviation ±15.3) μg/ml. At 45 to 50 min after injection, the mean serum concentration was 72.5 μg/ml. At 65 to 70 min after this dose, the serum concentrations ranged from 43.4 to 98.7 μg/ml, with a mean of 64.4 (standard deviation ±18.3) μg/ml. At 85 to 90 min after the 2-g dose, the mean concentration was 38.9 μg/ml. After 105 to 110 min, the mean serum concentrations were 19.6 μg/ml (12.4 to 33.0 μg/ml; standard deviation, ±9.3).

Table 1 shows the corresponding tissue concentrations, where the highest values were found 15 to 20 min after injection in the fascia with 11.5 μg/g. At the same time, the concentrations were 3.8, 2.7, and 0.4 μg/g in the skin, fat, and muscle, respectively. At 65 to 70 min after the injection, the concentrations in the gallbladder reached the maximum value of 8.7 μg/g. At the same time, the concentrations were 3.6, 2.1, and 1.4 μg/g in the fascia, muscle, and fat, respectively. With exception of the gallbladder (5.3 μg/g after 85 to 90 min), the concentrations of cefotaxime in all of the other tissues estimated were very low after 85 to 90 and 105 to 110 min, respectively.

Cefotaxime, a cephalosporin with broad-spectrum activity and low minimum inhibitory concentrations in vitro against most pathogenic gram-positive and gram-negative microorganisms, shows a good diffusibility into different human tissues. The results of this study indicate that the first 2-g i.v. dose of cefotaxime should be administered no more than 15 to 50 min before the operation is started to ensure an adequate antibiotic concentration in the tissues if the reason for the administration is to carry out chemoprophylaxis. To meet this requirement, the antibiotic should be given in the operating room, probably by the anesthesiologist, at the start of the surgical procedure. If the lag time between the entry of the antibiotic into the tissues and the onset of the operation is longer, an intraoperative dose must be given. A prospective double-blind study with cefamandole, done by Stone and co-workers (2), emphasizes the importance of adequate pre- and intraoperative levels of antibiotics in patients who under-

TABLE 1. *Cefotaxime concentrations in different tissues after a 2-g intravenous bolus injection*

Tissue	Concn (μg/g) at following time (min) after administration:				
	15–20	45–50	65–70	85–90	105–110
Skin	3.8	1.6		0.3	
Fat	2.7	2.0	1.4	0.3	0.1
Fascia	11.5	8.6	3.6		2.0
Muscle	0.4	5.4	2.1	0.3	
Gallbladder		5.1	8.7	5.3	0.4

went colon, gastric, and biliary surgery. It was found that the rate of wound infections was about 15% when the drug was administered after the operation or when no antibiotic was given. The infection rate dropped down to 4% when the drug was administered preoperatively.

1. **Burke, J. F.** 1961. The effective period of preventive antibiotic action in experimental incisions and dermal lesions. Surgery **50:**161–168.
2. **Stone, H. H., C. A. Hooper, L. D. Kolb, C. E. Geheber, and E. J. Dawkins.** 1976. Antibiotic prophylaxis in gastric, biliary and colonic surgery. Ann. Surg. **184:**443–452.

Penetration of Cefotaxime into the Human Eye

C. D. QUENTIN* AND R. ANSORG

Ophthalmology and Hygiene Departments, University of Göttingen, Göttingen, Federal Republic of Germany*

Recent studies have demonstrated that different cephalosporins show different rates of penetration into the eye (1). For this reason the present investigation was undertaken to determine the level of cefotaxime in the human aqueous humor.

Fifty-eight patients (aged 18 to 84 years) who were about to undergo routine cataract extraction under local anesthesia were selected for this study. The patients were divided into three groups. In the first group each of 17 patients was given 1.0 g of cefotaxime intravenously; in the second group each of 19 patients received 2.0 g of cefotaxime, whereas 27 patients in a third group received 0.5 g of cefotaxime subconjunctivally. The injections were given at time intervals scheduled to vary from 50 min to 4 h and 40 min. Since all patients received neomycin ointment as a routine procedure the night before surgery, a control group of five patients received no cefotaxime to test the aqueous humor antibacterial activity.

Patients were prepared for surgery with retrobulbar injection of 1% lidocaine, topical application of 0.4% oxybuprocain, and lid block. Just before the cataract operation was begun, the anterior chamber was entered with a 26-gauge needle on a Mantoux syringe and a sample of aqueous humor (0.1 to 0.2 ml) was removed. The chamber was reformed with Ringer solution, and the cataract surgery proceeded in routine fashion. The aqueous sample was stored at −40°C. Simultaneously, venous blood samples were also obtained and spun, and the serum was frozen at −40°C until analysis.

Cefotaxime activity was determined by the agar diffusion test, using Sulfonamid-Sensibilitätstest-Agar (E. Merck, Darmstadt, West Germany) and *Escherichia coli* V6311/65 as the test organism.

The aqueous humor levels after administration of 1.0 g of cefotaxime intravenously averaged 0.83, 1.85, 0.68, 0.67, 0.88, and 0.65 μg/ml after 1, 1.25, 1.5, 1.75, 2, and 2.25 h, respectively. The average serum concentrations were 146, 23, 14, 69.3, 26.6, and 130 μg/ml after 1, 1.25, 1.5, 1.75, 2, and 2.25 h. In the second group, in which the patients received 2.0 g of cefotaxime intravenously, the aqueous humor concentrations averaged 3.25, 3.95, 2.65, 1.78, 1.15, and 0.4 μg/ml after 50 min and 1, 1.25, 1.5, 2, and 3.6 h. The concentration maximum was reached after 1 h, which is 15 min earlier than after the administration of 1.0 g. The average serum concentrations in this group were 125, 122.5, 89, 65, 80, and 4 μg/ml after 50 min and 1, 1.25, 1.5, 2, and 3.6 h. In both groups (i.e., 1.0 and 2.0 g) the concentration peak in the aqueous humor had a delay of 15 to 10 min to the highest concentration found in the serum. The differences of the mean aqueous humor concentrations of the first and second groups were significant: $P < 0.05$ by Student's t test (Fig. 1).

In the third group, in which 0.5 g of cefotaxime was given subconjunctivally, the aqueous humor levels averaged 16.8 μg/ml after 18 min, 62.8 μg/ml after 28 min, and 107 μg/ml after 45 min, until a concentration peak of 482 μg/ml after 1 h was reached. A concentration plateau was then maintained with 363, 460, and 384 μg/ml after 1.75, 2.5, and 4.25 h (Fig. 2). Other than a slight edema of the conjunctiva for the first day, no side effects were noticed. In the aqueous humor of the control group, which received no cefotaxime but only neomycin ointment the night before the operation, no antibacterial activity was found.

This study revealed that significant levels of cefotaxime are achieved in the aqueous humor of the eye after 1.0 and 2.0 g intravenously. The levels obtained are greater than the MIC for the organisms most often responsible for bacterial

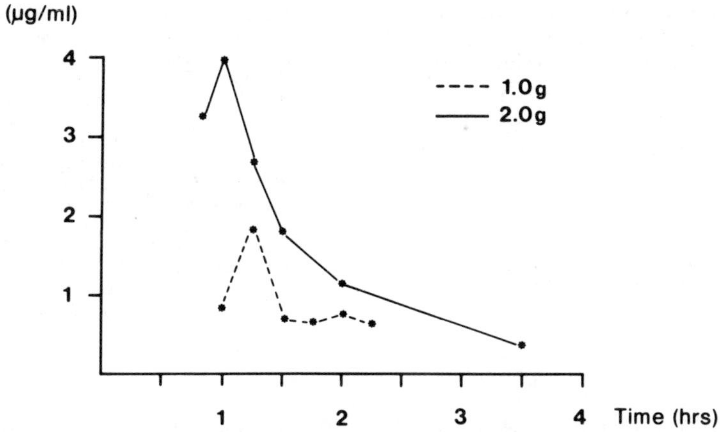

FIG. 1. *Comparison of average concentrations of cefotaxime in aqueous humor after administration of 1.0 and 2.0 g intravenously.*

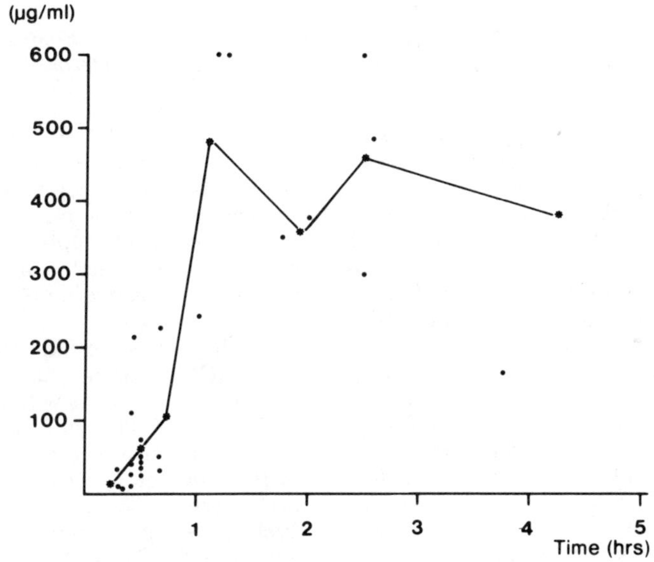

FIG. 2. *Average concentration of cefotaxime in aqueous humor after administration of 0.5 g subconjunctivally.*

endophthalmitis (4), except for *Pseudomonas aeruginosa.* It seems that cefotaxime penetrates the eye tissue more easily and therefore reaches higher levels more quickly in the aqueous humor than do other cephalosporins, but the concentration decrease appears to take place faster (1 , 5). There are no signs of a saturation point for penetration or a threshold at the blood-aqueous barrier, as was reported for cephalexin by Engels et al. (3). Since this study was carried out in uninflamed eyes, it is likely that in the presence of anterior segment inflammation of the eye, the breakdown of the blood-aqueous barrier permits an easier diffusion, probably with higher antibiotic concentrations.

After a subconjunctival injection of 0.5 g of cefotaxime, the concentration found in the aqueous humor was extremely high. At such high levels (above 350 µg/ml), which lasted nearly 5 h, even *P. aeruginosa* would be susceptible to cefotaxime. Compared with cefazolin, which has achieved particular popularity in the treatment of severe intraocular infections, the cefotaxime concentration in the aqueous humor is even higher (2).

Finally, we conclude that cefotaxime concentrations in the aqueous humor after intravenous administration reach the median MICs for most organisms responsible for eye infections, but that with a subconjunctival injection of cefotaxime, the level achieved in the aqueous humor will certainly eradicate even such critical bacteria as *P. aeruginosa*.

1. **Axelrod, J. L., and R. S. Kochman.** 1980. Cefoxitin levels in human aqueous humor. Am. J. Ophthalmol. **90**:388–393.
2. **Barza, M., A. Kane, and J. L. Baum.** 1979. Intraocular levels of cefamandole compared with cefazolin after subconjunctival injection in rabbits. Invest. Ophthalmol. Visual Sci. **18**:250–255.
3. **Engels, T., J. Ehrhorn, and H. Bleckmann.** 1979. Kammerwasser- und Serumkonzentration nach oraler Applikation von Cephalexin und Penicillin V beim Menschen. Graefes Arch. Opthalmol. **209**:249–255.
4. **Forster, R. K.** 1978. Etiology and diagnosis of bacterial postoperative endophthalmitis. Trans. Am. Acad. Ophthalmol. Otolaryngol. **85**:320.
5. **Richards, A. B., A. J. Bron, B. McLendon, M. R. K. Kennedy, and S. R. Walker.** 1979. The intraocular penetration of cefuroxime after parenteral administration. Br. J. Ophthalmol. **63**:687–689.

Comparison of Cefotaxime, Moxalactam, and Ceftriaxone Elimination in Varying Degrees of Renal Dysfunction

PETER WILLS, NOEL WRIGHT,* RICHARD BAX, AND RICHARD WISE

Departments of Medical Microbiology and Medicine, Dudley Road Hospital, Birmingham, B18 7QH, and Roussel Laboratories Limited, Wembley Park, Middlesex, HA9 0NF, U.K.*

Recently, three new cephalosporins have been introduced: cefotaxime, moxalactam, and ceftriaxone. Cefotaxime and ceftriaxone both have the same nucleus, whereas moxalactam has a substituent of a sulfur atom for oxygen in the I position. All three are stable to a variety of β-lactamases and have a broad spectrum of activity, particularly with respect to gram-negative organisms.

One of the more striking differences among these substances is the mode of elimination. Cefotaxime is partly eliminated unchanged in the urine and partly metabolized to a microbiologically active substance, desacetyl cefotaxime (DACM). Moxalactam is mainly eliminated unchanged by the kidneys, whereas ceftriaxone is 60% eliminated by the kidneys and the remainder is eliminated unchanged into bile. The consequent alteration in pharmacokinetics in patients with renal failure was investigated in a series of volunteer studies.

One gram of cefotaxime or 1 g of moxalactam or 0.5 g ceftriaxone was given intravenously as a bolus dose over 3 min to subjects with varying degrees of renal dysfunction. Renal function was assessed by creatinine clearances done before, during, and after the study in each patient. The causes of renal disease were varied, but included glomerulonephritis, hypertension, and pyelonephritis, and were comparable among the different groups. At least 15 subjects were used to study each drug, and selection ensured a wide scatter of renal function. Drug assays were performed by both bioassay and high-pressure liquid chromatography for all three substances, and a good correlation between the different methods was found. A two-compartment model was assumed, and drug half-lives and elimination constants were calculated by the least-squares method. Volumes of distribution were derived from analyses of the α and β phases. In all cases at least five points were used in each regression analysis.

Drug half-lives were less than 3 h for cefotaxime, DACM, and moxalactam and 7.2 h for ceftriaxone in subjects with normal renal function (Table 1). The half-lives became progressively longer with increasing renal dysfunction, but the lengthening as a multiple of half-life in normal subjects was greatest in those antibiotics which were eliminated by renal mechanism alone (i.e., DACM and moxalactam). This was particularly apparent for renal function in the range of 30 to 5 ml/min. The half-lives in subjects with clearances of less than 5 ml/min were extremely variable and less easy to assess.

TABLE 1. *Comparison of cephalosporin half-lives in patients with varying degrees of renal dysfunction*

GFR (ml/min)[a]	Half-life (h)			
	Cefotaxime	DACM	Moxalactam	Ceftriaxone
Normal	1.1	1.6	2.7	7.2
100–30	1.3	2.3	3.2	9.9
29–10	1.9	6.6	11.4	11.5
9–5	2.6	10	16.2	17.9
<5	5.6	18	19.9	46

[a] GFR, Glomerular filtration rate.

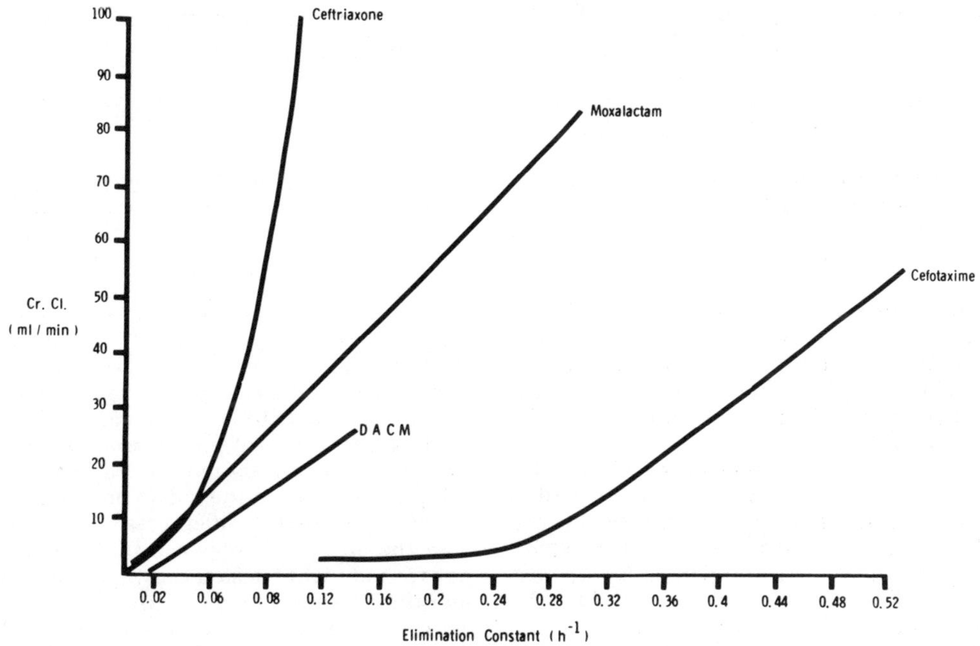

FIG. 1. *Plot of elimination constants against creatine clearance (Cr. Cl.).*

The calculated drug elimination constant was plotted against creatinine clearance (Fig. 1). Moxalactam and DACM showed a linear relationship which passed through the origin. This is compatible with the kidneys being the major route of elimination. The equation, clearance (total) = volume of distribution × elimination constant, becomes clearance (renal) = volume of distribution × elimination constant. The plots for ceftriaxone and cefotaxime were biphasic. The early phase, in which renal function was not seriously impaired, if extrapolated would not pass the origin, whereas the late phase tended to ultimately reach the origin. This could be interpreted as showing that the extrarenal mechanisms of elimination tended to become less effective in extreme renal failure, that is, when the clearances were less than 5 ml/min. The alternative is that the volume of distribution becomes considerably longer. There was little evidence for this on the calculated volumes of distribution from analysis of the α and β phases.

The implications for dosing in patients are clear: if accumulation of drug is to be avoided, then dosing should be reduced or the time interval should be increased when creatinine clearance falls below 30 ml/min for moxalactam. Change in dosing schedules need only occur when the clearance falls below 10 ml for ceftriaxone and 5 ml for cefotaxime. Drug levels are relatively unpredictable for patients with glomerular filtration rates of less than 5 ml/min; hence, in this group adequate drug concentrations, without excessive accumulation, can only be guaranteed if therapy is monitored by measurement of drug levels.

Single and Multiple Doses, Pharmacokinetics, and Bronchial Mucus, Bone, and Prostatic Tissue Levels of Cefotaxime

P. C. BRAGA,* F. SCAGLIONE, G. SCARPAZZA, F. APICELLA, M. GELOSA, V. GAGLIARDI, L. TESSARI, G. PAIOLA, G. BIELLA, AND F. FRASCHINI

Institute of Chemotherapy, Faculty of Medicine, and Department of Orthopaedy, St. Raffaele Hospital, University of Milan, Milan; INRCA Hospital, Castenovo, Como; and Urological Division, Treviglio Hospital, Bergamo, Italy*

Cefotaxime is a new powerful methoxycephalosporin, parenterally administrable, with a broad antimicrobial spectrum. The pharmacokinetic properties of cefotaxime have been determined in several studies, mainly in healthy human volunteers.

In the present study the pharmacokinetic behavior of cefotaxime has been investigated in serum and bronchial mucus after single- and multiple-dose administration (1 g/8 h intramuscularly per 7 days) in a group of patients suffering from acute exacerbation of chronic bronchitis with purulent expectoration.

In the morning of the first treatment day, blood samples were taken immediately before the injection and at 0.25, 0.50, 1, 2, 3, 4, 5, 6, and 8 h after administration. Each patient urinated immediately before drug intake, and all the urine passed thereafter was collected at 2-h intervals during an 8-h period.

Samples of bronchial mucus were collected by expectoration at 1, 2, 3, 4, 6, and 8 h after administration of the drug. The collection of samples was repeated with the same procedure on day 7 of treatment, until 12 h after the last administration.

Serum, urine, and sputum levels of cefotaxime were assayed by the Grove and Randall agar diffusion method, using *Bacillus subtilis* ATCC 6633 as the test organism.

A pharmacokinetic evaluation, based on the serum level data of each patient, was performed according to a first-order, one-comparment open model, using a curve-fitting computer program. For each subject the following parameters were estimated: K_a, K_e, $C_p{}^{\circ}$, $t_{1/2}$ (half-life), AUC (area under the curve), AVD, and Cl_{tot} (total clearance). The same calculations were carried out with bronchial mucus level data.

In a second and third group of volunteer patients, who had to undergo surgery, bone and prostatic levels were determined, using the microbiological method previously described, at progressive times from the last administration (1 g intramuscularly) of cefotaxime in correlation with serum levels.

The semilogarithmic plot of the mean serum and sputum concentrations of cefotaxime against time at days 1 and 7 of treatment is shown in Fig. 1. The decline in serum concentrations, after the peak, appears to be monoexponential at days 1 and 7 of treatment.

The mean values of the pharmacokinetic parameters for serum are reported in Table 1. The comparison between these data on days 1 and 7 showed no statistical differences.

In the study on bronchial mucus levels, we have found higher peak levels than those found by other authors. At day 7 the AUC and $t_{1/2}$ were significantly higher than at day 1. These data suggest that there is an accumulation of cefotaxime in the bronchial mucus. This accumulation could be explained by considering that the patients were treated with mucolitic agents, both to liquefy the dense and viscous bronchial mucus and to obtain more easily the amount of sputum needed to study the drug levels.

The penetration of the antibiotic from serum to sputum can be judged by comparing the AUC of serum with that of mucus. On day 1 this

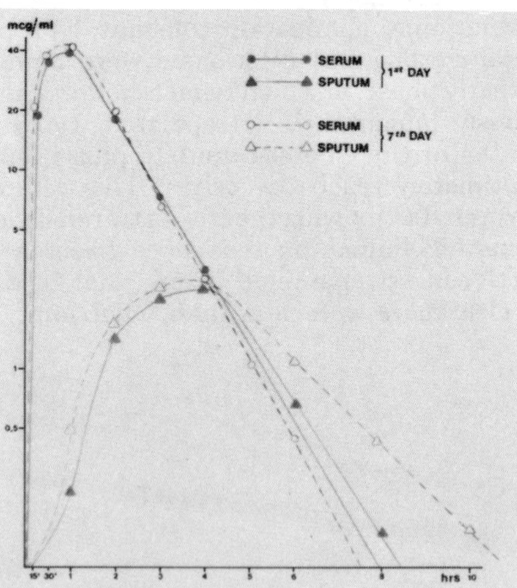

FIG. 1. *Semilogarithmic plot of the mean serum and sputum levels against time on days 1 and 7 of treatment with 1 g of cefotaxime intramuscularly per 8 h.*

TABLE 1. *Serum and sputum pharmacokinetic data for cefotaxime after single and multiple administration of 1 g intramuscularly per 8 h (mean ± SD)*

Parameter	Serum		Sputum	
	Day 1	Day 7	Day 1	Day 7
Peak	39.20 ± 3.25	41.33 ± 2.05	2.71 ± 0.45	3.25 ± 0.56
Time to peak (h)	1	1	4	4
C_p^o	125.21 ± 19.46	127.00 ± 18.71	63.18 ± 41.53	26.44 ± 10.25
K_a	0.95 ± 0.50	0.80 ± 0.44	1.5 ± 0.70	1.72 ± 1.10
K_e	0.99 ± 0.10	0.96 ± 0.09	0.73 ± 0.10	0.51 ± 0.08
$t_{1/2}$	0.70 ± 0.08	0.73 ± 0.07	0.96 ± 0.13	1.40 ± 0.27
AUC	53.42 ± 7.00	56.86 ± 6.29	5.72 ± 0.60	7.99 ± 0.56
AVD	19.28 ± 1.83	18.88 ± 1.77		
Cl_{tot}	18.71 ± 2.30	17.58 ± 2.12		

comparison gave a ratio of penetration of 10.70%, whereas on day 7 the ratio was 14.05%. It is noteworthy that the sputum at day 7 still contained, on average, 0.4 μg/ml 8 h after the 1,000-mg injection. This concentration is, for instance, about 8 to 10 times the MIC for most strains of *Haemophilus influenzae* and *Streptococcus pneumoniae*.

Urine excretion of cefotaxime was rapid, 40 to 45% of the dose being excreted in the first 4 h, whereas totals of 59 and 68%, respectively, were recovered in the urine during 8- and 12-h intervals on days 1 and 7.

The diffusion of cefotaxime in prostatic tissue was, on average, 45% of the corresponding serum level, whereas diffusion in bone was 16.7 and 12.5% of the corresponding serum level for cancellous and cortical bone, respectively.

Comparative Study on the Effectiveness of Cefotaxime and Cefazolin Against Respiratory Tract Infections

K. KOBAYASHI* AND O. KITAMOTO

Department of Internal Medicine, Kyorin University, School of Medicine, Tokyo, Japan

In comparison with the conventional cephalosporin antibiotics, cefotaxime (CTX) possesses a wider spectrum of antibacterial activity. This antibiotic is not only effective against gram-positive bacteria, but also shows particularly potent antibacterial activity against gram-negative organisms. CTX is, moreover, highly stable to the activity of β-lactamases.

In recent years, it has been recognized that gram-negative bacteria are often involved in chronic respiratory tract infections. To evaluate the efficacy and safety of CTX in the treatment of a wide range of such lower respiratory infections, a comparative study was performed using CTX and cefazolin (CEZ). CTX was used in a daily dosage of 2 g, whereas the CEZ dosage was 4 g/day. Both of these antibiotics were administered by intravenous drip infusion, generally for a period of 14 days. The clinical efficacies of these two drugs were then objectively compared. This study was carried out as a collaborative clinical trial at 45 research centers in Japan.

The patients consisted of cases of pneumonia, chronic lower respiratory tract infections, and secondary infections complicated with respiratory diseases. A total of 304 patients (154 in the CTX group and 150 in the CEZ group) were included in the analysis. Pneumonia, 200 cases in total, accounted for 97 of the CTX cases and 103 of the CEZ cases. Of those, 133 cases were diagnosed as bacterial pneumonia (63 in the CTX group and 70 in the CEZ group). There were 104 cases of chronic bronchitis and other diseases (57 in the CTX group and 47 in the CEZ group). There were no particularly significant differences between the CTX and CEZ groups in terms of the background factors.

The efficacy rate for all cases was 69.9% in the CTX group and 64.5% in the CEZ group. For the pnenumonia cases, the efficacy rate was 70.1% in the CTX group and 69.9% in the CEZ group. Against bacterial pneumonia, CTX gave an efficacy rate of 75.9%, whereas CEZ showed a rate of 75.4%. In the nonpneumonia cases, the efficacy rates were 69.6% (CTX) and 53.2% (CEZ).

In the stratified analysis, the efficacy rates

with CTX were significantly superior to those with CEZ in the nonpneumonia cases having no underlying diseases or complications, in all of the severe cases, and in the severe pneumonia cases.

Compared with CEZ, CTX generally brought about greater improvement in terms of the individual symptoms, clinical findings, and laboratory test results. Significant improvement was achieved in five categories in the CTX-treated patients: chest pains after day 3 in all cases and in bacterial pneumonia cases and sputum volume after days 3 and 14 and respiratory difficulty after day 7 in the nonpenumonia cases. In the CEZ-treated patients, significant improvement was recorded in three categories: sputum properties after day 14 in the pneumonia and bacterial pneumonia cases and sputum volume after day 14 in the bacterial pneumonia cases.

Concerning bacteriological effects, CTX showed an elimination rate of 50.0% for 2 strains of gram-positive bacteria and a rate of 80.0% for 31 strains of gram-negative bacteria. The corresponding rates with CEZ were 100% for 3 strains of gram-positive bacteria and 76.7% for 43 strains of gram-negative bacteria. Although replacement of bacteria by *Pseudomonas* was observed in two cases after the administration of CEZ, there were no such cases with CTX.

The incidence of side effects was 3.5% with CTX and 4.1% with CEZ. Abnormal laboratory results were observed at a rate of 24.9% in the CTX group and 23.6% with CEZ. The side effects included rash, elevated transaminase level, etc., and all of them were mild. There were no significant differences between the CTX and CEZ groups with regard to side effects. In addition, for both of the antibiotic administration groups, it was difficult to show clearly that there was a cause-effect relationship between the drug and the elevation in the transaminase level.

Compared with CEZ, CTX showed a higher score in the evaluation of usefulness in the nonpneumonia patients. However, the two antibiotics showed approximately the same scores in relation to the other stratified items. There were no significant differences between the two drug groups in this regard.

The efficacy rates according to the physicians in charge were 78.8% with CTX and 72.8% with CEZ when all of the cases were considered, and this difference was significant. The efficacy rates were 82.2% with CTX and 76.0% with CEZ for the pneumonia cases, 87.9% with CTX and 82.8% with CEZ for the bacterial pneumonia cases, and 73.2% with CTX and 66.0% with CEZ for the nonpneumonia cases.

It may be concluded from these results that, in the treatment of lower respiratory infections, 2 g of CTX per day produced effects which were equal or superior to the effects of 4 g of CEZ per day. In addition, CTX showed an incidence of side effects which was as low as that seen with CEZ. It can be expected that CTX will provide sufficient usefulness for the treatment of lower respiratory infections, especially severe cases.

Cefotaxime and Gentamicin in Empirical Treatment of Neutropenic, Febrile Patients

RODERIC E. WARREN,* ANNE HONG, CATHERINE E. HOGGARTH, JOHN K. H. REES, RODNEY M. SANDLER, DAVID M. SWIRSKY, HELEN V. SYKES, AND FRANK G. J. HAYHOE

Clinical Microbiology Laboratory and Department of Haematological Medicine, Addenbrookes Hospital, Cambridge, U.K. CB2 2QQ*

Cefotaxime's broad spectrum of in vitro activity, including *Pseudomonas aeruginosa* and some organisms resistant to carbenicillin, led us to assess it as an alternative to carbenicillin in empirical therapy of febrile (>38°C twice 4 h apart) patients with blood neutrophil counts of $<10^9$/liter. At the start patients were given gentamicin, 5 mg/kg per day, and either carbenicillin, 300 mg/kg per day, or cefotaxime, 100 mg/kg per day, as determined by opening a sealed envelope, with "first of pair" randomization. Antibiotics were given as 6-h bolus intravenous injections. No other antibacterials were given systemically or by mouth. Patients were not reentered as subsequent episodes if they had received trial antibiotics in the previous 24 h. Normal duration of therapy in the trial was fixed at 5 days. Patients were assessed clinically and by whether temperature was <38°C after 48 h of treatment. Patients who failed to respond at this stage were given all three antibiotics, and course length was extended to 7 days. Patients in the carbenicillin group who had responded to initial therapy, but had isolates from blood culture susceptible to ampicillin, penicillin, or cloxacillin after 48 h, were given one of these antibiotics instead of carbenicillin for a further 3 days.

One hundred episodes in 61 patients were treated. In 41 of these bacteremia was confirmed by blood culture, and an additional 12 localized bacterial infections were confirmed. Two episodes were withdrawn from analysis because of protocol violations, and in two other patients with no previous documented penicillin allergy carbenicillin was withdrawn at 24 h because of rashes.

In the carbenicillin group one death occurred from *Pseudomonas* septicemia, and a further nine patients were considered treatment failures at 48 h. Seven patients were changed to alternative penicillins and 29 continued with the inital regimen. In the cefotaxime group three deaths from septicemic shock occurred in the first 48 h (due to *Klebsiella*, *Klebsiella/Pseudomonas*, and *Escherichia coli*). In 10 patients carbenicillin was added, and in 1 cloxacillin was substituted because of treatment failure at 48 h. Only 1 of 10 cefotaxime treatment failures subsequently responded with carbenicillin, whereas 3 of 8 carbenicillin failures responded with cefotaxime (the ninth dying of mycobacterial infection). Five of 36 cefotaxime patients and 4 of 29 carbenicillin patients assessed as successes at 48 h were subsequently assessed as failures due to relapse or reinfection. Four of the late cefotaxime failures were associated with *Pseudomonas* infection. Late carbenicillin failures included cases of *Klebsiella* and *Acinetobacter* sepsis. Treatment failures in patients on all three drugs were associated with fatal *Clostridium difficile* colitis and *Bacteroides fragilis* septicemia (two cases), *B. fragilis* sepsis, one associated with *Pseudomonas* septicemia (two cases), staphylococcal sepsis, one with *Enterobacter cloacae* (two cases), and colonization with carbenicillin-resistant *Pseudomonas* (one case). In six additional episodes patients with susceptible infections responded only on marrow recovery. Only 12 of 99 treatments ended with neutrophil counts of $>10^9$/liter on stopping antibiotics.

Recurrent infection within 72 h of stopping antibiotics occurred in 3 of 36 of the cefotaxime-treated group but in 10 of 29 of the carbenicillin-treated group. *Acinetobacter* and *Enterobacter/Pseudomonas* septicemias occurred in the former group. The latter group was associated with a wide variety of carbenicillin-resistant gram-negative infections, especially *Klebsiella*. This finding correlates with changes in aerobic gram-negative flora of the throat and feces assessed at 5 days. *Enterobacteriaceae* or pseudomonads were detected in the throats of patients treated with cefotaxime alone in 2 of 36 episodes and in 2 of 17 treated with cefotaxime and carbenicillin. Corresponding figures for feces were 13 of 33 and 6 of 13. In contrast, the carbenicillin-treated group acquired these bacteria in the throat in 9 of 25 episodes assessed, and they were recovered from the feces in 21 of 27 episodes. *Candida* colonization did not apparently differ in the two groups, 60% of whom were receiving polyene antifungal prophylaxis.

Cefotaxime was well tolerated locally. The incidence of plasma potassium, <3 mmol/liter, was the same in the carbenicillin or cefotaxime group but was significantly higher and of greater severity in the group treated with both agents. One patient in the carbenicillin group with *Klebsiella* septicemia had carbenicillin suspended temporarily because of severe hypokalemia. Five patients in the cefotaxime group and one in the carbenicillin group died in acute renal failure. Three of the former patients had abnormal renal function from the outset. In one case the patient was developing amphotericin nephrotoxicity and in another the patient had diabetes mellitus and a coliform urinary infection. It is noteworthy that four of the cefotaxime and carbenicillin patients had *Pseudomonas* septicemia and that multiple predisposing factors were evident in all patients with this complication.

TABLE 1. *Range of MICs for causative organisms*

Organism	MIC (μg/ml)			
	Carbenicillin	Cefotaxime	Desacetyl cefotaxime	Gentamicin
Escherichia coli	2->512 (1)[a]	0.05–0.5	<0.1–2	<1
Klebsiella	64->512	0.05–0.5	<0.1–16 (1)	<1
Pseudomonas	16–64	1 (1)–32	>16	<1–4
Acinetobacter lwoffi	8	2	2	<1
Enterobacter	8–512	0.25–0.5	1	<1
Staphylococcus aureus	0.5 (1)–8	2–4	4–32	<1
Staphylococcus epidermidis	<0.5	1	16	<1
Viridans streptococci	<2	<0.05–05	0.5–2	>8
Fecal streptococci	512	>128	>16	>8

[a] (1), Only one strain showed an MIC of this value.

In 30 patients in each group, without raised plasma creatinine at any stage, antibiotic assays were carried out after 24 h of therapy. Peak and trough gentamicin levels were similar (mean peak, 6.6 mg/liter in the carbenicillin group, 6.9 mg/liter in the cefotaxime group). Mean peak levels (by high-pressure liquid chromatography) of cefotaxime and desacetyl cefotaxime were, respectively, 114 and 24 mg/liter. In 15 of 26 episodes cefotaxime and desacetyl cefotaxime levels immediately before repeat dosage were <5 mg/liter.

Six of seven patients with cefotaxime levels of >25 mg/liter immediately before repeat dosage had, or developed, renal failure or progressive creatinine rise. Although there was no difference in the mean peak cefotaxime level, mean peak desacetyl cefotaxime levels were three times higher in those patients (93 mg/liter) than in the 31 of 32 patients with trough cefotaxime levels of <25 mg/liter, who either never had raised plasma creatinine or whose original creatinine declined.

The MICs for causative pathogens in this study are shown in Table 1, and organisms identified in bacteremias are given in Table 2.

We conclude that the relative merits of choosing cefotaxime or carbenicillin with gentamicin as therapy for febrile neutropenic patients are finely balanced. Cefotaxime use is associated with a lower incidence of immediate recurrent infection if bowel sterilization routines are not used. It can be used to successfully treat some patients who fail to respond at 48 h to carbenicillin therapy, although the opposite rarely seems to be the case. Renal impairment may be commoner in cefotaxime–gentamicin-treated patients. Certainly caution should be exercised in treating patients with bacteremic shock due to *P. aeruginosa*. On a regime of 2 g of cefotaxime q.d.s., serum levels at 6 h after dosage are often inadequate to inhibit this organism in vitro.

TABLE 2. *Bacteremias*

Organism	No. of cases in:	
	Carbenicillin group	Cefotaxime group
Escherichia coli	5	7
Klebsiella	3 (1)[a]	4 (2)
Pseudomonas	2 (1)	5 (2)
Acinetobacter lwoffi	1	
Capnocytophaga		(1)
Staphylococcus aureus	3	2
Staphylococcus epidermidis		1
Viridans streptococci	3	
Fecal streptococci	1	(1)
Clostridium tertium		1

[a] Number in parentheses is number of times occurring as component of polymicrobial bacteremias.

Cefotaxime Therapy of Serious Infections in Hospitalized Patients

T. J. LOUIE,* B. ROBINSON, J. C. PECHERE, M. BERGERON, R. FELD, D. McNEELY, A. RACHLIS, AND S. I. VAS

University of Manitoba, Winnipeg, University of British Columbia, Vancouver, Laval University, Ste. Foy, Quebec, and University of Toronto, Toronto, Ontario, Canada*

Cefotaxime, a new third-generation extended-spectrum cephalosporin, was evaluated in an open nonrandomized trial in the treatment of serious infections in hospitalized patients. Seven university-affiliated medical centers in Canada participated in the trial. All patients were entered on the basis of clinical and laboratory evidence of established infection. Cultures from the infected site, blood cultures, and a biochemical and hematological laboratory profile were obtained before, during, and after therapy. In vitro susceptibilities were performed on aerobic isolates, using the Kirby-Bauer disk diffusion procedure, and MICs were determined by agar dilution, using a Steers replicator.

Three categories of clinical response were assessed: clinical and microbiological cure; improvement—when clinical evidence of infection resolves, but persistence or reappearance of the infecting organism is noted or where the nature of underlying disease obviates a cure; and failure—neither clinical nor microbiological response. Concurrent therapy directed at the same pathogen was termed unevaluable. Patients who were previously treated with other antibiotics were only evaluable if there was clinical and microbiological data to support infection unresponsive to the previous regimen. Microbiological evaluation was based on eradication, persistence, or relapse of the infecting organisms, superinfection with other organisms, or development of antibiotic resistance.

Ninety-nine patients were treated for 101 infections; 2 patients each had 2 infections. Thirty-one urinary tract, 20 lower respiratory tract, 21 soft-tissue, 15 bone, 9 intraabdominal, and 5 miscellaneous infections were treated. Sixty-one males and 38 females were treated; the mean age was 55 years (range, 18 to 94 years).

Of the 31 cases of urinary tract infection, 20 were cases of acute pyelonephritis, 7 were complicated by renal calculi or ureteric obstruction, and 5 were complicated by bacteremia (*Escherichia coli*, *Proteus mirabilis*, and three *Klebsiella pneumoniae*). Infecting organisms included *E. coli* in 6 cases, *Klebsiella* spp. in 6, indole-positive *Proteus* spp. in 3, *P. mirabilis* in 2, *Pseudomonas aeruginosa* in 2, and combined infection with *Citrobacter freundii* and *P. aeruginosa* in 1. All 20 cases responded to treatment; 16 were cured and 4 were classed as improvements because of relapse of the same organism within 30 days of stopping therapy.

The remaining 11 cases of urinary infection included 4 cases of urosepsis associated with obstructive uropathy (*K. pneumoniae* [1], *Serratia marcescens* [2], and *K. pneumoniae* with *Providencia stuartii* [1]), 4 cases of lower tract infection (*P. aeruginosa*, *P. aeruginosa* with *P. stuartii*, *K. pneumoniae*, and *C. freundii* [1 each]), 2 cases of epididymo-orchitis (*E. coli* and *S. liquifaciens*), and 1 case of *E. coli* bacteremia after a transrectal prostatic biopsy. Cure was achieved in the lower tract and epididymo-orchitis cases, in one case of urosepsis, and in the *E. coli* bacteremia secondary to a prostatic biopsy. Two cases of urosepsis were improved, and one was cured but unevaluable because of concurrent tobramycin therapy. Overall, all evaluable cases of urinary tract infection were cured (24) or improved (6).

Of the 20 cases of lower respiratory tract infection, there were 14 cases of pneumonitis, 2 lung abscesses, 1 *Staphylococcus aureus* empyema, and 3 cases that were unevaluable because of the inability to confirm an infective etiology for the pulmonary infiltrate in two patients and diagnosis of fungal infection in one. Of the 14 cases of pneumonitis, 7 were caused by gram-negative bacilli, including 2 *E. coli* and 5 *Klebsiella-Enterobacter* species; there were 4 cases of aspiration pneumonitis, one of which was complicated by an anaerobic empyema, 2 cases of *H. influenzae* type B, and a pneumococcal pneumonia. The diagnosis of gram-negative pneumonia was based on transtracheal aspiration and bronchoscopic, endotracheal, or lung aspirate specimens.

Twelve of 14 cases of pneumonitis were cured, including 5 of the 7 gram-negative pneumonias. Of the remaining two cases of gram-negative infection, one was improved and one failed. One patient with a *Pseudomonas* lung abscess was cured with 4 weeks of therapy; the other patient with a lung abscess caused by *P. aeruginosa* (MIC = 16 μg/ml) and *Acinetobacter calcoaceticus* var. *anitratus* (MIC = 8 μg/ml) failed on cefotaxime. Reculture of the abscess by transthoracic needle aspiration revealed that the *Acinetobacter* was eradicated, but the *Pseudomonas* persisted and became resistant to cefotaxime (MIC > 128 μg/ml). Overall, 15 of 17 evaluable patients responded to therapy.

Twenty-one soft-tissue infections, including 16 cases of cellulitis and 5 cases of aorto-femoral bypass graft infection, were treated. Two cases of cellulitis were unevaluable because of concurrent tobramycin treatment in one and amputation of the foot at 48 h in the other. All cases involved gram-negative bacilli: anaerobes were copathogens in eight cases and *S. aureus* in five cases. Cures were achieved in 10 of 14 evaluable cases of cellulitis, and 4 improved. Three of five cases of bypass graft infection were cured in association with surgical revision of the graft; two failed—one because the graft was left in situ and *Enterobacter cloacae* (MIC = 6.25 μg/ml) persisted, and the other because of rash on day 6 of treatment. Overall, 17 of 19 soft-tissue infections were cured or improved.

Of the 15 cases of osteomyelitis, 3 were due to *S. aureus* and 3 to *S. epidermidis* in association with orthopedic prosthetic devices, 6 were gram-negative contiguous osteomyelitis, and 3 were mixed aerobic-anaerobic infections secondary to decubitus lesions. The pathogens in gram-negative osteomyelitis included one case each of *E. coli* with *S. aureus*, *Proteus vulgaris* with *E. cloacae*, *K. pneumoniae*, and acute on chronic mastoiditis due to *P. aeruginosa*. There were two cases of infection with *A. calcoaceticus* var. *anitratus*. Biopsies were used to confirm the diagnosis in each case of gram-negative infection.

Cefotaxime therapy of osteomyelitis cured, improved, and failed in one case each of *S. aureus* infection. Two cases of *S. epidermidis* infection were cured in association with removal of the prosthetic device, and one failed to respond although the prosthesis was left in situ. Five of the six cases of gram-negative osteomyelitis were cured, one improved, and one failed. The failure, a case of *Pseudomonas* mastoiditis where the infecting organism had a cefotaxime MIC of 25 μg/ml, failed to respond to a 3-week course of treatment on a 2 g every 4 h schedule. Although two of the three cases of osteomyelitis secondary to decubitus ulcers were improved, severe underlying disease precluded any cures. Overall, 11 of 15 cases of osteomyelitis responded to treatment. The mean duration of therapy was 28 days (range, 22 to 52 days). The usual dosage regimen was 1 g on a 6-h schedule.

Nine intraabdominal infections, seven complicated by bacteremia and septic shock, were treated. Five had previously failed on parenteral antibiotic therapy. Infections included four cases of ascending cholangitis, one case of *Klebsiella* bacteremia associated with acute pancreatitis, and four cases of peritonitis. Bacteremic organisms included *E. coli* (2), *K. pneumoniae* (2), *P. aeruginosa* (2), and *Acinetobacter anitratus* (1). All bacteremias cleared with cefotaxime therapy alone. One case of nonbacteremic *Pseudomonas* peritonitis was cured with tobramycin plus cefotaxime therapy and was unevaluable. Overall, five of nine patients were cured, one improved (*Pseudomonas* bacteremia cleared, but the organism persisted in the bile), and two failed. Failures included one case of *E. coli* (MIC = 0.06 μg/ml) peritonitis secondary to surgery for hepatic rupture and one case of *P. aeruginosa* (MIC = 16 μg/ml) peritonitis, where the organism developed resistance.

Miscellaneous infections included two cases of mixed aerobic and anaerobic wound infection; both were cured. A case of enteric fever syndrome due to *Salmonella typhimurium* remained febrile on 10 days of intravenous chloramphenicol therapy; a 10-day course of cefotaxime resulted in defervescence by day 7. Relapse did not occur after treatment. A case of multiply antibiotic-resistant *E. coli* bacteremia occurred in a neutropenic patient on ticarcillin-plus-tobramycin treatment. Bacteremia and fever resolved on cefotaxime alone, but the patient subsequently died of disseminated candidiasis and marrow aplasia. In this series of 101 infections, all 14 bacteremias responded to treatment.

Adverse effects were monitored in 98 patients; antibiotic therapy given intravenously for a mean duration of 12 days (range, 5 to 52 days) in a dosage range of 1 to 2 g every 4 to 8 h resulted in side effects in 15 patients. Phlebitis occurred in nine patients; leukopenia with an absolute neutrophil count of 1,400/mm^3 on day 22 of treatment of osteomyelitis, in 1 patient; serum sickness at 28 days, in one patient; a maculopapular rash, in two patients; and *Clostridium difficile* pseudomembranous colitis, in two patients on cefotaxime therapy. However, prior penicillin therapy in both patients obviates a direct association of cefotaxime to the colitis.

TABLE 1. *Overall therapeutic outcome of cefotaxime treatment*

Type of infection	No. of infections[a]	No. evaluable	No. showing:		
			Cure[b]	Improvement[b]	Failure
Urinary tract	31	30	24	6	0
Respiratory	20	17	14	1	2
Soft tissue	21	19	13	4	2
Osteomyelitis	15	15	7	4	4
Intraabdominal sepsis	9	8	5	1	2
Miscellaneous	5	5	4	0	1

[a] There were 99 patients treated; 2 patients had two infections.

[b] Clinical response: 83 of 94 (88%).

The overall outcome of therapy is summarized in Table 1. Of the 94 evaluable infections, 83 (88%) responded to therapy. One hundred forty-seven isolates were identified as primary pathogens; 66% were ampicillin resistant, 43% were cephalothin resistant, and 13% were resistant to tobramycin or gentamicin or both. The overall bacteriological response was assessable for 141 isolates. Eight-five percent of pathogens were eliminated and 15% persisted or relapsed. Resistance developed in five cases of *P. aeruginosa* infection during cefotaxime therapy.

In conclusion, the results of an open nonrandomized experience in Canada with cefotaxime alone in the treatment of serious gram-negative infections shows that cefotaxime is a safe and effective drug. Although it may be effective alone in the treatment of *Pseudomonas* urinary infections, combined therapy with aminoglycosides may be desirable for therapy of susceptible *Pseudomonas* infections at other sites. This drug is effective in the treatment of infections caused by bacteria resistant to the first- and second-generation cephalosporins.

Cefotaxime: U.K. Trial Results in Treatment of Septicemia

R. P. BAX,* K. CONNELLY, R. BLOMER, AND J. P. W. YOUNG

Medical Department, Roussel Laboratories Limited, Wembley Park, Middlesex, U.K.; Medical Department, Hoechst AG, Frankfurt, Federal Republic of Germany; and Medical Department, Roussel UCLAF, Paris, France*

Cefotaxime is a new β-lactamase-stable cephalosporin antibiotic with high intrinsic activity against a wide range of important hospital pathogens. A total of 411 hospitalized patients in the United Kingdom, many with severe bacterial infections, were treated with cefotaxime during a phase III clinical trial program, including 111 patients with septicemia. Of these 111 patients, 31 were treated with a combination of cefotaxime and another antibiotic, usually gentamicin. The indications for combination treatment included severe infection in neutropenic patients or infections caused by pathogens of moderate susceptibility to cefotaxime, such as *Pseudomonas* spp. This paper details the clinical results of those 80 patients receiving cefotaxime monotherapy for the treatment of septicemia, diagnosed on clinical grounds and bacteriological evidence.

The patients were treated in 10 U.K. centers according to a standard protocol, and the data were recorded on a standard clinical trial record form. The concurrent use of metronidazole when infections caused by *Bacteroides fragilis* were suspected was allowed.

The indications for treatment included bacteriologically proven septicemia or a clinical suspicion of septicemia before the causative organism was known. A total of 80 patients had positive blood cultures diagnosing septicemia. Forty-eight percent of the patients were critically ill with severe infections, 43% of patients were in a poor general condition with moderate infections, and 9% of patients were classed as having a mild infection.

The average age was 61 years (range, 1 to 87). In 13 patients, cefotaxime replaced the use of the combination of gentamicin and a penicillin compound. Fifty-one patients (64%) received intravenous therapy, 25 (31%) received intramuscular therapy, and 4 received cefotaxime by both routes. The commonest dose used was 1.0 g every 8 h (43% of patients) for an average of 8 days, although 30% of patients received lower daily doses (1.5 to 2.0 g).

The commonest primary site of infection was the urinary tract (33 patients, including 15 patients who had had surgical procedures [prostatectomy, cystoscopy, etc.] performed). Eighteen patients had infection occurring in the abdomen, including peritonitis and abscesses, as the primary site of infection. Twelve patients developed septicemia after chest infections, eight patients developed it after cellulitis, and in nine patients no primary site was found. Seven patients were judged as clinically unassessable by the investigators because medical and surgical complications precluded a fair assessment of the antibiotic. Three of these patients died during therapy from complications after surgical anastomoses, and one patient died of hepatorenal failure, which was established before cefotaxime was administered. One patient died from multiple intraabdominal abscesses and a septicemia caused by *Proteus mirabilis* susceptible to cefotaxime.

The overall clinical results of treatment were very good, with 62 (85%) of the 73 assessable patients cured. Three patients (4%) relapsed, and there were 8 (11%) patients who failed treatment. Two of these patients with typhoid fever were changed to co-trimoxazole because of lack of clinical response, in spite of eradication of *Salmonella typhi* from the blood culture. One patient with endocarditis, caused by beta-hemolytic streptococci, required replacement of the aortic and mitral valves to control the infection. Another patient, with endocarditis caused by *Staphylococcus aureus*, was changed to specific antistaphylococcal treatment. Three patients died of overwhelming infection after immunosuppression, including one patient who developed a septicemia due to *Enterobacter cloacae* 5 days after treatment had finished. The last patient died of septicemia after a posterior mediastinitis caused by the breakdown of an esophagectomy for intractable achalasia. It is unlikely in those patients who died and the patient with endocarditis that antimicrobial therapy would have cured their infection. One patient with paratyphoid fever who was apparently successfully treated with cefotaxime relapsed 18 days after the end of treatment. A patient with pancreatitis and subphrenic abscess also relapsed after cefotaxime treatment. A patient who was apparently successfully treated with cefotaxime for a *Klebsiella* septicemia relapsed 7 days after the end of treatment. Surgery was required for a liver abscess. The bacteriological results of treatment were excellent, with 56 of the 67 (84%) assessable pathogens being eradicated. The commonest organism isolated from blood culture was *Escherichia coli* in 38 patients, followed by *Klebsiella* spp. in 14 patients and *Proteus* spp. in 7 patients (see Table 1). Other bacteria successfully eradicated included *Streptococcus pneumoniae*, *S. aureus*, and *Clostridium perfringens*. *Fusobacter mortiferens* and *Acinetobacter anitratus* persisted in the blood of the patient with mediastinitis; the latter organism became resistant to cefotaxime. Two patients developed superinfections, with *Streptococcus faecalis* cultured from the urine. *Candida* infection requiring local therapy occurred in four patients.

There were no patients who had impairment of renal function directly due to cefotaxime treatment. Cefotaxime was well tolerated by 65 (81%) of the patients. The commonest side effect noted was pain in 13 of the 29 patients who received intramuscular injections. Rashes occurred in four patients and phlebitis, thought to be specifically due to the intravenous use of cefotaxime, occurred in two patients.

In conclusion, this study shows that cefotaxime is an effective antibiotic against a wide range of those susceptible pathogens causing septicemia in U.K. hospitals. No serious toxicity was noted. Because of the very wide spectrum of activity, low incidence of side effects, and clinical effectiveness, cefotaxime should be considered for the initial treatment of severe infection before the causative organism is known.

TABLE 1. *Bacteriological results of treatment*

Organism	Bacteriological result (no.)		
	Eradicated (84%)	Persisted (16%)	Unassessable
E. coli	28	1[a]	9
Klebsiella spp.	9	1[b]	4
Proteus spp.	4	1[a]	2
S. typhi/S. paratyphi	4	1[a]	1
Pseudomonas spp.	2	1	2
Beta-hemolytic streptococci	4		
E. cloacae	2	(1)[c]	1
Others	3	3 (2)[a]	6

[a] Not from blood culture.
[b] Relapsed.
[c] Number in parentheses is number of superinfections.

Treatment of Gonorrhea with Cefotaxime

A. J. BOAKES,* D. BARLOW, AND I. PHILLIPS

St. Thomas' Hospital, London SE1, England

A total of 227 male patients presenting with gonorrhea at a teaching hospital department of genitourinary medicine were treated with an intramuscular injection of cefotaxime, 0.5 g in 2 ml of 1% lignocaine.

Of these patients, 221 (average age, 25.8 years; range, 16 to 62 years) were treated with apparent success; 210 had urethral, 9 had rectal, and 2 had combined urethral and rectal infections. Eleven of the patients had previously failed to respond to another drug (nine to ampicillin, one to benzylpenicillin, and one to co-trimoxazole). The diagnosis of gonorrhea was made by both positive microscopy and culture in 215 patients and by positive culture alone in 6 patients. Of these six latter patients, 3 occurred out of 212 urethral infections (1.4%) and 3 occurred out of 11 rectal infections (27.2%).

Penicillin sensitivity tests were performed by a standard three-disk technique, using disks with penicillin concentrations of 0.03, 0.25, and 1.0 mg/liter. The distribution of susceptibilities was as follows: 119 (53.8%) were susceptible to penicillin, 91 (41.1%) were moderately resistant, 9 (4.1%) were resistant, and 2 were not reported. When resistance to penicillin was found, there was further assessment for penicillinase (beta-lactamase) production by means of the Betatest, a commercially available indicator paper based on chromogenic cephalosporin. Five penicillinase-producing strains were identified from the nine resistant infections.

Patients were invited to reattend 2 days and 2 weeks after treatment for tests of cure by microscopy and culture. A total of 131, or 59.3% (average age, 26.5 years), completed full follow-up, 58, or 26.2% (average age, 25.0 years), had only one follow-up test, and 32, or 14.5% (average age, 24.2 years), failed to return for follow-up. Of those attending for only one follow-up test, 45 (77.6%) attended within 7 days, 5 (8.6%) attended between 7 and 13 days, and 8 (13.8%) attended 14 or more days after treatment.

Of the 131 patients who attended for full follow-up, 89 (68%) developed postgonococcal urethritis and were treated with a course of tetracycline. These cases represented 74% of the infections with penicillin-susceptible organisms, 59% of the moderately resistant infections, and 75% of the resistant infections. It might well be that this rather high incidence of postgonococcal urethritis is falsely inflated, for it takes no account of patients who failed to return for follow-up or those returning only once, who were presumably symptomless and probably free from residual urethritis.

All patients were questioned 1 h and again 2 days after treatment about pain at the site of injection. One patient complained of pain lasting for 5 min after injection, and one complained of pain lasting for the remainder of the day. No other side effects of treatment were observed or reported.

A further six patients (average age, 24.2 years; range, 19 to 31 years), all with urethral gonorrhea, received cefotaxime with apparent failure. Of these infections, two were reported as susceptible to penicillin, and four were moderately resistant. They were subsequently treated successfully with another drug (three with ampicillin and three with co-trimoxazole). At worst, this represents a failure rate of 2.6%. However, in two of the failures there had been sexual intercourse after treatment and probable reinfection, in two there was bodily contact with a sexual partner and possible reinfection, in one the infection was complicated by tysonitis and might not be expected reasonably to have responded to a single-dose regimen, and the sixth apparent failure was diagnosed by positive microscopy, but was not confirmed by culture, which was negative.

After this main study, the efficacy of cefotaxime was assessed in the management of infections caused by penicillinase-producing strains of *Neisseria gonorrhoeae* (PPNG). Since the first case reported by Phillips (2) from St. Thomas' Hospital in 1976, we have identified and treated 79 patients (25 females, average age 26.2 years; and 54 males, average age 30.7 years) who had infections caused by PPNG (up to the end of June 1981). Of these patients, 35 (10 females and 25 males) have been treated with cefotaxime with 100% success, as reported by Boakes et al. (1). These include one case which had shown clinical failure after treatment with spectinomycin, 2 g intramuscularly, although the organism was susceptible in vitro to spectinomycin (MIC, 15 mg/liter), and two cases with oropharyngeal in addition to genital infection. This latter result is of particular interest in view of the report by Walter et al. (3) of the poor response of oropharyngeal infection to spectinomycin therapy.

Thus, cefotaxime is safe, produces a high cure rate in uncomplicated gonorrhea, and is effective against penicillinase-producing and other penicillin-resistant strains of *N. gonorrhoeae*.

1. **Boakes, A. J., J. Barrow, S. J. Eykyn, and I. Phillips.** 1981. Cefotaxime for spectinomycin resistant *Neisseria gonorrhoeae*. Lancet **ii**:96.
2. **Phillips, I.** 1976. Beta-lactamase producing, penicillin resistant gonococcus. Lancet **ii**:656–657.
3. **Walter, W., M. Karney, and M. Pederson.** 1977. Spectinomycin versus tetracycline for the treatment of gonorrhoea. N. Engl. J. Med. **296**:889–894.

Treatment of Bone and Joint Infections with Cefotaxime

J. MADER,* J. LeFROCK, A. MOLAVI, AND J. REINARZ

University of Texas Medical Branch, Galveston, Texas 77550, and Hahnemann Medical College and Hospital, Philadelphia, Pennsylvania 19102, U.S.A.*

Cefotaxime (Claforan; HR-756), a new "third generation" cephalosporin, has substantial activity in vitro against numerous gram-negative aerobic bacteria, gram-positive aerobic bacteria including *Staphylococcus aureus*, and anaerobic bacteria (1–3). Consequently, it promises to be useful for the treatment of many diverse, serious infections. This clinical trial was initiated to evaluate the efficacy of cefotaxime for the treatment of osteomyelitis, among the most refractory of infections, and septic arthritis.

Patients with acute septic arthritis and acute or chronic osteomyelitis were referred to the University of Texas Medical Branch Hospitals or Hahnemann Medical College and Hospital. The individuals were 18 years or older, not pregnant, and capable of giving informed consent. There was no patient history of serious hepatic or renal disease (creatinine > 2.5 mg/dl) or type I hypersensitivity reaction to penicillin. The patient had received no antibiotic therapy within 3 days before cefotaxime therapy.

The diagnosis of osteomyelitis was confirmed by surgical biopsy with isolation of a causative aerobic or anaerobic pathogen from the bone lesion or a positive blood culture with a diagnostic X ray/bone scan. Whenever possible, the bone biopsy incision was made through uninvolved tissue in order to avoid wound flora and bacteria colonizing the sinus tract(s). The diagnosis of septic arthritis was confirmed by a clinical picture of an acute septic arthritis with a positive bacterial joint fluid culture.

A physical examination was performed on each patient at the beginning and completion of the study. A complete blood count, direct Coombs, SMA-12, serum protein electrophoresis, and urinalysis were obtained on the day preceding, at weekly intervals, and on the day after cessation of cefotaxime therapy. Vital signs were monitored daily while the patients were hospitalized. All patients with osteomyelitis were X-rayed before and after the completion of therapy.

A clinical response was considered satisfactory if no evidence of infection, pain, swelling, erythema, or draining sinus tracts (osteomyelitis) was noted at the completion of cefotaxime therapy or on subsequent follow-up. A clinical response was considered unsatisfactory if there was evidence of continued infection at the completion of cefotaxime therapy or if recurrence of the infection was noted at monthly follow-ups. Evaluation of clinical response was based primarily on resolution of signs and symptoms of the infection together with results of the post-treatment X rays (osteomyelitis).

Eleven patients with acute osteomyelitis (four females, seven males; mean age, 52 years) were treated with a mean dose of 10.2 g for a mean duration of 33.3 days of therapy. Ten of 11 (91%) patients had a satisfactory response. The mean duration of follow-up was 5 months.

Twenty-four patients with chronic osteomyelitis (7 females, 17 males; mean age, 49 years) were treated with a mean dose of 8.3 g for a mean duration of 30.5 days of therapy. All patients had at least one surgical debridement. Twenty-one of 23 (91%) patients had a satisfactory response. One patient could not be evaluated. The mean duration of follow-up was 5 months.

Five patients with acute septic arthritis (two females, three males; mean age, 42 years) were treated with a mean dose of 8.2 g for a mean duration of 15.4 days of therapy. Four of four patients (100%) had a satisfactory response. One patient could not be evaluated. The mean duration follow-up was 3.3 months.

Twenty patients had a single organism isolated, and 20 patients had multiple organisms isolated as the causative pathogens. *S. aureus* accounted for 30%, *Pseudomonas aeruginosa* accounted for 8%, and anaerobes accounted for 19% of the bacteria isolated. MICs of cefotaxime were determined for the bacterial isolates, and all were inhibited by 25.0 μg/ml or less.

Very few side effects were manifested during the study. Toxicity evaluation revealed a skin rash (one patient), phlebitis (two patients), eosinophilia of >500 mm^3 (two patients), a positive direct Coombs test (six patients).

The most severe side effect was a significant decrease in the absolute number of neutrophils in two patients. In the first patient, the total number of neutrophils decreased to 120 mm^3 on the 22nd day of cefotaxime therapy. A bone marrow revealed myeloid hyperplasia with a maturation arrest at the myelocytic state of development. Cefotaxime was discontinued, and the leukocyte count and differential returned to normal over the next 5 days. In the second patient, the absolute neutrophil count fell to 784 mm^3 on the 31st day of cefotaxime therapy. Cefotaxime was discontinued, and the leukocyte count and differential returned to normal over the next 4 days. Both patients had a positive direct Coombs test, but neither had evidence of hemolysis. A satisfactory treatment result was obtained in both patients.

On the basis of the results of this study, cefotaxime appears to be a clinically useful antibiotic for the treatment of acute and chronic osteomyelitis and of acute septic arthritis due to *S. aureus*, gram-negative bacteria, and anaerobes. Ninety-two percent (35 of 38) of the patients treated had a satisfactory response to cefotaxime therapy. Two patients could not be evaluated.

Cefotaxime was well tolerated in these patients. The only significant problem encountered was transient neutropenia in two patients, which occurred late in the course of cefotaxime therapy (mean, 26 days). This possible toxicity requires further study and should be considered when prescribing cefotaxime for longer than 3 weeks.

Evaluation for ultimate clinical and bacteriological cure in osteomyelitis will require prolonged clinical follow-up. Osteomyelitis is a difficult infection to evaluate, and it is often difficult to isolate the causative pathogen(s). It is even harder to ascertain efficacy of treatment, since evidence of continued infection may be occult and may not manifest for years. This study suggests that adequate debridement and 4 to 6 weeks of high-dose cefotaxime therapy results in a clinical arrest of both acute and chronic osteomyelitis.

1. **Hamilton-Miller, J. T. M., W. Brumfitt, and A. V. Reynolds.** 1978. Cefotaxime (HR 756), a new cephalo-

sporin with exceptional broad-spectrum activity *in vitro*. J. Antimicrob. Chemother. 4:437–444.

2. **Neu, H. C., N. Aswapokee, P. Aswapokee, and K. P. Fu.** 1979. HR-756, a new cephalosporin active against gram-positive and gram-negative aerobic and anaerobic bacteria. Antimicrob. Agents Chemother. **15**:273–281.

3. **Stephens, M., M. Potten, and A. J. Bint.** 1979. The sensitivity of gentamicin-resistant gram-negative bacilli to cefotaxime, other cephalosporins and aminoglycosides. Infection **7**:109–112.

Comparative Study of Cefotaxime and Ceftezole in the Treatment of Complicated Urinary Tract Infections

J. KUMAZAWA

Department of Surgery, Saga Medical School, Saga, Japan

We carried out a well-controlled study in which cefotaxime (CTX), a new cephalosporin antibiotic, was compared with ceftezole (CTZ) for clinical efficacy, usefulness, and safety in complicated urinary tract infections (UTI). CTX (1 g twice daily) or CTZ (2 g twice daily) was intravenously administered for 5 consecutive days.

Patients admitted to the Departments of Urology at hospitals of Kyushu and Fukuoka Universities and Miyazaki Medical College and 12 affiliated hospitals from September 1979 to February 1980 were enrolled into this study. The patients were at least 16 years of age.

The clinical efficacy and usefulness of the drugs were evaluated by the members of the Evaluation Committee (2) and investigators based on the UTI evaluation criteria (2).

Based on the overall improvement in UTI, the Evaluation Committee evaluated CTX to be significantly more effective than CTZ (Table 1). CTX was assessed to be excellent in 14.1% of the 85 patients, moderate in 52.9%, and poor in 32.9%, whereas CTZ was assessed to be excellent

TABLE 1. *Bacteriological response*[a]

Isolates	CTX			CTZ		
	No. of strains	Eradicated (%)	Persisted	No. of strains	Eradicated (%)	Persisted
Gram-positive cocci						
Streptococcus epidermidis	4	4 (100)	0	5	5 (100)	0
S. faecalis	5	3 (60)	2	9	6 (66.7)	3
S. pyogenes	3	3 (100)	0	1	1 (100)	0
Other	6	5 (83.3)	1	8	8 (100)	0
Subtotal	18	15 (83.3)	3	23	20 (87.0)	3
Gram-negative rods						
Escherichia coli	17	17 (100)	0	16	14 (87.5)	2
Klebsiella	2	2 (100)	0	5	3 (60)	2
Proteus mirabilis	4	4 (100)	0	2	1 (50)	1
P. vulgaris	1	0 (0)	1	0	0	0
P. morganii	3	3 (100)	0	0	0	0
P. rettgeri	3	3 (100)	0	5	3 (60)	2
Enterobacter	8	6 (75)	2	15	10 (66.7)	5
Citrobacter	10	9 (90)	1	5	2 (40)	3
Serratia	21	13 (61.9)	8	26	6 (23.1)	20
Pseudomonas aeruginosa	17	10 (58.8)	7	12	2 (16.7)	10
Other pseudomonas (*P. cepacia, P. maltophilia, P. alcaligenes*)	6	4 (66.7)	2	5	3 (60)	2
Acinetobacter	3	2 (66.7)	1	3	2 (66.7)	1
Flavobacterium	1	1 (100)	0	1	1 (100)	0
Subtotal	96	74 (77.1)	22	95	47 (49.5)	48
Total	114	89 (78.1)	25	118	67 (56.8)	51

[a] Statistical results: gram-positive cocci, $P_0 = 1.000$; gram-negative rods, $\chi_0^2 = 14.511$ ($P < 0.001$); total, $\chi_0^2 = 10.985$ ($P < 0.001$).

in 12.6% of the 87 patients, moderate in 27.6%, and poor in 59.8%.

The drug efficacy against infections caused by organisms other than *Serratia* and *Pseudomonas* was evaluated in 43 patients in the CTX group and 46 patients in the CTZ group. There was no significant difference between the two groups. However, CTX was significantly more effective than CTZ against mixed infections in these patients. No significant difference was detected in the efficacy against CTZ-susceptible organisms between the two treatment groups.

CTX was significantly of more clinical value than CTZ, in the investigators' judgment. CTX was assessed to be excellent in 32.5% of the 83 patients, good in 39.8%, fair in 14.5%, and poor in 13.3%, whereas CTZ was assessed to be excellent in 17.4% of the 86 patients, good in 32.6%, fair in 11.6%, and poor in 38.4%.

CTX was found to be significantly more useful than CTZ, with 90.0% of the CTX group and 66.6% of the CTZ group being assessed as responding at least satisfactorily. These results were in extremely good agreement with preclinical findings (1).

As for side effects, vomiting occurred in 1 of 103 patients receiving CTX (1.0%), and vomiting or nausea and/or eruption occurred in 3 of 103 patients receiving CTZ (2.9%). Abnormal laboratory findings attributable to treatment were noted in three cases in the CTX group and one in the CTZ group.

1. **Chabbert, Y. A., and J. Lutz.** 1978. HR 756, the syn isomer of a new methoxyimino cephalosporin with unusual antibacterial activity. Antimicrob. Agents Chemother. **14:**749–754.
2. **Ohkoshi, M., and Committee on Urinary Tract Infections in Japan.** 1980. Criteria for drug evaluation in urinary tract infection, 2nd report (Japanese). Chemotherapy **28:**324–341 and 1351–1358.

Cefotaxime in the Treatment of Infections in Hospitalized Patients

RAFAEL QUIÑONES-SOTO,* DORIS VERA, MINERVA NEVÁREZ, AND CARLOS H. RAMÍREZ-RONDA

Infectious Disease Program, University of Puerto Rico School of Medicine and Veterans Administration Medical Center; Departments of Research and Medicine, Veterans Administration Medical Center; and Department of Medicine, University of Puerto Rico School of Medicine, San Juan, Puerto Rico 00936, U.S.A.*

Cefotaxime is a third-generation cephalosporin with a broad range of antibacterial activity. In vitro it inhibits gram-positive cocci, including *Streptococcus pyogenes*, *Streptococcus pneumoniae*, and *Staphylococcus aureus*, and most of the members of the *Enterobacteriaceae* (2). It is also active against many strains of *Haemophilus influenzae* and *Neisseria gonorrhoeae*. High doses of cefotaxime can inhibit some strains of *Pseudomonas aeruginosa* and *Bacteroides fragilis* (1).

Thirty-six adult male hospitalized patients (age range, 24 to 75 years) with acute soft tissue, urinary tract, and lower respiratory tract infections were entered into the study after giving informed consent. All patients were treated with intravenous cefotaxime in a dose of 4 to 8 g per day. The infectious condition was documented by culture before initiation of drug administration. Cultures were taken before, during, and after treatment; culture sites included the site of infection and blood cultures. In the cases of lower respiratory tract infection, chest radiographs were taken before and after treatment. Hematological parameters as well as liver and renal function tests were monitored at regular intervals during the study, and every patient was followed closely for the development of any adverse effect. Serum levels were determined in several patients, using *Escherichia coli* 3989 as the test organism. Trough levels were taken before the next dose, and peak levels were taken 30 min after the end of a 30-min infusion.

Soft tissue infections. Twenty-four patients with acute soft tissue infections were entered into the study. Twelve patients received 2 g of cefotaxime every 6 h, and 12 received 1 g of cefotaxime every 6 h, for a median duration of treatment of 12 days. *Staphylococcus aureus* was the predominant organism recovered from this group of patients and was cultured from eight patients. The next most frequent organisms recovered were *E. coli* (five cases) and *Streptococcus pyogenes* (four cases). There were two cases of *P. aeruginosa*, two patients with *Proteus* infecting surgical wounds, and one of each of the following: *Staphylococcus epidermidis*, *Serratia marcescens*, *Enterobacter cloa-*

cae, *Providencia stuartii*, and *Neisseria gonorrhoeae*. Clinical cure was achieved in all patients with soft tissue infections (Table 1). Bacteriological cure was documented in 18 of 24 patients. In the rest, posttreatment culture could not be performed because of the complete disappearance of the original infection. Bacteriological cure was achieved in all of the 18 cases. In two instances, the anaerobic organisms *B. fragilis* and *Peptococcus asaccharolyticus* were recovered, both of them in mixed flora; the patients with these infections responded well to treatment.

Urinary tract infections. Seven patients with urinary tract infections were entered into the study. Four patients received 1 g of cefotaxime every 6 h, two patients received 2 g every 6 h, and one patient received 500 mg every 12 h, for a median duration of treatment of 12 days. *P. aeruginosa* was recovered from three of the patients. The others had urinary tract infection caused by *Klebsiella pneumoniae* (one patient), *E. coli* (one patient), *Serratia marcescens* (one patient), and *Acinetobacter calcoaceticus* (one patient). Clinical cure was achieved in all seven patients, and bacteriological cure was achieved in five patients; there were two instances of bacteriological failure (Table 1). One of the bacteriological failures was a patient with chronic prostatitis who received treatment for 8 days; the other was a patient with a recent surgical procedure for correction of a colovesical fistula. The latter patient failed to respond initially but responded later when his Foley catheter was removed.

Lower respiratory tract infections. Five patients with acute severe lower respiratory tract infections were entered into the study. All were treated with 2 g of cefotaxime intravenously every 6 h, for a median duration of treatment of 11 days. *K. pneumoniae* was cultured from two patients. *P. aeruginosa, E. coli,* and *H. influenzae*, respectively, were cultured from each of the other patients. Clinical cure with bacteriological cure was achieved in all of the patients (Table 1).

TABLE 1. *Response to treatment with cefotaxime of hospitalized patients with acute soft tissue, urinary tract, and lower respiratory tract infections*

Infection site	Response to treatment			
	Clinical cure	Clinical failure	Bacteriological cure	Bacteriological failure
Soft tissue	24/24	0/24	18/18	0/18
Urinary tract	7/7	0/7	5/7	2/7
Lower respiratory tract	5/5	0/5	5/5	0/5
Total	36/36	0/36	28/30	2/30

TABLE 2. *Serum concentrations of cefotaxime in patients with acute infections treated with two different dose regimens*[a]

Cefotaxime dose	Serum concn (μg/ml)			
	Peak		Trough	
	Mean	Range	Mean	Range
2 g every 6 h	63.55	54–88	5.05	1.6–10.5
1 g every 6 h	37.88	22–54	4.24	0.78–8

[a] Serum levels were determined after the third intravenous dose and before the ninth. Peak was obtained 30 min after an infusion lasting 30 min, and trough was obtained immediately before the next dose.

Pharmacokinetics. Serum levels were determined for patients receiving 2 g of cefotaxime every 6 h and in those receiving 1 g every 6 h by intravenous infusion lasting 30 min. For patients receiving 2 g, peak serum levels obtained 30 min after the infusion ended ranged from 54 to 88 μg/ml, with a mean concentration of 63.55 μg/ml, and trough levels ranged from 1.6 to 10.5 μg/ml, with a mean concentration of 5.05 μg/ml. For the patients receiving 1 g of cefotaxime every 6 h, peak concentrations ranged from 22 to 54 μg/ml, with a mean concentration of 37.38 μg/ml. Trough concentrations for this group ranged from 0.78 to 8 μg/ml, with a mean concentration of 4.24 μg/ml. All serum levels were determined after the third dose and before the ninth intravenous dose (Table 2).

Adverse effects. One patient developed a maculopapular rash while receiving the drug; the etiology of this rash remains unclear, since the patient had active systemic lupus erythematosus. Another patient developed nausea, vomiting, and diarrhea, but was receiving concomitantly adenine arabinoside. A third patient developed phlebitis on the arm where the intravenous line was placed. None of the patients had to abandon cefotaxime treatment because of these reactions. There were no significant function tests. None of the patients developed a positive Coombs test (3). This good tolerance of cefotaxime has been seen in other studies.

In summary, this study demonstrates that cefotaxime is a safe and effective agent in the treatment of acute soft tissue infections, complicated acute urinary tract infections, and severe acute lower respiratory tract infections caused by susceptible organisms.

1. **Neu, H. C., N. Aswapokee, P. Aswapokee, and K. P. Fu.** 1979. HR-756, a new cephalosporin active against gram-positive and gram-negative aerobic and anaerobic bacteria. Antimicrob. Agents Chemother. **15:**273–281.
2. **Neu, H. C., P. Aswapokee, and K. P. Fu.** 1980. Cefo-

taxime kinetics after intravenous and intramuscular injection of single and multiple doses. Clin. Pharmacol. Ther. **27**:677–685.

3. **Newsom, S. W. B., J. Mathews, S. J. Connellan, and V. R. Pearce.** 1980. Clinical studies with cefotaxime, p. 125–126. *In* J. D. Nelson and C. Grassi (ed.), Current chemotherapy and infectious disease, vol. 1. American Society for Microbiology, Washington, D.C.

Cefotaxime in the Treatment of Serious Gram-Negative Septicemia

R. G. FINCH* AND R. C. B. SLACK

The City and University Hospitals, Nottingham NG5 1PB, England

Cefotaxime is a new third-generation cephalosporin with high intrinsic activity and excellent β-lactamase stability. It is active against a wide range of bacteria, most notably *Haemophilus influenzae* and the *Enterobacteriaceae*, against which it is more active than the aminoglycoside antibiotics. It also possesses in vitro activity against *Pseudomonas aeruginosa* (1).

In this study cefotaxime was used in the most challenging of circumstances, namely, in the treatment of gram-negative septicemia in selected patients who were either at high risk from underlying disease, were elderly, or had failed to respond to other antibiotics. Cefotaxime was the only agent used that was active against the bloodstream isolate.

All patients consenting to enter the trial were carefully evaluated and assessed for the presence of shock, the source of the septicemic episode, and their underlying disease. All cultures were taken before treatment. The patients were monitored for their response to treatment by clinical examination and repeat microbiological evaluation where indicated. The severity of the infections were graded into mild, moderate, or severe, and the patients' general condition was assessed as good, poor, or critical.

The response to treatment was defined as (i) cure if treatment resulted in complete resolution of the infectious process, (ii) relapse if, after an initial clinical response, there was a subsequent deterioration of the clinical state due to infection, or (iii) failure if there was either no response or frank worsening of the clinical condition due to infection.

All patients were monitored closely for adverse reactions, with particular emphasis on assessing local intolerance, phlebitis, rash, or diarrhea. Stools were examined for the presence of *Clostridium difficile* toxin in patients who developed diarrhea. Blood samples were regularly monitored before, during, and after treatment for any alterations in hematological, renal, or liver function. Urine was also examined for the presence of casts, cells, sugar, and protein.

The MIC and MBC were determined in DST (Oxoid) broth with an inoculum of approximately 10^7 organisms per liter. The MBC was defined as a 99.9% reduction in growth.

A total of 19 patients (9 males and 10 females) with a mean age of 68 years (range, 22 to 87 years) were treated with cefotaxime in dosages ranging from 0.5 to 2.0 g, 6 to 12 hourly, by the intravenous or intramuscular route for periods ranging from 3 to 20 days.

Infections were judged as severe (8 cases),

TABLE 1. *Bacterial isolates and their MICs and MBCs of cefotaxime, cefuroxime, and gentamicin*

Antibiotic	Organism (no.) and susceptibility (mg/liter)				
	Pseudomonas aeruginosa (4)	*Citrobacter koseri* (2)	*Klebsiella aerogenes* (4)[a]	*Escherichia coli* (6)[b]	*Proteus mirabilis* (3)[a]
Cefotaxime					
MIC	8.0–16.0	0.1	0.06–0.1	0.03–1.0	0.06–0.1
MBC	16.0–64.0	0.1	0.06–1.0	0.03–0.12	0.06–1.0
Cefuroxime					
MIC	>512	16	2.0–16.0	2.0–32.0	32
MBC	>512	16	2.0–16.0	2.0–32.0	32
Gentamicin					
MIC	0.5–1.0	0.5	0.12–0.25	0.25–1.0	0.5
MBC	1.0	4.0	0.25	0.25–1.0	1.0

[a] One strain not tested.
[b] Two strains not tested.

moderate (10 cases), or mild (1 case). The general condition of the patients was judged as good (2 cases), poor (13 cases), or critical (4 cases). The underlying diseases included malignant disease (six cases), chronic renal failure (four cases), senile dementia (two cases), septic arthritis (one case), renal transplant (one case), diabetes mellitus (one case), intraabdominal sepsis (one case), burns (one case), alcoholism (one case), and hypersplenism (one case). Six patients had normal renal function before treatment, whereas the remaining patients (13) had serum creatinine levels ranging from 160 to 1,005 μmol/liter.

Table 1 indicates the pathogens isolated and their susceptibility to cefotaxime, cefuroxime, and gentamicin. The bacteria associated with a partial response were *Pseudomonas aeruginosa* (one case) *Escherichia coli* (one case), and *Proteus mirabilis* (one case). The one definite failure was due to *P. aeruginosa* causing multiple abscesses detected at autopsy.

Of the patients treated, 15 (79%) were cured, 3 (15.8%) showed a partial response, and 1 (5.2%) failed to respond. Adverse reactions were mild and included phlebitis (two cases), pain at the injection site (one case), and moderate diarrhea (two cases); both patients' stools were negative for the presence of *C. difficile* toxin. No patient suffered from skin rashes or superinfection; monitoring for hematological or biochemical abnormalities showed no alterations attributable to cefotaxime.

1. **Bax, R. P., and J. P. W. Young.** 1981. Cefotaxime: United Kingdom clinical trial results in the treatment of severe infections. Curr. Med. Res. Opin. **7**:401–409.

Cefotaxime or Ticarcillin with Gentamicin for Febrile Neutropenic Patients

P. J. HAMILTON,* A. J. BINT, J. CHARLTON, AND C. HILLER

Departments of Haematology and Bacteriology, Royal Victoria Infirmary, Newcastle upon Tyne, United Kingdom*

To minimize delay in combating sepsis, which once established leads to overwhelming infection and early death in patients with compromised bone marrows and impaired immunological defense mechanisms, treatment with high-dose broad-spectrum antibiotic chemotherapy is given to neutropenic patients at the first suspicion of infection. Cefotaxime is a new β-lactamase–stable cephalosporin with high intrinsic activity and a broad spectrum (1, 2). Ticarcillin is a broad-spectrum penicillin with useful activity against *Pseudomonas aeruginosa* (4). A combination of a penicillin or cephalosporin plus an aminoglycoside frequently produces in vivo synergy (3).

Because of difficulties in demonstrating pus or its clinical sequelae in neutropenic patients, infection is usually suspected on finding a persistently elevated temperature, a nonspecific marker of sepsis. In this report we detail our experience of treating 38 episodes of pyrexia (>38°C for at least 2 h) in 26 adult patients with a peripheral blood count of $< 10^9$ granulocytes per liter. Twenty-four such episodes were in patients undergoing intensive cytotoxic chemotherapy, 19 with acute leukemia, 5 with disseminated lymphoma, and 2 others with severe idiopathic aplastic anemia. Antibiotic chemotherapy for pyrexial episodes involved use of gentamicin, usually 120 mg intravenously every 8 h in all 38 episodes, combined with cefotaxime, 2 g intravenously every 8 h in 24 episodes, or ticarcillin, 5 g intravenously every 8 h by infusion in 14 episodes.

Treatment was successful, as judged by a sustained fall of temperature to normal, in 24 of 38 (63%) episodes. In 21 successful treatments the fall in temperature occurred within 4 days, but took up to 7 days in 3 septicemic patients. Only 10 of the 38 episodes were associated with bacterial isolates: 5 of these had positive blood cultures, there were 5 respiratory tract isolates, 2 had positive urine cultures, and there was one wound infection. In these grade 1 infectious episodes (significant positive bacteriology), six gram-positive bacteria (*Streptococcus pyogenes*, one; other streptococci, three; *Staphylococcus aureus*, one; pneumococcus, one) and seven gram-negative organisms (*Klebsiella pneumoniae*, three; *Escherichia coli*, one; *Enterobacter*, one; *Serratia* sp., one; *Pseudomonas aeruginosa*, one) were cultured. All the bacterial pathogens were susceptible to cefotaxime. In 13 episodes pyrexia was associated with chest radiograph appearances consistent with a pneumonic process, but no bacterial isolates were obtained.

Successful resolution of fever with use of the antibiotic combinations occurred in less than one-third (4 of 13) of these grade 2 episodes (site of infection identified but negative bacteriology). No localized infectious process could be identified on detailed retrospective analysis to account for the pyrexia in 15 of 38 episodes: antibiotic therapy, however, was associated with prompt lysis of fever in most of these grade 3 episodes (no localized site of infection found and negative bacteriology). Because of the small numbers in each grade and treatment group, it is invidious to contrast antibiotic combination performance other than to note that 17 of 24 (71%) gentamicin plus cefotaxime and 7 of 14 (50%) gentamicin plus ticarcillin treatments were successful and, in the 23 grade 1 and 2 episodes, 9 of 15 (60%) gentamicin plus cefotaxime and 2 of 8 (25%) gentamicin plus ticarcillin treatments were successful.

Failure to lyse fever did not appear to be associated with profound neutropenia: 17 of 28 (65%) pyrexial episodes with a profound neutropenia (granulocyte count of $<0.5 \times 10^9$/liter) on the fourth treatment day, the day by which most temperatures had resolved, lysed compared with 7 of 10 (70%) where the neutrophil count was higher. In 11 of 14 episodes responding successfully to gentamicin plus cefotaxime, there was a very profound neutropenia on the 4th day ($<0.1 \times 10^9$/liter). Analysis of the causes of failure of these antibiotic combinations to lower the temperature is given in Fig. 1. The diversity of explanations illustrates some of the difficulties of conducting antibiotic trials in this population. Attention is drawn to two patients in whom treatment of identified bacterial septicemia with appropriate antibiotics failed and unsuspected fungal pneumonia was identified postmortem. In addition, three deaths were associated with renal failure. These three patients had relapsed, uncontrolled leukemia but all three were receiving gentamicin plus cefotaxime. Careful review of the patients' charts leads us to attribute, in one case, the progressive renal failure to established *Klebsiella pneumoniae* septicemia in a 74-year-old man with severe marrow failure secondary to uncontrolled acute myeloid leukemia; in the second case, marked renal failure associated with lysozymuria and low potassium levels in acute myeloid leukemia was probably exacerbated by gentamicin plus cefotaxime. In this case, there was difficulty in obtaining correct gentamicin dosage, with trough and peak levels of 4.8 and 15.8 μg/ml being monitored on one occasion. In the third case, renal failure of modest degree ensued on the third day of gentamicin plus cefotaxime treatment (plasma creatinine, 65 rising to 203 μmol/liter) in a patient with relapsed acute myeloid leukemia and a high plasma lysozyme, who had been receiving co-trimoxazole. On discontinuing the antibiotics and substituting chloramphenicol on the fourth day with the temperature stable, she appeared to have improved, only to die on the fifth day of sudden clinical endotoxic shock. In 25 other episodes treated with gentamicin plus cefotaxime, 6 treatments were associated with rises in plasma creatinine of between 10 and 31 μmol/liter, 7 showed falls in creatinine of between 10 and 46 μmol/liter and in 12 there was little or no change. In the gentamicin plus ticarcillin treatments no rise in creatinine was seen.

As shown in Fig. 2, blood level estimations of cefotaxime and desacetyl cefotaxime were assayed by high-pressure liquid chromatography in some of our patients. The mean serum concentration of cefotaxime 1 h after 2 g intravenously was 59 mg/liter, falling to 1.9 mg/liter at

14/38 episodes (37%) did not lyse with antibiotics

Grade 1

3 of 10 : 2 died with post mortem fungal pneumonia
1 treated with resistant serratia

Grade 2

9 of 13 : 1 pneumocystis, 1 possible fungal. 1 herpes simplex.
6 terminal leukaemics died, 3 in renal failure

Grade 3

2 of 15 : 1 disease, 1 bleomycin infusion

FIG. 1. *Causes of failure of antibiotic therapy to lyse fever.*

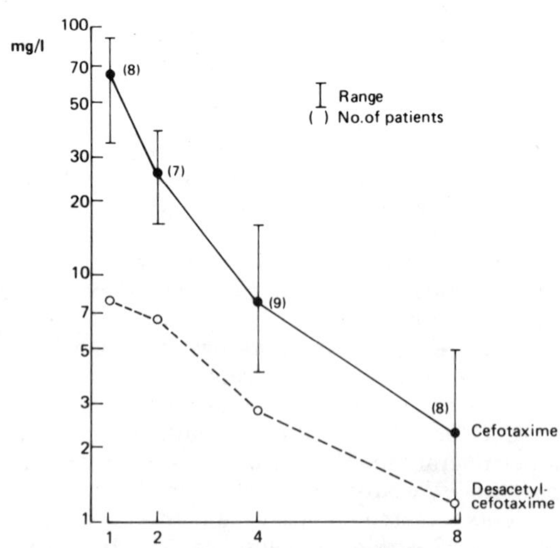

FIG. 2. *Serum concentrations of cefotaxime and desacetyl cefotaxime after 2 g intravenously.*

8 h. Concentrations of desacetyl cefotaxime at 1 and 8 h were 8.8 and 1.2 mg/liter, respectively. No accumulation of cefotaxime or desacetyl cefotaxime was seen in any patient. In this group of patients, all with normal renal function for their age, the mean half-lives were 2.0 h for cefotaxime and 3.5 h for desacetyl cefotaxime. Such estimates are slightly longer than those described in normal volunteers. A dose interval of 8 h would therefore seem to be satisfactory in these patients.

The combination of cefotaxime and gentamicin appears to be as effective as other reported combinations in the treatment of febrile, neutropenic patients. The very broad spectrum of cefotaxime is an added advantage. In some patients the combination may aggravate renal impairment caused by other factors.

1. **Drasar, F. A., W. Farrell, A. J. Howard, C. Hince, T. Leung, and J. D. Williams.** 1978. Activity of HR756 against *Haemophilus influenzae, Bacteroides fragilis* and Gram-negative rods. J. Antimicrob. Chemother. **4:** 445–450.
2. **Hamilton-Miller, J. M. T., W. Brumfitt, and A. V. Reynolds.** 1978. Cefotaxime (HR756) a new cephalosporin with exceptional broad spectrum activity *in-vitro*. J. Antimicrob. Chemother. **4:**437–444.
3. **Klastersky, J.** 1979. Combinations of antibiotics for therapy of severe infections in cancer patients. Eur. J. Cancer **15:** 3–13.
4. **Parry, M. F., and H. C. Neu.** 1976. Ticarcillin for treatment of serious infections with gram-negative bacteria. J. Infect. Dis. **134:**476–485.

Combined Action of Cefoperazone and Aminoglycosides on Gram-Negative Bacteria

ADOLF BAUERNFEIND

Max von Pettenkofer-Institut der Ludwig-Maximilians-Universität München, 8000 Munich 2, Federal Republic of Germany

The MIC of cefoperazone (CPZ) for most of our gram-negative clinical isolates was below 32 mg/liter. The frequency of resistant strains of *Escherichia coli* was 3 of 482, that of *Klebsiella pneumoniae* was 27 of 294, and that of *Pseudomonas aeruginosa* was 73 of 200 (unpublished data). Combined therapy may therefore be considered for treatment of undiagnosed and possibly polymicrobial nosocomial infections. Increased bactericidal activity should be expected for combinations with aminoglycosides. CPZ looks especially attractive for these combinations because of its predominantly (75%) biliary route of excretion. Therefore, the risk of potentiating nephrotoxicity in combinations with aminoglycosides should be lower with CPZ than with cephalosporins excreted mainly by the kidney. Extension of activity spectrum and possible synergism were investigated with 59 gram-negative isolates (Table 1). The effect of CPZ-aminoglycoside combinations was studied by the checkerboard-titration method. With the combinations, all the moderately susceptible or resistant strains became susceptible to one or both drugs. MBCs as well as MICs were determined. The fractional bactericidal concentrations are shown in Table 1. These values show that synergism is not obligatory but strain dependent (wide range of fractional inhibitory concentra-

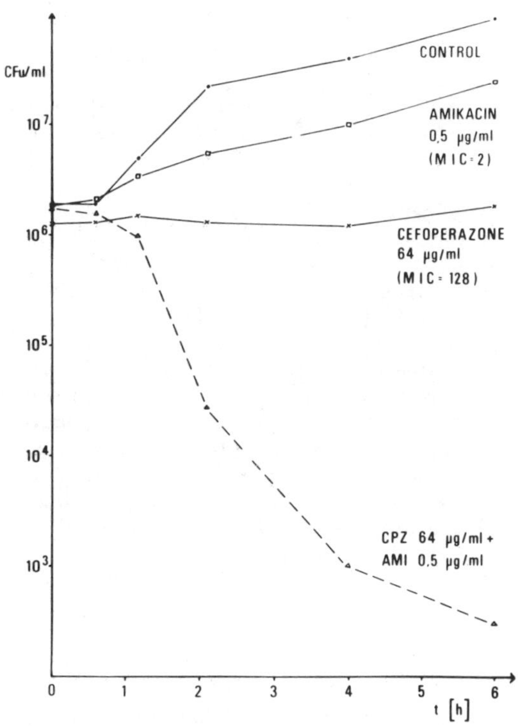

FIG. 1. *Killing curve showing CPZ–amikacin synergism against P. aeruginosa (ST 21311-79).*

TABLE 1. *Synergism of cefoperazone–aminoglycoside combinations*

Organism (no. of isolates)	Fractionary bactericidal concentrations							
	CPZ + gentamicin		CPZ + netilmicin		CPZ + tobramycin		CPZ + amikacin	
	Mean	Range	Mean	Range	Mean	Range	Mean	Range
Escherichia coli (13)	0.7	0.5–1.0	0.9	0.5–1.0	0.5	0.2–0.6	0.7	0.5–1.0
Klebsiella pneumoniae (12)	0.7	0.3–1.0	0.7	0.4–1.0	0.5	0.3–1.0	0.6	0.3–1.0
Proteus rettgeri (8)	0.7	0.3–1.0	0.8	0.3–1.0	0.4	0.3–0.6	0.4	0.1–0.6
Serratia marcescens (12)	0.6	0.3–1.0	0.6	0.2–1.0	0.5	0.1–0.8	0.5	0.2–0.6
Pseudomonas aeruginosa (14)	0.7	0.4–1.0	0.6	0.3–1.0	0.7	0.5–1.0	0.5	0.3–0.8
Mean	0.69		0.70		0.52		0.54	
Range		0.3–1.0		0.2–1.0		0.1–1.0		0.1–1.0

tions) and may be found in every species when optimal combinations are selected. The slightly better effect of the CPZ–tobramycin and CPZ–amikacin combinations was more pronounced when the fractional bactericidal concentrations were calculated. With part of the isolates for which fractional inhibitory concentrations were equal to or below 0.5, synergism could be confirmed by killing curves (e.g., Fig. 1). These in vitro data suggest that combined therapy with CPZ and aminoglycosides—apart from pharmacokinetic and toxicological considerations—may be useful in undiagnosed infections for safer coverage and higher bactericidal action when broad-spectrum effect and high bactericidal activity are necessary.

Pharmacokinetics of Cefoperazone in Neonates After a Single Intravenous Dose

EDWIN L. ANDERSON,* DONALD M. HILLIGOSS, AND ELLEN SZEGO

Schools of Medicine and Pharmacy, West Virginia University, Charleston Division, and Department of Pediatrics and Pathology, Charleston Area Medical Center, Charleston, West Virginia 25304, U.S.A.*

Meningitis in newborn infants caused by gram-negative bacilli has a high mortality rate, and many of the survivors are left with severe neurological impairment (3). Persistently positive cerebrospinal fluid (CSF) cultures have been shown to correlate with a poor prognosis in these patients. Antimicrobial agents that rapidly cure meningitis caused by coliform organisms may improve the outcome in neonates. Currently available antibiotics have several disadvantages: the aminoglycosides penetrate the CSF very poorly, chloramphenicol is not bactericidal against many gram-negative bacilli, and resistance to ampicillin is increasing (3).

Cefoperazone is an investigational cephalosporin. It is more active in vitro against bacterial pathogens than presently available β-lactam antibiotics (1). Laboratory studies have shown it to be active against coliform bacilli recovered from newborns with meningitis (4). It produced a rapid bacteriological response in the CSF in animal studies (2). In studies in normal adults, the serum half-life ($t_{1/2}$) of cefoperazone was twice that of cefamandole and slightly shorter than that of cefazolin (5).

To study the safety and pharmacokinetics of cefoperazone in neonates, we gave a single dose of 50 mg/kg intravenously to patients who were already being treated for suspected sepsis with antibiotics.

Twelve newborn infants, six females and six males, completed studies in the intensive care nursery at Charleston Area Medical Center. Written consent was obtained after informing the parents of the purposes, procedures, and potential hazards of the study.

All infants were being treated with antibiotics for suspected sepsis. The single dose of cefoperazone was substituted for one dose of the penicillin-like antibiotic in the therapeutic regimen. All other therapy was continued throughout the study.

Gestational ages of the study patients ranged from 28 to 40 weeks. Birth weights ranged from 880 to 3,510 g. Nine patients were classified as appropriate in weight for gestational age, and three were small for gestational age. Postnatal age on the study day ranged from 1 to 60 days.

Cefoperazone was reconstituted to a concentration of 250 mg/ml with sterile water for injection. Five percent dextrose in water was used for dilution to 25 mg/ml prior to administration. The dose of 50 mg/kg was intravenously infused over a 10-min period. Serum samples were obtained for cefoperazone assay by heelstick or through available arterial or venous lines. Sampling times were immediately at the end of infusion (zero time) and at 0.5, 1, 2, 4, 8, and 12 h postinfusion. Urine was collected for a 2- to 3-h period at 1 to 4 h after the infusion on four patients. CSF was obtained from four patients at 2 to 3 h postinfusion when lumbar punctures were performed for diagnostic purposes. Serum specimens were centrifuged after collection. All specimens were immediately frozen. Complete blood count, electrolytes, urinalysis, serum creatinine, albumin, total and direct bilirubin, alkaline phosphatase, serum glutamic oxalacetic transaminase, calcium, and phosphorus were obtained within 72 h before and again within 24 h after drug administration.

Cefoperazone concentrations in serum, urine, and CSF were initially determined by a reverse-phase, gradient elution, liquid chromatography procedure at Pfizer Quality Control Division, Groton, Conn. Later in the study, cefoperazone concentrations in serum and CSF were measured by an agar disk diffusion microbioassay method using a strain of *Escherichia coli* from our laboratory. Standards for serum samples were diluted in 25% human serum. Standards for CSF specimens were prepared in pH 6.0 phosphate buffer (4). Three percent sodium chloride was added to the media to inhibit aminoglycoside activity.

The postdistributional phases of the serum concentration time plots were fitted by least-squares exponential regression. Elimination rate constants (K_e) and $t_{1/2}$'s were obtained from this fit. Area under the curve (AUC) for the sampling period after the dose was calculated by the linear trapezoidal rule. AUC from the last serum concentration to infinity was estimated by dividing the last serum concentration by the K_e. Total body clearance (Cl_B) was obtained by dividing the dose by the total area under the curve; Cl_B = 50 mg per kg/AUC (total). Apparent volumes of distribution (V_d) were calculated by dividing the Cl_B by the K_e; $V_d = Cl_B/K_e$. Renal clearances (Cl_R) were obtained by dividing the average excretion rate (ER) for the urine collection interval by the interval midpoint serum concentration; $Cl_R = ER/C_p$ (midpoint).

No clinical or laboratory indications of adverse effects attributable to cefoperazone administration were noted in the study patients.

Correlation coefficients for the least-squares exponential fit of the postdistributional phases of the serum concentration time plots were greater than 0.90 for all reported patients. The mean and standard deviation (M ± SD) of the combined serum concentration time plots is depicted in Fig. 1. After a rapid distributional phase, serum concentrations declined in a monoexponential manner. At cessation of infusion, serum concentrations were (M ± SD) 131 ± 50 μg/ml. Twelve hours postinfusion, serum concentrations were 29 ± 16 μg/ml.

Pharmacokinetic analysis of data from the 12 patients yielded (M ± SD): $t_{1/2}$, 6.9 ± 2.7 h; Cl_B, 53.7 ± 15.6 ml/h per kg; and V_d, 491 ± 120 ml/kg. The individual data and mean values are depicted in Fig. 2. The individual values for Cl_B, V_d, and $t_{1/2}$ are fairly evenly distributed around the group mean with the exception of the single patient represented by open circles in Fig. 2. This patient was born at 28 to 29 weeks of gestation, weighed 880 g at birth, and was classified as small for gestational age. Cefoperazone was administered at 37 days of age. The low Cl_B (18.2 ml/h per kg) and prolonged $t_{1/2}$ (14.1 h) demonstrated by this patient cannot be related to any unique facet of her history, clinical course, or condition on the study day.

Cl_R of cefoperazone ranged from 15.9 to 37.7 ml/h per kg with a M ± SD of 27.9 ± 10.0 ml/h per kg. The proportion of Cl_B that was accounted for by Cl_R varied from 27 to 88%.

Cefoperazone concentrations present in CSF ranged from 1.8 to 5.7 μg/ml. These values represented 2 to 7% of the simultaneous serum concentrations. None of the patients had bacterial meningitis. Protein concentrations ranged from 122 to 310 mg/100 ml (mean, 209 mg/100

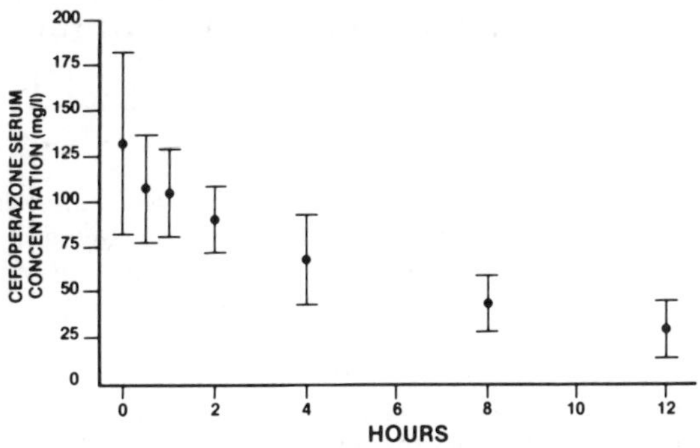

FIG. 1. *Neonatal serum concentrations of cefoperazone after a single intravenous 50-mg/kg dose (mean ± SD, n = 12).*

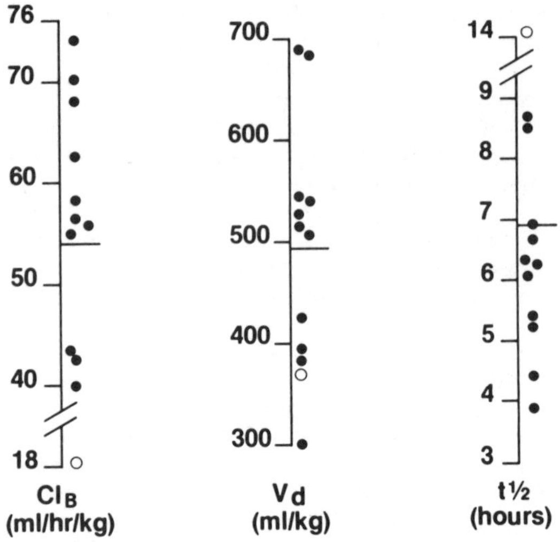

FIG. 2. *Ranges and mean values of the pharmacokinetic parameters for cefoperazone in neonates after a single intravenous 50-mg/kg dose. Open circles represent a patient with a Cl_B (18.2 ml/h per kg) and $t_{1/2}$ (14.1 h) that differed from the group mean by more than 2 SD.*

ml), and leukocytes varied from 0 to 110 cells per mm^3 (mean, 36 cells per mm^3).

The serum concentrations obtained throughout the 12 h of the study were well above the MIC for the more common bacterial pathogens of neonates. The concentrations of cefoperazone in CSF, although low, did exceed the MIC of many of the gram-negative bacilli that cause meningitis in newborn infants. Whether greater penetration of cefoperazone into CSF occurs in the presence of bacterial meningitis is not known. Further trials are needed to determine whether increased CSF concentrations of cefoperazone occur after multiple doses.

Significant amounts of cefoperazone appear to be cleared by neonates through mechanisms other than direct renal elimination. Similar observations have been made in adults (5). Whether these neonatal mechanisms involve metabolism, direct nonrenal elimination, or both is not known. Neonatal hepatic and renal function is considered to be immature relative to the same processes in older patients. Consequently, it is likely that some differences will exist in the pathways of disposition for cefoperazone in these two groups.

At the dose used in this study, cefoperazone did not cause adverse effects. Further trials are indicated to learn more of the safety and pharmacokinetics of cefoperazone in neonates.

1. **Pulliam, L., K. Hadley, and J. Mills.** 1981. In vitro comparison of third-generation cephalosporins, piperacillin, dibekacin, and other aminoglycosides against aerobic bacteria. Antimicrob. Agents Chemother. **19:** 490–492.
2. **Schaad, U. B., G. H. McCracken, C. A. Loock, and M. L. Thomas.** 1981. Pharmacokinetics and bacteriologic efficacy of moxalactam, cefotoxine, cefoperazone, and rocephin in experimental bacterial meningitis. J. Infect. Dis. **143:**156–163.
3. **Schaad, U. B., G. H. McCracken, N. Threlkeld, and M. L. Thomas.** 1981. Clinical evaluation of a new broad-spectrum oxa-beta-lactam antibiotic, moxalactam, in neonates and infants. J. Pediatr. **98:**129–136.
4. **Shelton, S., J. D. Nelson, and G. H. McCracken.** 1980. In vitro susceptibility of gram-negative bacilli from pediatric patients to moxalactam, cefotaxime, Ro 13-9904, and other cephalosporins. Antimicrob. Agents Chemother. **18:**476–479.
5. **Srinivasan, S., E. L. Francke, and H. C. Neu.** 1981. Comparative pharmacokinetics of cefoperazone and cefamandole. Antimicrob. Agents Chemother. **19:**298–301.

Single- and Multiple-Dose Pharmacokinetics and Tissue Levels After Intramuscular Administration of Cefoperazone

P. C. BRAGA,* G. CECCARELLI, F. SCAGLIONE, G. SCARPAZZA, V. GAGLIARDI, L. TESSARI, G. PAIOLA, AND F. FRASCHINI

Institute of Chemotherapy, Faculty of Medicine, and Department of Orthopaedy, St. Raffaele Hospital, University of Milan, Milan, Pediatric Department, University of Pavia, Pavia, INRCA Hospital, Casatenovo, Como, and Urological Division, Treviglio Hospital, Bergamo, Italy*

Cefoperazone is a third-generation semisynthetic parenteral cephalosporin. It has been reported that cefoperazone possesses β-lactamase resistance and quite a broad antimicrobial spectrum against many gram-positive and gram-negative microorganisms and most anaerobes. The pharmacokinetic profile of cefoperazone was examined, in the present study, in a group of patients suffering from chronic bronchopulmonary diseases, to investigate not only serum and urinary levels but also bronchial mucus levels and their correlations.

In the morning of the first treatment day, blood samples were taken immediately before

TABLE 1. *Serum and sputum pharmacokinetic data for cefoperazone after single and multiple administration of 1 g intramuscularly every 12 h (mean ± SD)*

Parameter[a]	Serum		Sputum	
	1st day	7th day	1st day	7th day
Peak (μg/ml)	65.08 ± 5.16	59.02 ± 3.80	0.34 ± 0.10	0.38 ± 0.15
Time to peak (h)	1	1	2	2
C^o_p (μg/ml)	122.72 ± 38.41	146.87 ± 53.03	1.55 ± 1.04	1.63 ± 0.26
K_a (h^{-1})	2.95 ± 2.15	2.60 ± 2.00	0.90 ± 0.58	0.86 ± 0.21
K_e (h^{-1})	0.60 ± 0.06	0.57 ± 0.05	0.63 ± 0.14	0.66 ± 0.50
Half-life (h)	1.22 ± 0.12	1.17 ± 0.09	1.12 ± 0.23	1.05 ± 0.93
AUC (g.h/ml)	150.95 ± 33.10	130.97 ± 35.36	0.80 ± 0.12	1.01 ± 0.22
AVC (liter)	14.16 ± 4.04	11.76 ± 3.07		
Cl_{tot} (liter/h)	8.05 ± 2.22	6.89 ± 1.54		

[a] C^o_p, Peak concentration at the endpoint of administration; K_a, absorption rate constant; K_e, elimination rate constant; AUC, area under the curve; Cl_{tot}, total clearance.

the injection and at 0.25, 0.50, 1, 2, 3, 4, 6, 8, 10, and 12 h after administration. Each patient urinated immediately before drug intake, and all the urine passed thereafter was collected at 2-h intervals during a 12-h period. Samples of bronchial mucus were collected by expectoration 1, 2, 3, 4, 6, 8, 10, and 12 h after administration of the drug.

The collection of samples was repeated with the same procedure at the seventh day of treatment until the 12th h after the last administration.

Serum, urine, and sputum concentrations of cefoperazone were assayed by the Grove and Randall agar diffusion method with *Bacillus subtilis* ATCC 6633 as the test organism.

Pharmacokinetic evaluation, based on the serum level data of each patient, was performed with a first-order one-compartment open model using a curve-fitting computer program.

For each subject the parameters listed in Table 1 were estimated.

The same calculations as above were carried out with the data for bronchial mucus levels.

In a second and third group of volunteers, patients who had to undergo a surgical operation, we determined by the microbiological method previously described bone and prostatic tissue levels at progressive times from the last administration (1 g intramuscularly) of cefoperazone in correlation with serum levels.

Figure 1 shows the semilogarithmic plot of the mean serum and sputum concentrations of cefoperazone against time at the first and seventh days of treatment.

The decline in serum concentrations after the peak appears to have a monoexponential decay at the first and seventh days of treatment.

The comparative plot shows that cefoperazone, at the dose of 1 g every 12 h, does not accumulate over a period of 7 days.

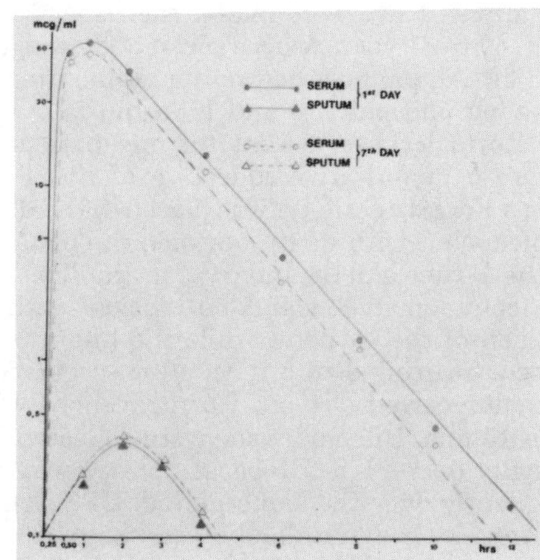

FIG. 1. *Semilogarithmic plot of the mean serum and sputum levels against time at the first and seventh days of treatment with 1 g of cefoperazone every 12 h intramuscularly.*

Pharmacokinetic parameters also reflect this similarity, and there are no statistical differences between data for the first and seventh days (Table 1).

The data on the bronchial mucus levels show that the disappearance curves for the first and the last dose have a monoexponential decay after the peak and are very similar (Table 1).

Cefoperazone reaches levels in bronchial mucus that are approximately the same as those obtained with other cephalosporins.

Urine excretion of cefoperazone was 23% of the administered dose for the first day and 26% for the last day. These amounts appear to be less than one-half of the amounts found for other cephalosporins.

The diffusion of cefoperazone in bone and prostatic tissue was, on average, 7% and 15% of the corresponding serum levels.

Biliary Excretion of Cefoperazone in Humans

B. KEMMERICH,* H. LODE, K. BORNER, G. BELMEGA, T. JENDROSCHEK, G. GOERTZ, AND P. KOEPPE

Medical Department, Klinikum Steglitz, Free University of Berlin, Federal Republic of Germany

Cefoperazone (CPZ) is a cephalosporin with a remarkably low renal elimination rate of 20 to 30% in normal subjects. High bile concentrations indicate the preponderant elimination of this drug via the bile (1, 3).

Six patients requiring T-tube drainage of their common bile duct were studied to assess the biliary tract excretion of CPZ. Four of them were females and two were males; their ages ranged from 40 to 81 years, with a mean body weight of 58.7 kg. All patients had normal renal function. Alkaline phosphatase and bilirubin lay within the normal range, except for one patient. To assure a quantitative collection of the T-tube bile, a Forgaty catheter was placed in the ductus choledochus with its tip between the distal end of the T-tube and the biliary tract papilla. Thus, the common duct could be blocked with the balloon of the catheter while the bile was collected. Starting 3 to 5 days after surgery each patient received 2.0 g of CPZ intravenously (i.v.) over 15 min. Bile and urine were collected fractionally over 24 h. Blood samples were taken frequently over the same period. CPZ concentrations were determined by means of an agar diffusion test and high-performance liquid chromatography (HPLC; values in parentheses). *Bacillus subtilis* ATCC 6633 and *Sarcina lutea* ATCC 9344 were used as test strains for the bioassay. The minimal detectable concentrations ranged from 0.1 mg/liter in bile to 0.6 mg/liter in serum. Relevant pharmacokinetic parameters were calculated by the relative least-squares method, using a digital computer. The program is based on a three-compartment, open-system kinetic model. The concentrations and kinetic parameters were compared with the results of a CPZ 2.0-g pharmacokinetic study in 10 healthy volunteeers. All values were recalculated for 70 kg of body weight. The mean total recovery rate of CPZ (Table 1) in urine and bile was 64.5 ± 15.3% (62.4 ± 15.5%) in 24 h. Of this amount, 18.6 ± 14.0% (11.5 ± 7.1%) was found in the bile, and 45.9 ± 16.2% (50.9 ± 19.7%) could be detected in urine. Peak bile concentrations were measured with 3,642 ± 2,975 mg/liter (2,259 ± 1,337 mg/liter) 2 to 3 h after application of CPZ. During the 10- to 24-h period, the mean bile concentration was 367 ± 368 mg/liter (187 ± 250 mg/liter) (Fig. 1). There seemed to be a compensatory renal elimination of CPZ in patients with biliary tract diseases compared with healthy subjects (45.9 versus 21.4%, 24-h urine recovery). Renal clearance of CPZ was within the same range for patients (mean, 17.9 ml/min) and normal subjects (18.3 ml/min).

The serum levels of CPZ showed a slow decrease in patients, with a long terminal half-life of 380 min ($t_{1/2\gamma}$) from 295 ± 90 mg/liter initially to 62.1 ± 23.6 mg/liter after 4 h, 15.9 ± 11.3 mg/liter after 12 h, and another 2.9 ± 2.8 mg/liter 24 h after injection of the antibiotic. In normal subjects, CPZ was eliminated from the serum with a terminal half-life of 143.5 ± 20 min. After

TABLE 1. *Recovery of CPZ in urine and T-tube bile after 2.0 g i.v. in six patients after cholecystectomy (bioassay, HPLC)*

Recovery of cefoperazone	Bioassay %	HPLC %
Urine	45.9 ± 16.2	50.9 ± 19.7
Bile	18.6 ± 14.0	11.5 ± 7.1
Total	64.5 ± 15.3	62.4 ± 15.5

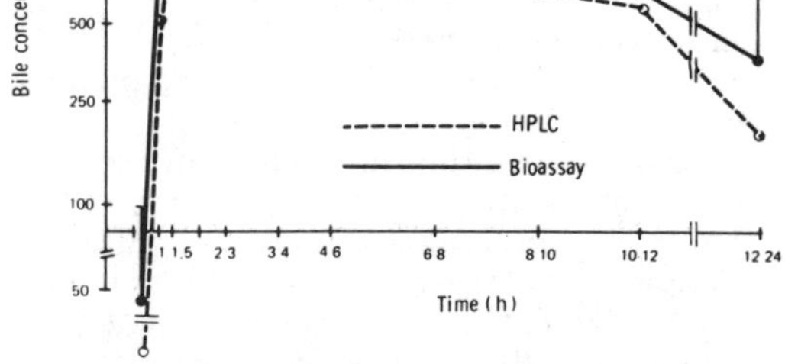

FIG. 1. *T-tube bile concentration of CPZ after 2.0 g i.v. in six patients after cholecystectomy (bioassay, HPLC; mean ± SD).*

the half-hour infusion, serum concentrations decreased much faster than in patients, from 232.8 ± 28.6 mg/liter to 28.5 ± 1.34 mg/liter after 4 h and to 0.28 ± 0.14 mg/liter after 12 h. The two test methods, bioassay and HPLC, showed a good correlation only when determinations were performed soon after the specimens were collected.

The apparent volume of distribution (V_{DSS}) showed comparable values for patients and healthy subjects, 15.7 and 14.5 liters/100 kg, respectively. There was a distinctly significant difference in the area under the serum level curve (AUC_{tot}) between patients (mean, 852 mg.h/liter) and normal subjects (389.7 mg.h/liter).

In summary, only a relatively low percentage of CPZ could be detected in T-tube bile, even by means of a blocking catheter in the common bile duct. The compensatory high urinary elimination and the slow decrease of serum levels with a long terminal half-life indicate the disturbance of hepatobiliary excretion of CPZ in patients with biliary tract diseases. Alkaline phosphatase, γ-glutamyltransferase, and bilirubin are not sensitive parameters for the estimation of the diminished biliary excretion and prolonged half-life of CPZ. The biliary excretion should be much higher in normal subjects.

The CPZ bile concentrations obtained in this study appear to be significantly higher than those of other cephalosporins like cephalothin, cefazolin, and cefamandole (2, 4). On the basis of its microbiological and pharmacokinetic properties, CPZ seems to be a valuable antibiotic for the treatment of biliary tract infections, but accumulation is possible and difficult to predict.

1. **Nakamura, R., I. Hashimoto, Y. Sawada, J. Mikami, E. Bekki, S. Hirasawa, H. Abe, and Y. Watanabe.** 1980. Cefoperazone concentrations in bile and gallbladder wall after intravenous administration. Antimicrob. Agents Chemother. **18:**980–982.
2. **Ratzan, K. R., H. B. Baker, and I. Lauredo.** 1978. Excretion of cefamandole, cefazolin, and cephalothin into T-tube bile. Antimicrob. Agents Chemother. **13:** 985–987.
3. **Shimizu, K.** 1980. Cefoperazone: absorption, excretion, distribution, and metabolism. Clin. Ther. **3**(special issue):60–79.
4. **Waterman, N. G., H. U. Eickenberg, and L. Scharfenberger.** 1976. Concentration of cefamandole in serum and interstitial fluid, bile, and urine. Antimicrob. Agents Chemother. **10:**733–735.

Concentrations of Cefoperazone in Bile and Gallbladder Wall After Intravenous Administration of One or Two Grams

A. KAZMIERCZAK, C. CHANDESRIS, J. P. FAVRE, P. POTHIER, H. PORTIER, AND R. JABOEUF

Faculté de Médecine, 21033 Dijon, France

After some preliminary studies (1, 3; A. Ducroux, P. Pothier, and H. Portier, Program Abstr. Intersci. Conf. Antimicrob. Agents Chemother. 20th, New Orleans, La., abstr. no. 115, 1980), we investigated the human biliary elimination of cefoperazone, a third-generation cephalosporin. Our study was concerned with 14 patients ranging in age from 25 to 80 years and undergoing cholecystectomy for cholelithiasis. These patients had no previous history of allergy to β-lactam agents, and at the time of the investigation they had normal renal and hepatic functions as confirmed by standard laboratory tests.

At the beginning of the operation, 1 g (seven patients) or 2 g (seven patients) of cefoperazone was given by intravenous bolus injection. About 30 min later, the cystic duct was ligated and the common duct was catheterized for manometric investigation and bile collection. In all cases, the gallbladder was removed after 1.5 h.

The gallbladder bile was collected after 1 h by gallbladder puncture. Bile was also collected after 1.5 h from the removed gallbladder when enough bile was present to be used for the determination of antibiotic concentrations. Likewise, common duct bile was collected at the same time, but in some cases the collection at 1.5 h was not possible because of surgical circumstances. The removed gallbladder was opened and cleaned with sterile gauze both before and after a gentle rinse with isotonic saline solution. It was cut into two or more fragments: one was used for histological study, and the other fragments were weighed before being used for antibiotic determination.

Blood samples were also collected at 1 and 1.5 h after injection. All samples were frozen at −20°C and assayed within 3 days.

Cefoperazone concentrations were determined both by microbiological assay with *Bacillus subtilis* ATCC 6633 as the test strain and by high-pressure liquid chromatography (HPLC). The method of extraction for HPLC (2) was based on cefoperazone's solubility in organic solvents when the pH of the medium was lower than the pK_a of cefoperazone (pK_a = 5). Thus, 1 ml of serum or bile or a crushed fragment of gallbladder was mixed with 0.5 ml of HCl (0.4 N) and 7 ml of a solution of chloroform-pentanol (3:1, vol/vol). After checking the pH (<3), the mixture was shaken for 5 min and then centrifuged at 3,000 rpm for 5 min. A volume of 5 ml of the organic layer was transferred into a new tube containing 0.35 ml of phosphate buffer (pH 7.2). After the pH was checked (>5.6), this mixture was again shaken for 5 min and centrifuged at 3,000 rpm for 5 min. The aqueous layer was removed for HPLC assay. HPLC was performed with an apparatus from Waters Associates. After preliminary studies, a solution of acetate buffer (pH 5) and methanol (6.5:3.5, vol/vol) was adopted as a mobile phase with a flow rate of 1.5 ml/min at a pressure of about 150 bars.

Under these experimental conditions, good separation of cefoperazone from the UV-absorbing components of serum, bile, and gallbladder wall was obtained. A good linear relationship was observed between peak height and drug concentration in the standards prepared with pooled human serum or bile.

All results presented in Table 1 were obtained by the HPLC method. It should be noted that similar results were also obtained by bioassay, which was performed on all bile samples and on a total of seven fragments of the four gallbladders which were large enough to be studied by both methods.

In all gallbladder bile samples but one, highest concentrations of cefoperazone were observed at 1 h after administration of the antibiotic. After the injection of 1 or 2 g of cefoperazone, the geometric mean levels in gallbladder bile at 1 h were 63.9 and 313.5 μg/ml, respectively, and in gallbladder wall samples collected at 1.5 h, the levels were 23.5 and 62.9 μg/ml, respectively. In some subjects, it was not feasible to collect common duct bile at 1.5 h; thus, only 1-h samples were available. The highest values may be observed at either 1 or 1.5 h. Therefore, it was not feasible to calculate and compare the geometric mean values of cefoperazone in common duct bile after 1- and 2-g doses. However, the results indicate that even with a 1-g dose very high levels were attained.

There was no direct relationship between concentrations of cefoperazone in the gallbladder bile, gallbladder wall, or blood. It may be hypothesized that the lack of a direct relationship is related to the passage of cefoperazone from the common duct bile (with its high concentrations) to the gallbladder bile because the cystic duct was ligated only 0.5 h after the cefoperazone injection. However, low concentrations were observed in gallbladder bile and high concentrations were observed in common duct bile and vice versa. Another possibility may be that the concentrations of cefoperazone in gallbladder bile come from the gallbladder blood supply. In this case the concentration of the antibiotic would be related to the vascular conditions of the gallbladder. Work is in progress to attempt to correlate our results in this study with histological findings. In conclusion, cefoperazone is a broad-spectrum antibiotic. Its concentrations in the biliary tract are well in excess of the concentrations required to inhibit the majority of the bacteria responsible for biliary tract infections, including bacteria which are β-lactamase pro-

TABLE 1. *Concentrations of cefoperazone after 1 and 2 g administered by intravenous bolus injection as determined by high-pressure liquid chromatography*

Dose (g)	Subject no.	Gallbladder bile (μg/ml)		Common duct bile (μg/ml)		Gallbladder wall (μg/g),	Serum (μg/ml)	
		1 h	1.5 h	1 h	1.5 h	1.5 h	1 h	1.5 h
1	1	2.1	13.2	3,106	3,412	30.9	84.4	62.2
	2	27.1	—	683.7	—	17.6	90.1	70.6
	3	30.0	—	1,888	—	11.0	—	—
	4	63.0	34.1	1,075	3,676	34.1	100.2	83.2
	5	178.8	—	4,016	—	22.5	—	—
	6	323.1	127.2	2,585	1,731	56.1	130.5	103.2
	7	683.2	512.3	2,197	1,562	16.9	93.7	90.2
2	8	55.0	38.1	2,840	6,598	68.1	166.1	148.2
	9	112.0	63.1	1,243	—	15.1	403.1	152.2
	10	254.5	177.4	553.5	800	67.3	84.2	62.6
	11	288.6	—	480.7	—	86.2	96.3	72.1
	12	426.0	—	100.3	2,308	200.3	126.4	87.8
	13	727.0	—	3,341	—	28.7	100.4	86.8
	14	2,262	1,681	2,780	1,603	124.9	80.6	73.3

ducers. Thus, the administration of cefoperazone seems particularly suitable for the treatment of biliary tract infections. Compared with the 1-g dose, the 2-g dose gave concentrations three times as high in the gallbladder wall and five times as high in the gallbladder bile. Thus, the 2-g dose is recommended.

1. **Aoki, N., O. Sekine, Y. Usuda, T. Shimizu, Y. Hirasawa, and T. Aoki.** 1980. Serum, urine and bile levels of cefoperazone (T-1551), p. 159–161. *In* J. D. Nelson and C. Grassi (ed.), Currrent chemotherapy and infectious disease. American Society for Microbiology, Washington, D.C.
2. **Brisson, A. M., and J. B. Fourtillan.** 1981. Determination of cephalosporins in biological material by reversed-phase liquid column chromatography. J. Chromatogr. **223:**393–399.
3. **Nakamura, T., I. Hashimoto, Y. Sawada, J. Mikami, E. Bekki, S. Hirasawa, H. Abe, and Y. Watanabe.** 1980. Cefoperazone concentrations in bile and gallbladder wall after intravenous administration. Antimicrob. Agents Chemother. **18:**980–982.

Lung Tissue Concentrations of Cefoperazone

J. AYARRA,* C. GARCIA IGLESIAS, J. LOSCERTALES, AND E. J. PEREA

Departments of Microbiology and Thoracic Surgery, University of Seville Medical School, Seville, Spain

We administered cefoperazone to 12 patients subjected to lung surgery, 10 males and 2 females (age range, 22 to 68; weight range, 68 to 78 kg). Cefoperazone was given in a dose of 1 g intravenously (i.v.) 1 h before taking the first lung biopsy. From each patient we removed two biopsies of lung tissue, separated by an interval of 1 h. All were considered macroscopically healthy. Samples of 10 ml of peripheral blood were collected at the same time. The lung biopsies were treated by trituration at 8,500 rpm in a Sorvall Omnimixer (1). Antibiotic levels were determined by a diffusion method, with *Sarcina lutea* ATCC 9341 as the reference strain and Mueller-Hinton agar.

The general distribution volume (GDV) was obtained by the exponential method, first applying the exponential formula $C = C_0 \cdot e^{-kt}$, where C is the concentration in time t, C_0 is the concentration at time zero, and e^{-kt} is the mathematical value of the curve. We then used the general formula $V = Q/C$, where Q is the dose of antibiotic, C is the serum concentration of antibiotic, and V is the distribution volume.

The relative histospecific volume distribution (RHVD) was obtained from the following formula:

$$\text{RHVD} = \frac{\text{tissue levels } (\mu\text{g/ml})}{\text{serum levels } (\mu\text{g/g})} = 1$$

and to adjusted values, for eliminating the fraction of antibiotic in the homogenate belonging to serum, the method of Lowry and Hastings (4) modified for us, was applied:

(i) Serum
concentration of antibiotic---Hb patient

X---Hb tissue

$$X = \frac{\text{Serum concentration of antibiotic} \times \text{Hb tissue}}{\text{Hb patient}}$$

(ii) Concentration obtained in tissue supernatant $- X =$ concentration of antibiotic in tissue (adjusted value)

In those patients treated with cefoperazone, very high serum levels were obtained at the 1st hour, varying from 23.73 to 40.1 μg/ml (mean, 32.18 ± 1.57 μg/ml). At the 2nd hour, the levels varied from 12.6 to 39.2 μg/ml (mean, 22.85 ± 2.36 μg/ml). The GDV obtained by using the exponential method for cefoperazone varied from 8.02 to 15.66 liters (mean, 11.83 ± 0.77 liters).

The unadjusted concentrations in lung tissue of cefoperazone varied in the 1st hour from 14.5 to 56 μg/g (mean, 30.37 ± 3.38 μg/g) and in the 2nd hour from 6 to 33 μg (mean, 15.74 ± 2.54 μg/g). The adjusted values varied in the 1st hour from 11.39 to 52.87 μg/g (mean, 27.78 ± 3.74 μg/g) and in the 2nd hour from 4.82 to 28.44 μg/g (mean, 13.83 ± 1.85 μg/g).

The unadjusted RHVD values in the 1st hour varied from 0.49 to 2 (mean, 0.96 ± 0.12), and in the 2nd hour they varied from 0.31 to 1.63 (mean, 0.70 ± 0.10). The adjusted values varied in the 1st hour from 0.34 to 1.76 (mean, 0.88 ± 0.12), whereas those in the 2nd hour varied from 0.22 to 1.54 (mean, 0.59 ± 0.11).

We have considered the body kinetically as a bicompartmental model. From all existing methods for measuring GDV, we believe the exponential method based on the formula $C = C_0 \cdot e^{-kt}$ to be more exact. For tissue values, we wish to differentiate between the unadjusted values obtained directly from the straight-line graph, without deducting the blood content of the homogenized lung tissue from the adjusted values obtained by allowing for the hemoglobin content the tissue, as we consider this latter value to be more accurate.

Also, we believe it to be of value to calculate the RHVD applied to the two types of values where a value of unity indicates uniform distribution of the antibiotic, as with cefoperazone. A value of greater than unity indicates that the concentration is higher in tissue, and a value of less than unity indicates that the concentration is greater in serum.

1. **Ayarra, J., C. Garcia Iglesias, J. Loscertales, and E. J. Perea.** 1980. Lung tissue concentrations of Cefoxitine. Abstr. III Mediterranean Congress of Chemotherapy, Nice.
2. **Brodie, B. B., and J. Axelrod.** 1950. The fate of antipyrine in man. J. Pharmacol. Exp. Ther. 87–98.
3. **Butler, I.** 1971. The distribution of drugs. *In* B. N. Ladu, H. G. Mandel, and E. L. Way (ed.), Fundamentals of drug metabolism and drug disposition. The Williams & Wilkins Co., Baltimore.
4. **Lowry, O. H., and A. R. Hastings.** 1942. Histochemical changes associated with aging. I. Methods and calculations. J. Biol. Chem. **145**:257–269.

Bone Concentrations of Six New β-Lactam Antibiotics

DIETMAR H. WITTMANN* AND HANS-H. SCHASSAN

Department of Surgery, Altona General Hospital, 2000 Hamburg 50, and Institute for Immunology and Medical Microbiology, University Hospital Hamburg Eppendorf, Hamburg University, 2000 Hamburg 19, Federal Republic of Germany*

The value of measurements of bone concentrations of drugs is impaired by methodological problems. One problem is the amount of blood within the bone sample which is measured with the bone concentration. This error leads to false-positive results. The blood originates from the intravascular bone compartment and additionally, to a higher degree, from contamination of the bone sample with operative blood at the time of sampling. Plaue et al. (2) were able to show with the dextran method that this error accounts for 5 to 10%. In our investigations special care was taken not to contaminate the spongy bone with additional blood at the time of surgery. The error resulting from intravascular blood of the bone specimen alone accounts in our investigations for only 2 to 3% false-positive results. Another methodological problem is the uncertainty of indirect measurements of the bone concentration in the eluate (1). In humans, bone concentration cannot be assessed directly in the bone itself. It is measured in a phosphate buffer into which antibiotics are eluted from small bone pieces until equilibrium between bone concentration and concentration in the supernatant fluid is reached. It has been questioned whether the concentration in the eluate is really representative of the actual concentration in bone (1). To date, all investigators related the concentration in the eluate to the total bone weight, which is expressed in milligrams per kilogram. The fact that some antibiotics do not penetrate into inorganic bone (hydroxylapatite) was not considered. This resulted in relatively low cortical bone concentrations compared with the results obtained in spongy bone. The reason for this is the relatively high specific weight of cortical bone due to its high content of minerals (hydroxylapatite).

The present study was designed to investigate the penetration of β-lactam antibiotics, gentamicin, and tetracyclines into inorganic bone. On the basis of these findings, bone concentrations were determined and, if there was no penetration into inorganic bone, the concentrations measured in the eluate were related to the organic bone compartment, which is expressed in units per volume (milligrams per liter) rather than in units per weight (milligrams per kilogram).

Bone samples were obtained during artificial hip joint replacements from the femoral head and the femoral trochanter. The following groups were investigated: 16 patients (mean age, 64.3 years) after 1.5 g of cefuroxime intravenously (i.v.), 12 patients (mean age, 63.8 years) after 2 g of cefoxitin (i.v.), 19 patients (mean age, 65.7 years) after 2 g of cefotaxime (i.v.), 8 patients (mean age, 71.3 years) after 2 g of moxalactam i.v., 10 patients (mean age, 69.1 years) after 2 g of cefoperazone i.v., and 12 patients (mean age, 58.4 years) after 2 g of ceftazidime i.v. The bone samples were frozen immediately after sampling, together with the serum samples, at −20 to −25°C. The standard for microbiological assay was prepared at the time of sampling to obviate any error which might have occurred as a result of loss of activity during storage. The test organisms for microbiological assay were *Sarcina lutea* ATCC 6633 for cefuroxime and cefoxitin and *Escherichia coli* 6311/65 for the other four antibiotics. The bone sample was divided, one part for microbiological assay and the other for the determination of the organic bone compartment by peroxide maceration (3). For this purpose the bone sample was dissolved in 6.5% sodium peroxide solution at 50°C for 2.5 h. After removal from the solution, the specimen was washed twice in distilled water for 2 h and a third time for 16 h and was then dried at 30°C for 24 h. The weight of the remaining specimen—pure hydroxylapatite—was then subtracted from the total bone weight, the difference representing the organic bone part. No hydroxylapatite was found in the solutions.

The first bone specimen was crushed with a mill at 2,000 rpm to small pieces and then eluted in phosphate buffer (pH 7) for 22 h until equilibrium was reached. The concentration in the eluate was then related to the organic bone part rather than to the entire bone, since we were able to show that β-lactam antibiotics do not penetrate into organic bone. For this purpose we reversed the elution. Hydroxylapatite from femoral head and also that available commercially (Merck no. 11490) were imbued with phosphate buffer containing 20 mg of the antibiotics per liter for 48 h. The concentrations in the supernatant fluid were then measured after 2, 4, 8, 24, and 48 h. It was found that after 8 h 50% of gentamicin and 87.5% of the tetracycline were lost from the fluid. The comparison with the standard showed that these substances must have been incorporated into hydroxylapatite. After 48 h, 85% of gentamicin and 99.75% of the tetracycline were lost, whereas the β-lactam antibiotics did not penetrate into inorganic mineral bone compartment. Therefore, we related the concentrations found with the β-lactam antibiotics to the organic bone part. As a consequence, the difference between concentrations of cortical and spongy bone was reduced to values without any statistical significance (Table 1).

In Fig. 1 the geometric means with SD of all bone concentrations measured within the first 2 h after i.v. bolus injection are presented for the six antibiotics investigated. Cefoperazone reached the highest concentrations of all antibiotics investigated. This is surprising since this substance is highly protein bound and poor tissue penetration is expected during the first period after the injection (4). Factors explaining this phenomenon are to be investigated further. The concentrations of ceftazidime and moxalactam were superior compared with the bone concentrations of cefuroxime, cefoxitin, and cefotaxime. Also, the SD with these newer β-lactam agents was low compared with the results with cefotaxime, cefuroxime, and cefoxitin. The reason for this is that we did measure the organic bone part for each individual sample in the cefoperazone, moxalactam, and ceftazidime study whereas with the other three antibiotics the results obtained and expressed in units per weight were multiplied by a factor giving the mean relation of total bone to organic bone which had been calculated from 73 samples. Therefore, the SD is that obtained with the first results in milligrams per kilogram. This SD was not reduced by computing each sample for measurements of organic bone concentration.

TABLE 1. *Geometric mean of bone concentrations in milligrams per liter after bolus injection of six β-lactam antibiotics*

Dose	Bone concn (mg/liter)					
	60 min after bolus injection			120 min after bolus injection		
	Sample *n*	Mean	SD	Sample *n*	Mean	SD
Cefuroxime, 1.5 g i.v.	48	15.0	2.27	26	8.5	2.24
Cefoxitin, 2.0 g i.v.	37	9.8	1.80	16	8.6	2.19
Cefotaxime, 2.0 g i.v.	28	8.4	2.22	41	5.7	2.75
Moxalactam, 2.0 g i.v.	10	19.4	1.43	10	19.1	1.16
Cefoperazone, 2.0 g i.v.	16	39.7	1.29	12	32.8	1.20
Ceftazidime, 2.0 g i.v.	18	31.1	1.49	30	23.4	1.37

From the serum concentrations of each antibiotic, pharmacokinetic parameters were evaluated by use of the computer program NONLIN of Metzler (1974) to facilitate nonlinear regression of the serum level/time data. The data fitted an open two-compartment model. The concentrations observed were slightly above those observed in young healthy volunteers. Therefore, the calculated elimination half-life ($T/2\ \beta$) was prolonged as follows: cefuroxime (n = 91 serum samples), $T/2\ \beta = 101$ min; cefoxitin ($n = 97$), $T/2\ \beta = 68$ min; cefotaxime ($n = 299$), $T/2\ \beta = 103$ min; moxalactam ($n = 249$), $T/2\ \beta = 184$ min; cefoperazone ($n = 110$), $T/2\ \beta = 429$

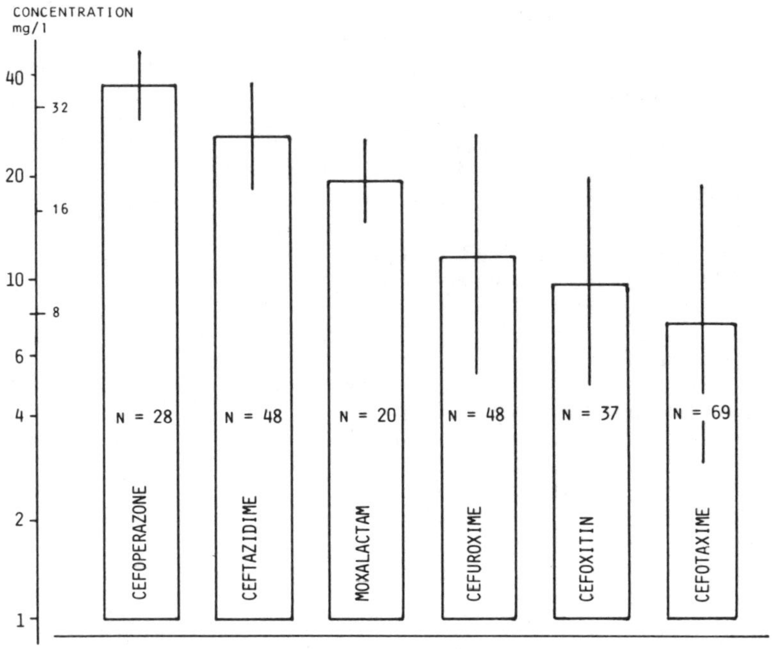

FIG. 1. *Bone concentration 30 to 120 min after i.v. bolus injection of six β-lactam antibiotics.*

min; and ceftazidime (n = 160), T/2 β = 121 min.

The prolonged serum half-life in older patients is a known phenomenon. However, the difference in the cefoperazone measurements is surprising. Whereas most β-lactam antibiotics are cleared from the body by renal excretion, cefoperazone's main route of elimination is biliary. Possibly in older patients the liver function is more impaired, as is known to be true of renal function, yielding extremely prolonged serum half-lives in the older age group. However, this different pharmacokinetic behavior is important with respect to the clinical use of the antibiotics, since most patients in hospitals suffering from infection are of the older age group. Therefore, the results presented here may be used as a guideline for the treatment of infections in this age group.

1. **Dornbusch, K., H. Hugo, and A. Lidstöm.** 1980. Antibacterial activity of cefuroxime in human bone. Scand. J. Infect. Dis. **12:**49–53.
2. **Plaue, R., R. O. Bethge, K. Fabricius, and O. Müller.** 1980. Kritische Untersuchungen zur Methodik von Antibiotika-Spiegelbestimmungen in menschlichen Geweben. Arzeneim. Forsch. Drug Res. **30:**1–5.
3. **Wittmann, D. H., H.-H. Schassan, F. Kohler, and H. Seidel.** 1981. Zur Frage der Penetration von Moxalactam in den Knochen. Unfallchirurgie **7:**142–146

Cefoperazone as a Prophylactic Antibiotic Regimen in Abdominal Hysterectomy

STANLEY A. GALL, W. ALLEN ADDISON, AND GALE B. HILL

Department of Obstetrics and Gynecology, Duke University Medical Center, Durham, North Carolina 27710, U.S.A.

Interest in antibiotic prophylaxis for obstetrical and gynecological surgery has been present for approximately 15 years. The basis for the rational use of prophylactic antibiotics was reported earlier by Burke (2). The reports of efficacy of prophylactic antibiotics in cesarean section has been studied at our institution (4) and has been summarized by Mead (5). This summary lists a febrile morbidity of 51% for placebo patients as compared with 21% for patients in the antibiotic group and a similar decrease in pelvic or wound infection of 30% versus 11% in the placebo and antibiotic groups.

Although an interest in the use of prophylactic antibiotics for abdominal hysterectomy exists, the published studies show less consistency in their support (1). The efficacy of the use of prophylactic antibiotics in modified radical gynecological surgery has been demonstrated (3).

The objectives of this investigation were to evaluate the safety and effectiveness of cefoperazone administration as a prophylactic regimen in patients undergoing abdominal hysterectomy. The study was a randomized blind investigation in which cefamandole and a placebo were included as additional study and control arms. Patients who were admitted to Duke University Medical Center for abdominal hysterectomy were given the opportunity to volunteer for this study. Complete blood count, urinalysis, automated Chemistry 18, direct Coombs test, and platelet count were obtained preoperatively and on the second day postoperatively. The medication was administered as follows: cefoperazone, 2.0 g intravenously (i.v.) on call to the operating room and 12 and 24 h postoperatively; cefamandole, 2.0 g i.v. on call and 6, 12, 18, and 24 h postoperatively; placebo i.v. on call and 6, 12, 18, and 24 h postoperatively.

The evaluation of the patients receiving the active drugs and placebo was based on febrile morbidity, serious infections, wound healing, number of postoperative days in the hospital, and number of patients requiring additional antibiotics. Febrile morbidity was defined as a temperature elevation of 38.0°C or greater on any 2 days excluding the first 24 h postoperative or other signs of obvious infection. Serious infections included wound infections, pelvic peritonitis, pelvic abscess, septicemia, and septic thrombophlebitis. Antibiotic concentrations were determined in uterine tissue and peripheral blood when the uterus was removed.

Forty-eight patients were included in this preliminary report, with 16 patients in each of the drug groups and the placebo group. The entire study will include 240 patients. No patient demonstrated hepatic, renal, or hematological aberrations due to the administration of either study drug. Minor side effects such as rash or pruritus or major side effects such as anaphylaxis were not observed.

The three groups were similar with respect to racial distribution, age, weight, and parity. Of the 16 patients in the cefoperazone and cefamandole groups, 3 (18.8%) developed febrile morbidity, but none developed serious infections, whereas patients in the placebo group developed febrile morbidity in 10 of 16 (62.5%) and serious infections in 4 of 16 (25%). The antibiotic groups showed significant differences in febrile morbidity as well as serious infections when compared with the placebo group ($P < 0.01$, chi square analysis).

The four serious infections in the placebo group included patients with the diagnosis of pelvic abscess, wound infection, vaginal cuff infection, and pelvic peritonitis. *Bacteroides bivius*, *Peptostreptococcus anaerobius*, *Peptococcus asaccharolyticus*, and group B beta-hemolytic streptococcus were cultured from the patient with a pelvic abscess at the time of surgical re-exploration. The wound infection yielded *Staphylococcus aureus* and group B beta-hemolytic streptococcus. The vaginal cuff infections and the pelvic peritonitis patients were not cultured.

The effect of prophylactic antibiotics was seen on postoperative hospitalization. The patients in the cefoperazone and cefamandole groups were hospitalized 5.8 ± 1.1 and 5.8 ± 0.9 days, respectively, whereas the patients in the placebo group stayed 8.5 ± 4.3 postoperative days ($P < 0.05$). No differences were noted in the patients who did not become infected.

The prevention of serious postoperative infections in patients undergoing major surgical procedures is an excellent goal. Since a major source of bacterial contamination, the vagina, is entered during abdominal hysterectomy, the opportunity for massive bacterial contamination exists. Since the results from previous studies employing prophylactic antibiotics in abdominal hysterectomy have been mixed, the results attained in the study may be important. The patients in the combined drug groups had significantly less febrile morbidity and fewer serious infections than the patients in the placebo group. The number of patients in this study is very small, and a final interpretation must be based on the entire study of 240 patients. The incidence of development of a serious infection by 4 of 16 patients receiving a placebo is consistent with other studies done at our institution.

This preliminary study suggests a significant benefit to the gynecological patient who undergoes preoperative administration of either cefoperazone or cefamandole when compared with a placebo. The incidence of febrile morbidity, serious infection, postoperative hospital days, and patients receiving postoperative antibiotics is significantly less in those receiving preoperative antibiotics. No adverse effects have been observed. This preliminary study supports the concept that cefoperazone and cefamandole are efficacious as a prophylactic agent in abdominal hysterectomy.

1. **Allen, J. L., J. F. Rampone, and C. R. Wheeless.** 1972. Use of a prophylactic antibiotic in elective major gynecologic operations. Obstet. Gynecol. **39**:218–224.
2. **Burke, J. F.** 1963. Preoperative antibiotics. Surg. Clin. North Am. **43**:665–676.
3. **Creasman, W. T., G. B. Hill, and S. A. Gall.** The use of prophylactic antibiotics in extended gynecological surgery. Obstet. Gynecol., in press.
4. **Gall, S. A.** 1979. The efficacy of prophylactic antibiotics in cesarean section. Am. J. Obstet. Gynecol. **134**:506–511.
5. **Mead, P. D.** 1977. Prophylactic antibiotics and antibiotic resistance. Semin. Perinatol. **1**:101–111.

Clinical Experience and In Vitro Activity of Cefoperazone Compared with That of Newer Cephalosporins

S. BREYER, W. GRANINGER, C. SCHMIDBAUER, C. SPISS, H. KOLLARITSCH, H. PICHLER, AND K. H. SPITZY

Department of Chemotherapy, Department of Anesthesia and General Intensive Care, University of Vienna, Vienna, Austria

The antibacterial spectrum of the recently developed cephalosporins has been remarkably extended to include most members of the *Enterobacteriaceae* family and, in the case of cefoperazone, *Pseudomonas aeruginosa* as well. We have compared the spectrum of activity of the newer cephalosporins against clinical isolates which were resistant to cephalothin, the classical cephalosporin. We have further applied cefoperazone in patients with severe infections who did not respond to therapy with conventional antibacterial drugs.

We compared the in vitro activity of cefoperazone with that of cefamandole, cefoxitin, and cefotaxime against a variety of 700 gram-positive and gram-negative bacterial strains. Susceptibility testing was carried out by agar diffusion test on DST agar. The antibiotic susceptibility disks used for the study were 30-μg disks of all cephalosporins and were provided by the manufacturers. The breakpoint for susceptibility was a zone 18 mm in diameter for cefamandole, cefoxitin, and cefoperazone and 25 mm for cefotaxime. The results of in vitro susceptibility testing are shown in Table 1. Against cephalothin-resistant *Staphylococcus aureus* strains, cefamandole was the most active compound, followed by cefoperazone. Against *Escherichia coli*, cefotaxime showed the highest activity. Cefoperazone and cefotaxime exhibited excellent activity against indole-positive *Proteus* species.

With regard to the susceptibility of *Enterobacter* strains, the low activity of cefoxitin was remarkable in contrast to the high activity of cefoperazone. *Serratia* species, which cause the most severe nosocomial infections in our intensive care units, show increasing resistance to the formerly very active cefoxitin. Cefotaxime and cefoperazone seem now to be the drugs of choice in infections due to *Serratia* species. Cefoperazone exhibited excellent activity against most gram-positive and gram-negative bacteria, but the susceptibility of *Klebsiella pneumoniae* strains to cefoperazone was surprisingly low. *Acinetobacter* strains, which represent a serious problem in our burn department because of mul-

TABLE 1. *In vitro susceptibility of clinical isolates resistant to cephalothin (n = 700)*

Bacterium	No. of strains	Susceptible strains (%)				
		Cefuroxime	Cefamandole	Cefoxitin	Cefotaxime	Cefoperazone
S. aureus	159	57	84	41	58	70
E. coli	77	88	86	75	99	91
P. mirabilis	81	89	68	81	97	91
Indole-positive *Proteus* spp.	95	60	71	87	98	98
Enterobacter spp.	127	60	44	16	73	83
S. marcescens	64	22	41	75	95	95
Klebsiella spp.	38	84	58	95	100	68
Acinetobacter spp.	43	35	19	49	70	74
Citrobacter spp.	16	40	40	33	73	80

tiresistance, were to a high degree susceptible to cefoperazone. Once again, cefamandole turned out to be the weakest of the newer cephalosporins with regard to cephalothin-resistant gram-negative bacteria. The activity of cefoperazone against *P. aeruginosa* was compared with that of carbenicillin, ticarcillin, azlocillin, cefsudolin, gentamicin, tobramycin and amikacin. Of 300 *P. aeruginosa* strains, 95% were susceptible to the two cephalosporins. The outstanding activity of the cephalosporins cefsulodin and cefoperazone against *P. aeruginosa* strains which were resistant to carbenicillin, the previous standard drug for *Pseudomonas* infections, was remarkable, with 83% of the strains susceptible.

Clinically, we treated a total of 70 patients with cefoperazone. The diagnoses are listed in Table 2. Fifty-five patients received 2 g of cefoperazone twice daily. Fifteen patients with life-threatening infections such as septicemia, peritonitis, and pancreatic abscesses were treated with 4 g twice daily. The average duration of treatment was 10 days in acute pyelonephritis, pneumonia, and cholangitis. In other infections treatment with cefoperazone was given until systemic and local signs of infection subsided, accompanied by eradication of the causative pathogens (median, 14 days). All patients were monitored daily by clinical assessment and control of laboratory parameters such as hemogram and liver and kidney function.

Of the 10 patients treated for septicemia, 8 patients showed a favorable response. Patient 1, a 65-year-old woman suffering from colon carcinoma, developed septicemia due to a complicated urinary tract infection. Her renal creatinine clearance was about 20 ml/min. She recovered within 2 days after a daily dose of 4 g. Patient 2, a 35-year-old man, had granulocytopenia due to a previous cytostatic treatment. He developed septicemia caused by *S. aureus* and was treated with 4 g of cefoperazone twice daily. In spite of clinical improvement, the organism could still be recovered from blood cultures until day 7 of therapy.

TABLE 2. *Overall clinical results of cefoperazone treatment*

Diagnosis	No.	Cure	Improved	Failure
Septicemia	10	7	1	2
Pneumonia	12	9	1	2
Cholangitis	6	6	—	—
Peritonitis and intraabdominal infection	8	6	1	1
Sinusitis and otitis	4	2	—	2
Osteomyelitis	1	—	—	1
Soft tissue infection	4	3	1	—
Upper urinary tract infection	25	17		8
Total	70	50	4	16

Case 3, a young man with bone marrow aplasia, had metastatic abscesses from which *P. aeruginosa* could be grown. He responded surprisingly well to 8 g per day. Patient 8, a young man with extensive burns, acquired pneumonia due to *P. aeruginosa*. This strain was resistant to all penicillins and aminoglycosides. Despite appropriate in vitro susceptibility to cefoperazone, the patient did not respond to therapy and died because of respiratory failure. In patients with purulent cholangitis whose pathogens were isolated from bile obtained by gastroscopy, excellent clinical effects were seen. A dosage of 2 g twice a day was sufficient in five of six patients. Patient 6, with multiple calculi in the biliary tract and infection due to *P. aeruginosa*, had clinical signs of sepsis and was cured by 8 g per day.

Twenty-five patients with urinary tract infection received cefoperazone, 2 g twice a day, for a period of 10 days. We defined urinary tract infection as significant bacteriuria, leukocyturia, and symptoms such as fever, granulocytosis, and pain in the renal region. Early morning urine was obtained by the midstream clean-catch method. Urine bacteriology was carried out before, during, and at the end of treatment. Therapy was assessed as successful if 6 weeks after the end of treatment no significant numbers of organisms could be demonstrated in urine. In 24 of 25 cases the causative pathogens could be eliminated. Seven patients showed a relapse within 6 weeks and were considered as failures. These 7 patients were all suffering from obstructive kidney disease. In one patient with *P. aeruginosa* infection, the bacteria could not be eliminated.

Nine of 12 patients with pneumonia were cured, and one patient improved after treatment with cefoperazone. In these patients the criteria for cure were based on clinical parameters such as defervescence and radiological improvement. No bacterial cultures could be obtained because of lack of cooperation and the advanced age of the patients.

Among the patients with peritonitis or intraabdominal infections, only one patient with liver abscesses due to *S. aureus* failed to respond to therapy with 4 g of cefoperazone per day.

With regard to our patients with sinusitis and otitis, we want to stress that in two patients the infection caused by *P. aeruginosa* could not be eradicated despite a dose of 8 g per day. The overall clinical results show that 77% of our patients were cured by treatment with cefoperazone.

Adverse effects of cefoperazone treatment

were diarrhea in eight patients and nausea in two patients. Two patients developed a macular rash, and three patients who drank wine secretly developed a disulfiram-like reaction with facial flush and nausea. The intravenous injections were well tolerated by all patients, and there were no complaints about local pain or phlebitis.

In conclusion, we consider cefoperazone, with its excellent in vitro antibacterial activity, particularly against *P. aeruginosa*, an interesting new compound. Clinically, good results were obtained in infections due to *Enterobacteriaceae*. Although we treated only five patients with infections due to *S. aureus*, the failure to eradicate this organism in four cases deserves further clarification. The cure rate in patients with infections due to *P. aeruginosa* was satisfying regarding the underlying diseases such as obstructive urinary tract infection, burns, and neoplasia. The high frequency of diarrhea which we found in our series might be due to the high biliary excretion of the drug.

Treatment of Gram-Negative Bacillary Septicemia with Cefoperazone

MARIO CRUCIANI, HJALMAR LAGAST, PHILIPPE VAN DER AUWERA, FRANÇOISE MEUNIER-CARPENTIER, AND JEAN KLASTERSKY

Department of Medicine, Institut Jules Bordet, Université Libre de Bruxelles, Brussels, Belgium

We report here our experience with cefoperazone used as empirical monotherapy of sepsis in cancer and neurosurgical patients. Cefoperazone is a third-generation cephalosporin which is active on a large number of gram-negative bacilli, some anaerobes (except *Bacteroides fragilis*), and *Staphylococcus aureus*. A long serum half-life allows the drug to be administered twice a day. Nephrotoxicity has not been described.

The open study described here at present includes 29 patients with gram-negative bacillary septicemia. Patients were randomized into two groups according to the method of administration of the daily dose of 4 g of cefoperazone. The first group received 2 g of cefoperazone twice daily. The antibiotic was dissolved in 50 ml of 5% dextrose in water and was infused over 15 min. This group received so called "intermittent therapy." The other group received "continuous therapy." Therapy was started with a loading dose of 1 g of cefoperazone dissolved in 50 ml of 5% dextrose in water, which was infused in 15 min and was immediately followed by a continuous infusion of cefoperazone. This additional dose of 3 g of cefoperazone was dissolved in 1 liter of 5% dextrose in water and administered via a constant-flow infusion pump for the remainder of the first 24 h. On the subsequent days of therapy, 4 g of cefoperazone was dissolved in 1 liter of 5% dextrose in water and infused continuously over 24 h. Therapy was completed when the patient made clinical recovery and was afebrile for at least 72 h.

There were 21 men and 8 women; ages ranged from 37 to 76 years, with a median of 60 years. Twenty-four patients had cancer as underlying disease, four had a noncancerous neurosurgical pathology, and one had hydronephrosis due to retroperitoneal fibrosis.

Twelve of the 29 septicemias had *Escherichia coli* as causative pathogen. *Proteus* spp. and *Klebsiella* spp. were also frequently isolated. Table 1 shows the various pathogens isolated from the blood cultures and their related primary focus of infection.

The initial site of infection was the urinary tract in 10 of 29 patients. All but one of these patients had a favorable outcome. Despite intensive research, most of the primary focuses of infection remained unknown.

Twenty-two of the 29 treatments (76%) were successful. There were 11 favorable outcomes in

TABLE 1. *Initial site of infection and related pathogens*

Site	No.	Pathogen	No.
Urinary tract	10	*Escherichia coli*	4
		Proteus mirabilis	3
		Acinetobacter sp.	1
		Proteus morganii	
		Klebsiella pneumoniae	1
Bronchopneumonia	1	*Enterobacter* sp.	
Endocarditis	1	*Escherichia coli*	
Venous catheter	1	*Citrobacter freundii*	
Unknown	16	*Escherichia coli*	7
		Salmonella typhimurium	2
		Acinetobacter sp.	1
		Edwardsiella tarda	1
		Klebsiella pneumoniae	2
		Pseudomonas aeruginosa	1
		Proteus morganii	1
		Proteus mirabilis	1

each therapy group: 14 patients randomized to an intermittent infusion and 15 to the continuous therapy.

Seven patients failed on cefoperazone therapy. Two patients died while on therapy; three underwent superinfections with pathogens resistant to cefoperazone, two of which were new septicemias (*Acinetobacter* sp., *Bacteroides fragilis*). Another patient deteriorated after 48 h of therapy, and the last patient who failed refused any intravenous administration of therapy on the eighth day. He relapsed with the same pathogen shortly thereafter.

We studied the MBCs of cefoperazone and gentamicin for the pathogenic gram-negative bacilli. The median MBC of cefoperazone was 0.2 μg/ml with a range of 0.09 to 200 μg/ml. Gentamicin had a median MBC of 0.185 μg/ml with a range of 0.09 to 50 μg/ml.

Serum samples were taken 1 and 11 h after the patient had received a total dose of 8 or 10 g of cefoperazone. These samples were assayed for serum bactericidal activity as described by Reller and Stratton (1), and results are shown in Table 2. Although with continuous therapy serum bactericidal activity constantly remained at a satisfactory level (≥1:8), this did not provide any advantage in terms of favorable outcome when compared with the intermittent therapy group.

TABLE 2. *Serum bactericidal activity (SBA) and final outcome*

Treatment	No. of patients with SBA ≥1:8		
	Peak SBA[a]	Trough SBA[a]	Successful outcome[b]
Intermittent infusion	10/12	7/12	11/14
Continuous infusion	10/10	10/10	11/15
Total			22/29 (76%)

[a] Number of patients/number tested.
[b] Number of patients/total patients.

Side effects of cefoperazone (one patient with skin rash and one with diarrhea) were minimal and doubtfully related to this compound.

In non-neutropenic cancer patients, cefoperazone appears to be a successful and safe alternative to antibiotic combinations in therapy of gram-negative bacillary septicemia.

1. **Reller, L. B., and C. W. Stratton.** 1977. Serum dilution test for bactericidal activity. II. Standardization and correlation with antimicrobial assays and susceptibility tests. J. Infect. Dis. **136:**196–204.

Mechanism of Action of Mezlocillin and Azlocillin, Semisynthetic Acylureidopenicillins, In Vitro

MICHIO MATSUHASHI,* SHIGEO TAMAKI, KOU HAYAKAWA, SHIGENORI UENO, AND FUMITOSHI ISHINO

Institute of Applied Microbiology, University of Tokyo, 1-1-1 Yayoi, Bunkyo-ku, Tokyo 113, Japan

Potencies of two semisynthetic acylureidopenicillins, mezlocillin and azlocillin, for binding to penicillin-binding proteins (PBPs) and for inhibiting their transpeptidase activity (cross-linking of peptidoglycan) were studied in *Escherichia coli*.

Binding to PBPs in *E. coli*. Binding of mezlocillin and azlocillin to PBPs of *E. coli* was estimated by two different methods for measuring the competition with ^{14}C-labeled penicillin G for the binding sites. In the first method, which we refer to as the "simultaneous competition assay," membranes were incubated with ^{14}C-labeled penicillin G (70 μM) in the presence of different concentrations of unlabeled acylureidopenicillins or penicillin G in control experiments, and inhibition of binding of ^{14}C-penicillin G to PBPs by the unlabeled antibiotic was measured (4).

In this method the concentration of the antibiotic required to inhibit binding of ^{14}C-penicillin G depends on the concentration of ^{14}C-penicillin G. Both acylureidopenicillins showed exceedingly high binding to PBP-3 (concentration of the antibiotics required for 50% inhibition of binding of ^{14}C-penicillin G being less than 17 μM) but low binding to PBP-4 (mezlocillin, >10,000 μM; azlocillin, 2,400 μM). Mezlocillin also showed comparatively low binding to PBP-1A (mezlocillin, 600 μM; azlocillin, 300 μM). Binding to other PBPs was intermediate (PBP-1Bs [mezlocillin, 130 μM; azlocillin, 100 to 140 μM], PBP-2 [mezlocillin, 60 μM; azlocillin, 40 μM], PBP-5 [mezlocillin, 220 μM; azlocillin, 120 μM], and PBP-6 [mezlocillin, 650 μM; azlocillin, 240 μM]). Similar low binding to PBP-1A and PBP-4 in the simultaneous competition assay has also been observed for apalcillin, an acylaminobenzylpenicillin (M. Fukasawa, H. Noguchi, T. Komatsu, F. Ishino, M. Matsuhashi and S. Mitsuhashi, manuscript in preparation). However, high binding of these penicillins to PBP-1A and PBP-4 was observed by another assay method, as described below.

In the second method, which we refer to as the "competition assay with prebound unlabeled antibiotic," the extent of binding of unlabeled antibiotics to PBPs during the preincubation was estimated by measuring the residual amounts of PBPs which are available for binding by ^{14}C-penicillin G added after the preincubation period. Concentrations of antibiotics required for 50% inhibition of ^{14}C-penicillin G binding are independent of the concentration of ^{14}C-penicillin G (5).

In this method, both acylureidopenicillins showed high binding to PBP-2 (mezlocillin, 2 μM; azlocillin, 3 μM), PBP-3 (2 μM for both penicillins), and also to PBP-1A (4 μM for both penicillins). Binding to other PBPs, including PBP-4, was moderate (PBP-1Bs [12 μM for both penicillins], PBP-5 [mezlocillin, 24 μM; azlocillin, 14 μM], PBP-6 [mezlocillin, 26 μM; azlocillin, 15 μM], and PBP-4 [mezlocillin, 60 to 200 μM; azlocillin, >100 μM]).

Inhibition of transpeptidase activities of PBP-1A, -1Bs, -3 and DD-alanine carboxypeptidase activities of PBP-4 and -5 in *E. coli*. By recent studies in our laboratory, methods for assaying transpeptidase activities (cross-linking of the peptidoglycan) of PBP-1A (1a), -1Bs (2, 3), and -3 (1) of *E. coli* with purified preparations of the respective PBPs became available. DD-Alanine carboxypeptidase activities of PBP-4 and -5 can be assayed either with purified proteins or crude membranes of *E. coli* strains which lack each of the activities of PBP-5 and -4 (4). The inhibitory effect of the two acylureidopenicillins and penicillin G in control experiments was measured for the enzymatic activities of the above PBPs. Concentrations of mezlocillin, azlocillin, and penicillin G required for 50% inhibition of the enzyme activities were, respectively: 0.5, 0.2, and 0.1 to 0.3 μM for PBP-1A; 4, 3, and 5 μM for PBP-1Bs; 0.2 to 0.3, 0.2 to 0.4, and 0.5 to 0.8 μM for PBP-3; 0.5, 0.2, and 0.03 μM for PBP-4; and 2, 1, and 3 μM for PBP-5. A method for estimating the inhibition of the transpeptidase activity of PBP-2, to which the two acylureidopenicillins showed high binding, is not yet available.

Conclusions. Among the seven major PBPs in *E. coli*, PBP-1A and -1Bs are presumed to function as wall peptidoglycan synthesis during cell elongation, and PBP-2 and -3 function as peptidoglycan synthesis during rod and septum formation, respectively, in the process of the cell cycle. Inhibition of one of these PBPs will cause lysis of cells after change of cellular phenotypes corresponding to the defect of its function. The above results indicate that inhibition of transpeptidase activities of both PBP-3 and PBP-1A occurs at low concentrations of the acylureidopenicillins. These proteins seem to be the most important targets of these penicillins for killing bacteria at low concentrations. These results are also compatible with the activity of these penicillins toward living cells, causing formation of unseptated filamentous cells and subsequent cell lysis. Concentrations required for inhibiting transpeptidase or DD-alanine carboxypeptidase activities of these and other PBPs were estimated to be considerably lower than those required for binding to the PBPs.

1. **Ishino, F., and M. Matsuhashi.** 1981. Peptidoglycan synthetic enzyme activities of highly purified penicillin-binding protein 3 in *Escherichia coli*: a septum-forming reaction sequence. Biochem. Biophys. Res. Commun. **101**:905–911.

1a. **Ishino, F., K. Mitsui, S. Tamaki, and M. Matsuhashi.** 1980. Dual enzyme activities of cell wall peptidoglycan synthesis, peptidoglycan transglycosylase and penicillin-sensitive transpeptidase, in purified preparations of *Escherichia coli* penicillin-binding protein 1A. Biochem. Biophys. Res. Commun. **97**:287–293.

2. **Matsuhashi, M., F. Ishino, J. Nakagawa, K. Mitsui, S. Nakajimi-Iijima, S. Tamaki, and T. Hashizume.** 1981. Enzymatic activities of penicillin-binding proteins of *Escherichia coli* and their sensitivities to β-lactam antibiotics, p. 169–184. *In* M. R. J. Salton and G. D. Shockman (ed.), β-Lactam antibiotics, mode of action, new developments, and future prospects. Academic Press, Inc., New York.

3. **Nakagawa, J., S. Tamaki, and M. Matsuhashi.** 1979. Purified penicillin binding proteins 1Bs from *Escherichia coli* membrane showing activities of both peptidoglycan polymerase and peptidoglycan cross-linking enzyme. Agric. Biol. Chem. **43**:1379–1380.

4. **Noguchi, H., M. Matsuhashi, M. Takaoka, and S. Mitsuhashi.** 1978. New antipseudomonal penicillin, PC-904: affinity to penicillin-binding proteins and inhibition of the enzyme cross-linking peptidoglycan. Antimicrob. Agents Chemother. **14**:617–624.

5. **Spratt, B. G.** 1977. Properties of the penicillin-binding proteins of *Escherichia coli* K12. Eur. J. Biochem. **72**: 341–352.

Comparison of Ticarbicillin-Azlocillin Serum Bactericidal Activity Against Gentamicin-Resistant *Pseudomonas aeruginosa*

EMIL TOMA, OLGA DOROBAT, VICTOR RUSU, AND LUDOVIC PAUN

Infectious and Tropical Diseases Clinic and Cantacuzino Institute, Bucharest, Romania

In a number of clinical situations, a bactericidal therapy is an important or even essential requirement (1, 2, 5). The bactericidal activity of a patient's serum against the offending organism during antibiotic administration is an accepted guide for assessing the efficacy of therapy (1, 4). Therefore, as part of the evaluation of new penicillin derivatives, we compared the serum bactericidal activity, during treatment, against the etiological agent as well as against other clinical isolates.

The purpose of this study was to compare the serum bactericidal activity, after ticarcillin and azlocillin administration, against gentamicin-resistant *Pseudomonas aeruginosa*. Infections caused by these strains have been reported with increased frequency in our laboratories.

A total of 14 strains of *P. aeruginosa* resistant to gentamicin, recently isolated from clinical material, were used in the tests. Ten patients received the two antibiotics on alternate days, in a crossover manner. Each antibiotic in 5-g doses was infused over 30 min.

Blood samples (two from each patient, one after each antibiotic) were drawn 30 min after the infusion. Serum bactericidal activity of these samples, against all 14 strains of *P. aeruginosa*, was determined by the method of Barry and Sabath with the modification of Stratton and Reller (1, 4). The medium used for culture and dilution was Mueller-Hinton broth supplemented with physiological concentrations of magnesium and calcium and combined with 50% pooled inactivated human serum (4). The bactericidal endpoint was defined as ≥99.9% killing of the initial inoculum of 5×10^5 colony-forming units per ml (4).

The MICs of ticarcillin and azlocillin for all the test strains of gentamicin-resistant *P. aeruginosa* were the same. Among the strains, 10 were susceptible (MIC ≤25 μg/ml) and 4 were resistant (MIC 400 μg/ml).

Serum bactericidal activities were encountered only against the strains that were susceptible to ticarcillin and azlocillin; as was expected, no serum bactericidal activity was noted against the resistant strains.

After the ticarcillin infusion, the serum bactericidal activities at a serum dilution equal to or greater than 1:2 (1:2 to 1:8) were encountered in 25 of the 140 determinations (i.e., 18%). The geometric mean titer of bactericidal activity was approximately 1:6.

After the azocillin infusion, serum bactericidal activity was seen in 15 instances, from the same number of determinations (i.e., 10.7%), at a serum dilution of 1:2 to 1:4. The geometric mean titer in the case of azlocillin was approximately 1:2.6.

A statistical analysis by the Student t test showed a significant difference, at $P < 0.01$, only among the geometric mean titers of serum bactericidal activity, the value for ticarcillin being significantly higher.

The difference between the number of instances or the percentage in which a serum bactericidal activity was achieved was not fully significant.

If the number of tests was increased by at least 50%, then the differences could be statistically significant.

Our results show a greater bactericidal activity of ticarcillin over azlocillin.

Differences in the bactericidal activity of the two antibiotics were also reported by other authors (2, 3, 5).

Such differences in bactericidal activity might be relevant in clinical situations in which a bactericidal effect is required. However, further clinical experience and well-controlled trials are necessary to assess this possibility.

1. **Barry, A. L., and L. D. Sabath.** 1974. Special tests: bactericidal activity and activity of antimicrobics in combination, p. 431–435. *In* E. H. Lennette, E. H. Spaulding, and J. P. Truant (ed.), Manual of clinical microbiology, 2nd ed. American Society for Microbiology, Washington, D.C.
2. **Basker, M. J., R. A. E. Edmondson, and R. Sutherland.** 1979. Comparative antibacterial activity of azlocillin, mezlocillin, carbenicillin, and ticarcillin and relative stability to beta-lactamase of Pseudomonas aeruginosa and Klebsiella aerogenes. Infection **7:**67–73.
3. **Coppens, L., and J. Klastersky.** 1979. Comparative study of antipseudomonas activity of azlocillin, mezlocillin, and ticarcillin. Antimicrob. Agents Chemother. **18:**182–189.
4. **Stratton, C. W., and L. B. Reller.** 1977. Serum dilution test for bactericidal activity. J. Infect. Dis. **136:**187–205.
5. **White, A. R., K. R. Comber, and R. Sutherland.** 1980. Comparative bactericidal effects of azlocillin and ticarcillin against *Pseudomonas aeruginosa*. Antimicrob. Agents Chemother. **18:**182–189.

Susceptibility Testing of New Broad-Spectrum Penicillins, Using the Agar Diffusion Method According to International Collaborative Study Standards

H. GRIMM

Institute for Medical Microbiology and Clinical Chemistry, D-7987 Weingarten, Federal Republic of Germany

The aim of the following study was to define interpretive criteria for the agar diffusion test with azlocillin, mezlocillin, and piperacillin for different laboratory methods and to examine the problem of optimum disk load. For this purpose, we examined 280 pathogens of different species, excluding *Staphylococcus aureus*, and 220 isolates of *S. aureus*. Agar dilution and agar diffusion tests with 30- and 100-μg disks on Mueller-Hinton agar were performed according to the International Collaborative Study (ICS) recommendations and the Kirby-Bauer method. Also, β-lactamase determinations, using the nitrocefin test, were done for the *S. aureus* strains.

The definition of zone diameter interpretive criteria for *Enterobacteriaceae*, *Pseudomonas aeruginosa*, and enterococci is based on regression line analyses. The correlation between inhibition zones and MICs was better with 30-μg disks than with 100-μg disks (with the exception of azlocillin) in the Kirby-Bauer method. By means of the regression equations, it was possible to calculate cutoff points of zone diameter for each recommended MIC breakpoint.

Assuming MIC breakpoints of 8 and 32 μg, respectively, the zone diameters compiled in Table 1 are necessary to separate the susceptibility categories. To evaluate the practical usability of the proposed cutoff points of zone diameter, it was vital to determine the ratio of error when interpreting the inhibition zone diameters with the MIC as the reference. This evaluation may also facilitate the decision as to which disk load should be used in the laboratory. A total of 86.1

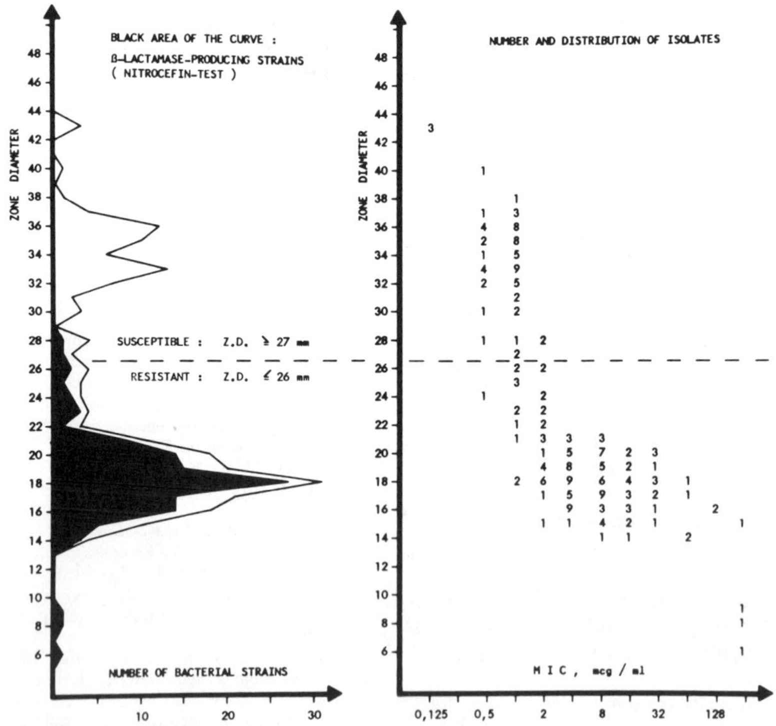

FIG. 1. *Interpretation of piperacillin zone diameter (30-μg disk, ICS method, Mueller-Hinton agar) of S. aureus (n = 220).*

TABLE 1. *Interpretation of acylureidopenicillin zone diameter on Mueller-Hinton agar*[a]

Antibiotic	Disk content (μg)	Method	n[b]	r	Regression equation	Zone diam (mm) at given MIC (μg/ml) correlates			Total zone diam correctly interpreted (%)	*S. aureus* zone diam cutoff point (mm)
						≥64 (resistant)	16–32 (intermediate)	≤8 (susceptible)		
Azlocillin	30	ICS	246	−0.8408	$x = -0.28\,y + 18.40$	≤15	16–22	≥23	88.2	≥29
Mezlocillin	30		275	−0.9424	$x = -0.35\,y + 19.35$	≤15	16–20	≥21	95.7	≥28
Piperacillin	30		274	−0.9124	$x = -0.33\,y + 18.58$	≤13	14–19	≥20	97.5	≥27
Azlocillin	30	Kirby-Bauer	242	−0.8663	$x = -0.32\,y + 18.17$	≤12	13–19	≥20	87.9	≥23
Mezlocillin	30		274	−0.9339	$x = -0.36\,y + 18.24$	≤11	12–17	≥18	95.7	≥24
Piperacillin	30		270	−0.9004	$x = -0.36\,y + 18.08$	≤11	12–16	≥17	95.4	≥22
Azlocillin	100	ICS	249	−0.8343	$x = -0.30\,y + 20.34$	≤20	21–27	≥28	86.1	≥32
Mezlocillin	100		277	−0.9223	$x = -0.38\,y + 21.40$	≤19	20–24	≥25	91.8	≥31
Piperacillin	100		277	−0.8780	$x = -0.34\,y + 20.28$	≤18	19–24	≥25	96.1	≥32
Azlocillin	100	Kirby-Bauer	249	−0.8871	$x = -0.32\,y + 19.58$	≤17	18–23	≥24	88.2	≥26
Mezlocillin	100		277	−0.9168	$x = -0.39\,y + 20.19$	≤15	16–20	≥21	94.3	≥26
Piperacillin	100		276	−0.8802	$x = -0.37\,y + 19.55$	≤14	15–20	≥21	95.4	≥26

[a] Statistical data for *Enterobacteriaceae*, *P. aeruginosa*, and enterococci.
[b] Not including strains with zone diameter of 6 mm or MICs of ≥256 μg/ml.

to 97.5% of the total zone diameters were correctly interpreted in this way depending on antibiotic, disk content, and method. For the ICS method, 30-μg disks were better than 100-μg disks. With the Kirby-Bauer method there were no great differences between the two disks.

In laboratory practice, very large inhibition zones often interfere with the readability of the antibiogram. It is self-evident that 100-μg disks produce larger inhibition zone diameters than 30-μg disks. The percentage of cultures with inhibition zones of >30 mm depends on antibiotic, disk content, and method. From this point of view, 30-μg disks are appropriate for the ICS method and 100-μg disks are better for the Kirby-Bauer method. In this way, for each of the three acylureidopenicillins tested, an almost identical percentage of zone diameters of >30 mm resulted.

The regression line analysis was not applicable for *S. aureus* because there was absolutely no linearity in the correlation of MIC and zone diameter (Fig. 1). An alternative way to get cutoff points for acylureidopenicillins is the β-lactamase production of *S. aureus*. A total of 51.8% of the *S. aureus* isolates tested were β-lactamase positive by means of the nitrocefin test. We suggest acylureidopenicillin zone diameter cutoff points which permit maximal 1% "false-susceptible" classifications regarding β-lactamase production. Thus, we get the cutoff points listed in Table 1.

The zone diameters necessary for acylureidopenicillin susceptibility of *S. aureus* are up to 7 mm larger than those obtained with *Enterobacteriaceae*, *P. aeruginosa*, and enterococci under the same conditions. The preferable acylureidopenicillin disk for the ICS method has a 30-μg loading capacity; that for the Kirby-Bauer method is 100 μg.

Dose-Dependent Elimination of Azlocillin in Healthy Volunteers

PIERRE SPRING* AND FERENC FOLLATH

Division of Clinical Pharmacology, Department of Medicine, Kantonsspital Basel, 4031 Basel, Switzerland

The pharmacokinetics of azlocillin were reevaluated by comparing the serum concentration–time curves and the urinary elimination rates of two different doses (5 g and 10 g) in six healthy volunteers aged 22 to 43 years and weighing 50 to 77 kg (mean, 61.8 kg). To avoid possible side effects, the low dose was given first, namely, 1 g as an intravenous bolus, followed by 1 g/h as an infusion for 4 h. The higher dose was administered at least 1 week later as a 2-g bolus and 2 g/h for 4 h. Multiple blood samples and urine portions were collected up to 12 and 24 h, respectively. Samples were kept at −80°C until assayed. Azlocillin concentrations were measured microbiologically, with *Bacillus subtilis* as test organism, the lower limit of the assay being 0.1 μg/ml.

A typical concentration–time curve is shown in Fig. 1 (subject 6). During the postinfusion phase on the lower dose, azlocillin concentrations fell exponentially with a half-life of 1.19 ± 0.08 h (mean ± SD), whereas after the high dose the serum concentration curve became nonlinear in all cases. In the first hour after the end of infusion, the azlocillin concentration decreased rapidly; then, in the concentration range between 120 and 60 mg/liter (up to about 3.5 h), the curve described a shoulder-like pattern. From azlocillin levels during this period an apparent half-life of 2.2 ± 0.15 h would have been obtained. However, the concentration curves also became linear after the high dose when azlocillin concentrations fell below 30 mg/liter. Half-lives calculated from the terminal slope were similar to those on the lower dose (1.20 ± 0.08 h).

The principal pharmacokinetic parameters (mean ± SD) and the corresponding *P* values for differences between the two doses are shown in Table 1. The steady-state serum concentration during the last hour of the infusion phase was proportional to the dose; the total clearance at steady state was practically identical in the two experiments, but the renal clearance at steady state was significantly smaller after the lower dose. Analyzing the areas under the serum concentration curves from hours 1 to 12 and the urinary excretion rates, we found that renal clearance and the amount of drug excreted unchanged in the urine increased significantly on the higher dose, whereas the extrarenal clearance and the total clearance decreased.

Seeking an explanation for the nonlinear azlocillin elimination on the higher dose, we also compared the hourly renal clearance values as a function of time and serum concentration.

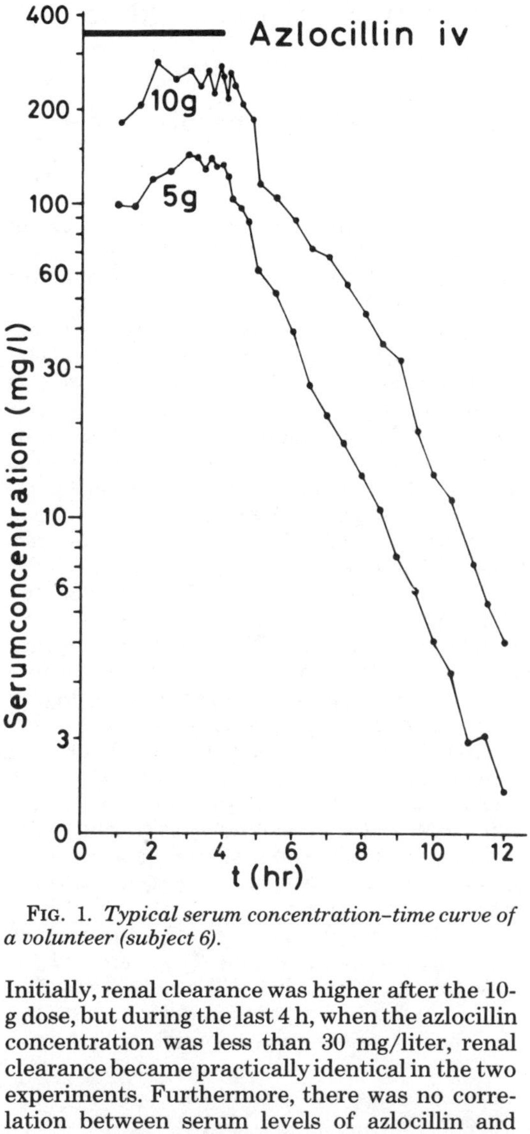

FIG. 1. *Typical serum concentration–time curve of a volunteer (subject 6).*

Initially, renal clearance was higher after the 10-g dose, but during the last 4 h, when the azlocillin concentration was less than 30 mg/liter, renal clearance became practically identical in the two experiments. Furthermore, there was no correlation between serum levels of azlocillin and renal clearance. This means that under the conditions of our experiment no evidence of a saturable tubular secretion could be demonstrated. On the contrary, our findings indicate a capacity-limited extrarenal elimination mechanism, with decreasing extrarenal clearance after administration of the higher dose. A clinically relevant drug accumulation, however, will not be observed, since there is a compensatory increase in the renally excreted dose fraction.

A dose-dependent elimination of ureidopenicillins was also found by other investigators.

TABLE 1. *Pharmacokinetic parameters for two doses of azlocillin*

Pharmacokinetic parameter[a]	Low dose (5 g)	High dose (10 g)	P
I. C_{ss} (mg/liter)	118.5 ± 9.3	247.0 ± 43.7	
$Cl_{tot,ss}$ (ml/min)	137.9 ± 20.0	141.3 ± 10.4	NS[b]
$Cl_{r,ss}$ (ml/min)	75.8 ± 23.0	107.8 ± 11.5	<0.01
II. Cl_{tot} (ml/min)	149.6 ± 14.9	127.2 ± 15.6	<0.06
Cl_r (ml/min)	92.9 ± 11.9	118.6 ± 12.2	<0.01
Cl_{er} (% of Cl_{tot})	38	7	<0.001
M_u (% of dose)	62.2 ± 5.7	90.5 ± 13.3	<0.005

[a] C_{ss}, Steady-state serum concentration during the last hour of the infusion; $Cl_{tot,ss}$, total clearance at steady state; $Cl_{r,ss}$, renal clearance at steady state; Cl_{tot}, total clearance; Cl_r, renal clearance; Cl_{er}, extrarenal clearance; M_u, amount of drug excreted unchanged in the urine.

[b] Not significant.

Leroy et al. (3) described a decrease of total clearance from 215 ± 50 to 152.9 ± 29.8 ml/min per 1.73 m^2 in five healthy volunteers receiving azlocillin doses of 2 and 5 g, respectively. Contrary to us, they also observed a decrease in renal clearance from 145.2 ± 48.5 to 94.1 ± 18.6 ml/min per 1.73 m^2. Comparable results were reported by Bergan (2) with mezlocillin after bolus injections of 1, 2, and 5 g. Total clearance decreased on the higher dose, but renal clearance showed no consistent changes. More recently, Aronoff et al. (1) also observed a nonlinear serum concentration curve, especially during the initial 4 h, after infusing 3 g of mezlocillin to patients with different degrees of renal impairment.

The exact cause of the dose dependency of azlocillin kinetics is at present unknown, but changes in protein binding or biliary excretion, or both, at high azlocillin levels may be responsible. The practical importance of the changing elimination mechanism of ureidopenicillins needs to be further investigated, especially in patients with impaired renal or liver function, or both.

1. **Aronoff, G. R., R. S. Sloan, F. C. Luft, R. L. Nelson, D. R. Maxwell, and S. A. Kleit.** 1980. Mezlocillin pharmacokinetics in renal impairment. Clin. Pharmacol. Ther. **28:**523–528.
2. **Bergan, T.** 1978. Pharmacokinetics of mezlocillin in healthy volunteers. Antimicrob. Agents Chemother. **14:** 801–806.
3. **Leroy, A., G. Humbert, M. Godin, and J. P. Fillastre.** 1980. Pharmacokinetics of azlocillin in subjects with normal and impaired renal function, p. 573. *In* J. D. Nelson and C. Grassi (ed.), Current chemotherapy, vol. 1. American Society for Microbiology, Washington, D.C.

Azlocillin and Mezlocillin: Pharmacokinetic Studies in Children

L. WEINGÄRTNER, U. SITKA, R. PATSCH, AND H. H. THIEMANN

Clinic of Pediatrics, Institute of Microbiology, Martin Luther University, Halle/Wittenberg, German Democratic Republic

The acylureidopenicillin azlocillin (Securopen) and mezlocillin (Baypen) were studied clinically and pharmacokinetically in 306 children (prematures, neonates, infants, and schoolchildren). The parameters investigated were first-order kinetics in an open one-compartment model: serum concentrations, elimination constant, half-life, distribution volume, excretion in bronchial secretions, and concentrations in meconium (azlocillin) and cerebrospinal fluid (mezlocillin).

Azlocillin and mezlocillin have bactericidal efficacy, the MBC usually being two- to fourfold the MIC. Stronger β-lactamase formation by the bacteria inhibits the efficacy. Resistance develops according to a multiple-step scheme. Both antibiotics must be given parenterally, intravenously (i.v.), but in children younger than 3 months intramuscular (i.m.) application is possible because of the smaller injection volume.

Azlocillin is active against gram-negative and -positive organisms, especially against *Pseudomonas aeruginosa*, including strains resistant to carbenicillin and gentamicin. Mezlocillin is also effective against gram-negative and -positive strains, including *Klebsiella, Serratia*, and anaerobes. Both antibiotics are monosodium salts with a small amount of sodium. This is an advantage, especially in young infants.

Serum concentrations were measured by an agar diffusion test with *Escherichia coli* 14 as test strain. The reference standards were diluted in pooled human serum. For determination of both antibiotics in meconium and bronchial secretions, dilutions for the standard were made in phosphate buffer.

Pharmacokinetic parameters of azlocillin are shown in Table 1. Included were 86 children who received doses of 50 to 100 mg/kg i.v. or i.m. The elimination constant rose from 0.157 in prematures to 0.745 in schoolchildren. The half-life, usually longest in prematures, decreased from 4.41 to 0.93 h in schoolchildren. The distribution volume showed a decrease from 0.344 liter/kg in prematures to 0.231 liter/kg in schoolchildren. The distribution volumes, 34% of the body-weight for prematures and 30% for neonates, were somewhat below the capacity of the extracellular space for age. The concentration-time integral (A) measured in neonates showed a dose proportionality. In a group receiving 50 mg/kg i.m., the concentrations after 5 min had already reached 64.0 ± 17.2 μg/ml. The peak was reached after 20 min, being 139.0 ± 40.7 μg/ml. In another group of neonates, monitored from 5 min to 14 h, the alpha phase was finished after 30 min; then followed a slower beta phase. A gamma phase or a deeper compartment was not detectable.

We studied eight neonates for azlocillin penetration into the meconium. They received one dose shortly after delivery. Except for the first hours of life, we always found the antibiotic, but the concentrations varied considerably, from a

TABLE 1. *Pharmacokinetic parameters for azlocillin (mean values, first-order kinetics, open one-compartment model)*[a]

Group	Dose (mg/kg)[b]	n	Monitored until (h)	k (h^{-1})	Half-life (h)	V_{ext} (liter/kg)	A (h × mg/liter)
Prematures	50 i.v.	7	12	0.157	4.41	0.344	—
Neonates	50 i.v.	7	8	0.204	3.40	0.395	428
	50 i.m.	11	8	0.236	2.94	0.271	630
	100 i.v.	6	12	0.262	2.65	0.288	1,020
	100 i.m.	7	12	0.270	2.57	0.309	1,134
	100 i.v.	6	14	0.270	2.43	—	—
Infants							
<3 months	100 i.v.	8	8	0.368	1.88	0.406	—
>3 months	100 i.v.	8	8	0.717	0.97	0.264	—
Schoolchildren	75 i.v.	9	6	0.745	0.93	0.231	321

[a] Parameters: k, elimination rate constant; V_{ext}, extracellular volume; A, concentration-time integral.
[b] Each dose was administered once.

TABLE 2. *Pharmacokinetic parameters for mezlocillin (mean values, first-order kinetics, open one-compartment model)*[a]

Group	Dose (mg/kg)[b]	*n*	Monitored until (h)	k (h^{-1})	Half-life (h)	V_{ext} (liter/kg)	A (h × mg/liter)
Prematures	50 i.v.	6	12	0.210	3.30	0.256	929
	75 i.v.	7	12	0.195	3.55	0.272	1,415
Neonates	100 i.v.	8	14	0.302	2.29	0.280	1,182
	100 i.v.	9	12	0.316	2.30	0.272	1,223
	150 i.v.	6	12	0.294	2.38	0.361	1,412
	200 i.v.	7	12	0.283	2.45	0.403	1,753
Infants							
<3 months	150 i.v.	7	12	0.364	1.93	0.489	578
>3 months	150 i.v.	6	6	0.782	0.89	0.344	596
Schoolchildren	100 i.v.	7	6	0.808	0.86	0.240	516

[a] Parameters are defined in footnote *a* of Table 1.
[b] Each dose was administered once.

few to 1,518 μg/ml. Part of the azlocillin reaches the gastrointestinal tract via the liver, unmetabolized.

Penetration of azlocillin into the bronchial secretions was studied in 30 patients who received a single i.v. injection of 75 mg/kg. The concentrations ranged between 25.9 and 287.0 μg/ml and lasted for 5 h. A relation to simultaneous concentrations does not exist.

Daily dosages of azlocillin are as follows: prematures and neonates, 100 mg/kg two times; infants, 100 mg/kg three times; schoolchildren, 75 mg/kg three times. In serious infections the dosage can be increased without risk.

Pharmacokinetic parameters of mezlocillin are shown in Table 2. The elimination constant rose from 0.210 in prematures to 0.808 in schoolchildren. The half-life was a little shorter than for azlocillin. It declined continuously from 3.55 h in prematures to 0.86 h in schoolchildren. The distribution volume was to 0.272 liter/kg in the prematures and 0.240 liter/kg in the schoolchildren. With regard to the extracellular space, azlocillin and mezlocillin showed no difference. In other respects as well the two antibiotics behaved similarly, but the concentration-time integral for mezlocillin did not have a distinct dosage proportionality as in the case of azlocillin.

The absorption of mezlocillin in nine neonates after 100 mg/kg i.m. 5 min after injection showed serum concentrations of 90.3 ± 40.6 μg/ml. The peak of 205.9 ± 69.4 μg/ml was reached 20 min after injection.

Samples of bronchial secretions from 77 patients who had received 75 to 150 mg of azlocillin per kg i.v. were selected. Four hours after the injection of 75 mg/kg, concentrations of about 50.9 μg/ml were still found.

In 10 patients with uninflamed meninges, cerebrospinal fluid could be studied. With one exception, the concentrations ranged between 1.2 and 13.7 μg/ml. Mezlocillin was given 1 to 2 h before sampling of the cerebrospinal fluid in a dosage of 100 mg/kg i.v.

Daily dosages of mezlocillin are as follows: prematures, 100 mg/kg two times; neonates 150 (to 200) mg/kg two times; infants, 150 (to 200) mg/kg three times; schoolchildren, 100 (to 150) mg/kg three times. In serious conditions the dosage can be increased without risk.

Azlocillin and mezlocillin are well-tolerated antibiotics. Serious side effects were not observed. Only slight nausea and abdominal pain during the injection occurred in a few children and there was an exanthema in one patient.

Pharmacokinetics of Azlocillin in Burned Patients

H. B. DRUGEON, M. PANNIER, AND A. L. COURTIEU

Laboratoire de Bactériologie et Secteur des Brûlés et de Chirurgie Plastique, Hotel-Dieu, Nantes, France

The *Pseudomonas* infection is an important complication often observed in burned patients. These illnesses are usually treated with two antibiotics: a β-lactam compound and an aminoglycoside. The β-lactam compound used is usually carbenicillin, but its activity is decreased because 15 to 50% of *P. aeruginosa* strains are now resistant.

New β-lactam compounds show activity against *P. aeruginosa*. Among these, azlocillin (an acylureidopenicillin) has produced good results. For carbenicillin-susceptible strains, MICs of azlocillin are between 2 and 8 mg/liter. Azlocillin is also active against a large part of the carbenicillin-resistant population. A few strains (10%) are azlocillin resistant (MIC ≥128 mg/liter), and these strains produce a high level of β-lactamase.

Because of the possible future use of azlocillin in the treatment of burn complications, we studied the pharmacokinetics of this molecule in burned patients. In this study, we have tried to observe the pharmacokinetic difference between the initial phase and the healing phase. Five subjects, ranging from 30 to 80 years old, were studied. The burn size was about 10 to 18% except for one patient (no. 2) with 50%. All subjects were studied during the initial phase, before the fifth day; two patients (no. 1 and 2) were studied again during the healing phase, after at least 15 days of evolution.

The patients were given a single intravenous infusion of 80 mg of azlocillin per kg over 30 min. Blood samples were taken at time zero and 0.25, 0.5, 1, 1.5, 2.5, 3.5, and 5.5 h after the end of the perfusion. The urine samples were collected every 2 h during an 8-h period.

Serum and urine concentrations of azlocillin were determined by the agar diffusion method with *Bacillus subtilis* as the test strain. Assays were performed in triplicate.

The pharmacokinetic parameters were calculated in the elimination phase by using a one-compartment open-body model. These parameters are the half-life, the serum concentration at time zero, the apparent volume of distribution, the serum clearance, the renal clearance, and the percentage of azlocillin excreted in urine. At the same time, creatinine concentrations were measured in the urine and the serum to determine the creatinine clearance.

Table 1 shows the different parameters calculated during the initial phase. The half-life of the elimination phase was 1.17 with creatinine clearance of 131 ml/min per 1.73 m^2. When the creatinine clearance decreased, the half-life increased. For subject 5, it was 3.3 h. These results are very similar to those found with unburned patients. The apparent volume of distribution was from 0.26 to 0.55 liter/kg. It was higher than that of unburned patients (1), usually being 0.22 liter/kg in normal subjects. The serum clearance was always above 100 ml/min per 1.73 m^2. In unburned patients, it is 150 ml/min per 1.73 m^2. The renal clearance varied from 30.9 to 128 ml/min per 1.73 m^2. The extrarenal clearance remained constant at 51 to 88 ml/min per 1.73 m^2, as in unburned patients (1), except for subject 2. In this patient the extrarenal clearance was 126 ml/min per 1.73 m^2. We could assume that this was connected with the burn size and the importance of the exudation.

TABLE 1. *Pharmacokinetic data during the initial phase*[a]

Subject no.	Creatinine clearance (ml/min per 1.73 m^2)	B (mg/liter)	$T_{1/2}\beta$ (h)	V_d-area (liters/kg)	C_s (ml/min per 1.73 m^2)	C_r (ml/min per 1.73 m^2)	$Fe = \frac{C_r}{C_s}$	Urine flow rate (ml/h)
1	131	230	1.17	0.29	196	128	65	237
2	111	115	1.4	0.38	194	37.6	19	97
3	94	180	1.78	0.34	148	76.3	51	132
4	60	190	1.73	0.26	107	38.9	36	94
5	14	128	3.3	0.56	118	30.9	26	73

[a] B, Serum concentration; $T_{1/2}\beta$, elimination half-life; V_d, apparent volume of distribution; C_s, serum clearance; C_r, renal clearance.

TABLE 2. *Differences in pharmacokinetic data between the initial and healing phases*[a]

Subject no.	Phase	Creatinine clearance (ml/min per 1.73 m^2)	B (mg/liter)	Half-life (h)	V_d (liters)	C_s (ml/min per 1.73 m^2)	C_r (ml/min per 1.73 m^2)	$Fe = \frac{C_r}{C_s}$	Urine flow rate (ml/h)
1	Initial	131	230	1.17	23.3	196	128	65	235
	Healing	176	220	1.14	21.8	190	136.6	71	250
2	Initial	111	115	1.4	26.1	194	36.6	19	97
	Healing	81	214	1.26	18.4	167	116	69	190

[a] Abbreviations as in Table 1.

Table 2 shows the results for the two subjects studied during the initial and the healing phases. For subject 1, whose burn size was 18%, the pharmacokinetic parameters were identical in the two phases. For the subject whose burn size was 50%, many differences can be noticed between the two phases. The serum concentrations were lower in the initial phase. The apparent volume of distribution was more important: about 8 liters. In the initial phase, he changed from 5 to 9 liters of hydrous volume a day. The renal clearance was much lower in this phase. This is usual in the healing phase when the urine flow rate has returned to normal. We can assume that in burned patients with small burn size the azlocillin pharmacokinetics are the same as in unburned patients. When the burn sizes are very large, serum concentrations of azlocillin should be checked regularly to maintain effective levels, as the dose may need to be increased.

1. **Leroy, A., G. Humbert, M. Godin, and J. P. Fillastre.** 1980. Pharmacokinetics of azlocillin in subjects with normal and impaired renal function. Antimicrob. Agents Chemother. **17**:344–349.

Pharmacokinetics of Intramuscularly Administered Mezlocillin in Normal Subjects and in Renal Impaired and Hemodialyzed Patients

JEAN-MARIE BROGARD,* MARIE-ODILE SPACH, FRANÇOISE COMTE, AND JEAN LAVILLAUREIX

Department of Internal Medicine and the Institute of Hygiene Hospitalo-University Center of Strasbourg, 67091 Strasbourg Cedex, France

Mezlocillin, a new semisynthetic derivative structurally related to the ureido penicillins, exhibits a broad spectrum of antibacterial activity, especially against *Streptococcus faecalis*, *Escherichia coli*, *Enterobacter* spp., *Klebsiella*, *Serratia*, *Proteus mirabilis*, strains of indole-positive *Proteus*, *Pseudomonas aeruginosa*, and *Bacteroides* (1–3). The present study was undertaken to determine the pharmacokinetic patterns of mezlocillin in patients with various degrees of renal insufficiency, including patients with end-stage renal disease submitted to repeated hemodialysis. Using these data, dosage guidelines for the use of mezlocillin in patients with renal failure could be formulated.

Mezlocillin concentrations were determined in serum and urine of 25 patients divided into 3 groups: group I, 10 healthy subjects (no. 1 to 10; creatinine clearance [Ccr] > 104 ml/min per 1.73 m^2); group II, 10 clinically stable patients with various degrees of renal insufficiency (no. 11 to 20; 68 ml/min per 1.73 m^2 > Ccr > 12 ml/min per 1.73 m^2); group III, 5 patients with end-stage renal disease requiring twice-weekly hemodialysis sessions (no. 21 to 25; 5.6 ml/min per 1.73 m^2 > Ccr > 0 ml/min per 1.73 m^2). Dialysis lasted 6 h and was performed on a Travenol Twin Coil apparatus, using Ultra-Flo cuprophane membranes.

Mezlocillin was given as a single 1.0-g intramuscular (i.m.) dose. Only patients undergoing hemodialysis were submitted to two injections of mezlocillin; the first was given at the start of a dialysis session, and the second was given 14 days later, at the beginning of an interdialytic period. Samples of peripheral venous blood were collected for assays at 0, 5, 15, and 30 min, at 1, 2, 3, 4, 5, 6, and 8 h, and even at 10, 12, 18, 24, and 48 h after antibiotic administration. Urine was collected during the 6 and 12 h after the administration of mezlocillin. Antibiotic activity was determined by the agar plate diffusion method with BBL medium no. 2 adjusted to pH 7.2 and *Bacillus subtilis* (ATCC 6633) as the test organism.

The serum concentration curves were analyzed with reference to a Bateman function, and a one-compartment model was assumed. Pharmacokinetic parameters were determined by applying formulas described elsewhere (5). The extraction coefficient (E) of mezlocillin during the dialysis process was established from the equation $E\% = A - V/A \times 100$, where A and V are the serum concentration of the blood samples taken from the arterial (A) and the venous (V) limbs of the hemodialysis circuit, respectively.

In normal subjects, resorption of the i.m.-injected mezlocillin began after a short lag time, t_0, of 1.2 min, and a calculated maximal serum concentration, C_{max}, of 24.7 μg/ml was reached after 43 min. The serum concentration curve was expressed by the formula $C = 64.57$ $(e^{-0.7908t} - e^{-2.3565t})$. The area under the serum concentration curve ($AUC_{0-\infty}$) averaged 37.87 μg.h/ml or 35.45 μg.h/ml by measurement or by calculation, respectively. The resorption rate constant, K_a, was 2.3565 h^{-1}, corresponding to a resorption half-life, $T_{a1/2}$, of 0.3 h; the overall elimination rate constant, K_e, was 0.7908 h^{-1}, corresponding to a biological half-life, $T_{b1/2}$, of 0.9 h. The initial theoretical serum concentration, B_0, was 42.9 μg/ml. The cumulative urinary excretion of mezlocillin amounted to 58.0 ± 3.9% during the first 6 h and to 72.2 ± 4.0% during the 12 h after injection of the drug. Renal clearance, Cr (263 ml/min per 1.73 m^2), accounted for 59.8% of the total clearance, Ct (449 ml/min per 1.73 m^2).

The patients of group II were nonhomogeneous enough with regard to renal function, not allowing the determination of mean values. The calculated maximal concentrations ranged between 27.0 and 113.5 μg/ml. The serum concentration decrease was slow (Table 1); biological half-lives ranged between 0.7 and 6.0 h, and values of K_e ranged between 0.1158 and 0.9997 h^{-1}. The values of $AUC_{0-\infty}$ rose considerably (55.78 to 482.62 μg·h/ml). The urinary excretion of mezlocillin was reduced (625 mg > U_{0-12h} > 253 mg), as were the total (278 ml/min per 1.73 m^2 > Ct > 130 ml/min per 1.73 m^2) and renal (170 ml/min per 1.73 m^2 > Ccr > 13 ml/min per 1.73 m^2) clearances.

The group of patients undergoing hemodialysis (Table 1) was sufficiently homogeneous to enable calculation of means. The following values were established when mezlocillin was injected at the beginning of the interdialytic period: C_{max} = 54.6 μg/ml (after 35 min); $T_{b1/2}$ = 9.7 h; K_e = 0.0712 h^{-1}; Ct = 22 ml/min per 1.73 m^2; Cr = 1.4 ml/min per 1.73 m^2; $AUC_{0-\infty}$ = 801.6 μg.h/ml.

When mezlocillin was administered at the start of a hemodialysis session, the serum concentration decrease was more pronounced than previously: from an initial theoretical level of 39.1 μg/ml, the mean serum concentration fell to 21.7 ± 2.8 μg/ml after 2 h, to 12.8 ± 2.7 μg/ml after 4 h, and to 7.2 ± 1.5 μg/ml after 6 h. The $T_{b1/2}$ mean value was 2.5 h, the AUC_{0-6h} mean value was 94.05 μg.h/ml, and the Ct mean value was 162 ml/min per 1.73 m^2. Mean hourly extraction of mezlocillin during hemodialysis, E, was 19.4 ± 1.3%. In the two patients where the mean antibiotic activity of the dialysate could be measured, it attained 1.15 and 1.30 μg/ml, respectively.

Using these results (Table 1), it was possible to demonstrate statistically significant correlations ($r = 0.6822$ to 0.8597 and $P < 0.001$ in every case) between the individual Ccr values of the patients on the one hand and their main determined pharmacokinetic parameters (K_e, $T_{b1/2}$, log $T_{b1/2}$, U_{0-12h}, $AUC_{0-\infty}$, Ct, log Ct, Cr, log Cr) on the other. Calculated with these correlations, the values of K_e, $T_{b1/2}$, U_{0-12h}, $AUC_{0-\infty}$, Ct, and Cr were, respectively, 0.673 h^{-1}, 1.05 h, 683 mg, 47 μg.h/ml, 360 ml/min, and 199 ml/min for a normal reference subject characterized by a CCr of 100 ml/min and 0.1973 h^{-1}, 4.72 h, 0 mg, 519 μg.h/ml, 40 ml/min, and 0 ml/min for a patient with a CCr of 0 ml/min. Applying the relation (6) $K_e = K_{nr} + K_r = 0.1973 + 0.0046$ Ccr ($n = 25$; $r = 0.771$; $P < 0.001$), where K_{nr} is the extrarenal elimination constant (= 0.1973) and K_r is the

TABLE 1. *Individual values of overall elimination rate constants (K_e), theoretical initial serum concentrations (C_o), and biological half-lives ($T_{b1/2}$) in the 25 patients under study*

PATIENTS		CREATININE CLEARANCE Ccr (ml/min/1.73 m2)	OVERALL ELIMINATION RATE CONSTANTS Ke (h^{-1})	THEORETICAL INITIAL CONCENTRATION Co (μg/ml)	BIOLOGICAL HALF-LIVES t 1/2 (hours)
WITH NORMAL RENAL FUNCTIONS	1	104	0.4813	57.8	1.44
	2	104	0.4874	18.1	1.42
	3	110	0.6292	18.2	1.10
	4	112	0.7243	38.2	0.96
	5	113	0.6505	49.2	1.07
	6	115	0.7617	17.8	0.91
	7	116	0.4210	15.9	1.65
	8	117	0.8523	52.7	0.81
	9	117	0.6985	20.7	0.99
	10	118	0.7908	63.6	0.78
WITH IMPAIRED RENAL FUNCTIONS	11	68	0.7045	82.4	0.98
	12	65	0.5216	74.3	1.33
	13	63	0.5331	182.1	1.30
	14	56	0.6538	180.1	1.06
	15	51	0.9997	79.4	0.69
	16	39	0.3951	33.3	1.75
	17	26	0.3865	45.2	1.79
	18	25	0.3553	52.0	1.95
	19	18	0.3677	41.3	1.89
	20	12	0.1158	58.3	5.99
ON HEMODIALYSIS	21	5,6	0.1137	20.1	6.10
	22	2,4	0.0836	54.2	8.29
	23	2,2	0.0754	63.7	9.12
	24	0	0.0686	47.1	10.10
	25	0	0.0904	121.5	7.67

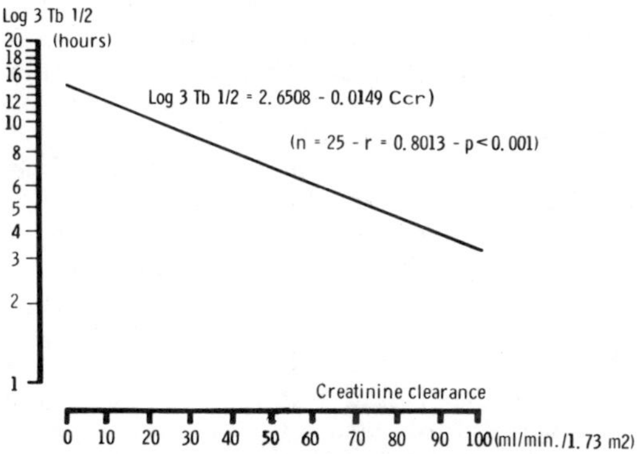

FIG. 1. *Direct determination of the adjusted dosage interval ($\tau = 3\ T_{b1/2}$) between two successive 1-g injections of mezlocillin from CCr values.*

renal elimination coefficient (= 0.0046 Ccr), a mezlocillin renal elimination rate of 70% and an extrarenal elimination rate of 30% could be calculated for the normal reference subject (Ccr = 100 ml/min per 1.73 m^2).

In patients with severe renal failure undergoing hemodialysis, $AUC_{0-6\ h}$ had a mean value of 271 or 94 μg.h/ml, according to whether the injection of mezlocillin was given at the beginning of the interdialytic or at the start of the dialytic period (ΔAUC = 177 μg.h/ml). Hemodialysis thus reduced the AUC by 62%; to compensate for this loss (corresponding to two-thirds of the quantity of mezlocillin present in the central compartment), it was necessary either to give a complementary dose (equivalent to half of the initial dose) at the end of the dialysis process or to administer the injection only at the end of the hemodialysis session.

Although renal excretion is lower than with most other beta-lactamines (4), urine is still the main excretion pathway for this antibiotic. It is thus advisable to adjust its dosage to the value of the renal function. This adaptation can be made by administering mezlocillin (1 g i.m.) at intervals τ, corresponding to three times the biological half-life, 3 $T_{b1/2}$. Adjusted 3 $T_{b1/2}$ durations adapted to the renal function can be read directly on Fig. 1, which expresses the linear relationship (log 3 $T_{b1/2}$ = 2.6508 − 0.0149 Ccr; $n = 25$; $r = 0.8013$; $P < 0.001$) between the values of log 3 $T_{b1/2}$ and those of Ccr.

Considering our former results, it appears that dosage modifications are in fact not really required in patients with Ccr of more than 40 to 50 ml/min. In practice, the dose could be reduced to one-half (or the dosage interval doubled) if 40 ml/min > Ccr > 10 ml/min. In patients with Ccr < 10 ml/min, the dose could be diminished to one-third.

1. **Bergan, T.** 1978. Pharmacokinetics of mezlocillin in healthy volunteers. Antimicrob. Agents Chemother. **14:** 801–806.
2. **Bergan, T., E. K. Brodwall, and E. Wiik-Larsen.** 1979. Mezlocillin pharmacokinetics in patients with normal and impaired renal function. Antimicrob. Agents Chemother. **16:**651–654.
3. **Bodey, G. P., and T. Pan.** 1977. Mezlocillin in vitro studies of a new broad-spectrum penicillin. Antimicrob. Agents Chemother. **11:**74–79.
4. **Brogard, J. M., F. Comte, J. P. Arnaud, and J. Lavillaureix.** 1981. Mezlocillin, serum and biliary concentrations. Level prediction with use of pharmacokinetics, p. 193–201. *In* Drugs under research, 1980–1982, vol. 4. Bioscience, Geneva, Switzerland.
5. **Brogard, J. M., M. Pinget, M. Dorner, and J. Lavillaureix.** 1976. Etablissement du profil pharmacocinétique d'un antibiotique. Intérêt pratique et application à l'étude comparative des céphalosporines. Bull. Inst. Pasteur Paris **74:**383–412.
6. **Dettli, L., P. Spring, and S. Ryter.** 1971. Acta Pharmacol. **29** (Suppl. 3):211–224.

Pharmacokinetic and Clinical Data of One-Dose Versus Three-Dose Mezlocillin Prophylaxis in Vaginal Hysterectomy

U. SIEKMANN,* F. DASCHNER, B. METZ, AND L. HEILMANN

Department of Obstetrics and Gynecology, University of Essen, Essen, and Department of Hospital Epidemiology, University of Freiburg, Freiburg, Federal Republic of Germany*

Postoperative infections in gynecology are usually mixed infections involving enterobacteria and anaerobes (3). Mezlocillin, a new broad-spectrum semisynthetic penicillin, shows high activity against those forms of infections. The efficacy of perioperative antibiotic prophylaxis in vaginal hysterectomy using a three-dose course of mezlocillin per day has been already demonstrated (1). Pharmacokinetic and clinical data of only one-dose mezlocillin prophylaxis at different times of administration have not been yet described. It was the purpose of our study to determine the levels of mezlocillin in sera and extirpated uterine myometria after preoperative administration of mezlocillin in a single dose of 5 g at different times before surgery. In addition, we compared the incidence rates of infectious morbidity in a prospective randomized clinical trial, which included 35 women receiving a one-dose course of mezlocillin prophylactic treatment and 31 women without any prophylaxis. Pharmacokinetic and clinical data of 15 patients receiving a three-dose course of mezlocillin were investigated before this randomized trial. All patients underwent vaginal hysterectomy, and in some cases anterior or posterior colporrhaphy, or both, was performed. Pertinent patient data (mean age, mean weight, mean operating time, and mode of operation) showed no remarkable differences. All patients had normal hepatic and renal function in preoperative examination.

Blood samples were collected before operation, simultaneously with ligation of the uterine vessels, and at the end of the operation. Serum and the biopsy of fundus myometrium were directly prepared, deep frozen, and stored at −70°C. Assay of mezlocillin was done by an agar diffusion method, using antibiotic medium no. 2 (Oxoid), pH 6.4, and *Bacillus subtilis* ATCC 6633 (BBL Microbiology Systems) as the test organism. The lower threshold of detection of mezlocillin was 2 mg/liter.

For the comparison of postoperative clinical data, we examined the standard febrile morbidity, serious pelvic infections, urinary tract infections, leukocytosis, and the mean length of hospital stay. Those cases with urinary tract infections were divided into patients with suprapubic and transurethral indwelling bladder catheter.

The serum levels after one-dose mezlocillin prophylaxis are shown in Fig. 1. The highest concentrations in the range from 306 to 138 μg/ml (average, 195.1 μg/ml) were measured 15 to 20 min after administration. Nearly 120 min after infusion, serum concentrations fell below the break point of 32 μg/ml (4).

In uterine tissue, the average content of hemoglobin was 0.74 g/100 ml. Peak mezlocillin levels in myometrial tissue of 120 to 72 μg/ml (mean, 86.7 μg/ml) were observed 25 to 30 min after one-dose administration (Fig. 1). The myometrial level of mezlocillin remained at or above the break point until 75 min after infusion. One tissue specimen extracted 250 min after administration showed no measurable myometrial concentrations of mezlocillin.

It is of interest that serum and myometrial levels of mezlocillin after the second dose of the

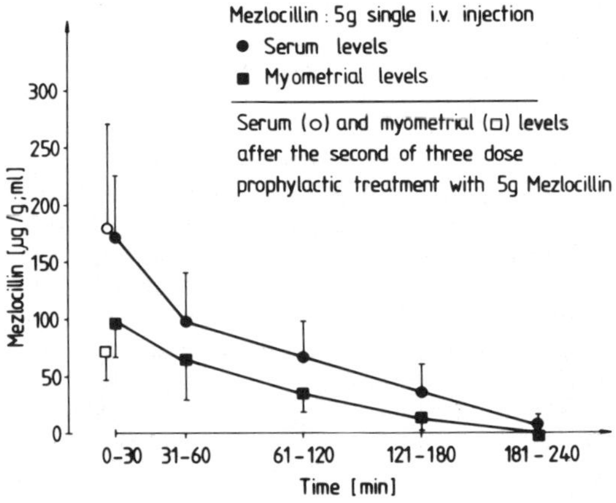

FIG. 1. *Serum levels after one-dose mezlocillin regimen.*

TABLE 1. *Incidence of infection and related parameters*

Group	Mean length of hosp. stay (days)	Serious pelvic infections	Standard febrile morbidity	Leucocytosis (days)	Urinary tract infections supra-pubic	Urinary tract infections trans-urethral
Single dose mezlocillin (n=35)	13.8 ± 3.6	0 / 35	1 / 35	4 / 35	3/14	2/21
Control group (n=31)	14.8 ± 3.5	2 / 31	5 / 31	13 / 31	3/10	7/21
Three dose mezlocillin (n=15)	13.8 ±3.2	0 / 15	1 / 15	1 / 15	0/5	1/10

perioperative three-dose course did not indicate any remarkable alterations in concentration within the first 30 min compared with the one-dose regimen.

There were no significant differences in the mean number of postoperative days in hospital between the three groups. Both groups receiving a prophylactic mezlocillin regimen had no severe pelvic infections. In contrast, there were two cases (6.4%) with severe pelvic infections in the control group. In those women without any antibiotic prophylaxis, the incidence of morbidity, including mild and moderate pelvic infections, was 25.9% and fell to 8.6% in the group receiving the one-dose mezlocillin regimen. Prophylactic antibiotics were of little value in preventing urinary tract infections. The clinical data are summarized in Table 1.

In a review of several studies concerning the role of antibiotic prophylaxis in vaginal hysterectomy, Duff and Park (2) found a distinct decrease in the number of postoperative severe infections in women undergoing an antibiotic prophylactic regimen. The pharmacokinetic as well as the clinical data of our study suggest that one dose of 5 g of mezlocillin 30 min before surgery appears to be effective in maintaining serum and uterine tissue antibiotic levels adequate to prevent severe pelvic infections.

1. **Decker, K., and R. Fleiner.** 1979. Behandlung geburtshilflich-gynäkologischer Infektionen mit Mezlocillin. 2. International Acylureido-Penicillin Symposium, Vienna.
2. **Duff, P., and R. C. Park.** 1980. Antibiotic prophylaxis in vaginal hysterectomy: a review. Obstet. Gynecol. **55**(suppl. 5):193S–202S.
3. **Hirsch, H. A.** 1978. Die antibiotische Behandlung gynäkologischer Erkrankungen. Immun. Infekt. **6:**140–145.
4. **Knothe, H.** 1979. Die antibakterielle Aktivität von Mezlocillin und Azlocillin. Arzneim. Forsch. **29:**1916–1920.

Mezlocillin Concentrations in Pancreatic Tissue and Serum After Intravenous Administration

W. RITZERFELD,* G. WITTRIN, AND W. GERLING

Hygiene-Institut und Chirurgische Klinik der Westfälischen Wilhelms-Universität, 4400 Münster, Federal Republic of Germany

The acylureidopenicillin mezlocillin, which has been used on a large clinical scale for some time, is marked by a broad antibacterial spectrum of action. Laboratory technical and clinical studies have furnished evidence for the substance's high activity against many pathogenic bacterial species. In our own routine determinations of bacterial resistance to mezlocillin in the first quarter of 1981, almost 5,000 pathogenic bacterial strains were examined. With the exception of organisms of *Pseudomonas* spp. and *Enterobacter*, the percentage of resistant pathogens was below 20%. Our preliminary results of in vivo studies were reported at the Ninth International Congress of Chemotherapy in London in 1975. An account of the serum levels of mezlocillin in children with serious renal damage was given at the Second Mediterranean Congress of Chemotherapy in Nice in 1980 (1). Although we found that mezlocillin can be prescribed over a prolonged period, we still do not know the answer to certain questions, one being the possible concentrations of mezlocillin in pancreatic tissue. Such findings would be of considerable clinical interest for prophylactic measures and possible treatment of bacterial infections of the pancreas. This paper reports on a number of studies aimed at determining the concentrations of mezlocillin in animal and human pancreatic tissue (and parallel concentrations in the serum) after single administration.

The concentrations of mezlocillin in serum and pancreatic tissue were determined according to the method of Grove and Randall (3). The test strain was *Bacillus subtilis* ATCC 6633, which has a lower limit of detectability of mezlocillin of 0.25 μg/ml. The standard curve was plotted on the basis of the following concentrations: 0.2, 0.4, 0.6, 1, 2, and 4 μg/ml. The reference value was 0.8 μg/ml; pooled serum was used as a solvent. The agar plates used for the determination of active substance levels had six punched holes: three for the concentrations of mezlocillin measured and three for the reference concentration. Three plates were prepared for each specimen so that nine values per specimen were always available. The findings were evaluated according to the scheme described by Dimmling (2).

The concentrations of mezlocillin in the pancreas and serum of three pigs were determined in preliminary studies. The substance was injected as an intravenous bolus at a dose of 5 g. The concentrations of mezlocillin were measured in the specimens collected intraoperatively 15, 30, and 60 min after administration. In another three animals, measurements were tried after 6, 7, and 8 h, but they were negative.

The subsequent studies on humans were carried out on 18 patients. The test persons received 5 g of mezlocillin intravenously pre- or intraoperatively. Serum levels had also been determined without prior medication before the operation. The specimens for examination were withdrawn 15 min to 6 h after medication, depending on the course of the operation.

Figure 1 shows the pancreas and serum levels found in the animals. For the three times of measurement, arithmetic means and standard deviation are plotted. Generally, serum levels were clearly higher than concentrations in pancreatic tissue. However, marked pancreas levels were demonstrable within the 1st hour; 15 min after medication, concentrations were 65 μg/ml in the serum and 25 μg/g in the pancreas. The concentrations then showed a rapid decline and had fallen to levels of around 30 μg/ml and just under 10 μg/g 12 h after medication. The half-lives for the serum specimens were 36.5, 38, and 42 min; those for pancreatic tissue specimens were 34, 34, and 35 min.

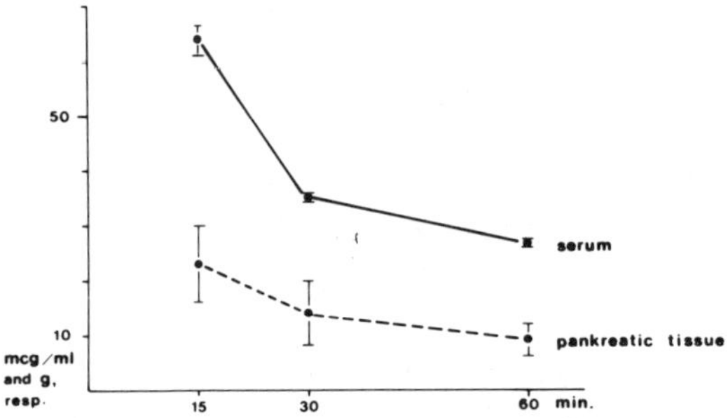

FIG. 1. *Pancreas and serum mezlocillin levels in three pigs.*

The following clinical diagnoses were established: chronic pancreatitis, 10 patients; pancreatic cancer, 6 patients; pancreatic cyst, 1 patient; and biliary duct cancer, 1 patient. These findings were histologically confirmed. The patients had not received any antibiotics before surgery. Mezlocillin had been given as a perioperative prophylaxis because of the massive interventions.

Figure 2 shows the values of 17 serum specimens (16 patients) and 12 pancreas specimens (11 patients). The discrepancy between the number of patients arises from the fact that specimens for examination were not available in every case. The values for each patient determined at the same time have been plotted below each other. The highest serum value measured about 10 min after the administration of mezlocillin was 65 μg/ml; the peak concentration in pancreatic tissue was 40 μg/g. Further pancreas specimens withdrawn during the first 30 min after medication were within the same order of magnitude. The difference between pancreas and serum values was reduced or no longer measurable 2 to 6 h after medication. At this time of determination, concentrations were around 10 μg/ml and g, respectively, later declining to 3 to 4 μg/ml and g, respectively.

These results generally indicate that mezlocillin is detectable at clearly antibiotically active

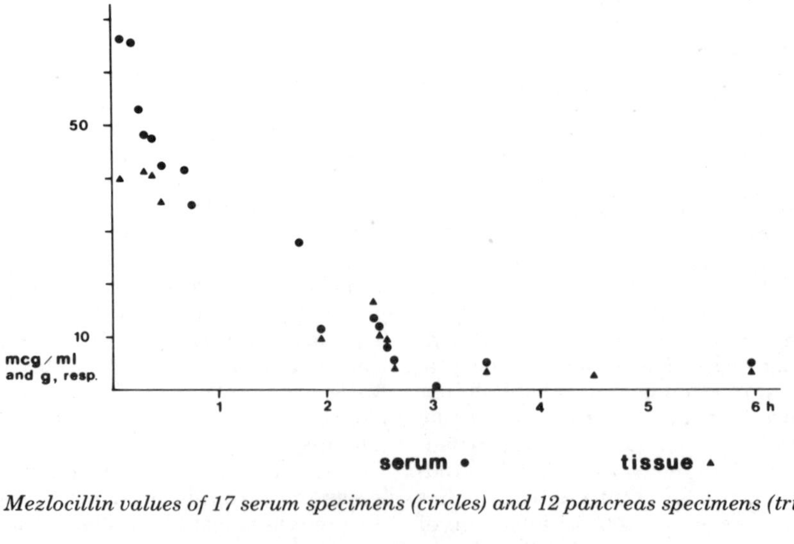

FIG. 2. *Mezlocillin values of 17 serum specimens (circles) and 12 pancreas specimens (triangles).*

levels during the first few hours after administration. Therefore, it will often be possible to exert a marked influence on the bacterial microorganism responsible for an inflammatory process in this operative field. The aspect of a perioperative prophylaxis must also be taken into account. It would certainly be worth considering the possibility of intensifying the mezlocillin medication to achieve adequately high antibacterial effects. Even though only a relatively small number of pancreatic tissue specimens were available to us, our findings indicate that mezlocillin has a quite remarkable significance for the indications described.

1. **Dieckmann, L., A. Niemann, and W. Ritzerfeld.** 1980. Serum mezlocillin levels in children with renal impairment. Second Mediterranean Congress of Chemotherapy, 13–16 October 1980, Nice, abstr. 224.
2. **Dimmling, T.** 1957. Ein Zylindertest zur quantitativen Bestimmung von Tetracyclin und seinen Derivaten in Körperflüssigkeiten. Drug Res. **7**:684–687.
3. **Grove, D. C., and B. A. Randall.** 1955. Assay methods of antibiotics, a laboratory manual. Antibiotic Monogr. no. 2. Medical Encyclopedia, Inc., New York.

Mezlocillin and Oxacillin Concentrations in Serum, Mammary Gland, and Fat

J. BORDT,* H. WAGNER, AND D. ADAM

Universitäts-Frauenklinik, D-4400 Münster, and Pediatric Clinic of the University, D-8000 Munich, Federal Republic of Germany*

The ability of an antimicrobial drug to reach bactericidal concentrations in body fluids and tissues is of special interest to surgeons, who use antibiotics as a perioperative prophylaxis to control postoperative infections. Therefore, the drug regimen must provide for adequate concentrations of the antimicrobial agent at the possible site of infection during the course of the operation (2, 3).

In this study, the concentrations of two simultaneously administered penicillins, mezlocillin and oxacillin, were examined in serum, mammary gland, and fat of 35 female patients with an average age of 42 years (range, 15 to 76) and an average weight of 71 kg (range, 51 to 100) undergoing major surgery of the breast. Doses of 4 g of mezlocillin and 2 g of oxacillin were given intravenously over a 30-min infusion period with a constant flow of 100 ml/h by means of a precision infusion pump. Samples of blood, mammary gland, and fat were taken at intervals of 0 (blood only), 20, 30, 45, 60, and 90 min and 2, 3, 6, and 8 h after the end of the infusion period. Blood, including samples from mammary gland and fat, was wiped off with a dry sterile swab. Serum was separated from whole blood by centrifugation at 2,000 rpm. All serum and tissue samples were frozen at −30°C and transported under refrigeration to the laboratory for further processing. The serum and tissue concentrations of the antibiotics were determined by biological assay with the agar diffusion method (1). Table 1 summarizes our findings.

In serum, the maximal concentrations of the two penicillins were found immediatey after the end of the infusion period: 281.0 μg/ml for mezlocillin and 107.8 μg/ml for oxacillin. The concentrations declined progressively according to their renal elimination, falling below the limit of detection (<2 μg/ml) after 6 h.

In mammary gland tissue, a steady increase in the mezlocillin concentration was measured, reaching its maximum of 52.3 μg/g at the 90-min interval, whereas oxacillin could not be detected in any of the samples examined.

In fat tissue, the maximal mezlocillin concentration was 38.3 μg/g, reached 20 min after the end of the infusion period, and declined to 0 within 3 h. The pattern paralleled that of mezlocillin in serum, but the average concentration was only about one-fifth the average mezlocillin concentration. Oxacillin in fat could not be detected in any of the samples examined.

In summary, we found the maximal concentrations of mezlocillin and oxacillin in serum and of mezlocillin in fat at the end of the infusion, whereas the peak concentrations of mezlocillin in mammary gland were found in the samples taken at the 90-min interval after the end of the infusion. This lag of distribution into the tissues to be operated on as the possible site of infection should be anticipated by clinicians when administering antibiotics as a perioperative prophylaxis to control postoperative infections. As oxacillin could not be detected in either mammary gland or fat, it may possibly be abandoned in the

TABLE 1. *Concentrations of mezlocillin (M) and oxacillin (O) after single intravenous infusion of 4 and 2 g, respectively, in serum, mammary gland, and fat*

Sample	Drug	Concn at given time[a] End of infusion	20 min	30 min	45 min	1 h	1.5 h	2 h	3 h	6 h	8 h
Serum	M	281.0 (135.7)	189.6 (111.5)	121.7 (36.8)	110.0 (0)	77.3 (31.9)	47.6 (40.3)	19.5 (7.8)	18.8 (9.8)	0	0
	O	107.8 (37.3)	62.2 (8.9)	51.5 (15.6)	52.5 (10.6)	29.5 (14.1)	12.0 (6.3)	4.8 (1.6)	2.0 (1.0)	0	0
Mammary gland	M			23.6 (7.5)		38.6 (20.8)	52.3 (6.1)	14.2 (12.2)	5.9 (4.1)	0	0
	O		0	0	0	0	0	0	0	0	0
Fat	M		38.3 (6.6)	32.6 (15.0)	25.5 (13.2)	20.5 (12.7)	21.0 (12.0)	8.5 (2.9)	0	0	0
	O		0	0	0	0	0	0	0	0	0

[a] Serum concentrations are given as micrograms per milliliter; mammary gland and fat concentrations are given as micrograms per gram. SD is given in parentheses.

regimen of preventive antibiotic therapy in major surgery of the breast.

1. **Bennett, I. V., I. L. Brodie, E. J. Benner, and W. M. M. Kirby.** 1966. Simplified accurate method for antibiotic assay for clinical specimens. Appl. Microbiol. **14:** 170–177.
2. **Stone, H. H., B. B. Haney, L. D. Kolb, C. E. Gehber, and C. A. Hooper.** 1979. Prophylactic and preventive antibiotic therapy. Timing, duration and economics. Ann. Surg. **189:**691–697.
3. **Stone, H. H., C. A. Hooper, L. D. Kolb, C. E. Gehber, and E. J. Dawkins.** 1976. Antibiotic prophylaxis in gastric, biliary and colonic surgery. Ann. Surg. **184:**443–448.

Influence of Protein Binding on Tissue Fluid Concentrations of Isoxalolyl- and Acylureidopenicillins

DIETMAR H. WITTMANN,* JOHANNA FEDDER, AND HANS-H. SCHASSAN

Altona General Hospital and Hamburg University, 2000 Hamburg 55, West Germany

In the present study, tissue fluid is defined as that fluid which is obtained from the periprosthetic space after hip joint replacement operations in humans, the hip joint being replaced by an artificial polyethylene cup and a femoral head. This fluid is similar to the tissue fluid obtained from subcutaneously implanted tissue cages in animals and humans (1, 2; D. Adam and B. Reichart, Program Abstr. Intersci. Conf. Antimicrob. Agents Chemother. 17th, New York, N.Y., abstr. 306, 1977). With respect to the albumin, protein, and electrolyte concentrations, similar ratios between tissue fluid and serum are found in all models. The protein and albumin concentrations are about 50% of the serum values in the tissue cage models, which represents the extravascular compartment better than does cantharide blister fluid (3); the latter has albumin content similar to that of serum and 62% of the serum protein concentrations.

There is some evidence that highly protein-bound antibiotics exhibit a different penetration pattern into the extravascular compartment than those of which less than 50% of the molecules are bound to serum proteins (3). The aim of the present study was to assess the antibiotic concentrations in tissue fluid after simultaneous administration of a highly protein-bound penicillin (i.e., oxacillin, 88 to 93% of which is bound to serum proteins) and a poorly protein-bound penicillin (i.e., mezlocillin, 38 to 48% of which is bound to serum proteins). In 20 patients, either 1 g of oxacillin and 2 g of mezlocillin or 2 g of oxacillin and 4 g of mezlocillin were administered intravenously as a bolus injection or a short infusion. The mean age of patients ranged from 59.4 (SD, 8.7) to 67.4 (SD, 8.2) years. All patients had normal renal and liver functions. The total protein concentrations, as well as the albumin concentrations, in the tissue fluid were between 51 and 56% of the corresponding serum values.

Tissue fluid together with serum samples were

obtained at defined intervals. The samples were frozen immediately at −21 to 25°C. The standard was prepared for microbiological assay at the time of sampling in pooled serum and tissue fluid from untreated patients. The samples were assayed with *Escherichia coli* 6311/65 for mezlocillin, the lowest traceable limit being 0.4 mg/liter in serum and 0.3 mg/liter in tissue fluid. Oxacillin was assayed with *Sarcina lutea* ATCC 9341 plus the penicillinase Penase (lot 784, Leo Pharmaceutical Products, Ballerup, Denmark) to inactivate mezlocillin. The lowest traceable limit in serum was 0.6 mg/liter and that in tissue fluid was 0.3 mg/liter.

From all serum concentrations measured, a mean concentration-time curve was calculated for each antibiotic and dosage. The R-squared value was above 0.95, which indicates that there is a good conformity between the mean calculated serum concentration-time curve and the concentrations measured.

In the 2-g dosage groups, the serum concentrations for oxacillin and mezlocillin were similar and therefore comparable, especially with respect to tissue fluid penetration of the two antibiotics. The prolonged half-life during the β-phase (all serum concentration-time curves fitted an open two-compartment model) with the 2-g dosage of oxacillin is probably due to competitive renal excretion mechanisms when two penicillins are given simultaneously. This half-life was similar to that observed with the 2-g mezlocillin dosage.

The results obtained with the simultaneous application of 1 g of oxacillin and 2 g of mezlocillin showed that the tissue fluid concentration-time curve crosses the serum concentration-time curve after 2.0 h with mezlocillin and after 2.5 h with oxacillin. The terminal half-life of oxacillin tissue fluid concentrations was calculated to be 216 min, whereas for mezlocillin it was only 69 min. This shows that highly protein-bound penicillin achieves the peak concentration in tissue fluid more slowly, and its pharmacokinetic behavior is characterized by a prolonged half-life in this extravascular compartment.

The simultaneous administration of 2 g of oxacillin and 4 g of mezlocillin showed substantially the same situation at a higher level. The cross-point of the tissue fluid concentration-time curve with the serum concentration-time curve was earlier with mezlocillin than with oxacillin. The terminal half-life was about the same as observed with the other dosages, i.e.,70 min for mezlocillin and 194 min for oxacillin.

The influence of protein binding upon tissue fluid penetration becomes even more obvious in comparing the concentrations after the 2-g dosages of both antibiotics (see Fig. 1). Whereas similar serum concentrations were observed, tissue fluid concentration-time curves were different.

Two hours after the injection, tissue fluid concentrations of oxacillin with 13.3 mg/liter was only 48% of the mezlocillin tissue fluid concentration with 27.5 mg/liter. After 4 h the oxacillin tissue fluid concentration was 56% of the mezlocillin tissue fluid concentration. After 6 h this ratio was 71%, and after 8 h higher oxacillin concentrations were found in tissue fluid than in mezlocillin tissue fluid concentrations (Table 1). The area under the curve for oxacillin was 70 mg.h/liter, whereas that for mezlocillin at the same dosage was 102 mg.h/liter with respect to tissue fluid concentrations. This indicates that the highly protein-bound substance has poor tissue fluid penetration compared with the less highly protein-bound mezlocillin. However, once

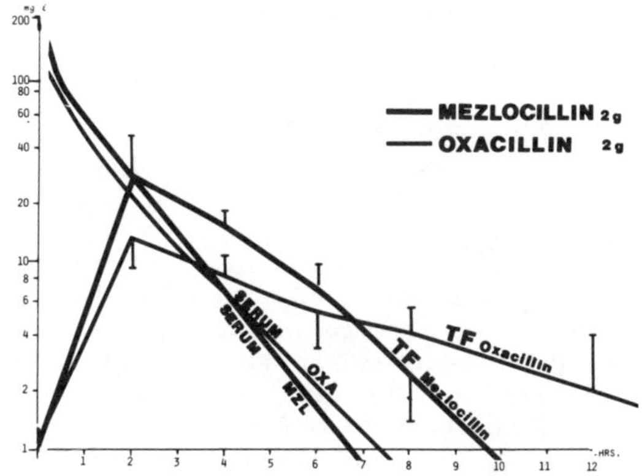

FIG. 1. *Serum and tissue fluid (TF) concentration-time curves after intravenous administration of oxacillin (OXA) and mezlocillin (MZL).*

TABLE 1. *Tissue fluid concentrations of oxacillin and mezlocillin*[a]

Time after injection (h)	Concn (mg/liter)				No. of samples	Ratio (oxacillin/mezlocillin)
	Oxacillin (2 g i.v.)		Mezlocillin (2 g i.v.)			
	Mean[c]	SD	Mean[c]	SD		
2	13.3	1.5	27.2	1.7	28	0.48
4	8.5	1.2	15.1	1.2	25	0.56
6	5.2	1.5	7.3	1.3	23	0.71
8	4.3	1.3	2.5	1.8	26	1.72
12	2.0	1.9	0.2[b]		12	8.00

[a] 93% of oxacillin was bound to serum proteins; 43% of mezlocillin was bound to serum proteins. i.v., Intravenous.

[b] Calculated.

[c] Geometric mean.

the molecule of oxacillin is trapped in the tissue fluid, it is released more slowly, supporting the theory that extracellular fluid has a protecting role toward highly protein-bound substances (4). Obviously the time for equilibrium between the bound and unbound molecule is responsible for both the slow penetration into tissue fluid and its protracted way back into the central compartment. This is in accordance with the findings of Henning and Holm (3), who found that the highly protein-bound substance is eliminated more slowly from the tissue cage.

With regard to the therapeutic consequences, our investigations indicate that the dosage of highly protein-bound substances should exceed that of poorly protein-bound antibiotics to achieve sufficient concentrations at the site of infection.

1. **Chisholm, G. D.** 1978. The tissue cage model in the distribution of antibacterial agents. Scand. J. Infect. Dis. Suppl. **14**:177–185.
2. **Eickenberg, H.-U.** 1978. What is interstitial fluid? Scand. J. Infect. Dis. Suppl. **14**:166–170.
3. **Henning, C., and S. E. Holm.** 1981. Penetration of ^{14}C-Ro 13-9904 into tissue cage fluid in rabbits. Chemotherapy **27** (Suppl. 1):32–36.
4. **Rotschild, M. A., M. Oratz, and S. S. Schreiber.** 1979. Extravascular albumin. N. Engl. J. Med. **301**:497–497.
5. **Wise, R., A. P. Gillet, B. Cadge, S. R. Durham, and S. Baker.** 1980. The influence of protein binding upon tissue fluid levels of 6 β-lactams. J. Infect. Dis. **142**:77–82.

Pharmacokinetic Studies and Results of a Clinical Trial with Combination Therapy with Mezlocillin and Oxacillin

J. STUTE,* H.-H. SCHASSAN, D. H. WITTMANN, AND J. KUECHLIN

Department of Dermatology, University Hospital, Hamburg-Eppendorf, Institute for Microbiology, and I Surgery Department, General Hospital of Hamburg-Altona, Hamburg, West Germany*

In dermatology there is often an indication for systemic antibiotic therapy of erysipelas, infected ulcers, impetigo, or furuncles, or as a perioperative protection of patients. In general, one cannot wait for the antibiogram. In more than 80% of the cases, the initial swab for bacteriological culture is followed by the initiation of antibiotic therapy. Therefore, it is definitely necessary to cover a wide spectrum of bacteria, and a combination therapy is indicated. The question arises as to what dosage of the antibiotic is necessary. The aim of this study was to measure the concentration in the tissues at its actual focus, i.e., in the skin. The skin concentrations were compared with the serum concentrations.

The substance was given only for a clinical indication. Of 21 patients we examined when we had to exchange a hip or a knee joint prosthesis, 10 patients were given 2 g of mezlocillin and 1 g of oxacillin simultaneously and 11 patients received 4 g of mezlocillin and 2 g of oxacillin given simultaneously for perioperative prophylaxis or therapy of a persisting infection. We examined the healthy skin which was connected with the scar. This part of the skin was microbiologically examined for its contents of mezlocillin and oxacillin. The mean age of the patients who received 2 g of mezlocillin and 1 g of oxacillin was 62.5 ± 18.5 years, and their weight was 61.7 ± 9.8 kg. The age of the patients who received 4 g of mezlocillin and 2 g of oxacillin was 66.0 ± 19.2 years, and their weight was 64.1 ± 7.1 kg. None of them had liver or renal impairment. There were no penicillin allergies.

Blood for determination of the serum concentrations was taken after 5, 10, 20, 30, 60, and 90 min, and tissue specimens were taken after 30, 60, and 90 min. The standard was always prepared at the time of sampling. The serum and tissue specimens were immediately frozen at −20 to −25°C. They were examined within 14 days after the time of application of the substance. The test organism for mezlocillin was *Escherichia coli* 6311/65 on Penassay agar, pH 7.0. The test organism for oxacillin was *Sarcina lutea* ATCC 9341 with addition of a penicillinase to degrade mezlocillin on Penassay agar, pH 7.0. The lowest detectable level was 0.3 mg/liter for mezlocillin and 0.6 mg/liter for oxacillin.

From all results the geometric mean and the SD were calculated.

We found that the concentration of both antibiotics in the skin showed a maximum 1 h after application (Table 1). It was noticeable that the concentration-time curve within 30 to 90 min was quite constant. There was a flat decline after 60 min.

We know that the protein binding of oxacillin in serum is 93%. In tissue fluid a lower binding

TABLE 1. *Mean values and SD of the serum and skin concentrations of mezlocillin and oxacillin*

Sample and drug	Dose (g)	Time (min)	No. of specimens	Concn (mg/liter)
Serum				
Mezlocillin	2	30	9	97.48 ± 1.35
Oxacillin	1	30	9	48.17 ± 1.44
Mezlocillin	4	30	11	168.65 ± 1.27
Oxacillin	2	30	11	70.35 ± 1.30
Skin				
Mezlocillin	2	30	10	22.55 ± 1.67
Oxacillin	1	30	10	7.62 ± 1.45
Mezlocillin	4	30	10	39.31 ± 1.39
Oxacillin	2	30	10	13.57 ± 1.40
Skin				
Mezlocillin	2	60	10	27.23 ± 1.48
Oxacillin	1	60	10	8.69 ± 1.49
Mezlocillin	4	60	10	48.26 ± 1.24
Oxacillin	2	60	10	16.45 ± 1.24
Skin				
Mezlocillin	2	90	6	22.38 ± 1.37
Oxacillin	1	90	6	7.42 ± 1.73
Mezlocillin	4	90	6	40.88 ± 1.21
Oxacillin	2	90	6	12.73 ± 1.17

of about 42% was found. This might mean that not all of the substance was available for antibacterial activity directly after infusion of the substance, but there was a high therapeutic potency. According to our investigations, successful antimicrobial chemotherapy with oxacillin requires the MIC for the bacteria involved to be below 4 mg/liter with the 1-g dosage and to be below 8 mg/liter with the 2-g dosage. Since oxacillin is directed against penicillinase-producing staphylococci, not all of our clinical isolates will be inhibited at the 1-g dosage. This is important with respect to the prominent role of staphylococci in skin and soft tissue infections. In our experience *Staphylococcus aureus* is responsible alone or in combination with gram-negative bacteria in mixed infections in about 60 to 70% of the cases.

The use of the combination of mezlocillin and oxacillin is—like all antibiotic therapy—to be made with caution to prevent selection of resistant organisms. The main indication is for the therapy of infections caused by unknown organisms because this combination covers a wide spectrum.

If a combination therapy has been chosen for the initiation of treatment, one has different alternatives for the further therapy after one knows the results of the microbiological investigations: (i) in monoinfections or mixed infections caused by susceptible organisms, one can exclude one combination partner, (ii) in mixed infections caused by susceptible organisms, one can continue the combination therapy; or (iii) in cases of resistance to both antibiotics, both substances have to be replaced.

Antibiotic Concentrations in Blood and Tissues: Intraoperative Ischemia as a Model for the Determination of Tissue Concentrations, with Mezlocillin and Oxacillin Used as Examples

D. ADAM,* K. WILHELM, AND V. CHYSKÝ

Pediatric Clinic and Surgical Clinic, University of Munich, Munich, and Bayer AG Pharmaceutical Research Center, Wuppertal, Federal Republic of Germany*

Antibiotic concentrations in tissues and organs determined in animal studies are more accurate than human data. The reason is that experimental animals can be completely bled after sacrifice. The blood remaining in ischemic tissues—the so-called blood error—is insignificant and can be disregarded. It has hardly any effect on the actual tissue and organ concentrations. However, if antibiotic concentrations are determined in intraoperatively removed human tissue, blood seepage is one of the main reasons for false results. The blood error increases with the amount of blood in the tissue or organ and with the shortness of time between administration and assay. Using as an example determination of mezlocillin and oxacillin concentrations, we present here a direct method for eliminating the blood error.

Twenty-four patients undergoing operations on the upper extremity were given an intravenous bolus injection during 5 min of 4 g of mezlocillin and 2 g of oxacillin (Optocillin). This amounted to an average dose of 60 mg of mezlocillin and 30 g of oxacillin per kg of body weight. The injection was given about 30 min before application of the Esmarch bandage. The interval between the end of the injection and the induction of ischemia was taken as the time for measurement of the tissue level of drug. No additional intervention was needed to collect the ischemic tissue. Venous blood was drawn from the contralateral vein when each ischemic tissue specimen was removed.

To ascertain to what extent blood contained in the tissue distorts antibiotic activity, we compared the hemoglobin content of the ischemic tissue with that of similar blood-perfused tissue specimens taken 10 min after removal of the Esmarch bandage. The hemoglobin was determined as described by Meijer (2).

To determine blood contained in the tissue homogenates, the tissue was processed in a Stomacher 80 in the same way as for determination of antibiotic concentrations.

TABLE 1. *Mean and range of hemoglobin content in ischemic and perfused tissue samples (milliliters per gram of tissue)*

Kind of tissue	Ischemia	Perfused tissue 10 min after removal of Esmarch bandage
Muscle (n = 6)	0.8 (0–2.5)	50.9 (7.9–76.8)
Fat (n = 6)	1.65 (0–3.5)	35.1 (17.2–70.9)
Muscle fascia (n = 1)	0.0	8.7
Ligament (n = 3)	1.4 (0–4.2)	30.7 (5.7–54.1)
Palmar fascia (n = 2)	1.85 (0.1–3.6)	10.85 (9.4–12.3)
Capsular tissue (n = 2)	1.05 (0–2.1)	33.1 (28.4–37.8)
Skin (n = 3)	3.13 (1.85–5.5)	38.9 (14.3–59.2)

This study confirmed that the application of the Esmarch bandage produces a very high degree of ischemia. The hemoglobin content of some types of tissue was either not measurable or so low that the error resulting from the antibiotic activity of residual blood in these tissue specimens could be discounted. The contrast of hemoglobin values of ischemic tissue and blood-perfused tissue is shown in Table 1. The blood concentrations in ischemic tissue varied between 0 and 10% of those in tissue with unrestrained blood flow.

The antibiotic concentrations were measured by the agar diffusion method (3).

The measurement time coincident with the induction of ischemia was selected, as there is no further elimination from the strangulated tissue, and on the assumption that the drug is not metabolized in the affected tissue.

The time between the injection of mezlocillin/oxacillin and application of the Esmarch bandage—the influx period—varied between 20 and 55 min (average, 33.6 min). The variation was due to the technical progress of the individual surgery.

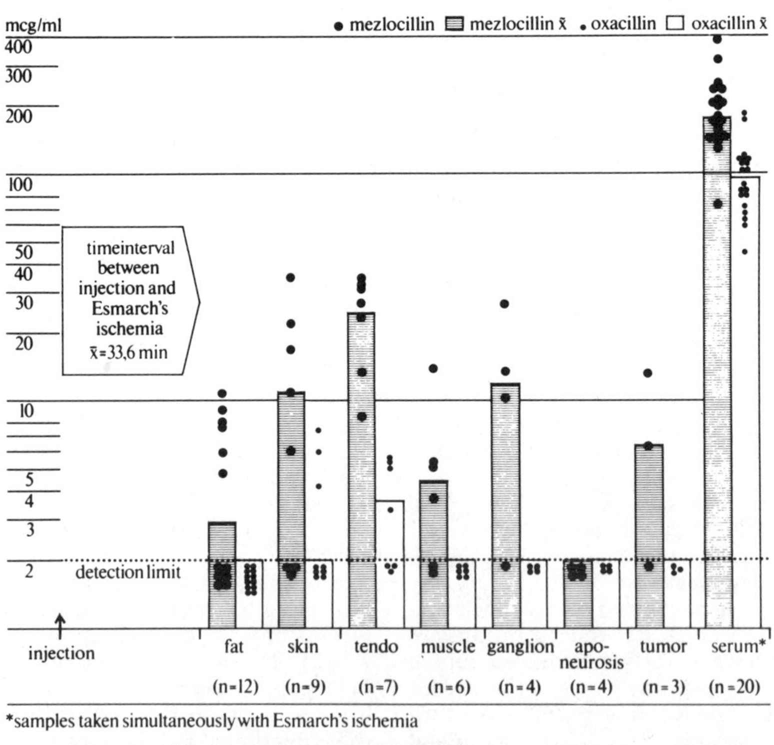

FIG. 1. *Concentrations of antibiotics in samples of ischemic tissues and serum taken 20 to 55 min (mean, 33.6 min) after a single simultaneous intravenous injection of 4 g of mezlocillin and 2 g of oxacillin (detection limit, 2 μg/ml).*

Figure 1 shows the mezlocillin and oxacillin concentrations in the individual tissue and the serum collected at the time of application of the Esmarch bandage. The tissue levels were highest in the tendon (median values), with 24.3 mg/kg for mezlocillin. High mezlocillin concentrations were also found in ischemic skin (10.8 mg/kg) and in ganglion (11.8 mg/kg). Mezlocillin concentrations detected were 4.4 mg/kg in muscle, 6.3 mg/kg in tumor, 11.2 mg/kg in ligamentum, and 7.3 mg/kg in sinovia. The oxacillin levels in many of the skin specimens and the other types of tissue were below the detection limit of 2.0 mg/kg.

The dose ratio of 4 g of mezlocillin to 2 g of oxacillin was reflected in the serum levels obtained. The round median values of mezlocillin and oxacillin concentrations in serum after the end of injection were as follows (milligrams per liter): 20 min, 208 and 97; 30 min, 187 and 107; 40 min, 169 and 85; 50 min, 147 and 52; 60 min, 123 and 48; 70 min, 80 and 35; 90 min, 78 and 23.

The serum levels of mezlocillin determined in this study are in accordance with the findings of other investigators who used a similar dose (1) as well as with our own results (P. Kratochvil, G. Brandstätter, D. Adam, and V. Chyský, in preparation).

1. **Helwing, E., M. Lux, W. Düben, J. Potel, and D. Tettenborn.** 1979. Mezlocillin: zur Gewebekonzentration und Wirksamkeit. Med. Klin. **74**:112–116.
2. **Meijer, A. E. F. H.** 1962. The quantitative determination of whole blood in homogenized tissue preparations. Clin. Chim. Acta **7**:638–641.
3. **Nauman, P., H. Lode, and E. Reintjens.** 1973. Zur Kombinationsbehandlung mit Penicillinen; Nachweisverfahren und Pharmakokinetik von Oxacillin und Ampicillin bei simultaner Verabreichung. Arzneim. Forsch. **23**:218–225.

Investigation into the Influence of Mezlocillin and Azlocillin on Plasmatic Blood Coagulation

W. BROCKHAUS,* H. SESSNER, G. HELD, AND C. HERZ

I. Medizin Klinik, Klinikum der Stadt Nürnberg, Nürnberg, Federal Republic of Germany

Clinical observations have given rise to the suspicion that semisynthetic penicillins could be responsible for disturbances of hemostasis. Investigations into this problem have yielded partly contradictory results, possibly as a result of different experimental designs (2, 6, 11).

Only a few investigators found no impairment of hemostasis when applying specific test methods (5, 10). The reason for this could be the different antibiotic dosages which caused plasma concentrations ranging from those produced by medium therapeutic dosage to many times the maximum levels attainable. In most of the cases, the hemostatic disturbances were found to be due to an impairment of the platelets (1, 3, 4, 6, 8, 9) which was reflected by a prolonged bleeding time and a disturbance of platelet aggregation, especially with ADP, perhaps as a consequence of a competitive inhibition of ADP receptors caused by a substance-induced platelet coating (3). The disturbance of aggregation was less pronounced with adrenalin, collagen, and thrombin. Since the disturbance was still demonstrable when the antibiotic had been discontinued, an additional impairment of the megakaryocytes was discussed (3, 4). However, our experimental conditions suggested that the platelets themselves are not adversely affected (6). The disturbances described are particularly often observed with ticarcillin and carbenicillin.

When fibrinogen is converted to fibrin, semisynthetic penicillins are assumed to interfere in cross-linking (1, 9). Several causes of a disturbed polymerization have been discussed: (i) a reduction or change in the coagulation factors of stage 1, (ii) a change in fibrinogen by accumulation or molecular rearrangement, and (iii) an interference with degradation products as a consequence of fibrinolysis.

The group tests for plasmatic coagulation (Quick methods, aPTT, and PTT) are only suited for the detection of massive deficits in factors. This may be the reason that changes in plasmatic coagulation are described only in individual cases (7). Individual investigators have seen changes in the activity of antithrombin III (1) which have not been confirmed by others (6, 7).

So far, only little experience has been gained regarding the influence of the acylureidopenicillins mezlocillin and azlocillin on plasmatic blood coagulation. Blood samples were withdrawn from four healthy male subjects and four patients subject to dialysis (creatinine above 10 mg/100 ml, urea above 200 mg/100 ml), treated with citrate buffer to prevent coagulation, and mixed with dilutions of mezlocillin and azlocillin (Bayer AG) 1:100 so that final concentrations of 5, 50, 500, and 1,000 μg/ml were present in the whole blood. The following parameters were examined immediately after an incubation period of 120 and 240 min at a temperature of 37°C: group tests (Quick, Normotest, aPTT), coagulation factors I–X, and antithrombin III; fibrin polymerization was examined by using reptilase time, thrombin coagulase time, thrombelastography, and two-dimensional electrophoresis as performed by Clark Freeman. Plasmatic coagulation was not found to be seriously impaired. However, aPTT was reduced in a concentration-dependent manner when dilutions with mezlocillin were used. With increasing duration of incubation, patients with impaired renal function showed a slight decrease in factors II–X, in contrast to individuals with a normal kidney. No such effect was observed with azlocillin. Mezlocillin possibly produces a mild activation by contact of the coagulation factors of stage 1. The two-dimensional electrophoresis of fibrinogen with the use of patient plasma indicated marked changes for both azlocillin and mezlocillin.

There was a second peak, but the exact cause is not clear: change in charge or molecular rearrangement or fibrinolysis via activation by contact?

In summary, there is no definite evidence that the acylureidopenicillins azlocillin and mezlocillin seriously impair plasmatic coagulation in vitro. However, there is evidence of changes in the fibrinogen molecule which might be the cause of the disturbance of polymerization discussed in connection with the use of semisynthetic penicillins.

1. **Andrassy, K., E. Weisschedel, D. Höffler, and E. Ritz.** 1980. Führen Ureido-Penicilline zu Hämostasestörungen und hämorrhagischer Kolitis? Therapiewoche **30:** 2777–2784.
2. **Baisch, C., U. Leopold, H. Grimm, D. Schmidt, V. Winter, and A. Suhayda.** 1980. Erfahrungen mit Azlocillin im Rahmen einer multizentrischen Studie, p. 183–186. International Symposium, Vienna, 1979, Acylureido-penicilline. Excerpta Medica, Amsterdam.
3. **Brown, C. H., III, E. A. Natelson, M. W. Bradshaw, C. P. Alfrey, and T. W. Williams.** 1975. Study of the effects of ticarcillin on blood coagulation and platelet function. Antimicrob. Agents Chemother. **7:**652–657.
4. **Brown, C. H., III, E. A. Natelson, M. W. Bradshaw, T. W. Williams, and C. P. Alfrey.** 1974. The hemostatic defect produced by carbenicillin. N. Engl. J. Med. **291:**265–270.
5. **Custer, G. M., B. R. Briggs, and R. E. Smith.** 1979. Effect of cefamandole nafate on blood coagulation and platelet function. Antimicrob. Agents Chemother. **16:** 869–872.
6. **Johnsson, H., and P. M. Niklasson.** 1977. Effects of some antibiotics on platelet function in vitro and in vivo. Thromb. Res. **11:**237–251.
7. **Matthiessen, W., and U. Kroening.** 1978. Phase II study on azlocillin for bronchopulmonary infections due to pseudomonas, p. 628–630. *In* W. Siegenthaler and R. Lüthy (ed.), Current chemotherapy, vol. 1. American Society for Microbiology, Washington, D.C.
8. **Nakahara, M.** 1978. Effect of antibiotics on platelet thromboplastic function and thrombin activity. J. Med. **9:**433–443.
9. **Natelson, E. A., W. T. Siebert, T. W. Williams, and M. W. Bradshaw.** 1979. Combined effects of ticarcillin and cefazolin on blood coagulation and platelet function. Am. J. Med. Sci. **278:**217–221.
10. **Schacht, P., H. Bruck, J. Dycka, R. Hullmann, and D. Tettenborn.** 1980. Ergebnisse der klinischen Prüfung von Azlocillin, p. 193–198. *In* International Symposium, Vienna, 1979, Acylureido-Penicilline. Excerpta Medica, Amsterdam.
11. **Tettenborn, D., P. Schacht, R. Hullmann, and H. Bruck.** 1979. Ergebnisse der klinischen Prüfung von Mezlocillin. Drug. Res. **29:**2009–2014.

Results of a Prospective, Randomized, Double-Blind Comparison of Mezlocillin and Ticarcillin for Treatment of Skin, Bone, and Soft Tissue Infections

RICHARD V. McCLOSKEY

Albert Einstein Medical Center, Daroff Division, Jefferson Medical College, Philadelphia, Pennsylvania 19147, U.S.A.

Ureidopenicillins (azlocillin, mezlocillin, and piperacillin) are a new class of broad-spectrum penicillins in which a substituted urea side chain appears instead of the α-amino group of ampicillin. The ureidopenicillins have greater activity against a wider range of gram-negative bacteria than currently used broad-spectrum penicillins (1, 4). In previous clinical studies, treatment of soft tissue infections with mezlocillin has been associated with failure in less than 5% of the treated cases (3). Similar results have been obtained in larger clinical trials with azlocillin (2).

The design of the study reported here was prospective, controlled, randomized, and third-party blinded. The study was performed from October 1978 to April 1980. As part of a larger clinical trial in which 178 patients were enrolled, 92 patients were treated for infection of the skin and supporting structures. Mezlocillin was compared with ticarcillin. Both antibiotics were given as an intravenous infusion over a 30-min period at a daily dose of 18 g in six divided doses. The duration of treatment for valid courses of therapy was 5 to 12 days for mezlocillin (mean, 11.1 days) and 4 to 25 days for ticarcillin (mean, 10.3 days). A course of therapy was accepted as valid for evaluation of drug effectiveness if the following criteria were met: (i) isolation and identification of one or more pathogens from pretreatment cultures obtained within 5 days of the initiation of therapy; (ii) susceptibility of at least one of the causative organisms to both study drugs; (iii) no concomitant administration of any other antimicrobial agent; (iv) duration of treatment of at least 3 days; and (v) appropriate cultures obtained after the conclusion of treatment except in those circumstances where skin structure infections had healed and no suitable material was available for culture. Mezlocillin was supplied as mezlocillin sodium monohydrate, and ticarcillin was supplied as ticarcillin disodium. The clinical investigator had no knowledge of which drug a patient received.

A random code with stratification for different sites of infection was used for enrollment of patients. The following conditions or clinical situations excluded patients from enrollment in the study: (i) pregnancy; (ii) history of allergy to penicillin; (iii) necessity to receive a concomitant antibiotic with a spectrum of activity similar to that of the study drug; and (iv) renal impairment (serum creatinine greater than 3 mg/100 ml). Mezlocillin or ticarcillin was administered intravenously to 92 patients: 47 patients received mezlocillin and 45 received ticarcillin. The mean doses were 287 mg/kg for mezlocillin and 271 mg/kg for ticarcillin. The treatment courses of 30 patients were deemed nonevaluable for the following reasons: violations of protocol, 12; primarily isolated organisms not susceptible to both mezlocillin and ticarcillin, 12; or no pathogen isolated from pretreatment cultures, 6. The evaluable patients treated for bone or skin and skin structure infections were 31 for both mezlocillin and ticarcillin. The number of valid bone infections treated was 5.

Table 1 displays the clinical response for the treatment of skin and skin structure infections. Failure rates of 7% and 8%, respectively, were observed for the mezlocillin and ticarcillin treatment groups. The numbers of patients undergoing complete resolution or improvement were not statistically different. The response of the infecting organisms is also shown in Table 1. Since some infections were polymicrobial, the number of bacteriological responses and clinical responses is not the same. The elimination of all organisms after treatment with mezlocillin was 80% as compared with ticarcillin at 75% (P = 0.05). Treatment with mezlocillin for skin and skin structure infections was at least as effective clinically and somewhat better bacteriologically than ticarcillin treatment for similar infections.

TABLE 1. *Randomized double-blind study of mezlocillin and ticarcillin in skin and skin structure infections*

Response	Mezlocillin		Ticarcillin	
	No.	%	No.	%
Clinical response				
Resolution	12	40	14	51
Improved	16	53	11	41
Failed	2	7	2	8
Total	30	100	27	100
Bacteriological response[a]				
Elimination	53	80	62	75
Reduction/ persistence	13	20	21	25
Total	66	100	83	100

[a] Some infections were polymicrobial.

Twelve patients (13% of the population) were infected by bacteria resistant to mezlocillin or ticarcillin before treatment. Four species were resistant to ticarcillin, and eight were resistant to mezlocillin. Seven of 12 patients were infected by staphylococci which were resistant to mezlocillin or ticarcillin. Six of the 34 strains which were not eliminated by mezlocillin or ticarcillin treatment were staphylococci. The remaining organisms which were not eliminated were gram-negative aerobic bacteria.

The number of valid bone infections treated was five. One patient with polymicrobial osteomyelitis improved on mezlocillin therapy, as did two patients who received ticarcillin. Two patients failed to respond to ticarcillin therapy, one with polymicrobial infection and one with *Proteus* species osteomyelitis.

Asymptomatic eosinophilia occurred in 10 of 47 mezlocillin-treated patients and 8 of 45 ticarcillin-treated patients. No other adverse hematological effects were noted. No deterioration in renal function was noted.

This randomized, prospective blind comparison of mezlocillin and ticarcillin for the treatment of skin and soft tissue infections showed that mezlocillin therapy was at least as effective clinically and somewhat better bacteriologically than ticarcillin treatment for these infections. *Staphylococcus aureus* was the most frequently encountered primarily resistant organism.

Staphylococci are likely to persist during treatment with these two drugs. Polymicrobial infections and soft tissue and skin infections in which gram-negative aerobic bacteria participate were treated satisfactorily with mezlocillin.

1. **Bodey, G. P., and T. Pan.** 1977. Mezlocillin: in vitro studies of a new broad-spectrum penicillin. Antimicrob. Agents Chemother. **11:**74–79.
2. **Schacht, P., H. Bruck, J. Dycka, R. Hullman, and D. Tettenborn.** 1980. Results of the clinical trial of azlocillin, p. 188–193. *In* W. Siegenthaler and H. Wenta (ed.), International Symposium Acylureidopenicillins, Vienna, 1979. Excerpta Medica, Amsterdam.
3. **Tettenborn, E., H. Bruck, J. Dycka, R. Hullman, and P. Schacht.** 1980. Results of large scale clinical studies with mezlocillin, p. 182–187. *In* W. Siegenthaler and H. Wenta (ed.), International Symposium Acylureidopenicillins, Vienna, 1979. Excerpta Medica, Amsterdam.
4. **Verbist, L.** 1978. In vitro activity of piperacillin, a new semisynthetic penicillin with an unusually broad spectrum of activity. Antimicrob. Agents Chemother. **13:** 349–357.

Mezlocillin Therapy for Serious Bacterial Infections

RODNEY K. KUSUMI* AND ROBERT J. FASS

Department of Medicine, The Ohio State University College of Medicine, Columbus, Ohio 43210, U.S.A.

Mezlocillin is an acylureidopenicillin with in vitro activity against most bacterial pathogens other than β-lactamase-producing *Staphylococcus aureus.* Because of this extended in vitro antimicrobial activity, a clinical trial was undertaken to evaluate efficacy and toxicity.

Informed consent was obtained from hospitalized patients suspected of having a severe bacterial infection for which mezlocillin was expected to be effective treatment. After obtaining appropriate cultures, mezlocillin was given intravenously in a regimen of 4 g every 6 h. The dose was modified for abnormal renal function. Nafcillin was given concomitantly if *S. aureus* was thought to be a possible pathogen and discontinued if cultures failed to confirm this possibility. Patients were evaluated clinically for response to treatment and for toxicity. Cultures during and after treatment were obtained to determine eradication of pathogens and possible superinfection. Laboratory evaluation for renal and liver toxicity was also performed. Determinations of MICs of mezlocillin for isolates were determined by a microdilution method. Peak and trough serum concentrations were determined by a microbiological assay. Cure was defined as a favorable course with clinical and laboratory evidence of eradication of infection.

A total of 28 patients were treated for 29 infection episodes. There were 22 men and 6 women. The overall mean age was 41 years, with a range of 17 to 85 years. Five patients received concomitant nafcillin therapy because *S. aureus* was isolated in mixed culture. In all instances, nafcillin was inactive against the primary pathogens.

There were 12 patients with complicated urinary tract infections (10 patients required bladder catheter drainage). Two patients were bacteremic with *Escherichia coli.* Five patients had mixed infections. The other pathogens were *E. coli, Pseudomonas aeruginosa, Providencia* sp., enterococci, *Proteus* sp., and *Enterobacter aerogenes.* Duration of treatment averaged 14 days. Clinical cure and eradication of pathogens was achieved in all cases. Five patients were reinfected within a 6-week follow-up period.

There were five patients with severe skin and soft tissue cellulitis. One patient was a drug addict who was treated on two separate occasions for subcutaneous abscesses. None of these patients was bacteremic. Three patients had mixed infections. Pathogens included *P. aeruginosa, Proteus mirabilis,* and *Streptococcus faecalis.* Another patient had pansinusitus with each of the following organisms cultured from a sinus aspirate: *Streptococcus* sp., *Peptococcus* sp., *Bacteroides thetaiotaomicron,* and *Veillonella parvula.* Overall duration of treatment averaged 19 days. All patients were cured.

There were four patients with pneumonia, one of whom had empyema and one of whom had bacteremia. Cultures were obtained by transtracheal aspiration. The pathogens were *Streptococcus pneumoniae* (bacteremic), *Haemophilus influenzae,* and *Neisseria meningitidis.* The patient with empyema had a pleural fluid Gram stain that showed gram-positive cocci and gram-negative bacilli; however, there was no growth in subcultures. Average duration of treatment was 14 days. All patients were cured.

There were four patients with bone infections. Three had sternal osteomyelitis, and one of these had bacteremia. The pathogens included *P. aeruginosa* and *Serratia marcescens* (bacteremic). The fourth patient had osteomyelitis in a congenitally abnormal foot. It was a mixed infection with *P. mirabilis, Streptococcus agalactiae, Bacteroides fragilis,* and *Peptostreptococcus* sp. Average duration of treatment was 38 days. Three patients were cured. The patient with *S. marcescens* infection failed. This patient had multiple systemic and metabolic abnormalities and also had unsatisfactory response to alternative antimicrobial therapy before and after mezlocillin therapy. This patient probably had an undrained mediastinal abscess.

One patient was bacteremic with *B. fragilis* associated with colon carcinoma. He was treated for 15 days and cured. Another patient, who was a drug addict, had *P. aeruginosa* endocarditis. He remained bacteremic on mezlocillin and required valve replacement. He did not respond to subsequent antimicrobial therapy including the combinations of ticarcillin and tobramycin and cefoperazone and tobramycin. He was bacteremic on these regimens and required a second valve replacement. At autopsy he had a myocardial abscess.

The MICs for streptococci were ≤0.13 to 2 μg/ml. For facultative gram-negative isolates, MICs were ≤0.13 to 64 μg/ml, and for anaerobic isolates the MICs were ≤0.13 to 128 μg/ml. The single anaerobe for which the MIC was 128 μg/ml was *V. parvula.* It was isolated in mixed culture from the patient with pansinusitis who was successfully treated with mezlocillin.

Serum concentrations of mezlocillin in 25 patients with normal renal function were as follows: mean peak (immediate postinfusion), 250 μg/ml with a range of 72.6 to 365 μg/ml; mean trough (immediate preinfusion), 13 μg/ml with a range of 1.7 to 35.3 μg/ml.

The following reversible side effects occurred once in different patients: hypokalemia, leukopenia, abnormal liver transaminases, diarrhea, and phlebitis at the intravenous site.

In summary, 93% of the patients were cured. The two who were not cured had unsatisfactory response to other appropriate antimicrobial agents. Mezlocillin appeared to be safe and effective treatment for serious bacterial infection.

Anaerobic Bacteria in Acute Appendicitis

TADEUSZ ORLOWSKI,* ELŻBIETA DACKA, AND ANDRZEJ LEWANDOWSKI

Institute of Surgery, Center of Postgraduate Medical Education, MMA, Warsaw, Poland

Patients with gangrenous or perforated appendices continue to pose a serious surgical problem. Septic complications after appendectomy are even life threatening (3). Anaerobic bacteria in acute appendicitis are underestimated because in routine bacteriological examinations the presence of anaerobes is often missed, leading to wrong conclusions and inadequate antibiotic treatment (2). Some authors found *Bacteroides fragilis* to be the commonest organism in infected appendectomy wounds (3). It seems also that the significance of clostridia is much greater than is generally recognized, so we have made an attempt to evaluate the role of sporeforming anaerobic bacteria in gangrenous appendicitis. Our present investigation has been carried out on 50 patients undergoing appendectomy. Patients were divided into three groups: I, 10 patients, 9 men and 1 woman, with chronic appendicitis; II, 10 patients, 6 men and 4 women, with acute purulent appendicitis; and III, 30 patients, 17 men and 13 women, with gangrenous appendicitis with a so-called "fulminant" course. Groups were comparable in respect to age and body weight. Specimens of all excised appendices were sent for bacteriological examination, and sporeforming anaerobes were cultured, isolated, and identified according to Bergey's taxonomy, using Tarrozi-Wrzosek, Zeissler, and Willis-Hobs media. The pyrogallol technique was used as the anaerobic method.

All identified anaerobes were tested for their susceptibility to 20 antibiotic substances by using the disk method.

In group I, the postoperative course was uneventful in seven patients; in three patients, a clinically nonsignificant wound infection occurred. Four strains of *Clostridium perfringens* were identified in this group.

In group II, the postoperative course was normal in nine patients; in 1 patient, a wound infection was noted. Twelve sporeforming anaerobic strains were identified, 11 strains of *C. perfringens* and 1 strain of *C. septicum.*

In group III, the postoperative course was normal in 14 patients; in 16 patients, various complications occurred, including wound infection, intraperitoneal abscess, and death, in one case. Thirty-eight anaerobic sporeforming strains were found in this group: 26 strains of *C. perfringens,* 4 strains of *C. septicum,* 3 strains of *C. histolyticum,* 2 strains of *C. sphenoides,* 2

TABLE 1. *Susceptibility of bacteria to various antibiotics*

Antibiotic	Susceptible strains (%)
Mezlocillin	96.3
Carbenicillin	94.5
Metronidazole	90.9
Rifampin	89.0
Cephalothin	87.2
Penicillin	85.1
Cephaloridine	81.8
Ampicillin	78.1
Oxytetracycline	76.3
Tetracycline	72.7
Rondomycin	54.5
Bacitracin	47.2
Clindamycin	45.4
Aureomycin	40.0
Erythromycin	14.4
Chloramphenicol	12.7

strains of *C. oedematiens,* and 1 strain of *C. tertium.* Gangrenous changes of the appendix were more intensive in patients in whom more than one anaerobic strain was isolated. The mean in-patient duration in this group increased to 17 days, as compared with 8.3 days in group II.

Susceptibility of identified strains is shown in Table 1. All anaerobes were resistant to aminoglycosides. The obtained results indicate that sporeforming anaerobes play an important role in the pathogenesis of gangrenous appendicitis.

We agree that the use of antibiotics in all cases of acute appendicitis is of questionable value. Based on the results of our study, we suggest that, if an inflamed appendix is found, appendectomy should not be followed by antibiotic therapy. If, however, the appendix is gangrenous, then a prophylactic antibiotic should be given, preferably before and during the operation, and two doses should be given after surgery.

The choice of drug remains very important, as resistance of *Bacteroides fragilis* to the majority of penicillins is well recognized (1) and abdominal infections are often mixed. In our opinion it is essential to choose an antibiotic or a combination of drugs which provides good aerobic and anaerobic coverage.

1. **Nord, C. E., K. Dornbusch, and B. Olsson.** 1980. Studies on beta-lactamase in Bacteroides fragilis. Infection (Suppl. 2). **8:**167–170.
2. **Peters, K., and W. Zilkens.** 1980. The importance of anaerobic infections in abdominal surgery. Infection (Suppl. 2) **8:**192–193.
3. **Pinto, D. J., and P. J. Sanderson.** 1980. Rational use of antibiotic therapy after appendicectomy. Br. Med. J. **281:**275–277.

Empiric Antibiotic Treatment of Infections in Myelosuppressed Cancer Patients: Preliminary Results

K. P. HELLRIEGEL,* J. KINDLER, C. WITTENBERG, M. KRESS, AND S. SPORS

Department of Internal Medicine, University of Cologne, D-5000 Cologne 41, Federal Republic of Germany

In myelosuppressed cancer patients, infection correlates with the degree and the duration of granulocytopenia. The risk of infection rises exponentially with the degree and duration of granulocytopenia. Infection has so far been a major cause of morbidity and mortality in granulocytopenic cancer patients.

One of the main problems of managing infections in granulocytopenic patients is the recognition of the infection. In this patient population, the cardinal symptoms of inflammation may be partially or completely missing. This is a result of the fact that granulocytes are unable to infiltrate the inflammatory tissue or unable to perform phagocytosis since they are missing. In addition, the cancer- and drug-induced immunosuppression makes the human organism incompetent to react adequately.

At onset of fever, it is necessary to start antibacterial therapy before bacteriological results are available. This empiric antibiotic therapy has to cover the wide range of gram-negative and gram-positive bacteria which can be expected from endogenous (physiological bacterial flora) or exogenous (hospitalization) sources. According to clinical experience, a combination of a β-lactam agent with an aminoglycoside covers this spectrum of bacteria to a high degree. To examine whether there are differences in efficacy and tolerability, two combinations, mezlocillin plus sisomicin (regimen A) and cefamandole plus tobramycin (regimen B), were compared in a prospective randomized controlled study (Fig. 1). Patients failing to respond to this treatment within 3 to 5 days either received the combination of cefotaxime, amikacin, and azlocillin (reg-

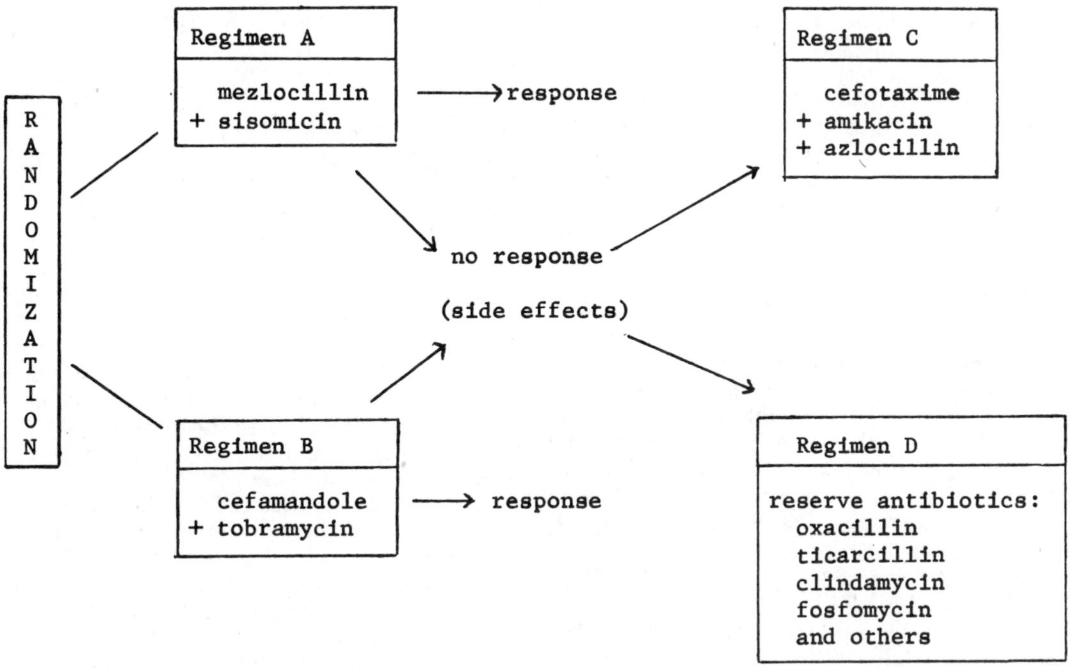

FIG. 1. *Strategy of antibacterial chemotherapy.*

imen C) or such antibiotics as oxacillin, ticarcillin, clindamycin, and fosfomycin according to clinical and bacteriological necessities (regimen D).

Forty-nine adult cancer patients suffering from infections during temporary myelosuppression have been included in the study up to now. The inclusion criteria were presence of fever of at least 38.5°C on two consecutive occasions and granulocyte counts less than 500/µl. Patients with known sensitization against β-lactam antibiotics or aminoglycosides were excluded. The underlying diseases of the 49 patients were acute nonlymphoblastic leukemia in 22, blastic crisis of chronic granulocytic leukemia in 4, acute lymphoblastic leukemia in 6, non-Hodgkin's lymphoma of high malignancy in 5, and other malignancies in 12 cases.

Before and when advisable during treatment, samples for bacteriological studies were taken: blood, midstream urine, sputum, feces, and swabs from pharynx and umbilicus. The patients were neither isolated nor treated prophylactically with antibiotics. All patients, however, received oral prophylactic antimycotic therapy with nystatin or ketoconazole, or both.

In the 49 patients, 61 episodes of documented infection occurred. For the 61 episodes, 81 courses of antibiotic therapy were applied. The 61 episodes of infection consisted of septicemia in 19, pneumonia in 17, and other localizations of infection in 25 instances. The most frequent bacterial isolates were *Pseudomonas aeruginosa* (n = 7), *Escherichia coli* (n = 6), *Streptococcus faecalis* (n = 6), and *Staphylococcus aureus* (n = 5). In half of the episodes the microorganisms responsible for the infectious process could not be isolated.

As initial antibiotic treatment, 27 episodes of infection were treated with regimen A and 34 with regimen B. The nonresponders (after 3 to 5 days of regimen A or B) were treated either with regimen C or with oxacillin, ticarcillin, clindamycin, fosfomycin, or others (regimen D).

The dosages used were as follows: mezlocillin, 5 g three times a day; sisomicin, 50 mg three times a day; cefamandole, 2 g three times a day; tobramycin, 40 mg three times a day; cefotaxime, 2 g three times a day; amikacin, 125 mg three times a day; azlocillin, 5 g three times a day. In renal insufficiency, the dosage of the antibiotics was reduced according to renal function. Antibiotic treatment was discontinued two days after disappearance of all clinical and laboratory signs of infection when the granulocyte count rose up to 1,000/µl.

Nineteen of the 27 episodes treated with regimen A and 22 of 34 episodes treated with regimen B responded to the antibacterial therapy. Eight patients treated with regimen A and 12 patients treated with regimen B failed to respond. These 20 episodes of infection were treated with regimen C or D. A response was observed in 13 instances. The remaining seven patients (7 episodes) died as a consequence of their underlying disease in four instances and of their infection in combination with the underlying disease in three instances.

The side effects seen in the 81 courses of antibacterial chemotherapy were impairment of renal function, exanthema, general symptoms of sensitization, and necrotizing enterocolitis (for details, see Table 1).

TABLE 1. *Side effects*

Side effect	Regimen		
	A	B	C + D
Impairment of renal function	3	1	2
Exanthema	2	2	2
General symptoms of sensitization	—	1	—
Necrotizing enterocolitis	—	—	1

Various antibiotic combinations were reported as effective empiric therapy for myelosuppressed cancer patients suffering from infections (1–5). The combination of ticarcillin plus an aminoglycoside in treating patients with granulocytopenia and cancer was shown to be effective in this patient population. In a recently published, randomized trial of ticarcillin plus gentamicin (group 1), ticarcillin plus amikacin (group 2), and ticarcillin plus netilmicin (group 3), Love et al. (4) showed a response rate for all infections of 97% in group 1, 91% in group 2, and 95% in group 3. Patients with septicemias improved in 93% (group 1), 78% (group 2), and 82% (group 3) of cases. Among patients with gram-negative septicemias, there was no statistically significant difference in response rate. In patients with resistant organisms and without evidence of granulocyte recovery, the failure rate was 67%. When the granulocyte count increased to 1,000/μl over the ensuing 14 days, the failure rate decreased to 20%, despite the presence of resistant organisms and persistent granulocytopenia (4).

In this study regimen A and regimen B appear to be equally efficacious, but only two-thirds of the infectious episodes responded to the initial antibacterial therapy. Among the nonresponders, however, a further two-thirds responded to regimens C and D. Thus, the overall response rate in our patients was also about 90%. In some nonresponders, the bacterial strains proved to be resistant against the administered antibiotic schedule, for example, *S. faecalis* in regimen B. Some other patients apparently did not respond to antibiotic therapy because of the missing granulocytes. Any evidence of granulocyte recovery, however, contributed significantly to patient improvement, even in patients with infections caused by antibiotic-resistant gram-negative bacteria. The numerous variants which play a role in the treatment of this patient population are attributable to the differences in the published results and impede the comparison of data of different authors.

In this trial, side effects of the antibiotic treatment were only rarely observed. When side effects occur in these seriously ill and intensively treated patients, it is often difficult to discriminate whether they are due to a distinct drug or due to the underlying disease.

In conclusion, the data suggest that febrile granulocytopenic cancer patients may profit from empirical, sequential antibiotic treatment of this type.

1. **Bodey, G. P.** 1975. Infections in cancer patients. Cancer Treat. Rev. **2:**89.
2. **EORTC Antimicrobial Therapy Project Group.** 1978. Three antibiotic regimens in the treatment of infection in febrile granulocytopenic patients with cancer. J. Infect. Dis. **137:**14.
3. **Lau, W. A., L. S. Young, R. E. Black, et al.** 1977. Comparative efficacy and toxicity of amikacin/carbenicillin versus gentamicin/carbenicillin in leukopenic patients. Am. J. Med. **62:**959.
4. **Love, L. J., S. C. Schimpff, D. M. Hahn, V. M. Young, H. C. Standiford, J. F. Bender, C. L. Fortner, and P. H. Wiernik.** 1979. Randomized trial of empiric antibiotic therapy with ticarcillin in combination with gentamicin, amikacin or netilmicin in febrile patients with granulocytopenia and cancer. Am. J. Med. **66:**603.
5. **Klastersky, J., C. Hensgens, and L. Debusscher.** 1975. Empiric therapy for cancer patients: comparative study of ticarcillin-tobramycin, ticarcillin-cephalothin, and cephalothin-tobramycin. Antimicrob. Agents Chemother. **7:**640.

Complicated *Pseudomonas* Urinary Tract Infections Treated with Intramuscular Azlocillin or Tobramycin: a Comparative Study

PAUL O. MADSEN* AND RENATE E. MADSEN

Urology Section, William S. Middleton Memorial Veterans Administration Hospital, Madison, Wisconsin 53705, and Department of Surgery, University of Wisconsin School of Medicine, Madison, Wisconsin 53792, U.S.A.*

Azlocillin, an acylureidopenicillin (2) which has a specific effect against *Pseudomonas,* and tobramycin, the aminoglycoside with the best effect against *Pseudomonas,* were compared in the treatment of complicated urinary tract infections in a prospective, randomized study of 23 male patients. Both drugs were administered intramuscularly to all patients. Azlocillin was administered in a dosage of 2 g every 8 h if the patient weighed >70 kg and 2 g every 6 h if the patient weighed <70 kg. The azlocillin was dissolved in 1% lidocaine to diminish the pain on injection. Tobramycin was administered in a dosage of 1 mg/kg every 8 h. All patients were treated for a total of 7 days. All patients had complicated urinary tract infections, and all were infected with *P. aeruginosa.* The patients were comparable as to age, weight, and the pathology of the urinary tract, which mainly consisted of benign prostatic hypertrophy, carcinoma of the prostate, bladder tumors, or urethral strictures. All cultures were carried out on a midstream, clean-catch urine specimen, and all treated patients had a count of $\geq 10^5$ colony-forming units per ml of urine. The culture results were all positive within 2 days before initiation of treatment. All urine cultures were considered susceptible to the two drugs as determined by a standardized disk susceptibility method (1). Urine cultures with colony counts were carried out before treatment, on the third and last days of treatment, and 1 week after treatment. MICs of the two drugs against *Pseudomonas* organisms were determined by an agar dilution technique.

One week after treatment, 8 of 12 patients in the azlocillin group (67%) and 9 of 11 patients in the tobramycin group (82%) had negative urines (Table 1), and this was considered as a cure. There was no statistical difference between the cure rate in the two patient groups.

The MICs of the two drugs for *P. aeruginosa* are shown in Table 2. The urine concentrations obtainable after administration of the two drugs were many times higher than the MICs of the two drugs, and this probably explains the good effect of these antibiotics.

Both drugs were well tolerated by the patients, and there were no changes in the laboratory values before and after 1 week of treatment in the two patient groups, including blood urea nitrogen, serum creatinine, serum glutamic oxalacetic transaminase, lactic dehydrogenase, alkaline phosphatase, hemoglobin, total leukocyte count, platelet count, and serum electrolyte levels.

TABLE 1. *Results of complicated Pseudomonas urinary tract infections treated with azlocillin or tobramycin*

Time of culture	Treatment group	Negative culture	Persistence or relapse[a]
Third day	Azlocillin	8/12 (67%)	4/12 (33%)
	Tobramycin	11/11 (100%)	0
Last day	Azlocillin	11/12 (92%)	1/12 (8%)
	Tobramycin	11/11 (100%)	0
1 week follow-up	Azlocillin	8/12 (67%)	4/12 (33%)
	Tobramycin	9/11 (82%)	2/11 (18%)

[a] There were no instances of super- or reinfection.

TABLE 2. *MICs of azlocillin and tobramycin against P. aeruginosa in urinary tract infections*

Agent	No. of patients	MIC (μg/ml)	
		Median	Range
Azlocillin	12	3.12	1.56–50
Tobramycin	8	4.68	0.78–12.5

1. **Bauer, A. W., W. M. M. Kirby, J. C. Sherris, and M. Turck.** 1966. Antibiotic susceptibility testing by a standardized single disk method. Am. J. Pathol. **43:**493–496.
2. **Fu, K. P., and H. G. Neu.** 1978. Azlocillin and mezlocillin: new ureidopenicillins. Antimicrob. Agents Chemother. **13:**930–938.

Combined Action of Azlocillin and Sisomicin Against *Pseudomonas aeruginosa* in a Kinetic In Vitro Model

I. HALLER

Institute for Chemotherapy, Bayer AG, 5600 Wuppertal-1, Federal Republic of Germany

When determining MICs or MBCs, the microorganisms to be tested are exposed to constant levels of antimicrobial agent. This in no way reflects the in vivo situation with permanently changing drug concentrations at the site of infection. To examine the effect of decreasing antibiotic concentrations in vitro, several test models simulating the in vivo serum kinetics

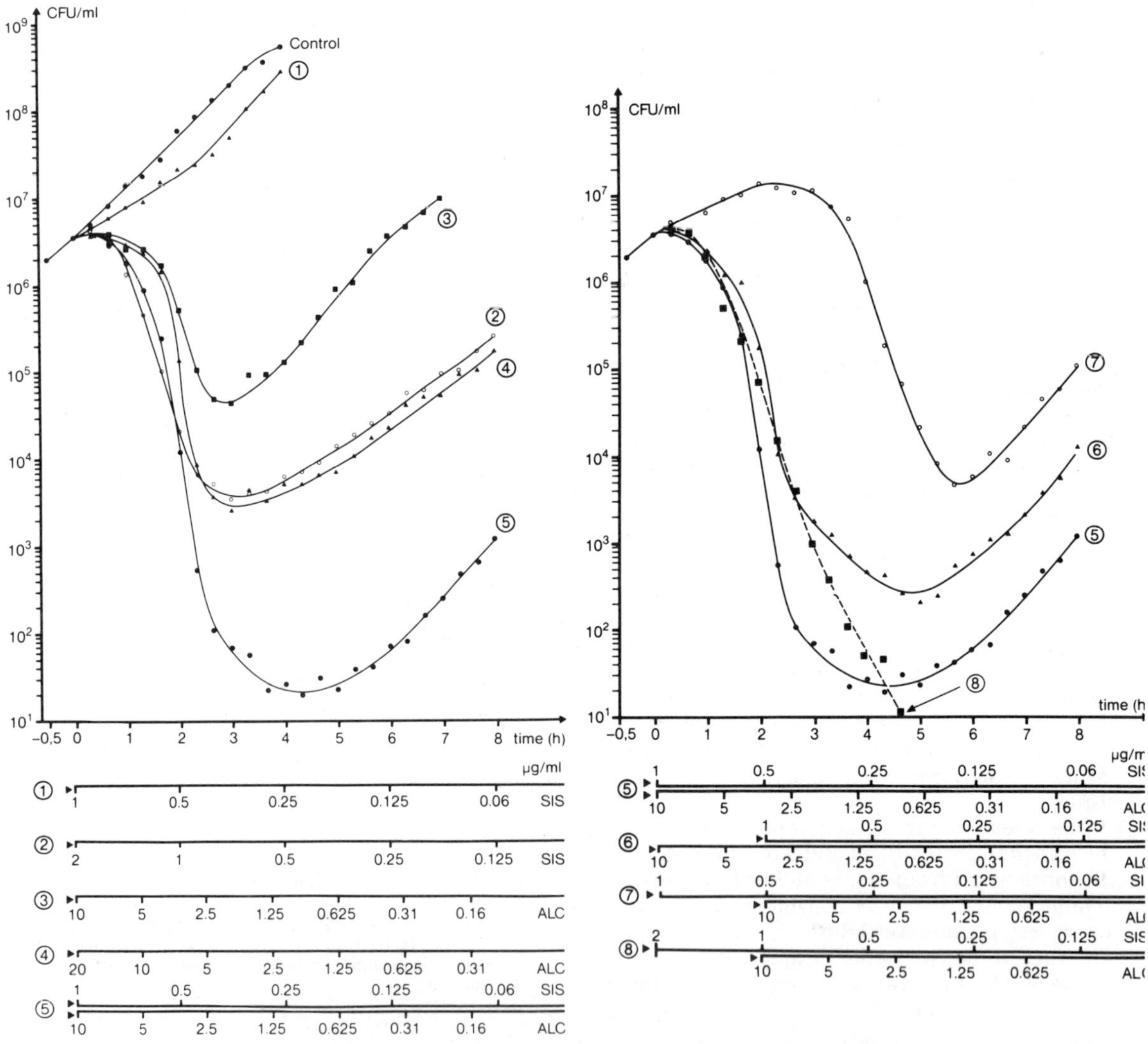

FIG. 1. *Growth and killing curves of P. aeruginosa obtained by the test model described. Decreasing concentrations of azlocillin (ALC) and sisomicin (SIS) were applied alone or combined simultaneously as well as at intervals. The initial concentrations can be seen from the gradients depicted below the diagram. The half-lives simulated were 75 min for azlocillin and 120 min for sisomicin.*

have been described (for references, see 1, 2). Using a modified technique, I was able to measure the combined action of independently decreasing gradients of azlocillin and sisomicin on *Pseudomonas aeruginosa.*

For each experiment a culture (800 ml) of the test strain was preincubated in an ultrafiltration cell (Amicon 2000C) while stirred until logarithmic growth was achieved. After addition of azlocillin, the culture was diluted every 20 min by adding about 160 ml of fresh broth to simulate the in vivo elimination rate of azlocillin with a half-life of 75 min. After dilution, the same volume of broth was eluted through a membrane filter (0.1-μm pore size) retaining the bacteria so that volume and cell density of the culture remained unchanged. When testing sisomicin, dilution was performed in exactly the same way so as to obtain comparable growth conditions. Small amounts of sisomicin, however, were added whenever diluting the medium to simulate a half-life of 120 min. For comparison of test methods, the susceptibility of the *Pseudomonas* test strain used was also assessed by conventional broth dilution technique: the MICs determined were 8 μg/ml for azlocillin and 1 μg/ml for sisomicin.

Some growth and killing curves resulting from the test model described are depicted in Fig. 1 together with the corresponding concentration gradients tested. Curves 1 through 4 illustrate the effect of various concentrations of azlocillin and sisomicin when tested alone. A kill rate of 99.9% was achieved by adding initial concentrations of 2 μg of sisomicin per ml (curve 2) or 20 μg of azlocillin per ml (curve 4). When half the amounts of both compounds were added simultaneously at time zero and eliminated with their specific elimination rates, a strong synergistic effect could be seen (curve 5). The viable-cell count was decreased by 5 logs, and regrowth of surviving bacteria was inhibited for almost 5 h.

When treating a patient with a combination of penicillin and aminoglycoside, the two drugs may be administered at different times because of practical reasons or different application schedules. Therefore, the effect of decreasing concentrations of azlocillin and sisomicin combined at different intervals was also examined. Initial concentrations were the same as in the case of simultaneous combination, i.e., 10 μg of azlocillin and 1 μg of sisomicin per ml. Application intervals of 40 min did not influence the results irrespective of the sequence of application (data not plotted). When azlocillin was administered first and sisomicin was added 120 min later, the synergistic effect was slightly reduced but still superior to the effect of double the concentration of each compound alone (curve 6).

When sisomicin was administered at time zero and azlocillin was added after an interval of 2 h, the number of viable bacteria was reduced to about the same level as with double the concentration of each agent alone (curve 7). It should be taken into account, however, that the bacterial culture continued growing during pretreatment with sisomicin so that addition of azlocillin resulted in a 99.95% killed rate. To be sure that pretreatment with higher concentrations of sisomicin would not block the effect of azlocillin, an initial sisomicin concentration of 2 μg/ml was also tested and 10 μg of azlocillin per ml was added 2 h later. By this treatment almost all bacteria were killed (curve 8).

The interpretation of the results described may be summarized briefly as follows. Strong synergistic effects may occur even when decreasing gradients of azlocillin and sisomicin act together at concentrations which exceed the individual MICs for only a short period of time. Alternating administration at intervals may reduce the period during which sufficient concentrations of both compounds can interact and therefore result in a reduced synergistic effect. In the test model used, neither pretreatment with sisomicin nor pretreatment with azlocillin blocked the antibacterial activity of the combination partner.

1. **Bergan, T., I. B. Carlsen, and J. E. Fuglesang.** 1980. An in vitro model for monitoring bacterial responses to antibiotic agents under simulated in vivo conditions. Infection **8**(Suppl. 1):96–102.

2. **Shah, P. M., and U. Hessberger.** 1981. Vergleichende Untersuchungen zur bakteriziden Aktivität von Ampicillin und Amoxycillin. Therapiewoche **31**:805–812.

Relative Efficacies of Ticarcillin and Ureidopenicillins (Azlocillin, Mezlocillin, Piperacillin) Against Experimental *Pseudomonas aeruginosa* Pyelonephritis Infections in Mice

ANGELA S. BEALE,* KEITH R. COMBER, AND ROBERT SUTHERLAND

Beecham Pharmaceuticals Research Division, Brockham Park, Betchworth, Surrey, United Kingdom

From the results of published studies, it is evident that there are pronounced differences between the α-carboxypenicillins and the acylaminopenicillins with regard to the antibacterial effects produced against *Pseudomonas aeruginosa*. For instance, the antipseudomonal activity of the latter group is influenced by inoculum size, and this has been correlated with instability to the β-lactamase of *P. aeruginosa*. In addition, the bactericidal activity of ureidopenicillins against *P. aeruginosa* has been reported to be much less than that of carbenicillin or ticarcillin, although in some studies little or no difference was observed in this respect between the two classes of penicillins. The purpose of this study was to compare the chemotherapeutic activities of ticarcillin and ureidopenicillins in the treatment of moderate and severe experimental *Pseudomonas* infections in mice. A kidney infection model was chosen for study because of the not infrequent appearance of *Pseudomonas* species in complicated urinary tract infections in humans.

Kidney infections were established in mice with three strains of *P. aeruginosa,* and the susceptibilities of the organisms to the penicillins were determined by serial dilution in Mueller-Hinton broth. The bacterial inocula employed (10^2 and 10^4 cells per ml) in the in vitro studies were representative of the numbers present in kidney tissue at the commencement of therapy of the mouse infections. Azlocillin and piperacillin showed similar activities (MICs, 1.5 to 3.1 μg/ml) against *P. aeruginosa* NCTC 10662 and *P. aeruginosa* 11 and were approximately fourfold more active than ticarcillin and mezlocillin. Strain D 47 was slightly more resistant to all four penicillins and the MIC values were twofold higher.

Administration of iron to mice infected intravenously with the three strains of *P. aeruginosa* consistently resulted in the development of progressive pyelonephritis, and the infection was restricted to the kidneys. Infection was initiated, after intavenous inoculation of approximately 2×10^6 cells per mouse, by intramuscular administration of 30 mg of iron per kg 18, 42, and 66 h after infection. Therapy was instituted either 19 or 43 h after infection and was continued four times a day for 3 days. Efficacy was assessed by macroscopic examination of the kidneys for the presence of abscesses and viable count determinations on kidney homogenates 7 days after infection.

Results in Fig. 1 illustrate the relative efficacies of azlocillin and ticarcillin in the treatment of *P. aeruginosa* 10662 kidney infections in mice. In this experiment, therapy with both penicillins was instituted either 19 h after infection, at which time the kidney bacterial population (geometric mean of five mice) was from 2×10^2 to 5×10^2 organisms per g of tissue and constituted a moderate infection, or 43 h after infection, at which time the geometric mean kidney bacterial population of a sample of five mice was approximately 10^5 organisms per g, and was considered to be representative of a severe infection.

Most (90%) of the control untreated mice had high bacterial kidney counts ($>10^8$ organisms per g of tissue), and kidney lesions were observed in all of these animals. Azlocillin therapy commenced 19 h after infection at a dose of 125 mg/kg was totally ineffective in the treatment of this infection. All 10 mice in this treatment group had high bacterial kidney counts, and abscesses were clearly visible on the cortical surface of all kidneys. Ticarcillin at the same dose (125 mg/kg) was effective in the treatment of 60% of the animals. Kidney homogenate counts from these mice were below the limit of detection and were free from macroscopic abscesses. At a higher dose level (500 mg/kg), azlocillin protected 60% of the animals, whereas ticarcillin produced complete protection, as judged by the absence of kidney homogenate counts and macroscopic abscesses.

When treatment was withheld for 43 h to allow time for bacterial multiplication and more widespread renal involvement, the therapeutic response to both penicillins was diminished. For example, both dose levels of azlocillin (125 and 500 mg/kg) and the lower dose of ticarcillin (125 mg/kg) had little effect on the course of the infection, large numbers of bacteria ($>10^7$/g) being recovered from 70 to 80% of kidneys of the animals in these treatment groups, with kidney abscesses present in these mice. It was apparent, however, that ticarcillin was more effective than

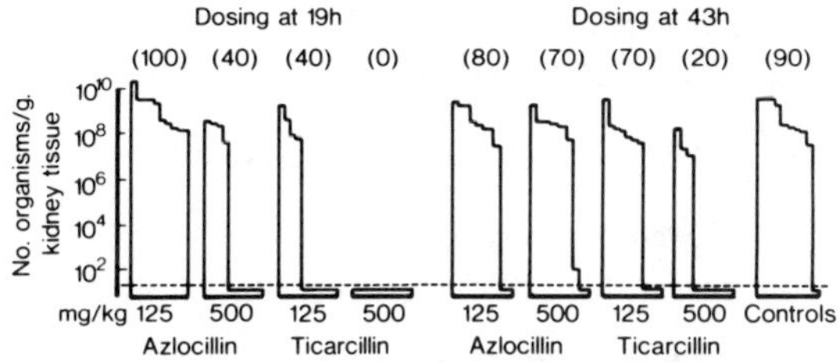

FIG. 1. *Comparative efficacies of azlocillin and ticarcillin against moderate and severe mouse pyelonephritis infections caused by P. aeruginosa NCTC 10662. Figures in parentheses show the percentage of mice with visible kidney abscesses.*

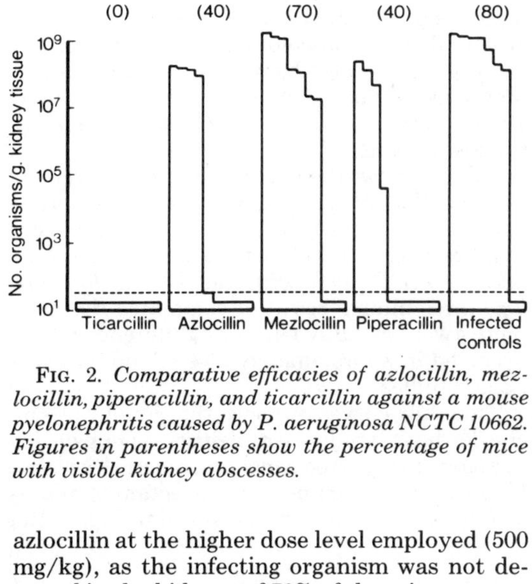

FIG. 2. *Comparative efficacies of azlocillin, mezlocillin, piperacillin, and ticarcillin against a mouse pyelonephritis caused by P. aeruginosa NCTC 10662. Figures in parentheses show the percentage of mice with visible kidney abscesses.*

azlocillin at the higher dose level employed (500 mg/kg), as the infecting organism was not detected in the kidneys of 70% of the mice nor was there evidence of macroscopic abscesses in the kidneys of these animals.

The comparative activities of ticarcillin and the ureidopenicillins azlocillin, mezlocillin, and piperacillin against an infection due to *P. aeruginosa* NCTC 10662 are shown in Fig. 2. Antibiotic therapy commenced 19 h after infection, and each of the penicillins was administered at 250 mg/kg. Ticarcillin was completely effective against the infection, and the infective strain of *Pseudomonas* was not isolated from any of the kidneys of the mice in this treatment group. Azlocillin was somewhat less effective and had activity similar to that of piperacillin. Forty percent of the mice treated with either of these penicillins showed evidence of persisting bacterial infection, with kidney homogenate bacterial counts of approximately 10^8 organisms per g and macroscopic kidney lesions. Mezlocillin was the least effective anti-*Pseudomonas* penicillin, with 70% of the mice in this treatment group having kidney homogenate counts of $>10^7$ organisms per g of tissue.

Similar results were obtained in the therapeutic studies with infections produced by the other test strains of *P. aeruginosa,* 11 and D 47. That is, ticarcillin was more effective in protecting the animals than were azlocillin and piperacillin, and mezlocillin was the least active of the compounds.

It is generally accepted that successful chemotherapy of uncomplicated urinary tract infections is determined to a large extent by the concentration of antibiotic excreted in the urine. It was considered therefore that large differences in the urinary excretion profiles of each of the penicillins in mice with pseudomonal kidney infections might have accounted for, or contributed to, the superior therapeutic efficacy observed for ticarcillin in these studies.

Accordingly, the urinary excretion profiles of ticarcillin, azlocillin, mezlocillin, and piperacillin were measured in infected mice. At a dose level of 50 mg/kg, high concentrations of all the penicillins were excreted in the urine, mostly during the first 2 h after dosing. The urinary concentration of ticarcillin (1,400 μg/ml) was approximately twice that of azlocillin (700 μg/ml) and piperacillin (900 μg/ml), and fourfold higher than that of mezlocillin (350 μg/ml). Although higher urinary concentrations of ticarcillin were measured in infected mice compared with the ureidopenicillins, it seems unlikely that differences in urinary excretion would have contributed substantially to the observed differences in therapeutic efficacy, as the urinary concentrations of all compounds were greatly in excess of MIC values.

In conclusion, the results of these studies with typical strains of *P. aeruginosa* showed that ticarcillin was consistently more effective than azlocillin, mezlocillin, and piperacillin in the treatment of kidney infections, although the organisms were more susceptible to the ureidopenicillins than to ticarcillin in serial dilution tests in vitro. The greater efficacy of ticarcillin in vivo may have been in part due to the higher urinary concentrations in infected mice, but other factors such as tissue distribution at the foci of infection or reported differences in in vitro characteristics, such as the greater stability to *Pseudomonas* β-lactamase and more rapid bacteriolytic effects exhibited by ticarcillin, would be more likely to play an important role.

Activity of Piperacillin Combined with Moxalactam or Cefotaxime Against *Pseudomonas aeruginosa* and Gram-Negative Enteric Bacilli

S. LANDESMAN,* A. GRUARIN, M. CORRADO, AND M. CUMMINGS

Department of Medicine, Downstate Medical Center, Brooklyn, New York 11357, U.S.A.

Moxalactam and cefotaxime are third-generation cephalosporin-type antibiotics that are highly active against most *Enterobacteriaceae* (MIC range, 0.06 to 1.0 μg/ml). These drugs are considerably less active against *Pseudomonas aeruginosa* (MIC range, 8 to 64 μg/ml). As a consequence, these drugs may have to be combined with antipseudomonal compounds to provide initial broad-spectrum coverage against gram-negative pathogens, including *P. aeruginosa*. Aminoglycosides such as amikacin, tobramycin, and gentamicin, although highly active against *P. aeruginosa*, are also nephrotoxic; their use, therefore, should be avoided when possible. The broad-spectrum penicillin piperacillin, being nontoxic and highly active against many gram-negative bacilli (including *P. aeruginosa*), is a reasonable alternative to aminoglycosides. Antibiotic combinations such as cefotaxime and piperacillin or moxalactam and piperacillin would be nontoxic and provide initial coverage for the septic patient against enteric pathogens and *P. aeruginosa*.

There is, however, evidence from several studies that suggest antagonism between piperacillin and cephalosporins. Kuck et al. (2) documented antagonism between cefoxitin and piperacillin or mezlocillin against strains of *P. aeruginosa*, *Serratia*, *Enterobacter*, and indole-positive *Proteus*. Other investigators, including Sanders and Sanders (5, 6) and Neu and Fu (4), have reported synergism, antagonism, or indifference with a variety of beta-lactam combinations tested against gram-negative bacilli.

We undertook a study, therefore, to examine the in vitro activity of piperacillin in combination with cefotaxime or moxalactam against *Enterobacteriaceae* and *P. aeruginosa*. The checkerboard technique, utilizing the microtiter broth dilution method, was used to evaluate the activity of the antibiotic combinations. Combinations were classified as synergistic, partially synergistic, indifferent, or antagonistic according to the fractional inhibitory concentration method of calculation (1). Time-kill curves were also performed. For the time-kill curves, antibiotic combinations and the concentrations used included piperacillin at its MIC against the test organism plus cefotaxime or moxalactam at one-fourth their MIC against the test organism. Tests were also done with moxalactam or cefotaxime concentrations equal to the MIC of the test organism plus piperacillin at a concentration one-fourth its MIC against the organism. Strains of *P. aeruginosa*, *Enterobacter*, *Serratia marcesens*, and *Providencia* were used for the time-kill curves. A total of 32 killing curves were performed. Synergy was defined as a 2-log or greater decrease in colony-forming units of the test organism occurring with the antibiotic combinations compared with the antibiotic used alone at a concentration equal to its MIC against the test organism.

Table 1 shows the results of the checkerboard studies. No antagonism was seen with either antibiotic combination against any organism. Synergy was seen only with a few strains of *P. aeruginosa*, *Providencia*, and *Escherichia coli*. The predominant result of combining the antibiotics was partial synergy or indifference, which occurred in approximately 85% of the checkerboard studies.

Time-kill curves support the results of the checkerboard studies; e.g., neither synergism nor antagonism occurred when piperacillin was combined with cefotaxime or moxalactam. A representative time-kill curve is shown in Fig. 1; the

TABLE 1. *Results of checkerboard studies with piperacillin-moxalactam and piperacillin-cefotaxime against gram-negative enteric bacilli*[a]

Organism (no. of strains tested)	No. of strains showing given result with:			
	Piperacillin-moxalactam		Piperacillin-cefotaxime	
	Synergy	Partial synergy-indifference	Synergy	Partial synergy-indifference
P. aeruginosa (20)	4	16	4	16
Enterobacter (9)		9		9
Providencia (7)	5	2		7
Serratia (9)		9		9
Klebsiella (10)		10		10
E. coli (10)		10	3	7

[a] None of the strains showed antagonism.

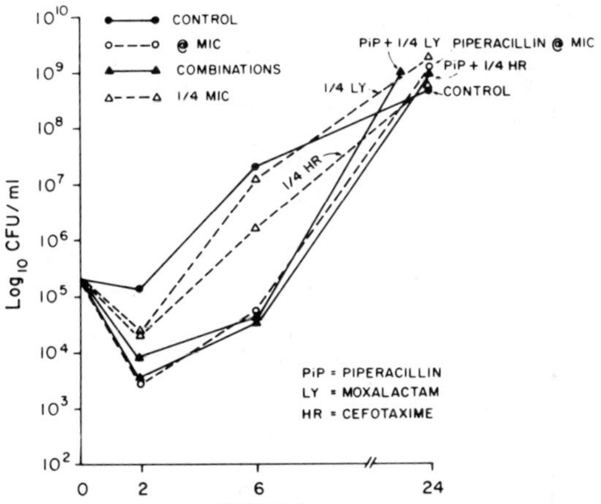

FIG. 1. *Kinetics of bacterial killing of P. aeruginosa by piperacillin in combination with moxalactam or cefotaxime. The piperacillin concentration is equal to its MIC against the organism (32 μg/ml). Moxalactam and cefotaxime concentrations (2 and 4 μg/ml, respectively) are one-fourth the MIC. CFU, Colony-forming units.*

killing of *P. aeruginosa* by piperacillin at a concentration equal to its MIC against the organism was not enhanced or inhibited by the addition of subinhibitory concentrations (one-fourth the MIC) of cefotaxime or moxalactam. A similar result was obtained when a subinhibitory concentration of piperacillin (equal to one-fourth the MIC) was added to cefotaxime or moxalactam at a concentration equal to the MIC against the test organism. Similar results were obtained when killing curves were done against *Enterobacter* spp., *S. marcesens*, and *Providencia* spp.

The results of these in vitro tests suggest that the antibiotic combinations of piperacillin-moxalactam and piperacillin-cefotaxime are neither synergistic nor antagonistic against *P. aeruginosa* or gram-negative enteric bacilli. In vitro methods of assessing antibiotic synergy or antagonism may not reflect in vivo activity because of a variety of technical and theoretical problems (3). Animal studies and clinical trials should therefore be done to fully evaluate the utility of these antibiotic combinations.

1. **Krogstad, D. J., and R. C. Moellering.** 1980. Combinations of antibiotics. Mechanisms of interaction against bacteria, p. 298–341. *In* V. Lorian (ed.), Antibiotics in laboratory medicine. The Williams & Wilkins Co., Baltimore.
2. **Kuck, N. A., R. A. Testa, and M. Forbes.** 1981. In vitro and in vivo antibacterial effects of combinations of beta-lactam antibiotics. Antimicrob. Agents Chemother. **19:** 634–638.
3. **Moellering, R., Jr.** 1979. Antimicrobial synergism—an elusive concept. J. Infect. Dis. **140:**639–641.
4. **Neu, H. C., and K. P. Fu.** 1978. Synergy of azlocillin and mezlocillin combined with aminoglycoside antibiotics and cephalosporins. Antimicrob. Agents Chemother. **13:**813–819.
5. **Sanders, C. C., and W. E. Sanders, Jr.** 1979. Emergence of resistance to cefamandole: possible role of cefoxitin-inducible beta-lactamases. Antimicrob. Agents Chemother. **15:**792–797.
6. **Sanders, C. C., and W. E. Sanders, Jr.** 1980. Antagonism of cefamandole by cefoxitin in routine disk susceptibility. Am. J. Clin. Pathol. **73:**562–563.

Pharmacokinetics and Therapeutic Effect of Piperacillin in Severely Ill Patients with and without Renal Impairment

K. UNERTL,* G. RUCKDESCHEL, W. KELLERMANN, AND U. JENSEN

Department of Anesthesia and Max v. Pettenkofer-Institute Klinikum Grosshadern, Ludwig-Maximilians-University, Munich, Federal Republic of Germany*

Piperacillin is a new semisynthetic penicillin with broad antimicrobial activity against both gram-positive and gram-negative bacteria including important pathogens of nosocomial infections. We report the pharmacokinetic properties as well as the clinical effectiveness and tolerability of the compound in 24 severely ill patients with a variety of infections.

Eleven males and 13 females, ages ranging from 15 to 84 years, with various degrees of renal function were included in the study. To establish the pharmacokinetics, three groups (Gp) of patients were defined according to renal function with mean creatinine clearances as follows: Gp 1 (12 patients), 94.9 ml/min; Gp 2 (5 patients), 34.1 ml/min; and Gp 3 (5 patients), 11.2 ml/min. The kinetic parameters were also obtained for two patients (single patient no. 1 and 2): patient 1 was anephric and patient 2 suffered from severe liver and moderate renal impairment due to amyloidosis. Piperacillin was administered by intravenous infusion over 30 min, via an infusion pump. Initial doses chosen were 4 g for the patients of Gp 1 and 2 g for the patients of Gp 2 and 3 and the two special patients. Serum samples were obtained at time zero, at 5 and 30 min, and at 1, 2, 3, 6, and 12 h after completing the infusion. Urine samples were obtained in 2-h intervals up to 12 h. Serum and urine concentrations were assayed by the agar well method, using *Sarcina lutea* ATCC 9341 as test organism. The individual patients fitted very well to the one-compartment pharmacokinetic model, which was therefore used for the calculation of the kinetic parameters. Response to therapy was assessed in 20 of the 24 patients who were treated for more than 4 days for 26 infections: bronchopulmonary, 13; urinary tract, 7; wound, 4; and central nervous system, 2. Duration of treatment averaged 9 days. Patients with normal renal function (Gp 1) received 12 g/day in three divided doses with the exception of four patients, who had 16 g/day (two patients) and 6 g/day (two patients). Of the patients with impaired renal function, 10 received 4 g/day in two divided doses, 1 patient received 12 g/day, and another patient received 8 g/day. In six patients we decided to combine piperacillin with other antibiotics, either to include all causative pathogens or to make up synergistic potential.

The serum concentration time curves are presented in Fig. 1. Peak concentrations averaged: Gp 1, 187 ± 67 (±SD) μg/ml; Gp 2, 155 ± 73 μg/ml; Gp 3, 106 ± 23 μg/ml. Serum levels declined almost monoexponentially, and after 12 h they were below detectable levels in Gp 1; in Gp 2 they were 0.85 μg/ml and in Gp 3, 12.7 μg/ml. Cumulative urinary recoveries after 6 h averaged: Gp 1, 49%; Gp 2, 40%; and Gp 3, 10%. After 12 h the recoveries averaged: Gp 1, 53%; Gp 2, 49%; and Gp 3, 14% of the administered doses, respectively. Pharmacokinetic parameters are presented in Table 1. Serum half-life ($t_{1/2}$) increased with increasing renal insufficiency to 6.43 h in the one anephric patient (Table 1, single patient 1). No strong correlation between serum half-life and creatinine clearance could be demonstrated. These findings, in combination with the marked difference between total body clearance and renal clearance of the drug, indicate that nonrenal mechanisms of drug elimination play an important role. The assumption that extrarenal excretion takes place primarily via the hepatobiliary pathway is supported by the data of the patient with severe liver and moderate renal insufficiency (Table 1, single patient 2). Serum half-life in this patient was 7.8 h, the highest value of all patients investigated.

The causative pathogens isolated from the infected sites were mainly *Enterobacter cloacae* (10×) and *Pseudomonas aeruginosa* (8×), followed by *Proteus mirabilis* (6×), *Streptococcus faecalis* (5×), *Escherichia coli* (4×), *Klebsiella pneumoniae* (2×), *Staphylococcus aureus* (2×), *S. pyogenes* (1×), *S. agalactiae* (1×), *Haemophilus influenzae* (1×), and *Serratia marcescens* (1×). With the exception of one strain of *E. cloacae* and the two *S. aureus* strains, all isolates were susceptible to piperacillin. Sixteen of the 20 patients suffered from polymicrobial infections, with two or more pathogens involved.

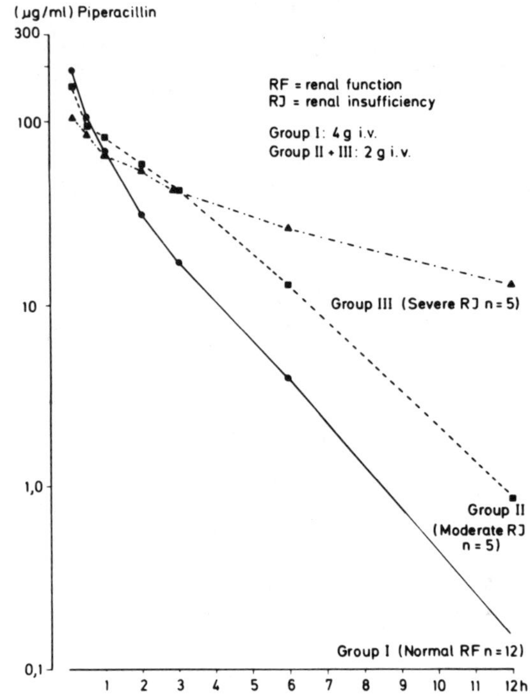

FIG. 1. *Mean serum concentrations of piperacillin after a 30-min intravenous infusion of 4 g in patients with normal renal function and of 2 g in patients with moderate and severe renal impairment.*

Thirteen patients had bronchopulmonary infections; all of them were intubated or had tracheostomy. Eight infections were considered to be severe and five were moderate. Nine were cured clinically, one improved, and three failed. The latter patients died, in spite of combination therapy, mainly because of severe underlying diseases with multiple organ failure, but pneumonia was considered to have contributed to fatal outcome. Seven patients suffered from urinary tract infections which had been acquired during prolonged catheterization of the bladder. Four infections were considered to be mild and three were moderate. The causative organisms were eradicated during treatment, but two pa-

TABLE 1. *Comparison of mean pharmacokinetic parameters of piperacillin in 12 patients with normal renal function (Gp 1), 5 patients with moderate renal impairment (Gp 2), 5 patients with severe renal impairment (Gp 3), a single anephric patient (single patient 1), and 1 patient with severe liver and moderate renal impairment (single patient 2)*

Parameter	Group			Single Patients	
				No	No
	I	II	III	1	2
Creat.-Clearance (ml/min)	94,9	34,1	11,2	0	23,5
t 1/2 (hrs)	1,0	1,6	4,2	6,43	7,8
V_d (liters)	18,9	11,7	23,2	26,7	24,7
AUC ($\mu g \cdot ml \cdot h^{-1}$)	320,1	420,2	544,5	693,5	910,1
Total body clearance (ml/min)	241,4	88,8	65,2	48,1	36,6
Renal clearance (ml/min)	122,9	38,9	11,3	--	13,4
K_{el} (h^{-1})	0,82	0,47	0,17	0,11	0,09

tients relapsed. Out of four patients with postoperative or posttraumatic wound infections, two were cured and two improved. Two patients with meningoencephalitis due to posttraumatic rhinorrhea were cured without neurological deficit.

Tolerability of piperacillin was good. One patient showed a transient pruritus and exanthem; one patient had mild diarrhea. These results suggest that piperacillin is a highly effective and well-tolerated antibiotic. The present dosage recommendations are supported by our data. As a routine, adults with normal renal function should be given 4 g three times daily, those with moderate renal impairment 2 g three times daily, and those with severe renal impairment 2 g twice daily.

1. **Evans, M. A. L., P. Wilson, T. Leung, and J. D. Williams.** 1978. Pharmacokinetics of piperacillin following intravenous administration. J. Antimicrob. Chemother. **4**:255–261.
2. **Fu, K. P., and H. C. Neu.** 1978. Piperacillin, a new penicillin active against many bacteria resistant to other penicillins. Antimicrob. Agents Chemother. **13**:358–367.
3. **Giron, J. A., B. R. Meyers, S. Z. Hirschman, and E. Srulevitch.** 1981. Pharmacokinetics of piperacillin in patients with moderate renal failure and in patients undergoing hemodialysis. Antimicrob. Agents Chemother. **19**:279–283.

Elimination of Piperacillin in Renal Impairment

H. LANGE,* R. BAIER, N. FLEISCHMANN, M. FREI, AND D. DAPPER

Department of Nephrology and Institute of Microbiology, University of Marburg, Marburg, and Department of Nephrology and Hypertension, Clinic "Old Mill", Wildungen-Reinhardshausen, Federal Republic of Germany*

Piperacillin is effective against most gram-positive and gram-negative organisms. Its pharmacokinetics have been studied in healthy subjects (3) and in patients with end-stage renal failure (4, 6). The present data are derived from investigations in patients with mild, moderate, and severe impairment of kidney function who were not being treated by dialysis. The kinetic parameters determined were the elimination rate constant, the elimination half-life, the distribution volume, and the percentage of the drug eliminated by urinary excretion. From these data dosage regimens were calculated for different degrees of renal failure.

The investigations were performed in 32 patients (21 males, 11 females) with chronic diseases of the kidney including glomerulonephritis, obstructive pyelonephritis, polycystic kidney disease, and drug nephropathy. According to their kidney function, the patients were divided into four groups, as shown in Fig. 1.

After a control sample of venous blood was drawn, 2 g of piperacillin was injected intravenously over 3 to 5 min. The piperacillin serum concentration was determined in venous blood specimens sampled at 15, 30, 60, 120, and 240 min, as well as after 24 h. After emptying the urinary bladder, 24-h urine was collected for determination of piperacillin and creatinine. Semilogarithmic graphs of serum concentration versus time data drawn for each patient showed that the distribution of piperacillin was completed within 30 to 60 min. The elimination rate constant (k_{el}) therefore was calculated from the piperacillin levels at 1, 2, 4, and 24 h according to the formula

$$k_{el} = \frac{\ln A - \ln B}{t}$$

and the data were subjected to linear regression analysis. Extrapolating the regression line to the ordinate yielded the initial theoretical concentration of piperacillin immediately after injection (A_i). The distribution volume of the drug was calculated by dividing the administered dose by A_i.

The elimination half-life in plasma was obtained by dividing the natural logarithm of two by the elimination rate constant. Dosage regimens for different degrees of renal failure were recommended on the basis of the corresponding half-life constant as described by Dettli (1). The cumulative peak serum concentration (A_{max}) expected under the recommended dosage regimen was determined with the formula

$$A_{max} = \frac{A_i}{1 - e^{-k_{el} \cdot t}}$$

Finally, the percentage of administered piperacillin excreted in the 24-h urine was estimated.

Concentrations of piperacillin in serum and urine were determined by a standard agar diffusion method with *Bacillus subtilis* (ATCC 6633) and *B. stearothermophilus* (Fa. Merck AG, Darmstadt, Germany) on Mueller-Hinton agar at pH 6.0. All samples were assayed in triplicate and calculated to the regression lines of standards in final concentrations of 160 to 2 μg/ml (*B. subtilis*) and 1 to 0.0078 μg/ml (*B. stearothermophilus*). The sensitivity of the assays was limited to 1 μg/ml (*B. subtilis*) and 0.0078 μg/ml (*B. stearothermophilus*), respectively.

Figure 1 shows the serum levels of piperacillin in the four groups of patients. From serum concentrations at 1, 2, 3, 4, and 24 h the elimina-

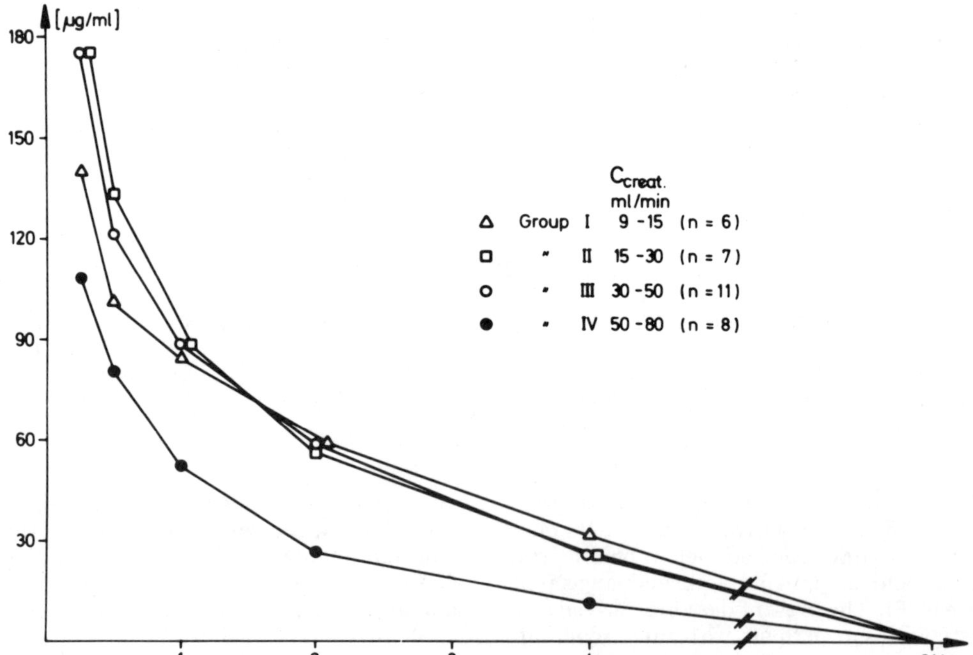

FIG. 1. *Serum levels after intravenous administration of 2 g of piperacillin.*

TABLE 1. *Elimination half-life of piperacillin*

Patients	Cl_{cr}[a] (ml/min)	Mean for each interval			Mean of entire interval	From regression analysis	% of drug in 24-h urine
		1-2 h	2-4 h	4-24 h			
Group IV (n = 8)	50–80	64.6 ± 10.3	102.5 ± 20.9	121.0 ± 8.4	96.6 ± 12.4	116.2 ± 8.0	45.1 ± 12.8
Group III (*n* = 11)	30–50	119.5 ± 33.4	137.5 ± 35.5	132.9 ± 24.3	133.0 ± 24.0	132.4 ± 23.8	44.7 ± 16.3
Group II (*n* = 7)	15–30	102.6 ± 30.2	158.8 ± 77.6	129.7 ± 32.0	130.4 ± 35.3	130.3 ± 32.1	35.8 ± 17.3
Group I (*n* = 6)	9–15	121.5 ± 23.7	179.5 ± 46.0	149.2 ± 12.4	150.1 ± 23.2	150.0 ± 13.1	18.6 ± 6.3

[a] Cl_{cr}, Creatinine clearance.

tion half-life was calculated and is shown for the different intervals in Table 1. In normal kidney function the half-life of piperacillin is 60 min (3). In this study patients with mild impairment of renal function had an elimination half-life of 96.03 ± 28.74 min, which increased to 133, 130, and 150 min in patients with more severe renal failure (Table 1). Using different methods for determination of the elimination half-life resulted in comparable data (Table 1). Only in group I patients was the half-life derived from single intervals significantly shorter than the half-life calculated by regression analysis. This was mainly due to larger differences during the early short time periods of drug elimination.

The theoretical initial concentration after 2 g of piperacillin in all 32 patients was $A_i = 100.75 \pm 40.6$ μg/ml on the average with an apparent distribution volume of 19.85 liters. The 24-h urinary excretion decreased from 45.0% in group IV patients to only 19% in patients with severe renal failure (Table 1).

In subjects with normal renal function the elimination half-life of piperacillin is 60 min and differs between 40 and 92 min (3). The present data show that patients with only mild renal insufficiency have a prolonged half-life of 96 min. With moderate renal failure (creatinine clearance, 15 to 50 ml/min), it increased to approximately 130 min and reached 150 min in severe renal insufficiency (creatinine clearance, 9 to 15 ml/min), an elimination half-life 2.5 times above normal. In patients with end-stage renal failure (creatinine clearance, 5 ml/min) a further increase to 200 min occurred (6). Thus, the diminution of kidney function to less than one-tenth of normal values is accompanied by only a threefold increase of the elimination half-life of piperacillin. This is in contrast to other semisynthetic penicillins such as carbenicillin and ticarcillin in which the prolongation of the half-life amounts to 10 times normal at comparable degrees of renal failure (2, 5). The relatively short half-life of piperacillin suggests an extrarenal route of excretion in addition to its renal elimination.

Calculations of the extrarenal elimination rate constant (1, 4) showed an increase from 0.0023 min^{-1} in healthy subjects to 0.0038 min^{-1} in patients with moderate to severe renal failure. It appears from these data that the extrarenal route of elimination does increase with deterioration of kidney function.

The prolongation of the elimination half-life of piperacillin in renal insufficiency requires an adjustment of the dosage regimen. In patients with normal kidney function 4 g is usually thought to be satisfactory. To ensure comparable antibiotic concentrations in patients with renal insufficiency, the dosage has to be reduced. Patients in groups I to IV should get 3.19 g/12 h, 3.70 g/12 h, 3.70 g/12 h, and 5.0 g/12 h, respectively. Using 3 g/12 h in group I patients (creatinine clearance, 9 to 15 ml/min) with a serum half-life of 150 min, the cumulative peak serum concentration does not exceed 155.6 μg/ml. The serum at the end of the dosage interval does not fall below 5.6 μg/ml. These concentrations ensure effective blood levels throughout the whole interval and avoid toxic side effects.

1. **Dettli, L.** Arneimitteldosierung bei Niereninsuffizienz, p. 83–91. *In* H. P. Kuemmerle, E. R. Garrett, and K. H. Spitzky (ed.), Klinische Pharmakologie und Pharmakotherapie, 3rd ed. Urban and Schwarzenber, Munich.
2. **Eastwood, J. B., and J. R. Curtis.** 1968. Carbenicillin administration in patients with severe renal failure. Brit. Med. J. **1:**486–487.
3. **Evans, M. A. L., P. Wilson, T. Leung, and J. D. Williams.** Pharmacokinetics of piperacillin following intravenous administration. J. Antimicrob. Chemother. **4:**255–261.
4. **Francke, E. L., G. B. Appel, and H. C. Neu.** 1979. Pharmacokinetics of intravenous piperacillin in patients undergoing chronic hemodialysis. Antimicrob. Agents Chemother. **16:**788–791.
5. **Parry, M. F., and H. C. Neu.** 1976. Pharmacokinetics of ticarcillin in patients with abnormal renal function. J. Infect Dis. **133:**46–49.
6. **Thompson, M. J. B., M. E. Russo, J. M. Matsen, and E. Atkin-Thor.** 1981. Piperacillin pharmacokinetics in subjects with chronic renal failure. Antimicrob. Agents Chemother. **19:**450–453.

Penetration of Piperacillin into Cerebrospinal Fluid in Patients with Bacterial Meningitis

GORDON DICKINSON,* RICHARD LEVINE, RICHARD GREENMAN, AND THOMAS HOFFMAN

University of Miami School of Medicine and Miami Veterans Administration Medical Center, Miami, Florida 33101, U.S.A.*

Piperacillin is reported to inhibit most gram-negative bacilli at levels of 12.5 μg or less per ml. Administration of large doses of this antibiotic is tolerated well; it has been shown that serum levels of more than 100 μg/ml can be achieved. It is likely that levels of piperacillin in the cerebrospinal fluid (CSF) could be achieved by intravenous administration that are sufficient to inhibit many gram-negative bacilli. This type of therapy would be an important advance in the treatment of patients with gram-negative bacillary meningitis who presently require intrathecal administration of antibiotics. A study using piperacillin as the single antibiotic in the treatment of gram-negative meningitis was undertaken to determine the penetrability of piperacillin into the CSF of patients with meningitis and to evaluate its efficacy as the sole antibiotic for treatment of patients with gram-negative meningitis.

Four adult patients with meningitis caused by gram-negative bacilli susceptible to piperacillin were studied. Susceptibility testing was initially performed by a standardized disk method using 100-μg piperacillin disks. A zone diameter of 23 mm or greater indicated susceptibility to piperacillin. Susceptibility to piperacillin was confirmed by a broth dilution method modified for use in a microtiter system. Therapy was initiated with piperacillin in a loading dose of 2 g infused intravenously over 20 min followed by a continuous infusion of 324 to 436 mg/kg of body weight per 24 h. A CSF sample was collected for piperacillin assay on days 1, 2, 3, and 10. Serum samples were collected hourly for 3 h prior to collection of the CSF specimens. The serum and CSF samples were frozen at −70°C and assayed within 4 weeks. The level of piperacillin in the samples was determined by an agar plate disk diffusion method with *Sarcina lutea* ATCC 9341 as the test organism. The average of the levels in the three serum samples was calculated for each day. The percent penetration was calculated by dividing the level of piperacillin in CSF by the average of the levels in the three serum samples collected on that day and multiplying the result by 100.

The age of the patients, the infecting organism, the MIC of piperacillin against the organism, and the outcome of treatment are shown in Table 1. The four patients, 16 to 64 years of age, were treated for 4 to 15 days with a continuous infusion of piperacillin; total duration of therapy, including intermittent infusions in two patients, was 10 to 37 days. Three of the infections had developed after the patients had undergone neurosurgical operations, and the fourth occurred in a patient hospitalized with alcoholic hepatitis. The causative organisms, *Pseudomonas aeruginosa* in three patients and *Flavobacterium meningosepticum* in one, were inhibited by levels of piperacillin that ranged from 1.56 to 6.25 μg/ml. All four patients treated with piperacillin improved, and two were cured of their infection. One of those considered improved had persistently positive CSF cultures until the ninth day of treatment, at which time a ventricular catheter was changed. One CSF sample collected the day after the catheter was changed was sterile; however, intrathecal aminoglycosides were subsequently administered in addition to continued intravenous piperacillin, and this patient was cured. The other patient had a parameningeal focus of infection which had not been eradicated by several neurosurgical operations and multiple courses of antibiotics prior to treatment with piperacillin. He responded to piperacillin, but relapsed after therapy was stopped. He eventually was placed on long-term suppressive therapy with another penicillin derivative and is presently doing well. The suppressive therapy has been continued for 2 years.

The mean leukocyte count in the CSF prior to administration of piperacillin was 4,000 cells per mm^3. The mean leukocyte counts in the CSF

TABLE 1. *Causative organisms and outcome of four cases of gram-negative meningitis treated with piperacillin*

Age (yr)	Infecting organism	MIC of piperacillin (μg/ml)	Outcome
50	*P. aeruginosa*	1.56	Cure
33	*P. aeruginosa*	3.13	Improvement[a]
64	*P. aeruginosa*	3.13	Improvement[b]
16	*F. meningosepticum*	6.25	Cure

[a] Intrathecal gentamicin administered on the tenth day.
[b] Presumed parameningeal focus of infection; the patient remained infected after multiple courses of treatment.

TABLE 2. *Piperacillin levels in serum and CSF of patients with meningitis given continuous intravenous infusions of 324 to 436 mg/kg of body weight per day*

Duration of infusion (days)	No. of patients	Mean CSF leukocytes (per mm³)	Mean piperacillin levels		Mean penetration (%)
			Serum (μg/ml)	CSF (μg/ml)	
1	4	2,130	73 (37–102)[a]	23 (13–35)	32
2	3	695	82 (21–121)	21 (4–33)	26
3	3	472	93 (81–110)	19 (7–30)	20
10	2	47	62 (59–64)	26 (21–31)	42

[a] Range of values.

samples collected for measuring drug levels are shown in Table 2. The levels of piperacillin in serum and CSF of four patients receiving a continuous infusion of piperacillin are also shown in Table 2. Samples were collected from four patients on the first day, from three patients on days 2 and 3, and from two patients on the tenth day of infusion. The mean serum levels of piperacillin on the days when samples were collected ranged from 62 to 93 μg/ml. The range of values for the individual patients studied is given in parentheses in Table 2. The mean level of piperacillin in the CSF was 23, 21, and 19 μg/ml on the first, second, and third days of infusion, respectively. Samples were collected from two patients on day 10, and the levels of piperacillin in CSF were 21 and 31 μg/ml. The mean percent penetration of piperacillin into the CSF was 32% on the first day, 26% on the second day, and 20% on the third day. The percent penetration for the two patients studied on the tenth day was 33% and 53%, with a mean of 42%.

In summary, high levels of piperacillin were maintained in the serum of these patients and the mean percent penetration of piperacillin into the CSF under steady-state conditions ranged from 20 to 42%. Two of the four patients were cured with this therapy and the other two were improved. These data indicate that piperacillin does penetrate well into the CSF of patients with meningitis. It appears to penetrate inflamed meninges as well as any of the penicillins currently available. Intermittent infusions of piperacillin are likely to yield high levels of this antibiotic in the CSF, too. Further studies of piperacillin in the treatment of meningitis caused by gram-negative bacilli are indicated.

This study was supported by a grant from Lederle Laboratories, Pearl River, N.Y.

Pharmacokinetics of Piperacillin in Newborn Infants

THOMAS RUBIO,* FREDERICK H. WIRTH, JR., AND EDWARD H. KAROTKIN

Eastern Virginia Medical School, Children's Hospital of The King's Daughters, Norfolk, Virginia 23507, U.S.A.

Piperacillin sodium is currently an investigational drug undergoing phase III clinical trials. The drug is a penicillin derivate with the following formula: [2S-[2α, 5α, 6β (S)]]-6[[[[(4-ethyl-2,3-dioxo-*l*-piperazinyl) carbonyl]amino]phenylacetyl]amino]-3,3-dimethyl-7 oxo-4-thia-*l*-azabicyclo[3.2.0]hepatane-2-carboxylate.

Piperacillin has been shown to be effective in the treatment of many serious infections (7). In vitro and in vivo studies demonstrate that piperacillin has a broad spectrum of activity. It is effective against most gram-positive and gram-negative organisms, including anaerobes. Its gram-negative spectrum includes *Escherichia coli, Enterobacter cloacae, Proteus mirabilis* (indole-negative *Proteus*), *Proteus vulgaris* (indole-positive *Proteus*), *Serratia marcescens, Klebsiella pneumoniae*, and *Haemophilus influenzae* (1, 2). It is four- to eightfold more active than carbenicillin in inhibiting *Pseudomonas aeruginosa* and fourfold more active against *Bacteroides fragilis* (4).

In vitro studies in our laboratory indicated that 79% of 142 strains of enteric gram-negative bacteria had an MIC of less than 1.9 μg/ml as compared to 58.5% for ampicillin. In 200 strains of *P. aeruginosa* the MIC for piperacillin was less than 1.9 in 99% of the strains.

The pharmacokinetics of piperacillin have been studied in adult patients with normal renal function, and dosage recommendations are fairly well established for this group of patients (6). This antibiotic has also been studied in patients with moderate renal failure and in patients undergoing hemodialysis (3), and, more recently, in adult patients with end-stage renal disease (5).

Although piperacillin has been studied in children of various ages, particularly by Japanese investigators (personal communication from Toyama Co., provided to us by Lederle Laboratories), and other groups, including our group, the pharmacokinetics studies of piperacillin in the newborn to our knowledge have not been reported to date in the English literature. The purpose of this study is to determine the pharmacokinetics of piperacillin sodium in newborn infants.

Forty-six infants were treated with conventional doses of ampicillin and amikacin for suspected or proven sepsis. A single dose of piperacillin was substituted for a dose of ampicillin.

Serum concentrations at 0.5, 2, 4, and 6 h after a single intravenous dose of 50 mg/kg, infused over a 5-min period, and a single intramuscular dose of 50 mg/kg were obtained from 36 and 10 patients, respectively. Piperacillin assays were done by a microbiological method using a strain of *P. aeruginosa* resistant to both ampicillin and amikacin.

The mean serum concentrations, in micrograms per milliliter, were as follows: 0.5 h, 115 (range 258 to 49); 2 h, 73 (range 118 to 31); 4 h, 49 (range 109 to 0); and 6 h, 33 (range 76 to <6). These data showed a great deal of intersubject variability as is generally observed in pharmacokinetic studies of newborn infants.

The pharmacokinetic parameters were calculated as follows. (i) The elimination half-life ($t_{1/2}$) = ln $2/K_{el}$. (ii) Extrapolation of the regression line (intravenous dose) to time zero allows an estimation of C'_0, the plasma concentration at zero time if distribution were rapid. This parameter is underestimated. (iii) The area under the intravenous serum concentration-time curve (AUC) was calculated from C'_0/K_{el}. This parameter is underestimated in proportion to the underestimation of C'_0. The AUC following intramuscular administration was calculated by the trapezoidal method and extrapolated to infinite time by the addition of C_{6HR}/K_{el}. (iv) The apparent volume of distribution (AVD) was calculated from dose/C'_0. This parameter is overestimated in proportion to the underestimation of C'_0. The AVDs are adjusted for body weight and reported as milliliters per kilogram. (v) The whole body clearance, Q_B, was calculated from dose/AUC. This parameter is overestimated in proportion to the underestimation of C'_0 (hence of AUC). The clearances were adjusted for body surface area and reported as milliliters per minute per 1.73 m^2.

The mean elimination half-life ($t_{1/2}$) was 3.5 h, which is two to four times that of the adult (approximately 60 min) (6). The serum concentrations of the subjects of this study fitted well to a one-compartment open model except for two of the patients, both of whom had higher 0.5-h serum concentrations than are compatible with the one-compartment model. Their kinetics indicated two-compartment behavior, but the data were insufficient to permit such treatment.

The subjects of this study were divided into three groups according to their postnatal age (Table 1). The mean elimination rate constant (K_{el}) was statistically greater (Students *t* test) and the $t_{1/2}$ shorter in the two groups of patients whose postnatal age was 6 days or greater compared to those whose ages were 5 days or fewer. There were no significant differences in the mean K_{el} or $t_{1/2}$ between the 6- to 10-day and greater than 10-day postnatal age groups.

There were no statistically significant correlations of K_{el} or $t_{1/2}$ with the gestational age, weight, or body surface area of the infant, nor were the whole body clearances (Q_B) or apparent volume of distribution (AVD) correlated with postnatal or gestational age of the infant. The

TABLE 1. *Piperacillin neonatal study: summary of pharmacokinetic parameters (mean ± SD)*

Dose	Age (days)	*N*	K_{el} (h^{-1})	$t_{1/2}$ (min)	AUC (μg.h ml^{-1})	V_d (ml kg^{-1})	Q_B (ml min^{-1}/1.73 m^2)	C'_0 (μg ml^{-1})
Intravenous								
	1–5	17	0.2042 ± 0.0514	217 ± 56	677 ± 252	404 ± 117	32.3 ± 15.2	129 ± 40
	6–10	12	0.2726 ± 0.0737[a]	162 ± 37[a]	536 ± 143	383 ± 119	40.5 ± 18.1	141 ± 39
	10	5	0.2989 ± 0.0672[a]	127 ± 67[a]	505 ± 188	396 ± 248	34.6 ± 13.3	154 ± 69
Intramuscular								
	1–5	3	0.1767 ± 0.0215	239 ± 27	606 ± 32	463 ± 36	27.4 ± 4.1	
	6–10	4	0.1973 ± 0.0422	244 ± 60	603 ± 116	427 ± 92	29.2 ± 9.5	
	10	3	0.1977 ± 0.0136	211 ± 15	446 ± 46	579 ± 17	34.8 ± 1.5	

[a] Statistically different from the 1- to 5-day group, $P < 0.01$.

mean Q_B was much smaller than the adult (approximately 250 mg $min^{-1}/1.73\ m^2$). The mean plasma concentration at zero time (C'_0) averaged 141 $\mu g\ ml^{-1}$, and the AVD averaged 101 ml kg^{-1}, indicating larger volume distribution in the infants than in the adults (approximately 300 ml kg^{-1}).

No adverse reactions associated with the administration of piperacillin were observed.

1. **Fu, K. P., and H. C. Neu.** 1978. Piperacillin, a new penicillin active against many bacteria resistant to other penicillins. Antimicrob. Agents Chemother. **13**:358–367.
2. **George, W. L., R. P. Lewis, and R. D. Meyer.** 1978. Susceptibility of cephalothin-resistant gram-negative bacilli to piperacillin, cefuroxime, and other selected antibiotics. Antimicrob. Agents Chemother. **13**:484–489.
3. **Giron, J. A., B. R. Meyers, S. Z. Hirschman, and E. Srulevitch.** 1981. Pharmacokinetics of piperacillin in patients with moderate renal failure and in patients undergoing hemodialysis. Antimicrob. Agents Chemother. **19**:279–283.
4. **Jones, R. N., P. C. Fuchs, E. H. Gerlach, and T. L. Gavan.** 1979. Piperacillin and carbenicillin: a collaborative in-vitro comparison against 10,838 clinical bacterial isolates. Cleveland Clin. Q. **46**:49–55.
5. **Thompson, M. I. B., M. E. Russo, J. M. Matsen, and E. Atkin-Thor.** 1981. Piperacillin pharmacokinetics in subjects with chronic renal failure. Antimicrob. Agents Chemother. **19**:450–453.
6. **Tjandramafa, T. B., A. Mullie, R. Verbesselt, P. J. DeSchepper, and L. Verbist.** 1978. Piperacillin: human pharmacokinetics after intravenous and intramuscular administration. Antimicrob. Agents Chemother. **14**:829–837.
7. **Winston, D. J., W. Murphy, L. S. Young, and W. L. Hewitt.** 1980. Piperacillin therapy for serious bacterical infections. Am. J. Med. **69**:255.

Piperacillin in the Treatment of Urinary Tract Infection: Effect on Renal Function

CLAUDIO BIANCHI,* CARLO DONADIO, GIANFRANCO TRAMONTI, GIUSEPPE GARCEA, PAOLO LORUSSO, AMALIA LUCCHETTI, ROBERTO GIORDANI, RITA PIEROTTI, AND GIUSEPPE FALCONE

Cattedra di Nefrologia, Clinica Medica 2, and Istituto di Microbiologia, University of Pisa, 56100 Pisa, Italy*

Piperacillin sodium (PIP) is a new semisynthetic penicillin derivative with a broad range of antibacterial potency against gram-positive and gram-negative bacteria. High renal clearances of PIP have been reported (1), but no exhaustive data are available concerning its effect on renal function in humans. This report evaluates efficacy and renal effects of moderate doses of PIP in patients with difficult urinary tract infections.

Six female patients aged 33 to 70 years (mean, 50.3 years), with body weights from 53 to 87 kg (mean, 63 kg), participated in this study. Creatinine clearances ranged from 48 to 98 ml/min (mean, 72.2 ml/min). The patients were free of hepatic or hematological disease and of allergy to penicillins. For each patient there was documentation of recurrent urinary tract infection during the preceding 5 years. Pyelography demonstrated pyelonephritic scarring in five of six cases. Routine diagnostic procedures allowed the diagnosis of chronic nonobstructive pyelonephritis in three patients, renal calculi in two patients, and ureteropelvic obstruction in one patient. Three patients had recently failed treatment with other antibiotics (cephaloridine, cotrimoxazole, pipemidic acid). No antimicrobial drug had been given within 30 days before the beginning of this study.

Before treatment, all patients had significant bacteriuria determined by the dilution pour-plate method in two consecutive clean-catch midstream urine samples collected within 7 days. *Escherichia coli* was isolated in three patients; *Proteus mirabilis*, *Pseudomonas aeruginosa*, and *Klebsiella pneumoniae* were isolated in one patient each. A disk susceptibility test showed that all of the isolated bacteria were susceptible to PIP.

In addition to urine cultures, the following tests were performed in the pretreatment period: urinalysis, renal concentrating ability, plasma urea, creatinine, uric acid and their renal clearances, glomerular filtration rate, and effective renal plasma flow. Glomerular filtration rate and effective renal plasma flow were determined by the noninvasive bladder cumulative method (2). In addition, urinary enzyme activities of *N*-acetyl-β-D-glucosaminidase (4), alanine aminopeptidase (5), and lysozyme (6) were measured. Routine hematological and hepatic tests were also carried out.

Urine culture and the above-mentioned tests were again performed on days 5 and 10 of treatment and 10 days after completion of therapy (except urinary concentrating ability, glomerular filtration rate, and effective renal plasma flow,

TABLE 1. *Effect of PIP on main parameters of renal function*[a]

Patient	Pre[b]	5th day	10th day	Post[c]	Pre	5th day	10th day	Post	Pre	5th day	10th day	Post
	Urine output (ml/min)				*Proteinuria (mg/dl)*				*Leukocytes in urine sediment*			
1	0.97	1.87	0.97	0.97	40	10	50	20	10–12	15–20	5–6	0
2	1.28	2.50	2.63	1.38	10	5	5	5	30–40	>50	25–50	>50
3	0.83	0.55	0.55	0.83	15	10	20	10	>100	>100	>50	>100
4	0.93	1.25	1.11	1.25	10	0	5	5	5–6	25–30	5–6	>50
5	0.48	0.55	0.27	0.35	10	5	20	10	50	5–6	8–10	6–7
6	0.67	0.78	0.83	0.97	5	0	5	10	0	1–2	0	15–20
Mean	0.86	1.25	1.06	0.96								
	Urine urea (mg/min)				*Urine creatinine (mg/min)*				*Urine uric acid (mg/min)*			
1	18.18	18.37	18.28	19.15	0.74	0.75	0.90	0.73	0.33	0.84	0.58	0.35
2	16.41	33.50	22.09	18.33	0.77	0.87	0.95	0.64	0.31	0.50	0.92	0.35
3	12.02	7.05	7.44	9.96	0.66	0.72	0.53	0.56	0.15	0.25	0.27	0.15
4	19.51	12.87	16.22	15.75	1.01	0.84	1.11	0.86	0.27	0.31	0.41	0.36
5	7.14	7.27	6.70	3.74	0.49	0.58	0.55	0.42	0.29	0.25	0.18	0.22
6	10.24	10.54	16.52	16.78	0.90	0.80	1.08	1.01	0.31	0.30	0.42	0.22
Mean	13.92	14.93	14.54	13.95	0.76	0.76	0.85	0.70	0.28	0.41	0.46	0.27
	Plasma urea (mg/dl)				*Plasma creatinine (mg/dl)*				*Plasma uric acid (mg/dl)*			
1	46	38	31	40	1.0	1.2	1.4	1.1	3.5	3.2	2.7	4.7
2	39	40	41	44	1.3	1.2	1.2	0.9	3.8	2.7	2.7	4.2
3	36	31	43	56	1.2	1.4	1.5	1.2	4.4	3.5	4.6	6.0
4	31	27	35	28	1.0	1.1	1.0	0.9	4.6	3.7	3.6	3.7
5	34	32	43	32	1.0	0.9	1.0	0.8	3.2	3.4	3.0	3.5
6	32	34	34	30	0.9	0.8	0.7	0.7	5.8	3.6	4.7	6.5
Mean	36.3	33.7	37.8	38.3	1.07	1.10	1.13	0.93	4.22	3.35[d]	3.55[d]	4.77
	Urea clearance (ml/min)				*Creatinine clearance (ml/min)*				*Uric acid clearance (ml/min)*			
1	43.5	48.2	58.8	47.8	74.0	62.3	64.4	66.1	9.4	26.3	21.5	7.9
2	41.4	83.7	54.0	41.7	61.4	72.9	79.1	71.0	8.1	18.5	34.2	8.3
3	32.9	22.7	17.3	17.8	54.6	51.6	53.4	46.3	3.3	7.1	7.7	2.5
4	61.9	47.7	46.3	56.2	96.4	76.1	111.0	95.8	5.8	8.4	11.4	9.8
5	21.0	22.7	15.6	11.7	48.4	64.2	55.5	52.5	8.9	7.4	5.8	6.2
6	32.0	31.0	48.6	55.9	98.5	99.4	152.9	144.1	5.2	8.2	9.0	3.4
Mean	38.78	42.67	40.10	38.52	72.22	71.08	86.05	79.30	6.78	12.65[d]	14.93	6.35
	Concentrating ability (s.g.)				*GFR (ml/min)*				*ERPF (ml/min)*			
1	1.018		1.018		45.2		45.2		194.6		175.8	
2	1.017		1.020		60.3		63.2		231.2		283.6	
3	1.012		1.014		38.0		52.7		222.7		329.9	
4	1.027		1.023		59.4		77.7		311.4		284.0	
5					51.4		40.2		233.2		194.6	
6	1.027		1.031		117.9		105.4		636.8		538.0	
Mean	1.020		1.021		62.03		64.07		304.98		300.98	
	Urine AAP (mU/mg of creatinine)				*Urine NAG (nmol/h/mg of creatinine)*				*Urine lysozyme (μg/mg of creatinine)*			
1	19.3	21.4	17.3	19.1	193.2	109.5	308.5	105.0	0	0	0	0
2	15.9	19.1	18.9	10.2	47.2	69.5	83.0	48.5	0	0	0	
3	8.3	9.5	10.1	14.2	165.0	190.0	146.0	108.0	0	0.23	0.27	1.67
4	12.7	9.6	9.5	16.7	39.0	25.0	41.0	62.3	0.10	0	0	0.18
5	14.0	14.5	11.7	12.0	20.9	29.0	33.3	36.3	0.16	0	0	0
6	12.0	12.4	13.1	13.2	21.9	30.0	37.0	50.5	0	0	0.06	0.81
Mean	13.70	14.42	13.43	14.23	81.20	75.50	108.13	68.43				

[a] Abbreviations: s.g., specific gravity; GFR, glomerular filtration rate; ERPF, effective renal plasma flow; AAP, alanine aminopeptidase; NAG, *N*-acetyl-*β*-D-glucosaminidase.
[b] Pre, Pretreatment values.
[c] Post, Posttreatment values (10 days after completion of therapy).
[d] $P < 0.05$ versus pretreatment value (*t* pair test).

which were repeated only on day 10). Urine output was measured daily in the base-line period and during therapy.

PIP (Lederle Laboratories), reconstituted with 0.5% lidocaine, was administered intramuscularly in all the patients in a total daily dose of 4 g (2 g every 12 h) for 10 days.

Patients were monitored daily for any evidence of allergic reactions, but no adverse effect was observed. A free diet was allowed.

Bacteriological response was satisfactory during therapy; urine cultures were negative on days 5 and 10 of treatment in all but one case. Ten days after completion of therapy, a relapse was observed in five patients and a reinfection was observed in one. This finding is not surprising considering that our patients had a history of difficult, recurrent urinary tract infections.

In a larger-population study, most having lower urinary tract infections, Van Blerk et al. obtained remarkably better results, using dosages equivalent to ours (7). Hypothetically, patients with upper tract infections, as in our case, would need a higher daily dose of PIP than we used.

PIP did not exhibit any negative effect on renal function. In particular, urine output, urinalysis, urinary concentrating ability, plasma urea and creatinine and their clearances, renal hemodynamics, and urinary enzyme activities all remained stable during treatment, indicating no nephrotoxicity of the drug, at least at the dosage schedule used (Table 1).

Unexpectedly, this study demonstrated an important uricosuric property of PIP. In fact, the mean value of uric acid output increased during treatment up to 64% above the mean base-line value. As a consequence, serum uric acid decreased by 21%. The net result was an increased renal clearance of uric acid of more than 2 times the base-line value during therapy. At the same time creatinine clearance remained unchanged (Table 1, Fig. 1). This uricosuric capacity of PIP is completely reversible, as 10 days after completion of therapy uric acid output returned to pretreatment values.

Antibiotics generally are not known to influence the renal handling of uric acid. The only exception seems to be penicillin G, which has been observed to inhibit uric acid uptake in separated rabbit renal tubules (3). PIP could induce uricosuria by either blocking reabsorption or enhancing tubular secretion of uric acid.

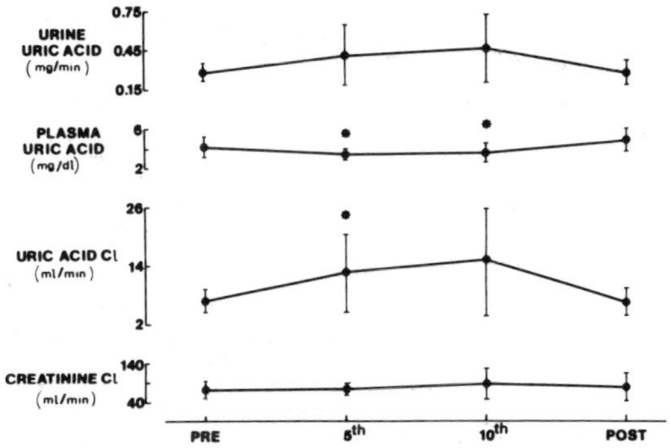

FIG. 1. *Urine uric acid, plasma uric acid, uric acid clearance (Cl) and creatinine clearance patterns (mean ± SD). Pre = pretreatment values; Post = posttreatment values (10 days after completion of therapy). 5th and 10th indicate progressive days of treatment. * $P < 0.05$ versus pretreatment value (t pair test).*

Therefore, keeping in mind the small number of patients studied, we can conclude that PIP seems to be a well-tolerated and non-nephrotoxic antimicrobial agent. Also, its strong uricosuric effect is of clinical interest and merits further investigation.

1. **Batra, V. K., J. A. Morrison, K. C. Lasseter, and V. A. Joy.** 1979. Piperacillin kinetics. Clin. Pharmacol. Ther. **26:**41–53.
2. **Bianchi, C.** 1980. Noninvasive methods for the measurement of renal function, p. 65–84. *In* C. Duarte, (ed.), Renal function tests—clinical laboratory procedures and diagnosis. Little, Brown and Co., Boston.
3. **Kippen, I., N. Nakata, S. Honda, and J. R. Klinenberg.** 1977. Uptake of uric acid by separated renal tubules of the rabbit. II. Effects of drugs. J. Pharmacol. Exp. Ther. **201:**226–232.
4. **Merle, L. J., M. M. Reidenberg, M. T. Camacho, B. R. Jones, and D. E. Drayer.** 1980. Renal injury in patients with rheumatoid arthritis treated with gold. Clin. Pharmacol. Ther. **28:**216–222.
5. **Peters, J. E., I. Schneider, and R. J. Haschen.** 1972. Bestimmung der l-Alanyl-peptidhydrolase (Alanin-aminopeptidase, Aminosäure-arylamidase) in menschlichen Harn. Clin. Chim. Acta **36:**289–301.
6. **Prockop, D. J., and W. D. Davidson.** 1964. A study of urinary and serum lysozyme in patients with renal disease. N. Engl. J. Med. **270:**269–274.
7. **Van Blerk, P. J. P., C. S. Block, E. Yourassowsky, E. Schoutens, S. Sander, and T. Bergan.** 1980. Efficacy, safety, and tolerance of piperacillin sodium in patients with urinary tract infections, p. 291–293. *In* J. D. Nelson and C. Grassi (ed.), Current chemotherapy and infectious disease, vol. 1. American Society for Microbiology, Washington, D.C.

Clinical Trial of Piperacillin in Children

B. MEYER* AND J. VIALATTE

Hôpital des Enfants Malades, 75730 Paris Cedex 15, France

Piperacillin is a new semisynthetic derivative of aminobenzyl-penicillin with an in vitro activity that covers the majority of gram-positive and gram-negative organisms. Within these two groups of organisms the activity of piperacillin, particularly against *Pseudomonas aeruginosa*, is superior to that of ampicillin and carbenicillin. The drug is for parenteral use only. We report the results of our clinical study carried out on 26 children.

Our 26 patients included 13 boys and 13 girls aged as follows: 5 months to 4 years, 9; 5 to 10 years, 10; and 11 to 15 years, 5. Various infections were treated, predominantly bronchopulmonary (18), urinary tract (5), meningitis (2), and otitis with mastoiditis (1). Among the bronchopulmonary infections, we treated five cases of exacerbated cystic fibrosis, one case of pneumonia with urinary infection, and one respiratory infection in an asthmatic child.

Microorganisms, single or multiple, were cultured in 17 patients and occurred as follows: *P. aeruginosa*, 7; *Staphylococcus aureus*, 3; *Escherichia coli*, 3; *Proteus* spp., 3; hemolytic streptococci, 3; *Meningococcus*, 2; and *Haemophilus influenzae*, 1.

Dosage of piperacillin, route of administration, and duration of treatment varied according to the severity of the infection: 50 to 100 mg/kg per day in 8 patients; 100 to 150 mg/kg per day, 9; 150 to 250 mg/kg per day, 9. The intramuscular route alone was used in eight patients, the intravenous route in 17, and 1 patient began with intravenous and was switched to intramuscular. Duration of treatment ranged from 4 to 10 days in 16 and from 11 to 26 days in 10 patients. Clinical cure or improvement occurred in 23 of 26 patients. Treatment failed in only three patients, one with pneumonia, and two cases of cystic fibrosis.

There are in these results several aspects: (i) that the indications treated responded well in 88.5% of patients, and (ii) that in the two cases of meningitis cured without complication, we used ampicillin as initial treatment, in one case for 4 days and in the second for 8 h. We felt this appropriate in view of the lack of prior knowledge on the patients with purulent meningitis. (iii) In one case of severe pneumonia caused by *P. aeruginosa* in an agammaglobulinemic child, we also gave immunoglobulin G. Lastly, two of five patients with exacerbated cystic fibrosis were failures, which should be viewed in light of pharmacokinetic data available in the literature. Table 1 presents microbiological data and results.

The microbiological failures (those persisting posttherapy) were essentially among the cases with cystic fibrosis.

Clinical tolerance of the drug was excellent, although pain at the site of intramuscular injections limits the use of this route in small children.

The concentrations of piperacillin achieved in the blood after intravenous or intramuscular injection show that high levels were obtained quickly which fell almost to nil at 4 h after dosing. Figure 1 shows the decline in serum levels against time. With either route of administration high concentrations of piperacillin were found in urine for prolonged times, often exceeding 6 h. The kinetics of piperacillin in the cases of cystic fibrosis seem to us most interesting insofar as they may explain the failure of antibiotic therapy to clear organisms which were susceptible and yet persisted through treatment in the sputum. We have looked at the serum concentrations in two cases of cystic fibrosis treated by intravenous route. In the first case, the levels were equivalent to the noncystic patients, whereas in the second case a slightly smaller dose of piperacillin gave only negligible serum concentrations. These levels are confirmed by studying the bactericidal capacity of

TABLE 1. *Microbiological data and results*

Microorganism	No.	Result	Associated treatment
S. aureus	3	Persistence	Tobramycin/gentamicin
H. influenzae	1	Eradication	
Meningococcus	2	Eradication	Ampicillin
E. coli	3	Eradication	
Proteus spp.	3	Eradication (1)	
		Persistence (2)	Gentamicin/tobramycin
Pseudomonas aeruginosa	7	Eradication (2)	Immunoglobulin G (1)
		Persistence (5)	Gentamicin/tobramycin/ampicillin
Hemolytic streptococci	3	Eradication	

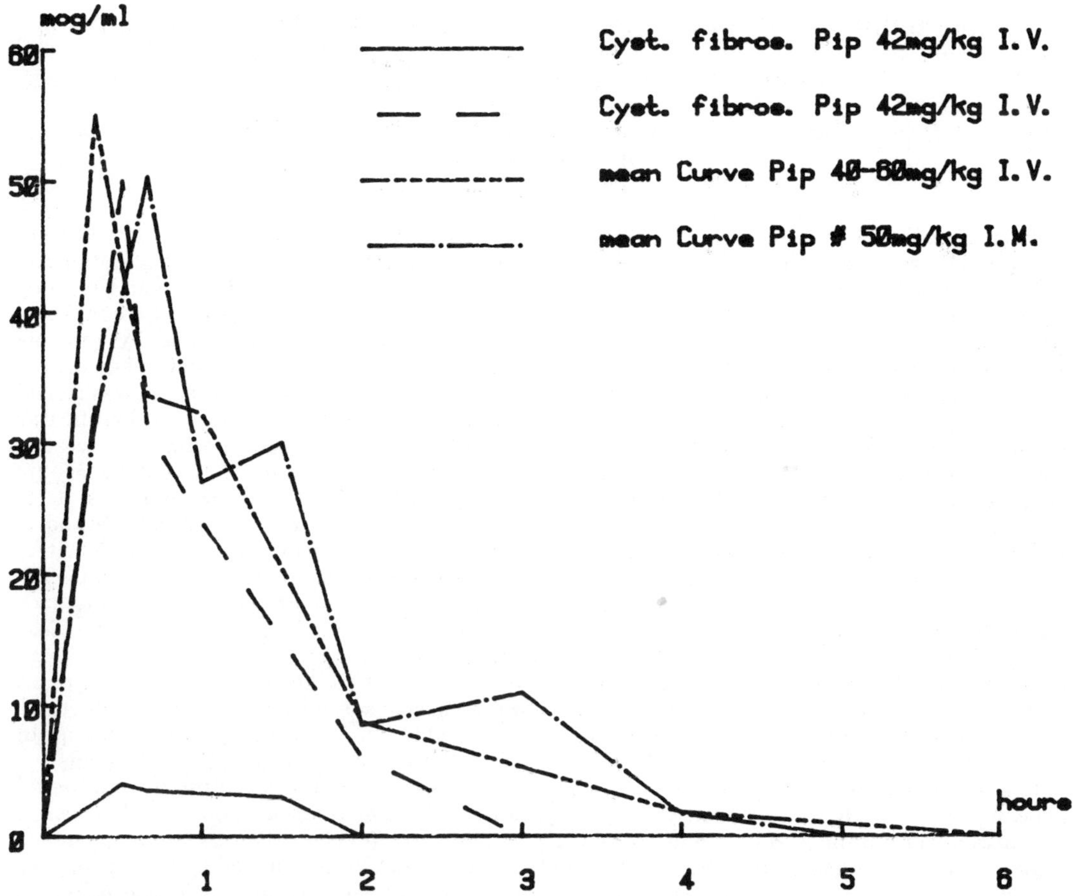

FIG. 1. *Serum concentrations against time in two patients with exacerbated cystic fibrosis treated with piperacillin (micrograms per milliliter) and mean curves in non-cystic fibrosis patients.*

serum taken 1 h after injections of piperacillin and gentamicin, on a strain of *Pseudomonas* isolated from the sputum of the patient which was susceptible in vitro to both antibiotics. The organism was 100% inhibited at a serum dilution of 1:2 but not at all at dilutions of 1:4 up to 1:28.

Thus, it appears that in some patients with cystic fibrosis the serum concentrations obtained after an average dose of piperacillin were inadequate for an antibacterial effect on susceptible microorganisms.

Piperacillin has proved highly effective against a variety of organisms, particularly *Proteus* and *Pseudomonas*. Its use in bacterial meningitis and in cystic fibrosis demands further study. Its tolerability is excellent, but in children utilization may be limited by the need for parenteral administration.

Piperacillin in the Treatment of Severe Urinary Tract Infections

OLE ZACHO, JØRGEN PRAEST,* AND BIRGITTE KORSAGER

Department of Surgery and Department of Clinical Bacteriology, Statens Seruminstitut, Aalborg Hospital, Aalborg, Denmark

Piperacillin is a new semisynthetic penicillin for parenteral administration. It has been shown to have a broad antibacterial spectrum, which includes clinically important gram-positive and gram-negative aerobic and anaerobic bacteria (3, 4), including many resistant to other penicillins, cephalosporins, or aminoglycoside antibiotics (2). Of special interest is its activity against *Pseudomonas*, *Proteus*, *Klebsiella*, *Serratia*, and *Escherichia coli*, pathogens often present in urine of patients with complicated urinary tract infections.

Drugs active against these bacteria may be hazardous to use, since many such patients also have impaired renal function. Thus aminoglycoside therapy carries a higher risk of toxicity in such patients compared to patients with normal renal function. In this study the object was to evaluate the efficacy and safety of piperacillin when used in the treatment of patients with severe urinary tract infections.

The study was performed as an open and noncomparative study and included 31 hospitalized patients in a urological unit. Patients with urinary tract infections caused by susceptible pathogens requiring a parenteral antibiotic agent were included in the study. Pregnant and nursing women, children, and patients with known hypersensitivity to penicillin were excluded. The material consisted of 27 male and 4 female patients, aged 27 to 85 years (mean, 67.5) weighing 49 to 97 kg (mean, 71.3). Table 1 shows infection site, initial microorganisms cultured, and clinical and microbiological response. Only one patient had no concomitant disease, while the remainder mostly had urological and/or cardiovascular disease. Nineteen patients had indwelling urinary catheters, and eight underwent some form of urological diagnostic procedure and/or surgery.

Piperacillin was administered by intravenous bolus injection of 4 g every 6 h, thus 16 g daily (mean 230 mg/kg per day), or by intramuscular injection of 2 g every 12 h, thus 4 g daily (mean 58 mg/kg per day), according to severity of infection. Lidocaine was administered as diluent in the case of intramuscular injection. Duration of treatment was 6 to 11 days (mean, 7.7). Urine cultures and routine hematological and biochemical tests were taken before and, repeatedly, during treatment as well as 1 day posttreatment, while fever, vital signs, and symptomatology were monitored daily throughout the study.

Bacteria in properly taken midstream specimens of urine were quantitated by the loop method on blood agar and MacConkey agar. A bacterial count of $\geq 10^5$ bacteria/ml was considered as significant bacteriuria. The identification of the bacterial strains was performed according to the routine procedure of the laboratory (5). The susceptibility to piperacillin was determined by the agar plate diffusion method on Danish blood agar using tablets (Neo-Sensitabs, Rosco, Denmark) containing 100 μg of piperacillin (diffusible amount). The IC_{50} values (50% inhibitory concentration) were estimated from the diameter of the zone of inhibition using a precalculated line. The following breaking points were chosen: susceptible ≤ 5 μg/ml, moderately susceptible 5 to 50 μg/ml, relatively susceptible 50 to 400 μg/ml, and resistant >400 μg/ml.

Initial microorganisms cultured were the following: *Pseudomonas aeruginosa*, 11; *E. coli*, 7; enterococci, 5; *Enterobacter cloacae*, indole-positive *Proteus*, and mixed flora, 2 each; coagulase-negative staphylococci, *Proteus mirabilis*, and *Klebsiella oxytoca*, 1 each. Negative pretreatment cultures were obtained in six patients, and only clinical judgments were made on these. Ninety percent of isolates were fully susceptible to piperacillin and 10% were moderately susceptible. IC_{50} values are shown in Table 2. Therapeutic responses were assessed at the end of treatment on the basis of clinical judgment (cure, improvement, relapse, or failure) and microbiological judgment (eradication or persistence; cases judged microbiologically unevaluable were assessed clinically and vice versa where possible, and the incidence of superinfection was noted).

Eighteen patients showed eradication of their infecting organisms, and two patients achieved eradication during therapy, but data were incomplete due to absence of follow-up. Persistence was seen in two cases, one with *P. aeruginosa* infection, and one with a double infection with *P. aeruginosa* and *Proteus*. The *P. aeruginosa* was eradicated, while the *Proteus* persisted. Nine cases were judged as indeterminate. Five of these showed a negative culture pretreat-

TABLE 1. *Clinical and microbiological data, therapy, and response*

Patient no.	Diagnosis	Pathogen	Clinical response	Bacterial response
1	Cystitis	*Proteus morganii*	Cure	Eradication
2	Cystitis	*P. aeruginosa*	Not evaluable	Persistence
3	Cystitis	*P. aeruginosa*	Cure	Eradication
4	Cystitis	*E. coli*	Cure	Eradication
5	Cystitis	No growth	Cure	Indeterminate
6	Cystitis	*P. aeruginosa*	Cure	Eradication
7	Cystitis	*P. aeruginosa*	Cure	Eradication
8	Cystitis	*Klebsiella oxytoca*	Cure	Eradication
9	Cystitis; obs.	No growth	Cure	Indeterminate
10	Cystitis	*E. cloacae*; enterococcus	Cure	Eradication
11	Cystitis	*P. aeruginosa*; enterococcus	Cure	Eradication
12	Cystitis	*P. aeruginosa*	Cure	Eradication
13	Cystitis	*P. aeruginosa*; enterococcus	Not evaluable	Indeterminate
14	Cystitis; obs.	Missing	Cure	Indeterminate
15	Cystitis; recurrent	*P. aeruginosa*	Not evaluable	Eradication
16	Cystitis	Mixed flora	Cure	Indeterminate
17	Cystopyelitis, urosepsis	*E. coli*	Not evaluable	Eradication
18	Cystitis	*E. coli*	Cure	Eradication
19	Urosepsis	*P. aeruginosa/P. mirabilis*	Cure	Eradication/persistence
20	Cystopyelitis	No growth	Cure	Indeterminate
21	Cystitis	Enterococcus	Not evaluable	Eradication
22	Cystopyelitis	No growth	Cure	Indeterminate
23	Cystitis	*E. coli*	Cure	Eradication
24	Cystitis; recurrent	*P. aeruginosa*; mixed flora	Not evaluable	Indeterminate
25	Cystitis	*P. aeruginosa*	Cure	Eradication
26	Cystitis	*E. coli*	Cure	Eradication
27	Cystitis	No growth	Cure	Indeterminate
28	Cystitis	*E. cloacae*; enterococcus	Cure	Eradication
29	Cystitis; urosepsis	*E. coli*	Cure	Eradication
30	Cystitis	*Proteus vulgaris*; enterococcus	Cure	Eradication
31	Cystopyelitis Urosepsis	*E. coli* Coagulase-negative staphylococci	Cure	Eradication

TABLE 2. *Bacterial susceptibility to piperacillin*

Pathogen	Susceptibility (IC_{50})	
	5–50 μg/ml	≤5 μg/ml
P. aeruginosa		11/11 (100%)
Proteus, indole negative		1/1 (100%)
Proteus, indole positive		2/2 (100%)
E. coli	1/7 (14%)	6/7 (86%)
Enterococcus	2/5 (40%)	3/5 (60%)
K. oxytoca		1/1 (100%)
E. cloacae		2/2 (100%)

ment and throughout the treatment. In one patient no culture was done pretreatment, but he was clinically cured. Treatment was stopped in one case. One patient was judged as indeterminate because of mixed flora pretreatment and one patient because of mixed flora posttreatment. However, six of these nine patients who were judged as indeterminate were clinically cured. Superinfection developed in one patient, in whom enterococci in significant amounts were isolated from the urine posttreatment.

Clinical cure was obtained in 25 out of 25 patients in which judgment of clinical efficacy was possible. Five of these patients had negative cultures pretreatment. Six patients were unevaluable regarding clinical response for various reasons. These results are according to earlier studies (6, 7).

Only one adverse reaction was seen, an erythematous rash on the lower body, and the treatment was stopped. In contrast to Bouza et al. (1), we found no episodes of phlebitis and our laboratory data showed no serious or unexpected events. Most of the minor changes seen could not with certainty be attributed to the antibiotic. Our objective was to examine the efficacy of this new penicillin in admitted patients with urological disease. These patients are especially prone to recurrent and severe urinary tract infection. Piperacillin is known to be excreted into the urine in high concentrations (8). The infecting organisms in these patients tend to be resistant gram-negative bacteria, and they normally require antibiotic therapy with agents known to be potentially toxic, i.e., aminoglycosides and polymyxin. Many such patients tend to have precarious renal function and thus nephrotoxicity is an added hazard. The in vivo results we have obtained, not withstanding the incidence of severe urological disease with indwelling catheters and the incidence of general debilitating nonurological disease, have been excellent on short-term review.

In conclusion, we believe that piperacillin is an antibiotic which will be of value in the treatment of severe urinary tract infections, particularly those caused by *P. aeruginosa* and *Proteus*. Low toxicity is an additional factor when selecting an appropriate agent for the treatment of such patients.

1. **Bouza, E., L. Buzon, J. Martinez-Beltran, M. Rodriques, I. Mneo, and C. Bergaleta.** 1979. Complications of the treatment of bacterial infections with piperacillin, p. 300–303. *In* Proceedings from 11th World Congress of Microbiology. Boston.
2. **Fu, K. P., and H. C. Neu.** 1978. Piperacillin, a new penicillin active against many bacteria resistant to other penicillins. Antimicrob. Agents Chemother. **13:**358–367.
3. **Gentry, L. O., R. T. Ives, and J. G. Jemsek.** 1979. Antibacterial activity of piperacillin against gram-negative baceria. Curr. Ther. Res. **26:**158–164.
4. **Kuck, N. A., and G. S. Redin.** 1978. In vitro and in vivo activity of piperacillin, a new broad-spectrum semisynthetic penicillin. Antibiotics **31:**1175–1182.
5. **Lautrop, H., N. Højby, A. Bremmelsgaard, and B. Korsager.** 1979. Bakteriologiske undersogelsmetoder. Fadl's Forlag, Copenhagen.
6. **Sander, S., T. Bergan, and E. Fossberg.** 1980. Piperacillin in the treatment of urinary tract infections. Chemotherapy **26:**141–144.
7. **Schoutens, E., C. Potvliege, and E. Yourassowsky.** 1979. Intramuscular piperacillin sodium in uncomplicated lower urinary tract infections. Evaluation of safety, clinical and bacteriological responses and blood levels. Curr. Ther. Res. **26:**848–855.
8. **Tjandramaga, T. B., A. Mullie, R. Verbesselt, P. J. de Schepper, and L. Verbist.** 1978. Piperacillin: human pharmacokinetics after intravenous and intramuscular administration. Antimicrob. Agents Chemother. **14:**829–837.

Comparative Study of Piperacillin Versus Cefoxitin in the Treatment of Female Pelvic Infection

RICHARD L. SWEET,* MARILYN O. ROBBIE, MARILYN OHM-SMITH, AND W. KEITH HADLEY

University of California, San Francisco, and San Francisco General Hospital, San Francisco, California 94110, U.S.A.*

Piperacillin sodium is a potent, semisynthetic penicillin with a wide spectrum of antibacterial activity which extends to many strains of microorganisms that are resistant to commonly used antimicrobial agents. In vitro studies with piperacillin have demonstrated a broad antibacterial spectrum against many clinically significant pathogens (2, 6, 7, 10). Piperacillin is active in vitro against most strains of the clinically important gram-negative facultative bacteria. Of significant importance in this extended spectrum are indole-positive *Proteus* species, *Klebsiella*, many *Serratia marcescens* strains, and *Pseudomonas aeruginosa*. Piperacillin exhibits activity against gram-positive aerobic bacteria, including enterococci. In addition, virtually all clinically important anaerobic organisms including *Bacteroides fragilis* and *Bacteroides bivius* are susceptible to piperacillin.

Recent investigations have identified the role of mixed aerobic and anaerobic bacteria in the pathogenesis of female genital tract infections (1, 3–5, 8, 9). These studies have yielded a pattern of microorganisms which are isolated from patients with pelvic infections. The commonly isolated aerobic organisms are gram-negative facultative bacteria, especially *Escherichia coli*, group B beta-hemolytic streptococci, nonhemolytic streptococci, and *Neisseria gonorrhoeae*. The anaerobic bacteria frequently isolated include *Peptococcus* species, *Peptostreptococcus* species, *Bacteroides* species, *B. fragilis*, and *B. bivius*.

The in vitro studies which demonstrated a broad antibacterial spectrum for piperacillin suggested that this agent might be an effective single agent for the treatment of mixed aerobic-anaerobic infections seen in obstetrics and gynecology.

This study was undertaken to compare the

clinical efficacy and safety of piperacillin and cefoxitin. We report herein the results for 49 female patients with upper genital tract infection. Twenty-four patients were treated with piperacillin in a dosage of 4.5 g intravenously every 6 h and 25 with cefoxitin, 2 g intravenously every 6 h, as determined by a computer-generated randomized protocol.

The piperacillin group included: acute salpingitis, 13; endomyometritis, 7; pelvic cellulitis, 2; and pelvic abscess, 1. The cefoxitin group included: acute salpingitis, 14; endomyometritis, 10; and pelvic abscess, 1.

From the 42 patients with recoverable organisms, 251 bacteria were isolated (Table 1), an average of 6 isolates per patient; 3 aerobes and 3 anaerobes per patient. Aerobic bacteria only were recovered from 8 patients (19%); anaerobic bacteria only were present in 4 (9.5%); and mixed aerobic and anaerobic bacteria were isolated in 30 patients (71.5%). The organisms isolated most frequently were: *Peptococcus* species, *Bacteroides* species, *Peptostreptococcus* species, *B. bivius*, *N. gonorrhoeae*, nonhemolytic aerobic streptococci, group B beta-hemolytic streptococci, *E. coli*, and *B. fragilis*.

Piperacillin susceptibility studies revealed that all of the strains of *N. gonorrhoeae*, group B streptococci, and *Staphylococcus aureus* were susceptible at levels of ≤0.06 μg/ml, 0.25 μg/ml, and 16 μg/ml, respectively; 100% of enterococci were susceptible at 2 μg/ml. Ninety-one percent of *E. coli* were susceptible at 128 μg/ml. All strains of *Bacteroides* spp., *B. bivius*, and *B. fragilis* were susceptible to 32 μg/ml. One-hundred percent of *P. prevotii, P. asaccharolyticus*, and *P. anaerobius* were susceptible to ≤0.06 μg/ml, 1.0 μg/ml, and 8 μg/ml, respectively.

Against cefoxitin, 100% of *N. gonorrhoeae, S. aureus, E. coli*, and group B streptococci were susceptible to 0.5 μg/ml, 4 μg/ml, 8 μg/ml, and 2 μg/ml, respectively. All enterococci were resistant at >128 μg/ml. All strains of *B. bivius* were susceptible to 8 μg/ml and all *B. fragilis* to 16 μg/ml. One-hundred percent of *P. prevotii, P. asaccharolyticus*, and *P. anaerobius* were susceptible to 0.125 μg/ml, 2 μg/ml, and 8 μg/ml, respectively.

Overall, 22 of 24 (92%) of the piperacillin treatment group and 23 of 25 (92%) of the cefoxitin group responded well and were cured. In the piperacillin group 13 of 13 salpingitis patients, 7 of 7 endomyometritis, 1 of 2 pelvic cellulitis, and 1 of 2 pelvic abscesses responded. The piperacillin failures were limited to a patient requiring additional antibiotics for treatment of pelvic cellulitis and a patient requiring surgical drainage of a pelvic abscess. In the cefoxitin group 13 of 14 salpingitis cases, 10 of 10 endomyometritis, and 0 of 1 pelvic abscesses responded. The cefoxitin failures included a pelvic abscess which required surgical drainage and a salpingitis patient who developed a tuboovarian abscess during treatment which required surgical intervention.

No hematological toxicity or nephrotoxicity occurred. A single piperacillin recipient developed a transient elevation in liver enzymes. No patients developed a rash, eosinophilia, diarrhea, or phlebitis. Both drugs were well tolerated by the patients.

TABLE 1. *Bacteria isolated from 49 women with pelvic infection*

Bacterium	No. of strains
Aerobic bacteria	
Gram-positive cocci	
Group B beta-hemolytic streptococci	7
Group D streptococci	5
Enterococci	4
Other nonhemolytic streptococci	23
S. aureus	5
S. epidermidis	14
Other gram-positive cocci	1
Gram-negative cocci	
N. gonorrhoeae	17
Other gram-negative cocci	1
Gram-negative rods	
E. coli	7
P. mirabilis	1
Gardnerella vaginalis	6
Gram-positive rods	
Lactobacillus	22
Diptheroids	7
Other gram-positive rods	2
Anaerobic bacteria	
Gram-positive cocci	
Peptococcus prevotii	16
P. asaccharolyticus	14
P. magnus	4
Peptococcus species	2
Peptostreptococcus anaerobius	15
P. productus	1
Micrococcus	2
Unidentified gram-positive cocci	7
Gram-negative cocci	
Veillonella species	4
Other gram-positive cocci	1
Gram-positive rods	
Clostridium perfringens	1
Clostridium species	2
Bifidobacterium species	6
Eubacterium species	3
Other gram-positive rods	4
Gram-negative rods	
Bacteroides species	16
B. bivius	13
B. fragilis	6
B. asaccharolyticus	7
Fusobacterium species	2
Other gram-negative rods	2

In summary, piperacillin appeared to be a safe and efficacious single drug for the treatment of female genital tract infections associated with a variety of aerobic and anaerobic bacteria. In 92% of the patients receiving piperacillin, a clinical cure was obtained without additional treatment. These results were similar to those achieved with cefoxitin.

1. **Cunningham, F. G., D. L. Hemsell, R. T. DePalma, S. Kappus, M. Roark, and B. Nobles.** 1981. Moxalactam for obstetric and gynecologic infections. Am. J. Obstet. Gynecol. **139**:915.
2. **Fu, K. P., and H. C. Neu.** 1978. Antimicrobial activity of piperacillin, p. 596–597. *In* W. Siegenthaler and R. Lüthy (ed.), Current chemotherapy. American Society for Microbiology, Washington, D.C.
3. **Gall, S. A., A. P. Kohan, O. M. Ayers, C. E. Hughes, W. A. Addison, and G. B. Hill.** 1981. Intravenous metronidazole or clindamycin with tobramycin for therapy of pelvic infections. Obstet. Gynecol. **57**:51.
4. **Gibbs, R. S., and R. W. Huff.** 1979. Cefamandole therapy of endomyometritis following cesarean section. Am. J. Obstet. Gynecol. **136**:32.
5. **Ledger, W. J., M. Norman, and C. Gee.** 1975. Bacteremia on an obstetric/gynecologic service. Am. J. Obstet. Gynecol. **121**:205–212.
6. **Monif, G. R. G., P. R. Clark, J. J. Shuster, and H. Baer.** 1978. Susceptibility of the aerobic bacteria, group D streptococci, *Enterobacteriaceae*, and *Pseudomonas* to semisynthetic penicillins: carbenicillin, piperacillin, and ticarcillin. Antimicrob. Agents Chemother. **14**:643–649.
7. **Roy, I., W. M. Abernathy, V. T. Bach, and H. Thadepalli.** 1978. In vitro activity of piperacillin against aerobic bacteria. Curr. Ther. Res. **23**:200–205.
8. **Sweet, R. L.** 1975. Anaerobic infections of the female genital tract. Am. J. Obstet. Gynecol. **122**:891.
9. **Sweet, R. L., and W. J. Ledger.** 1979. Cefoxitin: single-agent treatment of mixed aerobic-anaerobic pelvic infections. Obstet. Gynecol. **54**:193.
10. **Winston, D. J., D. Wang, L. S. Young, W. J. Martin, and W. L. Hewitt.** 1978. In vitro studies of piperacillin, a new semisynthetic penicillin. Antimicrob. Agents Chemother. **13**:944–950.

Polymicrobial Endometritis Treated with Piperacillin or Cefoxitin

D. A. ESCHENBACH,* K. A. ROSENE, G. P. WAGER, AND H. WATKINS

Department of Obstetrics and Gynecology, University of Washington, Seattle, Washington 98185, U.S.A.

We studied the microbiology and therapy of 46 nonconsecutive women who developed a fever after delivery. Patients were selected on the basis of severe clinical infection and the availability of the investigative team. The patients had to have a temperature of >38°C for 6 consecutive h more than 24 h after delivery, or a temperature >38.5°C within 24 h of delivery and clinical findings of abdominal and uterine tenderness. Patients who were breast-feeding, allergic to the antibiotics used, or treated with antibiotics in the past month were excluded.

All patients underwent a physical examination, including a pelvic examination, a leukocyte count, serum electrolyte, and liver and renal function tests. Urine cultures were placed on MacConkey medium; blood cultures were anaerobically incubated in peptone-enriched broth for bacterial isolates and in mycoplasma medium for genital mycoplasmal isolates. Cervical and endometrial cultures were transported in prereduced medium and plated in blood and MacConkey agar for aerobic and on prereduced blood agar for anaerobic bacterial isolation. The cervix was also cultured for mycoplasma and chlamydia.

Endometrial cultures were obtained through a triple-lumen system designed to reduce cervical flora contamination of endometrial samples. The cervix was prepped three times with iodine-alcohol, and a 14-mm sleeve was placed through the cervix into the lower uterine segment through which a 6-mm guide was placed. A Novak endometrial curette was placed through the inner cannula, and an endometrial biopsy was performed with a 10-cm^3 syringe. Endometrial samples were cultured for bacteria, mycoplasma, and chlamydia. Bacterial isolates were tested for susceptibility to piperacillin and cefoxitin by a disk diffusion method.

Patients were then assigned to a double-blind, randomized intravenous regimen of either piperacillin administered 4.5 g every 6 h or cefoxitin, 2.0 g every 6 h, for 4 to 7 days. Antibiotics were administered over a 1-h period. For this analysis, the two groups were separated, and all patients in group A received one drug and all patients in group B received the other drug. However, the blind code was not broken and the investigators did not know which drug was used for group A and which drug was used for group B.

Afebrile, vaginally delivered patients undergoing tubal ligation >24 h after delivery served as controls. After the tubal ligation, a 20-gauge spinal needle was placed, under direct visualization, through the anterior uterine fundus into the endometrial cavity, and endometrial material was recovered. Cervical and endometrial samples were cultured for bacteria and mycoplasma in the same manner as the samples from the patients.

Results. Bacteria were not recovered from the transfundal sample of seven afebrile controls. All of the cervical samples of controls had bacteria isolated. Two of seven controls had bacteria isolated from the transcervical triple-lumen sample. One was a laboratory *Staphylococcus aureus* contaminate from broth only and the other was an *S. epidermidis* cervical contaminate.

Endometrial organisms were recovered from 42 (91%) of 46 febrile postpartum women and from 2 (29%) of 7 afebrile postpartum women ($P < 0.005$). Forty-six febrile postpartum women were evaluated. A urinary infection was present in two patients who had $>10^5$ organisms isolated per ml of urine and sterile endometrial cultures. Two additional female patients had no organisms isolated from either the urine or endometrium. Endometrial organisms were recovered from the remaining 42 women (Table 1).

Forty-two women were considered to have postpartum endometritis. Several different endometrial organisms were isolated from these women, including bacteria alone in 9 (21%), bacteria combined with mycoplasma in 25 (60%), mycoplasma alone in 6 (14%), and bacteria combined with chlamydia and chlamydia alone in 1 each.

Bacteria were recovered from the blood of 14 (40%) of 35 patients with endometrial bacteria. *Mycoplasma hominis* was present in the blood of 1 of 25 patients with endometrial bacteria and mycoplasma. *Ureaplasma urealyticum* was isolated from the blood of two of six women that had ureaplasma alone present in the endometrium.

The most common aerobic, gram-positive endometrial bacteria recovered from the 42 women with postpartum endometritis included group B streptococci, *S. epidermidis*, enterococci, and *S. intermedius* MG. *S. epidermidis* was always recovered in low numbers, and it was always present together with virulent organisms. All virulent isolates were susceptible to piperacillin. The five enterococci and one *S. sangius* were resistant to cefoxitin in vitro. The most common aerobic, gram-negative endometrial bacteria were *Gardnerella vaginalis*, *Escherichia coli*, and *Enterobacter*. All isolates were susceptible to piperacillin, but both *Enterobacter* spp. were resistant to cefoxitin. The most common anaerobic isolates included *Bacteroides bivius*, *Peptostreptococcus asaccharolyticus*, *Peptococcus*, and *Peptostreptococcus* species. The anaerobes were susceptible in vitro to both antibiotics. The susceptibility of the mycoplasmal and chlamydial isolates to the two drugs has not yet been tested.

The most common blood isolate corresponded with the most common endometrial isolates: *G. vaginalis* (6), group B streptococci (2), *B. bivius* (4), *Bacteroides* species (4), and *P. asaccharolyticus* (2).

A favorable clinical response was noted in 43 of the 46 patients. One drug A patient had persistent uterine tenderness, a temperature of 37.8°C, and a leukocyte count of 26,000 after 22 doses. *G. vaginalis*, *B. bivius*, and a *Peptococcus* species were isolated from the endometrium after the 5 days of therapy. Two other patients receiving drug A had an improving clinical response, but were administered alternative antibiotics before becoming afebrile. Neither of these were considered drug failures. One patient became afebrile 12 h after drainage of a subcutaneous wound infection, and the second became afebrile 16 h after the antibiotic change.

The six patients with *U. urealyticum* only recovered from the endometrium initially had high temperatures but became afebrile at a mean time of 20 h after antibiotics were started. The 35 women with bacteria isolated from the endometrium became afebrile at a mean time of 26.6 h after antibiotics were started. The one patient with *Chlamydia trachomatis* became afebrile within 1 h after receiving drug A, but developed salpingitis 4 weeks later.

In summary, endometrial isolates from patients with endometritis included aerobic and anaerobic bacteria, genital mycoplasma, and *C. trachomatis*. All bacterial isolates were susceptible in vitro to piperacillin; eight were resistant to cefoxitin. A clinical response to therapy occurred in 43 (98%) of 44 patients treated with either piperacillin or cefoxitin who could be completely evaluated.

TABLE 1. *Recovery of organisms from 42 women with postpartum endometritis*

Endometrial isolate	No. of patients	Blood culture	
		Bacteria	Mycoplasma
Bacteria alone	9	2 (22%)	0
Bacteria and mycoplasma	25	12 (48%)	1 (4%)
Mycoplasma alone	6	0	2 (33%)
Bacteria and chlamydia	1	0	0
Chlamydia alone	1	0	0

Experiences with Piperacillin in Burn Wound Sepsis and Postoperative Surgical Infections

E. DIEM,* W. GRANINGER, J. KARNER, AND T. RATH

Department of Dermatology I, Department of Chemotherapy, and Department of Surgery I, University of Vienna, Vienna, Austria*

Piperacillin is a new semisynthetic piperazine derivative of ampicillin belonging to the acylureidopenicillin group. It has a broad spectrum of activity against a wide range of gram-positive and gram-negative organisms. Of particular interest is its activity against *Pseudomonas aeruginosa*, *Acinetobacter calcoaceticus*, *Streptococcus* species, and members of the *Enterobacteriaceae*.

To assess the clinical efficacy of this drug, we carried out a clinical trial on a group of 41 patients with severe life-threatening infections. Burn sepsis is a frequent, catastrophic, and often fatal complication for the burned patient. Commonly recovered bacteria in burn wound sepsis are *P. aeruginosa*, *Escherichia coli*, beta-hemolytic streptococci, and *Enterobacter*, which are in increasing numbers resistant to aminoglycosides and cephalosporins. Good tissue penetration and high biliary excretion rate make piperacillin a useful drug in the treatment of intraabdominal infection as well.

Our study was designed as an open noncomparative evaluation of the efficacy, safety, and tolerance of piperacillin sodium in the parenteral therapy of hospitalized adult patients with infections caused by susceptible strains of aerobic or anaerobic organisms, or both. Patients were eligible for inclusion if they had evidence of bacteremia or documented bacteriological evidence of invasive local infection.

Appropriate specimens for culture were obtained before piperacillin therapy, as were basic hematology and chemistry studies and urinalysis. All laboratory tests were repeated at 4-day intervals during treatment and 2 to 3 days after treatment. Cultures were repeated during treatment if indicated and 2 to 3 days after treatment. Standard isolation and identification procedures were employed by the hospital diagnostic microbiology laboratories. Routine antimicrobial susceptibility testing was performed by a modified Bauer-Kirby technique.

We treated 25 patients with burn sepsis. The mean amount of the total body surface area burned was 30% (third degree). Patients received 12 g of piperacillin per day. According to the bacteriological findings and at the discretion of the prescribing doctor, some patients received additional therapy with oxacillin or aminoglycosides, or both. Patients who received aminoglycosides were evaluated only if they had received therapy with the same aminoglycosides before the onset of piperacillin therapy. Therapy was continued until the patient showed clinical response or resistant organisms emerged. The most frequently isolated organisms were: *Staphylococcus aureus*, beta-hemolytic streptococci, *E. coli*, *Acinetobacter* spp., and *P. aeruginosa*. In 8 of 25 patients, repeated blood cultures revealed more than one organism. Excellent effectiveness was seen in patients with sepsis due to *E. coli*, *Proteus* species, and *Acinetobacter* species, as well as in infections due to streptococci. Noteworthy, however, was the persistence of two strains of *S. aureus*, one strain of *Enterobacter cloacae*, and one of *P. aeruginosa* in spite of appropriate in vitro susceptibility to piperacillin.

The second group which received piperacillin consisted of 10 patients with severe intraabdominal infections such as peritonitis and pancreatic and hepatic abscesses. The dosage of piperacillin was 150 to 200 mg/kg per day. In five patients with mixed infections due to resistant *Staphylococcus* and *Klebsiella* strains, piperacillin was given in combination with oxacillin or cephalothin. Causative organisms were mainly *Streptococcus faecalis*, *P. aeruginosa*, and *E. coli* (Table 1). Bacteria which could not be eliminated were *S. faecalis* in one, *Serratia marcescens* in one, *P. aeruginosa* in one, *Klebsiella* in two, and *S. aureus* in one case. Two patients had septicemia due to *Pseudomonas*, and three patients suffered from endocarditis due to *S. faecalis*. In one patient with septicemia due to *P. aeruginosa* and in one patient with endocarditis due to *S. faecalis*, the organism could not be eradicated by piperacillin monotherapy. The other patients, who received additional gentamicin (5 mg/kg per day), responded satisfactorily. Bacteria which emerged during therapy in burn patients were resistant *S. aureus* in six patients and resistant *P. aeruginosa* in five patients. In four of these patients, susceptible *P. aeruginosa* strains grew in the initial blood culture. During therapy resistant strains were recovered. It appeared as if these strains had developed resist-

TABLE 1. *Bacteriological effects of piperacillin (A) on causative organisms in burn sepsis and (B) in patients with intraabdominal infections and septicemia*

Study	Causative organism	Total	No. eradicated	No. that persisted
A	*S. aureus* (β-lactamase negative)	4	2	2
	Streptococcus group A	3	3	
	S. faecalis	2	2	
	E. coli	6	6	
	C. freundii	1	1	
	E. cloacae	3	2	1
	P. mirabilis	2	2	
	P. morganii	1	1	
	A. calcoaceticus	7	7	
	P. aeruginosa	5	4	1
	Total	34	30	4
B	*Peptostreptococcus*	1	1	
	E. coli	2	2	
	S. faecalis	6	4	2
	S. marcescens	2	1	1
	P. aeruginosa	6	4	2
	Enterobacter sp.	1	1	
	K. pneumoniae	2		2
	Citrobacter sp.	1	1	
	S. aureus	1		1
	Total	22	14	8

ance to piperacillin during therapy, as described by Simon et al. (4); however, we were not able to carry out *Pseudomonas* serotyping. Among the patients who had postoperative intraabdominal abscesses, five developed superinfection, with resistant strains of *Klebsiella* in three patients and *Enterobacter* sp. in two patients. The susceptible strains which occurred in surgical patients were regarded more as contamination since the patients recovered without a change of therapy.

The overall clinical effect of piperacillin in burn wound sepsis was satisfactory in 16 of 25 patients (Table 2). The remaining 9 patients with extensive thermal injuries and toxic complications failed to respond, 5 of them because of superinfection with resistant *P. aeruginosa* and *S. aureus*. In 4 patients the organisms persisted as shown above. Good results were obtained in intraabdominal infections. Only 2 patients showed no improvement; both patients suffered from infections due to *K. pneumoniae*. One patient with endocarditis due to *S. faecalis* showed initial response, but the original organisms were again grown after 18 days of treatment.

TABLE 2. *Clinical effect of piperacillin therapy*

Infection	No. of patients	No. excellent	No. good	No. poor
Burn wound sepsis	25	9	7	9
Hepatobiliary infection	4	2	1	1
Peritonitis or intraabdominal abscess	6	4	1	1
Septicemia and endocarditis	5	3	1	1
Endophthalmitis	1			1
Total	41	18	10	13

One patient with endophthalmitis due to *P. aeruginosa* received 24 g of piperacillin per day combined with 1 g of amikacin. However, only minimal clinical improvement was seen. After 2 weeks of this therapeutic regimen, fosfomycin was added with excellent success. The systemic and local tolerance of piperacillin was excellent. In three patients a macular rash developed (7.3%).

Piperacillin has been found to have a broader spectrum of antimicrobial activity than any of the other currently available penicillins (1, 3). In our study piperacillin proved to be an effective and safe antibiotic in treatment of severe infections such as sepsis and intraabdominal abscesses. Bacteria which could not be eliminated or which emerged during treatment were *S. aureus*, *K. pneumoniae*, and *P. aeruginosa*. Our findings of lack of effect against *K. pneumoniae* are in contrast to findings of Dickinson (2), who reported piperacillin to be effective against strains of these bacteria. Because there is a high incidence of mixed infections with *S. aureus* in burns, piperacillin should be given together with an antistaphylococcal agent such as oxacillin, cephalothin, or cefamandole. In septicemia due to *P. aeruginosa*, combination with an aminiglycoside is indicated to eradicate the organisms and to avoid the emergence of resistant *P. aeruginosa* strains.

1. **Daschner, F., H. Langmaack, M. Crohn, et al.** 1981. Chemotherapy (Basel) **27**:39–43.
2. **Dickinson, G. M., T. J. Cleary, and H. A. Hoffmann.** 1978. Comparative evaluation of piperacillin in vitro. Antimicrob. Agents Chemother. **14**:919–921.
3. **Prince, A. S., S. J. Pancoast, and H. C. Neli.** 1980. Efficacy of piperacillin in the therapy of serious infections, p. 295–296. *In* J. D. Nelson and C. Grassi (ed.), Current chemotherapy and infectious diseases. American Society for Microbiology, Washington D.C.
4. **Simon, G. L., D. R. Snydman, F. P. Tally, et al.** 1980. Clinical trial of piperacillin with acquisition of resistance by *Pseudomonas* and clinical relapse. Antimicrob. Agents Chemother. **18**:167–170.

Assessment of Piperacillin in the Treatment of Infection

J. HONORATO,* J. A. GARCIA-RODRIGUEZ, J. MONTERO, J. AZANZA, AND P. FERNANDEZ

Clinica Universitaria, Pamplona, and Hospital Clinico, Salamanca, Spain

There has been a reawakening of interest in the use of penicillins for the treatment of severe infections with the synthesis of new members of this class of antibiotics. Enhanced antimicrobial activity combined with the safety of penicillins makes the class once again as attractive for clinical use as it was with the appearance of ampicillin. In vitro studies have shown piperacillin to be the leading member of this group. It has an extended spectrum of activity which includes members of the family *Enterobacteriaceae*, *Pseudomonas* spp., enterococci, and anaerobic microorganisms. The currently available cephalosporins and aminoglycosides still have gaps in spectrum which may be relevant, especially in presumptive therapy. We have assessed piperacillin in vivo in infections of the respiratory and urinary tracts.

A total of 47 patients were enrolled in the study, 27 male and 20 female. Eleven patients were aged 16 to 49 years and the remainder were from 50 to 90 years. Mean ages were 62 years for males and 50 years for females. Forty-seven patients were suffering from a total of 49 infections including pneumonia in 7, acute or exacerbated bronchitis or bronchiectasis in 12, urinary infections in 24, acute or recurrent pyelonephritis in 3, infected surgical wounds in 2, and septicemia in 1. Twenty patients were classified as having severe infection, and 16 were moderately ill. Eleven patients, all with urinary infection, had milder symptomatology. In 49% of the patients, infections were acute; the remainder had exacerbations of chronic disease or recurrent infections. All patients had concomitant diseases of cardiovascular, pulmonary, urological, neoplastic, diabetic, or calculous origin.

Piperacillin was administered by intravenous bolus or by intramuscular injection according to severity of infection in the respiratory cases, whereas all cases of purely urinary tract infection were treated by intramuscular injection. Daily intravenous dosage ranged from 129 to 364 mg/kg, and intramuscular dosage ranged from 73 to 146 mg/kg. Unit doses were 2 g every 3 h in two patients, every 4 h in 14, every 6 h in 5, and every 8 h in 29. Only three patients had a change of route during treatment. Thus, 6 to 16 g piperacillin was given daily for therapy lasting from 5 to 24 days (mean, 8.3 days).

Single organisms were cultured initially in 25 patients and the remainder had multiple organisms. Table 1 shows the organisms cultured. All were susceptible to piperacillin as determined by diameter of inhibition (zone size). Twenty-two patients had been treated with other antibiotic regimens for these infections without success, including co-trimoxazole, ampicillin, and aminoglycosides.

Results are shown divided clinically and microbiologically in Table 2. Nearly 84% of the patients (41 of 49) were clinically cured or im-

TABLE 1. *Initial infecting organisms in 47 patients*

Organism	No. of isolations: Total	No. of isolations: As a single organism
Pseudomonas aeruginosa	22	15
Escherichia coli	12	10
Klebsiella spp.	6	4
Proteus mirabilis	6	4
Streptococcus faecalis	3	1
Serratia marcescens	3	2
Haemophilus spp.	2	—
Staphylococcus aureus	2	—
Streptococcus pneumoniae	1	—
Enterobacter sp.	1	1
Totals	58	37

TABLE 2. *Clinical and microbiological results in 47 patients*

Infection	No.	Clinical results: Cure/improvement	Clinical results: Failure	No. of organisms	Microbiological results: Eradication	Microbiological results: Persisted/reinfection
Bronchopulmonary	19	18 (95%)	1 (5%)	24	18 (75%)	6 (25%)
Urinary tract	27	20 (74%)	7 (26%)	30	23 (77%)	7 (23%)
Septicemia	1	1 (100%)	—	2	2 (100%)	—
Surgical wound	2	2 (100%)	—	2	2 (100%)	—
Totals	49	41 (83.7%)	8 (16.3%)	58	45 (77.6%)	13 (22.4%)

proved on follow-up. Only 8 patients (16%) failed to respond or relapsed posttherapy. Over 77% of microorganisms cultured initially (45 of 58) were eradicated by piperacillin treatment; 13 (22%) of the microorganisms persisted despite treatment or reappeared posttherapy. Superinfection with clinical signs occurred in five patients, but it should be noted that almost all of the clinical failures and superinfections occurred in patients with chronic urological disease and indwelling catheters.

Local adverse reactions were few, there being one episode of phlebitis and one of inflammation at intramuscular injection sites. No systemic adverse reactions were seen.

Laboratory hematological and biochemical tests carried out before, during, and after treatment did not show any clinically significant adverse changes.

Piperacillin has proved to be safe and effective in both respiratory and urinary tract infections. Organisms which had failed to respond to previous regimens in some cases and which were variably resistant to other antibiotics including ampicillin, carbenicillin, and some cephalosporins have in large measure been eradicated and the clinical responses have been gratifying. Intramuscular therapy was used mostly in the patients with urinary tract infection in view of the high concentrations of piperacillin excreted in the urine and has proved to be satisfactory in patients who all had urological complications. Intravenous therapy was used in the respiratory and other infections and has also given good results. We conclude that piperacillin has clinical efficacy commensurate with its in vitro superiority.

Use of Intravenous Piperacillin Sodium in Renal Unit Patients

JOHN F. DONOHOE,* ROSEMARIE HONE, FRANCIS WALKER, MARC LAHER, AND DAVID JACKSON

Departments of Medicine, Nephrology, and Microbiology, The Charitable Infirmary and Mater Hospital, Dublin, Ireland, and Lederle Laboratories, Gosport, United Kingdom*

Piperacillin sodium (PIP), a semisynthetic piperazine penicillin derivative, has a number of potential advantages for use in renal patients. Compared with carbenicillin, it contains less sodium, and its spectrum includes greater activity against *Pseudomonas* (2, 6), thus permitting the use of smaller doses. Both of these factors combine to lessen the risk of extracellular fluid volume expansion which may be significant in patients with compromised renal function. It has been suggested that in end-stage renal disease biliary excretion of PIP may be augmented and that serum half-life is not excessively prolonged (3, 5). Thus, only modest dose reduction policies may be necessary with renal failure in contrast to carbenicillin (1). The aminoglycosides also, because of their inherent ototoxic and nephrotoxic properties, require rigid dose reduction regimes in patients with renal failure, and monitoring of serum levels is mandatory.

We undertook an open, noncomparative, prospective trial to assess the efficacy, safety, and tolerance of PIP in the 13 patients whose clinical profiles are given in Table 1. All were hospitalized on the Renal Service. Informed consent was obtained from all adult patients and from parents in the case of minors. No deliberate dose reduction policy was followed despite wide variation in renal function (pretreatment glomerular filtration rate, 37 to 103% of normal). The majority of the patients had serious urinary tract infections (11 of 13), and 2 had *Pseudomonas* pulmonary infections. Factors acknowledged as impeding the action of antibiotics in clearing infection were present in several patients. Patients 1, 3, 9, and 12 were heavily immunosuppressed (three of them because of renal transplant rejection, and one was receiving an immunosuppressive "cocktail" for crescentic glomerulonephritis). Additionally, case 9 had ureteric reflux to her kidney transplant demonstrated by micturating cystogram. Patient 7 had xanthogranulomatous pyelonephritis with multiple intrarenal calculi in her solitary kidney. She had had several previous unsuccessful attempts to clear chronic infection, including long-term suppressive antibiotics. Other complicating features (see Table 1) included congestive cardiac failure, renal failure, bladder catheterization, and renal scarring of chronic pyelonephritis on intravenous urography.

In our experimental protocol PIP was diluted in 5% dextrose and water and infused over 30 min through an indwelling intravenous heparin lock. The drug was given in divided doses every 8 or 12 h; details of dosage and duration of therapy are given in Table 2. Midstream urine (or sputum) samples were tested each second study day and at 2 and 4 weeks after completion of therapy. Cure was defined as the absence of clinical and bacteriological infection by the end of treatment which was maintained at the time of these later cultures. Serum electrolytes, urea, creatinine, and liver enzymes, full blood count, and urinary microscopy were performed also on each second study day and thereafter if indicated. Ten patients had peak serum PIP levels measured on days 3 and 6. Six had 24-h urine collections on these days for determination of urinary potassium excretion.

Details of outcome are given in Table 2. All 13 patients achieved sterile cultures in the first few days after commencing PIP. Eleven patients achieved clinical and bacteriological "cure" when late cultures were examined. Two patients had persistence of infection. In one of these (no. 12) PIP was administered on the basis of disk susceptibility testing only, and later the organism was judged resistant at an MIC of 128 mg/liter. This patient was retained in the series although in retrospect persistence of infection is not unexpected. In the other persistent case (no. 10) PIP was withdrawn after day 3 because of the development of a typical allergic erythema multiforme skin eruption. This resolved promptly once PIP was discontinued. The drug was prematurely withdrawn also from patient 9, who showed a rising serum creatinine which subsequently settled back to base line. This patient received a daily dose of 400 mg/kg, the second highest dose in our series, and had chronic renal transplant rejection. It is notewor-

TABLE 1. *Clinical details of patients treated with piperacillin*[a]

Patient	Age (yr)	Sex	Base serum creatinine (μmol/liter)	Infection	Pathogen (MIC, mg/liter)	Complicating factors
1	45	M	260	Pyelonephritis	*Klebsiella pneumoniae* (16.0)	RTR, CCF, IMM
2	34	F	80	Pyelonephritis	*Escherichia coli* (8.0)	Renal scarring
3	13	F	110	UTI	*E. coli* (2.0)	Glomerulonephritis, IMM
4	63	F	50	UTI	*Pseudomonas aeruginosa* (16.0)	Bladder catheter, CCF
5	68	F	70	Pyelonephritis	*E. coli* (NA)	Renal scarring
6	71	M	135	UTI	*Proteus mirabilis* (0.5)	Bladder catheter, CCF
7	58	F	150	Xanthogranulomatous pyelonephritis	*E. coli* (0.25)	One kidney, multiple calculi
8	53	M	103	Lung abscess	*P. maltophilia* (8.0)	Bronchiectasis
9	13	F	310	Pyelonephritis	*E. coli* (0.25)	RTR, IMM
10	74	F	105	Pyelonephritis	*E. coli* (2.0)	Renal scarring
11	79	F	160	UTI	*E. coli* (1.0)	One kidney
12	16	F	182	Pyelonephritis	*E. coli* (128.0)	RTR, IMM
13	67	M	185	Pneumonia	*P. aeruginosa* (16.0)	Chronic lung disease

[a] RTR, Renal transplant rejection; IMM, immunosuppression; CCF, congestive cardiac failure; UTI, lower urinary tract infection; NA, not available.

TABLE 2. *Summary of intravenous piperacillin treatment and outcome*

Patient	Treatment			Clinical outcome	Clinically significant side effects[a]
	Daily dose (g)	Daily dose (mg/kg)	Duration (days)		
1	12	190	7	Cure	Mild CCF
2	16	290	9	Cure	Transient rise in SGOT/SGPT
3	18	360	7	Cure	None
4	18	430	8	Cure	None
5	18	330	6	Cure	None
6	18	250	8	Cure	None
7	18	220	6	Cure	Transient rise in SGPT
8	18	240	6	Cure	Frank hypokalemia
9	18	400	3	Cure	Raised serum creatinine
10	18	260	3	Persistence	Allergic skin rash
11	12	210	7	Cure	None
12	8	175	8	Persistence	None
13	18	280	8	Cure	None

[a] CCF, Congestive cardiac failure; SGOT, serum glutamic oxalacetic transaminase; SGPT, serum glutamic pyruvic transaminase.

thy that she achieved a cure despite this shortened duration of therapy.

Details of other side effects are stated concisely in Table 2. None of the patients, including those on concurrent immunosuppressives, experienced leukopenia. Patient 1 developed a mild exacerbation of prior congestive cardiac failure which responded to additional diuretics. Patients 2 and 7 experienced a transient increase in liver enzymes (serum glutamic pyruvic and oxalacetic transaminases) during therapy. Cumulating serum PIP levels (peak exceeding 250 mg/liter) were noted in Patients 3 and 11. A tendency toward clinically insignificant hypokalemia was commonplace, but in patient 8 serum potassium dropped to 2.5 mmol/liter. Mean pretreatment serum potassium of 4.05 mmol/liter fell to 3.51 after therapy ($P < 0.001$). Measurements of urine potassium excretion during therapy averaged 50 mmol/24 h. This inappropriate continuing potassium excretion at a time when serum potassium was decreasing suggests the possibility of urinary potassium wasting secondary to PIP. The mechanism may be similar to that seen with carbenicillin, which acts as a nonreabsorbable anion in the renal tubule (4). This hypokalemic effect was not more prominent in patients receiving corticosteroids. It is surprising, however, that this tendency was seen even in patients with moderately severe renal failure.

In conclusion, we believe that overall PIP was effective, safe, and well tolerated in the majority of these unusually complicated cases. Cure was achieved in 11 of 13 patients (84.6%) including several with significant renal function impairment. In two patients the drug was discontinued prematurely because of probable drug-related toxicity. The incidence of significant side effects in the other 11 was acceptably low. Further detailed observations of potassium balance during PIP therapy seem warranted.

1. **Eastwood, J. B., and J. R. Curtis.** 1968. Carbenicillin administration in patients with severe renal failure. Br. Med. J. **1**:486–487.
2. **Fu, K. P., and H. C. Neu.** 1978. Piperacillin, a new penicillin active against many bacteria resistant to other penicillins. Antimicrob. Agents Chemother. **13**:358–367.
3. **Giron, J. A., B. R. Meyers, S. Z. Hirschman, and E. Srulevitch.** 1981. Pharmacokinetics of piperacillin in patients with moderate renal failure and in patients undergoing hemodialysis. Antimicrob. Agents Chemother. **19**:279–283.
4. **Lipner, H. I., F. Ruzany, M. Dasgupta, P. D. Lief, and N. Bank.** 1975. The behaviour of carbenicillin as a nonreabsorbable anion. J. Lab. Clin. Med. **86**:183–194.
5. **Thompson, M. I. B., M. Russo, J. M. Matsen, and E. Atkin-Thor.** 1981. Piperacillin pharmacokinetics in subjects with chronic renal failure. Antimicrob. Agents Chemother. **19**:450–453.
6. **Winston, D. J., D. Wang, L. S. Young, W. J. Martin, and W. L. Hewitt.** 1978. In vitro studies of piperacillin, a new semisynthetic penicillin. Antimicrob. Agents Chemother. **13**:944–950.

Randomized, Comparative Evaluation of Piperacillin Versus Carbencillin-Gentamicin in Treating Serious Gram-Negative and Anaerobic Infections

RONICA M. KLUGE* AND R. BROOKS GAINER

West Virginia University Medical Center, Morgantown, West Virginia 26506, U.S.A.

Piperacillin sodium is an investigational semisynthetic penicillin which has in vitro activity against most gram-positive and gram-negative organisms, including anaerobes (2, 5, 6). Of particular importance is its activity against *Pseudomonas aeruginosa*, indole-positive *Proteus* species, and *Bacteroides fragilis*. Piperacillin has much greater inhibitory action than carbenicillin or ticarcillin against these organisms. Its pharmacokinetics are such that the inhibitory index of piperacillin for most organisms is much greater than that of carbenicillin or ticarcillin (1, 4). An open noncomparative evaluation of piperacillin done in our hospital (3) demonstrated its clinical safety and effectiveness in patients with serious gram-negative and anaerobic infections.

Therefore, we undertook a randomized, comparative evaluation of piperacillin versus the standard combination of carbenicillin and gentamicin in the therapy of hospitalized adult patients with serious infections caused by gram-negative and anaerobic organisms. Patients were eligible for the study if they had strong presumptive evidence of infection or documented bacteriological evidence of infection. Disease categories considered for inclusion were infections of the respiratory or genitourinary tract, bacteremia, bone and joint infections, skin and soft tissue infections, and deep abscesses. After informed consent was obtained, the patients were randomized to receive either piperacillin or a combination of carbenicillin and gentamicin.

Appropriate specimens for culture were obtained before the protocol antimicrobial therapy, as were basic hematology and chemistry studies and urinalysis. Direct and indirect Coombs tests were also performed. Laboratory tests were repeated at 4-day intervals during treatment and 2 to 3 days after treatment. Cultures were repeated during therapy as indicated and 2 to 3 days after treatment. Patients with urinary tract infections had additional cultures performed 8 to 10 days and 4 to 6 weeks post therapy. Standard isolation and identification procedures were employed by the hospital diagnostic microbiology laboratory. Routine antimicrobial susceptibility testing was performed by the Bauer-Kirby and standard MIC techniques.

Intravenous therapy was given in all instances. Patients randomized to piperacillin received 250 mg/kg per day in four to six divided doses. Those randomized to the standard combination received 450 mg of carbenicillin per kg per day in four to six divided doses *plus* 3 to 5 mg of gentamicin per kg per day in three to four divided doses. Patients were monitored closely for any evidence of allergic reactions and to assess local tolerance.

Thirty patients were entered into the study. Four were found subsequently to have sterile cultures and were not included in the analysis. There were 12 women and 14 men in the study group, ranging in age from 20 to 81 years (average, 50.7 years).

The sites of infection included: osteomyelitis, 8; cellulitis, 6; deep abscesses, 4; bacteremia, 2; genitourinary tract, 3; and one each, respiratory tract, joint, and myonecrosis.

A variety of organisms were isolated, and from 10 patients two or more organisms were recovered. There were eight *Pseudomonas aeruginosa* isolates, six of *Escherichia coli*, four each of *Serratia* species and *Enterobacter* species, three of *Klebsiella* species, two each of *Proteus mirabilis*, *Streptococcus faecalis*, and *Peptostreptococcus*, and one each of alpha-hemolytic streptococcus, *Hafnia*, *Eikenella corrodens*, *Clostridium perfringens*, *Bacteroides* species, and an unidentified anaerobic coccus.

All of the aerobic organisms were susceptible to piperacillin or to the combination of carbenicillin and gentamicin. MICs of piperacillin ranged from 1 to 32 μg/ml; those of carbenicillin, from 2 to 512 μg/ml; and those of gentamicin, from 0.3 to 10 μg/ml. For the three isolates of *Klebsiella*, one *Serratia* species, one *P. aeruginosa* isolate, and the *Hafnia* isolate, MICs of carbenicillin were high, but in each instance the MIC of gentamicin was well within therapeutic range. Anaerobes recovered in this study were not tested, but other investigators have reported that 78 to 95% of anaerobes are susceptible to clinically achievable concentrations of piperacillin (2, 6).

The duration of therapy for those patients receiving piperacillin was 4 to 38 days, with a mean of 18.5 days. Those patients receiving the combination of carbenicillin and gentamicin were treated for 6 to 45 days (mean, 18.6 days). The dose of piperacillin ranged from 9.8 to 25.2 g per day, that of carbenicillin ranged from 24 to 39 g per day, and that of gentamicin ranged from 180 to 370 mg per day.

Patients in each treatment group had excellent clinical and bacteriological responses. Eleven of 12 patients receiving piperacillin showed clinical cure, and there was clinical improvement in 1; in this group there were 10 bacteriological eradications and 2 patients with significant reduction in organisms. Patients receiving the combination of carbenicillin and gentamicin showed clinical cure in 10 of 14 and clinical improvement in the remaining 4; there were 13 bacteriological eradications in this group and 1 patient with a significant reduction in numbers of organisms.

Adverse reactions were noted in fewer of the patients receiving piperacillin than in those receiving the combination. Among piperacillin recipients, transient elevation of liver function tests were noted in one, increased eosinophils in two, one of whom also had a rash, and superinfection in two. Piperacillin therapy was discontinued on day 4 in the patient who developed rash and a 12% eosinophilia. Those patients receiving combination therapy with carbenicillin and gentamicin evidenced elevated liver function tests in six, increased eosinophils in three, and colonization with potential pathogens in three. Carbenicillin was discontinued in two patients because of marked elevations in liver function tests and clinical signs of hepatitis.

The two superinfections which occurred among the piperacillin recipients were due to *Staphylococcus*, one *S. epidermidis* and one *S. aureus*. These were treated satisfactorily with oxacillin. The potential pathogens which colonized patients treated with the carbenicillin-gentamicin combination included *E. coli*, *S. marcescens*, and *P. aeruginosa*. No local reactions or chemical thrombophlebitis were noted.

In summary, the 26 patients randomized to receive piperacillin or carbenicillin-gentamicin did well in terms of clinical and bacteriological responses. Side effects, however, were much more common in patients who received combination chemotherapy. Piperacillin given alone appears to be as efficacious as the combination of carbenicillin and gentamicin for treating serious infections caused by aerobic gram-negative organisms and anaerobic organisms, and it may produce fewer side effects.

1. **Evans, M. A. L., P. Wilson, P. Leung, and J. D. Williams.** 1978. Pharmacokinetics of piperacillin following intravenous administration. J. Antimicrob. Chemother. **4**:255–261.
2. **Fu, K. P., and H. C. Neu.** 1978. Piperacillin, a new penicillin active against many bacteria resistant to other penicillins. Antimicrob. Agents Chemother. **13**:358–367.
3. **Kluge, R. M., and R. B. Gainer.** 1980. Clinical effectiveness of piperacillin sodium in serious gram-negative and anaerobic infections, p. 290–291. *In* J. D. Nelson and C. Grassi (ed.), Current chemotherapy and infectious diseases. American Society for Microbiology, Washington, D.C.
4. **Meyers, B. R., S. Z. Hirschman, L. Strougo, and E. Srulevitch.** 1980. Comparative study of piperacillin, ticarcillin, and carbenicillin pharmacokinetics. Antimicrob. Agents Chemother. **17**:608–611.
5. **Shah, P. P., D. J. Briedis, H. G. Robson, and J. P. Conterato.** 1979. In vitro activity of piperacillin compared with that of carbenicillin, ticarcillin, ampicillin, cephalothin, and cefamandole against *Pseudomonas aeruginosa* and *Enterobacteriaceae*. Antimicrob. Agents Chemother. **15**:346–350.
6. **Winston, D. J., D. Wang, L. S. Young, W. J. Martin, and L. W. Hewitt.** 1978. In vitro studies of piperacillin, a new semisynthetic penicillin. Antimicrob. Agents Chemother. **13**:944–950.

Controlled Randomized Trial of Piperacillin Versus Gentamicin/Tobramycin plus Carbenicillin/Ticarcillin in Therapy of Serious Infections

MARIE J. GRIBBLE, CELIA V. McDONALD, WILLIAM R. BOWIE, STEPHEN L. SACKS, SHELLEY C. NAIMAN, LAWRENCE GROSSMAN, NOEL A. BUSKARD, JOHN A. SMITH, AND ANTHONY W. CHOW*

Divisions of Infectious Disease, Hematology, and Microbiology, Departments of Medicine and Pathology, University of British Columbia, and Vancouver General Hospital, Vancouver, British Columbia V5Z 1M9, Canada*

Piperacillin is a new semisynthetic piperazine penicillin derivative with a broad spectrum of activity against many gram-positive and -negative aerobic and anaerobic bacteria. Compared with carbenicillin and ticarcillin, it has superior activity against *Pseudomonas*, *Klebsiella*, *Enterobacter*, indole-positive *Proteus*, enterococcus, and *Bacteroides* species (1). Its activity against members of the *Enterobacteriaceae* family is comparable to that of gentamicin. At therapeutic doses, piperacillin has a lower sodium load than carbenicillin and may lead to less volume overload and hypokalemia (2). Piperacillin does not have the nephrotoxic or ototoxic potential associated with aminoglycosides. For these reasons, piperacillin may provide a single-drug alternative to combination aminoglycoside–β-lactam regimens, possibly resulting in equally effective and less toxic therapy.

This report presents the results of a prospective randomized study comparing efficacy and toxicity of piperacillin with that of gentamicin plus carbenicillin in therapy of serious infections.

Forty hospitalized adult patients with 50 separate episodes of infection known or suspected to be due to susceptible pathogens were randomized to receive either piperacillin or gentamicin plus carbenicillin. Piperacillin dosage was 250 mg/kg per day in six divided doses, except for urinary tract infection, for which the dose was 150 mg/kg per day. Carbenicillin dosage was 450 mg/kg per day in six divided doses (urinary tract infection, 200 mg/kg per day). Gentamicin dosage was 3 to 5 mg/kg per day in three divided doses; serum levels were monitored and doses were adjusted where necessary. At the discretion of the investigator, ticarcillin, 250 mg/kg per day, was substituted for carbenicillin, and tobramycin, 3 to 5 mg/kg per day, was substituted for gentamicin. Concomitant antistaphylococcal therapy was given if indicated.

Of the 50 episodes, 46 episodes in 37 patients were considered evaluable for efficacy. Four episodes were excluded because therapy was given for less than 3 days (three patients) or because infection was proved to be fungal (one patient with *Candida* urinary tract infection). Twenty-three episodes were treated with piperacillin and 23 received combination therapy. There were no significant differences in the demographic characteristics of the two groups (Table 1).

Rapidly fatal underlying disease (McCabe-

Jackson classification) (3) was present in 10 of the piperacillin group and 17 of the combination group. All of these were neutropenic. Infections were clinically and bacteriologically proved in 19 episodes in the piperacillin group and 15 in the combination group. Clinical proof alone was present in 4 episodes in the combination group. Febrile neutropenia with presumed infection but no bacteriological proof of infection occurred in 4 episodes treated with piperacillin and 4 treated with combination therapy. These were included in the analysis for efficacy.

Two episodes in each group were bacteremic prior to initiation of therapy. In addition, three patients in the combination group developed bacteremia during therapy, and two patients in the combination group were bacteremic 24 h after completion of therapy. Of these 5 bacteremias, three were "breakthrough bacteremias" with the original causative organism, one was a transient asymptomatic bacteremia requiring no further therapy, and one represented treatment failure and resulted in infection-related death.

Pseudomonas aeruginosa was isolated in 8 piperacillin (35%) and 9 combination (39%) episodes. Infection was polymicrobial in 11 piperacillin (48%) and 8 combination (35%) episodes. Aerobic gram-positive cocci including enterococci were present in most of these polymicrobial infections (Table 1).

The clinical response to therapy (Table 2) was judged to be cure or improvement in 17 episodes in each group and failure in 6 episodes in each group. Death due to infection occurred in two patients treated with piperacillin and three in the combination group. Both infection-related deaths in the piperacillin group and one of three in the combination group had rapidly fatal underlying diseases. Bacteriological response was comparable in the two groups. However, it is noted that breakthrough bacteremia occurred three times in the combination group but in none in the piperacillin group.

Emergence of resistant isolates was noted in the piperacillin group seven times, and in the carbenicillin group three times. This phenomenon was associated with two of the six clinical failures (including one infection-related death) in each group, with three of seven bacteriological failures in the piperacillin group, and three of five bacteriological failures in the combination group. Organisms which acquired resistance associated with clinical failure were *P. aeruginosa*, *Enterobacter cloacae*, *Escherichia coli*, and *Klebsiella pneumoniae*.

Hypokalemia judged probably or definitely related to therapy was seen in 4 episodes in the piperacillin group and 11 episodes in the combination group ($P < 0.05$). The serum potassium fell by ≥1.0 mg/100 ml during therapy in 1 patient receiving piperacillin versus 9 patients receiving combination therapy ($P < 0.005$).

Nephrotoxicity due to antimicrobial therapy was seen in two episodes treated with combination therapy. In the piperacillin group, one case of mild interstitial nephritis occurred. Eosinophilia in two patients in the piperacillin group,

TABLE 1. *Demographic characteristics of episodes evaluated for efficacy*[a]

Characteristic	Piperacillin	Combination
No. of episodes	23	23
Mean age and range (yr)	49 (16–75)	46 (16–80)
Sex (M:F)	15:8	14:9
Underlying disease:		
Rapidly fatal	10	17
Ultimately fatal	3	2
Nonfatal	10	4
Failed previous therapy	7	5
Concomitant antistaphylococcal therapy	7	5
Bacteriologically proven infection	19	15
Anatomic site:		
Skin and soft tissue	5 (1)	10 (1)
Pneumonia	3	4 (1)
Oropharyngeal	4 (1)	1 (1)
Urinary tract	4	1 (1)
Intraabdominal	1	3 (3)
Bone	2	0
Bacteremia pretherapy	2	2
Bacteremia during/after therapy	0	5
Organism:		
Pseudomonas	8	9 (2)
Klebsiella	3	1 (1)
E. coli	2 (1)	2 (1)
Other gram-negative aerobic rods	4	9
Aerobic gram-positive cocci	14 (1)	13 (3)
Bacteroides	2	4 (1)
Peptococcaceae	2	2
Other	2	5 (1)
Polymicrobial infection	11	8

[a] Numbers in parentheses indicate bacteremias.

TABLE 2. *Outcome of therapy in 23 episodes treated with piperacillin and 23 treated with a drug combination*

Regimen	Clinical			Bacteriological		
	Cure or improved	Failure	Died[a]	Cure	Failure	Indeterminate
Piperacillin	17	6	2	10	7	6
Combination	17	6	3	8	5	10

[a] Related to infection.

diarrhea in two patients in each treatment group, and hemolytic anemia and hepatitis each in one patient with combination therapy were also encountered.

We conclude that in this group of patients with serious infections piperacillin was as effective as conventional combination therapy. Piperacillin was associated with significantly less (and less severe) hypokalemia. Piperacillin may provide a single-drug alternative to combination carbenicillin plus gentamicin therapy of serious infections. Emergence of resistant isolates during therapy with either regimen should be carefully monitored.

1. **Bodey, G. P., and B. LeBlanc.** 1978. Piperacillin: in vitro evaluation. Antimicrob. Agents Chemother. **14**:78–87.
2. **Lederle Laboratories.** 1977. Clinical investigator's brochure. Lederle Laboratories, American Cyanamid Co., Pearl River, N.Y.
3. **McCabe, W. R., and G. G. Jackson.** 1962. Gram-negative bacteremia. I. Etiology and ecology. Arch. Intern. Med. **110**:847–855.

Piperacillin or Cefotaxime plus Amikacin: Result of Empirical Antibiotic Therapy for Febrile Episodes in Granulocytopenic Patients

P. DUPREZ AND J. L. MICHAUX*

UCL Hospital, Brussels, Belgium

Most infections occurring in patients suffering from hematological malignancy are caused by gram-negative organisms, especially *Escherichia coli, Klebsiella* spp., and *Pseudomonas*. Piperacillin and cefotaxime represent advances among the new antibiotics because of enhanced activity against such organisms and potential synergy when used in combination with aminoglycosides. Because of this greater activity, especially against gram-negative organisms resistant to carbenicillin, and lower incidence of side effects, we opted to perform a controlled comparison of each drug in combination with amikacin in immunologically suppressed patients.

Piperacillin has greater activity against *Pseudomonas*, and cefotaxime has pronounced activity against *Klebsiella* and is β-lactamase stable. Amikacin has been shown to have a lesser incidence of microbial resistance than other aminoglycosides.

One hundred six patients, including 24 children, were admitted to the study. Age and sex were comparable in the two groups. Most had leukemia with neutropenia and were treated with cytostatic drugs. Infection diagnoses included septicemia and chest, soft tissue, and urinary infections. Microorganisms isolated consisted of various gram-negative species and several *Staphylococcus* spp. Microbiological monitoring by the Kirby-Bauer disk method was performed prior to treatment and thereafter once weekly. The average daily dose of piperacillin or cefotaxime was 170 mg/kg per day, usually given as 4 g every 8 h, with amikacin, 70 mg/kg per day. Drugs were administered intravenously as a 30-min infusion three times a day diluted in normal saline.

Patients were carefully examined for clinical and biological responses, being considered cured when they became afebrile and when signs of infection had disappeared. Tables 1 and 2 summarize the clinical and microbiological results.

Piperacillin plus amikacin (P+A) achieved 76% favorable responses, and cefotaxime plus amikacin (C+A) had 78% favorable responses in proved infections. The true failures consisted of those patients whose infections failed to respond rapidly, who relapsed, or in whom superinfection occurred, even if caused by a resistant organism.

In the P+A group, a resistant *Escherichia coli* septicemia developed, complicating abdominal sepsis, a staphylococcal pneumonia occurred in a patient treated successfully for septicemia, and a staphylococcal septicemia forced a change

TABLE 1. *Clinical data on patients in the P + A group*

Infection	No. of patients	Cured/improved	Relapse/failure
Septicemia	14	9	5
Pneumonia	7	6	1
Soft tissue infection	9	8	1
Urinary tract infection	4	3	1
Bacterial causes	34	26 (76%)	8 (24%)
Fever of unknown origin	23	16 (69%)	7 (31%)
Total response	57	42 (74%)	15 (26%)

TABLE 2. *Clinical data on patients in the C + A group*

Infection	No. of patients	Cured/improved	Relapse/failure
Septicemia	20	15	5
Pneumonia	6	4	2
Soft tissue infection	6	5	1
Urinary tract infection	5	5	—
Bacterial causes	37	29 (78%)	8 (22%)
Fever of unknown origin	24	15 (62%)	9 (38%)
Total response	61	44 (72%)	17 (28%)

of regimen. Similarly, in the C+A group, a *Klebsiella* infection developed while on treatment, and one pneumonia and two additional septicemias failed to respond.

The overall rate of therapeutic success in febrile episodes with negative microbiological culture was judged on a clinical basis and was similar for each antibiotic regimen.

The bacteriological data show that in the P+A group 77% of the microorganisms were eradicated. Organisms persisted or reappeared in six patients, and four could not be evaluated for lack of follow-up. In the C+A group 43 organisms were considered to be responsible for infection. Eradication was achieved in 35; organisms persisted in only 2 instances, and 6 could not be assessed. Of the microorganisms isolated, 65% were gram-negative in type, and susceptibility testing showed that 87% were susceptible to piperacillin, 90% to cefotaxime, and 93% to amikacin.

Local adverse reactions were few, and there was a small incidence of phlebitis (only two occurring in each group). We attributed this to the use of central venous catheters via subclavian vein entry in preference to prolonged infusion in small veins. We also observed systemic adverse reactions. Five skin rashes occurred in the P+A group, three of them being possibly drug related; in the C+A group seven rashes occurred, four of which could be drug related. Pseudomembranous colitis occurred in two instances, one as a result of ampicillin therapy, and P+A followed by C+A failed to influence the condition. The second case occurred in a C+A patient. Both patients responded to oral vancomycin. *Clostridium difficile* and toxin were identified in both cases.

Most patients had abnormal laboratory values as a result of underlying disease. In each group, 15 patients had moderate elevation of transaminases that may have been drug related. Such elevation was not considered clinically important. Four patients were shown to have slight deterioration of renal function. Association with a drug was not established.

In summary, both combinations have cured a variety of infections occurring in severely compromised patients, including several young children. Neither combination was associated with untoward toxicity.

Piperacillin Alone or in Combination in the Treatment of Intraabdominal Sepsis

H. FREDLUND,* J. BARR, O. GUSTAVSSON, AND J. KJELLANDER

Departments of Infectious Diseases and Bacteriology, Central County Hospital, Örebro, Sweden*

The treatment of intraabdominal infection is frequently complicated by the presence of mixed gram-negative aerobic and anaerobic organisms, and few antibiotics have a broad enough spectrum to cope singly. The presence of *Staphylococcus aureus*, often β-lactamase producing, may be a further complication. Clindamycin has been used because of its activity against anaerobic organisms and more recently metronidazole, but neither of these is active against gram-negative aerobic organisms, and aminoglycosides are often added in view of increasing resistance to ampicillin. Piperacillin is a new semisynthetic penicillin with proven in vitro activity against both types of organisms, although not against β-lactamase-producing staphylococci. We have studied the effect of piperacillin in intraabdominal sepsis and some other severe infections, combining it when necessary with a suitable anti-staphylococcal antibiotic.

Twenty-seven patients (15 male, 12 female) aged 23 to 93 years (mean, 62.1) were included in an open study of parenteral piperacillin therapy. Most were suffering from intraabdominal infection, pre- or postoperative, and several had infections of other sites. The majority had, in addition, concomitant diseases of various organs including malignant disease, peptic ulceration, and diabetes mellitus, and some required other medication as well. Twenty of 27 patients had had previous unsuccessful antibiotic therapy, alone or in combination, for this infection without improvement, or prophylactically. New or resistant strains had emerged during the previous treatment in several patients.

Before treatment, cultures were taken from available sources for both aerobic and anaerobic organisms and these were repeated at intervals throughout treatment and for follow-up after treatment in all patients. Blood and urine samples were also taken before, during, and after treatment to monitor drug safety, and a close watch was kept for signs of adverse reaction as well as clinical improvement.

Piperacillin was administered by short intravenous infusion in a dose of 3 to 7 g every 8 h. Clindamycin was given in combination initially and later this drug was changed to cloxacillin so as to cover possible staphylococcal infection and not to obscure the assessment of piperacillin. The mean daily dose of piperacillin was 203 mg/kg, of clindamycin, 31 mg/kg (9 patients), and of cloxacillin, 100 mg/kg (14). Concomitant antibiotics were also given by short intravenous infusion.

Fifty-five microorganisms judged to be pathogenic were cultured initially in 22 out of 27 patients. Other strains were cultured during therapy, and these, added to the initial cultures, gave a total of 99 strains (Table 1), of which 69 were wholly susceptible to piperacillin (MIC ≤16 μg/ml) and 12 were intermediate in susceptibility. Of the remaining 18 strains resistant to piperacillin, 14 were β-lactamase-producing staphylococci. Eighteen anaerobic strains were cultured, and 17 of these were wholly susceptible to piperacillin.

Infections diagnosed numbered 35 occurring in 27 patients. There were 20 episodes of intraabdominal sepsis, pre- or postoperative, and 10 had septicemia. Urinary tract infection occurred twice; pneumonia, osteitis due to crush injury, and septic arthritis occurred once each. Seven infections could not be evaluated clinically, and 10 could not be evaluated microbiologically (Table 2). Of these, three patients died of severe surgical complications, whereas three had obvious clinical infection but negative cultures. One patient developed an allergic response immediately after the first dose. Drug fever, probably related to piperacillin, was observed in two patients, one with eosinophilia and one with elevated transaminases. Allergic rashes were seen in four patients on combination therapy, one probably caused by previous therapy but all leading to discontinuation of therapy. Mild insignificant diarrhea was seen in four patients, one occurred during previous therapy, but therapy was not discontinued in these patients. In all, therapy was discontinued due to adverse reactions in six patients. Biochemical changes were not clinically significant, and local venous tolerance was excellent.

Ampicillin, gentamicin, clindamycin, metronidazole, cephaloridine, cefazolin, and, more re-

TABLE 1. *Susceptibilities of isolates to piperacillin*

Isolated pathogen	MIC: Susceptible (≤16 μg/ml)	MIC: Intermediate	MIC: Resistant >128 μg/ml
Aerobes			
Gram-positive			
Streptococcus spp.	4	0	0
Enterococci	12	0	1
Staphylococcus (β-lactamase producing)	0	0	14
Gram-negative			
E. coli	17	3	0
Klebsiella	5	0	1
Enterobacter	0	2	2
Citrobacter	2	4	0
Proteus mirabilis	4	0	0
Proteus morganii	0	1	0
Proteus vulgaris	2	1	0
P. aeruginosa	5	0	0
Aeromonas hydrophila	1	0	0
Anaerobes			
Bacteroides fragilis	10	1	0
Bacteroides spp.	5	0	0
Gram-positive rods	2	0	0

TABLE 2. *Clinical and microbiological responses by infection*

Infection	Clinical response[a] C/I	Clinical response[a] R/F	Microbiological response[b] E/MR	Microbiological response[b] P
Intraabdominal	10 (71%)	4 (29%)	9 (75%)	3 (25%)
Septicemia	9 (100%)	0	8 (100%)	0
Other	5 (100%)	0	4 (80%)	1 (20%)
Overall	24 (86%)	4 (14%)	21 (84%)	4 (16%)

[a] C/I, Cure/improvement; R/F, relapse/failure.

[b] E/MR, Eradication/marked reduction; P, persistence.

cently, cefoxitin have all been tried alone and in various combinations in the treatment of intraabdominal sepsis (3, 4). The fact that the combinations of treatment appear to differ from center to center suggest that no clear definitive therapy has yet emerged for this condition. Indeed, all the antibiotics mentioned have gaps in their antibacterial spectra that make recommendations difficult and some have, in addition, problems of toxicity. Pinto and Sanderson (3) compared ampicillin and metronidazole in the treatment of patients with perforated or gangrenous appendicitis and concluded that while metronidazole helped, another antibiotic was necessary to manage such patients.

Similarly Willis (4) has shown that metronidazole cuts the incidence of anaerobic postoperative adbominal infections dramatically. The microbiological population in our seriously ill patients yielded on initial culture 22% anaerobes and 55% gram-negative aerobic pathogens, including *Escherichi coli* and *Pseudomonas aeruginosa*. Enterococci were also cultured in seven patients. Piperacillin has been shown to have a broad in vitro spectrum (1, 5), covering *E. coli*, *Klebsiella*, *Pseudomonas*, enterococci, and *B. fragilis*, the organisms that form the expected polymicrobial population of intraabdominal infections (2). Our results in patients with severe abdominal sepsis, including several cases with failure on other antibiotic therapy, show that piperacillin has contributed substantially to their management. The drug has been safe and well tolerated. Cloxacillin has been added safely and effectively in deference to possible staphylococcal infection. We conclude that piperacillin, particularly because of its lower toxicity, may have advantages over existing treatment for intraabdominal infection and, thus, a role as part of recommended therapy for the condition.

1. **Monif, G. R. G., P. R. Clark, J. J. Schuster, and H. Baer.** 1978. Susceptibility of the anaerobic bacteria, group D streptococci, *Enterobacteriaceae*, and *Pseudomonas* to semisynthetic penicillins: carbenicillin, piperacillin, and ticarcillin. Antimicrob. Agents Chemother. **14**:643–649.
2. **Pieper, R., L. Kaeger, A. A. Lindberg, and C. E. Nord.** 1979. Acute appendicitis and *B. fragilis*. Scand. J. Infect. Dis. **19** (Suppl.):92–97.
3. **Pinto, D. J., and P. J. Sanderson.** 1980. Rational use of antibiotic therapy after appendicectomy. Br. Med. J. **280**:275–277.
4. **Willis, A. T.** 1979. Metronidazole in the prevention and treatment of anaerobic sepsis. Scand. J. Infect. Dis. **19** (Suppl.):98–104.
5. **Winston, D. J., D. Wang, L. S. Young, W. J. Martin, and W. L. Hewitt.** 1978. In vitro studies of piperacillin, a new semisynthetic penicillin. Antimicrob. Agents Chemother. **13**:944–960.

Clinical Experience with Piperacillin in Combination Therapy in Surgical Intensive Care Medicine

E. THIES,* W. SCHWARZ, AND H. FREIESLEBEN

Departments of Surgery and Medical Microbiology, School of Medicine, Luebeck, Federal Republic of Germany*

Patients admitted to surgical intensive care units are frequently suffering from severe infections (e.g., peritonitis and cholangitis), or are highly prone to hospital infections as a consequence of invasive therapeutic measures (e.g., respiratory assistance) and impaired immunological responsiveness due to severe underlying disease. Besides methods of hygiene, antibiotic therapy is still the mainstay in intensive care units for controlling infection. Because of the high frequency of mixed and severe infections caused by hospital-acquired organisms, the introduction of the newer broad-spectrum antibiotics is of great interest. Another indication for antibiotic treatment in surgical intensive care is perioperative prophylaxis in the prevention of postoperative infection. Opinions vary substantially in this area.

Over a period of 6 months we treated 48 patients admitted to the surgical intensive care unit (of the School of Medicine, Luebeck) with the recently developed semisynthetic, broad-spectrum penicillin derivative piperacillin. Thirty-eight patients were suffering from severe infections, and 10 patients received piperacillin as prophylactic treatment. In 47 patients, piperacillin was given in combination with other antibiotics.

Most frequently, piperacillin was combined with the newer cephalosporins, or with aminoglycosides: in the first case, to expand the antimicrobial spectrum and in the second case to make use of the known synergistic potency. In all cases piperacillin was administered as short-time intravenous infusion through a central venous catheter. The daily dose was 12 g given in three single injections, both as treatment and as prophylaxis. The average duration of treatment was 10 days. In the case of impaired renal function, the daily dose was reduced according to the serum creatinine values. Of the 48 patients treated, 58% underwent abdominal surgery, 21% vascular surgery, and 2% each thoracic and urological surgery. Sixteen percent were suffering from multiple injuries.

The mean age of the 38 patients treated for severe infections was 57.6 years (range, 11 to 96 years). In 81.6% the infection was associated with previous surgery. All patients had indwelling urinary catheters as well as central venous catheters. Forty-six percent of patients required respiratory assistance. Underlying conditions in these patients are shown in Table 1, which shows that patients with abdominal surgery infections are most often concerned with postoperative infectious problems.

TABLE 1. *Diagnoses of piperacillin-treated patients in the surgical intensive care unit of the School of Medicine, Luebeck*

Diagnosis	No.
Diffuse purulent peritonitis	6
Circumscribed peritonitis/intraabdominal abscess	11
Carcinoma of stomach/gallbladder/rectum	3
Hemorrhagic pancreatitis	2
Esophageal variceal bleeding	1
Sacculated kidney, urosepsis	2
Occlusion of iliac artery/stenosis of renal arterial/mesenteric infarction	4
Necrosis of amputation-stump	1
Thigh bone fracture	1
Multiple injury	7
Lung collapse	1

To summarize the data, 43% of patients suffered from severe pulmonary infections with hospital-acquired pathogens, and 43% of patients showed diffuse or local peritonitis. The mortality rate of 53% in patients with pneumonia and only 27% in patients with other infections confirms the clinical experience that secondary pneumonia in patients admitted to intensive care has a bad prognosis. In 84% of our patients organisms could be cultured; these are presented in Table 2 correlated to the samples.

Because of the high frequency of abdominal operations, most cultures were taken from drainage material and wounds. According to the high frequency of artificial ventilation, 18 patients had positive tracheal swabs. Sixty-eight percent of patients suffered from infections of mixed etiology. In 19 patients septicemia occurred during the course of the infection as judged by clinical criteria. Eight patients had positive blood cultures. Approximately 74% of all organisms cultured were susceptible to piperacillin.

A separate evaluation was done for all strains isolated from blood cultures during a 10-month period. The organisms recovered were gram-negative (93), gram-positive (40), and anaerobes (10). The number of strains susceptible to piperacillin was 78, 21, and 8, respectively. Twenty-one of 38 patients survived; 17 patients died, and in 13 of these infection still played a major role. Eight patients of these 13 died of severe hospital-acquired pulmonary infection after long-term artificial ventilation. One patient died because of severe mediastinitis and pneumonia after insufficiency of a esophagojejunostomy. Four patients died of abdominal diseases despite surgical and antibiotic therapy as a consequence of severe infections which had already induced organ failure in the moment of operation. Diagnoses were: hepatic abscess following cholangitis and

TABLE 2. *Organisms acquired from different swabs in 38 patients in the surgical intensive care unit, Luebeck*

Isolate	Culture site						
	Urine	Blood	Trachea	Drainage	Wound	Catheter	Fluid
Streptococcus	6	1	9	6	7	1	1
E. coli	5	2	3	5	1		
Proteus	1		4	2	2		
Staphylococcus epidermidis		4	1	1	1	3	1
S. aureus			1	1	2		
Enterobacter		1	5			2	
Klebsiella			2	3	2		
Pseudomonas			5		1		1
Bacteroides spp.				6	2		
Acinetobacter				1			
Clostridium					1		
Serratia					1		

necrotizing cholecystitis, perforation of rectum, and pancreatitis with gangrene of colon. This may show the severity of underlying diseases and explain the problems of surgical and antibiotic therapy.

Nevertheless 13 of 17 cases with peritonitis, 8 of 17 cases with bronchopulmonary infection, and 7 of 19 cases with clinical signs of sepsis were cured. In five of seven surviving septic patients, surgery contributed to clinical cure and only one patient died subsequently. In the other 14 patients, surgery was not necessary or could not be or was not performed because of various reasons. In this group only three patients survived.

Side effects were observed in only two patients. These were mild allergic reactions which led to discontinuation of the medication. One patient showed signs of allergic illness on day 21 of treatment, and the second showed systemic allergic reaction shortly after the first dose. This patient had a history of penicillin allergy which was not known at the time of administration.

Ten patients received piperacillin as perioperative prophylaxis. The mean age of these patients was 59.3 years. Five patients underwent abdominal surgery and five patients vascular surgery. In none of these patients could pathogens be isolated before operation. In all patients piperacillin was combined with cefuroxime, and, in addition, in two patients undergoing abdominal surgery, metronidazole was added. Daily dose was 12 g/day given as short-time intravenous infusions. During the postoperative period no patient suffered from clinical infection. Wound healing was by primary intention. No side effects were observed in this group. We conclude that piperacillin has given good results in our cases with severe infection as well as where prophylaxis was desired. As expected, those infections where adjuvant surgery was successful also had the best prognosis.

The clinical outcome of patients suffering from nosocomial infections depends mainly on the underlying conditions and the ability to respond immunologically. In this situation antibiotic treatment can only be supportive so as to improve the prognosis for these severely ill patients. Prophylactic administration of antibiotics can decrease the rate of postoperative wound infections in certain indications. A prophylactic prevention of pulmonary infection with antibiotics does not seem possible. In our field we have seen the advantage of piperacillin in its broad spectrum, so necessary for the treatment of potentially fatal infections, mixed infections, and wound infections with high incidence of *Pseudomonas*. This is especially so when beginning treatment, which has to be presumptive. Piperacillin is also suitable for prophylaxis in the perioperative period.

Treatment of Severe Neonatal Infections with Piperacillin with or without Gentamicin

J. A. A. HOOGKAMP-KORSTANJE

Laboratory for Public Health, 8917 EN Leeuwarden, The Netherlands

Gram-negative bacteria and group B streptococci are the major causative organisms in severe neonatal infections including septicemia and meningitis. The mortality is high (50 to 90%) in those infections, and the choice of antibiotics is limited because of the toxicity of some drugs in the newborn and the increasing resistance of the infecting agents, especially gram-negative organisms, to currently available antibacterial drugs. Usually, broad-spectrum bactericidal antibiotics, often in combination, are used, and the therapy of first choice in acute severe neonatal infections of unknown etiology is the combination of a penicillin and an aminoglycoside. Many data are available about combinations of the older penicillins and aminoglycosides in newborns, but there is little or no information about the efficacy of piperacillin with or without aminoglycosides in neonatal infections. As piperacillin has been found to be very active in vitro against gram-negative organisms, especially *Pseudomonas aeruginosa*, and appears to be highly synergistic with gentamicin, it was desirable to test this therapy in our patients.

We have studied a number of neonates treated with piperacillin with or without gentamicin to ascertain the effectiveness, safety, and pharmacokinetics of this drug. Twelve neonates, all hospitalized because of clinical signs of severe, life-threatening infections, were included in the study. Seven babies were premature, five were females and seven males. Their age ranged from

TABLE 1. *Sites of infection, bacteriology, previous therapy, and response to therapy with piperacillin (P) with or without gentamicin (G) in 12 neonates*

Patient	Infection	Bacteriology	Previous therapy	Therapy	Response
1	Meningitis	*P. aeruginosa*	Penicillin + gentamicin	P + G	Cured
	Septicemia	*P. aeruginosa*			Cured
2	Meningitis	*E. coli*	Chloramphenicol	P + G	Cured
	Septicemia	*E. coli/S. aureus*			Cured
	Urinary tract	*E. coli*			Cured
	Soft tissue	*E. coli*			Cured
3	Meningitis	*E. coli*	Chloramphenicol	P + G	Cured
	Septicemia	*E. coli*			Cured
	Urinary tract	*E. coli*			Cured
	Soft tissue	*S. aureus*			Cured
4	Septicemia	—[a]	Cephalothin + gentamicin	P + G	Cured
	Pneumonia	*P. aeruginosa*			Improved[b]
5	Septicemia	—	Penicillin	P + G	Cured
6	Septicemia	*S. epidermidis*	Penicillin + kanamycin	P + G	Cured
7	Pneumonia	—		P	Cured
8	Septicemia	—		P	Cured
	Pneumonia	—			Cured
9	Pneumonia	—	Penicillin + cloxacillin	P + G	Relapse
	Soft tissue	—			Cured
10	Pneumonia	*P. aeruginosa*	Penicillin + kanamycin	P + G	Improved[b]
11	Septicemia	—		P	Cured
12	Pneumonia	—		P	Cured
	Soft tissue	—			Cured

[a] —, Negative culture.
[b] Persistence of *P. aeruginosa* in bronchial aspirate, despite clinical and radiological improvement.

1 to 24 days, their weight from 1.2 to 3.1 kg. A total of 23 infections were diagnosed (Table 1). Of the 12 infants, 6 had bacteriologically proven infections, including septicemia in 4, meningitis in 3, and pneumonia, urinary tract infection, and soft tissue infections in 2 infants. Four infants had clinical, radiologically defined pneumonia, four had clinical septicemia with negative blood cultures, and two had soft tissue infections with negative cultures. Eight infants had had previous antibiotic therapy for their infections, including penicillin, cephalothin, chloramphenicol, kanamycin, and gentamicin, without response: *P. aeruginosa* and *Escherichia coli* were mainly the organisms in the bacteriologically proven infections. The MIC and MBC of piperacillin and gentamicin determined for these organisms were well within the therapeutic range.

Eight infants were treated with piperacillin and gentamicin, four infants (three with pneumonia and one with clinical septicemia) with piperacillin alone. Piperacillin was given in intravenous doses of 100 to 150 mg/kg per day every 12 h in 10 infants. Two infants with meningitis (patient 2 and 3) received 250 to 300 mg/kg per day. Gentamicin was given in intramuscular doses of 2.5–5 mg/kg per day every 12 h.

The infants were monitored with various laboratory tests before, during, and after treatment; clinical examination was carried out several times a day. Serum samples were taken at regular intervals to study the kinetics of piperacillin in neonates. Figure 1 shows the mean levels in serum corrected to a standard dose of 100 mg

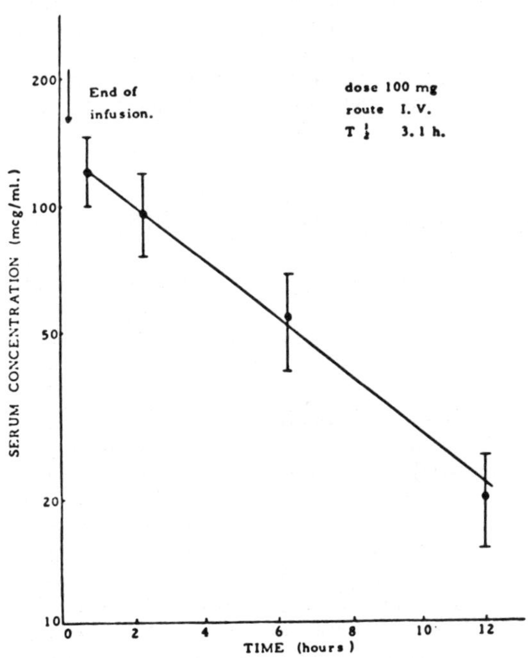

FIG. 1. *Mean serum levels ± SE for neonates after intravenous injection of 100 mg of piperacillin.*

intravenously. The peak levels ranged from 100 to 150 μg/ml, with an average of 122 μg/ml, occurring 0.5 h after the end of infusion. After 2 h the mean level was 98 μg/ml, after 6 h 54 μg/ml, and the trough level was 10 to 25 μg/ml. These levels were well above the MICs of the infecting organisms during the whole period between two dosages. Half-life time approximated 3.1 h, ranging from 3.7 h in the premature to 2.28 h in the full-term infants. From the serial trough levels obtained, no significant accumulation was seen.

Meningitis, septicemia, soft tissue infections, and urinary tract infections were treated successfully with cure and eradication of pathogens. Pneumonia was also cured in three babies. In two babies, both treated with piperacillin and gentamicin, the chest X rays and the clinical signs of pneumonia improved, but *P. aeruginosa* persisted in the bronchial aspirate. In one baby, also treated with the combination, a relapse was observed after initial improvement (Table 1).

Of special interest were the three infants with meningitis and septicemia, caused by *E. coli* in two cases and by *P. aeruginosa* in one case. They all responded well and quickly to systemic therapy of piperacillin and gentamicin. In two patients cerebrospinal fluid levels and serum levels could be determined at the same time. The patient with meningitis due to *P. aeruginosa* (MIC for piperacillin = 3.1 μg/ml) was treated with 150 mg/kg per day for 6 days and with 300 mg/kg per day the following 19 days. On day 5 of therapy the piperacillin levels in the cerebrospinal fluid and in the serum determined 1 h after the dosage were 20.5 μg/ml and 120 μg/ml, respectively. Patient 3 had meningitis caused by *E. coli* and was treated with 280 mg/kg per day. The MIC for piperacillin was 0.8 μg/ml. The cerebrospinal fluid level and serum level determined 5 h after the dosage, on day 6 of treatment, were 7.0 μg/ml and 50 μg/ml, respectively. So the cerebrospinal fluid levels were about 15% of the serum levels and exceeded many times the MICs of the microorganisms. There was no need for intrathecal or intraventricular administration of the drug. After 6 days of treatment the cerebrospinal fluid was sterile (in one patient after 2 days) and the neutrophil count in the fluid dropped from about 4,000/mm^3 to normal values.

Piperacillin was well tolerated in all patients. No adverse reactions or drug-related changes in hematological and biochemical analyses of blood and urine were noted. An additional advantage was to be able to give the drug in a small volume of diluent with low sodium loading.

In conclusion, piperacillin is a safe drug in neonates, effective in gram-negative infections, with adequate blood levels and adequate cerebrospinal fluid levels. The combination with gentamicin is very effective in severe neonatal infections and may be advised as therapy of first choice in neonatal infections of unknown origin.

Pharmacokinetics of Flucloxacillin in the Presence of Piperacillin

D. ADAM, A. NEISS,* AND U. KISSLINGER

Childrens Hospital of the University, Munich, West Germany

In various circumstances it is desirable to combine antibiotics either to enhance activity or to broaden the spectrum. Piperacillin is a penicillin with a broad antimicrobial spectrum encompassing gram-negative and gram-positive organisms. The drug is sensitive to hydrolysis by staphylococcal penicillinase, and is ineffective in treatment of infections caused by these organisms. For the treatment of mixed-bacterial infections where *Staphylococcus aureus* cannot be excluded, it is advisable to combine piperacillin with a penicillinase-stable isoxazolyl derivative, such as flucloxacillin.

In our investigations we determined serum concentration and urinary recovery as well as pharmacokinetic parameters after intravenous injection of either 2 g of piperacillin or 1 g of flucloxacillin and after simultaneous administration of both substances in 12 volunteers. These 12 volunteers were given either 2 g of piperacillin or 1 g of flucloxacillin after randomization and then in combination, both substances as intravenous bolus injections.

Blood samples were taken before administration of the medications and 5, 10, 20, 40, 90, 120, 240, and 360 min after administration. Urine was collected in 2-h samples over a period of 8 h. Determination of serum and urine concentration was performed using the agar well method. The test organism for piperacillin was *Escherichia coli* no. 6311/65, which is flucloxacillin resistant. For determination of flucloxacillin concentrations, *Sarcina lutea* ATCC 9341 was used. The piperacillin portion in the combination investigation was inactivated by adding penicillinase. The semilog plot of serum concentration allows the data to be calculated, using either one- or two-compartment models. The Wilcoxon signed rank test for matched pairs was used, which is applicable also when the samples are not normally distributed.

When flucloxacillin is administered simultaneously, it is obvious that there is a competitive inhibition by piperacillin of tubular transport. Piperacillin has a higher total renal clearance (TRC), the TRC for 2 g of piperacillin being 143.96 ml/min and the TRC for 1 g of flucloxallin being 85.54 ml/min. For this reason the serum concentrations of flucloxacillin in the combination are significantly higher beyond 90 min (Table 1). There is a corresponding increase in the area under the curve for flucloxacillin in both models, the values being 12.014 μg.min/ml (12.030 μg.min/ml in two-compartment model) and 13.816 μg.min/ml (13.699 μg.min/ml). The decreased elimination results in an increase in plasma half-lives of 13 and 11 min, respectively.

In accordance with the significant decrease of elimination constant K_2 and β (K_2 of -0.0230 to -0.0160, β of -0.0191 to -0.0146 min^{-1}), the initial concentration (C_o) is lower in both models. There is a reciprocal increase in the distribution volume (V_p). In both models TRC was decreased, the values being 85.54 ml/min (85.27 ml/min for two-compartment model) and 74.62 ml/min (175.51 ml/min for two-compartment model), respectively.

During an 8-h period the urinary excretion of flucloxacillin following combined administration decreased by 24%. This is mainly due to reduced recovery of administered drug in the first 2-h period, whereas in the later periods, more flucloxacillin is excreted per period. Calculation of accumulated drug excretion shows a significantly higher amount in M_o for plasma half-life and a higher initial urinary excretion when compared with the excretion of 1 g of flucloxacillin administered alone. Average plasma clearance, CL_8, is significantly lower for flucloxacillin in combination, the values being 61.6 ml/min in combination and 35.6 ml/min alone. When administered simultaneously, flucloxacillin did not inhibit the excretion of piperacillin, but, on the contrary, led to an increased excretion of piperacillin. This led to lower serum concentrations of piperacillin beyond 40 min, which is not significant (Table 1).

From these findings serum half-life is only 3.5 and 6 min shorter in each model.

The corresponding elimination constants increased, to K_2 of 0.0172 to 0.0184 and β of 0.0130 to 0.0149, and the area under the curve was slightly decreased, the values being 15.144 μg.min/ml (14.719 μg.min/ml for two-compartment model) and 13.890 μg.min/ml (13.453 μg.min/ml), respectively. TRCl increased in accordance with the increased elimination, the values being 134.96 ml/min (138.80 ml/min for two-compartment model) and 147.76 ml/min (151.93 ml/min for two-compartment model), respectively. The central distribution volume was in both models slightly increased in combination, the initial concentration C_o being almost identical.

The increased elimination of piperacillin into the urine in combination was also reflected in all urine-collecting periods, where larger amounts of piperacillin were recovered. According to that finding, the limit of M_o for the cumulative amount of drug in combination is significantly higher, the rate of excretion nevertheless being identical. The average plasma clearance (CL_8) for piperacillin in combination was significantly higher, the values being 52.93 and 77.58 ml/min for each model.

Discussion. Piperacillin and flucloxacillin are not metabolized and are rapidly excreted via the kidney. Inhibition of tubular excretion by different substances (e.g., caronamid, probenecid) and a corresponding increase in serum concentra-

TABLE 1. *Serum concentrations of flucloxacillin and piperacillin, alone and in combination*

Drug	Serum concn (mg/liter) after:							
	5 min	10 min	20 min	40 min	90 min	120 min	240 min	360 min
Flucloxacillin (1 g)	347	237.3	143.2	91.1	29.5	17.8	1.1	0.0
Flucloxacillin (1 g) in combination	293	198.1	137.1	97.6	48.2	29.9	5.1	0.0
Piperacillin (2 g)	408.1	252.5	163.8	104.4	40.1	25.5	5.0	0.5
Piperacillin (2 g) in combination	371.6	245.3	166.1	97.6	37.2	22.3	4.0	0.0

tions and area under the curve of penicillin and other antibiotics, which are mainly excreted via tubular filtration and tubular secretion, is a well-known finding.

When two penicillin derivatives are administered simultaneously via intravenous injection, a probenecid-like situation may arise. There is competitive inhibition of excretion of the penicillin derivative which has the higher renal clearance. According to the capacity of the active transport system to be saturated, both substances will be excreted differently. The effect is similar to a dose increase of the single substance. In comparable investigations using other penicillin derivatives we made similar findings.

In the present trial after simultaneous administration of flucloxacillin and piperacillin, flucloxacillin excretion is inhibited by piperacillin, which has a higher TRCl. Therefore, the serum concentrations of flucloxacillin in a combination are significantly higher. In accordance with this finding, the area under the curve of flucloxacillin concentration in both compartment models is increased. The reduced elimination leads to a longer plasma half-life of 13 and 11 min, according to the model. The urine collected during an 8-h period yielded 24% less flucloxacillin in combination compared with the single administration. On the other hand, 1 g of flucloxacillin in combination does not inhibit the excretion of piperacillin.

Mode of Action of MK 0787 (*N*-Formimidoyl Thienamycin): Microcalorimetric and Morphological Study

E. SEMENITZ, G. GSTRAUNTHALER, AND W. PFALLER

Institute of Hygiene and Institute of Physiology, University of Innsbruck, Innsbruck, Austria

Thienamycin, a β-lactam antibiotic, exhibits broad-spectrum activity in vitro against gram-negative and gram-positive bacteria (1, 4–6). This was substantiated in this study by a decrease in heat production determined with a flow microcalorimeter. Upon addition of thienamycin at concentrations below the MIC values, remarkable structural changes could be observed by phase-contrast and electron microscopy for *Escherichia coli*, *Serratia*, and *Proteus*.

Microcalorimetry measures the minimal temperature changes produced during the multiplication of bacteria in a fluid nutrient medium. This method allows new insights into the metabolic properties of bacterial substances. The addition of an antibiotic to an outgrowing culture gives characteristic changes in the kinetics of heat production. Simultaneously, the multiplication of bacteria can be monitored continuously by turbidimetric measurements. With these two techniques, the antimicrobial activity of chemotherapeutic agents can be continuously monitored and continuously registered (3).

As far as the structural alterations of bacteria by β-lactam antibiotics are concerned, only a few studies have been carried out (2, 7).

In the present study we tried to find out whether MK 0787 produces similar changes in different strains of the *Enterobacteriaceae* as found with other β-lactam antibiotics.

E. coli 279, *S. marcescens* 104, and *P. morganii* 8 were grown in Columbia bouillon. MK 0787 (*N*-formimidoyl thienamycin) was dissolved in distilled water and added to the log culture in the concentrations indicated. Microcalorimetry and turbidimetry were carried out as described earlier (3). For electron microscopy, cultures were fixed in 3.5% buffered glutaraldehyde, postfixed in OsO_4, dehydrated with acetone, and embedded in Durcupan ACM (Fluka). The ultrathin sections were stained with uranylacetate and lead citrate. Phase-contrast microscopy was carried out parallel to the microcalorimetric measurements to get information about the time course of structural changes.

In a second series of experiments, MK 0787 was added to Mueller-Hinton agar, which was inoculated with the strains indicated above at 10^5 cells per ml. During the outgrowth, the dose-dependent structural changes were studied by phase-contrast microscopy.

Microcalorimetry and turbidimetry showed that MK 0787 has a marked effect on the shape of the kinetic curve. Turbidity initially increased as a result of an increase of the cell numbers in the logarithmic phase of growth; in the presence of MK 0787, however, at the concentrations used, a rapid decrease of turbidity due to the lysis of cells could be observed. The microcalor-

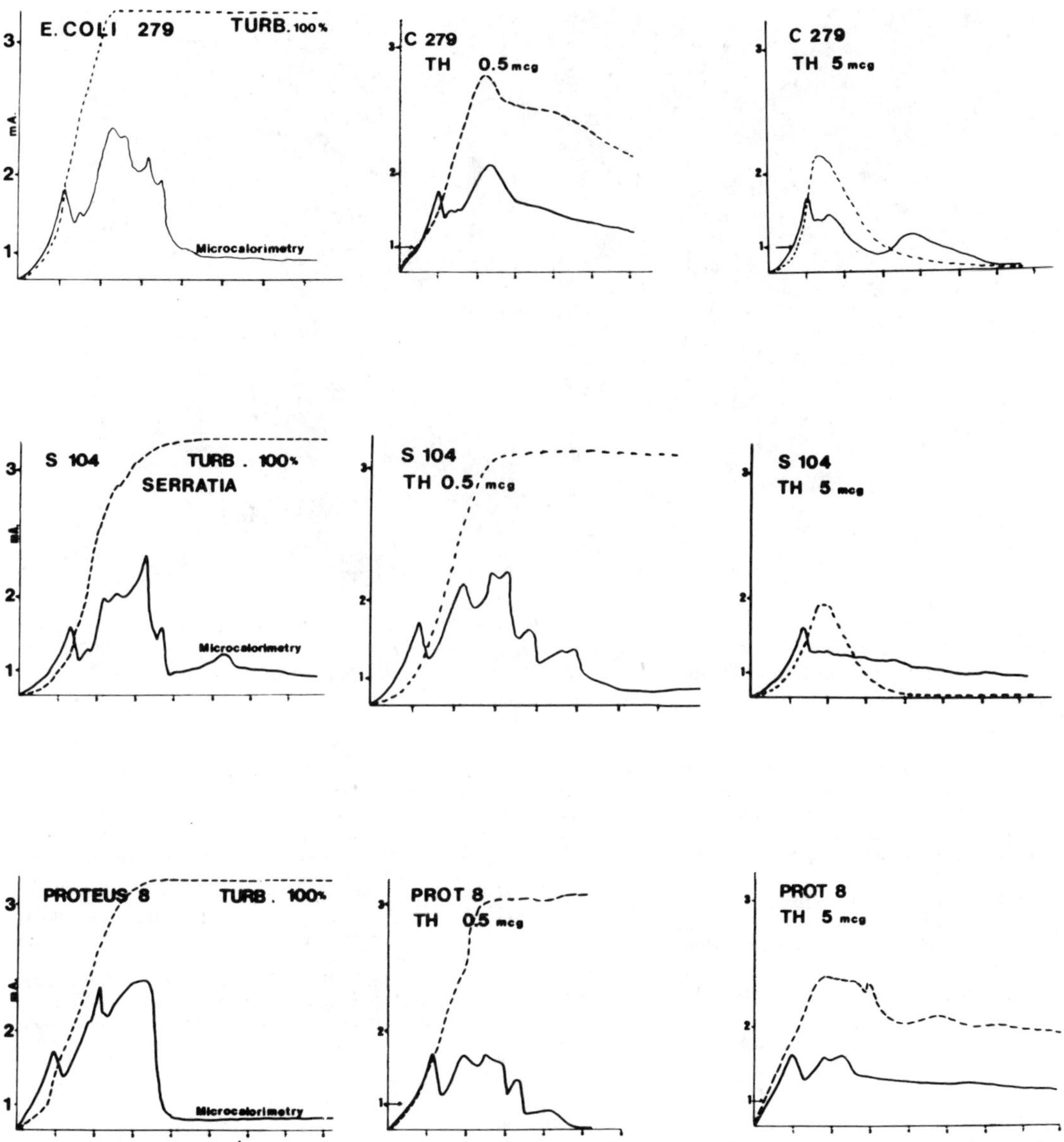

FIG. 1. *Microcalorimetry and turbidimetry of E. coli 279, S. marcescens 104, and P. morganii 8. The first column shows untreated cultures in Columbia broth. The other columns show cultures treated with 0.5 or 5.0 μg of MK 0787 per ml.*

imetric activity decreased with increasing concentrations of MK 0787 (Fig. 1).

Phase-contrast microscopy revealed that drastic structural changes of bacterial cells may occur when MK 0787 concentrations below MIC values are used. One hour after addition of MK 0787 (0.5 μg/ml), cells became rounded up and lysis occured (Fig. 1).

Electron microscopic studies of treated cells demonstrated a change in cell shape, possibly induced by osmotic swelling. The cell wall was separated from the protoplast and displayed large folds. The periplasmic space (Fig. 2) appeared remarkably widened. These changes were found to be identical in all strains of *Enterobacteriaceae* which we tested so far.

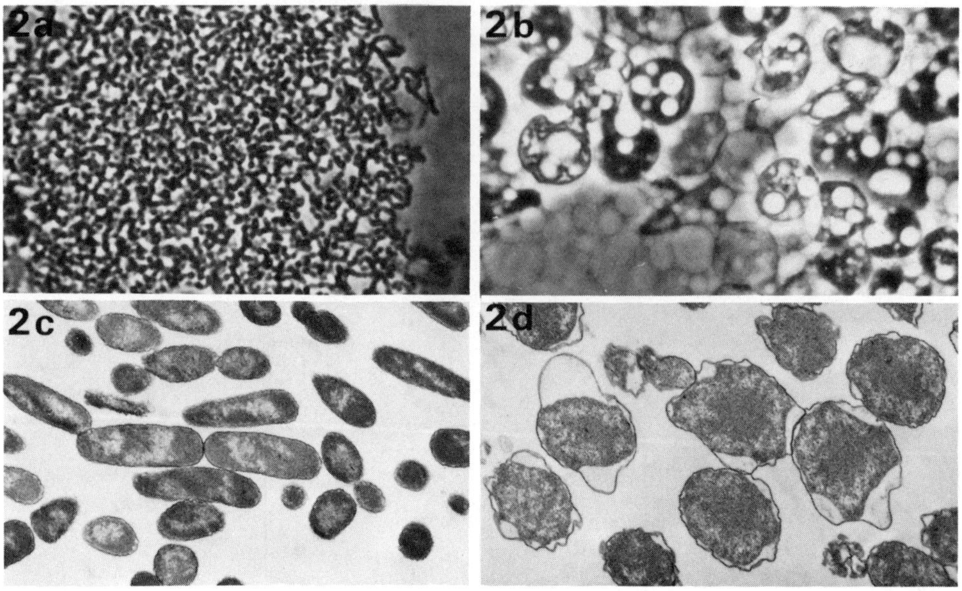

FIG. 2. *Phase-contrast and electron microscopy of E. coli 279. (a and b) Phase-contrast microscopy of E. coli on Mueller-Hinton agar: (a) untreated culture, (b) culture treated with MK 0787, 0.5 μg/ml. ×1,000. (c and d) Electron microscopy of E. coli in Columbia broth: (c) untreated culture, (d) culture treated with MK 0787, 0.5 μg/ml. ×10,000.*

1. **Hanslo, D., A. King, K. Shannon, C. Warren, and I. Phillips.** 1981. *N*-Formidoyl thienamycin (MK 0787): in-vitro antibacterial activity and susceptibility to beta-lactamases compared with that of cefotaxime, moxalactam and other beta-lactam antibiotics. J. Antimicrob. Chemother. **7**:607–617.
2. **Ryan, D. M., and D. Monsey.** 1981. Bacterial filamentation and in vivo efficacy: a comparison of several cephalosporins. J. Antimicrob. Chemother. **7**:57–63.
3. **Semenitz, E.** 1980. Mikrokalorimetrie zur Aktivitätsbestimmung von Chemotherapeutika. Thermochim. Acta **40**:99–107.
4. **Tally, F. P., N. V. Jacobus, and S. L. Gorbach.** 1978. In vitro activity of thienamycin. Antimicrob. Agents Chemother. **14**:436–438.
5. **Weaver, S. S., G. P. Bodey, and B. M. Le Blanc.** 1979. Thienamycin: new beta-lactam antibiotic with potent broadspectrum activity. Antimicrob. Agents Chemother. **15**:518–521.
6. **Wise, R., J. M. Andrews, and N. Patel.** 1981. *N*-Formimidoyl-thienamycin a novel β-lactam: an in-vitro comparison with other β-lactam antibiotics. J. Antimicrob. Chemother. **7**:521–529.
7. **Zimmerman, S. B., and E. O. Stapley.** 1976. Relative morphology effects induced by cefoxitin and other β-lactam antibiotics in vitro. Antimicrob. Agents Chemother. **9**:318–336.

Activity of *N*-Formimidoyl Thienamycin (MK 0787) Against β-Lactam–Resistant Enterobacteria and Pseudomonads and Its Sensitivity to β-Lactamases

DAVID HANSLO,* IAN PHILLIPS, KEVIN SHANNON, ANNA KING, AND CHRISTINE WARREN

St. Thomas's Hospital Medical School, London, England

The in vitro activity of *N*-formimidoyl thienamycin (MK 0787) was assessed against clinical isolates of *Enterobacteriaceae* and *Pseudomonas aeruginosa* by determination of MICs. Agar dilution was used for *P. aeruginosa*, but broth dilution, with an MIC 2000 dispenser and inoculator (Dynatech Laboratories Ltd., Billingshurst, West Sussex, England), was used for enterobacteria (1).

N-Formimidoyl thienamycin was active against all enterobacteria tested, though less so than cefotaxime and moxalactam against most isolates (Table 1). The compound was less active against *Morganella morganii*, *Proteus* spp., and *Providencia* spp. than it was against other genera. Enterobacteria that were resistant (MICs ≥ 16 μg/ml) to ampicillin, cephaloridine, or both compounds were almost as susceptible to *N*-formimidoyl thienamycin as fully susceptible isolates.

N-Formimidoyl thienamycin was also active against *P. aeruginosa* (Table 1). It was equally active against isolates that were susceptible to carbenicillin (MICs ≤ 64 μg/ml) and against those that were moderately resistant to this compound (MICs 128 to 512 μg/ml), but it was slightly less active against isolates that were highly resistant to carbenicillin (MICs > 1,024 μg/ml). In contrast, cefotaxime and moxalactam were more active against highly carbenicillin-resistant isolates than against isolates that were moderately resistant (Table 1).

The activity of *N*-formimidoyl thienamycin was also tested against strains of *Escherichia coli* and *P. aeruginosa* that produced plasmid-mediated β-lactamases. All were susceptible to the compound, as were *Klebsiella* 1082E and strains that produced chromosomally determined cephalosporinases (Table 2). The stability of *N*-formimidoyl thienamycin to these β-lactamases was assessed by the UV spectrophotometric method (4) at a wavelength of 300 nm. *N*-Formimidoyl thienamycin was highly resistant to β-lactamases. There was very slow hy-

TABLE 1. *In vitro activity of N-formimidoyl thienamycin*

Organism (no. of isolates)	Antibiotic	MICs (μg/ml) Range	For (% of isolates) 50	75	90
Enterobacteria other than *M. morganii*, *Proteus* spp., and *Providencia* spp.[a]					
Ampicillin- and cephaloridine-susceptible (49)	*N*-Formimidoyl thienamycin	0.03–1	0.25	0.25	0.5
	Cefotaxime	0.004–0.12	0.06	0.06	0.12
	Moxalactam	0.016–0.5	0.12	0.12	0.25
Ampicillin-resistant, cephaloridine-susceptible (72)	*N*-Formimidoyl thienamycin	0.06–1	0.25	0.5	1
	Cefotaxime	0.004–0.5	0.03	0.06	0.12
	Moxalactam	0.03–0.5	0.12	0.12	0.25
Ampicillin-susceptible, cephaloridine-resistant (17)	*N*-Formimidoyl thienamycin	0.12–2	0.5	0.5	1
	Cefotaxime	0.06–0.5	0.12	0.25	0.25
	Moxalactam	0.06–4	0.12	0.25	0.5
Ampicillin- and cephaloridine-resistant (102)	*N*-Formimidoyl thienamycin	0.06–4	0.25	0.5	1
	Cefotaxime	0.016–128	0.12	0.25	0.5
	Moxalactam	0.016–32	0.25	0.25	0.5
***M. morganii*, *Proteus* spp., and *Providencia* spp.[b]**					
Ampicillin- and cephaloridine-susceptible (35)	*N*-Formimidoyl thienamycin	0.25–8	2	4	4
	Cefotaxime	0.004–0.12	0.03	0.03	0.06
	Moxalactam	0.03–0.25	0.12	0.12	0.12
Ampicillin- and cephaloridine-resistant (114)	*N*-Formimidoyl thienamycin	0.25–8	2	4	4
	Cefotaxime	0.008–16	0.06	0.12	1
	Moxalactam	0.03–16	0.12	0.12	0.25
P. aeruginosa					
Carbenicillin-susceptible (33)	*N*-Formimidoyl thienamycin	0.5–4	2	4	4
	Cefotaxime	4–16	8	16	16
	Moxalactam	2–16	8	8	16
Moderately carbenicillin-resistant (12)	*N*-Formimidoyl thienamycin	0.5–8	2	4	4
	Cefotaxime	16–64	64	64	64
	Moxalactam	16–64	32	32	64
Highly carbenicillin-resistant (13)	*N*-Formimidoyl thienamycin	1–8	4	8	8
	Cefotaxime	1–128	8	8	8
	Moxalactam	4–>32	8	8	8

[a] *Citrobacter koseri* (20 isolates), *C. freundii* (20 isolates), *Escherichia coli* (50 isolates), *Enterobacter aerogenes* (25 isolates), *E. cloacae* (35 isolates), *Klebsiella* spp. (65 isolates), and *Serratia* spp. (25 isolates).

[b] *Morganella morganii* (20 isolates), *Proteus mirabilis* (47 isolates), *P. vulgaris* (26 isolates), *Providencia alcalifaciens* (8 isolates), *P. rettgeri* (17 isolates), and *P. stuartii* (31 isolates).

TABLE 2. *Sensitivity of N-formimidoyl thienamycin to β-lactamases*

Organism (enzyme)	MICs (μg/ml)			β-Lactamase activity[a]	Hydrolysis relative to cephaloridine (100)		
	N-Formimidoyl thienamycin	Cefotaxime	Moxalactam		*N*-Formimidoyl thienamycin	Cefotaxime	Moxalactam
E. coli (TEM-1)	0.25	0.03	0.06	7.9	—[b]	—	—
E. coli (TEM-2)	0.25	0.06	0.06	34.7	0.02	0.2	—
E. coli (SHV-1)	0.25	0.06	0.12	0.8	—	—	—
E. coli (OXA-1)	0.25	0.12	0.12	0.4	—	45	—
E. coli (OXA-2)	0.25	0.03	0.12	0.3	—	—	—
E. coli (OXA-3)	0.5	0.06	0.12	0.08	—	—	—
Klebsiella 1082E	0.25	1	0.12	43.0	0.04	6	—
E. cloacae P99	0.25	64	8	19.5	—	—	—
E. cloacae 4.37.76	0.25	16	16	53.5	0.1	0.3	—
M. morganii 1036.3	4	0.5	0.25	17.4	—	—	—
P. vulgaris PC 37	4	1	0.25	18.9	—	0.7	—
Serratia sp. 9.2.75	0.25	0.12	0.25	0.4	—	—	—
P. aeruginosa (TEM-1)	4	4	4	Not tested			
P. aeruginosa (PSE-1)	2	16	16	0.5	—	—	—
P. aeruginosa (PSE-2)	2	16	16	0.02	—	—	—
P. aeruginosa (PSE-3)	2	16	16	0.04	—	—	—
P. aeruginosa (PSE-4)	2	8	8	1.4	—	—	—
P. aeruginosa NCTC 10662	4	16	8	1.3	—	—	—

[a] Nanokatals per milligram of protein with cephaloridine as substrate.
[b] Not detected.

drolysis by a few enzymes, but this was not sufficient to confer resistance to the compound (Table 2).

N-Formimidoyl thienamycin has also been found to be active in vitro against most other bacteria of medical importance, with the exception of *P. maltophilia* (1–3, 5). Some methicillin-resistant staphylococci have also been found to be less susceptible than other staphylococci to *N*-formimidoyl thienamycin, especially when large inocula were tested (1, 3, 5).

We are grateful to Merck Sharpe & Dohme Research Laboratories for financial support and for providing *N*-formimidoyl thienamycin.

1. **Hanslo, D., A. King, K. Shannon, C. Warren, and I. Phillips.** 1981. *N*-Formimidoyl thienamycin (MK 0787): in-vitro antibacterial activity and susceptibility to beta-lactamases compared with that of cefotaxime, moxalactam and other beta-lactam antibiotics. J. Antimicrob. Chemother. **7**:607–617.
2. **Kesado, T., T. Hashizume, and Y. Asahi.** 1980. Antibacterial activities of a new stabilized thienamycin, *N*-formimidoyl thienamycin, in comparison with other antibiotics. Antimicrob. Agents Chemother. **17**:912–917.
3. **Kropp, H., J. G. Sundelof, J. S. Kahan, F. M. Kahan, and J. Birnbaum.** 1980. MK 0787 (*N*-formimidoyl thienamycin): evaluation of in vitro and in vivo activities. Antimicrob. Agents Chemother. **17**:993–1000.
4. **O'Callaghan, C. H., P. W. Muggleton, and G. W. Ross.** 1969. Effects of β-lactamase from gram-negative organisms on cephalosporins and penicillins, p. 57–63. Antimicrob. Agents Chemother. 1968.
5. **Wise, R., J. M. Andrews, and N. Patel.** 1981. *N*-Formimidoyl thienamycin a novel β-lactam: an in vitro comparison with other β-lactam antibiotics. J. Antimicrob. Chemother. **7**:521–529.

N-Formimidoyl Thienamycin Activity Against Aerobes and Anaerobes: Effect of Inoculum Size, pH Variation, and Different Culture Medium

E. J. PEREA,* E. MARTIN, M. C. NOGALES, A. PASCUAL, AND M. V. BOROBIO

Department of Microbiology, Medical School, University of Seville, Seville-9, Spain

The in vitro activity of *N*-formimidoyl thienamycin (MK 0787) was determined against 100 anaerobic bacteria: 50 *Bacteroides* strains (26 *B. fragilis*, 8 *B. distasonis*, 5 *B. ovatus*, 7 *B. vulgatus*, and 5 *B. thetaiotaomicron*), 25 being β-lactamase producers and 25 nonproducers; 25

Clostridium strains (13 *C. perfringens*, 8 *C. bifermentans*, 2 *C. sordellii*, and 2 *C. septicum*); 13 *Peptococcus* strains (2 *P. indolicus*, 3 *P. saccharolyticus*, 4 *P. prevotii*, 2 *P. magnus*, 2 *P. asaccharolyticus*); and 12 *Peptostreptococcus* strains (8 *P. productus*, 4 *P. parvulus*). Activity was also determined against 210 aerobic bacteria: 30 *Salmonella* spp., 30 *Shigella* spp., 15 *Klebsiella* spp., 15 *Serratia* spp., 15 *Escherichia coli* strains, 15 *Proteus* spp., 15 *Enterobacter* spp., 15 *Pseudomonas aeruginosa* strains, 30 *Staphylococcus aureus* strains, and 30 *Streptococcus faecalis* strains. The activity was evaluated by the agar dilution method.

Three different culture media were used in susceptibility tests for anaerobes: brucella agar (BA), Wilkins-Chalgren agar (W-C), and brain heart agar (BHA). Two different media were used for aerobes: Mueller-Hinton agar (MH) and diagnostic sensitivity test agar (DST). All media were without cysteine. The effect of the pH on the antibiotic activity was evaluated at three pH levels, 6, 7, and 8, and the effect of the inoculum density with 30 anaerobes was tested by using 10^3, 10^5, and 10^7 colony-forming units.

β-Lactamase production was determined in all *Bacteroides* strains by the plate method.

A laboratory standard of MK 0787 was kindly supplied by Merck Sharp & Dohme.

Anaerobes. The MICs for 50 *B. fragilis* strains were lower than 0.125 μg/ml, the lowest concentration tested. There was no difference between the β-lactamase producers and nonproducers. The MICs for *Clostridium* strains were also less than 0.125 μg/ml. Among the *Peptococcaceae*, there were two different groups: the isolates of the genus *Peptococcus* were inhibited at 0.125 μg/ml whereas those of the genus *Peptostreptococcus* were inhibited only at 1 μg/ml (Table 1).

The MBCs for *Bacteroides, Clostridium*, and *Peptococcus* strains were 0.125 μg/ml, and that for *Peptostreptococcus* was 4 μg/ml (Table 1).

There were no significant differences between MIC and MBC values obtained in the different media tested; however, the MIC for *Peptostreptococcus* was three dilutions higher in BHA than in W-C or BA.

The initial pH of the medium and the inoculum size had no appreciable effect on MK 0787 activity on anaerobes.

Aerobes. The MICs for 90% of strains (MIC_{90}) were as follows: *S. faecalis*, 8 μg/ml; *S. aureus*, 0.125 μg/ml; *Salmonella, Shigella, Klebsiella*, and *Enterobacter*, 0.5 μg/ml; *Serratia*, 1 μg/ml; *Proteus*, 2 μg/ml; and *P. aeruginosa*, 4 μg/ml (Table 1).

The MBCs for 90% of strains (MBC_{90}) were 8 μg/ml for *S. faecalis*, 0.25 μg/ml for *S. aureus*, 0.5 μg/ml for *Shigella* and *E. coli*, 1 μg/ml for *Salmonella, Serratia, Klebsiella*, and *Enterobacter*, and 4 μg/ml for *Proteus* and *Pseudomonas* (Table 1).

TABLE 1. *N-Formimidoyl thienamycin activity in BA and MHA at pH 7 against 310 anaerobic and aerobic bacteria*

Bacteria	No. of strains	Range of MIC (μg/ml)	MIC_{90} (μg/ml)	MBC_{90} (μg/ml)
Bacteroides fragilis	50	0.125	0.125	0.125
Clostridium spp.	25	0.125	0.125	0.125
Peptococcus spp.	13	0.125	0.125	0.125
Peptostreptococcus spp.	12	1	1	4
Streptococcus faecalis	30	0.015–8	>8	>8
Staphylococcus aureus	30	0.03–0.125	0.125	0.125
Salmonella	30	0.25–0.5	0.5	1
Shigella	30	0.125–0.5	0.5	0.5
Serratia	15	0.03–2	1	1
Klebsiella	15	0.125–0.5	0.5	1
Enterobacter	15	0.125–0.5	0.5	1
Proteus	15	0.25–4	2	4
Escherichia coli	15	0.125–0.5	0.25	0.5
Pseudomonas aeruginosa	15	0.25–8	4	4

There were no significant differences between MIC and MBC values obtained in the different media tested; however, the MIC_{90} for *Enterobacter* at pH 7 was two dilutions higher in DST than in MH, and the MBC for *Klebsiella, Serratia*, and *S. faecalis* in DST at pH 7 was three dilutions greater than the MIC.

In general, the slight differences found in MIC and MBC values for anaerobes and aerobes in the different media are not significant because they generally fell within the range of the experimental error of the procedure.

The initial pH of the medium had no appreciable effect on the activity of MK 0787 on aerobes, except with *Salmonella, E. coli*, and *S. faecalis*, for which the MIC_{90} was two dilutions higher at pH 8 than at pH 6.

Our results with *N*-formimidoyl thienamycin on 50 *B. fragilis* isolates were similar to those obtained by Tally et al. (2), who used thienamycin on 7 *Bacteroides* spp., but we disagree on the MIC for clostridia. They found an MIC of 4 μg/ml for 5 *Clostridium* spp., and our results, with 25 *Clostridium* spp., gave MICs of 0.125 μg/ml. They also studied 7 anaerobic gram-positive cocci and found an MIC of 0.125 μg/ml. We obtained the same results with the genus *Peptococcus*, but not with the genus *Peptostreptococcus*.

There are no studies on the susceptibility on the genera *Salmonella* and *Shigella*. We found these organisms to be highly susceptible, the MIC_{90} for both being 0.25 μg/ml.

Our results with *N*-formimidoyl thienamycin on members of the *Enterobacteriaceae* are similar to those obtained by others (1; H. Kropp, J. S. Kahan, J. Sundelof, G. Darland, and J. Birnbaum, Program Abstr. Intersci. Conf. Antimicrob. Agents Chemother. 15th, Chicago, Ill., abstr. no. 228, 1976) for *E. coli*, *Enterobacter*, *Klebsiella*, *Proteus*, and *Serratia*. We agree with Tadataka et al. (1) on the MICs for *Pseudomonas*.

Among the gram-positive organisms, *Staphylococcus* shows MICs ranging from 0.015 to 0.5 μg/ml (1; Kropp et al.). The MICs for *S. faecalis* ranged from 1 to 8 μg/ml. These results agree with those of Tadataka (1).

These results, when compared with those obtained with the original thienamycin, show the new derivative to have at least equal, and often superior, in vitro activity (2, 3).

The effect of inoculum size on the activity of thienamycin was to increase fivefold or more the MIC and MBC against *Enterobacteriaceae* with an inoculum increase from 10^5 to 10^7 colony-forming units (2). In our study with the new compound, variation of inoculum between 10^3 and 10^7 colony-forming units yielded similar MICs and MBCs with the 30 anaerobe strains tested.

The original instability of thienamycin to pH variations has been avoided with the new MK 0787 because its MICs are not affected by variations of pH between 6 and 8.

We conclude that the new thienamycin derivative is more active than the original compound against anaerobes and aerobes; its activity against anaerobes is not affected by pH, culture medium composition, inoculum size, or by β-lactamase of *B. fragilis*. When tested against aerobes, the MICs and MBCs are not affected by pH or composition of culture medium.

1. **Tadataka, K., H. Terutaka, and A. Yoshinaki.** 1980. Antibacterial activities of a new stabilized thienamycin, *N*-formimidoyl thienamycin, in comparison with other antibiotics. Antimicrob. Agents Chemother. **17**:912–917.
2. **Tally, F. P., N. V. Jacobus, and S. L. Gorbach.** 1978. In vitro activity of thienamycin. Antimicrob. Agents Chemother. **14**:436–438.
3. **Weaver, S., G. P. Bodey, and B. M. LeBlanc.** 1979. Thienamycin: new β-lactam antibiotic with potent broad-spectrum activity. Antimicrob. Agents Chemother. **15**:518–521.

Susceptibility of Ampicillin-Resistant Strains of Enterobacteria and *Pseudomonas* to Thienamycin

W. CULLMANN, M. STIEGLITZ, U. WERKMEISTER, AND W. OPFERKUCH

Department of Medical Microbiology and Immunology of the Ruhr-Universitaet, Bochum, Federal Republic of Germany

N-Formimidoyl thienamycin (MK 0787), a novel β-lactam compound, exhibits a broad spectrum of antibacterial activity against gram-positive and gram-negative bacteria (1). It was the purpose of this study to evaluate its activity against ampicillin-resistant bacteria in comparison with that of mezlocillin, cefuroxime, cefotaxime, ceftizoxime, cefoperazone, and moxalactam. Moreover, as β-lactamase production is one mechanism of resistance to β-lactam antibiotics, its influence on the MIC was investigated.

Three hundred seventy-eight strains of ampicillin-resistant enterobacteria (MIC > 16 mg/liter), 50 *Pseudomonas aeruginosa* strains, 28 *Acinetobacter* strains, 50 *Streptococcus faecalis* strains, and 7 oxacillin-resistant *Staphylococcus aureus* strains, all recently isolated from clinical specimens, were included in this study. Susceptibility tests were performed in Mueller-Hinton broth with twofold serial dilutions (from 0.032 to 1,024 mg/liter). For thienamycin the bactericidal concentration was determined by plating clear tubes to CLED agar (Oxoid Ltd., Basingstoke, England). To investigate β-lactamase production, all strains of enterobacteria, *Pseudomonas*, and *Acinetobacter* species were subjected to ultrasonic disruption. A color change of the chromogenic cephalosporin nitrocefin (compound 87/312, Glaxo Ltd., Greenford, England) from yellow to red at room temperature within 5 min was considered positive (3).

Most of the ampicillin-resistant isolates of enterobacteria were inhibited by low concentrations of cefotaxime, ceftizoxime, and moxalactam (Table 1). Moreover, all these drugs remained unaffected by β-lactamases. Cefuroxime and cefoperazone, however, were less active against the isolates and were attacked by β-lactamases (Table 2). In addition, the well-known instability of mezlocillin with respect to β-lactamases was seen (Table 2).

Among the 378 strains of enterobacteria, resistance to cefotaxime (MIC > 16 mg/liter) was observed in 26 strains and to moxalactam (MIC > 32 mg/liter) in 7 isolates. Strains resistant to cefotaxime showed elevated MICs of ceftizoxime as well. All these strains were inhibited by thienamycin (MIC ranged from 0.25 to 4 mg/liter).

TABLE 1. *In vitro activity of N-formimidoyl thienamycin against ampicillin-resistant enterobacteria and P. aeruginosa: comparison of the MICs of various β-lactam compounds*[a]

Species	No.	Mezlocillin		Cefuroxime		Cefoperazone		Cefotaxime		Ceftizoxime		Moxalactam		Thienamycin	
		50%	90%	50%	90%	50%	90%	50%	90%	50%	90%	50%	90%	50%	90%
E. coli	50	128	1,024	2	8	2	64	<0.032	1	<0.032	1	0.125	0.5	0.25	0.5
Klebsiella spp.	50	32	>1,024	2	16	1	512	<0.032	0.125	<0.032	0.063	0.125	0.5	0.25	1
Enterobacter spp.	50	8	1,024	8	512	2	256	0.5	64	0.25	128	0.25	16	1	2
Serratia spp.	44	32	>1,024	128	1,024	2	512	0.25	1	0.063	0.5	0.25	2	4	4
Citrobacter spp.	43	>1,024	>1,024	8	256	128	1,024	0.125	64	0.25	128	0.25	16	2	2
Proteus mirabilis	41	1,024	>1,024	2	1,024	32	>1,024	<0.032	0.063	<0.032	<0.032	0.125	0.5	4	8
P. vulgaris	43	4	>1,024	512	>1,024	1	32	0.063	4	<0.032	<0.032	0.25	0.5	4	8
P. morganii	45	2	512	32	64	1	64	0.125	2	0.5	4	0.25	0.5	4	4
P. rettgeri	13	1,024	>1,024	4	128	512	1,024	0.063	0.5	0.063	0.5	0.25	4	4	4
				Azlocillin											
Pseudomonas aeruginosa	50	32	1,024	8	512	8	128	16	32	32	64	32	64	1	2

[a] MICs (milligrams per liter) for 50 and 90% of strains are shown. With the exception of oxacillin-resistant staphylococci, the action of thienamycin is bactericidal at twice the MIC or lower.

TABLE 2. *Influence of β-lactamase production on the antimicrobial activity of thienamycin and other β-lactam compounds (the geometric mean values are collated)*

Species[a]	No.	Mezlocillin	Cefuroxime	Cefoperazone	Cefotaxime	Ceftizoxime	Moxalactam	Thienamycin
E. coli								
+	45	93	3.1	4.9	0.13	0.08	0.22	0.40
−	5	111	1.7	1.1	0.29	0.04	0.13	0.29
Klebsiella spp.								
+	28	205	4.5	16.0	0.06	0.04	0.27	0.34
−	22	21	3.4	0.46	0.05	0.04	0.19	0.42
Enterobacter spp.								
+	29	94	46	9.7	2.2	20	1.7	1.1
−	21	3.9	7.8	0.7	0.53	0.26	0.35	1.0
Serratia spp.								
+	23	110	153	16	0.64	0.15	0.49	3.1
−	21	7.8	141	2.3	0.35	0.08	0.44	1.7
Citrobacter spp.								
+	30	446	20	147	1.1	2.9	0.91	1.45
−	13	12	6.5	0.95	0.16	0.24	0.31	0.56
P. mirabilis								
+	20	462	3.6	274	0.06	0.03	0.18	5.7
−	21	19	8.3	4	0.08	0.03	0.18	4.9
P. vulgaris								
+	3	25	102	645	0.03	0.03	0.20	8
−	40	20	197	2.4	0.18	0.05	0.36	2.9
P. morganii								
+		790	76	128	0.60	2.6	0.25	4
−	36	4.7	35	1.6	0.18	0.55	0.28	4
P. rettgeri								
+	9	813	8.6	376	0.29	0.13	0.40	2.7
−	4	45	4.0	1.4	0.08	0.04	0.25	3.3
			Azlocillin					
P. aeruginosa								
+	5	388	147	446	42	37	28	1.4
−	45	45	13	12	17	35	25	1.3

[a] β-Lactamase producers and nonproducers are indicated by + and −, respectively. In the *Acinetobacter* strains included in this study, no β-lactamase production could be detected.

With the exception of some strains of *Proteus* species, we did not observe any strain of enterobacteria for which the MIC was more than 4 mg/liter (Table 1). Some strains of *Proteus* species required a concentration of 8 mg/liter for inhibition, which is consistent with recently reported findings (1). The action of thienamycin is bactericidal, at least with twice the MIC.

N-Formimidoyl thienamycin proved to be the most effective drug against *Pseudomonas aeruginosa*; even in strains exhibiting β-lactamase production, the MIC never exceeded 4 mg/liter. MICs of other antibiotics known to be very effective against *Pseudomonas*, such as azlocillin, piperacillin, and cefsulodin, are approximately 10 times that of thienamycin (4).

With respect to *Streptococcus faecalis*, thienamycin proved to be at least as effective as ampicillin: both showed MICs between 1 and 2 mg/liter. Cefoperazone was less active: for inhibition of 90% of the strains, 64 mg/liter was required.

Thienamycin showed MICs ranging from 0.032 to 1 mg/liter against *Acinetobacter* species, thus exceeding the antibacterial effect of other β-lactam compounds.

Oxacillin-resistant isolates of *Staphylococcus aureus* were inhibited by *N*-formimidoyl thienamycin at 0.063 to 0.25 mg/liter, a level much lower than that required in the case of other β-lactam antibiotics. However, the bactericidal activity was markedly impaired in these strains: they required approximately 100 times the MIC. This phenomenon is well known in other β-lactam compounds and is probably influenced by the media and procedures employed (2).

These data make it apparent that *N*-formimidoyl thienamycin can be regarded as a highly active agent against both gram-positive and gram-negative bacteria. Its action is bactericidal, corresponding to other β-lactam antibiotics. It is also very active against isolates of *P. aeruginosa*, *S. faecalis*, and *Acinetobacter* species; its bactericidal action is limited only in the case of oxacillin-resistant staphylococci.

1. **Hanslo, D., A. King, K. Shannon, C. Warren, and I. Phillips.** 1981. N-Formimidoyl thienamycin (MK 0787): in-vitro antibacterial activity and susceptibility to beta-lactamases compared with that of cefotaxime, moxalactam, and other β-lactam antibiotics. J. Antimicrob. Chemother. **7**:607–618.
2. **Norden, C. W., and E. Keleti.** 1981. Antibiotic tolerance in strains of Staphylococcus aureus. J. Antimicrob. Chemother. **7**:599–606.
3. **O'Callaghan, C. H., A. Morris, S. M. Kirby, and A. H. Shingler.** 1972. Novel method for detection of β-lactamases by using a chromogenic cephalosporin substrate. Antimicrob. Agents Chemother. **1**:283–288.
4. **Slack, M. P. E., D. B. Wheldon, R. A. Swann, and E. Perks.** 1979. Cefsulodin a cephalosporin with specific antipseudomonal activity; in vitro studies of the drug alone and in combination. J. Antimicrob. Chemother. **5**:687–691.

Susceptibility of *Bacteroides* to Eight Beta-Lactam Compounds (Including *N*-Formimidoyl Thienamycin [MK 0787]): Study of Resistant Strains

JEFFREY P. MASKELL,* MASARU NASU, AND J. DAVID WILLIAMS

The London Hospital Medical College, London, England

Organisms of the *Bacteroides fragilis* group are relatively resistant to many chemotherapeutic agents. This resistance is often associated with beta-lactamase production (3). Several compounds with beta-lactamase stability, such as cefoxitin, have been developed, and reports have described a high percentage of strains to be susceptible to this compound (1, 3). MK 0787 is a carbapenem which, like cefoxitin, is beta-lactamase stable and therefore of potential use in the treatment of infections where *Bacteroides* species are implicated. In this study, we compared the activity of MK 0787 and several newer cephalosporins with that of cefoxitin, lincomycin, and metronidazole. We investigated both inhibitory effects and beta-lactamase stability of the compounds. Isoelectric points of the beta-lactamases of some of the more resistant strains were determined by isoelectric focusing, and the influence of beta-lactamase inhibitors on MICs to each beta-lactam compound were studied.

MIC determination. MICs were estimated by an agar dilution technique with an approximate inoculum of 10^3 colony-forming units. Incubation was for 48 h at 37° C in an anaerobic atmosphere with 5% carbon dioxide.

The compounds tested were kindly supplied by the following companies: MK 0787 and cefoxitin (Merck Sharp & Dohme), ceftriaxone (Roche), cefotaxime (Hoechst Roussel), ceftazidime (Glaxo), moxalactam (Lilly), cefoperazone (Pfizer), cefsulodin (Ciba-Geigy), metronidazole

(May & Baker), lincomycin (Upjohn), and clavulanic acid (Beecham).

Table 1 shows susceptibility of strains to each of the compounds tested. MK 0787 inhibited all strains at 1 μg/ml, and metronidazole was the only other compound with similar activity. Cefoxitin inhibited all strains at 64 μg/ml; cefsulodin and ceftazidime were of lowest activity, whereas moxalactam and cefotaxime showed high activity against most strains, with 93 and 87%, respectively, susceptible to 16 μg/ml, although a proportion of strains were very resistant to these compounds. In general, *B. thetaiotaomicron* and *B. distasonis* were more resistant than the other species tested to most of the beta-lactams investigated. MK 0787 was, as reported by others (2), extremely active against this group of organisms, with much lower MICs than with cefoxitin.

Stability of beta-lactam compounds to beta-lactamases of resistant *Bacteroides* strains. The stability of several beta-lactams to beta-lactamase hydrolysis was determined by adding sonicated cultures of resistant beta-lac-

TABLE 1. *Antimicrobial activity of eight beta-lactam antibiotics, lincomycin, and metronidazole to Bacteroides strains*

Species	No. of strains	Antibiotic	Range of MIC (μg/ml)	MIC$_{50}$[a]	MIC$_{90}$[b]
B. fragilis	38	Cefoperazone	1->128	4	32
		Moxalactam	≤0.5->128	≤0.5	8
		Ceftazidime	1->128	8	128
		Cefotaxime	≤0.5->128	2	32
		Ceftriaxone	≤0.5->128	2	64
		Cefsulodin	≤0.5->128	8	64
		MK 0787	≤0.5-1	≤0.5	≤0.5
		Cefoxitin	2-64	8	32
		Lincomycin	≤0.5-8	2	4
		Metronidazole	≤0.5-2	≤0.5	2
B. thetaiotaomicron	19	Cefoperazone	4->128	32	32
		Moxalactam	≤0.5-128	4	16
		Ceftazidime	16->128	64	>128
		Cefotaxime	1-128	16	32
		Ceftriaxone	4->128	32	64
		Cefsulodin	32->128	>128	>128
		MK 0787	≤0.5	≤0.5	≤0.5
		Cefoxitin	2-32	8	16
		Lincomycin	≤0.5-16	4	8
		Metronidazole	≤0.5-1	≤0.5	1
B. distasonis	11	Cefoperazone	4-64	32	64
		Moxalactam	1-64	8	64
		Ceftazidime	8->128	32	>128
		Cefotaxime	2-16	8	16
		Ceftriaxone	≤0.5-64	32	64
		Cefsulodin	16->128	>128	>128
		MK 0787	≤0.5-1	≤0.5	≤0.5
		Cefoxitin	8-32	16	32
		Lincomycin	2-32	4	8
		Metronidazole	≤0.5-1	≤0.5	1
B. fragilis group, other[c]	14	Cefoperazone	4->128	8	64
		Moxalactam	≤0.5-8	2	4
		Ceftazidime	4->128	32	>128
		Cefotaxime	≤0.5-128	1	32
		Ceftriaxone	1->128	2	64
		Cefsulodin	2->128	32	>128
		MK 0787	≤0.5	≤0.5	≤0.5
		Cefoxitin	2-32	16	32
		Lincomycin	≤0.5-8	2	4
		Metronidazole	≤0.5-1	≤0.5	1

[a] Lowest concentration inhibiting 50% of strains tested.

[b] Lowest concentration inhibiting 90% of strains tested.

[c] Included 13 strains of *B. vulgatus* and one of *B. ovatus*.

TABLE 2. *Inactivation after 1 h at 37°C of 10-µg/ml solution of beta-lactam compound by sonicated cultures of Bacteroides spp.*

Culture		Ceftazidime		Moxalactam		Cefoxitin		MK 0787	
Species[a]	No.	MIC	% Inactivation	MIC	% Inactivation	MIC	% Inactivation	MIC	% Inactivation
F	3	128	60	>128	78	32	0	≤0.5	0
F	5	>128	>94	>128	>94	64	71.5	1	0
F	7	>128	>94	4	0	2	0	≤0.5	0
F	10	>128	90	>128	>94	64	0	1	0
V	6	>128	>94	4	0	8	0	1	0
V	17	>128	0	4	0	16	0	≤0.5	0
T	11	>128	62	>128	>94	32	0	1	0
T	J25	>128	0	16	0	16	0	≤0.5	0
T	B209	>128	0	2	0	16	0	≤0.5	0
O	12	>128	61	16	0	32	0	≤0.5	0

[a] F, *B. fragilis*; V, *B. vulgatus*; T, *B. thetaiotaomicron*; O, *B. ovatus*.

tamase-producing *Bacteroides* strains to solutions containing known concentrations of each compound. Residual antibiotic activity was determined after 1 h of incubation at 37°C, using a standard well diffusion assay procedure.

Table 2 shows the stability of each compound tested to the enzymes of 10 *Bacteroides* strains. Cefoperazone and ceftriaxone showed total inactivation by all 10 strains. MK 0787 was completely stable to all preparations, whereas cefoxitin was stable to all except for one preparation of a strain of *B. fragilis* with an MIC of 64 µg/ml. Moxalactam was inactivated by resistant strains but unaffected by susceptible ones. Ceftazidime was completely hydrolyzed by the sonic extracts of three highly resistant strains but unaffected by three other strains which were equally resistant, indicating non-beta-lactamase-mediated resistance in these strains. This was confirmed by the fact that the effect of beta-lactamase inhibitors on the ceftazidime MICs of these strains was less marked than on strains producing substantial hydrolysis of this compound.

Effect of clavulanic acid on MICs to beta-lactam compounds. The influence of clavulanic acid on the MICs of 20 strains of *Bacteroides* was investigated by comparing MICs on media containing the compound alone or combined with clavulanic acid (2 µg/ml). All MICs to cefotaxime and ceftriaxone were reduced substantially, indicating pure enzymatic resistance to these compounds, whereas only 25% of strains showed a dramatic reduction in MIC to cefoperazone, ceftazidime, and cefsulodin, the remainder showing only a slight reduction. The four moxalactam-resistant strains showed a substantial MIC reduction in the presence of clavulanic acid; other strains were influenced to a much lesser degree. Although enzyme-mediated resistance to beta-lactams is of great significance in *Bacteroides*, other factors such as permeability barriers preventing access of drugs to the target site also play an important role with some compounds (5).

Isoelectric focusing of beta-lactamases. Isoelectric focusing was used to determine the isoelectric points of beta-lactamases produced by the resistant strains under investigation. An LKB multiphor system was used in conjunction with both narrow (pH 4 to 6.5)- and wide (pH 3.5 to 9.5)-range ampholine gels. Isoelectric points of the beta-lactamases produced by the 10 strains used for stability studies are shown in Table 2. Four strains which had high resistance to most of the beta-lactams tested, including moxalactam, produced two beta-lactamases with pI values of 4.9 and 8.0 (4). Although enzymes with a pI of 4.9 are common in this group of organisms and are normally associated with *B. fragilis*, beta-lactamases of pI 8.0 have not previously been reported in these organisms.

1. **Darland, G., and J. Birnbaum.** 1977. Cefoxitin resistance to beta-lactamase: a major factor for susceptibility of *Bacteroides fragilis* to the antibiotic. Antimicrob. Agents Chemother. **11**:723–734.
2. **Kropp, H., J. G. Sundelof, J. S. Kahan, F. M. Kahan, and M. Birnbaum.** 1980. MK 0787 (*N*-formimidoyl thienamycin): evaluation of in vitro and in vivo activities. Antimicrob. Agents Chemother. **17**:993–1000.
3. **Leung, T., and J. D. Williams.** 1978. Beta-lactamases of subspecies of *Bacteroides fragilis*. J. Antimicrob. Chemother. **4**:47–54.
4. **Maskell, J. P., and M. Nasu.** 1981. Enzyme-mediated resistance of *Bacteroides fragilis* to moxalactam. Lancet **i**:733.
5. **Olsson, B., K. Dornbusch, and C. E. Nord.** 1979. Factors contributing to resistance to beta-lactam antibiotics in *Bacteroides fragilis*. Antimicrob. Agents Chemother. **15**:263–268.

Bactericidal Activity of a Thienamycin Against *Pseudomonas aeruginosa*

ROSAMUND J. WILLIAMS* AND DAVID M. LIVERMORE

The London Hospital Medical College, London, England

Thienamycin, a recently discovered β-lactam antibiotic, has the broadest spectrum of antibacterial activity yet reported for a β-lactam. However, this activity is considerably hampered by the chemical instability of the compound. The preparation of a crystalline derivative, *N*-formimidoyl thienamycin (MK 0787), has largely overcome the problem of instability of the parent compound while retaining its antibacterial activity. In this study, we examined the activity of MK 0787 against *Pseudomonas aeruginosa* in terms of both MICs and killing curves. The susceptibility of MK 0787 to pseudomonal β-lactamases was also investigated.

MICs. The MICs of MK 0787 for 95 well-characterized clinical isolates of *P. aeruginosa* were determined by the agar dilution method, using Oxoid DST agar (CM 261) and an inoculum of approximately 5×10^3 organisms. The results were compared with those obtained with the newer cephalosporins and moxalactam tested on the same strains (Table 1). Results with gentamicin and carbenicillin are included for comparison. All isolates were susceptible to MK 0787; the MICs ranged from ≤0.5 to 8 mg/liter, with a mode MIC of 2 mg/liter. Thus the activity of MK 0787 compared very favorably with that of the new cephalosporins.

Killing curves. Killing curves were determined by inoculating 1 ml of an overnight culture of *P. aeruginosa* into 200 ml of Oxoid nutrient broth (no. 2). Cultures were incubated for 2 h at 37°C on an orbital shaker before addition of antibiotics. This resulted in an initial viable count of approximately 10^6 organisms per ml. MK 0787, gentamicin, cefsulodin, and ceftazidime solutions were prepared at concentrations such that addition of 1 ml to 200 ml of culture resulted in 4 × MIC for the test strain. Incubation was continued under the above conditions for 24 h. Viable counts were made at timed intervals by preparing 10-fold dilutions of culture samples, and 5 × 0.2-ml volumes were dropped onto nutrient agar plates and incubated overnight. Colony counts were made at suitable dilutions. Typical results are shown in Fig. 1. The viable count of MK 0787-treated cultures fell more rapidly than that of cefsulodin-treated cultures but more slowly than that of gentamicin-treated cultures. Ceftazidime inhibited growth even more slowly than cefsulodin.

Hydrolysis of MK 0787 by β-lactamases. β-Lactamases were extracted from six *P. aeruginosa* strains from our collection. These strains had previously been studied in detail, and their β-lactamases had been identified by isoelectric focusing (D. M. Livermore, R. J. Williams, and D. Williams, in press). Three strains produced type Id (Sabbath & Abraham) enzymes; the other strains produced type Vd (PSE 1), Vd (PSE 4), and IIIa (TEM 2) enzymes, respectively. β-Lactamases of type Vd (PSEs 1, 2, and 4) and type Ve (PSE 3) were also extracted from reference strains of *P. aeruginosa* kindly provided by Glaxo Group Research. For completeness, the stability of MK 0787 to hydrolysis by β-lactamase types Ia, IIIa (TEM 1), and IV was also studied by using enzyme extracts from reference strains of *Enterobacter cloacae*, *Escherichia coli*, and *Klebsiella aerogenes*, respectively. Two methods of detecting β-lactamase hydrolysis of MK 0787 were used: (i) the spectrophotometric assay of O'Callaghan et al. (2) and (ii) a bioassay system in which enzyme extract was incubated with MK 0787 for 4 h at 37°C and the mixture was placed in wells cut in agar seeded with *E. coli* 10418. The plates were incubated overnight, and β-lactamase hydrolysis was detected by comparing zones of inhibition obtained with treated and untreated MK 0787.

MK 0787 was found to be extremely stable to hydrolysis by the β-lactamases tested when examined by both methods. Enzymes of types Ia, Id, Vd, and Ve had no detectable activity against MK 0787. Only one type of β-lactamase extracted from *P. aeruginosa* was found to be active. This was a type III (TEM 2) enzyme, and

TABLE 1. *MICs of MK 0787, new cephalosporins, carbenicillin, and gentamicin for P. aeruginosa*

Antibiotic	% of *P. aeruginosa* inhibited by a concentration (mg/liter) of:									
	≤0.5	1	2	4	8	16	32	64	128	>128
MK0787	8	39	44	7	2					
Cefotaxime	0	1	0	5	27	32	15	11	8	1
Cefoperazone	1	1	30	28	15	12	11	2		
Cefsulodin	1	15	33	24	9	11	4	2	1	
Ro 13-9904	5	2	22	43	17	4	6	1		
Ceftazidime	19	41	19	15	1	5				
Moxalactam	0	1	0	14	27	21	22	9	4	2
Carbenicillin	1	0	0	0	0	2	22	29	24	22
Gentamicin	43	24	8	6	9	3	2	2	2	1

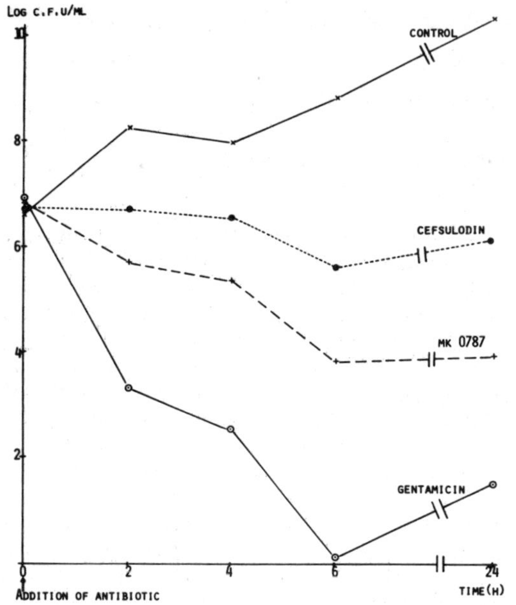

FIG. 1. *Comparative killing of P. aeruginosa by MK 0787, gentamicins, and cefsulodin.*

the degree of hydrolysis it produced was minimal. Similarly, minimal hydrolysis was detected with a TEM 1 and TEM 2 enzyme from strains of *E. coli* and a type IV enzyme from *K. aerogenes*. These results are in agreement with the findings of Richmond (3).

A 3 to 4% decomposition of MK 0787, due to chemical instability, was detected over the 40-min spectrophotometric assay. This is slightly greater than the 1% at 23°C quoted by Wildonger et al. (K. J. Wildonger, W. J. Leanza, T. W. Miller, and B. G. Christensen, Program Abstr. 11th Int. Congr. Chemother. and 19th Intersci. Conf. Antimicrob. Agents Chemother., Boston, Mass., abstr. 232, 1979) and is probably due to the temperature in the spectrophotometer (about 30°C). This was accounted for when calculating comparative rates of hydrolysis.

Relationship between susceptibility of *P. aeruginosa* to carbenicillin and MK 0787. Our collection of clinical isolates of *P. aeruginosa* could be subdivided into groups according to carbenicillin susceptibility: group A comprised susceptible strains with MIC (carbenicillin) of ≤64 mg/liter; group B comprised strains with moderate resistance, with MIC (carbenicillin) usually of 128 to 320 mg/liter; group C comprised highly resistant strains with MICs of ≥2,560 mg/liter. Resistance in group C was demonstrably due to β-lactamase production, whereas strains in group B did not produce carbenicillinases and their resistance was probably due to intrinsic mechanisms. When tested against the newer cephalosporins, group B strains showed enhanced resistance to all the cephalosporins and moxalactam, whereas group C strains showed increased resistance only to cefoperazone and cefsulodin, which are hydrolyzed by their β-lactamases, while remaining susceptible to the other new cephalosporins and moxalactam (Livermore et al., in press).

However, we found no correlation between MIC of MK 0787 and MIC of carbenicillin for *P. aeruginosa*. This is important since it suggests that MK 0787 will be active against *P. aeruginosa* strains that are resistant to carbenicillin (and the newer ureidopenicillins azlocillin, mezlocillin, and piperacillin) and against strains resistant to the antipseudomonal cephalosporins. The results also suggest that the interaction between MK 0787 and its target site on the bacterial cell differs significantly from that of the penicillins and cephalosporins. It will be interesting to see whether MK 0787 bears out its in vitro activity in vivo.

1. **Brown, A. G.** 1981. New naturally occurring β-lactam antibiotics and related compounds. J. Antimicrob. Chemother. **7**:15–48.
2. **O'Callaghan, C., P. W. Muggleton, and G. W. Ross.** 1969. Effects of β-lactamase from gram-negative organisms on cephalosporins and penicillins, p. 57–63. Antimicrob. Agents Chemother. 1968.
3. **Richmond, M. H.** 1981. The semi-synthetic thienamycin derivative MK 0787 and its properties with respect to a range of β-lactamases from clinically relevant bacterial species. J. Antimicrob. Chemother. **7**:279–285.

In Vitro Activity of *N*-Formimidoyl Thienamycin Compared with Beta-Lactamase–Stable Compounds Against Clinical Strains of *Acinetobacter calcoaceticus*

EUGÉNIE BERGOGNE-BEREZIN,* MARIE-LAURE JOLY-GUILLOU, FRANCIS MEGRAUD, AND CATHERINE VERIN

Department of Microbiology, Bichat Hospital, Paris 75877 Cedex 18, France

Thienamycin was described in 1976 (4) as a new beta-lactam antibiotic with a markedly extended spectrum of activity in vitro against both aerobic and anaerobic bacteria. Preliminary studies showed that thienamycin was very active against *Acinetobacter calcoaceticus*, an organism normally highly resistant to most beta-lactam antibiotics (2, 6). *N*-Formimidoyl thienamycin (MK 0787), a congener of thienamycin, was shown to be more stable than the parent compound and also more active than the latter (3, 8), which had been reported to be insufficiently effective when used in high concentrations. The present study was undertaken to evaluate the activity of *N*-formimidoyl thienamycin against multiresistant strains of *A. calcoaceticus*, obtained from clinical sources, compared with that of other beta-lactamase–stable cephalosporins and cephamycins.

The study included 161 *Acinetobacter* strains and 50 other clinical strains (36 *Enterobacteriaceae*, 6 *Pseudomonas aeruginosa*, and 8 *Staphylococcus aureus*). All were clinical isolates except for four reference strains of *Acinetobacter*, including three *A. calcoaceticus* var. *anitratus* (ATCC 1704, 17903, 7013) and one *Acinetobacter* var. *lwoffi* (ATCC 9036).

Acinetobacter clinical strains were isolated mainly from wounds and pus, from the respiratory and urinary tracts (123 strains), and from blood cultures (25 strains). Nine isolates were obtained from environmental sources such as ventilation equipment and catheters. The strains tested had been collected between 1971 and 1981, a decade that saw the increasing resistance of these bacteria to antibiotics (1), which hindered the therapeutic management of infectious processes due to these organisms. The strains tested in this study had been saved because of the resistance that they had shown to multiple antibiotics. Sterile standardized powders of antimicrobial agents were kindly supplied by their respective manufacturers: *N*-formimidoyl thienamycin and cefoxitin by Merck Sharp & Dohme Research Laboratories; cefamandole and moxalactam by Eli Lilly and Co.; cefotaxime by Hoechst-Roussel Pharmaceuticals, Inc.; ceftazidime by Glaxo Laboratories; and cefotiam by Ciba-Geigy Laboratories.

The MICs were determined by using the agar dilution technique: antibiotic solutions were freshly prepared every day, and serial dilutions were prepared in Mueller-Hinton agar, obtaining final concentrations of from 128 to 0.016 μg/ml, following the criteria of C. Ericsson and J. Sherris (ICS). All plates were inoculated with a multiple replicating device (Dynatech AM 80) which permits the simultaneous testing of 50 strains. The MIC was defined as the lowest concentration of drug that suppressed visible growth of the strains to be tested after incubation at 37°C for 18 h.

N-Formimidoyl thienamycin showed excellent activity against most of the resistant strains tested in this study. The geometric mean MIC was less than 0.5 μg/ml for all the groups tested except for *Pseudomonas* (6.34 μg/ml) and *Proteus* (1 μg/ml). For the 161 strains of *A. calcoaceticus*, 50% of the strains were inhibited at 0.27 μg/ml and 90% were inhibited at 0.75 μg/ml. The same values were valid for the 137 strains of *Acinetobacter* of the variety *anitratus*, whereas for *A. calcoaceticus* var. *lwoffi*, 50 and 90% of the strains were inhibited at 0.15 and 0.5 μg/ml, respectively. The geometric mean MIC for all *Acinetobacter* strains was 0.317 μg/ml, being slightly higher (0.34 μg/ml) for *A. calcoaceticus* var. *anitratus* and lower (0.2 μg/ml) for *A. calcoaceticus* var. *lwoffi*. This last result was predictable, since *Acinetobacter* var. *lwoffi* is known to be more susceptible than *A. calcoaceticus* var. *anitratus*.

The distribution of *Acinetobacter* strains inhibited at various concentrations of MK 0787 was bimodal and exhibited two peaks of susceptibilities, at 0.125 μg/ml (30.5% of the strains) and at 0.5 μg/ml (30.5% of the strains). This bimodal susceptibility to *N*-formimidoyl thienamycin had been reported in previous studies with *Acinetobacter* strains when tested with beta-lactam antibiotics, corresponding with beta-lactamase production (5). It is interesting to note that a few strains of *A. calcoaceticus* var. *anitratus* were, from the very start, less susceptible: five strains were inhibited at 2 μg/ml; one strain was inhibited at 4 μg/ml; and one strain was totally resistant at 128 μg/ml. This particular strain was examined for the presence

TABLE 1. *MICs against Acinetobacter clinical strains*

Strain	No. of strains	Antibiotic	MIC range (μg/ml)	MIC (μg/ml) for 50%	MIC (μg/ml) for 90%	Geometric mean
A. calcoaceticus	161	MK 0787	0.032–4	0.27	0.75	0.317
A. calcoaceticus var. *anitratus*	137	MK 0787	0.016–4	0.27	0.75	0.34
A. calcoaceticus var. *lwoffi*	24	MK 0787	0.016–1	0.15	0.5	0.2
A. calcoaceticus var. *anitratus*	96	Ceftazidime	0.064–128	4	42	7
	63	Cefotaxime	0.032–128	11	43	10.77
	64	Moxalactam	0.032–128	17	42	15
	64	Cefamandole	0.025–>128	80	128	57
	96	Cefotiam	0.125–>128	90	122	88.5
	64	Cefoxitin	0.25–>128	51	112	43

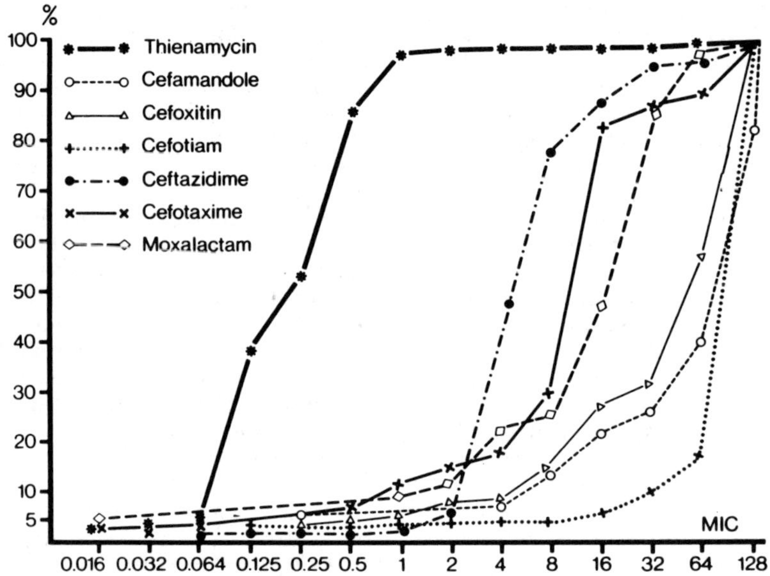

FIG. 1. *Cumulative distribution curves of susceptibilities of Acinetobacter isolates to N-formimidoyl thienamycin and six other beta-lactam antibiotics.*

of beta-lactamase, but the enzyme has not yet been characterized. MK 0787 has been described as a compound relatively stable to beta-lactamase hydrolysis and as a significant inhibitor of at least two enzymes (7). Our results suggest that at least one strain hydrolyzed *N*-formimidoyl thienamycin, possibly by means of an inducible beta-lactamase which was shown to closely resemble that of *Proteus*, *C. freundii*, and *P. aeruginosa* (5). Otherwise, the comparison of the activity of MK 0787 with that of six other cephalosporins or cephamycins showed a much higher susceptibility of *Acinetobacter* to *N*-formimidoyl thienamycin (Table 1 and Fig. 1).

In summary, this study demonstrates that *N*-formimidoyl thienamycin is a very promising new beta-lactam antibiotic. It is highly active especially against resistant strains of *A. calcoaceticus* derived from clinical sources. *N*-Formimidoyl thienamycin inhibits bacteria resistant or less susceptible to several new cephalosporins or cephamycins. Comparable results were recently published (9). Even though our results suggest a possible hydrolysis of the compound by one beta-lactamase–producing strain, MK 0787 is currently the only beta-lactam compound really active in vitro against *Acinetobacter*.

1. **Bergogne-Berezin, E., M. L. Joly, N. Moreau, and F. Le Goffic.** 1980. Aminoglycoside-modifying enzymes in clinical isolates of *Acinetobacter calcoaceticus*. Curr. Chemother. **4**:361–364.
2. **Glew, R. H., R. C. Moellering, and L. J. Kunz.** 1977. Infections with *Acinetobacter calcoaceticus* (*Herellea*

vaginicola): clinical and laboratory studies. Medicine **56:**79–87.

3. **Horadam, V. W., J. D. Smilack, C. L. Montgomery, and J. Werringloer.** 1980. In vitro activity of *N*-formimidoyl-thienamycin (MK 0787), a crystalline derivative of thienamycin. Antimicrob. Agents Chemother. **18:**4, 557–561.
4. **Kropp, H., J. S. Kahan, J. Sundelof, G. Darland, and J. Birnbaum.** 1976. Thienamycin: in vitro and in vivo evaluation. Program Abstr. Intersci. Conf. Antimicrob. Agents Chemother. 15th, Chicago, abstr. no. 228.
5. **Morohoshi, T., and T. Saito.** 1977. Beta-lactamase and beta-lactam antibiotic resistance in *Acinetobacter anitratus* (syn. *A. calcoaceticus*). J. Antibiot. **30:**969–973.
6. **Retailliau, H. F., A. W. Hightower, R. E. Dixon, and J. R. Allen.** 1979. *Acinetobacter calcoaceticus*: a nosocomial pathogen with an unusual seasonal pattern. J. Infect. Dis. **139:**371–375.
7. **Richmond, M. H.** 1981. The semi-synthetic thienamycin derivative MK 0787 and its properties with respect to a range of β-lactamases from clinically relevant bacterial species. J. Antimicrob. Chemother. **7:**279–285.

Antibacterial Activity of Thienamycin Against Clinical Isolates

P. M. SHAH, G. JUST, AND W. STILLE*

Zentrum der Inneren Medizin, J.W.-Goethe-Universität, D-6000 Frankfurt am Main 70, Federal Republic of Germany

Thienamycin is a novel β-lactam antibiotic. The in vitro activity of its *N*-formimidoyl derivative was determined against clinical isolates. Multiresistant strains were selected, and minimum inhibitory activity was determined in Mueller-Hinton agar. Viable counts were performed to evaluate the drug's bactericidal activity.

Table 1 gives the concentrations required to inhibit 50 and 90% of the strains tested in com-

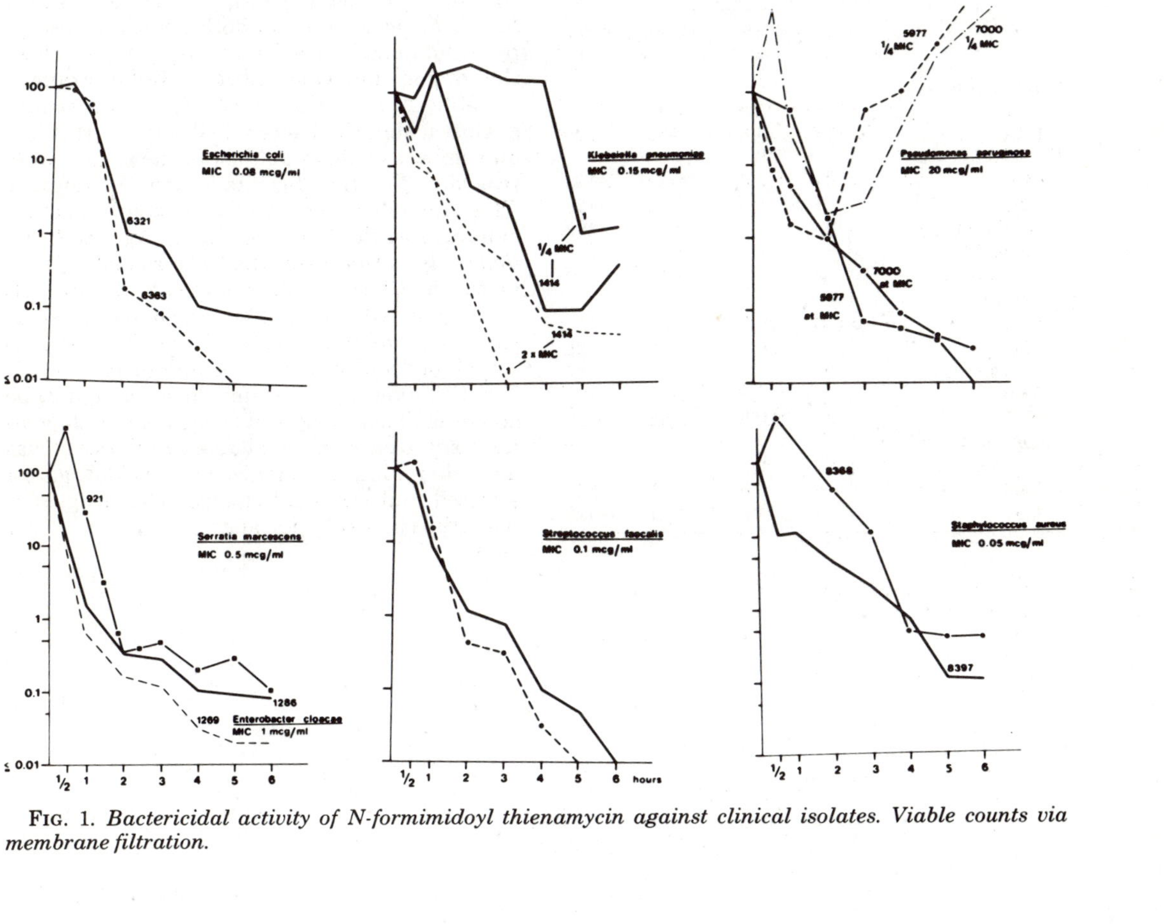

FIG. 1. *Bactericidal activity of N-formimidoyl thienamycin against clinical isolates. Viable counts via membrane filtration.*

TABLE 1. *Concentrations required to inhibit 50 and 90% of the strains studied*

Species	MIC (μg/ml)					
	Thienamycin		Cefoxitin		Cefotaxime	
	50%	90%	50%	90%	50%	90%
E. coli (*n* = 100)	0.06	0.06	8	32	0.1	1
K. pneumoniae (*n* = 50)	0.05	0.05	8	32	0.5	4
Enterobacter spp. (*n* = 50)	1	2	>64	>64	32	>64
Proteus spp. (*n* = 50)	1	2	1	2	0.125	0.125
S. aureus (*n* = 25[a])	<0.06	0.03	4	8	4	8
P. aeruginosa (*n* = 50)	2	2	ND[b]	ND	32	>64

[a] Twenty strains resistant to penicillin G.
[b] ND, Not done.

TABLE 2. *MICs of strains against which bactericidal activity of thienamycin was evaluated*

Strain	MIC (μg/ml)			
	Cefoxitin	Cefotaxime	Gentamicin	Azlocillin
K. pneumoniae				
1	>128	8	>32	>128
1414	>128	16	>32	>128
Escherichia coli				
6321	64	8	>32	>128
6363	4	0.1	2	>128
Serratia marcescens	>128	32	>32	>128
Enterobacter cloacae				
1286	>128	>32	>32	>128
1269	>128	>32	>32	>128
P. aeruginosa				
7000		>128	>32	>128
5977		>128	>32	>128
Staphylococcus aureus				
8368	8	8	1	>128
8397	8	8	1	>128

TABLE 3. *Time needed to kill 99% of the inoculum by thienamycin at 2× MIC and at one-fourth MIC*

Strain	Time (min)	
	2× MIC	¼ MIC
K. pneumoniae		
1414	120	200
1	90	300
E. coli		
6363	105	
6321	120	
Serratia marcescens	105	
E. cloacae		
1286	75	
1269	52	
P. aeruginosa		
7000	120	
5977	125	105
Staphylococcus aureus		
8368	225	
8397	217	
Streptococcus faecalis		
1602	135	
3578	105	

parison with other antibiotics. Against these strains, thienamycin was the most active compound on a weight basis. Its activity against *Staphylococcus aureus* (both penicillin susceptible and penicillin resistant) was comparable to that of penicillin G against susceptible strains.

Table 2 lists the susceptibility of strains against which the bactericidal activity of thienamycin was evaluated. Most of the strains were resistant to the β-lactams and gentamicin. Thienamycin at 2× MIC was rapidly bactericidal against these strains (Fig. 1). Against *Pseudomonas aeruginosa*, the bactericidal activity at the MIC was evaluated. Even at sub-MIC levels (1/4 MIC against *Pseudomonas* and *Klebsiella pneumoniae*), 99% of the three strains were killed within 105 to 300 min (Table 3).

N-Formimidoyl thienamycin was found to be active against a variety of nosocomial pathogens resistant to currently available antibiotics. It was not only inhibitory, but also bactericidal against selected multiresistant strains. The drug is of potential clinical importance.

In Vitro Activity of *N*-Formimidoyl Thienamycin Against *Pseudomonas* and Staphylococci Associated with Endocarditis

CHARLES KALLICK,* THOMAS RICE, JEANETTE NORSEN, K. RAJASHEKARAIAH, DAYLE MARSH, DORIS McCULLEY, AND KALOO THADHANI

Division of Infectious Disease, Department of Medicine, Cook County Hospital, Chicago, Illinois 60612, U.S.A.

Major organisms causing endocarditis in drug addicts, especially those at Cook County Hospital, are *Pseudomonas aeruginosa* and *Staphylococcus aureus*. Clinical experience at this hospital and elsewhere suggests that only one third of all cases caused by *P. aeruginosa* are curable by conventional medical therapy. Therapy for *Pseudomonas* endocarditis has traditionally consisted of an aminoglycoside with carbenicillin or ticarcillin. Virtually no patients with left-sided involvement caused by *Pseudomonas* will survive without surgical intervention. The mortality rate associated with surgical intervention is extremely high (50%) (1–3).

The reasons for increased morbidity with *Pseudomonas* infection are not known, although speculations have been made in regard to concentrations of bactericidal antibiotics beneath the fibrin vegetations of the lesions of infective endocarditis. Carbenicillin with an aminoglycoside may not achieve optimal bactericidal concentrations in what amounts to a sequestered space. *N*-Formimidoyl thienamycin (NFTM) appears potentially more active against *Pseudomonas* than alternative β-lactam antibiotics. We undertook to study the growth inhibition, bactericidal activity, and killing kinetics of this agent to ascertain whether it held promise in treatment of endocarditis caused by these organisms. Twenty-seven strains of *P. aeruginosa* and 19 strains of *S. aureus* were available, having been isolated from patients with infective endocarditis at this institution. MICs were determined by the agar dilution method with the use of Mueller-Hinton agar and an inoculum of approximately 5×10^5 colony-forming units per ml. Bactericidal concentrations were determined by the macrotube dilution method with the use of Trypticase soy broth and an inoculum of 5×10^5 colony-forming units per ml. Killing curves on these isolates were determined with 5-ml Trypticase soy broth cultures. Subcultures were taken at 0, 2, 5, and 24 h. Tenfold serial dilutions were plated to obtain viable counts. Antibiotic stability was determined by utilizing NFTM at an initial concentration of 5 μg/ml in Trypticase soy broth incubated at 37°C. Samples were taken and the activity was determined by agar diffusion bioassay at 0, 2, 4, 8, and 24 h.

For *P. aeruginosa* the modal MICs of the antibiotics tested were as follows: tobramycin, 1.0 μg/ml; NFTM, 2 μg/ml; piperacillin, 8 μg/ml; moxalactam, 16 μg/ml; ticarcillin, 32 μg/ml; and carbenicillin, 64 μg/ml. For *S. aureus* the modal MICs of the antibiotics tested were as follows: oxacillin, 0.25 μg/ml; clindamycin, 0.12 μg/ml; and NFTM, $\leq$0.015 μg/ml. Macrotube dilution susceptibility testing of NFTM revealed that for most strains of *S. aureus* and *P. aeruginosa*, the MBC was significantly higher than the MIC.

Killing kinetics were determined for selected strains of *P. aeruginosa* and *S. aureus*. The strains of *P. aeruginosa* selected were ones which were least susceptible to the bactericidal activity of NFTM. During the initial phase (5 h), killing was more rapid with NFTM at 8 μg/ml than with carbenicillin (50 μg/ml) or tobramycin (1 μg/ml). However, all tubes showed visible growth after 24 h of incubation. This was

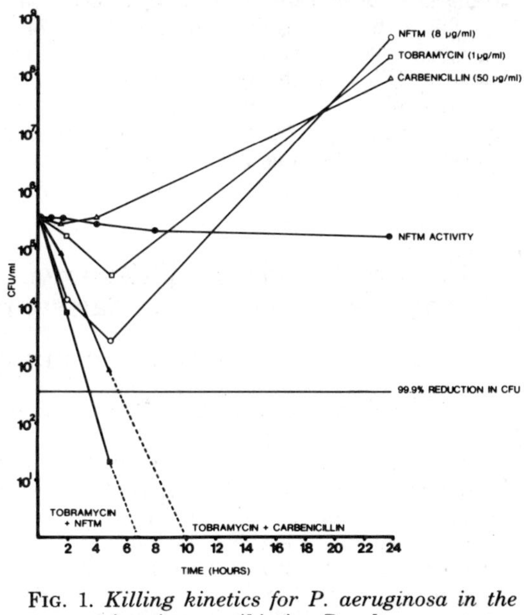

FIG. 1. *Killing kinetics for P. aeruginosa in the presence of various antibiotics. Results are average values for nine strains. Dashed lines represent projections. All 24-h subcultures with tobramycin plus carbenicillin or tobramycin plus NFTM had* $\leq 10^1$ *colony-forming units per ml.*

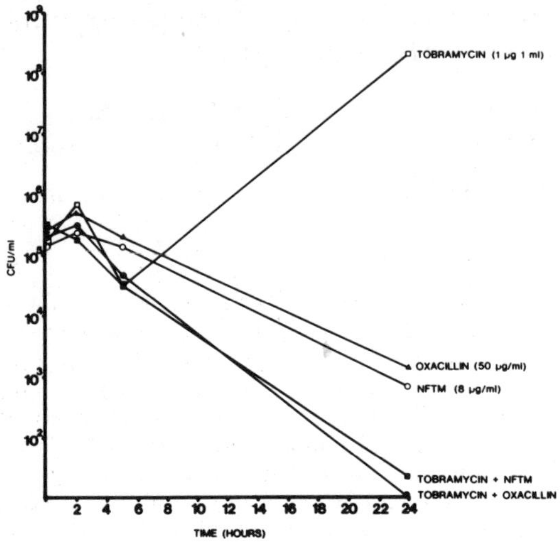

FIG. 2. *Killing kinetics for a representative tolerant strain of S. aureus in the presence of various antibiotics.*

apparently due (in the case of NFTM) to the appearance in broth of organisms with intermediate susceptibility to NFTM (16 μg/ml), although the MIC of other β-lactam antibiotics was not altered. NFTM in combination with tobramycin (1 μg/ml) was more rapidly bactericidal than carbenicillin plus tobramycin for all strains of *P. aeruginosa* tested, showing at least a 99.9% reduction in viable organisms at 24 h (Fig. 1). For selected strains of *S. aureus*, killing rates for NFTM were similar to those obtained with oxacillin. Enhanced killing against *S. aureus* was observed when tobramycin was combined with NFTM (Fig. 2).

We conclude from these data that NFTM is 32 times more active in growth inhibition than carbenicillin and 4 times more active than piperacillin for *P. aeruginosa* isolates from our endocarditis patients. NFTM is 10 to 20 times more active in growth inhibition than oxacillin or clindamycin for *S. aureus* isolates from endocarditis patients. The majority of *S. aureus* strains tested were tolerant to the bactericidal activity of NFTM. A combination of NFTM and tobramycin was bactericidal for the selected tolerant strains tested. The majority of *P. aeruginosa* strains were not completely killed by NFTM (8 μg/ml) at 24 h. This was due to the appearance in broth of moderately resistant organisms. A combination of NFTM plus tobramycin was rapidly bactericidal for all strains tested. We conclude that NFTM is a potentially effective agent for treatment of bacterial endocarditis caused by *S. aureus*, and in combination with tobramycin is potentially effective against *P. aeruginosa* strains causing this syndrome. This drug with an aminoglycoside offers hope for an improvement in the proportion of medical cures in endocarditis caused by *P. aeruginosa*. This combination may be of value as initial broad-spectrum therapy for endocarditis in all patients with this syndrome.

1. **Cohn, P. S., J. H. McGuire, and L. Weinstein.** 1980. Infective endocarditis caused by gram negative bacteria. A review of the literature, 1945–1977. Progr. Cardvasc. Dis. **22**:205–242.
2. **Reyes, M. P., W. J. Brown, and M. Lerner.** 1978. Treatment of patients with high dose aminoglycoside and carbenicillin therapy. Medicine (Baltimore) **57**:57–67.
3. **Saroff, A. L., D. Armstrong, and W. D. Johnson.** 1973. Pseudomonas endocarditis. Am. J. Cardiol. **32**:234–237.

In Vitro Activity of Thienamycin and Cefoxitin Against *Bacteroides fragilis* and Other Cephalosporinase-Positive *Bacteroides* Species

H. WERNER,* C. KRASEMANN, AND R. HAMMANN

Institute of Medical Microbiology and Immunology, Bonn, Federal Republic of Germany

Bacteroides fragilis and *B. thetaiotaomicron*, which account for about 90% of anaerobic infections in humans, are the most resistant of all anaerobes to antimicrobial agents. Both species as well as many other members of the *Bacteroides* group (e.g., *B. bivius*) are able to produce beta-lactamases, which are especially active against cephaloridine and most other cephalosporins (4, 5). Inactivation of broad-spectrum beta-lactam antibiotics by *Bacteroides* enzymes might well be a crucial point in the treatment of aerobic-anaerobic polymicrobial infections, and substances with good activity against *B. fragilis* and other beta-lactamase-producing *Bacteroides* species are needed.

The first beta-lactam antibiotic to have high stability against *Bacteroides* enzymes was cefoxitin. Quite recently, the new beta-lactam antibiotic thienamycin was also found to be resistant against beta-lactamases of anaerobes (1, 2). We therefore investigated the antibacterial activity of thienamycin against a total of 132 fresh clinical isolates of *Bacteroides* spp. in comparison with that of cefoxitin and cephalothin. With *B. fragilis* and other saccharolytic species, agar dilution and broth dilution tests, described in detail elsewhere (6, 7), were simultaneously performed to study the influence of the method on the outcome of the test. *B. splanchnicus*, members of the *B. oralis/B. bivius* group, *B. melaninogenicus*, and *B. asaccharolyticus* were exclusively studied in agar dilution tests. Additionally, MBCs were determined by subculturing the several suspensions of the broth dilution test after reading the MICs.

The high resistance of *B. fragilis*, *B. thetaiotaomicron*, and related saccharolytic species as well as certain strains of the *B. oralis/B. bivius* group to cephalothin was confirmed. The MICs ranged from 4 to >256 μg/ml. All strains of *B. melaninogenicus* and *B. asaccharolyticus* were susceptible to cephalothin (MICs from ≦0.125

TABLE 1. *In vitro activity of thienamycin against Bacteroides species*

Species	No.	Test[a]	No. of strains inhibited at each concentration (μg/ml)									
			≦0.015	0.03	0.06	0.125	0.25	0.5	1	2	4	8
B. fragilis	27	A				1	5	18	1	1	1	
		B		1	1	7	12	4			1	1
B. thetaiotaomicron	51	A						17	33	1		
		B		1	6	13	27	3		1		
B. vulgatus	12	A						6	4	2		
		B				1	3	8				
B. distasonis	5	A							2	3		
		B					2	2	1			
B. variabilis	7	A						3	2	2		
		B		1		1		4		1		
B. uniformis	5	A				1	1	1	2			
		B			2	1	1	1				
B. splanchnicus	2	A			1	1						
B. oralis group	6	A		1	3	2						
B. melaninogenicus subsp. *melaninogenicus*	4	A	1	1	2							
B. melaninogenicus subsp. *intermedius*	3	A		3								
B. asaccharolyticus	10	A	6	2	2							

[a] A, Agar dilution test; B, broth dilution test.

TABLE 2. *In vitro activity of cefoxitin against Bacteroides species*

Species	No.	Test[a]	No. of strains inhibited at each concentration (μg/ml)										
			≦0.125	0.25	0.5	1	2	4	8	16	32	64	128
B. fragilis	27	A							6	19	2		
		B					4	17	4	2			
B. thetaiotaomicron	51	A						1		2	21	27	
		B					1	1	2	18	15	11	3
B. vulgatus	12	A				1		3	7	1			
		B				1	4	6		1			
B. distasonis	5	A							1		4		
		B					1		3	1			
B. variabilis	7	A						4	2			1	
		B				2	2	2		1			
B. uniformis	5	A						2	1	2			
		B					2	3					
B. splanchnicus	2	A				2							
B. oralis group	6	A				1	4	1					
B. melaninogenicus subsp. *melaninogenicus*	4	A		1	1	1	1						
B. melaninogenicus subsp. *intermedius*	3	A		2	1								
B. asaccharolyticus	10	A	3	3	3		1						

[a] A, Agar dilution test; B, broth dilution test.

to 4 μg/ml). The results obtained for thienamycin and cefoxitin are given in Tables 1 and 2. Against all strains tested, thienamycin showed a better antibacterial activity than cefoxitin. Most strains of *B. fragilis* were inhibited in agar dilution tests by 0.25 to 0.5 μg of thienamycin per ml compared with cefoxitin MICs of 8 to 16 μg/ml. *B. thetaiotaomicron* exhibited slightly to moderately higher MICs, namely, 0.5 to 1 μg of thienamycin per ml and 32 to 64 μg of cefoxitin per ml, in agar dilution tests. However, the difference between *B. fragilis* and *B. thetaiotaomicron* was virtually unrecognizable in the broth dilution tests.

Good susceptibility to both substances was found in members of *B. splanchnicus*, *B. oralis*/*B. bivius*, *B. melaninogenicus*, and *B. asaccharolyticus*. The agar dilution MICs did not exceed 4 μg/ml for cefoxitin and 0.125 μg/ml for thienamycin (Tables 1 and 2).

With both cefoxitin and thienamycin, as a rule the broth dilution technique yielded lower MICs than the agar dilution technique, the difference mostly being one to two dilution steps. The comparatively higher broth dilution MICs determined with other cephalosporins, which are sensitive to *Bacteroides* β-lactamases, can at least in part be attributed to the larger amount of enzyme in the fluid medium (3). The opposite phenomenon with cefoxitin and thienamycin cannot, however, be explained by the stability of these substances to the *Bacteroides* β-lactamases: with moxalactam, a substance stable to the *Bacteroides* β-lactamases, broth MICs were regularly found to be higher than the corresponding agar MICs (6).

The MBCs varied over a wide range. For some strains the MICs and MBCs of thienamycin, cefoxitin, and cephalothin were either identical or very close together. Certain strains showed MBCs which were up to five or more dilution steps higher than the MIC. Whether these latter strains are susceptible or resistant to cefoxitin and thienamycin in vivo remains to be elucidated.

With regard to its in vitro activity, thienamycin seems to be a promising substance for the therapy of anaerobic or mixed anaerobic-aerobic infections, which are frequently encountered in gynecology and colon surgery.

1. **Brown, J. E., and V. E. Del Bene.** 1980. In vitro activity of *N*-formimidoyl thienamycin and other beta-lactam antibiotics against *Bacteroides fragilis*: contribution of beta-lactamase to resistance. Program Abstr. Intersci. Conf. Antimicrob. Agents Chemother. 20th, New Orleans, abstr. no. 261.
2. **Butler, T., F. P. Tally, and S. L. Gorbach.** 1980. The interaction of *Bacteroides* with moxalactam, cefoperazone, thienamycin, cefoxitin, and cephalothin. Intersci. Conf. Antimicrob. Agents Chemother. 20th, New Orleans, abstr. no. 268.
3. **Krasemann, C., and H. Werner.** 1978. Susceptibility of *Bacteroidaceae*, *Peptococcaceae*, and *Clostridium* spp. to cefazoline and cefamandole, p. 293–295. *In* Current chemotherapy. American Society for Microbiology, Washington D.C.
4. **Leung, T., and J. D. Williams.** 1978. β-lactamases of subspecies of *Bacteroides fragilis*. J. Antimicrob. Chemother. **4**:47–54.
5. **Saylers, A. A., J. Wong, and T. D. Wilkins.** 1977. Beta-lactamase activity in strains of *Bacteroides melaninogenicus* and *Bacteroides oralis*. Antimicrob. Agents Chemother. **11**:142–146.
6. **Werner, H., and C. Krasemann.** 1980. In-vitro-Aktivität des Oxa-Beta-Laktams LY 127 935 gegenüber Bacteroides fragilis und anderen anaeroben gramnegativen Stäbchen. Infection **8**(Suppl. 3):342–346.

In Vitro Activity of *N*-Formimidoyl Thienamycin (MK 0787) Alone and Combined with Other β-Lactam Compounds and Gentamicin

STEPHEN H. ZINNER* AND JEAN KLASTERSKY

Department of Medicine, Roger Williams General Hospital, Brown University, Providence, Rhode Island 02908, U.S.A., and Departement of Medicine, Laboratoire de Investigation Clinique de H. Tagnon, Institut Jules Bordet, Université Libre de Bruxelles, Brussels, Belgium*

N-Formimidoyl thienamycin (NFT) is a crystalline derivative of the new β-lactam, thienamycin (1). This agent has potent activity against a broad range of organisms including *Staphylococcus aureus* and *Pseudomonas aeruginosa* (1). Combinations of β-lactam antibiotics plus aminoglycosides as well as combinations of two β-lactam agents have been used clinically, especially in the treatment of bacteremia in neutropenic patients with cancer. This study was designed to evaluate the in vitro activities of NFT alone and in combination with four other new β-lactam antibiotics and gentamicin.

In vitro checkerboard assays using microtiter plates were performed in Mueller-Hinton broth supplemented with calcium (50 mg/liter) and magnesium (20 mg/liter). Five strains each of *Escherichia coli*, *Serratia marcescens*, *Klebsiella pneumoniae*, and *Proteus* species were studied at a final inoculum of 10^5 organisms per ml, and five strains each of *S. aureus* and *P. aeruginosa* were studied at an inoculum of 10^6 organisms per ml. The MICs and MBCs were determined for NFT and for azlocillin, cefoperazone, cefotaxime, moxalactam, and gentamicin alone and in combination with NFT. MICs were read as the lowest concentrations of antibiotic inhibiting growth as determined by visualization of the wells after overnight incubation at 37°C. MBCs were determined by replicate inoculation of approximately 0.02 ml onto antibiotic-free solid media and subsequent overnight incubation at 37°C. The MBC was read as the lowest concentration producing a 99.9% reduction in the original inoculum. All assays were performed in duplicate, and the average of the two determinations was used in the calculations.

To assess the presence of synergism or antagonism with the antibiotic combinations, fractional inhibitory concentration (FIC) and fractional bactericidal concentration (FBC) indices were calculated (2):

$$\Sigma FIC \text{ (FIC index)} = \text{MIC of antibiotic A in presence of antibiotic B/MIC of A alone} + \text{MIC of B in presence of A/MIC of B alone}$$

Synergism is present if the FIC or FBC index is <1, and antagonism is present if these index values exceed 2. Indifference or an additive effect is represented by an index value of 1 to 2.

Most of the organisms were susceptible to all of the antibiotics although one strain of *P. aeruginosa* was resistant to gentamicin (MIC = 6 μg/ml) and three strains of *P. aeruginosa* were resistant to cefotaxime and moxalactam. One strain of *E. coli* was resistant to azlocillin and one strain each of *S. marcescens* and *S. aureus* was resistant to gentamicin.

Of the β-lactam agents, NFT was most active against *P. aeruginosa* (MIC = 0.8 to 2.7 μg/ml) and *S. aureus* (MIC = 0.016 to 0.18 μg/ml), and the MIC of NFT was not greater than 2.7 μg/ml for any of the 30 organisms tested.

Median FIC and FBC indices are presented in Table 1. Synergism was found with double β-lactam combinations primarily against *Proteus* species and *S. aureus*. High FIC and FBC indices suggestive of marked antagonism were found

TABLE 1. *Median FIC and FBC indices for NFT (MK 0787) with other antibiotics*

Organism (no.)	MK 0787									
	Azlocillin		Cefoperazone		Cefotaxime		Moxalactam		Gentamicin	
	ΣFIC	ΣFBC	ΣFIC	ΣFBC	ΣFIC	ΣFBC	ΣFIC	ΣFBC	ΣFIC	ΣFBC
E. coli (5)	0.75	0.75	0.97	0.75	1.0	1.5	1.0	1.0	2.0	2.0
P. aeruginosa (5)	8.5	4.3	4.7	4.5	4.5	4.5	2.5	2.0	1.0	1.0
S. marcescens (5)	1.0	1.0	2.0	1.0	2.0	1.5	2.0	2.0	1.5	1.5
K. pneumoniae (5)	1.0	0.83	0.85	0.81	1.0	1.0	0.75	0.75	2.0	2.0
Proteus spp. (5)	0.75	0.75	0.5	0.5	0.63	0.59	0.42	0.46	2.0	2.0
S. aureus (5)	0.75	0.75	0.75	0.75	0.75	0.75	1.0	1.0	1.0	2.0

TABLE 2. *Number of strains showing synergism[a] (bactericidal) with NFT (MK 0787) and other antibiotics*

Organism (no.)	MK 0787														
	Azlocillin			Cefoperazone			Cefotaxime			Moxalactam			Gentamicin		
	S	I	A	S	I	A	S	I	A	S	I	A	S	I	A
E. coli (5)	4	1	0	3	2	0	0	5	0	1	4	0	0	5	0
P. aeruginosa (5)	0	1	4	1	1	3	0	1	4	0	3	2	1	4	0
S. marcescens (5)	2	1	2	1	2	2	0	4	1	0	5	0	2	3	0
K. pneumoniae (5)	3	2	0	5	0	0	1	4	0	3	2	0	0	5	0
Proteus spp. (5)	5	0	0	5	0	0	3	2	0	5	0	0	0	3	2
S. aureus (5)	4	1	0	4	1	0	5	0	0	1	4	0	1	4	0
Total	18[f]	6	6	19[f]	6	5	9	16	5	10	18	2	4[f]	24	2

$P < 0.05$ (Azlocillin S vs. Cefotaxime S)

$P < 0.05$ (Cefoperazone S vs. Cefotaxime S)

$P < 0.05$ (Cefoperazone S vs. Moxalactam S)

[a] S (synergism) = FBC index <1; I (indifference) = FBC index of 1 to 2; A (antagonism) = FBC index >2. Superscript f: $P < 0.001$.

with NFT plus other β-lactam agents against *P. aeruginosa*. Most other organisms were affected indifferently by the tested combinations.

The number of strains affected synergistically or antagonistically by the combinations in a bactericidal assay is presented in Table 2. Synergism was more frequent with thienamycin plus azlocillin and thienamycin plus cefoperazone than with the other combinations. Antagonism was found with double β-lactam combinations only against *P. aeruginosa* and *S. marcescens*. Thienamycin plus gentamicin was antagonistic against two strains of *Proteus*.

These data suggest that NFT is very active in vitro against *E. coli*, *P. aeruginosa*, *S. marcescens*, *K. pneumoniae*, *Proteus* species, and *S. aureus*. Azlocillin, cefoperazone, cefotaxime, and moxalactam were also active against these organisms, but their activities against *P. aeruginosa* and *S. aureus* were less than that of NFT.

These results also suggest that thienamycin combined with other new β-lactam agents or gentamicin does not produce much in vitro synergism. The high degree of antagonism found when NFT was combined with these β-lactam agents against *P. aeruginosa* suggests that double β-lactam combinations should not be used to treat infections with these organisms.

1. **Kropp, H., J. G. Sundelof, J. S. Kahan, F. H. Kahan, and J. Birnbaum.** 1980. Evaluation of in vitro and in vivo activity (MK-0787) N-formimidoyl thienamycin. Antimicrob. Agents Chemother. **17**:93–1000.
2. **Parsley, T. L., R. B. Provonchee, C. Glicksman, and S. H. Zinner.** 1977. Synergistic activity of trimethoprim and amikacin against gram-negative bacilli. Antimicrob. Agents Chemother. **12**:349–352.

In Vitro Comparison of Newer β-Lactam Antibiotics Against Aerobic Blood Culture Isolates

KEVIN R. FORWARD, GODFREY K. M. HARDING,* GLORIA GRAY, BARBARA URIAS, TERYL WADE, AND ALLAN R. RONALD

Departments of Medical Microbiology and Medicine, University of Manitoba, and the Health Sciences Centre, Winnipeg, Manitoba, Canada*

The recent development of extended-spectrum β-lactam antibiotics and their availability for clinical investigation offer the prospect of single-agent management of life-threatening infections associated with bacteremia. The broad antimicrobial spectra and high therapeutic indices of these newer agents are desirable for initial empirical therapy of severe infections. Numerous previous in vitro studies have documented the extended antimicrobial spectra of newer agents including cefotaxime (HR-756), moxalactam (LY 127935), cefoperazone (T-1551) and ceftazidime (GR 20263) (1, 3). Azlocillin, a newer ureidopenicillin, is not yet available in North America, but has been undergoing extensive clinical trials and has a very broad spectrum of activity. *N*-Formimidoyl thienamycin (MK 0787), a novel β-lactam agent, also has activity against a remarkably broad range of organisms (2). Although the spectrum of activity of each of these agents has been defined for routine clinical isolates and for selected samples of resistant organisms, available data for comparing the relative efficacy of these six agents are limited. We therefore compared the activity of the above agents with that of seven presently available antibiotics against 693 aerobic blood culture isolates recovered between 1 January 1978 and 30 June 1980.

Over the 30-month period, 2,903 blood culture isolates were recovered consecutively from 2,013 patients. Isolates from postmortem cultures and other organisms judged to be likely contaminants were not tested. Only a single agent was selected when multiple cultures from the same patient were positive for the same organism. Of the 1,076 organisms deemed suitable for antimicrobial susceptibility testing, random samples were chosen of species of frequently occurring organisms. In all, 693 aerobic blood culture isolates were tested.

MICs were determined by the agar dilution technique with the use of a Steers replicator device. The strains isolated included 77 strains of *Haemophilus influenzae*, 150 strains of *Staphylococcus aureus*, 141 strains of *Streptococcus pneumoniae*, and 66 strains of viridans streptococci, of which smaller random samples were selected. There were 77 anaerobic isolates which were not tested, and 58 aerobic isolates were not retrievable from stock cultures.

The comparative inhibitory activities of six newer agents and six other agents which are presently available are shown in Tables 1 and 2.

TABLE 1. *Comparative activity of N-formimidoyl thienamycin (NFT) and other agents against aerobic gram-negative bacilli isolated from blood cultures*

Organism (no.) and antibiotic	MIC (μg/ml) Range	50%[a]	90%
***Escherichia coli* (188)**			
NFT	0.06–32	0.25	0.5
Cefotaxime	<0.03–1	0.06	0.125
Moxalactam	0.03–8	0.125	0.25
Ceftazidime	0.03–2	0.25	0.5
Cefoperazone	0.03–128	0.125	2
Cefoxitin	0.03–>64	4	8
Cefamandole	0.03–>64	0.5	4
Cefazolin	0.03–>64	1	4
Azlocillin	0.125–>256	8	>256
Ticarcillin	0.125–>256	4	>256
Ampicillin	0.125–>64	8	>64
Tobramycin	0.03–8	1	2
***Klebsiella* spp. (71)**			
NFT	<0.03–2	0.25	1
Cefotaxime	0.03–0.06	0.03	0.06
Moxalactam	0.03–0.5	0.125	0.5
Ceftazidime	0.03–1	0.25	0.5
Cefoperazone	0.03–32	0.25	2
Cefoxitin	0.03–>64	8	16
Cefamandole	0.03–32	0.5	2
Cefazolin	0.03–64	2	4
Azlocillin	0.125–>256	32	128
Ticarcillin	0.125–>256	128	>256
Ampicillin	0.25–>64	>64	>64
Tobramycin	0.03–4	1	2
***Acinetobacter* spp. (16)**			
NFT	<0.03–0.5	0.25	0.5
Cefotaxime	0.125–64	16	64
Moxalactam	8–256	32	128
Ceftazidime	2–64	8	32
Cefoperazone	0.5–128	64	128
Cefoxitin	16–>64	>64	>64
Cefamandole	16–>64	>64	>64
Cefazolin	>64	>64	>64
Azlocillin	8–64	64	64
Ticarcillin	4–256	16	256
Ampicillin	8–128	64	64
Tobramycin	0.06–64	1	4
***Proteus mirabilis* (23)**			
NFT	0.25–16	4	8
Cefotaxime	0.06–16	0.06	0.5
Moxalactam	0.125–>64	0.125	>64
Ceftazidime	0.25–32	0.25	16
Cefoperazone	0.25–64	1	8
Cefoxitin	1–>64	4	>64
Cefamandole	0.25–>64	2	8
Cefazolin	2–>64	16	>64
Azlocillin	1–>256	64	>256
Ticarcillin	0.25–>256	8	>256
Ampicillin	2–>64	64	>64
Tobramycin	0.25–16	0.5	16
***P. aeruginosa* (39)**			
NFT	<0.03–256	2	4
Cefotaxime	2–64	8	32
Moxalactam	4–32	8	16
Ceftazidime	0.03–8	2	4
Cefoperazone	2–64	4	16
Cefoxitin	8–>64	>64	>64
Cefamandole	8–>64	>64	>64
Cefazolin	8–>64	>64	>64
Azlocillin	0.125–32	4	16
Ticarcillin	1–>256	16	32
Ampicillin	16–>64	>64	>64
Tobramycin	0.03–32	0.5	1
***Pseudomonas* spp. (15)**			
NFT	<0.03–>256	4	>256
Cefotaxime	0.03–>128	64	256
Moxalactam	0.03–128	16	128
Ceftazidime	0.03–>128	16	64
Cefoperazone	0.03–128	64	128
Cefoxitin	8–>64	>64	>64
Cefamandole	8–>64	>64	>64
Cefazolin	8–>64	>64	>64
Azlocillin	0.125–>256	32	256
Ticarcillin	0.5–>256	256	>256
Ampicillin	8–>64	64	>64
Tobramycin	0.03–64	32	64
***Enterobacter* spp. (16)**			
NFT	<0.03–2	0.25	1
Cefotaxime	0.03–0.5	0.06	0.5
Moxalactam	0.03–25	0.06	0.25
Ceftazidime	0.03–1	0.5	0.5
Cefoperazone	0.03–1	0.125	1
Cefoxitin	0.03–>64	>64	>64
Cefamandole	0.03–>64	1	8
Cefazolin	0.03–>64	64	>64
Azlocillin	0.125–128	8	64
Ticarcillin	0.125–128	1	128
Ampicillin	0.125–>64	64	>64
Tobramycin	0.03–2	0.5	1
***Serratia marcescens* (6)**			
NFT	0.25–32	0.25	32
Cefotaxime	<0.03–2	0.125	2
Moxalactam	0.125–5	0.25	0.5
Ceftazidime	0.125–.5	0.25	0.5
Cefoperazone	0.125–64	0.5	64
Cefoxitin	8–>64	8	>64
Cefamandole	2–>64	32	>64
Cefazolin	>64	>64	>64
Azlocillin	4–256	16	256
Ticarcillin	0.5–8	2	8
Ampicillin	32–>64	>64	>64
Tobramycin	0.5–4	1	4
***H. influenzae* (39)**			
NFT	1–>8	2	8
Cefotaxime	0.03–0.25	0.03	0.06
Moxalactam	0.03–1	0.03	0.25
Ceftazidime	0.03–0.5	0.06	0.25
Cefoperazone	0.03–1	0.03	0.5
Cefoxitin	2–>16	4	8
Cefamandole	0.03–0.25	0.06	0.125
Cefazolin	4–32	4	8
Azlocillin	0.06–2	0.125	2
Ticarcillin	0.06–1	0.125	1
Ampicillin	0.25–8	0.5	4
Tobramycin	0.5–32	4	4
Miscellaneous aerobes (27)			
NFT	<0.03–4	0.25	0.5
Cefotaxime	0.03–0.125	0.03	0.125
Moxalactam	0.03–8	0.125	0.25
Ceftazidime	0.03–1	0.25	0.5
Cefoperazone	0.03–8	0.125	1
Cefoxitin	0.03–>64	1	32
Cefamandole	0.03–8	0.25	4
Cefazolin	0.03–>64	1	>64
Azlocillin	0.03–>256	4	256
Ticarcillin	0.03–>256	2	128
Ampicillin	0.125–>64	8	>64
Tobramycin	0.03–8	1	4

[a] Percentage of strains.

TABLE 2. *Comparative activity of N-formimidoyl thienamycin (NFT) and other agents against aerobic gram-positive cocci and anaerobic blood culture isolates*

Organism (no.) and antibiotic	MIC (μg/ml) Range	50%[a]	90%
S. aureus (49)			
NFT	<0.03–1	0.03	0.06
Cefotaxime	<0.03–8	2	4
Moxalactam	<0.03–>32	16	16
Ceftazidime	<0.03–32	16	32
Cefoperazone	<0.03–8	2	4
Cefoxitin	<0.03–16	2	8
Cefamandole	0.03–4	0.25	0.5
Cefazolin	<0.03–2	0.25	1
Azlocillin	0.125–>64	2	8
Ticarcillin	0.125–32	2	8
Ampicillin	0.125–32	2	16
Tobramycin	<0.03–32	0.06	0.5
Cloxacillin	<0.125–8	<0.125	0.5
S. epidermidis (44)			
NFT	0.03–32	0.125	0.5
Cefotaxime	0.25–64	2	16
Moxalactam	8–>128	32	64
Ceftazidime	8–128	16	32
Cefoperazone	0.5–8	1	4
Cefoxitin	1–64	4	16
Cefamandole	0.06–2	0.25	1
Cefazolin	0.125–2	0.25	1
Azlocillin	0.125–16	2	8
Ticarcillin	0.5–>64	4	16
Ampicillin	0.25–64	4	16
Tobramycin	<0.03–>64	0.06	64
Cloxacillin	<0.125–64	0.5	2
S. faecalis (22)			
NFT	2–8	2	2
Cefotaxime	>128	>128	>128
Moxalactam	>64	>64	>64
Ceftazidime	>128	>128	>128
Cefoperazone	16–64	32	64
Cefoxitin	32–>64	>64	>64
Cefamandole	32–64	32	32
Cefazolin	16–>64	16	32
Azlocillin	1–8	1	4
Ticarcillin	32–128	32	64
Ampicillin	2–8	2	2
Tobramycin	16–>64	32	64
Cloxacillin	16–>64	32	64
S. pyogenes (18)			
NFT	<0.03	<0.03	<0.03
Cefotaxime	<0.03	<0.03	<0.03
Moxalactam	0.5–1	1	1
Ceftazidime	0.03–0.5	0.125	0.25
Cefoperazone	<0.03–0.125	0.06	0.125
Cefoxitin	0.5–2	1	2
Cefamandole	<0.03	<0.03	<0.03
Cefazolin	<0.03–0.06	<0.03	0.06
Azlocillin	<0.125	<0.125	<0.125
Ticarcillin	0.125–0.05	0.125	0.25
Ampicillin	<0.125	<0.125	<0.125
Tobramycin	2–8	2	8
Cloxacillin	<0.125–1	<0.125	0.5
S. agalactiae (23)			
NFT	<0.03–0.06	<0.03	0.06
Cefotaxime	<0.03	<0.03	<0.03
Moxalactam	1–8	8	8
Ceftazidime	0.25–0.5	0.5	0.5
Cefoperazone	0.125–0.25	0.25	0.25
Cefoxitin	1–8	8	8
Cefamandole	<0.03–0.06	<0.03	0.06
Cefazolin	<0.03–0.125	0.125	0.125
Azlocillin	<0.125	<0.125	<0.125
Ticarcillin	0.25–2	2	2
Ampicillin	<0.125	<0.125	<0.125
Tobramycin	8–32	16	16
Cloxacillin	<0.125–1	1	1
S. pneumoniae (40)			
NFT	<0.03–0.25	0.03	0.03
Cefotaxime	<0.03–0.125	0.03	0.03
Moxalactam	0.5–8	1	2
Ceftazidime	0.06–2	0.125	0.25
Cefoperazone	0.03–0.5	0.03	0.06
Cefoxitin	0.5–8	1	2
Cefamandole	0.03–1	0.06	0.125
Cefazolin	0.06–0.25	0.06	0.125
Azlocillin	0.03–0.5	0.125	0.125
Ticarcillin	0.125–4	0.25	0.5
Ampicillin	0.03–0.125	0.03	0.06
Tobramycin	4–32	8	32
Cloxacillin	0.25–8	0.25	0.5
Viridans streptococci (32)			
NFT	<0.03–0.25	0.03	0.125
Cefotaxime	0.03–2	0.06	0.125
Moxalactam	0.06–>32	8	32
Ceftazidime	0.03–8	0.5	2
Cefoperazone	0.03–8	0.5	2
Cefoxitin	0.03–>32	8	32
Cefamandole	<0.03–2	0.125	0.5
Cefazolin	0.03–2	0.25	0.5
Azlocillin	<0.125–1	<0.125	0.25
Ticarcillin	0.5–32	2	8
Ampicillin	<0.125–8	<0.125	0.25
Tobramycin	0.5–32	4	16
Cloxacillin	0.125–32	1	2
Miscellaneous *Streptococcus* spp. (25)			
NFT	<0.03–>16	0.125	4
Cefotaxime	<0.03–>32	0.25	>32
Moxalactam	<0.03–>32	8	>32
Ceftazidime	0.03–>32	1	>32
Cefoperazone	0.03–>32	2	>32
Cefoxitin	0.03–>32	32	>32
Cefamandole	<0.03–>32	5	32
Cefazolin	0.03–>32	2	32
Azlocillin	<0.125–8	0.125	1
Ticarcillin	0.125–16	0.5	8
Ampicillin	<0.125–4	0.25	1
Tobramycin	0.03–>64	4	64
Cloxacillin	0.125–>64	2	>64

[a] Percentage of strains.

Of agents tested, *N*-formimidoyl thienamycin was most active, inhibiting 99% of strains at 16 μg/ml. The MICs of *N*-formimidoyl thienamycin were >32 μg/ml for only six isolates: five strains of *Pseudomonas maltophilia* and a single strain of *P. aeruginosa*. The agent was highly active against all currently important genera tested. At 16 μg/ml, cefotaxime, cefoperazone, ceftazidime, and moxalactam inhibited 95, 95, 94, and 90% of all isolates, respectively. Newer cephalosporins were highly active against strains of *P. aeruginosa* but, like second-generation cephalosporins, were generally inactive against *S. faecalis*. Compared with cefazolin and cefamandole, newer cephalosporins were less active against both *S. aureus* and *S. epidermidis*. Most genera were slightly more susceptible to azlocillin than to ticarcillin.

The breakpoints chosen for designation of susceptibility for newer cephalosporins were arbitrarily chosen to facilitate comparison with first- and second-generation agents. However, many other factors other than in vivo MIC data determine the efficacy of these antimicrobial agents in vivo, and interpretation of such MIC data requires appreciation of many other parameters, including the achievable serum levels, tissue distribution, bactericidal properties, and perhaps such other factors as the degree of protein binding. Similarly, for *N*-formimidoyl thienamycin the interpretation of the impressive MIC data must await the results of human pharmacokinetic studies. The broad range of activity of all newer agents tested has been confirmed, and clinical investigations are required to define the place of each agent in our antibiotic armamentarium. Further study of comparative pharmacokinetics and clinical efficacy is necessary to define the role of each of the newer β-lactam agents in various circumstances.

1. **Hall, W. H., B. J. Opfer, and D. N. Gerding.** 1980. Comparative activities of the oxa-β-lactam LY127935, cefotaxime, cefoperazone, cefamandole, and ticarcillin against multiply resistant gram-negative bacilli. Antimicrob. Agents Chemother. **17**:273–279.
2. **Horadam, V. W., J. D. Smilack, C. L. Montgomery, and J. Werringloer.** 1980. In vitro activity of N-formimidoyl thienamycin (MK0787), a crystalline derivative of thienamycin. Antimicrob. Agents Chemother. **18**:557–561.
3. **Verbist, L., and J. Verhaegen.** 1980. GR-20263: a new aminothiazolyl cephalosporin with high activity against *Pseudomonas* and *Enterobacteriaceae*. Antimicrob. Agents Chemother. **17**:807–812.

Comparative In Vitro Activity of MK 0787 (*N*-Formimidoyl Thienamycin) and Ten Other β-Lactam Antibiotics Against *Pseudomonas aeruginosa*

M. O. SANTOS FERREIRA* AND J. A. MONIZ PEREIRA

Microbiology Laboratory, Faculty of Pharmacy, University of Lisbon, Lisbon, Portugal

Thienamycin is a β-lactam antibiotic that exhibits a high order of potency against many important pathogenic species. Its potential usefulness was limited by poor stability, both in concentrated solutions and as an amorphous solid. Of the many derivatives and analogs synthesized to overcome this problem, the crystalline monohydrate of *N*-formimidoyl thienamycin (MK 0787) proved especially convenient (1, 4).

The present report is part of a joint study on hospital strains of *Pseudomonas aeruginosa* isolated in Portugal. In previous papers, we have analyzed the distribution of serotypes, lysotypes, and pyocinotypes (2, 3, 5) as well as their susceptibility to aminoglycosides and β-lactam antibiotics (J. F. Moniz Pereira and M. O. Santos Ferreira, Mediterranean Congress of Chemotherapy, Symposium no. VI, Abstr. p. 35, 1980). Here we present the results of a study on the in vitro activity of MK 0787 against 300 hospital strains of *P. aeruginosa*, using as comparative agents apalcillin, piperacillin, azlocillin, ticarcillin disodium, carbenicillin, mezlocillin, cefsulodin sodium, cefoperazone, moxalactam, and cefotaxime.

The MICs of the different antibiotics were determined by an agar dilution technique. The test medium used was Mueller-Hinton agar (Difco Laboratories), at pH 7.4, according to the recommendations of the World Health Organization working group. The bacterial inoculum was prepared from a 1:1,000 dilution of an 18-h culture at 37°C in brain heart infusion (Difco), without stirring, and contained an average of 10^6 bacteria per ml. It was applied on the agar surface by means of a Steers replicator that permitted the simultaneous deposit of 52 different strains. Each drop of the bacterial suspensions had a diameter of 6 to 7 mm and contained an average of 10^4 bacteria.

All antibiotic solutions were prepared fresh on

the day of use, following the product's information inserts or special recommendation supplied. Solutions of MK 0787 were prepared in 10 mM MOPS 3-(*N*-morpholino)propanesulfonic acid, pH 7.1. The results were read after an incubation period of 18 h at 37°C.

Apalcillin, cefsulodin sodium, and MK 0787 were the most potent antibiotics tested in this study (Fig. 1), inhibiting 97.2% of the strains used at concentrations of 4, 8, and 16 μg/ml, respectively. All of the strains were inhibited when these agents were tested at 32 μg/ml. Concentrations of the other agents that inhibited all strains were as follows: cefotaxime, 64 μg/ml; piperacillin, azlocillin, moxalactam, and ticarcillin, 128 μg/ml; mezlocillin and cefoperazone, 256 μg/ml; and carbenicillin, 512 μg/ml.

Piperacillin and azlocillin had similar inhibitory activity and were superior to carbenicillin, ticarcillin, mezlocillin, cefoperazone, and moxalactam. At a concentration of 32 μg/ml, piperacillin was able to inhibit 80% of the carbenicillin-resistant strains. Higher concentrations (32 to 128 μg/ml) of ticarcillin, mezlocillin, moxalactam, and cefotaxime were required to obtain the same inhibition of carbenicillin-resistant strains. Cefoperazone and ticarcillin showed similar activities and inhibited carbenicillin-resistant strains at concentrations between 4 and 256 μg/ml. MK 0787 inhibited carbenicillin-resistant strains at concentrations of 4 to 16 μg/ml.

The more resistant strains were found in urinary specimens, and the most susceptible strains belonged to the "several infected sites" group.

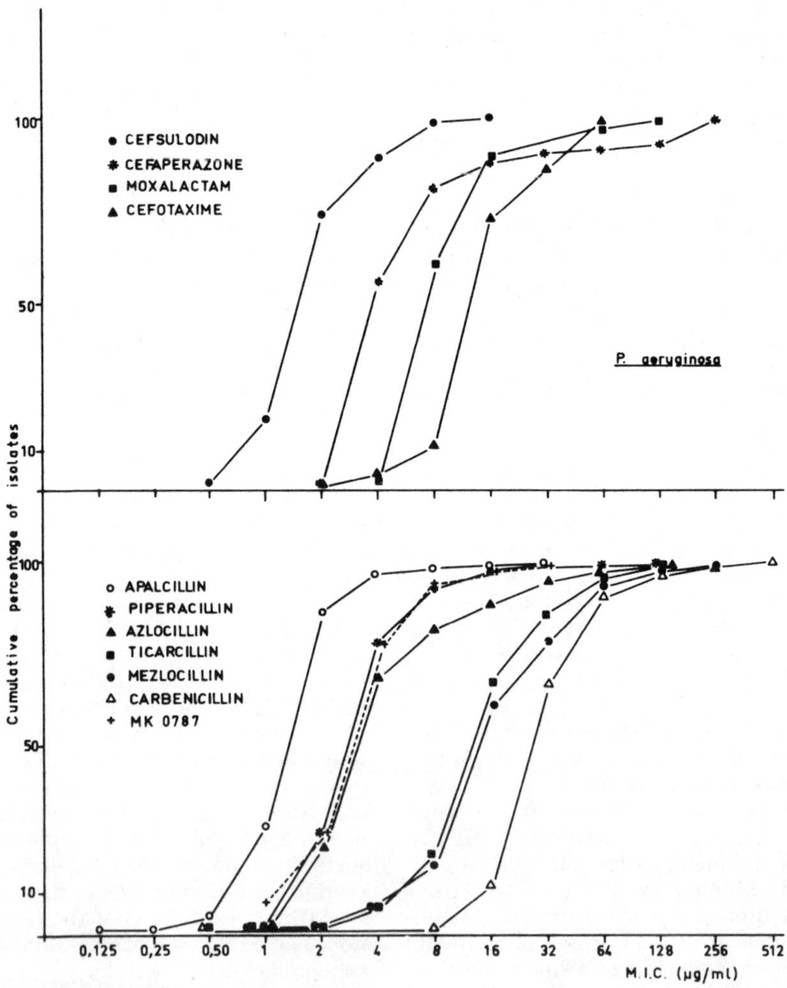

FIG. 1. *Susceptibility of 300 strains of P. aeruginosa to 11 β-lactam antibiotics. Cumulative percentage of isolates inhibited by increasing concentrations.*

The O:11 serotype appeared predominantly in urinary and tracheal specimens (pyocinotype 1, subtype a or b).

The results obtained confirm that MK 0787 has excellent in vitro activity against *P. aeruginosa*. Of particular importance was its activity against isolates exhibiting resistance to other β-lactam antibiotics.

1. **Kahan, J. S., F. M. Kahn, et al.** 1979. Thienamycin a new β-lactam antibiotic. I. Discovery, taxonomy, isolation and physical properties. J. Antibiot. **32:**1–12.
2. **Santos Ferreira, M. O., Y. M. Darmon, and J. F. Vieu.** 1976. Lysotypie complémentaire de *Pseudomonas aeruginosa*. Ann. Microbiol. (Paris) **127B:**189–193.
3. **Santos Ferreira, M. O., and J. F. Vieu.** 1977. Marqueurs epidemiologiques de *Pseudomonas aeruginosa*: isolement de quatre nouveaux pyocinotypes. Ann. Microbiol. (Paris) **128B:**487–494.
4. **Spratt, B. G., V. Jobranputra, and W. Zimmerman.** 1977. Binding of thienamycin and clavulanic acid to the penicillin-binding proteins of *Escherichia coli* K12. Antimicrob. Agents Chemother. **12:**406–409.
5. **Toucas, M., M. O. Santos Ferreira, and J. F. Vieu.** 1975. Recherche d'anticorps antipyocyaniques dans la population normale en France et au Portugal. Med. Mal. Infect. **5:**465–468.

Activity of Thienamycin (MK0787) in Comparison with Cefotaxime, Moxalactam, Ceftazidime, and Other Beta-Lactams Against Clinically Important Gram-Negative Nonfermenters and *Enterobacteriaceae*

H. H. SCHASSAN,* R. HÖRNING, R. MALOTTKE, AND J. POTEL

Institute of Medical Microbiology, University of Hamburg, and Med. Hochschule, Hannover, Federal Republic of Germany*

Thienamycin is a new beta-lactam antibiotic produced by cultures of *Streptomyces cattleya* and differs chemically from the penicillins and cephalosporins by lacking the sulfur in the secondary ring, which bears a thioethylamine moiety (1, 2). From this structure of the 5-member ring the name thienamycin was derived. Thienamycin is the first representative of a new family of antibiotics. It is structurally very similar to clavulanic acid; however, it shows, in addition to its beta-lactamase-inhibiting properties, a broad antimicrobial activity against gram-positive and gram-negative aerobic and anaerobic bacteria (5, 6). The efficacy of thienamycin against *Bacteroides fragilis* and other anaerobes is comparable to that of clindamycin and metronidazole (5).

The aim of this study was to compare the in vitro activity of *N*-formimidoyl thienamycin (MK0787), which is chemically 5 to 10 times more stable and twice as active as thienamycin, with those of cefotaxime, ceftazidime, moxalactam, cefoperazone (T-1551), piperacillin, azlocillin, and ticarcillin. Cefsulodin was additionally tested against *Pseudomonas aeruginosa* and netilmicin against *Pseudomonas maltophilia*. We used the microdilution technique with an inoculum of 10^5 colony-forming units/ml of Mueller-Hinton broth, standardized by an Eppendorf photometer.

The activity of thienamycin and the other antibiotics against the nonfermentative gram-negative bacilli is shown in Table 1. Thienamycin was most active against *Acinetobacter calcoaceticus* var. *anitratum*, of which 90% were inhibited by 0.5 mg/liter. *A. calcoaceticus* var. *lwoffi* was a bit less susceptible to thienamycin, which inhibited 90% of the strains at 2 mg/liter. The MBCs of thienamycin against both *Acinetobacter* species were 1.6 and 1.8 mg/liter, respectively, which means a 10-fold-higher bactericidal potency compared with cefotaxime. Behind thienamycin the most effective drugs were ceftazidime and cefotaxime, whereas cefoperazone was least active against *Acinetobacter*.

Thienamycin and ceftazidime exhibited an extraordinarily high efficacy against *P. aeruginosa*; 100% of the strains were inhibited by 4 mg of both drugs per liter. The median bactericidal effectiveness of these antibiotics against *P. aeruginosa* was estimated with 5.6 mg/liter for thienamycin and 8.5 mg/liter for ceftazidime. Both are twofold more active than cefsulodin; the bactericidal potency of thienamycin was even threefold better than that of cefsulodin, the most effective antipseudomonal β-lactam available today. Cefotaxime and moxalactam were fourfold less active than cefsulodin in *P. aeruginosa*. Cefoperazone, piperacillin, and azlocillin are nearly of the same value, but they did not reach the activity of thienamycin, ceftazidime, and cefsulodin.

The *Pseudomonas fluorescens-P. putida* group was especially susceptible to ceftazidime,

TABLE 1. *Activity of thienamycin, cefotaxime, moxalactam, ceftazidime, cefoperazone, piperacillin, azlocillin, and ticarcillin against nonfermentative gram-negative bacilli*

Organism	Antibiotic	MIC_{90} (mg/liter)	MIC range (mg/liter)	Geometric mean (mg/liter)	
				MIC	MBC
Acinetobacter anitratus (20)	Thienamycin	0.5	0.125–1	0.27	1.6
	Ceftazidime	8	0.5–32	5.3	42.2
	Cefotaxime	16	4–32	6.5	19.7
	Moxalactam	64	2–64	21.1	64
	Cefoperazone	64	2–>128	18.4	59.7
	Piperacillin	32	2–64	10.9	27.8
	Azlocillin	64	0.5–>128	13	39.4
	Ticarcillin	32	1–64	13	29.8
Acinetobacter lwoffi (20)	Thienamycin	2	0.06–4	0.3	1.8
	Ceftazidime	8	0.03–128	1.8	10.5
	Cefotaxime	32	0.03–64	1.6	13.9
	Moxalactam	64	1–>128	5.3	18.4
	Cefoperazone	64	4–64	11.3	59.7
	Piperacillin	64	0.125–>128	6.9	14.9
	Azlocillin	64	0.125–>128	5.3	22.6
	Ticarcillin	128	0.06–128	3	22.6
Pseudomonas aeruginosa (50)	Thienamycin	4	1–4	1.5	5.6
	Ceftazidime	4	0.5–4	1.8	8.5
	Cefsulodin	8	0.5–64	2.8	18.4
	Cefotaxime	32	2–>128	18.4	84.5
	Moxalactam	32	8–>128	14.9	42.2
	Cefoperazone	32	2–64	8.5	36.7
	Piperacillin	64	2–>128	9.5	64
	Azlocillin	64	2–>128	14.9	48.5
	Ticarcillin	>128	8–>128	39.4	78.8
Pseudomonas fluorescens and *P. putida* (18)	Thienamycin	16	0.25–32	2.4	6
	Ceftazidime	8	0.5–16	1.8	4.3
	Cefotaxime	64	8–64	14.9	48.5
	Moxalactam	128	32–>128	55.7	128
	Cefoperazone	64	2–>128	11.3	17.1
	Piperacillin	64	0.5–>128	9.2	17.1
	Azlocillin	>128	4–>128	16	24.2
	Ticarcillin	>128	64–>128	>128	>128
Pseudomonas cepacia (20)	Thienamycin	32	8–>128	14.9	26
	Ceftazidime	8	0.5–64	1.7	4
	Cefotaxime	8	2–>128	5.3	16
	Moxalactam	8	2–16	7.4	10.5
	Cefoperazone	32	4–32	14.9	18.4
	Piperacillin	4	1–8	2.4	8.5
	Azlocillin	16	4–16	6.9	12.1
	Ticarcillin	>128	>128	>128	>128
Pseudomonas maltophilia (25)	Thienamycin	>128	>128	>128	>128
	Ceftazidime	>128	2–>128	39.4	78.8
	Cefotaxime	>128	32–>128	>128	>128
	Moxalactam	32	1–64	8.5	42.2
	Cefoperazone	>128	8–>128	59.7	119.4
	Piperacillin	>128	64–>128	>128	>128
	Azlocillin	>128	16–>128	>128	>128
	Ticarcillin	>128	32–>128	>128	>128
	Netilmicin	32	2–32	6.9	39.4

as 90% of the strains were inhibited by 8 mg of ceftazidime per liter compared with 16 mg of thienamycin per liter. Two to three steps less active were piperacillin, cefoperazone, and cefotaxime. Azlocillin and moxalactam yielded a low activity and ticarcillin no activity against *P. fluorescens* and *P. putida*.

The gentamicin-resistant *Pseudomonas cepacia* was inhibited by piperacillin in a range of 1 to 8 mg/liter and by ceftazidime in a range of

TABLE 2. *Activity of thienamycin, ceftazidime, cefotaxime, moxalactam, cefoperazone, piperacillin, azlocillin, and ticarcillin against Enterobacteriaceae*

Organism	Antibiotic	MIC_{90} (mg/liter)	MIC range (mg/liter)	Geometric mean (mg/liter)	
				MIC	MBC
E. coli (50)	Thienamycin	2	0.125–2	0.28	8.5
	Ceftazidime	0.25	0.06–1	0.16	3.7
	Cefotaxime	1	0.008–2	0.10	1.4
	Moxalactam	0.125	0.008–1	0.07	0.35
	Cefoperazone	8	2–32	4	13
	Piperacillin	2	0.06–4	0.75	12.1
	Azlocillin	128	4–>128	26	78.8
	Ticarcillin	>128	4–>128	78.8	>128
Klebsiella pneumoniae (50)	Thienamycin	16	2–16	7.4	13
	Ceftazidime	0.5	0.06–2	0.21	4.6
	Cefotaxime	0.125	0.008–0.5	0.03	0.66
	Moxalactam	0.5	0.03–4	0.15	4.9
	Cefoperazone	128	0.125–>128	9.2	17.1
	Piperacillin	>128	1–>128	45.2	>128
	Azlocillin	>128	16–>128	111.4	>128
	Ticarcillin	>128	16–>128	>128	>128
Enterobacter aerogenes (20)	Thienamycin	2	0.125–2	0.87	1.8
	Ceftazidime	128	1–>128	29.8	64
	Cefotaxime	64	0.13–128	2.8	8.5
	Moxalactam	16	1–64	4.3	9.8
	Cefoperazone	128	0.25–>128	6.9	16
	Piperacillin	>128	2–>128	52	104
	Azlocillin	>128	4–>128	111.4	>128
	Ticarcillin	>128	2–>128	64	84.5
Enterobacter cloacae (40)	Thienamycin	1	0.125–2	0.66	2.8
	Ceftazidime	64	0.5–>128	19.7	55.7
	Cefotaxime	64	0.008–>128	1.2	12.1
	Moxalactam	1	0.03–32	0.16	0.57
	Cefoperazone	128	0.25–>128	2.4	4.9
	Piperacillin	128	1–>128	5.3	48.5
	Azlocillin	>128	4–>128	24.2	111.4
	Ticarcillin	>128	2–>128	22.6	97
Serratia marcescens (40)	Thienamycin	2	0.5–2	1	10.5
	Ceftazidime	0.25	0.03–0.25	0.04	6
	Cefotaxime	16	0.015–64	1.2	97
	Moxalactam	1	0.125–32	0.53	6.9
	Cefoperazone	128	0.5–>128	5.3	45.2
	Piperacillin	>128	0.25–>128	13	45.2
	Azlocillin	>128	8–>128	48.5	119.4
	Ticarcillin	>128	2–>128	119.4	>128
Proteus mirabilis (50)	Thienamycin	32	8–64	18.4	34.3
	Ceftazidime	0.06	0.015–0.125	0.04	0.20
	Cefotaxime	1	0.008–2	0.10	0.5
	Moxalactam	0.125	0.015–2	0.14	0.46
	Cefoperazone	2	0.125–4	0.66	8
	Piperacillin	2	0.06–>128	0.5	5.6
	Azlocillin	8	1–128	3.2	22.6
	Ticarcillin	16	1–>128	2	39.4

TABLE 2. *Continued*

Organism	Antibiotic	MIC_{90} (mg/liter)	MIC range (mg/liter)	Geometric mean (mg/liter)	
				MIC	MBC
Morganella morganii (40)	Thienamycin	8	1–8	3	6
	Ceftazidime	1	0.06–16	0.25	1.4
	Cefotaxime	4	0.015–16	0.23	3.4
	Moxalactam	0.125	0.06–0.25	0.10	0.23
	Cefoperazone	2	0.25–16	1.4	5.3
	Piperacillin	2	0.125–32	0.61	11.3
	Azlocillin	>128	2–>128	18.4	119.4
	Ticarcillin	16	0.5–>128	4.3	34.3
Proteus rettgeri (30)	Thienamycin	16	1–32	5.6	18.4
	Ceftazidime	2	0.25–4	0.61	19.7
	Cefotaxime	4	0.06–8	0.25	5.3
	Moxalactam	0.25	0.015–4	0.11	0.33
	Cefoperazone	32	1–>128	6.9	22.6
	Piperacillin	>128	0.125–>128	2.6	5.3
	Azlocillin	>128	0.5–>128	22.6	97
	Ticarcillin	>128	1–>128	12.1	30.4
Proteus vulgaris (40)	Thienamycin	16	4–32	12.1	17.1
	Ceftazidime	0.06	0.015–0.125	0.038	0.21
	Cefotaxime	64	0.015–>128	1.6	18.4
	Moxalactam	0.25	0.06–0.25	0.19	0.71
	Cefoperazone	32	0.125–>128	2.1	9.8
	Piperacillin	2	0.06–>128	0.40	13.9
	Azlocillin	>128	0.25–>128	12.1	78.8
	Ticarcillin	16	1–>128	4.6	52

0.5 to 64 mg/liter; however, 85% of the strains were inhibited by 2 mg of ceftazidime per liter. Also cefotaxime, moxalactam, and azlocillin showed sufficient effectiveness, inhibiting 90% of the strains by 8 and 16 mg/liter, respectively. *Pseudomonas maltophilia* was highly resistant to the majority of the beta-lactams and aminoglycosides. Also thienamycin was totally ineffective against this *Pseudomonas* species. Of the beta-lactams tested only moxalactam showed a therapeutically realizable effectiveness; the range of activity reached from 1 to 64 mg/liter. The behavior of netilmicin deserves special attention, for 84% of the strains were inhibited by 8 mg/liter, which will be regarded as the breakpoint of netilmicin. The drug of choice against *P. maltophilia* is moxalactam, inhibiting 96% of the strains by 32 mg and killing 50% of the strains by 42.2 mg/liter; these concentrations of moxalactam are in a therapeutically feasible range.

The efficacy of thienamycin and the other drugs against the *Enterobacteriaceae* is illustrated in Table 2. Moxalactam was the most active drug against *Escherichia coli*; 90% of the strains were inhibited by 0.125 mg/liter. Comparable were the activities of ceftazidime and cefotaxime (MIC_{90} = 0.25 and 1 mg/liter, respectively). Thienamycin followed in the fourth position for *E. coli* (MIC_{90} = 2 mg/liter), exceeding the activity of cefoperazone, piperacillin, azlocillin, and ticarcillin.

Superior to all drugs against *Klebsiella pneumoniae* was cefotaxime, for 90% of the strains were killed by 0.125 mg/liter. Also the bactericidal effect of cefotaxime was excellent (median MBC, 0.66 mg/liter). Similar were the activities of moxalactam and ceftazidime; both inhibited 94% of the strains at a concentration of 0.5 mg/liter. Thienamycin was more active than the penicillins. All piperacillin-resistant strains proved susceptible to thienamycin.

Against *Enterobacter cloacae* moxalactam was most effective, especially with regard to its bactericidal potency (median MBC, 0.57 mg/liter). Cefotaxime inhibited 90% of the strains at a concentration of 0.5 mg/liter; 10% were resistant to cefotaxime. Thienamycin showed a narrow range of MIC from 0.125 to 2 mg/liter, but the bactericidal efficacy was better than that of cefotaxime. A total of 70 to 80% of the *Enterobacter* strains were in the therapeutic range of cefoperazone and piperacillin.

Against *Serratia marcescens* ceftazidime proved the most effective drug; all strains were inhibited by 0.25 mg/liter and approximately

50% of the strains were killed by 6 mg/liter. Moxalactam and thienamycin also exhibited high effectiveness with MIC_{90} inhibition values of 1 and 2 mg/liter, respectively, and a very similar bactericidal activity (median MBC of 6.9 and 10.5 mg/liter). A total of 75% of the *Serratia* strains were susceptible to cefoperazone and 60% to piperacillin; their bactericidal potencies were identical (median MBC of 45.2 mg/liter).

Against indole-negative and -positive *Proteus* species, including *Morganella morganii*, moxalactam and ceftazidime exceeded all other antibiotics; the activity of thienamycin was less remarkable against the *Proteus* species. The *Proteus* strains with resistance to cefoperazone, piperacillin, azlocillin, and ticarcillin, however, all proved susceptible to thienamycin.

Although thienamycin is structurally different from penicillins and cephalosporins, it shows the same mode of action as typical β-lactams with high affinity for penicillin-binding proteins, especially for protein 2 (4). The major target for β-lactam action is a membrane-bound transpeptidase, which catalyzes the cell wall peptidoglycan synthesis, and thienamycin was found to be a more potent inhibitor than ampicillin of this peptidoglycan transpeptidase from *E. coli* (3). In conclusion, thienamycin is a most promising, novel β-lactam antibiotic with a broad activity against aerobic and anaerobic problem pathogens and a high bactericidal potency against *Acinetobacter* species, *P. aeruginosa*, *P. fluorescens* and *P. putida*, *E. aerogenes*, *E. cloacae*, and *Serratia marcescens*.

1. **Cama, L. D., and B. G. Christensen.** 1978. Total synthesis of thienamycin analogues. 1. Synthesis of the thienamycin nucleus and dl-decysteaminylthienamycin. J. Am. Chem. Soc. **100:**8006–8007.
2. **Kahan, J. S., F. M. Kahan, R. Goegelman, S. A. Curri, M. Jackson, E. O. Stapley, T. W. Miller, A. K. Miller, D. Hendlin, S. Mochales, S. Hernandez, H. B. Woodruff, and J. Birnbaum.** 1979. Thienamycin, a new β-lactam antibiotic. I. Discovery, taxonomy, isolation and physical properties. J. Antibiot. **32:**1–12.
3. **Moore, B. A., S. Jevons, and K. W. Brammer.** 1979. Inhibition of transpeptidase activity in *Escherichia coli* by thienamycin. Antimicrob. Agents. Chemother. **15:** 831–833.
4. **Spratt, B. G., V. Jobanputra, and W. Zimmermann.** 1977. Binding of thienamycin and clavulanic acid to the penicillin-binding proteins *Escherichia coli* K-12. Antimicrob. Agents Chemother. **12:**406–409.
5. **Tally, F. P., N. V. Jacobus, and S. L. Gorbach.** 1978. In vitro activity of thienamycin. Antimicrob. Agents Chemother. **14:**436–438.
6. **Weaver, S. S., G. P. Bodey, and B. M. LeBlanc.** 1979. Thienamycin: new beta-lactam antibiotic with potent broad-spectrum activity. Antimicrob. Agents Chemother. **15:**518–521.

Activity of *N*-Formimidoyl Thienamycin (MK 0787) Against *Haemophilus influenzae* and *Streptococcus pneumoniae*

ANTHONY J. HOWARD† AND CAROL J. HINCE

Department of Medical Microbiology, London Hospital Medical College, London E1 2AD, Great Britain

N-Formimidoyl thienamycin (*N*-f. thienamycin) is a crystalline derivative of thienamycin which exhibits both greater stability (K. J. Wildonger, W. J. Leanza, T. W. Miller, and B. G. Christensen, Program Abstr. Intersci. Conf. Antimicrob. Agents Chemother. 19th, Boston, Mass., abstr. no. 232, 1979) and enhanced antimicrobial activity (1). In this study, the activity of *N*-f. thienamycin against *Streptococcus pneumoniae* and *Haemophilus influenzae* was evaluated and, in the latter case, compared with the activity of ampicillin.

Forty strains of *S. pneumoniae* and *H. influenzae* were studied. MICs were determined by agar dilution methods, using Oxoid DST agar supplemented with 4% lysed horse blood for *S. pneumoniae* or with 10 mg of NAD per liter and 0.25% lysed horse blood for *H. influenzae*. Inocula of 10^4 and 10^6 colony-forming units (CFU) were applied with a multipoint inoculator. *N*-F. thienamycin was supplied by Merck Sharp & Dohme, and ampicillin was supplied by Beecham Research Laboratories. For the determination of broth dilution MICs, serial dilutions of antibiotics were made in Oxoid nutrient broth no. 2 supplemented with 5% Fildes extract. One-milliliter portions of broth were inoculated with either 10^4 or 10^6 CFU/ml and incubated overnight at 37°C. MBCs were determined by subculturing the broths onto chocolate agar.

Six strains of *H. influenzae* were selected for experiments to determine the rate of antibacterial activity. These comprised two ampicillin-

†Present address: Department of Medical Microbiology, Area Pathology Laboratory, Caernarvon and Anglesey Hospital, Bangor, Gwynedd LL57 2HW, North Wales.

susceptible strains, two beta-lactamase producers, and two non-beta-lactamase–producing, ampicillin-resistant strains. For these studies, 100-ml quantities of sterile Oxoid nutrient broth no. 2 were supplemented with 5% Fildes extract. Ampicillin or *N*-f. thienamycin was added to final concentrations corresponding to 1/5, 1× MIC, and 10× MIC. Flasks were inoculated with between 10^6 and 10^7 CFU of the organism under test per ml, and cultures were incubated in a shaking water bath at 37°C. Viable counts were determined at 0, 2, 4, 6, 8, and 24 h by preparing serial dilutions and subculturing known volumes onto chocolate agar. The morphology of the bacterial cells removed with each sample was examined by phase-contrast microscopy. The stability of *N*-f. thienamycin in Fildes broth was determined by removing samples at intervals and assaying them by a plate method, using standards freshly prepared on each occasion in Fildes broth. The half-life was found to be approximately 18 h. This was unaffected by the presence of organisms in the medium, whether they were beta-lactamase producing or not.

The MICs of *N*-f. thienamycin for *S. pneumoniae* and two groups of *H. influenzae*, determined by an agar dilution method, are illustrated in Table 1. It can be seen that the compound exhibited a high degree of activity against *S. pneumoniae*. For *H. influenzae*, ampicillin exhibited greater intrinsic activity against susceptible strains (MICs of ampicillin, 0.06 to 0.5 mg/liter; mode, 0.25 mg/liter). However, *N*-f. thienamycin was more active against beta-lactamase producers (MICs of ampicillin, 4 to 8 mg/liter; mode, 4 mg/liter). Increasing the inoculum size to 10^6 CFU did not result in any significant increase in the MICs of *N*-f. thienamycin for *S. pneumoniae* (range, 0.003 to 0.015 mg/liter; mean, 0.057 mg/liter; mode, 0.007 mg/liter). However, the degree of background growth observed with *H. influenzae* at this inoculum rendered end points impossible to determine. Table 2 includes the MICs of *N*-f. thienamycin and ampicillin for three strains of *H. influenzae* exhibiting a reduced susceptibility to ampicillin in the absence of beta-lactamase production (MICs of ampicillin, 2.0 to 8.0 mg/liter). It can be seen that one strain, 1115, demonstrated marked resistance to *N*-f. thienamycin when tested by an agar method, though results for broth dilution tests were unremarkable. From Table 2 it can also be seen that for *H. influenzae*, MICs of ampicillin determined by agar or broth dilution correlated well, that beta-lactamase–producing strains exhibited the expected inoculum effect when tested in broth, and that few differences were observed between the values representing MICs and MBCs. For *N*-f. thienamycin there was again little difference between the values representing MICs and MBCs, but in this case no inoculum effect was observed for the beta-lactamase–producing strains studied.

Experiments to determine the rate of antibacterial activity of *N*-f. thienamycin produced similar results for all six strains tested. Exposure to the MIC produced a marked bactericidal effect over the first 8 h of incubation, though some regrowth occurred by 24 h. No regrowth was observed at 10× MIC. At 1/5 MIC, a bacteriostatic effect was observed over the first 8 h of incubation. For the non-beta-lactamase–produc-

TABLE 1. *MICs (in mg/liter) of N-f. thienamycin against S. pneumoniae and H. influenzae measured by an agar dilution technique and an inoculum of 10^4 CFU*

Strain	No.	MIC (mg/liter)		
		Range	Mean	Mode
S. pneumoniae	40	0.003–0.015	0.0053	0.007
H. influenzae				
Ampicillin susceptible	25	0.25–2	1.03	1.0
Ampicillin resistant, β-lactamase producing	10	0.5–4	1.2	1.0

TABLE 2. *Susceptibility of six strains of H. influenzae to N-f. thienamycin and ampicillin*

Strain	MIC (mg/liter)									
	Ampicillin					*N*-f. thienamycin				
	Agar dilution (10^4 CFU)	Broth dilution				Agar dilution (10^4 CFU)	Broth dilution			
		10^4 CFU/ml		10^6 CFU/ml			10^4 CFU/ml		10^6 CFU/ml	
		MIC	MBC	MIC	MBC		MIC	MBC	MIC	MBC
334	0.25	0.25	0.5	0.5	1.0	2.0	2.0	2.0	2.0	4.0
314	2.0	4.0	4.0	4.0	8.0	0.25	0.25	1.0	0.5	4.0
960	2.0	2.0	2.0	2.0	2.0	8.0	2.0	4.0	4.0	8.0
1115	8.0	4.0	4.0	2.0	4.0	32.0	2.0	2.0	2.0	2.0
1435[a]	8.0	4.0	8.0	>256	>256	4.0	0.25	1.0	0.5	2.0
2453[a]	8.0	2.0	4.0	128	>256	0.5	0.5	0.5	1.0	1.9

[a] Beta-lactamase producer.

ing strains studied, ampicillin was noted to have a bactericidal effect at 1× and 10× MIC. Viable counts from cultures exposed to 1/5 MIC of ampicillin corresponded to those obtained in drug-free controls. Exposure of beta-lactamase-producing strains to 20 mg of ampicillin per ml resulted in some reduction in viable count at 4 h though the counts corresponded to drug-free controls at 8 h. Morphological studies demonstrated the formation of large, pleomorphic, bulbous cells and some ovoid forms on exposure to 0.2× MIC of *N*-f. thienamycin. Higher concentrations induced round forms, spheroplasts, and cell lysis. Exposure to ampicillin produced filaments, spheroplasts, and cell lysis, depending on the concentration. Morphological studies with the non-beta-lactamase–producing, ampicillin-resistant strain 1115 demonstrated that this produced neither filaments in response to ampicillin nor bulbous forms when exposed to a sub-MIC of *N*-f. thienamycin. In each case, round cells were the predominant cell type. This strain corresponds to the type two form of *H. influenzae* described by Sykes et al. (2), i.e., a strain that readily produces stable spheroplasts at low inocula and gives a false impression of a raised MIC, especially using solid media. This indicates that care should be taken in interpreting the results of susceptibility studies with such strains for this antibiotic as well as for other beta-lactams.

In summary, *N*-f. thienamycin was found to exhibit good activity against the two bacterial species studied. Against *H. influenzae*, susceptibility was little affected by inoculum size and unaffected by beta-lactamase production. In addition, marked inhibitory activity was noted at 1/5 MIC.

1. **Kropp, H., J. G. Sundelof, J. S. Kahan, F. M. Kahan, and J. Birnbaum.** 1980. MK 0787 (N-formimidoyl thienamycin): evaluation of in vitro and in vivo activities. Antimicrob. Agents Chemother. **17**:993–1000.
2. **Sykes, R. B., A. Griffiths, and D. M. Ryan.** 1977. Comparative activity of ampicillin and cefuroxime against three types of *Haemophilus influenzae*. Antimicrob. Agents Chemother. **11**:599–604.

Recovery Period of Bacteria After Brief Exposure to *N*-Formimidoyl Thienamycin and Other Antibiotics

PETER J. McDONALD,* PAUL HAKENDORF, AND HENDRIK PRUUL

School of Medicine, Flinders University, and Flinders Medical Centre, Adelaide, South Australia*

Antibiotic-induced changes in bacterial growth occur not only while bacteria are in direct contact with the antibiotic but also for a period after removal or inactivation of the antibiotic. This persistent growth suppression or post-antibiotic effect (PAE) has been clearly documented (1). Staphylococci which have been treated with various inhibitors of protein synthesis and β-lactam antibiotics may take up to 4 h to resume normal growth after 2 h of antibiotic treatment. Gram-negative bacteria recover more rapidly from nonlethal antibiotic damage. However, only a few antibiotics have been studied in this regard, and the present investigation reviews the ability of β-lactam antibiotics to produce PAE.

Typical, susceptible strains of *Staphylococcus aureus*, *Escherichia coli*, and *Pseudomonas aeruginosa* in logarithmic growth were treated at 37°C for 1 or 2 h with 5× MIC of *N*-formimidoyl thienamycin (FTH), moxalactam (MOX), cefoperazone (CPZ), cefotaxime (CTX), amoxicillin (AMX), ampicillin (AMP), or carbenicillin (CAR) (*Pseudomonas* only). Antibiotic concentrations (5× MIC, expressed as micrograms per milliliter) used for *S. aureus*, *E. coli*, and *P. aeruginosa* experiments were, respectively: FTH, 1, 2, and 20; MOX, 20, 2, and 20; CPZ, 4, 2, and 10; CTX, 4, 2, and 10; AMX, 1, 20, and not applicable (NA); AMP, 2, 20, and NA; CAR, NA, NA, and 40.

Antibiotic was removed by centrifugation and washing twice in drug-free medium, and the kinetics of bacterial growth and recovery was followed by regular viable counts. All experiments and washings were undertaken in tryptic soy broth (Difco Laboratories), and at least a 1: 10,000 dilution of antibiotic was achieved.

An example of the kinetics of recovery of *P. aeruginosa* treated for 2 h with 5× MIC of FTH is provided in Fig. 1. After removal of antibiotic, sequential viable counts varied unpredictably for a limited period of time. In some instances killing continued, whereas in other circumstances there was an initial acceleration in viable counts after antibiotic removal (Fig. 1). Nevertheless, after an initial recovery period, the treated cultures resumed a rate of growth which was the same as the control rate of growth. In all instances, by the time the treated cultures had increased by 1 $\log_{10}$ after antibiotic removal, a normal (equivalent to control) rate of growth had resumed. Thus, a calculation which enables comparison of PAE between different organisms and antibiotics is: PAE (hours) = (time for treated culture to increase by 1 $\log_{10}$ after antibiotic removal) − (time for control culture to increase by 1 $\log_{10}$). The PAE values for treatment of *S. aureus*, *E. coli*, and *P. aeruginosa* with 5× MIC of the antibiotics listed above are outlined in Table 1.

All antibiotics produced PAE after 1 and 2 h

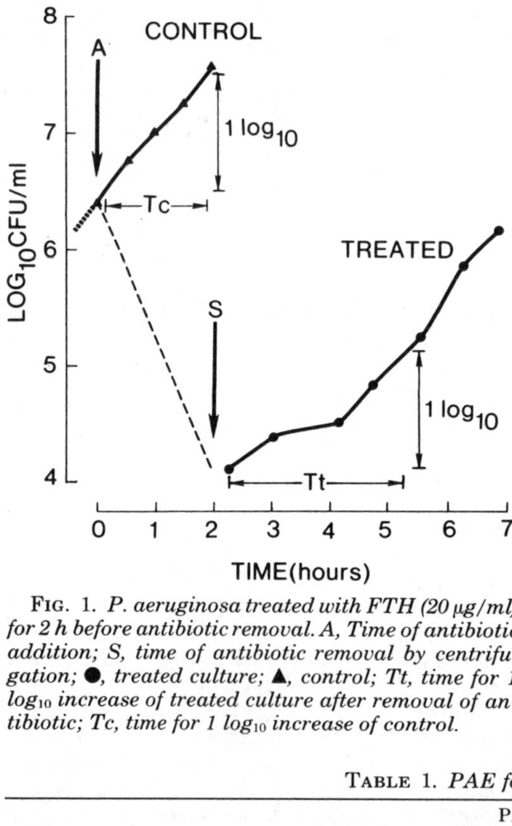

FIG. 1. *P. aeruginosa treated with FTH (20 μg/ml) for 2 h before antibiotic removal. A, Time of antibiotic addition; S, time of antibiotic removal by centrifugation; ●, treated culture; ▲, control; Tt, time for 1 $\log_{10}$ increase of treated culture after removal of antibiotic; Tc, time for 1 $\log_{10}$ increase of control.*

of treatment of *S. aureus*. Using the Newman Keuls method of analysis (3), no significant difference at the 5% level could be detected between antibiotics. A shorter PAE was consistently detected with all antibiotics against *E. coli*. However, FTH, AMX, and AMP produced significantly longer PAE values than the other antibiotics acting against *E. coli* ($P < 0.05$). The only antibiotic tested which demonstrated PAE with *P. aeruginosa* was FTH, and this effect was most evident with 2 h of treatment. Considerable interexperimental variation was noted with *Pseudomonas*.

PAE with any antibiotic could be demonstrated only if cultures were in logarithmic growth at the time of antibiotic addition. In the *Pseudomonas* experiments where minimal PAE was demonstrated by FTH, the growth rate of the test culture was comparatively slow at the time of antibiotic addition, and the kill observed during treatment was less than with cultures treated in maximal growth phase.

PAE was related to the bactericidal capacity of the antibiotic. Also, those antibiotics (FTH and AMX) which demonstrated greatest bactericidal capacity and PAE produced ghost cells and side-wall disruptions. This was in contrast to CTX, MOX, and CPZ, which induced gross elongation of gram-negative bacteria and even macroscopic turbidity before killing commenced.

We believe that PAE is another useful in vitro parameter to compare antibiotic efficacy. Also, PAE may assist in providing a basis for determining dosage intervals. While bacteria are in the recovery phase, they are more susceptible to phagocytosis and intracellular killing (2). Thus, estimation of PAE may allow more precise determination of optimal dosage schedules. These experiments indicate that the total antibiotic effect (killing during exposure plus PAE) varies significantly between antibiotics and bacteria. Staphylococci regularly demonstrate PAE, whereas gram-negative bacteria respond differ-

TABLE 1. *PAE for various antibiotics*

Antibiotic	PAE (h ± SEM)[a]					
	S. aureus		*E. coli*		*P. aeruginosa*	
	1 h	2 h	1 h	2 h	1 h	2 h
FTH	1.08 ± 0.16 (3)	1.16 ± 0.26 (3)	0.55 ± 0.08 (4)	1.37 ± 0.28 (3)	0.35 ± 0.16 (4)	0.81 ± 1.08 (4)
AMP	0.83 ± 0.02 (3)	1.07 ± 0.15 (3)	0.64 ± 0.03 (4)	1.35 ± 0.20 (3)	NA	NA
AMP	0.77 ± 0.06 (3)	1.17 ± 0.14 (4)	0.68 ± 0.02 (5)	1.35 ± 0.43 (3)	NA	NA
MOX	0.65 ± 0.1 (3)	1.16 ± 0.18 (4)	0.28 ± 0.07 (5)	0.26 ± 0.07 (3)	0.09 ± 0.07 (3)	−0.13 ± 0.21 (3)
CTX	0.78 ± 0.09 (3)	1.41 ± 0.04 (4)	0.43 ± 0.09 (5)	0.73 ± 0.13 (3)	0.16 ± 0.08 (3)	−0.04 ± 0.31 (3)
CPZ	0.67 ± 0.07 (3)	1.15 ± 0.10 (4)	0.22 ± 0.08 (5)	0.61 ± 0.17 (3)	0.27 ± 0.19 (3)	0.08 ± 0.13 (4)
CAR	NA	NA	NA	NA	0.22 ± 0.18 (3)	−0.15 ± 0.28 (3)

[a] 1 h and 2 h refer to antibiotic treatment time before separation of bacteria from antibiotic. Number of experiments is given in parentheses.

ently to various antibiotics. Perhaps dosage intervals can be prolonged with antibiotic-bacterium combinations which demonstrate PAE. In vivo studies are required to validate this hypothesis.

1. **McDonald, P. J., W. A. Craig, and C. M. Kunin.** 1977. Persistent effect of antibiotics on *Staphylococcus aureus* after exposure for limited periods of time. J. Infect. Dis **135**:217–223.
2. **Pruul, H., B. L. Wetherall, and P. J. McDonald.** 1981. Enhanced susceptibility of *Escherichia coli* to intracellular killing by human polymorphonuclear leukocytes after in vitro incubation with chloramphenicol. Antimicrob. Agents Chemother. **19**:945–951.
3. **Snedecor, G. W., and W. G. Cochran.** 1967. Statistical methods, 6th ed., p. 273. Iowa State University Press, Ames.

Enhanced Urinary Recovery of *N*-Formimidoyl Thienamycin (MK 0787) on Administering an Inhibitor of the Renal Dipeptidase Responsible for Antibiotic Metabolism

S. RAGNAR NORRBY,* KJELL ALESTIG, FRANCOISE FERBER, FREDRICK M. KAHAN, JEAN S. KAHAN, HELMUT KROPP, AND MELVIN A. P. MEISINGER

Department of Infectious Diseases, University of Umeå, Umeå, and Department of Infectious Diseases, University of Gothenburg, Gothenburg, Sweden; Merck Sharp & Dohme Research Laboratories, Zurich, Switzerland; and Merck Sharp & Dohme Research Laboratories, Rahway, New Jersey 07065, U.S.A.*

N-Formimidoyl thienamycin (TF) is a β-lactamase-resistant carbapenam antibiotic with an unusually broad antibacterial spectrum, covering both gram-positive and gram-negative aerobic and anaerobic bacterial species, including pathogens such as *Pseudomonas aeruginosa* and enterococci (1, 2). Animal pharmacokinetic studies have demonstrated that TF is metabolized to a varying degree by a renal dipeptidase, dehydropeptidase I, resulting in a relatively low urinary recovery (Kropp et al., Program Abstr. Intersci. Conf. Antimicrob. Agents Chemother. 20th, New Orleans, La., abstr. no. 272, 1980). The enzyme has been located to the luminal face of the proximal tubular cells and can be inhibited by dehydropeptidase inhibitors (Ashton et al., 20th ICAAC, abstract no. 271, 1980).

The present study was undertaken to investigate the pharmacokinetics of TF administered alone or in combination with a dehydropeptidase inhibitor [DHI; *Z*-2-(*S*-2,2-dimethylcycloproylcarboxamido)*C*-propenoate] as single doses to healthy male volunteers. Fifteen subjects with a mean age of 24 years (range, 19 to 30 years) and a mean body weight of 73 kg (range, 62 to 88 kg) were chosen for the study and gave their written informed consent to participate. Each of the volunteers received three test doses: one dose of 150 mg of TF (MK 0787, Merck Sharp & Dohme Research Laboratories, Rahway, N.J.); one dose of 25 mg (five subjects, group A), 75 mg (five subjects, group B), or 150 mg (five subjects, group C) of DHI (MK 0789, Merck Sharp & Dohme); one dose of 150 mg of TF plus 25 mg (group A), 75 mg (group B), or 150 mg (group C) of DHI. All doses were administered as intravenous bolus injections over 3 min with the substances dissolved in 15 ml of sterile saline. A wash-out period of at least 1 week was allowed between each of the three doses.

After each dose, plasma was collected for assays of TF and DHI before and at 0.1, 0.2, 0.5, 0.75, 1, 1.5, 2, 3, 4, 5, and 6 h after the beginning of the bolus injection. Urine was collected before and 0 to 1, 1 to 2, 2 to 3, 3 to 4, 4 to 5, 5 to 6, and 6 to 8 h after the administration. TF was assayed with a bioassay technique, using *Bacillus subtilis* ATCC 12432 as a test strain, and DHI was assayed by its inhibition of purified dehydropeptidase by a spectrophotometric technique. All samples were quick-frozen at −80°C and kept at that temperature until analyzed. Pharmacokinetic analyses of the dispositions of TF and DHI were performed by using a two-compartment open model. Both TF and DHI were well tolerated by the subjects, and no clinical or laboratory adverse reactions attributed to the drugs were noted.

There were very small variations between the 15 subjects in the plasma concentrations of TF obtained after administration of 150 mg of TF alone (Fig. 1). The mean plasma TF concentration 6 min after the start of the injection was 12.1 μg/ml. Co-administration of DHI resulted in slightly higher plasma concentrations of TF, still with minimal intersubject variability (Fig. 1). The disappearance of TF from plasma was characterized by a short half-life ($t_{1/2}$ in the α-phase irrespective of whether TF was given alone ($t_{1/2} = 0.19 \pm 0.05$ h, SD) or in combination with DHI ($t_{1/2}$ = 0.20 ± 0.05 h, SD). $t_{1/2}$ in the β-phase was about 1 h when TF was given both alone and in combination with DHI (Table 1). DHI caused small increases of the areas under the plasma concentration curves ($AUC_{0-\infty}$) and corresponding small decreases of the apparent volume of distribution (V_d) and the plasma clearance (PlCl) of TF (Table 1). These differences seemed to be more pronounced when 75 or 150 mg of DHI was administered than when 25 mg of DHI was given, indicating a dose-response relationship.

The plasma pharmacokinetics of DHI was characterized by a $t_{1/2}$ in the β-phase very similar to that of TF (1.0 ± 0.1 h, SD, after 150 mg of DHI alone or in combination with TF). The $AUC_{0-\infty}$ was consistently higher for DHI than for TF (7.3 ± 0.7 μg.h/ml per mg/kg, SD, for 150 mg of DHI alone and 7.1 ± 0.5 μg.h/ml per mg/kg, SD, for 150 mg of DHI given with TF). In the results obtained with DHI, there was no indication of any significant differences when DHI was given alone or when it was combined with TF.

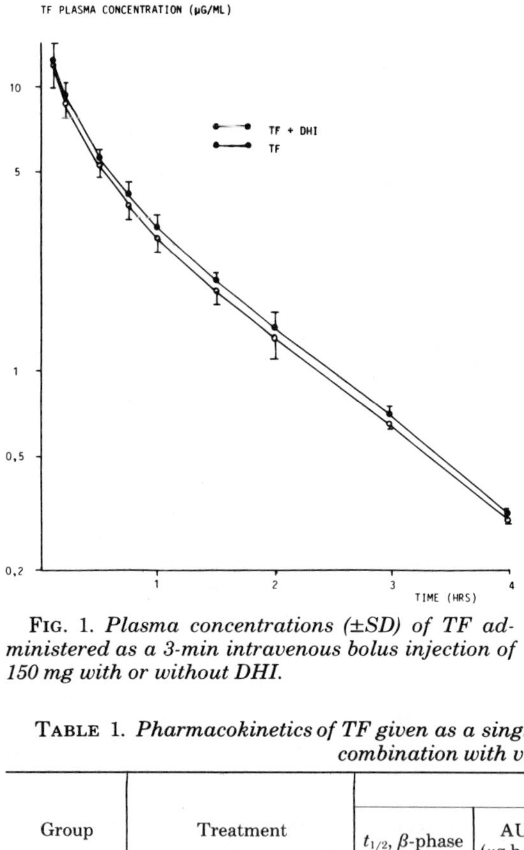

FIG. 1. *Plasma concentrations (±SD) of TF administered as a 3-min intravenous bolus injection of 150 mg with or without DHI.*

Whereas minimal intersubject variations were observed in the plasma pharmacokinetics of TF, considerable variations were found for urinary recovery (UR_{0-8}) and renal clearance (RCl). Thus, administration of TF alone resulted in urinary recoveries varying from 5.5 to 33.8% of the dose, with RCl of 0.21 and 1.04 ml/min per kg, respectively. As demonstrated by Table 1, co-administration of TF with DHI reduced these intersubject variations to a considerable extent, increasing the urinary recoveries of TF to 48 to 76% of the dose. This increase was more marked in the volunteers who received 75 or 150 mg of DHI than in those receiving the lower dose of 25 mg of DHI. Also, the UR_{0-8} of DHI was highly varying (5.6 to 33.0% of the dose) but with no correlation to the degree of metabolism of TF nor to co-administration with TF.

The results obtained in this study correlated well with the previously reported results in chimpanzees (Kropp et al., 20th ICAAC, 1980). Thus, the systemic bioavailibility seems unaffected by metabolism, and high plasma concentrations are achieved with an elimination pattern from plasma similar to that of many other nonmetabolized β-lactam antibiotics with a $t_{1/2}$ of about 1 h. However, the bioavailability of TF in urine showed large variations in the subjects studied, and in no case could more than 34% of the dose be recovered. That observation indicated the existence of a renal metabolism similar to the one described in several animal species, i.e., a degradation of TF by a dipeptidase located to the luminal face of the proximal tubular cells. The existence of such a metabolic pathway was

TABLE 1. *Pharmacokinetics of TF given as a single 3-min intravenous injection of 150 mg alone or in combination with various doses of DHI*

Group	Treatment	Measurement (mean ± SD)					
		$t_{1/2}$, β-phase (h)	$AUC_{0-\infty}$ (μg.h/ml per mg/kg)	V_d (liters/kg)	PlCl (ml/min per kg)	RCl (ml/min per kg)	UR_{0-8} (% of dose)
A	TF	0.93 ± 0.09	4.82 ± 0.56	0.24 ± 0.02	3.50 ± 0.41	0.56 ± 0.22	19.0 ± 8.0
	TF + 25 mg of DHI	0.99 ± 0.15	5.31 ± 0.47	0.22 ± 0.02	3.14 ± 0.25	1.71 ± 0.12	55.0 ± 4.3
B	TF	0.98 ± 0.14	4.29 ± 0.60	0.25 ± 0.03	3.94 ± 0.53	0.42 ± 0.13	11.2 ± 4.8
	TF + 75 mg of DHI	0.95 ± 0.11	4.73 ± 0.83	0.23 ± 0.01	3.6 ± 0.60	2.12 ± 0.13	61.1 ± 3.2
C	TF	1.03 ± 0.13	5.05 ± 0.56	0.23 ± 0.03	3.33 ± 0.40	0.65 ± 0.37	19.9 ± 12.3
	TF + 150 mg of DHI	0.96 ± 0.08	5.50 ± 0.75	0.21 ± 0.03	3.08 ± 0.44	1.90 ± 0.34	62.1 ± 7.9
A + B + C	TF	0.98 ± 0.12	4.72 ± 0.62	0.24 ± 0.03	3.59 ± 0.50	0.54 ± 0.26	16.7 ± 9.0

strongly supported by the markedly enhanced UR_{0-8} observed when TF was given together with DHI, which not only increased the UR_{0-8} but also markedly reduced the observed intersubject variability in renal metabolism.

1. **Kropp, H., J. G. Sundelof, J. S. Kahan, F. M. Kahan, and J. Birnbaum.** 1980. MK 0787 (*N*-formimidoyl thienamycin): evaluation of in vitro and in vivo activities. Antimicrob. Agents Chemother. **17**:993–1000.
2. **Livingston, W. K., A. M. Elliot, and C. G. Kobbs.** 1981. In vitro activity of *N*-formimidoyl thienamycin (MK 0787) against recent strains of *Pseudomonas aeruginosa*, *Staphylococcus epidermidis*, *Serratia marcescens*, and *Enterococcus* spp. Antimicrob. Agents Chemother. **19**:114–116.

Structure, Regulation, and Evolution of Cephalosporinase Genes in Gram-Negative Bacteria

SVEN BERGSTRÖM,* OLOF OLSSON, THOMAS GRUNDSTRÖM, BENGTÅKE JAURIN, AND STAFFAN NORMARK

Department of Microbiology, University of Umeå, S-901 87 Umeå, Sweden

Many gram-negative bacteria produce a chromosomally mediated β-lactamase. In general these enzymes show substrate specificity for cephalosporins. Some are inducible by β-lactams, but the majority are constitutively produced (3).

The chromosomal β-lactamase of *Escherichia coli* K-12 is the most well-characterized representative of these cephalosporinases. Its structural gene, *ampC*, has been cloned and DNA sequenced (1, 2). The deduced amino acid sequence showed no significant homologies with other sequenced β-lactamases (1). The serine residue at position 61 of *ampC* β-lactamase reacts with cloxacillin (V. Knott-Hunziker, S. G. Waley, B. Jaurin, and T. Grundström, Biochem. J., in press). Interestingly, the region around this serine residue exhibited an extensive homology with an active site fragment of *Pseudomonas aeruginosa* cephalosporinase (Knott-Hunziker et al., in press). A DNA fragment carrying the major part of the *ampC* structural gene was used as a probe in Southern blotting experiments using endonuclease digests of chromosomal DNA from a number of gram-negative species. The probe hybridized to a DNA segment of the same size in *E. coli*, *Shigella flexneri*, *Shigella sonnei*, *Klebsiella pneumoniae*, *Salmonella typhimurium*, and *Serratia marcescens*. No hybridization was found with DNA from *Neisseria gonorrhoeae* (Fig. 1). The hybridization was most pronounced using DNA from *E. coli* and *Shigella*, suggesting that the *ampC* gene of *Shigella* is more closely related to that of *E. coli* than the other gram-negative *ampC* genes.

Expression from the *ampC* gene of *E. coli* K-12 is low. However, like many other components, e.g., in the translatory machinery, the level of *ampC* β-lactamase increases with growth rate. The metabolic regulation of *ampC* is not restricted to *E. coli* K-12, but is also found in clinical isolates of *E. coli* as well as in *S. sonnei*. Possibly this regulation is a common feature of constitutively expressed cephalosporinases.

The DNA segment immediately adjacent to the *ampC* structural gene of *E. coli* K-12, previously called *ampA*, was found to contain the *ampC* promoter, and an efficient transcription terminator located within the 59-base pair (bp)-long *ampC* leader. In vitro, 94% of all initiated transcripts terminated after base 41 (2). One type of mutation weakened the thermodynamic strength of the terminator stem in the nascent transcripts and abolished transcription termination in vitro completely. Such attenuator mutations increased *ampC* β-lactamase production by a factor of four when cells were grown in rich media. Interestingly, in these attenuator mutants, the *ampC* β-lactamase level was invariant with growth rate, showing that this mode of regulation is exerted by antitermination of transcription. Except for mutants of *E. coli* K-12, mutants of *S. sonnei* and clinical isolates of *E. coli* producing elevated levels of *ampC* β-lactamase were found that had lost this growth rate-dependent response. However, most in vivo-selected *ampC* hyperproducing *E. coli* isolates had retained their growth rate control. Thus, in only one isolate out of six the growth rate-dependent regulation was abolished (Fig. 2). Our belief is that the cephalosporinase genes in many gram-negative genera are metabolically controlled by antitermination of transcription.

The *ampC* promoter consists of a −10 and a −35 region that show a 5 out of 6 bp homology

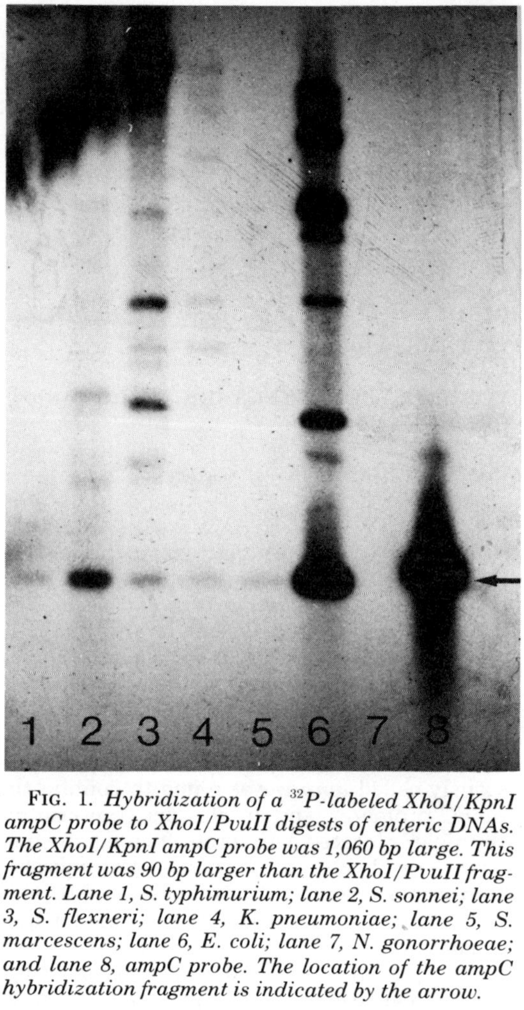

FIG. 1. *Hybridization of a ³²P-labeled XhoI/KpnI ampC probe to XhoI/PvuII digests of enteric DNAs. The XhoI/KpnI ampC probe was 1,060 bp large. This fragment was 90 bp larger than the XhoI/PvuII fragment. Lane 1, S. typhimurium; lane 2, S. sonnei; lane 3, S. flexneri; lane 4, K. pneumoniae; lane 5, S. marcescens; lane 6, E. coli; lane 7, N. gonorrhoeae; and lane 8, ampC probe. The location of the ampC hybridization fragment is indicated by the arrow.*

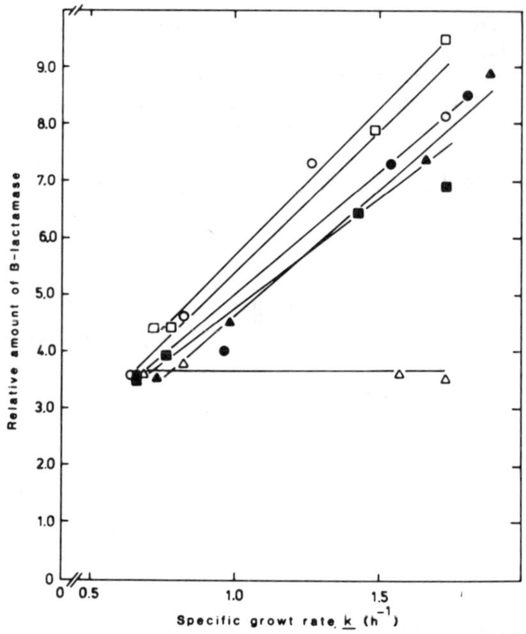

FIG. 2. *Relative amount of β-lactamase at different growth rates at 37°C in clinically isolated E. coli strains;* □, *C11,* △, *C13,* ○, *C14,* ■, *C15,* ▲, *C16, and* ●, *C17. The relative amount of β-lactamase per total protein was determined with rocket immunoelectrophoresis and plotted as a function of the first-order constant for growth (k), as calculated from the expression k=ln 2/mass doubling time in hours. The media used were as follows: medium E+glycerol, medium E+glucose, medium E+glucose+Casamino Acids, and LB medium. A relative amount of β-lactamase of 1.0 is found in an uppromoter mutant of E. coli K-12 grown in minimal glycerol medium.*

with the consensus sequences found among *E. coli* promoters (1). The distance between these conserved regions was 16 bp, which is 1 bp shorter than the distance most often found for *E. coli* promoters. We have studied an uppromoter mutation of *E. coli* K-12 that increases the frequency of transcription initiation by a factor of 15, leading to a corresponding increase in β-lactamase production and β-lactam resistance. DNA sequencing revealed that an insertion of a G-C bp had occurred between the −10 and the −35 regions of the *ampC* promoter. This mutation will affect the sterical arrangement of the *ampC* promoter, and we believe that it results in an improved fitness between the −10 and the −35 regions and the RNA polymerase.

Five clinical *E. coli* isolates that we have studied produce about 50 times more *ampC* β-lactamase than the wild type. Such high β-lactamase levels are also found in *E. coli* K-12 mutants carrying both the G-C insertion in the *ampC* promoter and an attenuator mutation. However, in the five clinical isolates the β-lactamase production increased with growth rate, suggesting that they had an intact attenuator. The *ampA* region of one such isolate has been DNA sequenced. Only one difference from *E. coli* K-12 wild type was found in the leader region. This alteration, however, occurred downstream the attenuator close to the *ampC* initiation codon. The *ampC* attenuator was, therefore, structurally intact in this clinical isolate. Likewise, no differences were found between the isolate and *E. coli* wild type in the first 200 bp of the *ampC* gene. However, both base substitutions and insertions were found in the *ampC* promoter. This indicates that a number of alterations are needed in the *ampC* promoter in order to increase its efficiency to the degree found in the isolate.

It is intriguing that *ampC* attenuator mutants

are so rare among clinical *E. coli* isolates despite the fact that they are easily obtained in batch cultures. However, the *ampC* attenuator serves as the transcriptional terminator for the preceding fumarate reductase operon (Grundström and Jaurin, Proc. Natl. Acad. Sci. U.S.A., in press). The DNA sequencing and expression analyses have demonstrated that the *ampC* promoter is part of the coding sequence for the last protein of this operon. A single insertion in the *ampC* promoter as found in the uppromoter mutant of *E. coli* K-12 results in a frame-shift mutation in this 13,000 protein. It will be interesting to see if such frame-shift mutations may also be selected for in the in vivo situation.

Taken together, our data demonstrate that gram-negative cephalosporinase genes show sequence homologies and code for a distinct class of serine β-lactamases. Mutations leading to elevated β-lactamase production in *E. coli* have been shown to occur in either the *ampC* promoter or the *ampC* attenuator.

This work was supported by grants from the Swedish Natural Science Research Council (Dnr 3373) and from the Swedish Medical Research Council (Dnr 5428).

1. **Jaurin, B., and T. Grundström.** 1981. *ampC* cephalosporinase of *Escherichia coli* K-12 has a different evolutionary origin from that of β-lactamases of the penicillinase type. Proc. Natl. Acad. Sci. U.S.A. **78:**4897–4901.
2. **Jaurin, B., T. Grundström, T. Edlund, and S. Normark.** 1981. The *E. coli* β-lactamase attenuator mediates growth rate dependent regulation. Nature (London) **290:**221–225.
3. **Sykes, R. B., and M. Matthew.** 1976. The β-lactamases of gram-negative bacteria and their role in resistance to β-lactam antibiotics. J. Antimicrob. Chemother. **2:**115–157.

Distribution and Characterization of β-Lactamase-Producing Strains Isolated in the Southern Part of the Netherlands

ELLEN E. STOBBERINGH,* ANTON W. HOUBEN, AND CEES P. A. VAN BOVEN

Department of Medical Microbiology, State University of Limburg, 6200 MD Maastricht, The Netherlands

To monitor the occurrence and mechanism of bacterial resistance to antibiotics in the region of South Limburg, the Netherlands (population ca. 900,000), a random sample of 487 gram-negative strains isolated in the six regional hospitals was collected in the months of April and May 1980. In this study comprising strains of *Escherichia coli* (n = 158), *Proteus* spp. (n = 125), *Klebsiella* spp. (n = 114), and *Pseudomonas* spp. (n = 90), the MIC for several cephalosporins was determined and the prevalent β-lactamase types were characterized. The cephalosporins included in the study were cephaloridine, a representative of the first-generation cephalosporins; cefamandole, cefoxitin, and cefuroxime, representatives of the second generation; cefotaxime of the third generation; and the newer semisynthetic derivatives cefotiam, cefsulodin, cefoperazone, moxalactam, and ceftazidime. All compounds were generous gifts of their respective manufacturers.

The MIC values were determined by a microbroth dilution method, using an inoculum size of a 1:100 diluted overnight culture (i.e., 10^5 colony-forming units/ml). The plasmid-mediated β-lactamases were characterized by isoelectric focusing, substrate profiles, and K_m and V_{max} values (1, 3). Because of the transferability of plasmids, the plasmid-mediated β-lactamases are, from an epidemiological point of view, of greater interest than the strain- and (sub)-species-specific chromosomally mediated β-lactamases (2).

The MIC 50 and MIC 90 values of the different cephalosporins are given in Table 1. Ceftazidime was the most active compound against *Pseudomonas* spp. with a MIC 50 value of 2 μg/ml. Ceftazidime was also active against *E. coli* and *Klebsiella* spp. with MIC 50 values of 0.125 and 0.25 μg/ml, respectively. Cefotaxime was even more effective against the two latter species as shown by MIC 50 values of 0.06 and 0.125 μg/ml, respectively.

Cefotaxime and cefoperazone were the two most active compounds against *Proteus* spp. *E. coli* strains were susceptible to all the tested cephalosporins, even to a certain extent to cephaloridine, a compound of the first generation (MIC 50 and MIC 90 value of 4 and 128 μg/ml, respectively).

The distribution of the different β-lactamase types, within each species and within the total population, is shown in Table 2. Seventy percent of the strains showed a distinct β-lactamase activity. In 62% of these strains a plasmid-mediated β-lactamase was found. TEM 1 was the

TABLE 1. *Comparative activity of different cephalosporins*

Drug	Activity against:							
	E. coli		*Proteus* spp.		*Klebsiella* spp.		*Pseudomonas* spp.	
	MIC 50	MIC 90	MIC 50	MIC 90	MIC 50	MIC 90	MIC 50	MIC 90
Cephaloridine	4	128	16	128	16	128	128	>128
Cefamandole	1	128	16	128	8	128	128	>128
Cefoxitin	8	32	32	128	8	128	128	>128
Cefuroxime	4	16	16	128	8	128	128	>128
Cefotaxime	0.06	0.5	4	32	0.125	8	32	>32
Cefotiam	0.5	8	32	>32	1	32	32	>32
Cefsulodin	32	>32	32	>32	32	>32	4	16
Cefoperazone	0.125	32	4	32	8	32	4	16
Moxalactam	0.25	1	8	32	0.5	4	32	>32
Ceftazidime	0.125	0.5	32	>32	0.25	4	2	8

TABLE 2. *Percent distribution of different β-lactamase types*

Organism	β-Lactamase									
	TEM 1	TEM 2	SHV 1	OXA 1	OXA 2	OXA 3	PSE 1	PSE 2	PSE 3	PSE 4
E. coli	81.3	2.7	5.3	1.3	8.0	1.3				
Proteus spp.	40.2	3.7	7.3	17.1	11.0	20.7				
Klebsiella spp.	64.8	15.9	11.4	2.3	2.3	3.4				
Pseudomonas spp.	61.9	4.8	9.5	2.4	2.4	2.4	4.8	1.2	1.2	9.5
Total population	62.1	6.8	8.4	5.6	5.9	7.0	1.2	0.3	0.3	2.4

most prevalent β-lactamase type, followed by SHV 1, OXA 3, and TEM 2. No HMS type was found throughout the tested bacterial population.

In this study a similar distribution was found for the MIC values and the β-lactamase types of the isolates from the different hospitals. Further analysis to correlate the resistance patterns with the different types of β-lactamases seems worthwhile. Furthermore, monitoring on a regular basis of the resistance patterns in the region might answer the question as to what extent antibiotic usage influences the resistance parameters.

1. **Matthew, M., A. M. Harris, M. J. Marshall, and G. W. Ross.** 1975. The use of analytical isoelectric focusing for detection and identification of β-lactamases. J. Gen. Microbiol. **88**:169–178.
2. **Matthew, M., and A. M. Harris.** 1976. Identification of β-lactamases by analytical isoelectric focusing: correlation with bacterial taxonomy. J. Gen. Microbiol. **94**:55–67.
3. **Samuni, A.** 1975. A direct spectrophotometric assay and determination of Michaelis constants for the β-lactamase reaction. Anal. Biochem. **63**:17–26.

Purification and Characterization of a *Proteus vulgaris* Beta-Lactamase that Hydrolyzes Methoxyiminocephalosporins

J. CHRISTENSON,* E. SQUIRES, R. GEIGER, AND M. TALBOT

Hoffmann-La Roche Inc., Nutley, New Jersey 07110, U.S.A.

Methoxyiminocephalosporins, such as ceftriaxone and cefotaxime, are resistant to hydrolysis catalyzed by most β-lactamases from *Enterobacteriaceae.* However, strains of *Proteus vulgaris,* including *P. vulgaris* 1028, have been reported to produce an enzyme capable of inactivating these and other β-lactams (1). A constitutive mutant of this strain was isolated by R. Then by serial passage in the presence of increasing concentrations of ceftriaxone. We report here the purification and characterization of the β-lactamase produced by this mutant, *P. vulgaris* 1028 β-c.

The enzyme was purified from a sonic extract by centrifugation, protamine sulfate treatment, gel filtration on Sephadex G-75, negative adsorption on QAE-Sephadex A-50, and rechromatography on Sephadex G-75. This resulted in a

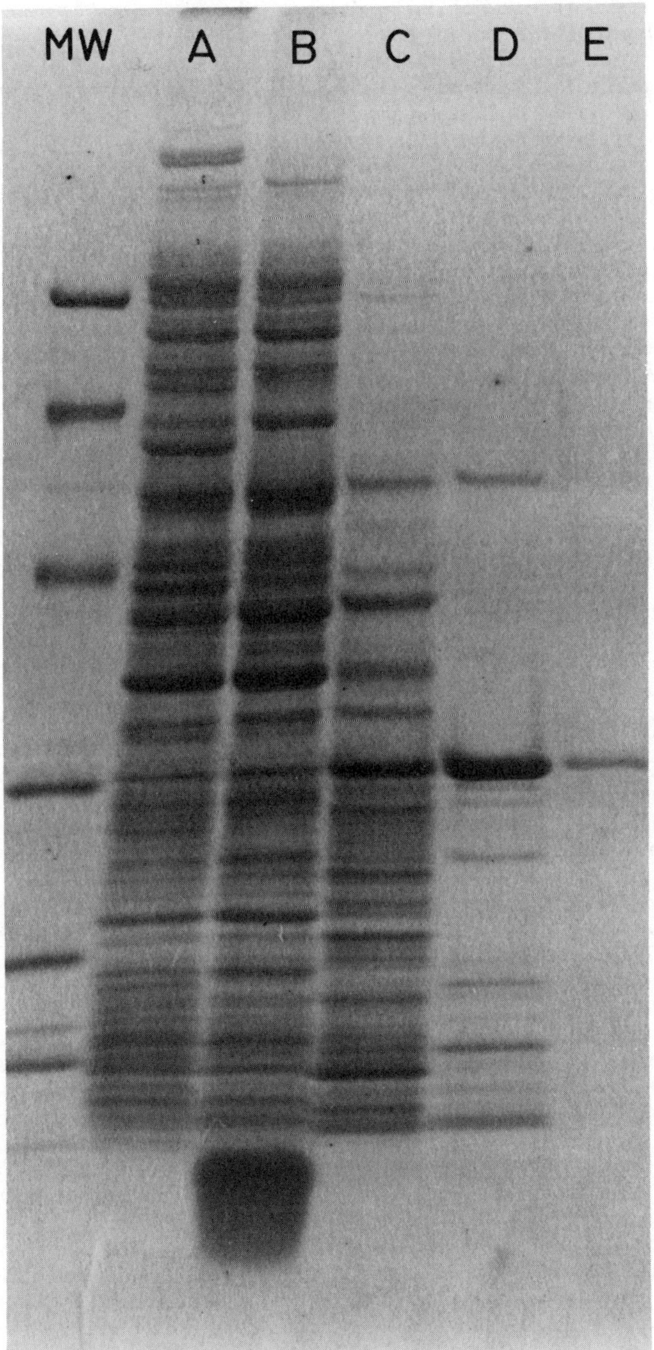

FIG. 1. *Sodium dodecyl sulfate-polyacrylamide gel electrophoresis of the enzyme at various stages of purification. Samples were fractionated on an 8 to 18% gradient gel. (MW) Molecular weight standards; (A) crude supernatant (22 μg of protein); (B) protamine sulfate supernatant (20 μg of protein); (C) Sephadex G75 (12 μg of protein); (D) QAE-Sephadex (6.25 μg of protein); (E) second Sephadex G75 (0.65 μg of protein). Molecular weight standards were: phosphorylase B (94,000 daltons), bovine serum albumin (68,000), ovalbumin (45,000), carbonic anhydrase (30,000), soybean trypsin inhibitor (21,000), and lysozyme (14,300).*

preparation with a specific activity of 79.1 μmol of nitrocefin hydrolyzed per min per mg of protein (71-fold purification compared with crude supernatant). The purified enzyme gave only a single band on sodium dodecyl sulfate-polyacrylamide slab gel electrophoresis (Fig. 1), but at the low protein concentration, minor contaminants may have escaped detection. Most of the experiments reported below were done with enzyme purified through the QAE-Sephadex step, which was highly purified, though not homogeneous (Fig. 1). The enzyme had a molecular weight of 30,000 by sodium dodecyl sulfate-polyacrylamide gel electrophoresis (Fig. 1).

Isoelectric focusing was carried out in polyacrylamide gels, which were then stained for β-lactamase activity by immersion in 0.1 mM nitrocefin solution. Under various conditions, a major band appeared at pH 8.6 to 8.8. This correlated well with the major band of β-lactamase activity found in crude extracts of *P. vulgaris* 1028 β-c as well as of the parent strain, *P. vulgaris* 1028. The major band of enzyme activity coincided with the single protein band (separately stained).

The substrate profile of the enzyme in a crude supernatant from a sonic extract under standard assay conditions was as follows: benzylpenicillin, 100; ampicillin, 152; mecillinam, 26; cloxacillin, ~0; nitrocefin, 1,012; cefazolin, 3,029; cephaloridine, 1,053. The enzyme thus appeared to be mainly a cephalosporinase, but also hydrolyzed penicillins at a significant rate. More detailed kinetic studies with a highly purified preparation are described below.

The rate of enzymatic hydrolysis of nitrocefin was optimal at pH 7.5. However, the rate at pH 7.0 was at least 90% of the rate at pH 7.5 and nonenzymatic hydrolysis was negligible at pH 7.0, so the standard assay conditions utilized sodium phosphate buffer, pH 7.0. The hydrolysis of nitrocefin was inhibited 93 to 97% by 0.1 mM cloxacillin, clavulanic acid, and penicillanic acid sulfone (CP-45,899). *p*-Chloromercuribenzoate (0.5 mM) inhibited the enzyme only 19%.

Significant departures from Michaelis-Menten kinetics were observed with all substrates tested except nitrocefin and mecillinam (Table 1). Substrate inhibition occurred with cephaloridine, ceftriaxone, benzylpenicillin, ampicillin, and cloxacillin. With ceftriaxone, the substrate inhibition was so severe that no hydrolysis was detectable at a substrate concentration of 0.2 mM. Cloxacillin was hydrolyzed only at a very slow rate. Because of its relatively strong affinity for the enzyme (K_m = 5.5 μM) and its slow rate of hydrolysis, cloxacillin would be expected to act as an inhibitor of the hydrolysis of better substrates.

TABLE 1. *Kinetic parameters of purified β-lactamase from P. vulgaris 1028 β-c*

Substrate	Parameter		Remark
	K_m (μM)	V_{max} (μmol/min·mg)	
Nitrocefin	27	111	
Cephaloridine	243	288	Substrate inhibition
Cefazolin			Non-Michaelis-Menten
Cefotaxime			Non-Michaelis-Menten
Ceftriaxone	29	66	Substrate inhibition
Benzylpenicillin	7.4	29	Substrate inhibition
Ampicillin	9.1	29	Substrate inhibition
Mecillinam	131	7.7	
Cloxacillin	5.5	0.2	Substrate inhibition

Angehrn et al. (1) reported that *P. vulgaris* 1028 was susceptible to ceftriaxone in vitro and in vivo. We found the constitutive mutant to be relatively resistant in vitro (MIC 16 μg/ml) and in vivo (PD_{50} > 250 mg/kg, single subcutaneous treatment immediately after infection). Although CP-45,899, ceftriaxone, and cefotaxime were all inactive against *P. vulgaris* 1028 β-c at a dose of 250 mg/kg, combinations of the β-lactamase inhibitor with the cephalosporins had good in vivo activity (PD_{50} 43+43 and 71+71 mg/kg, respectively).

Although the purified enzyme was not conclusively demonstrated to be homogeneous, it is clear from the isoelectric focusing experiments that the β-lactamase activity resided in the major protein component and not some minor contaminant.

Since *P. vulgaris* 1028 β-c was isolated by multiple passages in the presence of increasing concentrations of ceftriaxone, it is possible that the enzyme described here is structurally different from the wild-type enzyme produced by the parent strain. The simplest hypothesis, however, is that *P. vulgaris* 1028 β-c is a regulatory mutant of *P. vulgaris* 1028, producing the same enzyme at a higher, constitutive rate. The similarity in substrate profile and isoelectric point would tend to support this hypothesis, but further studies will be necessary to establish the point conclusively.

In the Richmond and Sykes classification of gram-negative β-lactamases (3), type Ic enzymes were characterized as having high activity against cephaloridine, moderate activity against penicillin and ampicillin, and low activity against cloxacillin. Both examples listed were from *P. vulgaris* strains. The enzyme described here and that described recently by Matsubara et al. (2) would appear to belong to this class. These two enzymes were similar to each other in terms of source, predominant cephalosporinase activity, molecular weight, pH optimum, isoelectric point, and inhibition by cloxacillin and clavulanic acid.

1. **Angehrn, P., P. J. Probst, R. Reiner, and R. L. Then.** 1980. Ro 13-9904, a long-acting broad-spectrum cephalosporin: in vitro and in vivo studies. Antimicrob. Agents Chemother. **18:**913–921.

2. **Matsubara, N., A. Yotsuji, K. Kumano, M. Inoue, and S. Mitsuhashi.** 1981. Purification and some properties of a cephalosporinase from *Proteus vulgaris*. Antimicrob. Agents Chemother. **19:**185–187.

3. **Richmond, M. H., and R. B. Sykes.** 1973. The β-lactamases of gram-negative bacteria and their possible physiological role, p. 31–88. *In* A. H. Rose and D. W. Tempest (ed.), Advances in microbial physiology. Academic Press, Inc., New York.

Isolation and Characterization of a β-Lactamase from *Escherichia coli* with an Unusual Substrate Profile

GERHARD SEIBERT* AND MICHAEL LIMBERT

Hoechst AG, D-6230 Frankfurt/Main, Federal Republic of Germany

Many β-lactamases from gram-negative bacteria are known which hydrolyze predominantly cephalosporins. Most of these enzymes have a rather poor activity against the cephalosporins of the third generation, for example cefotaxime or ceftizoxime. Enzymes hydrolyzing these compounds are mainly isolated from *Pseudomonas* (1), *Proteus* (2), or *Bacteroides* (3) species. Here the isolation and characterization of a β-lactamase from an *Escherichia coli* strain, which hydrolyzes some of the newly introduced cephalosporins very rapidly, is described.

The enzyme-producing strain *E. coli* 984 was isolated from clinical material. The strain is resistant to ampicillin, carbenicillin, and penicillin G. Table 1 shows the MICs of various cephalosporins for *E. coli* 984 determined in the serial dilution test with Mueller-Hinton broth. It is obvious that the activity of the majority of the antibiotics is dependent on the inoculum size. With increasing density the MICs of the different antibiotics rise up to 12 to 25 μg/ml. Only cefoxitin and desacetyl-cefotaxime do not show this marked inoculum effect with *E. coli* 984.

E. coli 984 produces a very active, noninducible β-lactamase. This β-lactamase is responsible for the dependence of MIC on the inoculum size. It was purified by ammonium sulfate precipitation, gel chromatography on Sephacryl S200 superfine (Pharmacia), and affinity chromatography on cefotaxime-Sepharose 4B. The enzyme could be enriched nearly 500-fold. The final preparation had a specific activity of 600 U/mg of protein. The highly purified β-lactamase migrated in sodium dodecyl sulfate-gel electrophoresis as a single band, indicating a molecular weight of approximately 39,000. The determination of the molecular weight by high-performance gel chromatography (Sephadex blue column, Pharmacia) confirmed this result in the same order of magnitude. The isoelectric point was pH 7.2. Optimal pH was about 8.4, and the optimal temperature was about 40°C, determined with cephaloridine as substrate. The β-lactamase possessed nearly no activity (V_{max} = 0.01) against penicillin G, ampicillin, cloxacillin, dicloxacillin, and carbenicillin. In contrast to clavulanic acid, cloxacillin, dicloxacillin, cefoxitin, and CP-45,899 do not inhibit the enzyme.

Table 2 shows the kinetics of hydrolysis of

TABLE 1. *Dependence of the MIC on the inoculum size of E. coli 984*

Antibiotic	MIC (μg/ml) with different inoculum sizes (CFU/ml):				
	10^7	10^6	10^5	10^4	10^3
Cephaloridine	25	6.25	3.13	1.56	1.56
Cefamandole	12.5	6.25	3.13	0.78	0.19
Cefotaxime	12.5	6.25	1.25	0.31	0.31
Desacetyl-cefotaxime	1.56	0.78	0.78	0.78	0.78
Ceftizoxime	25	12.5	1.25	0.62	0.31
Cefoxitin	12.5	12.5	3.13	3.13	3.13

TABLE 2. *Kinetics of hydrolysis of some cephalosporins by the β-lactamase from E. coli 984*

Antibiotic	Parameter	
	K_m (μM)	V_{max}[a]
Cephaloridine	220	100
Ceftizoxime	180	140
Cefotaxime	210	75
Desacetyl-cefotaxime	200	3
Cefoxitin	200	4
Cefuroxime	18	70
Cefazolin	23	38
Cefotiam	22	61
Cefoperazone	18	3

[a] V_{max} is expressed by the relative rate of hydrolysis; cephaloridine hydrolysis was taken as 100.

some cephalosporins by the β-lactamase from *E. coli* 984. K_m and V_{max} were determined from Lineweaver-Burke plots. The cephalosporins tested can be divided in two groups: one group with high affinity substrate to the enzyme and K_m values of about 20 μM, and one group with low affinity to the enzyme with values of about 200 μM for K_m. Among the antibiotics from the second group, ceftizoxime, cephaloridine, and cefotaxime are degraded with high velocity. Desacetyl-cefotaxime and cefoxitin are hydrolyzed only to a small extent by the *E. coli* 984 β-lactamase.

The data on ceftizoxime, cefotaxime, and its metabolite desacetyl-cefotaxime show that obviously the substituent in 3-position of the cephalosporin nucleus, which represents the only difference between these derivatives, is responsible for the susceptibility of the three molecules to an enzymatic attack. Ceftizoxime with a hydrogen in 3-position is degraded very rapidly (V_{max} = 140); cefotaxime with its acetoxy-methyl residue in 3-position is destroyed only with half of the velocity of ceftizoxime. In contrast the main metabolite of cefotaxime with its 3-methyl group is a very poor substrate for the *E. coli* 984 β-lactamase.

We are grateful to J. Conrady for technical assistance.

1. **Hirai, K., S. Iyobe, M. Inoue, and S. Mitsuhashi.** 1980. Purification and properties of a new β-lactamase from *Pseudomonas cepacia*. Antimicrob. Agents Chemother. **17**:355–358.
2. **Matsubara, N., A. Yotsuju, K. Kumano, M. Inoue, and S. Mitsuhashi.** 1981. Purification and some properties of a cephalosporinase from *Proteus vulgaris*. Antimicrob. Agents Chemother. **19**:185–187.
3. **Sato, K., M. Inoue, and S. Mitsuhashi.** 1980. Activity of β-lactamase produced by *Bacteroides fragilis* against newly introduced cephalosporins. Antimicrob. Agents Chemother. **17**:736–737.

Beta-Lactamase-Producing *Bacteroides* spp. in the Oral Cavity in Relation to Penicillin Therapy

CARL E. NORD,* ANDERS HEIMDAHL, AND LARS KONOW

Department of Bacteriology, National Bacteriological Laboratory, and Huddinge University Hospital, Karolinska Institute, Stockholm, Sweden*

The frequency of carriage of beta-lactamase-producing *Bacteroides* strains in the oral cavity is unknown. The effect of penicillin therapy on the resistance of oral *Bacteroides* strains has not been investigated, although reports suggest that increased use of penicillin influences the number of penicillin-resistant strains. Although an increasing proportion of penicillin-resistant strains among clinical isolates of *Bacteroides* species has been reported, penicillin is still considered to be the drug of choice in case of oral infections with *Bacteroides*. Recently, however, clinical failures with penicillin therapy of orofacial infections have been reported to be associated with beta-lactamase-producing *Bacteroides* species (1). The present study reports the incidence of carriage of penicillin-resistant *Bacteroides* species in the oral cavity, their production of beta-lactamase, their susceptibility patterns to different antibiotics, and their occurrence in relation to previous penicillin therapy.

Collection of specimens. Mixed-saliva samples were collected in glass tubes from 104 healthy persons. None of them was on medication at the time of sampling. Any history of penicillin treatment during the preceding 6 months was recorded.

Processing of specimens. Undiluted mixed-saliva samples (0.2 ml) were inoculated onto kanamycin-vancomycin-penicillin blood agar plates (kanamycin, 100 μg/ml; vancomycin, 7.5 μg/ml; benzylpenicillin, 2 μg/ml). All manipulations of the anaerobic medium were performed in an anaerobic chamber (Coy, Ann Arbor, Mich.) under a 90% (vol/vol) nitrogen and 10% (vol/vol) hydrogen atmosphere. The plates were incubated for 48 h anaerobically (GasPak Anaerobic Jars, BBL Microbiology Systems, Cockeysville, Md.). *Bacteroides* species were identified by Gram stain, biochemical tests, and gas-liquid chromatographic analysis of metabolic end products according to Holdeman et al. (2).

Carriage of penicillin-resistant strains. Fifty-seven penicillin-resistant *Bacteroides* species were isolated from 44 (42%) of the 104 participants. The most commonly found species were *B. melaninogenicus*, *B. ruminicola*, and *B. oralis* (Table 1). Twelve of 44 persons who harbored penicillin-resistant species in the oral cavity had been on penicillin therapy during the

TABLE 1. *Fifty-seven penicillin-resistant oral Bacteroides isolates and their production of β-lactamase*

Bacteroides species	No. of isolates	No. of isolates producing β-lactamase detected by:		β-Lactamase activity[a] (U/mg of bacterial dry wt)	
		Slide iodometric assay[b]	Nitrocefin assay[a]	Mean value	Range
B. melaninogenicus	27	27	27	0.004	0.001–0.010
B. ruminicola	14	14	14	0.006	0.002–0.012
B. oralis	5	5	5	0.002	0.001–0.004
B. ovatus	3	3	3	0.005	0.003–0.013
B. multiacidus	2	2	0	ND[c]	
B. hypermegas	1	1	0	ND[c]	
Bacteroides species	5	5	5	0.002	0.001–0.005

[a] Activity measured spectrophotometrically, using nitrocefin assay according to Olsson et al. (4).
[b] Detected by slide iodometric assay according to Murray and Rosenblatt (3).
[c] Not detected.

6 months preceding the saliva sampling. In contrast, only 5 out of the 60 persons from whom no penicillin-resistant *Bacteroides* strains were isolated had received penicillin during the corresponding time ($P < 0.01$).

Antibiotic susceptibilities. The MICs of phenoxymethylpenicillin, benzylpenicillin, ampicillin, clindamycin, erythromycin, doxycycline, and tinidazole were determined for the different strains by the agar dilution method. All strains isolated were resistant (MIC ⩾ 4 μg/ml) to phenoxymethylpenicillin, benzylpenicillin, and all but one strain (MIC = 2 μg/ml) were resistant to ampicillin. About 45% of the strains were resistant to erythromycin (MIC ⩾ 4 μg/ml). Most strains were found to be rather susceptible (MIC ⩽ 2 μg/ml) to doxycycline, but 12 strains were resistant (MIC ⩾ 4 μg/ml). Tinidazole and clindamycin inhibited all strains at low concentrations (Fig. 1).

Beta-lactamase production. Nitrocefin (Glaxo, Greenford, England) was used as substrate for determination of beta-lactamase activity spectrophotometrically (4). The strains were also tested for production of beta-lactamase by the iodometric assay (3). Beta-lactamase was detected in all strains by slide iodometric assay (Table 1). *B. melaninogenicus*, *B. ruminicola*, and *B. ovatus* strains produced the highest amounts of beta-lactamase.

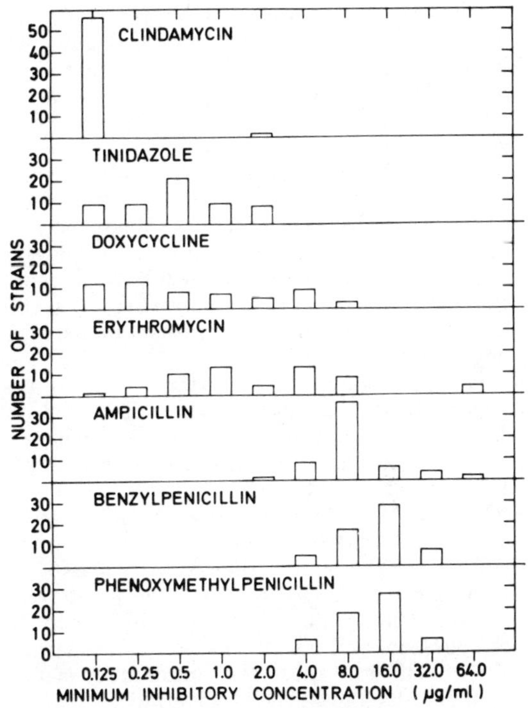

FIG. 1. *MICs of phenoxymethylpenicillin, benzylpenicillin, ampicillin, erythromycin, doxycycline, tinidazole, and clindamycin for 57 penicillin-resistant Bacteroides strains isolated from the oral cavity.*

Conclusions. Since *Bacteroides* species are the dominating pathogens in orofacial infections, resistance to penicillin could be of clinical importance. Clinical failures in the treatment of orofacial infections with penicillin have recently been reported. The *Bacteroides* strains which were resistant to phenoxymethylpenicillin were also resistant to benzylpenicillin and ampicillin, and accordingly other antimicrobial agents must be chosen in cases of infection with such bacteria. All strains were susceptible to clindamycin and tinidazole, but several strains were resistant to doxycycline and or erythromycin. The drug of choice in such infections should, therefore, be clindamycin or nitroimidazoles.

1. **Heimdahl, A., L. von Konow, and C. E. Nord.** 1980. Isolation of β-lactamase-producing *Bacteroides* strains

associated with clinical failures with penicillin treatment of orofacial infections. Arch. Oral Biol. **25:**689–692.
2. **Holdeman, L. V., E. C. Cato, and W. E. C. Moore.** 1977. Anaerobe laboratory manual, 4th ed. Virginia Polytechnic Institute and State University, Blacksburg.
3. **Murray, P. R., and J. E. Rosenblatt.** 1977. Penicillin resistance and penicillinase production in clinical isolates of *Bacteroides melaninogenicus*. Antimicrob. Agents Chemother. **11:**605–608.
4. **Olsson, B., C. E. Nord, and T. Wadström.** 1976. Formation of beta-lactamase in *Bacteroides fragilis*: cell-bound and extracellular activity. Antimicrob. Agents Chemother. **9:**727–735.

Role of Plasmid-Mediated Beta-Lactamases in the Resistance of *Pseudomonas aeruginosa* to New Beta-Lactams

DAVID M. LIVERMORE* AND ROSAMUND J. WILLIAMS

The London Hospital Medical College, London, United Kingdom

Virtually all *Pseudomonas aeruginosa* strains produce a chromosomally mediated inducible beta-lactamase, the Sabath and Abrahams (Id) enzyme (7). This is active against many earlier beta-lactams but not carbenicillin (5). Occasional isolates of *P. aeruginosa*, however, carry plasmids specifying additional beta-lactamases active against carbenicillin. Seven such carbenicillinases are listed by Matthew (3) as occurring in *P. aeruginosa*. Clinical isolates producing these enzymes are infrequent (2) but can cause therapeutic problems, especially where plasmids also encode resistance to antipseudomonal aminoglycosides.

We investigated the importance of these enzymes in resistance to carbenicillin and to several new antipseudomonal beta-lactams, namely: the cephalosporins cefoperazone (T-1551; Pfizer), cefotaxime (Roussel), cefsulodin (Ciba-Geigy), ceftazidime (Glaxo), and ceftriaxone (Roche); the 1-oxa beta-lactam moxalactam (Lilly); *N*-formimidoyl thienamycin (MK0787) (Merck Sharp & Dohme); and the monocyclic beta-lactam Squibb 26,776 (Squibb). Excepting cefoperazone and ceftriaxone, which are marginally unstable, all these antibiotics are resistant to Id beta-lactamase (D. M. Livermore, in press). Two experimental approaches were used.

Beta-lactamase hydrolysis studies. Beta-lactamase-producing organisms were grown overnight at 37°C, with shaking, in 500-ml volumes of nutrient broth (Oxoid no. 2). Cells were harvested at 5,000 × *g*, washed, and ultrasonically disrupted. Debris was removed by ultracentrifugation at 100,000 × *g*. Identity of beta-lactamases in these extracts was confirmed by isoelectric focusing (4), and their activity against new beta-lactams was assayed spectrophotometrically and by a considerably more sensitive bioassay method.

Spectrophotometric assay. The assay was based on the methods of Waley (8) (carbenicillin) and O'Callaghan et al. (5) (cephalosporins). Volumes (25 μl) of enzyme extracts were added to 2.5 ml of 0.1 mM (1 mM in case of carbenicillin) beta-lactam in 0.1 M phosphate buffer, pH 7.2. Absorbance was scanned from 300 to 230 nm (cephalosporins and moxalactam), 250 to 220 nm (carbenicillin), and 330 to 270 nm (MK0787) at 5-min intervals to 40 min. Scans were compared to those for intact and totally hydrolyzed antibiotic, and hydrolysis rates were thus calculated.

Bioassay. For this assay, 100 μl of enzyme extract was added to 900 μl of beta-lactam solution in 0.1 M phosphate buffer, pH 7.2 to give a final antibiotic concentration of 20 mg/liter. After 4 h of incubation at 37°C, residual antibiotic was assayed, in comparison to identically incubated (no enzyme) standards, in bioassay plates seeded with 10^7 colony-forming units of indicator organism per ml (Table 1). Inhibition zones were measured after 18 h of incubation at 37°C. Hydrolysis results are given in Table 1.

Degree of resistance conferred by plasmid-coded beta-lactamases. Plasmids coding TEM 1, TEM 2, OXA 3, and PSE 2 were transferred into the auxotrophic *rif*^{r} *str*^{r} *P. aeruginosa* mutant PU21 (1) as follows: 0.1-ml volumes of overnight (37°C) cultures of donor (isolate producing beta-lactamase) and recipient (PU21) were mixed with 2.5 ml of fresh nutrient broth. After overnight incubation (37°C), mixtures were plated onto diagnostic sensitivity test agar (Oxoid DST) containing 500 mg of carbenicillin plus 100 mg of rifampin per liter. Colonies growing were purified and confirmed as transconjugants. PU21 transconjugants producing PSE 1, PSE 2, and PSE 3 were obtained from Glaxo Group Research. We were unable to transfer PSE 4 enzyme.

Beta-lactam MICs against PU21R$^-$ and its exconjugants were determined by the agar dilu-

TABLE 1. *Hydrolytic activity of plasmid-mediated beta-lactamases occurring in P. aeruginosa*

Enzyme	Hydrolytic activity (% activity vs. cephaloridine)[a]								
	Carbenicillin	Cefoperazone	Cefsulodin	Ceftriaxone	Cefotaxime	Ceftazidime	MK0787	Moxalactam	Squibb 26,776
TEM 1	481	85	5	B	B	O	B	O	O
TEM 2	547	29	B	B	B	O	B	O	O
OXA 3	475	25	13	B	B	B/O	O	O	O
PSE 1	1,709	27	10	O	O	O	O	O	O
PSE 2	2,976	388	19	5	B	O	O	O	B/O
PSE 3	2,820	B	80	B	B	B/O	O	B/O	O
PSE 4	820	20	19	O	O	O	O	O	O

[a] B, Hydrolysis undetectable by spectrophotometry but detectable by high-enzyme long-time bioassay method. O, No hydrolysis detectable by either method. Bioassay indicators: ceftriaxone, *Sarcina lutea* 8430; cefsulodin, *P. aeruginosa* 799/61; others, *Escherichia coli* 10418; carbenicillin, not done.

TABLE 2. *MICs of new beta-lactams against PU21R⁻ and its plasmid-coded beta-lactamase-producing exconjugants*

Organism	MIC[a]								
	Carbenicillin	Cefoperazone	Cefsulodin	Ceftriaxone	Cefotaxime	Ceftazidime	MK0787	Moxalactam	Squibb 26,776
$PU21R^-$	40	4	1	4	16	2	1	16	4
$PU21(TEM\ 1)^+$	640	64	8	8	8	2	1	8	8
$PU21(TEM\ 2)^+$	5,210	32	32	4	16	2	1	8	4
$PU21(OXA\ 3)^+$	1,280	128	32	8	16	8	1	8	2
$PU21(PSE\ 1)^+$	5,120	32	16	8	16	2	1	16	8
$PU21(PSE\ 2)^+a$	1,280	256	32	64	32	2	1	8	16
$PU21(PSE2)^+b$	160	32	4	8	8	1	1	8	4
$PU21(PSE\ 3)^+$	5,120	16	8	8	8	2	1	16	4

[a] Differences of 1 dilution greater or less than PU21 were considered to be within experimental variation for purposes of the discussion.

tion technique with doubling antibiotic dilutions in DST agar. Inoculum used was about 10^5 colony-forming units. Results are shown in Table 2.

Because the degree of resistance to a beta-lactam conferred by beta-lactamase production depends on the physiological efficiency of the enzyme, the amount of enzyme, and the rate of antibiotic penetration, a direct quantitative relationship between enzymic activity and resistance conferred would not be expected. However, an increase in resistance to labile compounds would be expected in enzyme producers, with the proviso that, below a certain activity, this increase would be insignificant. This indeed was observed.

All six transferred beta-lactamases hydrolyzed cefoperazone, cefsulodin, and carbenicillin; PU21 transconjugants producing these enzymes showed increased resistance to these agents. PSE 2 was also active against ceftriaxone and $PU21(PSE\ 2)^+a$ was resistant to this agent. Although slight activities of TEM enzymes against cefotaxime, ceftriaxone, and MK0787 and of PSE 3 and OXA 3 against ceftriaxone and cefotaxime were detected, these were below the significant level and did not affect resistance to these agents.

A few anomalies were evident: PSE 2 showed negligible hydrolysis of Squibb 26,776, yet $PU21(PSE\text{-}2)^+a$ showed resistance to this agent; OXA 3 production conferred ceftazidime resistance although hydrolytic activity against this agent was also barely detectable (Table 2). These observations may indicate the plasmids carried further markers determining resistance by other mechanisms or may reflect inherent weaknesses in in vitro hydrolysis studies.

Comparison of MIC data against the two PSE 2-producing PU21 exconjugants indicates $PU21(PSE\text{-}2)^+a$ showed higher resistance to PSE 2 labile agents than did PU21(PSE-2)b. Preliminary results suggest this is consequent on greater enzyme production by $PU21(PSE\text{-}2)^+a$ during log-phase growth. Genetically this difference may depend on plasmid copy number or degree of gene expression.

We thank manufacturers as stated for their antibiotics. Our thanks also to Glaxo Group Research for PU21 exconjugants specifying PSE beta-lactamases.

1. **Jacoby, G. A.** 1974. Properties of R plasmids determining gentamicin resistance by acetylation in *P. aeruginosa*. Antimicrob. Agents Chemother. **6**:239–252.
2. **King, T. D., T. Farmer, C. Reading, and R. Sutherland.** 1980. Sensitivity to carbenicillin and ticarcillin and the beta-lactamases of *P. aeruginosa* in the UK in 1978–9. J. Clin. Pathol. **33**:297–301.
3. **Matthew, M.** 1971. Plasmid-mediated beta-lactamases of Gram-negative bacteria: properties and distribution. J. Antimicrob. Chemother. **5**:349–358.
4. **Matthew, M., A. Harris, M. Marshall, and G. W. Ross.** 1975. The use of analytical isoelectric focussing for the detection and identification of beta-lactamases. J. Gen. Microbiol. **88**:169–178.
5. **O'Callaghan, C. H., P. W. Muggleton, and G. W. Ross.** 1969. Effects of beta-lactamase from gram-negative organisms on cephalosporins and penicillins, p. 57–63. Antimicrob. Agents Chemother. 1968.
6. **Ohmori, H., A. Azuma, Y. Suzuki, and Y. Hashimoto.** 1977. Factors involved in beta-lactam resistance in *P. aeruginosa*. Antimicrob. Agents Chemother. **12**:537–538.
7. **Sabath, L. D., M. Jago, and E. P. Abraham.** 1965. Cephalosporinase and penicillinase activities of a beta-lactamase from *P. aeruginosa*. Biochem. J. **96**:739–752.
8. **Waley, S.** 1974. A spectrophotometric assay of beta-lactamase action on penicillins. Biochem. J. **139**:789–790.

Practical Significance of Resistance to β-Lactamases Among New and Established β-Lactam Antibiotics

SYDNEY SELWYN* AND MOHAMMAD BAKHTIAR

Department of Medical Microbiology, Westminster Medical School, University of London, London SW1P 2AR, England

Resistance to β-lactamases has become the major prerequisite for new cephalosporins or comparable β-lactam antibiotics. Unfortunately, however, the remarkable range of these agents introduced recently has led to inevitable confusion due both to the lack of adequate comparative data and the absence of a comprehensive assessment of the part played by β-lactamase resistance in the in vitro and in vivo activity of these antibiotics. To resolve the first problem we have determined in parallel, using two independent methods, antibiotic stabilities against β-lactamases from *Staphylococcus aureus* (PC 1), *Escherichia coli* class III2(TEM), *Klebsiella aerogenes* class IVc (K 1), and *Enterobacter cloacae* class Ia (P 99), as well as the two enzymes from *Bacillus cereus* (569/H/9) which are widely used as a mixture in the laboratory. The antibiotics studied included moxalactam, ceftazidime, cefotaxime, cefsulodin, cefuroxime, cefamandole, cefoxitin, the earlier derivatives cefazolin, cephalexin, and cephradine, and the enzyme-resistant penicillins methicillin and cloxacillin.

Using a recently developed solid test system, which allows the direct comparison of 12 or more antibiotics on a single agar plate (1), and converting the reductions of zone sizes summarized in Table 1 into actual losses of antibiotic activity, ceftazidime was found to possess the highest degree of resistance to β-lactamase from *S. aureus*. Moxalactam was the next most stable at moderate enzyme concentrations, followed by cefotaxime; but this sequence was reversed at high concentrations (Fig. 1). Then in descending order of resistance were cefoxitin, methicillin, cephradine, cefuroxime, cefsulodin, cloxacillin, cephalexin, and—very far behind—cefamandole and cefazolin. In additional tests, the resistance of isoxazolylpenicillins was, in descending order, cloxacillin, dicloxacillin, flucloxacillin, and oxacillin (2). Similarly, further cephalosporins of the first and second generations were—with decreasing resistance after cephalexin—cefadroxil (at high enzyme concentrations), cephaloglycin, cefaclor (the most unstable of oral cephalosporins), cephacetrile, cephalothin, cephapirin, and, finally, cephaloridine, which was as unstable as cefazolin (4). The same order was obtained using a conventional enzyme assay system (2), except that cloxacillin then appeared marginally more resistant than cephradine.

With class IIIa (TEM) enzyme, the sequence was the same except for greater stability of cefuroxime and cloxacillin. The order was also similar with class IVc (K 1) enzyme, apart from the paradoxical finding that cefuroxime was remarkably unstable in this case.

The two enzymes of special value for destroying β-lactamases in laboratory samples—class Ia(P 99) and *B. cereus* type II—fortunately showed broadly reciprocal activities. Thus moxalactam was highly resistant to P 99 and so, to a lesser extent, were cefsulodin, ceftazidime, cefotaxime, and cefuroxime; all, however, were susceptible to *B. cereus* II (Table 1). The reverse was seen with cefoxitin, cephradine, and cephalexin. Therefore a mixture of the two enzymes

TABLE 1. *Effects of β-lactamases on 12 β-lactam antibiotics in a solid test system*

Antibiotics	Reduction of inhibition zone (%) due to action of β-lactamase from:									
	S. aureus (PC 1)		*B. cereus* (569/H/9)		*E. coli* (TEM)		*Klebsiella* (K 1)		*E. cloacae* (P 99)	
	100[a]	20[a]	100	20	100	20	100	20	100	20
Methicillin	33	20	100	100	100	100	100	100	86	46
Cloxacillin	75	20	95	75	100	100	100	100	35	0
Cefamandole	100	92	100	80	100	100	100	100	100	95
Cefazolin	100	95	95	70	100	100	100	100	100	100
Cefotaxime	20	15	100	100	80	40	100	80	87	60
Cefoxitin	20	15	13	0	73	33	13	8	100	80
Cefsulodin	64	28	100	79	100	100	100	71	64	21
Ceftazidime	10	0	100	50	0	0	12	10	75	25
Cefuroxime	38	20	100	72	83	44	100	100	88	61
Cephalexin	71	35	43	8	100	83	86	64	100	100
Cephradine	33	16	26	0	86	73	80	47	100	86
Moxalactam	20	0	60	20	10	0	0	0	20	0

[a] Percentage of enzyme stock solution used.

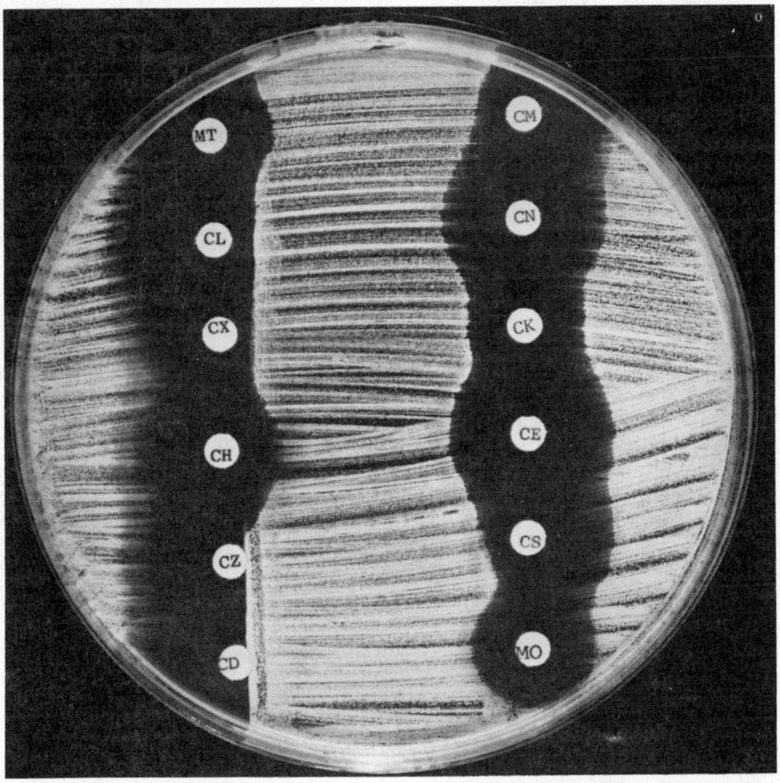

FIG. 1. *Action of staphylococcal β-lactamase (1.5 IU/cm² of central band) on 12 β-lactam antibiotics. Paper disks containing 10 μg of, from the top, (left) methicillin (MT), cloxacillin (CL), cephalexin (CX), cephradine (CH), cefazolin (CZ), cefamandole (CD); (right) cefuroxime (CM), cefoxitin (CN), ceftazidime (CK), cefotaxime (CE), cefsulodin (CS), and moxalactam (MO). Outer zones are free of enzyme and act as controls in each case. (This culture plate corresponds to the first column of Table 1, which refers to undiluted enzyme solution.)*

remains ideal for laboratory use (2). An additional amount of *B. cereus* II enzyme will, however, be needed for moxalactam.

The studies were extended to a novel monocyclic β-lactam "monobactam" Squibb 26,776 (6), which was found to have a high order of stability except to class IVc. Although like cefsulodin, Squibb 26,776 has useful activity only against gram-negative species, its resistance to staphylococcal enzyme will protect against its destruction in mixed infections involving staphylococci.

The clinical significance of β-lactamase production has been controversial for many years. However, in the case of *S. aureus* recent detailed studies (which did not include the newest derivatives) have confirmed that antibiotic stability was positively correlated with clinical efficacy (3). Paradoxically, the highly enzyme-resistant new β-lactams have less anti-staphylococcal activity than most earlier compounds.

With the gram-negative bacilli, the correlation is most evident in the case of bacteria such as *E. coli*, *Haemophilus influenzae*, and gonococci that produce the plasmid-mediated class IIIa enzyme. Nevertheless, in all gram-negative infections the antibacterial efficacy of β-lactam therapy depends largely on the ability of the drug to penetrate the cell wall permeability barriers. These features must, moreover, be combined with satisfactory tissue distribution. Unfortunately, conventional in vitro tests greatly underestimate the effects of β-lactamase production and ignore protein binding of antibiotics. Technical modifications and correction factors have, therefore, recently been introduced to improve the predictive value of laboratory tests (5).

The results of our studies on β-lactamase resistance and antibacterial activity in vitro and in vivo, together with the available data on pharmacokinetics, form the basis for the antibiotic policy and recommended strategy in our group of University Hospitals. The classical indications remain for benzylpenicillin—notably infection with *Streptococcus pyogenes*, pneumococci, gonococci, and spirochetes. Staphylococcal infections are treated primarily with either an isoxazolylpenicillin or a cephalosporin. Our routine choice of cephalosporin here and in a range of infections due to gram-negative bacilli, notably klebsiellae, remains cephradine on account of its uniformly good enzyme resistance (the most stable of oral β-lactams), its availability by all routes, and its excellent pharmacokinetics. However, in relatively resistant gram-negative infections we substitute cefuroxime or, increasingly, cefotaxime. In *Pseudomonas* infections our recent findings have led us to prefer piperacillin or azlocillin to carbenicillin or ticarcillin because of greater activity and lower sodium content. Similarly, in severe gram-negative infections due to nonproducers of β-lactamase we favor piperacillin for intravenous use rather than a carboxypenicillin, often combined with aminoglycoside. We have not yet found any requirements for moxalactam or cefsulodin, nor have we had recourse to ceftazidime, although the latter may prove a useful reserve drug against pseudomonads and other bacteria resistant to our first-line antibiotics.

We thank J. Melling and Glaxo Laboratories for supplying β-lactamases, and R. B. Sykes, Squibb Research Institute, for supplying SQ 26,776.

1. **Selwyn, S.** 1977. Susceptibility of penicillins and cephalosporins to β-lactamases assessed by a new test. J. Antimicrob. Chemother. **3:**161–168.
2. **Selwyn, S.** 1980. Beta-lactamases in practice, p. 180–206. *In* The beta-lactam antibiotics: penicillins and cephalosporins in perspective. Hodder and Stoughton, London.
3. **Selwyn, S.** 1980. Comparative stabilities of penicillins and cephalosporins to staphylococcal β-lactamase and activities against *Staphylococcus aureus*. J. Antimicrob. Chemother. **6:**794–795.
4. **Selwyn, S., and M. Bakhtiar.** 1979. Comparative studies on beta-lactamase susceptibility using a two-dimensional solid system. Drugs Exp. Clin. Res. **5:**13–21.
5. **Selwyn, S., and M. Bakhtiar.** 1981. New correction factors to improve the predictive value of in vitro tests. Drugs Exp. Clin. Res. **7:**163–168.
6. **Williams, J. D., et al.** 1981. Monobactams: naturally-occurring monocyclic beta-lactam antibiotics produced by bacteria, p. 55–56. Abstr., 12th Int. Cong. Chemother.

Correlation of β-Lactamase Production and Resistance to β-Lactam Antibiotics in *Enterobacteriaceae*

W. OPFERKUCH,* W. CULLMANN, T. FLENSBERG, M. STIEGLITZ, AND B. WIEDEMANN

Department of Medical Microbiology and Immunology, Ruhr-Universität Bochum, and Department of Medical Microbiology, University of Bonn, Federal Republic of Germany*

Production of β-lactamases in *Enterobacteriaceae* can be regarded as one resistance mechanism (4). Recently developed β-lactam compounds exhibit great stability against the attack of β-lactamases. However, a number of bacteria can develop resistance to the new β-lactam antibiotics. Therefore, it was of interest to examine to what extent the production of different β-lactamases influences the resistance of gram-negative bacteria.

A total of 284 strains of ampicillin-resistant strains of *Enterobacteriaceae*, recently isolated from clinical specimens and identified by the API 20 system, were investigated. The MIC against various β-lactam antibiotics was determined using a microdilution method, with two-fold serial dilutions in Mueller-Hinton broth. The strains exhibiting the following MICs were considered resistant: ampicillin, >16 mg/liter; ticarcillin, >64 mg/liter; piperacillin, >8 mg/liter; mezlocillin, >16 mg/liter; cephalothin, >8 mg/liter; cefoxitin, >8 mg/liter; cefuroxime, > 8 mg/liter; and cefotaxime, >4 mg/liter.

TABLE 1. *β-Lactamase profiles of Enterobacteriaceae*

Species	No. of strains	Production of: No production	TEM 1	TEM 2	Non-classified
E. coli	50	3	43	2	2
Klebsiella	50	17	16	4	30
Enterobacter	50	25	12	2	18
Serratia	50	23	21	5	3
Proteus mirabilis	20	9	3	8	
Proteus vulgaris	33	29	1	1	2
Proteus morganii	18	14	2		2
Proteus rettgeri	13	1		12	
Total	284	121	98	34	57
% of total number		42.6	34.5	12.0	20.1
% of lactamase-positive strains			60.1	20.8	35.0

All strains were investigated for their β-lactamase production using the chromogenic cephalosporin 87/312 (Nitrocefin) (Glaxo Research Ltd.). The cell-free supernatant of bacterial lysates was incubated with Nitrocefin for 5 min at room temperature. A color change to red was taken as an indication of β-lactamase production (3). To classify the enzymes, the cell-free supernatants of the lactamase-positive strains were subjected to analytical isoelectric focusing on polyacrylamide gel, according to the method described by Matthews et al. (2).

As revealed by the semiquantitative Nitrocefin test, 120 of the 284 strains investigated lacked spontaneous production of β-lactamases (Table 1). From Table 1 it can be seen that 42.2% of the strains did not produce any lactamase at all; 34.5% of the strains, or 60.1% of the lactamase-positive strains, produced TEM 1; 12% (or 20.8% of the positive strains) produced TEM 2; and 20.1% (or 35.0%) produced non-TEM enzymes. These figures show that 9.5% of all strains or 15.5% of the lactamase-positive strains produced an additional lactamase to a TEM enzyme.

To gain further information on the influence of β-lactamase production on the resistance pattern against various β-lactam compounds, our strains were classified according to their resistance pattern. For the 7 β-lactam antibiotics, 21

TABLE 2. *Geometric mean values of β-lactamase-producing and nonproducing strains of ampicillin-resistant Enterobacteriaceae*

Species	No. of strain	Production of lactamase	Mean MIC (μg/ml): Mezlocillin	Piperacillin	Ticarcillin	Cephalothin	Cefoxitin	Cefuroxime	Cefotaxime
E. coli	47	+	74.2	118.9	576	14.2	2.3	2.4	<1
	2	0	16	16	362	4	1.5	1.5	<1
Klebsiella	18	+	29.6	27.4	323	8.3	3.5	3.7	<1
	17	0	5.8	6.5	128	2.4	1.7	1.3	<1
Enterobacter	19	+	19.9	27.7	107	330	59.4	20.7	2.8
	26	0	3.5	4.1	8.4	196	41.8	6.3	1.3
Serratia	25	+	105	120	194	1,024	18.9	99.7	0.44
	23	0	8.0	4.8	16.5	1,024	13.4	70.0	0.38
Proteus mirabilis	11	+	398	481.0	512	82.4	4.5	4	0.25
	9	0	18.7	20.1	47.0	40.3	4.7	8.0	0.25
Proteus vulgaris	3	+	323	81	813	203	2.5	2.0	0.28
	28	0	2.0	4.3	14.1	512	4.2	297	0.28
Proteus morganii	4	+	256	152	107	1,024	11.3	32	0.84
	14	0	2.0	2.1	2.6	1,024	8	26.2	0.58
Proteus rettgeri	10	+	724	223	776	128	3.5	1.7	0.31
	1	0	256	512	1024	16	2	1	0.25
No. of strains	257								
Lactamase positive		137							
Lactamase negative		120							

different resistance patterns were found. When correlated with the β-lactamase production, some species showed identical resistance patterns in several strains independent of lactamase production and the type of enzyme produced. Strains which lacked β-lactamase production more frequently showed resistance to cephalosporins. However, a close relationship between resistance pattern and lactamase production could not be observed.

To quantify the effect of lactamase production on resistance the geometrical mean values of the MICs of the lactamase-producing and the nonproducing strains were compared (Table 2). As can be seen, the production of β-lactamases is often associated with an increase in the MIC values. However, this phenomenon cannot be observed, e.g., in the case of *Serratia* and cephalothin, *Enterobacter* and cefoxitin, or *Proteus morganii* and cefuroxime. In these cases it is obvious that a specific, lactamase-independent intrinsic resistance must be assumed.

Consequently, the production of β-lactamases cannot be regarded as the sole determinant of resistance to β-lactam antibiotics in ampicillin-resistant strains of *Enterobacteriaceae* (4).

Four other mechanisms must also be considered: (i) the production of different amounts of β-lactamase; (ii) an impaired affinity of the enzyme to various antibiotics (5); (iii) an impaired penetration of the outer membrane; and/or (iv) an impaired affinity to penicillin-binding proteins (1).

1. **Crowlesmith, J., and T. G. B. Howe.** 1980. Characterization of β-lactamase-deficient (*bla*) mutants of the R-plasmid R1 in *Escherichia coli* K-12 and comparison with similar mutants of RP. Antimicrob. Agents Chemother. **18:**667–674.
2. **Matthews, M., A. M. Harris, M. J. Marshall, and G. W. Ross.** 1975. The use of analytical isoelectric focusing for detection and identification of β-lactamases. J. Gen. Microbiol. **88:**169–178.
3. **O'Callaghan, C. H., A. Morris, S. Kirby, and A. H. Shingler.** 1972. Novel method for determination of β-lactamases by using a chromogenic cephalosporin substrate. Antimicrob. Agents Chemother. **12:**126–128.
4. **Richmond, M. H., and N. A. C. Curtis.** 1974. The interplay of β-lactamase and intrinsic factors in the resistance of gram negative bacteria to penicillins and cephalosporins. Ann. N.Y. Acad. Sci. **235:**553–563.
5. **Spratt, B. G.** 1978. Escherichia coli resistance to β-lactam antibiotics through the decrease in the affinity of a target for lethality. Nature (London) **274:**713–715.

Inactivation of β-Lactam Molecules in *Citrobacter diversus* Related to Unusual Chromosomal Penicillinases

ROBERT LETARTE,* ROBERT DELAGE, CLAUDE ASSELIN, AND JEAN-CLAUDE PECHERE

Department of Microbiology, Faculty of Medicine, Laval University, Quebec, Canada G1K 7P4

β-Lactamases appear to play a major role in bacterial resistance to β-lactam antibiotics (5). Many enzymes have been characterized among gram-negative bacteria, and according to their substrate profile, they have been classified into three groups: penicillinases, cephalosporinases, and broad-spectrum β-lactamases.

Citrobacter diversus is known to be distinct from *C. freundii* in its resistance profile to antibiotics. In fact, *C. diversus* is usually penicillin, ampicillin, and carbenicillin resistant but remains cephalothin susceptible. To explain that resistance pattern, we undertook a study to identify the β-lactamase in *C. diversus* strains and to evaluate its activity on various β-lactam drugs, including newer cephalosporins.

Crude enzymatic extracts were prepared from 10 clinical isolates of *C. diversus*. Extracts were obtained by sonication of the cells collected from an 18-h culture in brain heart infusion broth supplemented with 100 μg of penicillin G per ml.

TABLE 1. *Substrate profile activity (K_m and V_{max}) of the C. diversus 4.9 and 5.4 penicillinases*

Substrate	*C. diversus* MULB 650, pI 4.9		*C. diversus* MULB 662, pI 5.4	
	K_m (m)	V_{max}[a]	K_m (m)	V_{max}[a]
Penicillin G	4.3×10^6	100	2.0×10^6	100
Ampicillin	2.1×10^6	31	3.3×10^6	83
Carbenicillin	1.2×10^6	14	2.6×10^6	14
Methicillin	1.5×10^6	13	2.0×10^6	2
Oxacillin	NM[b]	NM	2.0×10^6	6
Cloxacillin	NM	NM	2.0×10^6	1
Cephalothin	3.0×10^6	7	2.2×10^6	4
Cephaloridine	2.1×10^6	5	1.3×10^6	15
Cefoxitin	NM	NM	NM	NM
Cefamandole	NM	NM	NM	NM
Cefotaxime	1.8×10^6	3	1.4×10^6	2

[a] V_{max} values are expressed as the ratio from 100 for penicillin G.

[b] NM, Not measurable. The antibiotic is a poor substrate. No hydrolysis.

TABLE 2. *Inhibition assays of Citrobacter β-lactamases by four β-lactam derivatives*[a]

Strain	CP-45899	Cefoxitin	Moxalactam	GR 20263
C. diversus MULB 650, pI 4.9	3.8×10^{-2}	No inhibition	23	No inhibition
C. diversus MULB 662, pI 5.4	2.3×10^{-2}	No inhibition	3	No inhibition
C. freundii MULB 601, pI 8.7	No inhibition	No inhibition	2.8×10^{-3}	Not done

[a] Values are expressed as the K_i/K_m ratio.

All extracts showed β-lactamase activity in the nitrocefin assay correlated with a microacidimetric test.

Isoelectric focusing on density gradient was performed on all strains. Isoelectric values clearly demonstrated that all the β-lactamases tested could be classified into two groups: seven strains, represented by *C. diversus* MULB 650, had a pI of 4.9, and three strains, represented by *C. diversus* MULB 662, had a pI value of 5.4.

Kinetic determinations (K_m and V_{max}) were measured with each of the representative group by a computerized microacidimetric method. Data illustrated in Table 1 suggested strong similarities between the 4.9 and 5.4 β-lactamases. Penicillin G, ampicillin, and carbenicillin were easily hydrolyzed by both enzymes. The 4.9 enzyme showed a better hydrolysis of methicillin than that observed with the 5.4 enzyme. The MULB 662 β-lactamase showed a weak but measurable hydrolysis of oxacillin and cloxacillin, but these molecules appeared unaffected by the 4.9 β-lactamase. Both enzymes showed a poor hydrolyzing activity on cephalosporins with the exception of cephaloridine, which was destroyed at the same rate as carbenicillin by the 5.4 enzyme. The K_m and V_{max} values indicated that the β-lactamases found in *C. diversus* shared a penicillinase profile. It is important to note that cefotaximine, which is highly resistant to β-lactamase action (2), was slowly hydrolyzed by the *C. diversus* penicillinases. This uncommon situation can be compared with the 4.9 β-lactamase already described in *Bacteroides fragilis* (3).

Inhibition assays of the enzymatic activity were performed by a spectrophotometric method using various concentrations of nitrocefin as a substrate and four β-lactam molecules including cefoxitin, moxalactam, CP-45,899, and GR 20263. Results are summarized in Table 2. CP 45,899 appeared as an excellent inhibitor of *C. diversus* penicillinases, but moxalactam acted as a poor inhibitor. The opposite inhibition pattern of activity has already been reported in the case of *C. freundii* β-lactamases (1). Both 4.9 and 5.4 penicillinases had no affinity for cefoxitin or GR 20263.

Characterization of the β-lactamase activity in *C. diversus* strains clearly demonstrates the presence of at least two penicillinases in that species. The description of the 4.9 β-lactamase correlates with a previous report in *Levinea malonatica* (4). According to substrate profiles and inhibition patterns, the *C. diversus* β-lactamases are very different from the enzymes of *C. freundii*, which are known as chromosomal cephalosporinases (pI range, 8 to 9). Induction studies with pencillin G (100 and 500 μg/ml) show that the *C. diversus* penicillinases are uninducible.

Previous experiments on plasmid detection have shown an absence of plasmid material in at least three penicillinase-producing strains of *C. diversus*. These results are indicative that these penicillinases are chromosomally mediated. The constant distribution of these penicillinases among *C. diversus* strains also favors a chromosomal support. The poor activity of these enzymes toward cephalosporins maintains interest in using these antibiotics in clinical infections due to *C. diversus*.

1. **Guay, R., R. Letarte, J. C. Pechere, and B. Roy.** 1980. Comparative efficiency of inhibitors on beta-lactamases produced by Gram-negative bacteria. IRCS Med. Sci. **8**:209.
2. **O'Callaghan, C. H.** 1979. Description and classification of the newer cephalosporins and their relationship with the established compounds. J. Antimicrob. Chemother. **5**:635–673.
3. **Pechere, J. C., R. Guay, J. Dubois, and R. Letarte.** 1980. Hydrolysis of cefotaxime by a beta-lactamase from *Bacteroides fragilis*. Antimicrob. Agents Chemother. **17**:1001–1003.
4. **Philippon, A., G. Paul, M. Barthelemy, R. Labia, and P. Nevot.** 1980. Properties of the beta-lactamase (penicillinase) produced by *Levinea malonatica*. FEMS Microbiol. Lett. **8**:191–194.
5. **Sykes, R. B., and M. Matthew.** 1976. The beta-lactamase of Gram-negative bacteria and their role in resistance to beta-lactam antibiotics. J. Antimicrob. Chemother. **2**:115–157.

High Frequency of β-Lactamases Related to the PSE-1 Type of *Pseudomonas aeruginosa* Strains

MICHÈLE JOUVENOT,* PATRICE BONIN, AND YVON MICHEL-BRIAND

Unité de Recherches de Biochimie Hormonale et des Régulations INSERM, 25000 Besançon-Chateaufarine, France

Pseudomonas aeruginosa normally produces an inducible β-lactamase which is active against cephaloridine, benzylpenicillin, and ampicillin, but not against carbenicillin (7). One mechanism for enhanced resistance in *P. aeruginosa* is the production of additional constitutive β-lactamases that hydrolyze carbenicillin and that are determined by plasmids. These β-lactamases have been divided into seven types, differing in substrate range, molecular weight, isoelectric point, and other properties (2). Four of these types have been defined as *Pseudomonas*-specific or PSE types (1). Because carbenicillin resistance in *P. aeruginosa* strains isolated at the Besançon Medical School Hospital has increased, we have been particularly interested in the β-lactamase activity of these strains.

From cell disruption by ultrasonication, we obtained crude enzymatic preparations and tested the β-lactamase activity by an acidimetric or iodometric method. We also used isoelectrofocusing (IEF) on polyacrylamide gel slabs to identify β-lactamases that were present (5).

In a first study for 10 highly carbenicillin-resistant strains isolated in 1975 to 1976, we could distinguish three groups of enzymes. A first group included three broad-spectrum β-lactamases which had the same IEF pattern as the TEM-1 enzyme. In the second group, there was one β-lactamase from the HL strain (4). This enzyme was a penicillinase (PCase) with the same IEF pattern as the PSE-4 type. The third group included six PCases which we defined previously as "atypical penicillinases" (3). Since then, we have compared by IEF these PCases with the PSE-1 enzyme from the PU21 (RPL11) strain. These enzymes had a main band at pH 5.9 (Fig. 1). However, our photo was taken 5 min after the detection of β-lactamase activity, and at this time a second band appeared at approx-

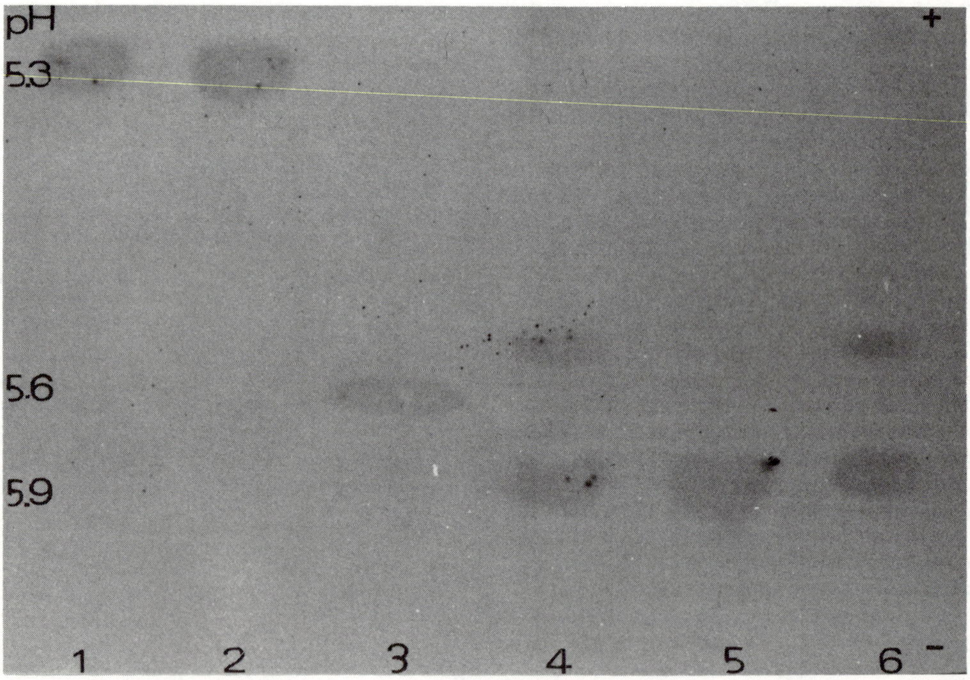

FIG. 1. *IEF pattern on polyacrylamide gel slabs. Crude enzymatic extracts from: 1, HL wild-type strain; 2, Dalgleish strain; 3, PAO8 (RP1); 4, S18 wild-type strain with PCase activity; 5, PU21 (RPL11); and 6, T21 wild-type strain with PCase activity.*

TABLE 1. *Different types of β-lactamases in 50 carbenicillin-resistant P. aeruginosa strains*

No. of strains	Characteristic of enzyme: pI	Characteristic of enzyme: Analogy with β-lactamase reference	Associated resistances[a]
2	5.3	PSE-4 from Dalgleish strain	None
7	5.4	TEM-1 from *Escherichia coli* (R6K)	None
35	5.9	PSE-1 from PU21	Gm/Tm
1	5.9	(RPL11)[b]	None
5	7.7	Cephalosporinase	None

[a] χ^2 test > 0. Gm/Tm, Gentamicin/tobramycin.
[b] Strain provided by G.A. Jacoby, Massachusetts General Hospital, Boston.

imately pH 5.6 for the PCases, but not for the PSE-1 reference. Thus, it would appear that our PCases are related to the PSE-1 reference enzyme in IEF because of the main band at pH 5.9 (6). We observed another slight difference between our PCases and the PSE-1 type: this latter type hydrolyzed mecillinam, whereas the PCases did not. In view of the high frequency of PCases related to the so-called rare PSE-1 type (2), an epidemiological study appeared necessary to complete our first results.

Among 300 *P. aeruginosa* strains isolated in 1980, 29% were carbenicillin resistant. We observed that, among these 87 carbenicillin-resistant strains, 61 presented a β-lactamase activity. In other words, 20% of the wild strains were carbenicillin resistant and β-lactamase positive. Among the carbenicillin-resistant strains having a β-lactamase activity, we chose 50 strains as different as possible in their origins and serotypes. Crude enzymatic preparations from these strains were tested in IEF simultaneously with β-lactamase references (Table 1). It appeared that 72% of the β-lactamases focused in the same way as the PSE-1 enzyme or as our "PCases related to the PSE-1 type" (defined in the first study and shown in Fig. 1).

We must point out the correlation between the nature of the β-lactamases and the nature of the bacterial resistances in the corresponding strains (Table 1). We detected enzymes related to the PSE-1 type in strains that presented multiple resistances, particularly gentamicin and tobramycin resistances (except for one strain). On the contrary, the other types of β-lactamases were found in gentamicin- and tobramycin-susceptible strains.

Until 1980, the PSE-1 β-lactamase was considered as uncommon and having a plasmidic nature. Our β-lactamases related to this type by IEF could be due to R plasmids carrying multiple resistances. Such plasmids could diffuse easily in the hospital environment, and this fact could explain the high frequency of enzymes related to the so-called rare PSE type. So far, we have used only the IEF technique to identify these enzymes. However, we feel that these results must be interpreted with care, and we are now trying to determine the hydrolysis activities as well as other properties of these enzymes. The characterization of the supposed plasmids is also in progress.

This work was supported by INSERM under grant 811040.

1. **Hedges, R. W., and M. Matthew.** 1979. Acquisition by *Escherichia coli* of plasmid-borne β-lactamases normally confined to *Pseudomonas* spp. Plasmid **2**:269–278.
2. **Jacoby, G. A., and M. Matthew.** 1979. The distribution of β-lactamase genes on plasmids found in *Pseudomonas*. Plasmid **2**:41–47.
3. **Jouvenot, M., and Y. Michel-Briand.** 1980. Six atypical β-lactamases from *Pseudomonas aeruginosa*, p. 771–773. *In* J. D. Nelson and C. Grassi (ed.), Current chemotherapy and infectious diseases. American Society for Microbiology, Washington, D. C.
4. **Jouvenot, M., Y. Michel-Briand, and J. M. Laporte.** 1978. Argument en faveur de la localisation plasmidique du gène β-lactamase chez une souche de *Pseudomonas aeruginosa* hautement résistante à la Carbénicilline. C.R. Acad. Sci. Ser. D **287**:1067–1070.
5. **Matthew, M., A. M. Harris, M. J. Marshall, and G. W. Ross.** 1975. The use of analytical isoelectric focusing for detection and identification of β-lactamases. J. Gen. Microbiol. **88**:169–178.
6. **Matthew, M., and R. B. Sykes.** 1977. Properties of the beta-lactamase specified by the *Pseudomonas* plasmid RPL11. J. Bacteriol. **132**:341–345.
7. **Sykes, R. B., and M. H. Richmond.** 1971. R factors, beta-lactamase and carbenicillin-resistant *Pseudomonas aeruginosa*. Lancet **ii**: 342–344.

In Vitro Activity of Sulbactam (CP-45,899), a Beta-Lactamase Inhibitor, in Combination with Beta-Lactam Antibiotics

ANNA KING,* MARTIN MOULSDALE, KEVIN SHANNON, AND IAN PHILLIPS

St. Thomas's Hospital Medical School, London, England

The in vitro activities of ampicillin, mezlocillin, cephaloridine, cefamandole, and cefoperazone (T-1551) were assessed alone and in combination with sulbactam sodium (CP-45,899, sodium penicillanate sulfone) against enterobacteria by chessboard determinations of MICs with an MIC 2000 dispenser and inoculator (Dynatech Laboratories Limited, Billingshurst, West Sussex, England). The activities of ampicillin and sulbactam were also assessed against *Bacteroides* spp.

Alone sulbactam had poor activity against enterobacteria (MICs mostly 32 to 128 μg/ml). Most of the enterobacteria tested were resistant (MICs ≥ 16 μg/ml) to ampicillin and cephaloridine, but many were susceptible to mezlocillin, cefamandole, and cefoperazone (Table 1). Against *Proteus vulgaris*, sulbactam had a dramatic effect on the MICs of ampicillin, cephaloridine, and cefamandole, to which this species is generally resistant, but little effect on the MICs of mezlocillin and cefoperazone to which it is usually susceptible (Table 1). The activity of ampicillin and cephaloridine against other

TABLE 1. *Effect of sulbactam on MICs of β-lactam antibiotics for enterobacteria*

Organism	Antibiotic	Cumulative % of isolates inhibited at MIC (μg/ml):													
		0.03	0.06	0.12	0.25	0.5	1	2	4	8	16	32	64	128	>128
Proteus vulgaris (6 isolates)															
	Ampicillin												17		100
	+ Sulbactam (4 μg/ml)							67	100						
	+ Sulbactam (8 μg/ml)							83	100						
	Cephaloridine														100
	+ Sulbactam (4 μg/ml)								50	100					
	+ Sulbactam (8 μg/ml)								50	100					
	Mezlocillin				17	100									
	+ Sulbactam (4 μg/ml)				50	100									
	+ Sulbactam (8 μg/ml)				50	100									
	Cefamandole								23					50	100
	+ Sulbactam (4 μg/ml)					83	100								
	+ Sulbactam (8 μg/ml)				17	100									
	Cefoperazone				50	66	100								
	+ Sulbactam (4 μg/ml)			17	66	100									
	+ Sulbactam (8 μg/ml)			17	66	100									
Other *Enterobacteriaceae* (50 isolates)[a]															
	Ampicillin								10	20	30	40	50	52	100
	+ Sulbactam (4 μg/ml)							6	12	36	48	64	68	74	100
	+ Sulbactam (8 μg/ml)					2		12	22	42	60	76	82	84	100
	Cephaloridine								4	8	14	22	28	38	100
	+ Sulbactam (4 μg/ml)							14	16	24	42	58	72	76	100
	+ Sulbactam (8 μg/ml)						6	20		34	56	64	80	84	100
	Mezlocillin					2	13	28	56	59		63	74	80	100
	+ Sulbactam (4 μg/ml)					7	20	43	72	76	83	87	91	93	100
	+ Sulbactam (8 μg/ml)					4	32	61	74	80	85	89	91	98	100
	Cefamandole			2		4	20	36	62	70	80	88	94	96	100
	+ Sulbactam (4 μg/ml)			2	4	22	40	62	80	82	88	94	96		100
	+ Sulbactam (8 μg/ml)			2	6	36	50	66	76	84	90	96		98	100
	Cefoperazone			14	22	47	55	63	76	90	98	100			
	+ Sulbactam (4 μg/ml)		10	20	41	57	65	73	86	96	98	100			
	+ Sulbactam (8 μg/ml)	4	16	29	47	59	65	78	88	96	100				

[a] *Citrobacter freundii* (4 isolates), *Enterobacter aerogenes* (5 isolates), *E. cloacae* (4 isolates), *Escherichia coli* (5 isolates), *Klebsiella* spp. (4 isolates), *Morganella morganii* (5 isolates), *Proteus mirabilis* (5 isolates), *Providencia rettgeri* (7 isolates), *P. stuartii* (6 isolates), and *Serratia* spp. (5 isolates).

TABLE 2. *Effect of sulbactam on MICs of ampicillin for Bacteroides spp.*[a]

Antibiotic	Cumulative % of isolates inhibited at MIC (μg/ml):											
	0.06	0.12	0.25	0.5	1	2	4	8	16	32	64	>64
Ampicillin					10	15		26	58	63		100
+ Sulbactam (0.5 μg/ml)			42	58		63	73	95	100			
+ Sulbactam (1 μg/ml)		10	52	58	63	79	100					
+ Sulbactam (2 μg/ml)	5	26	52	73	100							

[a] *Bacteroides fragilis* (7 isolates), *B. ovatus* (3 isolates), *B. thetaiotaomicron* (3 isolates), *B. uniformis* (3 isolates), and *B. vulgatus* (3 isolates).

enterobacteria considered as a whole was increased to some extent by 4 or 8 μg of sulbactam per ml, but even with 8 μg of the compound per ml, only 34% were susceptible to cephaloridine and 42% susceptible to ampicillin (Table 1). However, the species differed somewhat in their behavior with this compound, in that MICs of ampicillin were reduced four- to eight-fold by 8 μg of sulbactam per ml for *Citrobacter freundii*, *Enterobacter aerogenes*, *Morganella morganii*, and *Proteus mirabilis*, whereas its effect was generally less marked and somewhat variable for *Enterobacter cloacae*, *Escherichia coli*, *Klebsiella* spp., *Providencia rettgeri*, and *Providencia stuartii*. The effects of sulbactam on MICs of mezlocillin, cefamandole, and cefoperazone were generally somewhat lower (Table 1).

The MICs of ampicillin for *Bacteroides* spp. were greatly reduced by sulbactam (Table 2). Lower concentrations of sulbactam were tested in combination with ampicillin against these organisms because they were more susceptible than enterobacteria to sulbactam (MICs mostly 8 μg/ml).

The ability of sulbactam to inhibit β-lactamases was assessed with the UV spectrophotometric method (3). Hydrolysis of 100 μM ampicillin (at 235 nm) or cephaloridine (at 260 nm) was measured in the presence of 1, 10, or 100 μM sulbactam, and the percentage inhibition relative to hydrolysis in the absence of the inhibitor was calculated. For each enzyme preparation, inhibition was measured when sulbactam and the antibiotic were added at the same time and also when sulbactam was added to the enzyme 5 min before the antibiotic (for convenience, henceforth called preincubation). The cephalosporinase from *P. vulgaris* PC37 was exquisitely sensitive to sulbactam, with total inhibition by 1 μM sulbactam without preincubation. The enzyme from *Bacteroides fragilis* also was highly sensitive to sulbactam, with 90% inhibition by 10 μM sulbactam without preincubation and complete inhibition when this concentration of inhibitor was preincubated with the enzyme. The plasmid-mediated β-lactamases TEM 1, TEM 2, OXA 2, OXA 3, PSE 1, and PSE 4 were sensitive to sulbactam with at least 50% inhibition by 10 μM sulbactam without preincubation and nearly complete inhibition when 100 μM sulbactam was preincubated with the enzyme. OXA 1 was less sensitive as were most cephalosporinases (apart from those from *P. vulgaris* and *B. fragilis* mentioned above). However, there was at least 85% inhibition of nearly all enzymes if they were preincubated with 100 μM sulbactam. The exceptions were a cefoxitin-hydrolyzing enzyme from *E. cloacae* 4.37.76 (48% inhibition) and the enzyme from *P. stuartii* (70% inhibition).

Our results confirm previous reports (1, 2, 4) that sulbactam enhances the activity of β-lactam antibiotics against β-lactamase-producing bacteria, though not always sufficiently to render them susceptible to the compounds.

We are grateful to Pfizer Central Research, Sandwich, Kent, for providing sulbactam and for financial support.

1. **English, A. R., J. A. Retsema, A. E. Girard, J. E. Lynch, and W. E. Barth.** 1978. CP-45,899, a beta-lactamase inhibitor that extends the antibacterial spectrum of beta-lactams: initial bacteriological characterization. Antimicrob. Agents Chemother. **14:**414–419.
2. **Hunter, P. A., and J. R. Webb.** 1980. Comparative in vivo and in vitro activity of two novel β-lactamase inhibitors—clavulanic acid and CP-45,899, p. 340–342. *In* J. D. Nelson and G. Grassi (ed.), Current chemotherapy and infectious disease. American Society for Microbiology, Washington, D.C.
3. **O'Callaghan, C. H., P. W. Muggleton, and G. W. Ross.** Effects of β-lactamase from gram-negative organisms on cephalosporins and penicillins, p. 57–63. Antimicrob. Agents Chemother. 1968.
4. **Wise, R., J. M. Andrews, and K. A. Bedford.** 1980. Clavulanic acid and CP-45,899: a comparison of their in vitro activity in combination with penicillins. J. Antimicrob. Chemother. **6:**197–206.

Efficacy of Different Beta-Lactam Antibiotics and Beta-Lactamase Inhibitors in the Treatment of Experimentally Induced Intraabdominal Sepsis

GORDON LAHNBORG AND CARL E. NORD*

Department of Surgery, St. Görans Hospital, and National Bacteriological Laboratory, Stockholm, Sweden*

In most cases of intraabdominal sepsis a mixture of aerobic and anaerobic bacteria is found (3). For the antibiotic treatment of these infections, antibiotics covering both aerobic and anaerobic bacteria are recommended (3). The different approaches in the antibiotic treatment vary, and it has been difficult to evaluate the clinical outcome of many studies since variables in the patient exist, including underlying conditions and the degree and origin of the contaminating bacterial flora. A reproducible experimental model of intraabdominal infection in rats has been worked out in order to simulate intraabdominal sepsis in humans. The efficacy of different beta-lactam antibiotics and beta-lactamase inhibitors in the treatment of experimentally induced intraabdominal sepsis has been investigated using this model.

Experimental design. The model used in these experiments consisted of Sprague-Dawley rats undergoing abdominal surgery. The cecum and terminal part of ileum were mobilized out of the abdomen. A 1-cm segment of ileum was isolated on its bascular pedicle, which was interrupted with a single ligature. The intestine was divided at each end of the segment, and intestinal continuity was reestablished by a one-layer end-to-end anastomosis of the two ends of the ileum. The anastomosis was checked for leakage and passage before the intestine and devascularized segment of ileum were returned to the abdominal cavity. The abdominal wall was closed in two layers. All animals were autopsied and examined for abscesses, and cultures of purulent collections were obtained for bacteriological assessment.

Antibiotic administration. Each experiment group consisted of 18 rats. Antimicrobial agents were given by subcutaneous injection initially 1 h after surgery and then at 12 h intervals for 12 days. The agents used were benzylpenicillin, 15 mg; CP-45,899, 15 mg (Pfizer, Sandwich, England); cefoxitin, 20 mg; and benzylpenicillin, 15 mg + CP-45,899, 15 mg. The control group received 0.9% sterile saline.

Collection and processing of specimens. The specimens were taken with sterile swabs and transported to the laboratory immediately. Each specimen was streaked on 2 blood agar plates and 10 selective media (1). The aerobic plates were incubated for 24 h and the anaerobic plates for 48 h at 37°C. The plates were then examined, and different colony types were isolated in pure cultures and identified by the methods described elsewhere (2). The results with the beta-lactam compounds are shown in Fig. 1. Mortality rates in the different treatment groups ranged from 7 to 88% compared with 77% in untreated controls.

Benzylpenicillin. During the first 24 h, 13% of the rats died, and for each day up to day 5 the mortality rate was 18 to 19% of the total number of rats. All rats that died had signs of peritonitis. In the peritoneal fluids a polymicrobial flora with a predominance of *Escherichia coli*, *Proteus mirabilis*, *Streptococcus faecalis*, and *Bacteroides fragilis* was found.

CP-45,899. The mortality rate (71%) was similar to that found in the control group. *E. coli*, *P. mirabilis*, *S. faecalis*, and *B. fragilis* were recovered from the peritoneal fluids.

Cefoxitin. All rats but one survived. The rats not surviving died because of ileus due to a stricture of the anastomosis. All specimens except three showed no growth. *S. faecalis* in pure culture was isolated from these three rats. No signs of previous peritonitis were observed at autopsy.

Benzylpenicillin + CP-45,899. The mortal-

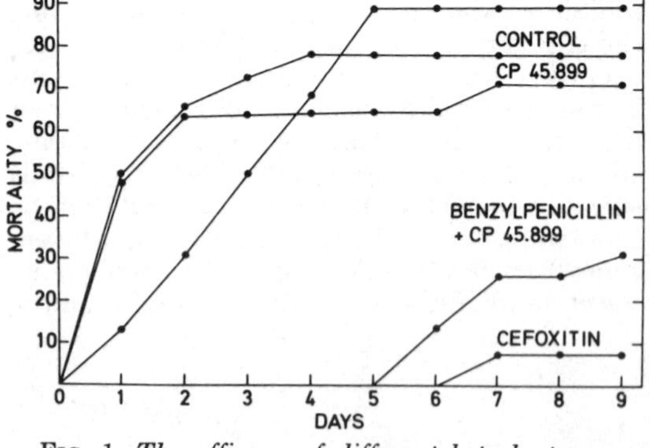

FIG. 1. *The efficacy of different beta-lactams on the mortality in rats after experimentally induced intraabdominal sepsis.*

ity rate was 32%. All animals survived the first 5 days. In all infected rats an abscess in connection to the anastomosis was found. Growth of *E. coli*, *P. mirabilis*, *S. faecalis*, and lactobacilli was observed in the abscesses. As in the cefoxitin group the abdominal cavity was macroscopically normal in the surviving rats.

Conclusions. The study indicates that superior results were obtained with cefoxitin in this animal model. Comparable results were noted with benzylpenicillin plus CP-45,899 (a beta-lactamase inhibitor) for the treatment of peritonitis but not for preventing abscess formation in this model.

1. **Heimdahl, A., and C. E. Nord.** 1979. Effect of phenoxymethylpenicillin and clindamycin on the oral, throat and faecal microflora of man. Scand. J. Infect. Dis. **11:** 233–242.
2. **Kager, L., I. Ljungdahl, A. S. Malmborg, C. E. Nord, R. Pieper, and P. Dahlgren.** 1981. Antibiotic prophylaxis with cefoxitin in colorectal surgery. Ann. Surg. **193:**277–282.
3. **Nichols, R. L.** 1977. Intraabdominal sepsis: characterization and treatment. J. Infect. Dis. **135**(Suppl.):54–57.

Comparative Activity of Ticarcillin and Ticarcillin Plus Clavulanic Acid Against β-Lactamase-Producing Clinical Isolates

HERMAN W. VAN LANDUYT,* BART DENOLF, AND ANNEMIE LAMBERT

Department of Microbiology, A. Z. St. Jan, B-8000 Brugge, Belgium

Clavulanic acid, a naturally occurring metabolite of *Streptomyces clavuligerus*, possesses a broad spectrum of β-lactamase inhibition (2). In combination with other β-lactam antibiotics, it shows a marked in vitro synergy against a wide range of β-lactamase–producing bacteria (1, 3).

We investigated the in vitro activity of ticarcillin in combination with clavulanic acid in fixed concentrations of 5 and 10 mg/liter compared with ticarcillin alone against 468 recent clinical isolates. These included 32 *Haemophilus influenzae*, 41 *Bacteroides* spp., 77 *Staphylococcus aureus*, 278 *Enterobacteriaceae*, 28 *Pseudomonas aeruginosa*, 9 *Acinetobacter* spp., and 3 *Aeromonas hydrophila* isolates. All isolates were β-lactamase–producing as determined by the rapid chromogenic cephalosporin method and resistant to carbenicillin as determined by the Kirby-Bauer technique. The MICs of the strains were determined by an agar dilution technique. After overnight incubation for 48 h for the *Bacteroides* strains, the strains were further diluted and inoculated with an automatic multipoint inoculator (Denley, Billingshurst, England) to deliver a final inoculation spot of 2 × 10^5 to 4 × 10^5 colony-forming units (CFU). The test medium was Mueller-Hinton medium (Difco Laboratories, Detroit, Mich.) for the *Enterobacteriaceae* and *S. aureus* strains, Mueller-Hinton medium supplemented with 1% PolyViteX enrichment (Bio Mérieux, Marcy-l'Etoile, France) and 1% hemoglobin (Oxoid Ltd., London, England) for the *Haemophilus* strains, Isosensitest agar (Oxoid Ltd.) for the *Pseudomonas* strains, and Wilkins Chalgren medium for the *Bacteroides* strains. The incubation was 18 h at 37°C for the *Enterobacteriaceae*, *Pseudomonas*, and *S. aureus* strains, 24 h at 37°C in 10% CO_2 for the *Haemophilus* strains, and 48 h at 35°C in an anaerobic chamber (Forma Scientific, Marietta, Ohio) for the *Bacteroides* strains. The activity of the compounds was checked by comparison of the MIC ranges, the MICs to inhibit 50 and 90% of the strains (MIC_{50} and MIC_{90}), and the geometric mean MICs (Table 1). On 10 selected strains, the inoculum effect with three different inocula, 10^3, 10^5, and 10^7 CFU/ml, was determined with a macrobroth dilution method, using the same media in broth form as those used for the MIC determinations. Finally, the minimal lethal concentration (MLC), defined as the lowest concentration which yielded 99.9% killing, was determined on these 10 selected strains from the tubes containing an inoculum of 10^5 CFU/ml (Table 2).

The geometric mean MIC as well as the MIC_{90} for both combinations, ticarcillin plus 5 mg of clavulanic acid per liter and ticarcillin plus 10 mg of clavulanic acid per liter, was equal to or lower than 0.25 mg/liter for the *H. influenzae* and *Bacteroides* strains, with the one exception of the MIC_{90} of ticarcillin plus 5 mg of clavulanic acid per liter, against the *Bacteroides* strains, which was 1 mg/liter. The same parameters were equal to or lower than 4 mg/liter for the *S. aureus* and *Proteus* strains. The geometric mean MICs were lower than 16 mg/liter for both combinations or at least for ticarcillin plus 10 mg of clavulanic acid per liter for the *E. coli*, *Klebsiella*, *Citrobacter*, *Morganella morganii*, *Provi-*

TABLE 1. *In vitro activity of ticarcillin, ticarcillin plus 5 mg of clavulanic acid per liter, and ticarcillin plus 10 mg of clavulanic acid per liter against β-lactamase-producing bacteria*

Species (no. of strains tested)	Drug[a]	MIC (mg/liter of medium)			
		Range	For % of strains		Geometric mean
			50	90	
Staphylococcus aureus (77)	TC	4->128	16	16	12.89
	TC5CA	1->128	4	4	3.28
	TC10CA	1->128	2	4	2.5
Escherichia coli (116)	TC	16->128	>128	>128	235.45
	TC5CA	4->128	32	128	28.9
	TC10CA	2->128	16	32	14.54
Klebsiella spp. (96)	TC	32->128	>128	>128	193.17
	TC5CA	1->128	4	128	8.53
	TC10CA	1->128	2	64	5.18
Citrobacter spp. (13)	TC	128->128	>128	>128	185.91
	TC5CA	2->128	64	>128	20.88
	TC10CA	1->128	32	>128	15.16
Enterobacter spp. (7)	TC	16->128	>128	>128	172.27
	TC5CA	8->128	64	>128	64
	TC10CA	4->128	32	>128	31.99
Serratia spp. (18)	TC	32->128	>128	>128	181.01
	TC5CA	1->128	>128	>128	97.75
	TC10CA	2->128	128	>128	83.8
Proteus spp. (18)	TC	16->128	>128	>128	181.01
	TC5CA	0.5–4	1	2	1.21
	TC10CA	0.25–1	0.5	1	0.6
Morganella morganii (3)	TC	>128	>128	>128	256
	TC5CA	2–32	4	32	6.34
	TC10CA	1–32	4	32	5.03
Providencia spp. (7)	TC	>128	>128	>128	256
	TC5CA	0.5–128	4	128	6.56
	TC10CA	0.125–32	4	32	4
Aeromonas hydrophila (3)	TC	32->128	128	>128	101.59
	TC5CA	32->128	64	>128	80.63
	TC10CA	8–32	16	32	15.99
Acinetobacter spp. (9)	TC	16->128	32	>128	54.86
	TC5CA	16->128	32	>128	40.31
	TC10CA	8->128	16	>128	25.39
Pseudomonas aeruginosa (28)	TC	32->128	64	>128	79.97
	TC5CA	32->128	64	128	74.24
	TC10CA	32->128	64	128	78.01
Haemophilus influenzae (32)	TC	0.5–8	2	8	2.59
	TC5CA	0.125–0.25	0.25	0.25	0.19
	TC10CA	0.125–0.25	0.25	0.25	0.18
Bacteroides spp. (41)	TC	4->128	32	64	27.95
	TC5CA	≤0.03–8	0.125	1	0.17
	TC10CA	≤0.03–8	≤0.03	0.25	0.05

[a] TC, Ticarcillin; TC5CA, ticarcillin plus 5 mg of clavulanic acid per liter; TC10CA, ticarcillin plus 10 mg of clavulanic acid per liter.

TABLE 2. *Inoculum effect on and MLC of ticarcillin, ticarcillin plus 5 mg of clavulanic acid per liter, and ticarcillin plus 10 mg of clavulanic acid per liter against 10 selected strains*

Organism (strain no.)	Drug[a]	MIC (mg/liter) with an inoculum[b] of:			MLC with 10^5
		10^3	10^5	10^7	
B. fragilis (17)	TC	32	64	128	128
	TC5CA	0.06	0.06	0.5	0.06
	TC10CA	≤0.03	≤0.03	1	≤0.03
H. influenzae (4)	TC	2	4	128	8
	TC5CA	0.12	0.12	0.25	0.25
	TC10CA	0.12	0.12	0.25	0.25
S. aureus (560)	TC	4	4	>128	8
	TC5CA	0.5	0.5	2	2
	TC10CA	0.5	0.5	2	0.5
E. coli (14)	TC	>128	>128	>128	>128
	TC5CA	8	16	16	16
	TC10CA	4	8	8	16
K. pneumoniae (13)	TC	>128	>128	>128	>128
	TC5CA	2	2	2	8
	TC10CA	2	2	2	8
P. mirabilis (3)	TC	128	>128	>128	>128
	TC5CA	0.25	0.25	0.25	8
	TC10CA	0.12	0.12	0.25	16
P. vulgaris (168)	TC	2	16	>128	32
	TC5CA	0.5	0.5	1	2
	TC10CA	0.5	0.5	0.5	1
M. morganii (480)	TC	>128	>128	>128	>128
	TC5CA	4	4	8	8
	TC10CA	2	4	4	8
P. rettgeri (247)	TC	>128	>128	>128	>128
	TC5CA	2	2	2	2
	TC10CA	1	2	2	2
P. alcalifaciens (584)	TC	>128	>128	>128	>128
	TC5CA	2	4	4	8
	TC10CA	2	4	4	8

[a] TC, Ticarcillin; TC5CA, ticarcillin plus 5 mg of clavulanic acid per liter; TC10CA, ticarcillin plus 10 mg of clavulanic acid per liter.

[b] Inocula given in CFU per milliliter.

dencia, and *Aeromonas* strains. In contrast, the MIC_{90} was equal to or above 32 mg/liter for these strains. Both the geometric mean MIC and MIC_{90} were equal to or greater than 32 mg/liter with both combinations against the other strains tested, with exception of the geometric mean MIC for ticarcillin plus 10 mg of clavulanic acid per liter, which was 25.39 mg/liter against the *Acinetobacter* strains.

The inoculum effect was minimal for ticarcillin plus 5 mg of clavulanic acid per liter and ticarcillin plus 10 mg of clavulanic acid per liter against the *H. influenzae* strains and the selected *Enterobacteriaceae* strains, with no increase in MIC or with an augmentation of only one twofold dilution when the inoculum varied from 10^3 to 10^7 CFU/ml. The MIC increased by two twofold dilutions for both combinations with the same inoculum variation against the *S. aureus* strain and by three twofold dilutions and even five twofold dilutions for the combination of, respectively, ticarcillin plus 5 mg of clavulanic acid per liter and ticarcillin plus 10 mg of clavulanic acid per liter against the *B. fragilis* strain.

There was no difference or only a difference

of one twofold dilution between the MIC and MLC of ticarcillin plus 5 mg of clavulanic acid per liter and ticarcillin plus 10 mg of clavulanic acid per liter against the *B. fragilis*, *H. influenzae*, *E. coli*, *M. morganii*, *Proteus rettgeri*, and *Providencia alcalifaciens* strain. There was a difference of two twofold dilutions for one or both of the combinations between the MIC and MLC against the *S. aureus*, *K. pneumoniae*, and *Proteus vulgaris* strains and even a difference of five and six twofold dilutions between MIC and MLC for, respectively, the combination of ticarcillin plus 5 mg of clavulanic acid per liter and ticarcillin plus 10 mg of clavulanic acid per liter against the *Proteus mirabilis* strain.

1. **Neu, H. C., and K. P. Fu.** 1978. Clavulanic acid, a novel inhibitor of β-lactamases. Antimicrob. Agents Chemother. **14:**650–655.
2. **Reading, C., and M. Cole.** 1977. Clavulanic acid: a beta-lactamase-inhibiting beta-lactam from *Streptomyces clavuligerus*. Antimicrob. Agents Chemother. **11:**852–857.
3. **Wise, R., J. M. Andrews, and K. A. Bedford.** 1978. In vitro study of clavulanic acid in combination with penicillin, amoxycillin, and carbenicillin. Antimicrob. Agents Chemother. **13:**389–393.

Interaction of R46 β-Lactamase with Inhibitors

J. W. DALE,* C. MONAGHAN, S. HOLLAND, AND C. READING

Department of Microbiology, University of Surrey, Guildford, and Beecham Pharmaceuticals Research Division, Brockham Park, Betchworth, Surrey, United Kingdom*

Some plasmid-mediated β-lactamases in gram-negative bacteria have the unusual property of preferentially hydrolyzing isoxazolyl penicillins such as oxacillin (3). Of these, the R46 β-lactamase, which belongs to the OXA-2 group, has other unusual properties which make it worth investigation. First, it is unique among those penicillinases which have been characterized as having a dimeric structure (4). Second, it is inhibited by the anthraquinone dye cibacron blue (Fig. 1), which is more commonly known as a probe for the dinucleotide fold, a structural feature often found in nucleotide-requiring enzymes (6).

Studies of inhibitors of β-lactamases are useful both for possible therapeutic applications and also because of the information that can be gained about structure-function relationships. We have therefore characterized the inhibition of the R46 β-lactamase by various anthraquinone derivatives as well as by β-lactam inhibitors.

The enzyme was purified as described by Dale and Smith (2), and the K_i values were determined by means of the microiodometric assay with benzylpenicillin as the substrate, using reciprocal (Lineweaver-Burk) plots at different concentrations of inhibitor. Cibacron blue showed a typical competitive pattern of inhibition, with the plots intersecting on the $1/v$ axis, and this was also true for most of the other inhibitory anthraquinones tested. The K_i values were therefore calculated by assuming the inhibition to be competitive. In the few cases where there was some evidence for a reduced value of V_{max} at high concentrations of inhibitor, reinterpretation of the data on the basis of a mixed type of inhibition did not give significantly different results.

Examination of the inhibition by the series of related dyes differing only in the nature of the side chain on the C-4 amino group (Table 1, lines 1–7) shows that the nature of this side chain had little effect on the affinity for the enzyme, this being essentially a property of the anthraquinone moiety. This is borne out by the inhibition shown by alizarin saphirol and alizarin red S, which are simple anthraquinones. However, the nature of the substituents on the anthraquinone nucleus is important. Thus, Solway blue SE, which is very closely related to alizarin saphirol, was a very much weaker inhibitor. This result was initially suspect, as Solway blue SE reacts with the iodine reagent. However, the use of a different assay system (direct UV spectrophotometric assay, with cephaloridine or benzylpenicillin as the substrate) confirmed that Solway blue SE was a comparatively poor inhibitor, although it was not possible to determine a K_i value for comparison. It is also significant that the 1-amino-2-sulfonic acid was only weakly inhibitory, and the 2,6-disulfonic acid showed no inhibition. It is not yet possible to formulate a general rule as to which groups and which positions are required for inhibition.

It has been claimed (5) that cibacron blue is a structural analog of NAD, with the anthraquinone and terminal phenylsulfonate rings resem-

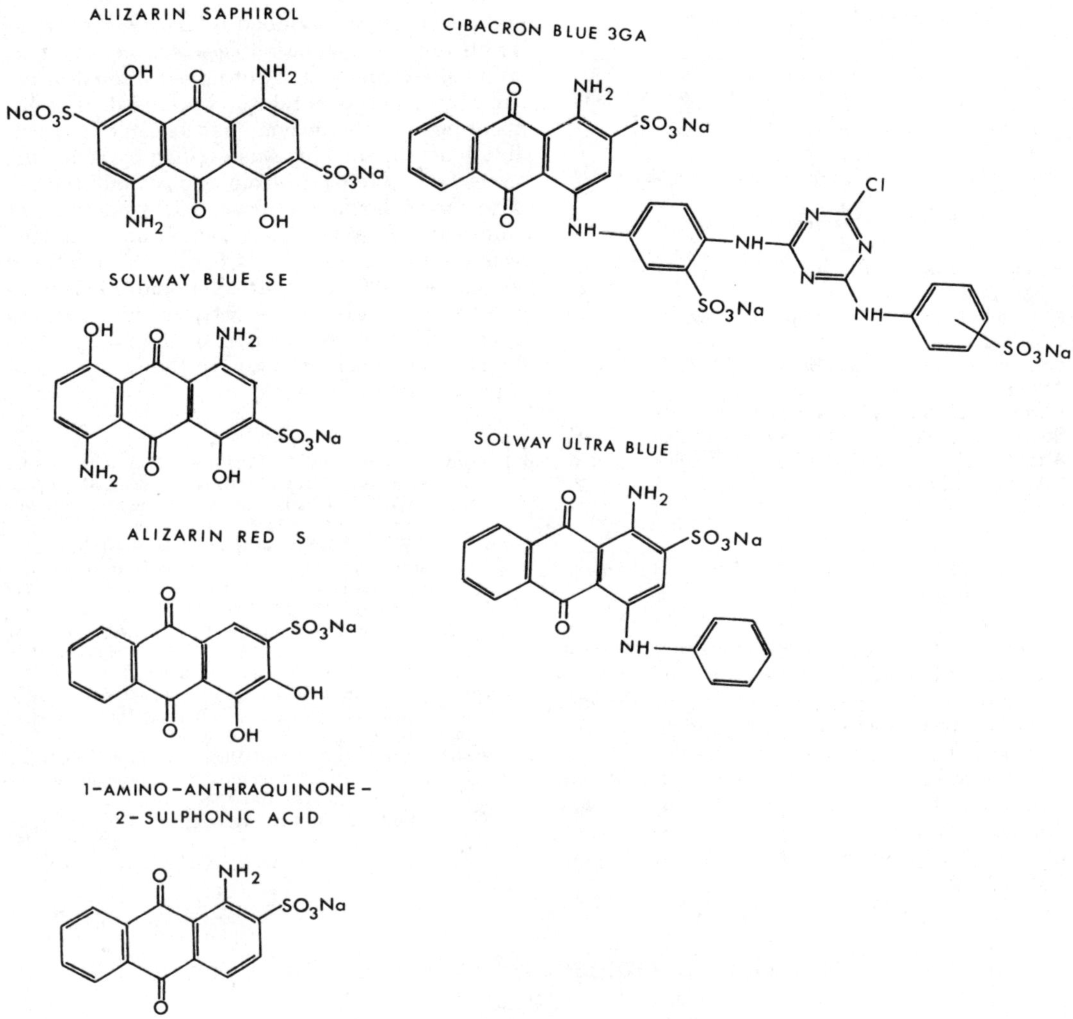

FIG. 1. *Structure of cibacron blue and some related anthraquinone dyes.*

bling the adenine and nicotinamide rings of NAD, and that there is also a resemblance to the structures of ATP and coenzyme A. These structural similarities are supposed to account for the competitive inhibition of nucleotide-requiring enzymes. However, there is no evidence that the R46 β-lactamase required any nucleotide coenzymes or has any affinity for them. This would support the suggestion made by Ashton and Polya (1) that the interaction between these dyes and the enzymes that are affected by them is not due to specific conformational relationships.

Stellwagen (5) showed that interaction of cibacron blue with lactate dehydrogenase caused a red shift in the absorption spectrum of the dye, with the difference spectrum having a positive maximum at 660 nm and an isosbestic point at 584 nm. A similar effect was seen with the R46 β-lactamases: the maximum difference was at 670 nm, and the isosbestic point was at 584 nm. This result indicates that the nature of the interaction between the penicillinase and the dye may be the same as that which occurs with the nucleotide-requiring enzymes.

If the enzyme can be inhibited in vivo by anthraquinone derivatives, then treating a bacterial culture with a dye such as cibacron blue would result in abolishing or reducing the ampicillin resistance of cells containing the R46 plasmid. This would provide a system for examining the function of this enzyme in vivo and would also enable rapid identification of this type of enzyme. However, tests so far have failed

TABLE 1. *Inhibition of R46 β-lactamase by anthraquinone derivatives*

Commercial name	*Colour Index* generic name	*Colour Index* no.	K_i (μM)
Cibacron blue 3GA	Reactive blue 2	61211	1.2
Procion blue H-GR	Reactive blue 5	61205:1	2.7
Procion blue MX-R	Reactive blue 4	61205	1.0
Remazol brilliant blue R	Reactive blue 19	61200	0.5
Nylomine blue B-3G	Acid blue 40	62125	2.7
Solway ultra blue	Acid blue 25	62055	1.0
ASSO[a]			4.0
Alizarin saphirol	Acid blue 45	63010	1.2
Solway blue SE	Acid blue 43	63000	>20
Alizarin red S	Mordant red 3	58005	3.0
1-Amino-anthra-quinone-2-sulfonic acid			>20

[a] 1-Amino-4-(4^1-aminophenylamino)-anthraquinone-2,3′-disulfonic acid.

to show any significant reduction in ampicillin resistance of cibacron blue-treated cells, probably due to lack of penetration of the dye. Further work is in progress to establish conditions under which such an effect could be observed.

Inhibition of the R46 β-lactamase by β-lactam inhibitors was also examined. The enzyme was inhibited by both clavulanic acid and penicillanic acid sulfone, with a maximum level of inhibition being obtained with a few minutes preincubation. In neither case was any regeneration of enzyme activity observed when limiting concentrations of inhibitor were used, thus indicating that the enzyme had become irreversibly inactivated. This was verified by removing excess clavulanic acid from a fully inhibited enzyme and following return of enzyme activity at different pH values. No regeneration of enzyme was obtained. However, treating the inhibited enzyme with 20 mM hydroxylamine did produce 50% recovery of enzyme activity, which shows that at least the major part of the inactivation by clavulanic acid was due to the formation of an acyl-enzyme complex.

1. **Ashton, A. R., and G. M. Polya.** 1978. The specific interaction of Cibacron and related dyes with cyclic nucleotide phosphodiesterase and lactate dehydrogenase. Biochem. J. **175**:501–506.
2. **Dale, J. W., and J. T. Smith.** 1971. The purification and properties of the β-lactamase specified by the resistance factor R-1818 in *Escherichia coli* and *Proteus mirabilis*. Biochem. J. **123**:493–500.
3. **Dale, J. W., and J. T. Smith.** 1974. R-factor mediated β-lactamases that hydrolyze oxacillin: evidence for two distinct groups. J. Bacteriol. **119**:351–356.
4. **Dale, J. W., and J. T. Smith.** 1976. The dimeric nature of an R-factor mediated β-lactamase. Biochem. Biophys. Res. Commun. **68**:1000–1005.
5. **Stellwagen, E.** 1977. Use of Blue Dextran as a probe for the nicotinamide adenine dinucleotide domain in proteins. Acc. Chem. Res. **10**:92–98.
6. **Thompson, S. T., and E. Stellwagen.** 1976. Binding of Cibacron blue F3Ga to proteins containing the dinucleotide fold. Proc. Natl. Acad. Sci. U.S.A. **73**:361–365.

Activity of Three Beta-Lactamase Inhibitors on Characterized Beta-Lactamases

F. MOOSDEEN,* J. D. WILLIAMS, AND J. T. LI

Department of Microbiology, The National University of Malaysia, Kuala Lumpur, Malaysia, and The London Hospital Medical College, London E1, England; and Institute of Clinical Pharmacology, Beijing Medical College, Beijing, China*

The use of beta-lactamase inhibitors with beta-lactam antibiotics is an alternative to using beta-lactamase-stable antibiotics against resistant organisms. There are many different beta-lactamases, and they seem likely to show varying susceptibility to inhibitors. A number of new beta-lactamase inhibitors have been reported in recent years, e.g., by Cole (1). We have studied three such inhibitors, clavulanic acid, penicillanic acid sulfone (CP-45,899), and 6-beta-iodo penicillanic acid (UK-38,006), for their activity on enzymes produced by gram-negative rods, both as extracts and with the enzyme present in intact cells. The enzymes studied were PSE 1,

TABLE 1. *Activity of enzyme inhibitors on beta-lactamases: spectrophotometric method*

Enzyme	Concn of inhibitors (μg/ml)	% Enzyme activity inhibited		
		Clavulanic acid	CP-45,899	UK-38,006
Whatman	5.0	45	31	92
TEM 1	1.0	60	0	87
TEM 2	0.5	85	19	83
K 1	0.5	68	2	3
SHV 1	0.5	91	7	84
Bacteroides J5	1.0	51	36	58
Bacteroides J6	0.05	73	9	45

TABLE 2. *Effect of combinations of inhibitors with beta-lactam compounds on different bacterial species*

Organism	Enzyme	Drug combination[a]								
		Ampicillin			Carbenicillin			Cephaloridine		
		+CA	+CP	+UK	+CA	+CP	+UK	+CA	+CP	+UK
E. coli	TEM 1	+	−	+	+	−	+	+	−	+
Proteus morganii	TEM 1	+	+	+	+	−	+	+	−	+
Klebsiella pneumoniae	TEM 1	+	−	+	+	−	−	+	−	+
Citrobacter freundii	TEM 1	−	−	−	+	−	−	−	−	−
E. coli	TEM 2	+	−	+	+	−	−	+	−	+
Pseudomonas aeruginosa	PSE 1	−	−	−	−	−	−	−	−	−
Serratia liquefaciens	PSE 1	−	−	−	+	−	−	+	+	+
Klebsiella oxytoca	K 1	+	−	−	−	−	−	+	−	−
E. coli	OXA 1	+	−	+	+	−	−	+	−	+
E. cloacae	P 99	−	−	−	−	−	−	−	−	−

[a] +, Reduction in MIC of 5 log 2 or more; CA, clavulanic acid; CP, CP-45,899; UK, UK-38,006.

OXA 1, TEM 1, TEM 2, SHV 1, K 1, P 99, Whatman beta-lactamase, and enzymes obtained from *Bacteroides* spp.

Cephaloridine was used as the substrate for spectrophotometric study of hydrolysis and inhibition. Ampicillin was used as the substrate in the biological assay. Susceptibility of the organisms to ampicillin, cephaloridine, and carbenicillin in the absence and presence of inhibitors was also tested. In the spectrophotometric method, portions of the inhibitor were added to cephaloridine to give final concentrations of 5 μg/ml or fractions of this; the enzyme was then added, and absorbance curve was recorded at different time intervals. The percentage of enzyme activity inhibited by each inhibitor was calculated from hydrolysis of the cephaloridine by enzyme alone and by enzyme-inhibitor mixture by using the change in optical density at 255 nm in 12 min. Both clavulanic acid and UK-38,006 showed greater inhibitory activity than CP-45,899 (Table 1). CP-45,899 was more active against Whatman enzyme and enzymes produced by *Bacteroides.*

In the bioassay method, portions of logarithmic dilutions of enzyme preparations were incubated for 15 min at room temperature with the inhibitors at concentrations of 1 and 10 μg/ml. After incubation, a volume of the mixture was added to 1 ml of phosphate buffer containing 8 μg of ampicillin. After incubation for 15 min at room temperature, the residual ampicillin was assayed. Clavulanic acid and UK-38,006 effectively inhibited TEM 1, TEM 2, K 1, OXA 1, PSE 1, SHV 1, and *Bacteroides* enzymes. CP-45,899 showed poor activity against all enzymes compared to the other two inhibitors. The three inhibitors produced little inhibition of P 99 hydrolysis of enzymes, similar to the report by Wise et al. (3).

Against cephaloridine, ampicillin, and carbenicillin, all the strains used required high MICs (≥2,048 μg/ml). The combination of clavulanic acid with carbenicillin resulted in a marked fall of MIC of most of the strains studied, whereas clavulanic acid and UK-38,006 in combination with cephaloridine or ampicillin resulted in fall of MIC with *Escherichia coli*, *Proteus*, and *Klebsiella* producing strains containing TEM 1, TEM 2, K 1, and OXA 1 enzymes. The MICs of antibiotics of *Enterobacter* strains containing P 99 enzyme were not reduced by any of the inhibitors (Table 2).

The study showed that most beta-lactamases can be inhibited at concentrations of clavulanic acid and UK-38,006 of less than 1 μg/ml. CP-45,899 is less active than these compounds and P 99 enzyme from *Enterobacter cloacae* was only marginally affected by the inhibitors. There are differences among various bacteria and among strains of the same species in their response to beta-lactamase inhibitors. The effect of inhibitors depends on the type and amount of the beta-lactamase produced and penetration of the inhibitors into the cell. The inhibitor also needs to be combined with a beta-lactam antibiotic which must be able to reach the site of action to be effective.

We thank Beecham Research Laboratories for having kindly supplied clavulanic acid; Pfizer Research for supplying CP-45,899 and UK-38,006; and Glaxo Research Laboratories for making available some of the bacterial strains used in the study.

1. **Cole, M.** 1979. Inhibitors of antibiotic-inactivating enzymes, p. 99–135. *In* J. D. Williams (ed.), Antibiotic interactions. Academic Press, London.
2. **Matthew, M., A. Harris, M. Marshall, and G. W. Ross.** 1975. The use of analytical isoelectric focussing for the detection and identification of beta-lactamases. J. Gen. Microbiol. **88:**169–178.
3. **Wise, R., J. M. Andrews, and N. Patel.** 1981. 6-Beta-bromo and 6-beta-iodo penicillanic acid, two novel beta-lactamase inhibitors. J. Antimicrob. Chemother. **7:**531–536.

Distribution and Bactericidal Activity of BRL 25000 (Augmentin) in Localized β-Lactamase–Producing Infections in the Rat Granuloma Pouch

LINDA W. MIZEN* AND ELAINE J. CATHERALL

Beecham Pharmaceuticals Research Division, Betchworth, Surrey, England

The distribution and bactericidal activity of BRL 25000 (Augmentin; Beecham Pharmaceuticals) was studied in the rat granuloma pouch, a distribution model simulating a localized infection (2). BRL 25000 formulations contain the broad-spectrum penicillin amoxicillin and the β-lactamase inhibitor clavulanic acid (1). In the studies described, two oral formulations were used, BRL 25000A (2 parts amoxicillin free acid equivalent as the trihydrate to 1 part clavulanic acid as the potassium salt) and BRL 25000G (4 parts amoxicillin free acid equivalent as the trihydrate to 1 part clavulanic acid as the potassium salt).

The granuloma pouches were formed dorsally by a subcutaneous injection of air followed immediately by an injection of 1 ml of a 1% solution in olive oil of the phlogistic agent croton oil. Rats were used 7 days later, after which time the pouches were lined with granulomatous tissue and contained approximately 10 ml of inflammatory exudate. The pouches were inoculated with a dilution of an overnight culture of one of three β-lactamase–producing organisms, *Escherichia coli* E96, *Klebsiella pneumoniae* T767, or *Staphylococcus aureus* 1555, which was administered in the presence of mucin (hog gastric mucin; American Laboratories Inc., Omaha, Neb.). Groups of four to six animals received oral doses of BRL 25000G (250 mg/kg), BRL 25000A (150 mg/kg), amoxicillin trihydrate alone (100 or 200 mg of free acid equivalent per kg), or potassium clavulanate (50 mg of free acid equivalent per kg) at 0.5 h after infection. In addition, included in each study was a similar-sized group of infected but untreated animals which served as controls.

Studies in which the pouches were left uninfected showed that, after oral administration, both components of the amoxicillin/clavulanic acid formulation penetrated equally well into the inflammatory exudate (L. Mizen et al., Drugs Exp. Clin. Res., in press). Peak exudate concentrations were between 40 and 50% of those in serum and generally occurred later, at around 2 h compared with 1 h in serum. Clavulanic acid concentrations fell more rapidly than those of amoxicillin, and both compounds were eliminated more slowly from the pouch than from serum. Half-lives for clavulanic acid in serum and exudate were around 0.6 h and 2.9 h, respectively, compared with half-lives for amoxicillin of around 1.5 h in serum and 4.0 h in exudate.

After oral administration of the formulations to rats with pouches infected with *E. coli* E96, *S. aureus* 1555, or *K. pneumoniae* T767, it was found that the distribution kinetics of amoxicillin and clavulanic acid described above for rats with uninfected pouches were unchanged in the presence of infection. The similarity of the amoxicillin concentrations in infected and uninfected pouches after dosing with the formulations would imply that the exudate concentrations of clavulanic acid were sufficient to prevent the degradation of amoxicillin by the β-lactamase produced in vivo. This observation has been substantiated in the following series of studies.

In groups of rats with pouches infected with *E. coli* E96, a potent producer of the plasmid-mediated R TEM β-lactamase, BRL 25000A, BRL 25000G, or amoxicillin alone was administered orally. Pouch exudate samples were taken at 0.5 h after infection, and at 2, 4, and 6 h after dosing. Viable counts were performed on all samples, and concentrations of amoxicillin and clavulanic acid in 2-, 4-, and 6-h samples were measured by the large-plate microbiological assay technique. Blood samples were also removed at 1.0 h after dosing to check that serum levels were similar in rats receiving either the formulations or amoxicillin alone and, in addition, to confirm that they were of the same order as those in rats with uninfected pouches. Studies with the 4:1 formulation, BRL 25000G, are illustrated in Fig. 1. After administration of the formulation, exudate concentrations of amoxicillin were in the region of 3 to 4 μg/ml at 6 h, in contrast to levels of only 0.1 μg/ml after administration of amoxicillin alone.

The more rapid fall in concentrations when amoxicillin alone was administered would be a consequence of degradation by the rising levels of β-lactamase in the pouch as the bacterial numbers increased. The growth rate in these pouches was similar to that in untreated rats. However, in the presence of amoxicillin and clavulanic acid, after administration of the formulation, bacterial numbers had dropped sig-

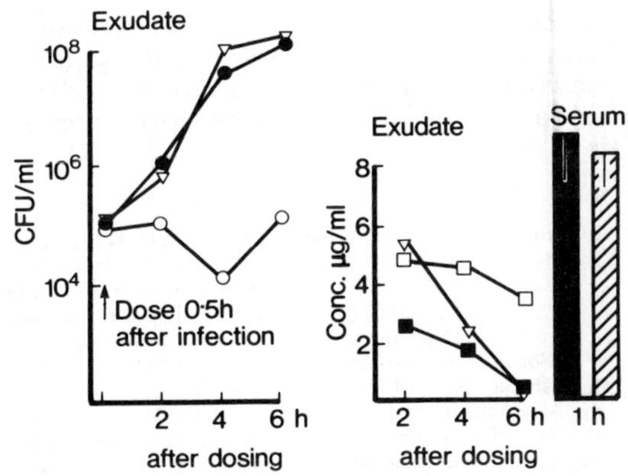

FIG. 1. *Distribution and bactericidal activity of BRL 25000G and amoxicillin trihydrate in pouches infected with E. coli E96. Symbols for colony-forming units per milliliter: ○, BRL 25000G; ▽, amoxicillin trihydrate; ●, untreated rats. Symbols for exudate concentrations: ▽, amoxicillin trihydrate; □, amoxicillin; ■, clavulanic acid, after BRL 25000G. Symbols for serum concentrations (µg/ml) of amoxicillin: solid bar, BRL 25000G; shaded bar, amoxicillin trihydrate.*

nificantly by 4 h, although levels were subinhibitory for this strain (MIC of BRL 25000, 25 µg/ml). From 4 h onwards, there was a resumption of growth as a result of elimination of both compounds from the animal.

A similar order of results was obtained when rats were dosed with the BRL 25000A formulation and amoxicillin alone. After a single dose of the formulation, exudate concentrations of amoxicillin were considerably more prolonged than in pouches of rats receiving amoxicillin alone, in which levels declined rapidly and were barely detectable at 6 h. A bactericidal effect was observed after treatment with BRL 250000A, with numbers dropping to 1.8×10^4 colony-forming units per ml at 4 h whereas in rats receiving only amoxicillin the growth rate was similar to that in untreated rats.

Studies in which the pouches were infected with *K. pneumoniae* T767, which produces a chromosomally mediated β-lactamase, were undertaken with the same experimental procedures described above. Studies with the BRL 25000A formulation (2:1) are shown in Fig. 2. In the absence of clavulanic acid, exudate concentrations of amoxicillin tended to decline more rapidly than in animals receiving the formulation. The degradation of amoxicillin was not so marked as that observed with *E. coli* E96, but amoxicillin alone was totally ineffective, and bacterial numbers increased at a rate similar to that in untreated rats or in rats receiving potassium clavulanate alone. After administration of BRL 25000A, exudate concentrations reached levels of the same order as the MIC of this formulation (2.5 µg/ml), and the observed bactericidal effect was marked and sustained, resulting in a 99% kill by 6 h. The BRL 25000G formulation also gave rise to a marked bactericidal effect, with bacterial counts being generally lower than those observed after administration of BRL 25000A. Bacterial growth was uninterrupted after administration of amoxicillin alone at the higher dose of 200 mg/kg and proceeded at the same rate as in the untreated animals.

Results for studies in rats with pouches infected with *S. aureus* 1555 clearly showed that, after administration of BRL 25000A, clavulanic acid was highly effective in protecting amoxicillin from degradation by the β-lactamase produced by this strain. After treatment with the formulation, exudate concentrations of amoxicillin were similar to those seen in rats with uninfected pouches injected with mucin alone, whereas in the amoxicillin-treated animals exudate concentrations were barely detectable at 1 h after dosing (0.10 µg/ml) and were <0.01 µg/ml thereafter. In animals receiving either amoxicillin or potassium clavulanate, the bacterial counts increased slowly but at the same rate as in untreated rats, with numbers rising 10-fold over 24 h. This slow growth rate in the pouch was in accordance with the observations of Nishida and Murakawa (2) for *S. aureus* strains. Under these circumstances the bactericidal activity of β-lactam antibiotics would be expected to be diminished; nevertheless, the formulation produced a distinct bactericidal effect, with a 10-

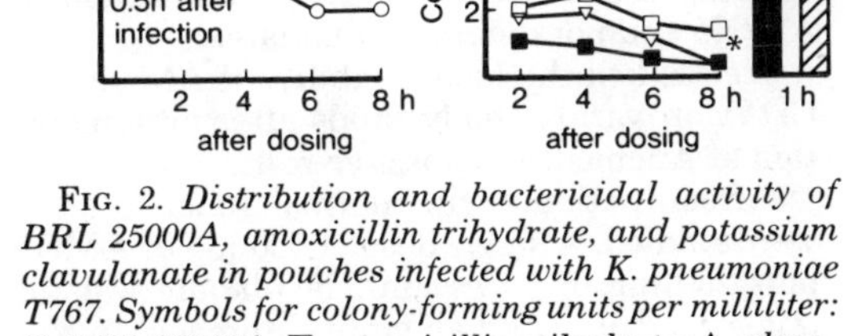

FIG. 2. *Distribution and bactericidal activity of BRL 25000A, amoxicillin trihydrate, and potassium clavulanate in pouches infected with K. pneumoniae T767. Symbols for colony-forming units per milliliter: ○, BRL 25000A; ▽, amoxicillin trihydrate; ▲, clavulanic acid; ●, untreated rats. Symbols for exudate concentrations: □, amoxicillin, and ■, clavulanic acid, after BRL25000A; ▽, amoxicillin trihydrate. Symbols for serum concentrations (µg/ml): solid bar, BRL 25000A; shaded bar, amoxicillin trihydrate. Asterisk indicates that results are significantly different.*

fold reduction in counts at 2 h after dosing. Bacterial counts fell to a similar extent in all rats within the group, and numbers remained down over the following 4 h.

In conclusion, these studies have demonstrated the ability of both components of the BRL 25000 formulations to penetrate into inflammatory exudate infected with either gram-positive or gram-negative organisms, with the subsequent protection of amoxicillin by clavulanic acid from inactivation by the β-lactamases produced in vivo. This was demonstrated not only by the presence of higher exudate concentrations of amoxicillin after administration of BRL 25000A or BRL 25000G compared with concentrations observed after separate administration of amoxicillin but also by the superior bactericidal activity of the amoxicillin/clavulanic acid formulations compared with amoxicillin alone.

1. **Comber, K. R., R. Horton, L. Mizen, A. R. White, and R. Sutherland.** 1980. Activity of amoxicillin/clavulanic acid (2:1) (BRL 25000 AUGMENTIN) in vitro and in vivo, p. 343. *In* J. D. Nelson and C. Grassi (ed.), Current chemotherapy and infectious disease, vol. 1. American Society for Microbiology, Washington, D.C.
2. **Nishida, M., and T. Murakawa.** 1977. Exudate levels and bactericidal activity of cefazolin in a new local infection system using rat granuloma pouches. Antimicrob. Agents Chemother. **11:**1042.

Pharmacokinetic Studies with Augmentin, a Combination of Amoxicillin and Potassium Clavulanate

JOHN KOSMIDIS,* CHARALAMPOS STATHAKIS, DEMETRIOS KOTILIS, AND GEORGE K. DAIKOS

First Department of Propedeutic Medicine, Athens University School of Medicine, King Paul's Hospital, Athens, 609, Greece

Clavulanic acid (CLAV) is a β-lactam compound produced by *Streptomyces clavuligerus*. It has a weak antibacterial activity but is an effective inhibitor of β-lactamases of Richmond types II, III, IV, and V (2). It has marked in vitro synergism with various β-lactam compounds against many β-lactamase-producing bacteria.

A clinical trial of a 2:1 combination of amoxicillin (AMOX) and sodium clavulanate in a variety of infections due to amoxicillin-resistant bacteria resulted in a 76.5% cure rate (1). The use of the sodium salt has since been discontinued, and the potassium salt, which is better tolerated by the gastrointestinal tract, has been substituted. The name Augmentin now corresponds, therefore, to a 2:1 combination of AMOX and potassium clavulanate.

We studied the bioavailability of AMOX and CLAV in various body fluids after administration of Augmentin potassium salt.

Fifteen patients with normal renal function were studied. A single dose of 500 mg of AMOX plus 250 mg of potassium clavulanate was administered orally on an empty stomach. In four patients a full profile of serum and urine levels was studied. In three patients with exacerbation of chronic bronchitis, sputum was collected every 2 h for 6 h after the first dose as above, which was then repeated every 8 h. On the fourth day of treatment, sampling was repeated after the morning dose. In four patients with normal cerebrospinal fluid (CSF) undergoing lumbar puncture for diagnostic purposes, specimens of CSF were taken after a dose. Finally, in four patients with pleurisy, one or more specimens of pleuritic fluid were collected after a dose. A specimen of blood was taken simultaneously with every sputum, CSF, or pleuritic fluid sample.

Concentrations of AMOX were measured by a microbiological well-plate technique, with *Sarcina lutea* as indicator organism; CLAV was assayed by a technique which measures β-lactamase inhibitory activity (1).

The results presented in Table 1 show that the mean concentration of AMOX in serum reached a peak of 8.1 mg/liter 2 h after a dose and was 1.6 mg/liter at 6 h and 0.76 mg/liter at 8 h. Terminal serum half-life averaged 1.5 h. The highest mean level of CLAV was 5.2 mg/liter at 1 h; at 6 h the mean level was 0.34 mg/liter and at 8 h it was 0.12 mg/liter. Half-life was 1.4 h.

Mean urine levels of AMOX reached a peak of 810 mg/liter at the 2- to 4-h collection period and were 154 mg/liter from 6 to 8 h. Urinary recovery averaged 51% of dose. Corresponding values of CLAV were 580 mg/liter for the peak reached at the 0- to 2-h collection period and 46 mg/liter for the 6- to 8-h period. Mean urinary recovery was 41.2%.

Levels of AMOX in sputum reached a mean

TABLE 1. *Concentration of AMOX and CLAV in various fluids after administration of 750 mg of Augmentin (potassium salt)*

Fluid	Mean concn (mg/liter) at indicated times (h) after a dose						Half-life (h)
	1	2	3	4	6	8	
Serum							
AMOX	5.3	8.1	6.0	4.2	1.6	0.76	1.5
CLAV	5.2	2.6	1.6	0.85	0.34	0.12	1.4
Sputum, 1st day							
AMOX	0.44	0.21		0.05	0.03		
CLAV	0.92	0.35		0.16	0.08		
Sputum, 4th day							
AMOX	0.08	0.12		0.12	0		
CLAV	0.74	0.45		0.23	0.04		
CSF							
AMOX	0.12	0	0.18	0.34			
CLAV	0.18	0.11	0.17	0.19			
Pleuritic fluid							
AMOX	0.98	0.79	0.77	5.00	2.14		
CLAV	0.48	1.05	1.40	2.40	1.18		
		0–2		2–4	4–6	6–8	Recovery (%)
Urine							
AMOX		685		810	228	154	51
CLAV		580		240	59	46	41.2

peak of 0.44 mg/liter 1 h after the first dose, and at 6 h they were 0.03 mg/liter. Those of CLAV were 0.92 mg/liter at 1 h and 0.08 mg/liter at 6 h after the first dose. On the fourth day, levels of AMOX and CLAV in sputum were considerably lower.

In CSF AMOX levels were 0.12 mg/liter at 1 h and 0.34 mg/liter at 4 h after a dose. Corresponding CLAV levels were 0.18 mg/liter at 1 h and 0.19 mg/liter at 4 h. In pleuritic fluid individual values for AMOX levels ranged from 0.28 to 5.00 mg/liter, reaching a peak at 4 or 6 h after a dose. Those of CLAV ranged from 0.10 to 2.4 mg/liter, peaking somewhat earlier.

Levels of both components of Augmentin in serum and especially in urine were many times higher than those necessary for synergistic action against most pathogens. Levels in sputum were quite satisfactory on the first day, but on the fourth day levels of AMOX were much lower. It seems that sputum purulence is an important factor for passage of AMOX into sputum, whereas CLAV passes easier, even in mucoid sputum. Levels in normal CSF were rather low, as expected for a penicillin, although even at those levels synergistic inhibitory action against *Haemophilus influenzae* should be expected. Finally, levels in pleuritic fluid were quite high, certainly sufficient for killing of most pathogens responsible for pneumonia.

The kinetics of AMOX and CLAV were quite compatible. Very similar serum half-life and urinary recovery were found. In various body fluids AMOX and CLAV seemed to be present at the same time, as is necessary for their synergistic action. CLAV seemed to reach a peak somewhat earlier than AMOX, a desirable property, since this would enable CLAV to inhibit any β-lactamase present at the infection site before arrival of AMOX, which would then kill the infecting organism unmolested.

1. **Kosmidis, J., A. Anyfantis, C. Stathakis, K. Mantopoulos, and G. K. Daikos.** 1980. Augmentin (amoxicillin plus sodium clavulanate, a beta-lactamase inhibitor) is active in amoxicillin-resistant infections, p. 330–331. *In* J. D. Nelson and C. Grassi (ed.), Current chemotherapy and infectious disease. American Society for Microbiology, Washington, D.C.
2. **Neu, H.C., and K. P. Fu.** 1980. Clavulanic acid, a novel inhibitor of β-lactamases. Antimicrob. Agents Chemother. **14**:650–655.

Comparative Pharmacokinetics of Amoxicillin, Clavulanic Acid Potassium, and Their Combination

GERT HÖFFKEN,* G. WITKOWSKI, H. LODE, AND P. KOEPPE

Medical and Radiological Departments, Klinikum Steglitz, Berlin, and Institute for Biology, Technical University, Berlin, Federal Republic of Germany

One of the most important mechanisms of bacterial resistance to cephalosporins and penicillins is the production of β-lactamases, which hydrolyze the antibiotic molecules (8). The destruction of the β-lactam ring leads to a loss of antibacterial activity of these antibiotics. The concomitant use of a β-lactamase inhibitor is a modern attempt to lower the frequency of bacterial resistance to β-lactam antibiotics. Clavulanic acid is a naturally occurring substance produced by *Streptomyces clavuligerus*, which, although possessing only a small degree of antibacterial activity itself, progressively and irreversibly inhibits the β-lactamases which are of greatest clinical importance (6). In the present study, the pharmacokinetics of amoxicillin, clavulanic acid potassium and their combination were tested in 10 healthy volunteers.

Amoxicillin (500 mg), clavulanic acid potassium (125 mg), and their combination as 625 mg of Augmentin were administered orally to 10 fasting subjects, 5 men and 5 women, at intervals of 1 week. The average age was between 25 and 44 years (mean, 32.3 years). Body weight was between 51 and 86 kg (mean body weight, 67.4 kg). First food intake was permitted 2 h after administration of the test substance. As a point of reference for determination of the absolute bioavailability, a bolus injection of 500 mg of amoxicillin was given intravenously.

Blood sampling was done before administration of the substances and up to 8 h thereafter. The recovery rate in urine was determined for four collection periods from 0 to 24 h.

An agar diffusion test served as bioassay for measurement of the serum and urine concentrations (4, 5). Test species were *Sarcina lutea* ATCC 9341 for low and *S. lutea* ATCC 8340 for high concentrations of amoxicillin, as well as *Klebsiella aerogenes* NCTC 11228 for clavulanic acid potassium. The lower limit of detection was 0.03 mg/liter for amoxicillin in serum at a pH of 6.5 and 0.015 mg/liter in the buffer at a pH of 6.5. For clavulanic acid potassium the lower limit of detection was 0.2 mg/liter in serum at a pH of 7.0 and 0.1 mg/liter in the buffer at a pH of 7.0. The bioassay of the two individual substances was not influenced by the simultaneous presence of the other.

Computation of the regression curves of serum concentrations (Fig. 1) was based on an open two-compartment model (9). The pharmacokinetic parameters determined included the peak serum level, the area under the serum concentration time curve after oral administration and after intravenous injection, the absorption coefficient, and the half-life in the elimination phase (Table 1). They were related to an average body weight of 70 kg.

The data computations were made with the least relative squares method by use of a digital computer and a FORTRAN program as described by Koeppe and Hamann (3). The statistical significance computations were done with the Wilcoxon test for paired differences, which is independent of the distribution.

After intravenous administration of 500 mg of amoxicillin, the serum concentration dropped, with a half-life of 75.5 ± 10.1 min, from 38.0 ± 6.4 mg/liter at 5 min to 0.1 ± 0.07 mg/liter after 8 h, the area under the curve being 27.8 ± 5.5 mg.h/liter. After oral administration of amoxicillin, a maximal serum concentration of 6.5 ± 1.6 mg/liter was reached. The elimination half-life was 68.5 ± 20.0 min, which corresponds to the results of Verbist et al. (10). At 19.5 ± 5.4 mg.h/liter, the area under the serum concentration curve after oral administration of amoxicillin was 70% of the AUC after intravenous administration of amoxicillin. This coincides with the results published by Brogden et al. in 1979

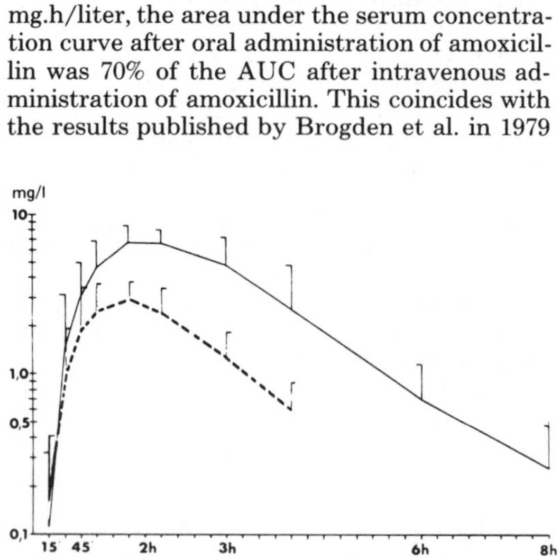

FIG. 1. *Mean serum concentrations (milligrams per liter) of amoxicillin (solid line) and clavulanate potassium (dashed aline) after administration as Augmentin in 10 fasting subjects.*

TABLE 1. *Pharmacokinetic parameters*[a]

Drugs and application form	Y max (mg/l)	AUC tot. (h · mg/l)	AUC oral / AUC i.v.	t 1/2 ß (min.)	Urine recovery 0-24 h (% of dose)	T max (min.)
1. Amoxicillin i.v.	---	27.8 ± 5.5	----	75.5 ±10.1	73.8 ± 3.6	----
2. Amoxicillin orally	6.5 ±1.6	19.5 ± 5.4	0.70 ±0.12	68.5 ±20.0	50.1 ±15.4	77.1 ±13.8
3. Amoxicillin in augmentin orally	6.5 ±1.4	23.2 ±10.6	0.83 ±0.13	79.9 ±25.7	52.0 ±13.7	88.7 ±19.1
4. Clavulanate- K^+ orally	3.4 ±1.4	7.8 ±3.2	----	78.6 ±42.2	36.3 ±18.3	56.6 ±10.3
5. Clavulanate- K^+ in augmentin orally	2.8 ±1.1	7.3 ±2.0	----	51.1 ± 8.9	43.4 ±15.6	77.6 ±17.2

[a] Y max, Peak serum level; AUC tot., area under the serum concentration-time curve; AUC oral and AUC i.v., area under the serum concentration-time curve after oral and intravenous administration; $t_{1/2\beta}$, half-life in the elimination phase; T max, time of the maximum serum concentration.

(2). Simultaneous administration of amoxicillin and clavulanic acid potassium as Augmentin did not influence the characteristics of the serum kinetics of amoxicillin. Almost identical maximal serum concentrations were reached in the test group, at 6.5 ± 1.4 mg/liter. The elimination half-life was 79.9 ± 25.7 min. At 23.2 ± 10.6 mg.h/liter, the area under the curve, a sensitive parameter for determination of the bioavailability of a substance, was also slightly, but not significantly, below the area under the curve after administration of amoxicillin alone, corresponding to a bioavailability of 83%.

It was not possible to detect any substantial difference between the serum concentration characteristics of clavulanic acid potassium alone and in Augmentin. However, for administration of clavulanic acid potassium alone, a serum maximum of 3.4 ± 1.4 mg/liter was reached, which statistical confirmation does show to be above the maximum of 2.8 ± 1.1 mg/liter for clavulanic acid potassium in Augmentin. Ball et al. (1) reported a serum maximum of 2.55 ± 0.97 mg/liter after administration of 125 mg of clavulanic acid sodium; the elimination half-life was 69 min. Furthermore, at 56.6 min, the maximum was reached statistically earlier ($P <$ 0.01) than in combined administration, for which the maximum was 77.9 ± 17.2 min. The remaining pharmacokinetic data, such as the area under the curve data, revealed no significant differences.

Likewise, in determining the recovery rate in urine for amoxicillin alone and in Augmentin, as well as for clavulanic acid potassium alone and Augmentin, no differences were found which could be confirmed as statistically significant. The urine recovery rates for clavulanic acid potassium were under 50% in 24 h for both groups, which, in accordance with the results of Münch et al. (5) and Ball et al. (1), could indicate extrarenal elimination, e.g., as a result of instability of the substance.

Taking into account the maximal serum concentrations, the time elapsed before the maximal serum concentration was reached, and the elimination half-life, the serum concentration curves of amoxicillin and clavulanic acid potassium run to a great extent parallel after administration of Augmentin.

In summary, the bioavailability of oral amoxicillin, computed from the quotient of the oral and intravenous area under the curve values, was 0.70 ± 0.12. The bioavailability of oral amoxicillin was not impaired by simultaneous administration of clavulanic acid potassium in Augmentin (0.83 ± 0.13). The serum concentration characteristics of clavulanic acid potassium alone and in Augmentin were to a great extent identical. The serum kinetics of amoxicillin and clavulanic acid potassium had the same characteristics.

1. **Ball, A. P., P. G. Davey, A. M. Geddes, and I. D. Farrell.** 1980. Clavulanic acid and amoxicillin: a clinical bacteriological and pharmacological study. Lancet **i:** 620–623.
2. **Brogden, R. N., R. C. Heel, T. M. Speight, and G. S. Avery.** 1979. Amoxicillin injectable: a review of its antibacterial spectrum, pharmacokinetics and therapeutic use. Drugs **18:**169–184.
3. **Koeppe, P., and C. Hamann.** 1978. Zwei Methoden zur Parameterschätzung nichtlinearer Regressionsfunktionen bei fehlerhaften Messdaten. EDV Med. Biol. **9:** 112–117.
4. **Lode, H., P. Janisch, G. Küppen, and H. Wenta.** 1974. Comparative clinical pharmacology of three ampicillins and amoxicillin administered orally. J. Infect. Dis. **129**(Suppl.):156–168.
5. **Münch, R., R. Luthy, J. Blaser, and W. Siegenthaler.** 1980. Clavulanic acid: human pharmacokinetics and penetration into cerebrospinal fluid, p. 345–347. *In* J. D. Nelson and C. Grassi (ed.), Current chemotherapy and infectious disease, vol 1. American Society for Microbiology, Washington, D.C.
6. **Reading, C., and M. Cole.** 1977. Clavulanic acid: a beta-lactamase-inhibiting beta-lactam from *Streptomyces clavuligerus*. Antimicrob. Agents Chemother. **11:**852–857.
7. **Reeves, D. S., P. J. Elliott, H. A. Holt, Z. Mojaddedi, and S. T. Chapman.** 1979. Clinical trial of clavulanic acid/amoxicillin formulation in urinary tract infections, p. 347–349. *In* J. D. Nelson and C. Grassi (ed.), Current chemotherapy and infectious disease, vol. 1. American Society for Microbiology, Washington, D.C.
8. **Richmond, M. H.** 1978. β-Lactamases. Int. J. Clin. Pharmacol. Biopharmacol. **17:**135–136.
9. **Ritschel, W. A.** 1980. Handbook of basic pharmacokinetics, 2nd ed. Drug Intelligence Publications, Inc., Publisher, City.
10. **Verbist, C.** 1976. Triple crossover study on absorption and excretion of ampicillin, talampicillin, and amoxicillin. Antimicrob. Agents Chemother. **10:**113–115.

Augmentin (Amoxicillin/Clavulanic Acid Formulation) in the Treatment of Urinary Tract Infections

H. KOLLARITSCH, H. PICHLER, E. JESCHKO, S. BREYER, AND W. GRANINGER

Kaiser Franz Josefs-Hospital, Infectious Disease Unit, Clinic of Chemotherapy, University of Vienna, Vienna, Austria

The frequent occurrence of urinary tract infections caused by penicillinase-producing gram-negative bacilli poses an increasing clinical problem. Clavulanic acid (CA) has been shown to be an irreversible inhibitor of most β-lactamases (3, 4). In combination with amoxicillin (AMX), CA protected the antibiotic agent from destruction by β-lactamase-producing bacteria when tested in vitro and in vivo (5–7). CA per se has only weak intrinsic antibacterial activity. Absorption and peak serum levels of AMX and CA are quite similar; in urine, however, the amount of CA detected is less than that of AMX but far in excess of that required to inhibit most β-lactamases (1, 2). Greenwood et al. (3) performed an in vitro study with low concentrations of CA (about 8 μg/ml) and got good results in inhibiting β-lactamase activity. Ball et al. (1) showed that AMX in combination with CA (at a dose of 625 mg three times daily [t.i.d.] or 750 mg t.i.d.) was effective in approximately 70% of cases in eradicating the causative organisms in urinary tract infections. Whereas in the group treated with 625 mg t.i.d. no intolerance was noted, 8 of the 20 patients treated with 750 mg t.i.d. complained of nausea; two of these had to be withdrawn from the trial because of vomiting. In the other six patients, the nausea was reduced by administering Augmentin with meals. The same authors showed also that the dose of CA given seems to be critical in terms of patient tolerance. Overall, in the studies done in Great Britain at 750 mg t.i.d. the incidence of vomiting was much lower.

The purpose of our investigation was to examine the cure rate and tolerance of a dose of two tablets of 625 mg of Augmentin (4:1) given twice daily. Patients were selected only if they had significant bacteriuria, proven by at least two midstream urine specimens.

Complete bacteriological investigation and susceptibility testing of the organisms causing the UTI was done twice. The immunofluorescence test for detection of antibody-coated bacteria to define upper or lower UTI was performed. The Betatest to detect β-lactamase-producing bacteria was done in each case. Urine bacteriology was again carried out at the end of treatment and 1 and 2 weeks afterwards. An intravenous pyelogram was performed in every patient, and whenever there was proof or suspicion of complicated UTI a urological investigation was carried out. Complete erythrocyte, leukocyte, and differential counts, as well as liver and kidney function tests, were carried out before and after treatment. Side effects and tolerance were noted by daily clinical assessment of patients.

TABLE 1. *Organisms causing UTI in 33 patients treated with Augmentin (4:1)*

Species	No.	AMX susceptible	AMX resistant	β-Lactamase producer
Escherichia coli	19	17	2	2
Proteus mirabilis	6	4	2	2
Klebsiella pneumoniae	4	0	4	4
Staphylococcus epidermidis	1	1	0	0
Providencia stuartii	1	0	1	1
Staphylococcus aureus	1	0	1	1
Streptococcus faecalis	1	1	0	0
Total	33	23	10	10

The following criteria excluded patients from treatment: known penicillin allergy, pregnancy, renal impairment (serum creatinine > 2.5 mg/100 ml), indwelling urinary catheter, and severe gastrointestinal diseases which could influence enteral absorption of the drug.

Thirty-three patients (mean age, 58 years; range, 18 to 84 years), 27 women and 6 men, were selected for treatment with Augmentin. Twelve of the 33 suffered from underlying disease: 3 had diabetes, 1 had cirrhosis, 1 had systemic lupus erythematosus, 1 had asthma (both were on long-term corticosteroid treatment), 1 had hypokalemia, 1 had colon cancer, 3 had chronic cystitis, and 1 had a diverticulum of the bladder. Twenty-one had acute UTI without underlying disease. There were 14 outpatients and 19 inpatients.

Augmentin (containing 500 mg of AMX and 125 mg of potassium clavulanate) was given in a dosage of two tablets twice daily. The length of treatment in patients with lower UTI (20 patients) was 7 days; in patients with upper UTI (13 patients), it was 14 days. Causative organisms are shown in Table 1. Cure was defined as eradication of causative organisms and no reappearance of the same organism in significant numbers within 2 weeks after the end of treatment.

Thirty patients received full treatment with Augmentin; 3 had to be withdrawn from the study because of vomiting. Of 30 patients treated, 25 were cured according to our criteria, a cure rate of 81%. In 9 of 10 patients with UTI caused by β-lactamase–producing bacteria, the infecting organism was eliminated.

In five patients we found a relapse within 14 days after end of treatment. In four of the patients with relapse, the causative organisms were *Escherichia coli*, none of which was a β-lactamase producer. One *E. coli* strain causing relapse became Augmentin resistant after the end of treatment. The other isolates remained susceptible. Three patients with relapse due to *E. coli* had recurrent UTI for several months. In only one case were we unable to find an explanation for failure of treatment. The fifth patient with a relapse had an infection due to *Klebsiella pneumoniae*. The isolate was a β-lactamase producer and became Augmentin resistant during therapy.

TABLE 2. *Side effects in 33 patients treated with Augmentin (4:1)*

Side effects	No. of patients
Nausea, diarrhea (therapy continued)	3
Vomiting (therapy discontinued)	3
Penicillin rash	2
Total	8

Eight of 33 patients complained of side effects, as shown in Table 2. Three who suffered from vomiting were withdrawn from the study. Two patients got a penicillin rash, both on the last day of therapy so that they were able to remain in the study. Three patients complained of minor side effects, such as nausea in two cases and diarrhea in one case. In these three patients treatment could be completed. Biochemical and hematological screening tests performed before and after treatment did not show any abnormalities attributable to the antibiotic treatment.

The combination of amoxicillin and clavulanic acid in a ratio of 4:1 proved to be effective in eradicating β-lactamase–producing bacteria causing upper and lower UTI. It is interesting to note that vomiting, which occurred in three patients in this trial, was very rare in other European trials in which the same or similar doses of Augmentin were used.

1. **Ball, A. P., A. M. Geddes, P. G. Davey, I. D. Farrell, and G. R. Brookes.** 1980. Clavulanic acid and amoxicillin, a clinical, bacteriological and pharmacological study. Lancet **i:**620–623.
2. **Goldstein, F. W., M. D. Kitzis, and J. F. Acar.** 1979. Effect of clavulanic acid and amoxicillin formulation against β-lactamase producing gram-negative bacteria in urinary tract infection. J. Antimicrob. Chemother. **5:**705–709.
3. **Greenwood, D., F. O'Grady, and P. Baker.** 1979. An in vitro evaluation of clavulanic acid, a potent broad spectrum β-lactamase inhibitor. J. Antimicrob. Chemother. **5:**539–547.
4. **Neu, H. C., and K. P. Fu.** 1978. Clavulanic acid, a novel inhibitor of β-lactamase. Antimicrob. Agents Chemother. **14:**650–655.
5. **Philippon, A. M., G. C. Paul, and P. A. Nevot.** 1981. Synergy of clavulanic acid with penicillin against ampicillin and carbenicillin-resistant gram-negative organisms, related to their type of β-lactamase, p. 327–329. *In* J. D. Nelson and C. Grassi (ed.), Current chemotherapy and infectious disease, vol. 1. American Society for Microbiology, Washington, D.C.

6. **Sjöberg, B., B. Ekström, U. Forsgren, L. Magni, and B. G. Pring.** 1978. Synergy of mecillinam and clavulanic acid with other β-lactam antibiotics. Infection **6**(Suppl. 1):17–23.

7. **Wise, R., J. M. Andrews, and K. A. Bedford.** 1978. In vitro study of clavulanic acid in combination with penicillin, amoxicillin, and carbenicillin. Antimicrob. Agents Chemother. **13**:389–393.

Augmentin, Cefotaxime, and Rocephin in Genitourinary and Hepatobiliary Tract Infections by β-Lactamase–Producing Bacteria

D. TANPHAICHITRA,* A. BUSAYANON, O. SUKATHAT, AND P. CHAIPRASITTIGUL

Ramathibodi Hospital, Paolo, and PhyaThai Hospitals, Bangkok, Thailand*

Augmentin (BRL 25000) is a new orally absorbed broad-spectrum antibacterial agent comprising amoxicillin trihydrate and potassium clavulanate. In vitro and in vivo studies have shown that clavulanic acid protects amoxicillin from inactivation by many β-lactamase–producing bacteria, thus allowing the intrinsic activity of amoxicillin against that organism to be manifested (3).

Rocephin is a new broad-spectrum semisynthetic cephalosporin with marked stability to enterobacterial β-lactamase and penicillinase-producing *Neisseria gonorrhoeae* (PPNG). It possesses an expanded spectrum of activity and an increased potency against a wide range of both gram-positive and gram-negative bacteria (G. Beskid, Program Abstr. Intersci. Conf. Antimicrob. Agents Chemother. 20th, Atlantic City, N.J., abstr. no. 70, 1980).

Cefotaxime is a new cephalosporin that has been shown in vitro to inhibit both gram-positive and gram-negative organisms. It is more active on a milligram per liter basis against *Streptococcus pneumoniae* and *Klebsiella* than many other cephalosporins and also exhibits a much lower protein binding (1).

These characteristics prompted us to investigate further the effectiveness of these compounds in the treatment of human infections caused by β-lactamase–producing bacteria.

For assay of β-lactamase, a chromogenic method using compound 87/312 and a novel method for detection of β-lactamase by using a chromogenic cephalosporin, described by O'Callaghan (2), were used.

Patients were divided into three groups (Table 1): (A) Augmentin, 18 patients (13 inpatients and 5 outpatients); (B) Rocephin, 32 patients (20 inpatients and 12 outpatients); (C) cefotaxime, 18 patients (6 inpatients and 12 outpatients).

In group A, the patients suffered from various diseases. Laboratory investigation indicated an impaired hepatobiliary function in 6 patients with moderate to marked elevation of serum bilirubin and alkaline phosphatase. The infections treated were urinary tract infections (7 patients), PPNG urethritis (5 patients), and hepatobiliary tract infections (6 patients). Of the 18 patients 16 had received other antibiotics prior to Augmentin. Previous therapy included ampicillin, amoxicillin, tetracycline, and aminoglycosides. Most of these patients had either failed on their previous treatment or had infecting organisms resistant to the antibiotic used. All patients were given 375 to 750 mg (250 mg of amoxicillin and 125 mg of clavulanic acid per tablet) of Augmentin three times a day for 10 to 14 days except for the use of a single dose in PPNG urethritis.

Twenty patients in group B received the Rocephin by the intramuscular route as a single injection of 250 mg for the treatment of PPNG urethritis. Furthermore, 12 patients received repeated intravenous/intramuscular injections of 500 to 1,000 mg every 12 h for 5 to 10 days. These infections comprised urinary tract infections (8 patients) and typhoid fever (4 patients).

In group C 12 patients received cefotaxime by the intramuscular route as a single injection of 500 mg for the treatment of PPNG urethritis. Furthermore, 4 patients with typhoid fever and 2 patients with pneumonitis due to *Pseudomonas aeruginosa* and *Klebsiella* species received repeated intravenous/intramuscular injections of 500 to 1,000 mg every 12 h for 10 to 21 days.

All patients except 8 with typhoid fever had

TABLE 1. *Age and sex of patients*

Group	Sex	Age			
		16–35 yr	36–45 yr	46–55 yr	56–75 yr
A. Augmentin	Male	5	2	2	1
	Female	1	6	1	
B. Rocephin	Male	15	3	2	1
	Female	6	2	1	2
C. Cefotaxime	Male	9	1	1	
	Female	4	1	2	

TABLE 2. *Clinical and bacteriological outcome*

Group	Type of infection	No.	Result: Cure	Result: Failure	Result: Unassessable
A. Augmentin	Urinary tract infection, *E. coli*	3	3		
	Klebsiella	4	4		
	PPNG urethritis	5	4	1	
	Hepatobiliary	6	—	2	4
B. Rocephin	Urinary tract infection, PPNG urethritis	20	18	2	
	Serratia	4	4		
	Citrobacter	4	4		
	S. typhi	4	4		
C. Cefotaxime	Urinary tract infection, PPNG urethritis	12	12		
	Sepsis-pneumonia	2	2		
	S. typhi	4	4		

infections caused by β-lactamase–producing organisms.

The clinical and bacteriological response of patients in group A to Augmentin therapy is shown in Table 2. In most cases relief was reported in 3 days. The only failures were two cases of hepatobiliary tract infections and one case of PPNG urethritis; four cases of hepatobiliary infections were unassessable. Bacterial counts in the bile were undertaken at 0, 4, 8, and 24 h in two patients. Despite the presence of clavulanic acid, the Augmentin could not eradicate β-lactamase–producing *E. coli* and *Klebsiella* species.

In group B all patients except 4 with typhoid fever had infections caused by β-lactamase–producing organisms. Of 20 cases of PPNG urethritis, 18 were cured by Rocephin. All patients with urinary tract infections (*Serratia marcescens*, 4 patients; *Citrobacter* species, 4 patients; typhoid fever, 4 patients) were cured by Rocephin. The only failures were 2 cases of PPNG urethritis.

In group C all patients except 4 with typhoid fever had infections caused by β-lactamase–producing organisms. In most patients clinical improvement was reported in 3 days. All patients with typhoid fever (4 cases), PPNG (12 cases), and pneumonia 2 (cases) were cured by cefotaxime.

Augmentin, cefotaxime, and Rocephin have been shown in the study to be effective in the treatment of infections caused by β-lactamase–producing bacteria and *Salmonella*. All patients treated with cefotaxime were found to recover rapidly from their illness with no evidence of relapses. No notable side effects occurred during therapy with these cephalosporins and Augmentin. Two treatment failures in hepatobiliary infections were treated successfully with a combination of cefoxitin and amikacin.

This study shows that cefotaxime and Rocephin are highly active bactericidal cephalosporins with a broad antibacterial spectrum. In general, the activity of these compounds against *Enterobacteriaceae*, *N. gonorrhoeae*, and *Salmonella* species was greater than that of amoxicillin. Of greater interest was the activity of cefotaxime and Rocephin against *Salmonella* infections. The study indicates that all three agents show considerable stability to a wide range of infections, mostly due to β-lactamase–producing organisms.

1. **Hamilton-Miller, J. M. T., W. Brumfitt, and A. V. Reynolds.** 1978. Cefotaxime. J. Antimicrob. Chemother. **4**:437–444.
2. **O'Callaghan, C. H., A. Morris, S. M. Kirby, and A. H. Shingler.** 1972. Novel method for detection of β-lactamases by using a chromogenic cephalosporin substrate. Antimicrob. Agents Chemother. **1**:283–288.
3. **Wise, R., J. M. Andrews, and K. A. Bedford.** 1978. In vitro study of clavulanic acid in combination with penicillin, amoxicillin, and carbenicillin. Antimicrob. Agents Chemother. **13**:389–393.

Recent Trends in Gonorrheal Urethritis and Its Therapeutic Treatment in Japan

SHOICHI ONODERA,* TOYOHEI MACHIDA, TAKEJIRO OKAZAKI, AND SUSUMU MITSUHASHI

Department of Urology, Jikei University School of Medicine, Tokyo, Department of Urology, Taito Municipal Hospital, Tokyo, and Department of Microbiology, Gunma University, Gunma Prefecture, Japan*

The number of patients with gonorrheal urethritis reached a peak shortly after World War II, in 1948. As venereal disease control measures became effective, it decreased gradually and leveled off, except for a temporary surge in 1966 after the Vietnam War. However, the number of gonorrhea sufferers apparently started increasing again from 1979. This upswing is characterized by an increasing number of cases resistant to treatment with antibiotics such as ampicillin, cephalexin, and tetracycline. We conducted epidemiological and bacteriological studies of gonorrheal urethritis to clarify these trends, using male patients in two hospitals which are of a different character, one being a university hospital situated in central Tokyo and the other a metropolitan hospital located in an amusement area.

Jikei University Hospital and Taito Hospital received a total of 1,293 patients with gonorrheal urethritis between 1965 and 1980. In Taito Hospital, the number of patients peaked at 102 cases in 1966 and thereafter dropped to a low of 23 in 1978. However, a sharp increase has been seen, 44 cases in 1979 and 88 cases in 1980. On the other hand, in Jikei University Hospital, which tends to receive fewer cases with gonorrheal urethritis because of its institutional character, a remarkable increase in patient numbers was also noted for the past 2 years, that is, 41 cases in 1979 and 55 cases in 1980, when compared with an annual average level of 20 cases until 1978.

Under these circumstances, we investigated the source of infection to clarify the epidemiological aspect of the problem. The infection sources for male patients with gonorrheal urethritis were prostitution, foreign prostitution, other (including infection from sexual consorts other than prostitutes), and unknown. There were no major annual shifts in the proportion of one source to another until 1978. However, an increase has been noticed in infection from prostitutes since 1979, especially from employees at Japan's "turkish bath," a possible cause of the recent spread of venereal disease in Japan. The prevailing source of transmission varies somewhat from one city to another. For example, the number of teen-age patients with gonorrheal urethritis was reported to have increased in one city as a result of consorts met at discotheques.

We reviewed the results of the therapeutic treatment of 180 patients who visited the two hospitals between January 1979 and December 1980. Table 1 shows the results. Administration of ampicillin was effective in 19 of the 28 patients; that is, the failure rate was about 30%. Cephalexin and doxycycline were each administered to 9 patients and were found to be ineffective in about 70% of the cases. A combination of a single dose of kanamycin injected intramuscularly and an oral dose of ampicillin or doxycycline was administered to 19 patients and was found to be effective in 18. A combination of dibekacin with the above oral agent was also found to be effective in 15 of 16 patients. Spectinomycin alone and a combination with an oral agent were administered to 23 and 17 patients, respectively. Both were found to be 100% therapeutically effective. BRL 25000, a formulation comprising the antibiotic amoxicillin and the β-lactamase inhibitor potassium clavulanate is under development in Japan, and it is known that BRL 25000 is a strong inhibitor of β-lactamase–producing *Neisseria gonorrhoeae* (2). We ob-

TABLE 1. *Dosing method and clinical efficacy of antimicrobial agents in gonorrheal urethritis*

Treatment[a]	No. of cases	Effective rate
Ampicillin (1.5 g)	28	19/28 (68%)
Cephalexin (1.5 g)	9	3/9 (33%)
Doxycycline (0.2 g)	9	3/9 (33%)
BRL 25000 (1.5 g)	59	58/59 (98%)
Kanamycin (1 g) + oral agents[b]	19	18/19 (95%)
Dibekacin (0.1 g) + oral agents	16	15/16 (94%)
Spectinomycin (2 g)	23	23/23 (100%)
Spectinomycin (2 g) + oral agents	17	17/17 (100%)

[a] Ampicillin, cephalexin, doxycycline, and BRL 25000 were administered orally in the daily doses shown for 5 to 10 days. Kanamycin, dibekacin, and spectinomycin were administered as one intramuscular dose.

[b] The oral agents were ampicillin, cephalexin, doxycycline, and BRL 25000 at the daily doses indicated above.

TABLE 2. *In vitro susceptibility of 101 N. gonorrhoeae strains to six antimicrobial agents*

Antimicrobial agent	No. of strains requiring MIC (μg/ml) of													
	≦0.0125	0.025	0.05	0.1	0.2	0.4	0.8	1.6	3.13	6.25	12.5	25	50	100≦
Penicillin G	2	3	4	11	14	13	12	13	12	9	2			6
Ampicillin	4	3	6	9	15	10	21	14	8	4	1			6
BRL 25000	1	2	7	13	14	25	17	17	5					
Spectinomycin								2	10	66	8	8	5	2
Kanamycin								1	33	37	10	2	9	9
Tetracycline				5	6	17	13	30	12	1	4	10	3	

tained a 98% (58 of 59) efficacy rate with gonorrheal urethritis. No serious side effects were seen.

The MICs of six drugs against 101 viable strains obtained from the patients with gonorrheal urethritis were measured (Table 2). The antibacterial potency was measured by the agar plate dilution method employing a GC culture medium containing 10% horse blood. The amount of inoculum was adjusted to 10^8/ml with a 0.5 McFarland standard, diluted 100-fold, and inoculated over the agar plate. MIC values were determined after 24 h of incubation. The MICs of benzylpenicillin were found to be distributed over a wide range, from 0.0125 to 100 μg/ml. Resistance to 0.8 μg/ml or higher concentrations was observed in 54 of the 101 strains, including 6 strains with a high resistance to 100 μg/ml or higher. Ampicillin was similar to benzylpenicillin in MIC distribution, drug resistance being observed in half the strains studied. BRL 25000 had a susceptibility peak at 0.4 μg/ml, and its highest MIC value was 3.13 μg/ml. This result indicates the high antibacterial potency of the drug compared with benzylpenicillin and ampicillin. Spectinomycin at a concentration of 6.25 μg/ml inhibited the growth of 78% (78 of 101) of the strains investigated. Although this result may suggest the susceptibility of most of the strains to the drug, an MIC of 100 μg/ml was observed with two strains. In the kanamycin-susceptibility curve the MICs for about 70% of the strains lay within the range 3.13 to 6.25 μg/ml. Resistance to 25 μg/ml or higher concentrations was found in 20% of the strains. The curve for tetracycline had two peaks, one at 1.6 and another at 25 μg/ml. Resistance to the drug was observed in over half the strains studied.

The activity of β-lactamase was measured in 68 of the strains studied by using the chromogenic cephalosporin method (1). Six of the 68 strains (9%) were found to be β-lactamase positive. These 6 strains required 100 μg/ml as the MIC of penicillin G and ampicillin.

As mentioned above, a remarkable increase in the number of cases of gonorrheal urethritis has been observed in Japan over the past 2 years, and the clinical efficacy of current antibiotic therapy has declined. The deterioration of the clinical results caused by resistance to ampicillin, cephalexin, and doxycycline, as demonstrated by the MIC measurements, will be a social problem. Spectinomycin and BRL 25000 treatment yielded good results clinically and bacteriologically, and these agents would be effective in the treatment of clinical infections due to *N. gonorrhoeae* hereafter.

1. **O'Callaghan, C. H., A. Morris, S. M. Kirby, and A. H. Schingler.** 1972. Novel method for detection of β-lactamase by using a chromogenic cephalosporin substrate. Antimicrob. Agents Chemother. **1**:283–288.
2. **Wise, R., J. M. Andrews, and K. A. Bedford.** 1978. In vitro study of clavulanic acid in combination with penicillin, amoxicillin, and carbenicillin. Antimicrob. Agents Chemother. **13**:389–393.

Therapy of Genital Ulcer Disease: Comparison of Amoxicillin Alone with Amoxicillin Combined with Clavulanic Acid

H. NSANZE, P. KARASIRA, P. KABULEETA, L. J. D'COSTA, M. FAST, F. PLUMMER, I. MACLEAN, Y. GIROUARD, AND A. R. RONALD*

*Department of Medical Microbiology, University of Nairobi, and Nairobi City Council, Health Department, Nairobi, Kenya; and Department of Medical Microbiology, University of Manitoba, Winnipeg, Canada**

Haemophilus ducreyi, the presumed etiological agent for the genital ulcer disease chancroid, can now be isolated from the majority of patients suspected to have this venereal disease. Some doubt however, continues as to its role as the sole primary pathogen. For many years the sulfonamides and tetracyclines have been effective agents for the treatment of chancroid. Recently, Nsanze et al. (2) have reported that many patients in Nairobi, Kenya, fail to respond to therapy with these agents.

Most *H. ducreyi* isolates in Nairobi produce beta-lactamase, and presumably, if *H. ducreyi* is an important pathogen in the lesion, the penicillins would not be effective therapy. Recently, a specific beta-lactamase inhibitor, clavulanic acid, has been developed as an agent designed to be combined with the penicillins as a treatment for infections caused by beta-lactamase-producing organisms.

The present study was undertaken as a randomized single-blind study to compare the efficacy of amoxicillin alone with amoxicillin plus two different dosage formulations of clavulanic acid. We intended to determine if the clinical response of chancroid to treatment would correlate with the bacteriological response and antimicrobial susceptibility and whether clavulanic acid would permit amoxicillin to be effective in patients infected with beta-lactamase-producing *H. ducreyi*.

Eighty patients with genital ulcer disease suspected to be chancroid were treated at the Special Treatment Clinic, Nairobi, Kenya, between January and May 1981. The ulcers were investigated by both cultural and serological studies as previously outlined by Nsanze et al. (2).

Patients were randomized to one of three drug regimens; amoxicillin, 500 mg three times a day (t.i.d.) (A); amoxicillin, 500 mg, plus clavulanic acid, 125 mg, t.i.d. (AC 375); and amoxicillin, 500 mg, plus clavulanic acid, 250 mg, t.i.d. (AC 750). Patients were followed up on days 4, 7, 10, 14, and 28. If on day 7 the ulcers were either unchanged or worse, patients were declared treatment failures and changed to an alternate antimicrobial agent. If the ulcer was healing, no further antimicrobial therapy was given.

All *H. ducreyi* isolates throughout the course of this study were tested for beta-lactamase and were positive by the chromogenic cephalosporin method of O'Callaghan et al. (3). Susceptibilities to amoxicillin, clavulanic acid, and amoxicillin plus clavulanic acid were determined by techniques described by Girouard et al. (1).

H. ducreyi was isolated from the ulcers of 54 of the 80 men entering the study. The bacteriological and clinical responses of the patients to the three treatment regimens are shown in Table 1. Of particular interest, 12 patients were treated with amoxicillin alone. All 11 patients examined on day 4 on this regimen continued to have positive cultures, and all 9 patients who returned on day 7 had shown no improvement. In contrast, none of the patients treated with amoxicillin and either of the two regimens of clavulanic acid were bacteriological or clinical failures at either day 4 or day 7. After this initial failure of amoxicillin alone to eradicate *H. ducreyi* from the lesion or result in ulcer healing, this regimen was discontinued and all patients were subsequently randomized to either of the two amoxicillin regimens combined with clavulanic acid.

Overall, 25 patients (including 6 failures from group A) were treated with AC 375, and 23 patients were treated with AC 750. At the end of the 1-week course of therapy, 8 of 23 treated with AC 375 and 8 of 19 treated with AC 750 had resolved completely. All but one patient in each of the two clavulanic acid groups showed some improvement at or before the 7th day of therapy. The average time to complete healing of the ulcer was 11.2 days for AC 375 and 9.7 days for AC 750 for 15 and 16 patients, respectively, who were adequately followed.

Twenty-six males with genital ulcers were culture negative for *H. ducreyi*. Seven were ultimately diagnosed as syphilitic and were treated with long-acting penicillins. In three, *Neisseria gonorrhoeae* was the only pathogen isolated from the ulcer, and 16 had no microbiological diagnosis. Of the latter patients, one was treated with amoxicillin alone, six were treated with AC 375, and seven were treated with AC 750. No failures were noted in any group.

All but one of the *H. ducreyi* isolates tested

TABLE 1. *Therapeutic response of patients with H. ducreyi-positive genital ulcer disease to three drug regimens*

Regimen	No. treated	Day 7				Day 10				Day 14			
		No. seen	No. cured	No. improved	No. +Hd[a]	No. seen	No. cured	No. improved	No. +Hd	No. seen	No. cured	No. improved	No. +Hd
A	12	9	0	0	9								
AC 375	25	23	8	15	0	22	15	7	0	21	20	1	0
AC 750	23	19	8	11	0	17	10	6	0	16	16	0	0

[a] +Hd, *H. ducreyi* positive.

from these patients was amoxicillin resistant (MIC $\geq$ 8 μg/ml). All isolates became susceptible to amoxicillin in the presence of clavulanic acid with an MIC of 4 μg/ml or less.

This study has demonstrated that *H. ducreyi*-positive genital ulcers fail to heal during treatment until the organism is eradicated. A close correlation is evident between organism eradication and response to treatment, further evidence for a primary pathogenic role of *H. ducreyi* in genital ulcer disease.

Although amoxicillin was of no value in the treatment of *H. ducreyi*-positive chancroid, the combination of amoxicillin and clavulanic acid (either 125 mg or 250 mg of clavulanic acid t.i.d.) successfully eradicated *H. ducreyi* from the ulcer and resulted in rapid healing. Clavulanic acid is an effective potentiator of amoxicillin in soft tissue infections due to *H. ducreyi*, and further trials are indicated for infections outside the urinary tract due to other beta-lactamase-producing organisms.

1. **Girouard, Y. G., I. W. Maclean, A. R. Ronald, and W. L. Albritton.** Synergistic antibacterial activity of clavulanic acid and amoxicillin against β-lactamase producing strains of *Haemophilus ducreyi*. Antimicrob. Agents Chemother. **20:**144–145.
2. **Nsanze, H., M. V. Fast, L. J. D'Costa, P. Tukei, J. Curran, and A. R. Ronald.** 1981. Genital ulcers in Kenya: a clinical and laboratory study of 97 patients. Br. J. Vener. Dis., in press.
3. **O'Callaghan, C. H., A. Morris, S. M. Kirby, and S. H. Shingler.** 1972. Novel method for detection of β-lactamases by using a chromogenic cephalosporin substrate. Antimicrob. Agents Chemother. **1:**283–288.

Interest in the Use of a Beta-Lactamase Inhibitor, Clavulanic Acid, in the Assay of Amoxicillin in Ischemic Leg Ulcers

Y. JUILLET,* M. D. KITZIS, J. N. FIESSINGER, J. F. ACAR, AND E. HOUSSET

Hôpital Broussais and Hôpital Saint-Joseph, Paris, France*

Ischemic leg ulcers are superinfected in more than 75% of cases (2). Empirical use of antibiotics in the treatment of these infections has been much debated; one of the criticisms made about this treatment is that the antibiotic diffuses badly into an ischemic area.

A preliminary study in nine patients showed that 3 h after oral administration of 1 g of ampicillin, it was impossible to measure the quantity of antibiotic because of the presence of bacteria secreting a beta-lactamase at the wound site. The purpose of this study was to illustrate that the joint use of a beta-lactamase inhibitor, clavulanic acid (CA), and amoxicillin (AMX) made it possible to measure the antibiotic at the site of the wound, thus allowing a demonstration of its diffusion.

Twelve patients with trophic skin changes complicating arteritis of the lower limbs were included in this study. The antibiotics used were Augmentin (250 mg of AMX plus 125 mg of CA per tablet) and AMX (250 mg per tablet). The total daily dosage administered was two tablets of Augmentin and two tablets of AMX, one of each given morning and evening (i.e., 1 g of AMX and 250 mg of CA). The treatment lasted 5 days.

Blood and pus samples were taken daily at various times to establish the kinetics of each substance. Simultaneously a bacteriological study of the wound site was made each day. The local pus sample was treated in the following way: after the weight of pus was determined, the pus was placed in phosphate buffer, pH 7.0, stirred, and centrifuged; the assays were carried out on the resulting supernatant fluid. The assays of AMX and CA were carried out according to previously described microbiological methods (1).

Measurable quantities of antibiotics were

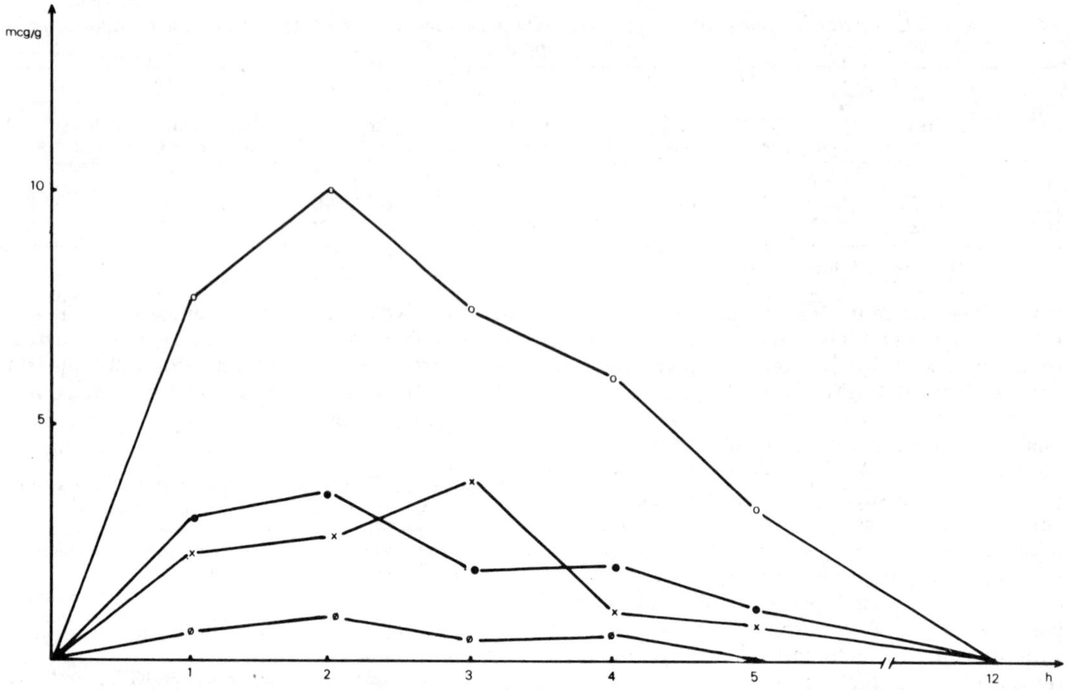

FIG. 1. *Concentrations of AMX and CA in serum and wound pus. Symbols:* ○, *serum AMX concentration;* ×, *local (wound) concentration of AMX;* ●, *serum CA concentration;* ∅, *local (wound) CA concentration.*

found in the pus samples from 10 of 12 patients. A curve of AMX and CA concentrations in the serum and wound pus versus time was obtained (Fig. 1). A correlation was found between the serum and pus levels 3 h after AMX administration and 2 and 4 h after CA administration. There was no change in the bacteriological flora except in a case of sterilization, as the study was very short (5 days).

As a result of the protective effect of CA, it was possible to establish the penetration of AMX into ischemic ulcers when the drugs were administered by the oral route. Serum and wound site kinetics for the two antibiotics were made possible.

1. **Brown, A. G., D. Butterworth, M. Cole, G. Hanscomb, J. D. Hood, C. Reading, and G. N. Rolinson.** 1976. Naturally occurring β-lactam inhibitors with antibacterial activity. J. Antibiot. **29:**668–669.
2. **Dagher, F. J., S. V. Alongi, and A. Smith.** 1978. Bacterial studies of leg ulcers. Angiology **29:**641–653.

Beta-Lactamase Inhibitors, Clavulanic Acid and CP-45,899: In Vitro Comparative Evaluation

O. PANIARA,* A. SIMA, G. SAROGLOU, K. KOLTSIDA, P. PARASKEVOPOULOU, AND P. KONTOMICHALOU

Department of Clinical Therapeutics, Athens University, "Alexandra" Hospital, Athens 611, Greece

Beta-lactamases of bacteria contribute significantly to their resistance to beta-lactam antibiotics. Initially, penicillins with inhibitory activity produced by structural modification of the basic penicillin nucleus were used to overcome the intracellular hydrolytic activity of beta-lactamases. Recently, natural or semisynthetic beta-lactam compounds have been used as inhibitors in combination with antibiotics sensitive to beta-lactamases. Two of those are clavulanic acid and penicillanic acid sulfone or CP-45,899. Both have weak antibacterial but potent beta-lactamase inhibitory activity (1, 4).

In our hospital, resistance to amoxicillin is very high, approximately 80% among *Enterobacteriaceae*. Therefore, alternative therapeutic schemes are required. We studied the activity of clavulanic acid and CP-45,899 against 57 *Enterobacteriaceae* clinical isolates resistant to amoxicillin and ampicillin. The combinations were: amoxicillin plus clavulanic acid in proportion 2:1 and ampicillin plus CP-45,899 in 1:1 and 3:1 ratios. In 33 of the isolates beta-lactamase production and characterization were investigated to determine the activity of beta-lactamase produced (2). We thought this was important since it has been reported that the activity of beta-lactamase inhibitors varies, depending on the type of beta-lactamase produced (2, 3).

In all *Enterobacteriaceae* strains tested a decrease in the MIC of amoxicillin plus clavulanic acid or ampicillin plus CP-45,899 was found, compared to the activity of those antibiotics alone. MIC_{90} of amoxicillin and ampicillin in all combinations and all species dropped to concentrations between 25 and 125 μg/ml. MIC_{50} for all combinations was below 25 μg/ml. The lowest values of MIC_{50} (≤16 μg/ml) were obtained with amoxicillin plus clavulanic acid in proportion 2:1 for all species except *Enterobacter*. In the combinations of ampicillin and CP-45,899 the 3:1 ratio was less effective than the 1:1 ratio, particularly for *Escherichia coli* and *Klebsiella* strains.

Results of beta-lactamase production and characterization are shown in Table 1; also shown is the effect of the inhibitors on the antimicrobial activity of amoxicillin and ampicillin in relation to the type of enzyme produced. Eight out of the nine *E. coli* strains produced TEM 1 beta-lactamase. For those strains the MIC of amoxicillin in the presence of clavulanic acid dropped significantly from over 1,000 μg/ml to 16 or 32 μg/ml. The MIC of ampicillin in the presence of CP-45,899 (ratio, 1:1) dropped from over 800 μg/ml to a range between 6.5 and 100 μg/ml. In one *E. coli* strain which produced an unusual cephalosporinase, clavulanic acid had no effect on amoxicillin susceptibility, whereas CP produced an eightfold decrease of ampicillin susceptibility. The seven *Klebsiella* strains tested produced a variety of most unusual beta-lactamases. In five of six strains the beta-lactamase inhibitors reduced significantly the MIC of the two antibiotics. In one *Klebsiella* strain, which produced two different beta-lactamases (one cephalosporinase and one TEM 2), there was significant reduction. Clavulanic acid did not reduce the amoxicillin MIC, whereas in another *Klebsiella* strain, which produced an unusual penicillinase, CP-48,899 had no effect on ampicillin susceptibility. Three of five *Enterobacter* strains produced cephalosporinases, and two produced TEM 1 beta-lactamases. The drop in amoxicillin MIC in the presence of clavulanic acid seems less significant in the *Enterobacter* strains which produced cephalosporinases, whereas for the same strains the ampicillin ac-

TABLE 1. *Beta-lactamase type in relation to activity of beta-lactamase inhibitors*

Strain	No.	Beta-lactamase: pI	Beta-lactamase: Type	MIC (μg/ml): Amoxicillin	MIC (μg/ml): Amoxicillin + clavulanic acid (2:1)	MIC (μg/ml): Ampicillin	MIC (μg/ml): Ampicillin + CP-45,899 (1:1)
E. coli	8	5.4	TEM 1	1,000	16–32	800	6.5–100
E. coli	1	8.8	Cephalosporinase	125	125	100	12.5
Klebsiella	2	7	Unusual broad spectrum	250	2–8	25–200	6.2–200
Klebsiella	1	5.9	TEM 2	1,000	500	800	25
Klebsiella	1	7.5	Penicillinase hydrolyzing cefoxitin	1,000	4	800	50
Klebsiella	2	8	Cephalosporinase	64–1,000	8–500	50–125	2–12.5
Klebsiella	1	7.8	Cephalosporinase, unusual	64	4	50	12.5
Enterobacter	2	5.4	TEM 1	500–1,000	62	50–800	12.5–25
Enterobacter	3	7.8	Cephalosporinase	250–100	500–62	100	25–50
Proteus spp.	5	5.6	TEM 2	1,000–1,000	8–32	800	50–12.5
Proteus spp.	1	5.4	TEM 1	1,000	32	800	25
Proteus spp.	1	6.6	Unusual penicillinase hydrolyzing cefoxitin	250	125	800	25
Proteus spp.	1	7.9	Cephalosporinase	500	500	800	50
Proteus spp.	1	8.5	Unusual broad spectrum				
Proteus spp.	2	ND[a]	Unusual broad spectrum	500	2	200	3–25

[a] ND, Not detectable.

tivity was potentiated in the presence of CP-45,899.

Five of 10 *Proteus* species tested produced TEM 2 beta-lactamases: one strain a TEM 1, one strain a cephalosporinase, and four strains unusual beta-lactamases. For the strains producing TEM 2 the drop of ampicillin MIC in the presence of CP-45,899 was constant at 25 μg/ml, whereas the effect of clavulanic acid on amoxicillin MIC varied between 8 and 62 μg/ml. In three of four strains producing unusual beta-lactamases both combinations reduced the MIC of the beta-lactam drugs to therapeutic levels, and for the fourth the ampicillin–CP-45,899 combination had better results than the amoxicillin-clavulanic acid. In Table 2 we summarize the results of potentiation of beta-lactam drugs by the beta-lactamase inhibitors. We show separately the number of strains producing each type of beta-lactamase for which the inhibitor caused either an eightfold drop of MIC or a decrease to ≤25 μg/ml.

For strains producing TEM 1, TEM 2, and unusual beta-lactamases, both inhibitors were found to be equally active. For cephalosporinase producers, the difference between the two inhibitors was pronounced in favor of CP-45,899. In eight of nine strains there was an eightfold or more decrease in MIC in the CP-45,899 combination as compared to four of nine strains for the clavulanic acid combination. A similar drop of the therapeutic levels occurred in six of nine strains in the presence of CP-45,899 as compared to three of nine in the presence of clavulanic acid. Reports in the literature on clavulanic acid action indicate that cephalosporinases are less sensitive to clavulanic acid inhibition than the other types of beta-lactamases (1, 3). Similar findings concerning cephalosporinases have also been reported for the combination of ampicillin and CP-45,899 (4). In our strains we found that the presence of CP-45,899 in cephalosporinase-producing *E. coli*, *Enterobacter*, and *Proteus* species had considerably more effect on ampicillin susceptibility than amoxicillin plus clavulanic acid. The unsatisfactory synergistic activity of clavulanic acid with beta-lactam drugs against cephalosporinase producers might be attributed to a combination of factors, i.e., a low affinity or an inacessibility of clavulanic acid to chromosomal enzymes.

Conclusions. Ampicillin- or amoxicillin-resistant *Enterobacteriaceae* clinical isolates from our hospital gave quite satisfactory and promising results when tested in vitro for susceptibility to amoxicillin plus clavulanic acid and ampicillin plus CP-45,899.

TABLE 2. *Potentiation of amoxicillin and ampicillin by clavulanic acid and CP-45,899, respectively, in relation to beta-lactamase type*

Beta-lactamase		Effect of beta-lactamase inhibitors[a]:			
Type	No. of strains	CA + amoxicillin (drop of MIC)		CP − ampicillin (drop of MIC)	
		≥8-fold	≤25 μg/ml	≥8-fold	≤25 μg/ml
TEM 1	11	11	5	10	5
TEM 2	7	6	4	5	6
Cephalosporinases	9	4	3	8	6
Unusual beta-lactamases	6	5	5	4	4

[a] CA, Clavulanic acid; CP, CP = 45,899.

These findings apply to all four species, *E. coli*, *Klebsiella*, *Enterobacter*, and *Proteus*, tested. However, we have to point out that the MIC_{90} for the beta-lactam drugs did not drop, in the presence of the inhibitors, to therapeutic levels. Therefore susceptibility tests should be performed before administering the combinations in infections with beta-lactam-resistant *Enterobacteriaceae*.

There was no difference, overall, in activity between the two inhibitors for the randomly selected strains investigated for beta-lactamase production. In individual strains, however, potentiation of beta-lactam drugs was more profound with one inhibitor than with the other. This apparently indicates that the problem of intracellular inhibition of beta-lactamase by the new inhibitors is a multiple-parameter phenomenon. CP-45,899 was a more potent inhibitor than clavulanic acid for cephalosporinase-producing *Enterobacteriaceae*.

The new beta-lactamase inhibitors clavulanic acid and CP-45,899 are promising compounds for expanding the antimicrobial activity of beta-lactam drugs against beta-lactamase-producing *Enterobacteriaceae*.

1. **Fu, K. P., and H. C. Neu.** 1979. Comparative inhibition of β-lactamases by novel β-lactam compounds. Antimicrob. Agents Chemother. **15:**171–176.
2. **Matthew, M., A. M. Harris, M. J. Marshall, and G. W. Ross.** 1975. The use of analytical isoelectrical focusing for detection and identification of β-lactamases. J. Gen. Microbiol. **88:**169–176.
3. **Neu, H. C., and K. P. Fu.** 1978. Clavulanic acid, a novel inhibitor of β-lactamases. Antimicrob. Agents Chemother. **14:**650–655.
4. **Wise, R., J. M. Andrews, and K. A. Beford.** 1980. Clavulanic acid and CP-45,899: a comparison of their in vitro activity in combination with penicillins. J. Antimicrob. Chemother. **6:**197–206.